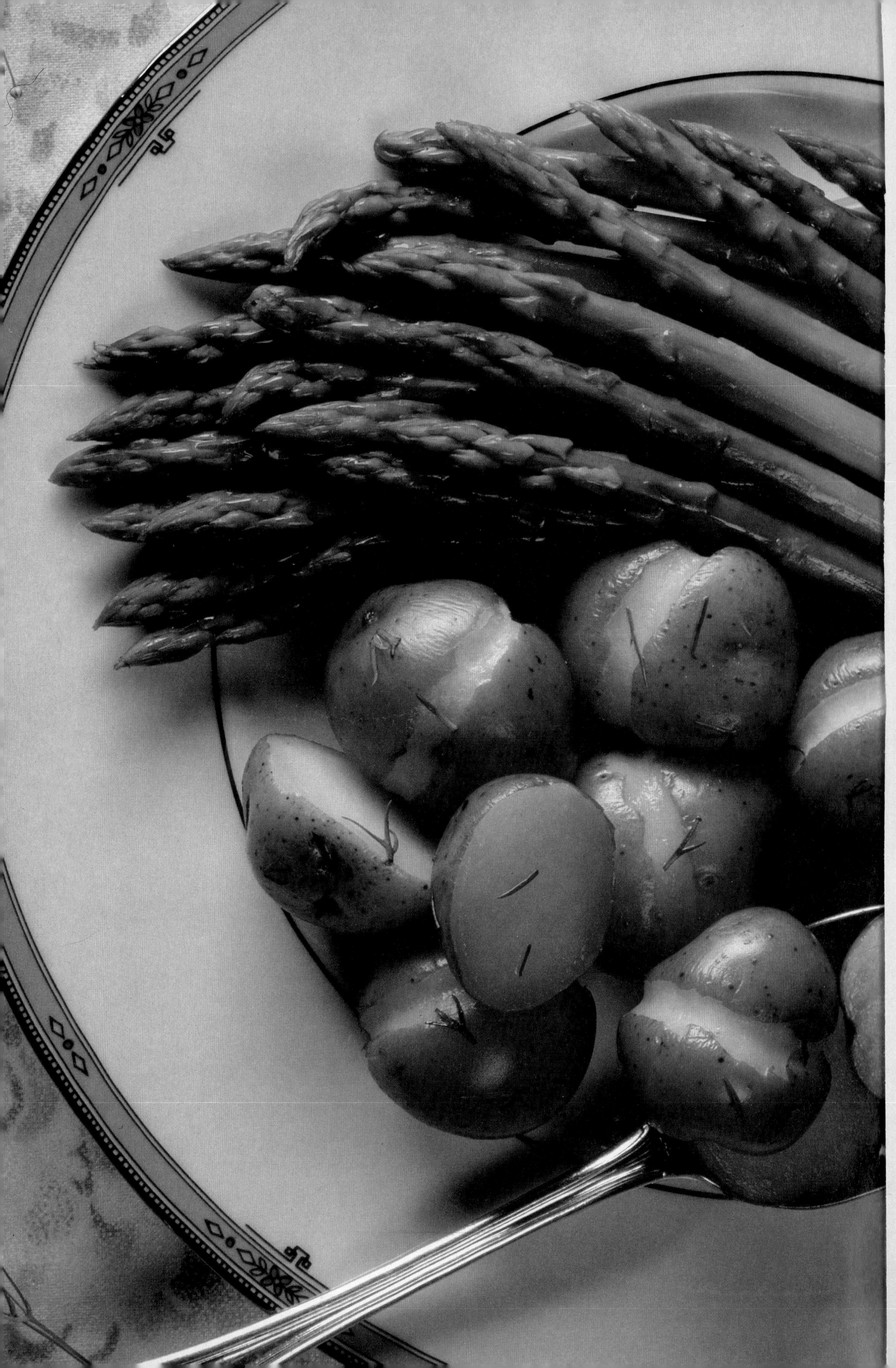

Designed for the maintenance of good nutrition of practically all healthy people in the United States

Water-Soluble Vitamins							Minerals						
Vitamin C (mg)	Thiamin (mg)	Riboflavin (mg)	Niacin (mg NE)[f]	Vitamin B_6 (mg)	Folate (μg)	Vitamin B_{12} (μg)	Calcium (mg)	Phosphorus (mg)	Magnesium (mg)	Iron (mg)	Zinc (mg)	Iodine (μg)	Selenium (μg)
30	0.3	0.4	5	0.3	25	0.3	400	300	40	6	5	40	10
35	0.4	0.5	6	0.6	35	0.5	600	500	60	10	5	50	15
40	0.7	0.8	9	1.0	50	0.7	800	800	80	10	10	70	20
45	0.9	1.1	12	1.1	75	1.0	800	800	120	10	10	90	20
45	1.0	1.2	13	1.4	100	1.4	800	800	170	10	10	120	30
50	1.3	1.5	17	1.7	150	2.0	1,200	1,200	270	12	15	150	40
60	1.5	1.8	20	2.0	200	2.0	1,200	1,200	400	12	15	150	50
60	1.5	1.7	19	2.0	200	2.0	1,200	1,200	350	10	15	150	70
60	1.5	1.7	19	2.0	200	2.0	800	800	350	10	15	150	70
60	1.2	1.4	15	2.0	200	2.0	800	800	350	10	15	150	70
50	1.1	1.3	15	1.4	150	2.0	1,200	1,200	280	15	12	150	45
60	1.1	1.3	15	1.5	180	2.0	1,200	1,200	300	15	12	150	50
60	1.1	1.3	15	1.6	180	2.0	1,200	1,200	280	15	12	150	55
60	1.1	1.3	15	1.6	180	2.0	800	800	280	15	12	150	55
60	1.0	1.2	13	1.6	180	2.0	800	800	280	10	12	150	55
70	1.5	1.6	17	2.2	400	2.2	1,200	1,200	320	30	15	175	65
95	1.6	1.8	20	2.1	280	2.6	1,200	1,200	355	15	19	200	75
90	1.6	1.7	20	2.1	260	2.6	1,200	1,200	340	15	16	200	75

[c] Retinol equivalents. 1 retinol equivalent = 1 μg retinol or 6 μg ß-carotene.

[d] As cholecalciferol. 10 μg cholecalciferol = 400 IU of vitamin D.

[e] α-Tocopherol equivalents. 1 mg d-α tocopherol = 1 α-TE.

[f] 1 NE (niacin equivalent) is equal to 1 mg of niacin or 60 mg of dietary tryptophan.

Estimated Safe and Adequate Daily Dietary Intakes of Selected Vitamins and Minerals[a]

		Vitamins	
Category	Age (years)	Biotin (μg)	Pantothenic Acid (mg)
Infants	0–0.5	10	2
	0.5–1	15	3
Children and adolescents	1–3	20	3
	4–6	25	3–1
	7–10	30	4–5
	11+	30–100	4–7
Adults		30–100	4–7

		Trace Elements[b]				
Category	Age (years)	Copper (mg)	Manganese (mg)	Fluoride (mg)	Chromium (μg)	Molybdenum (μg)
Infants	0–0.5	0.4–0.6	0.3–0.6	0.1–0.5	10–40	15–30
	0.5–1	0.6–0.7	0.6–1.0	0.2–1.0	20–60	20–40
Children and adolescents	1–3	0.7–1.0	1.0–1.5	0.5–1.5	20–80	25–50
	4–6	1.0–1.5	1.5–2.0	1.0–2.5	30–120	30–75
	7–10	1.0–2.0	2.0–3.0	1.5–2.5	50–200	50–150
	11+	1.5–2.5	2.0–5.0	1.5–2.5	50–200	75–250
Adults		1.5–3.0	2.0–5.0	1.5–4.0	50–200	75–250

[a] Because there is less information on which to base allowances, these figures are not given in the main table of RDA and are provided here in the form of ranges of recommended intakes.

[b] Since the toxic levels for many trace elements may be only several times usual intakes, the upper levels for the trace elements given in this table should not be habitually exceeded.

Perspectives in Nutrition

Perspectives in Nutrition

Gordon M. Wardlaw, Ph.D., R.D., L.D.
The Ohio State University

Paul M. Insel, Ph.D.
Stanford University School of Medicine

with 400 *illustrations*

Illustrations by
Medical and Scientific Illustration:
William C. Ober, M.D.
Claire Garrison
Margaret B. Ober

Times Mirror / Mosby College Publishing
St. Louis • Toronto • Boston 1990

Publisher: Edward F. Murphy
Acquisitions Editor: Pat Coryell
Developmental Editor: Vicki Van Ry
Project Manager: Mark Spann
Production Editor: Gina Gay Chan
Designer: Liz Fett
Photographic Researcher: Francine Kohnen

We would like to thank the National Cancer Institute for the beautiful photograph that appears on the cover of this text.

A division of The C.V. Mosby Company
11830 Westline Industrial Drive
St. Louis, MO 63146

Printed in the United States of America

ISBN 0-8016-2847-4

C/CD/VH 9 8 7 6 5 4 3 2

About the Authors

Gordon M. Wardlaw, Ph.D., R.D., L.D., teaches nutrition to both majors and non-majors at The Ohio State University. The author of numerous articles in prominent nutrition, biology, physiology, and biochemistry journals, Dr. Wardlaw was the 1985 recipient of the prestigious Mary P. Huddleson Award from the American Dietetic Association and has received research grants from many major corporations.

Paul M. Insel, Ph.D., is currently Clinical Associate Professor at the Stanford University School of Medicine. He has been the principal investigator of numerous NIH studies, is the senior author of a leading introductory health text, and is Editor-in-Chief of *Healthline,* a leading health journal.

Contents in Brief

Contents

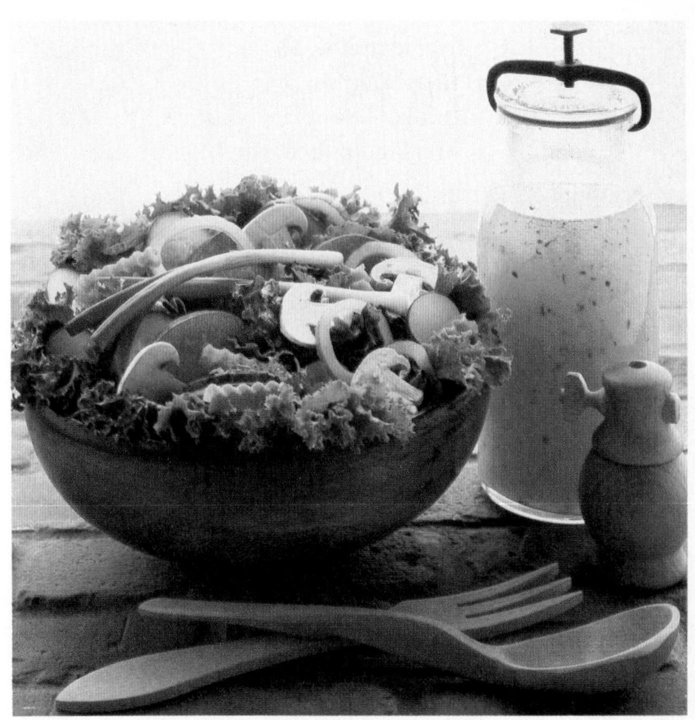

Part II The Energy-Yielding Nutrients

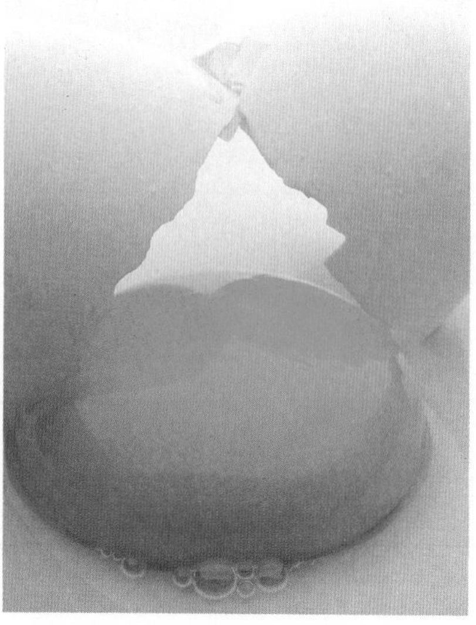

Part III Energy Production and Energy Balance

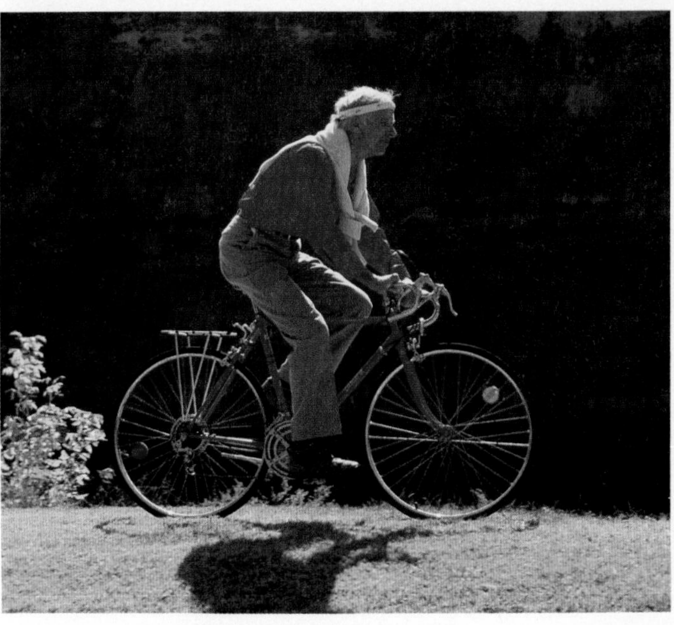

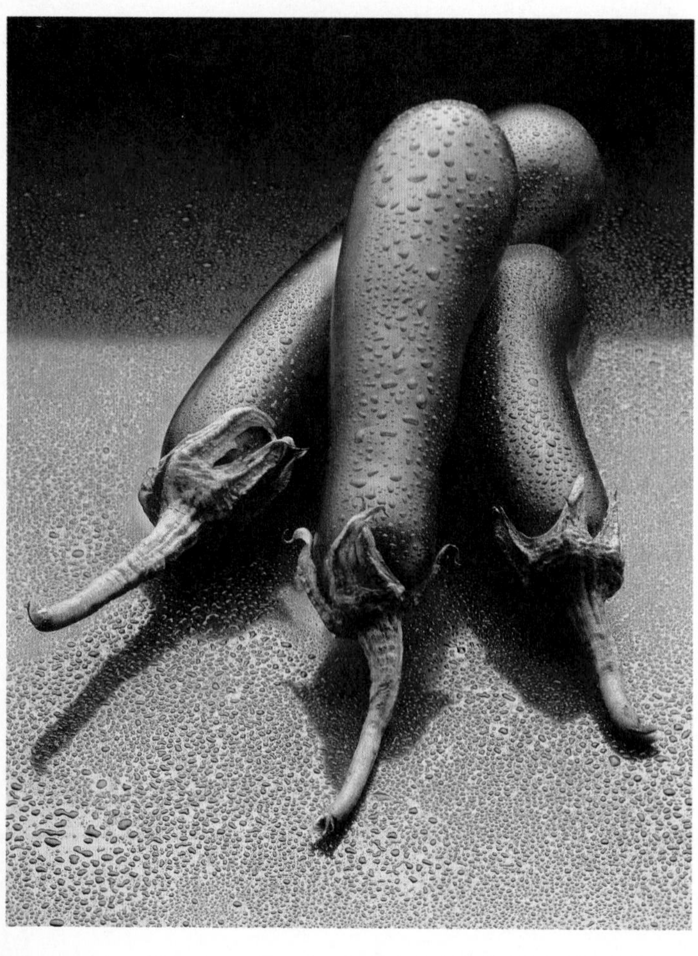

Part V Nutrition Applications in the Life Cycle

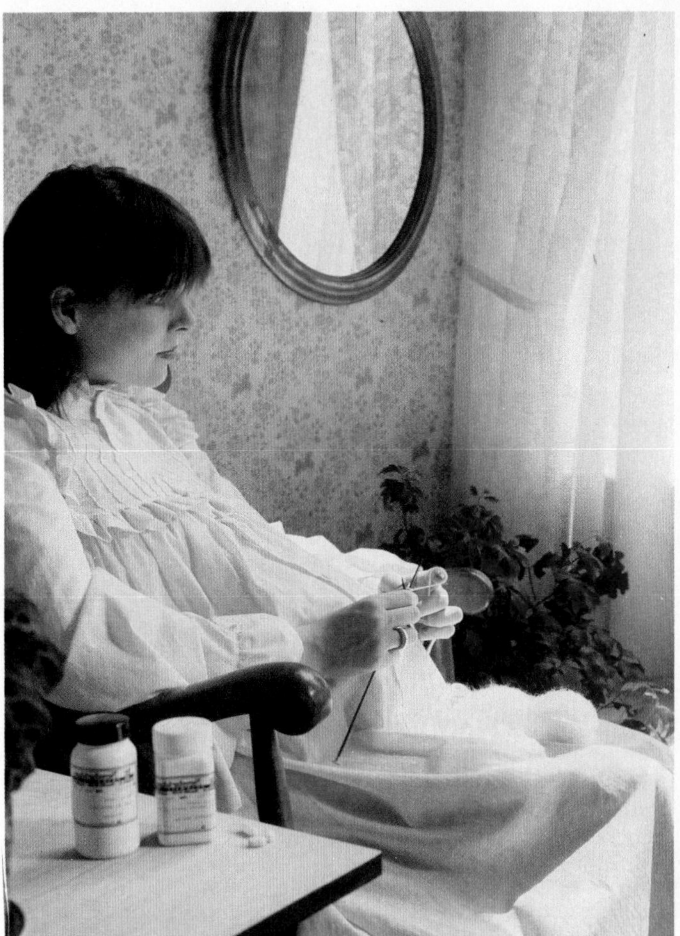

Part VI Putting Nutrition Knowledge to Practice

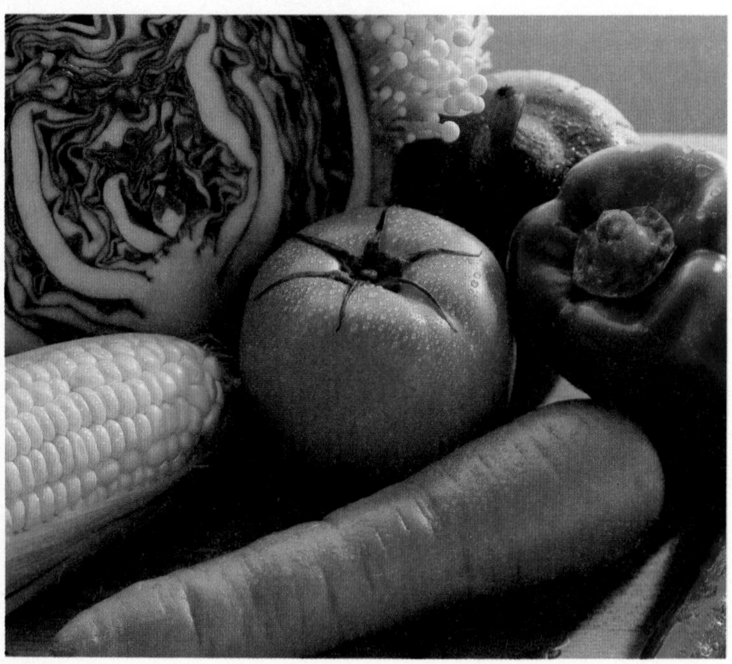

Preface to the Instructor

As a professor, you undoubtedly already find nutrition a fascinating topic. However, it can also be quite frustrating to teach. Claims and counter-claims abound about the need for certain constituents in our diet, such as dietary fiber. One group of researchers promotes fiber as an effective preventive measure for colon cancer, while other groups show that high levels of wheat bran increase the risk of colon cancer in animals.

We, too, are frustrated by conflicting data in our field, and so have attempted to draw on as many sources as possible in writing this textbook. Since we began in December of 1987, major publications have appeared, such as the *Surgeon General's Report on Nutrition and Health* and the latest *National Academy of Sciences Report on Diet and Health and the 10th edition of the RDA.* We have incorporated much of the material from those sources, especially the new RDA values, as well as many current review articles and basic scientific reports. We also have consulted with a number of experts and provide their opinions of the current state of nutrition research.

This textbook makes a break from all others in the field. Like other textbooks, it focuses on the latest research in nutrition but it goes further to document important research studies throughout the chapters, list those references at the back of the chapters, and provide Expert Opinions in each chapter to re-examine the most controversial issues in the chapter. In all, we provide you with many perspectives of current nutrition research so that you and your students can more clearly understand and take part in the debate of the nutrition issues in our time.

PERSONALIZING NUTRITION

One overriding theme in nutrition research today is **individuality.** Not all of us find that the cholesterol in our diets raises our blood cholesterol levels over recommended standards. Sodium does not raise everyone's blood pressure above current guidelines. We often respond in an idiosyncratic manner to nutrients, and that is something we constantly point out in this textbook.

Even at this basic level we do not try to put every nutrition student through the same square hole. We constantly ask your students to learn more about themselves and their health status and apply the information in a manner appropriate to improving their own health. After reading this textbook, students will have a much clearer understanding of how the nutrition information given on the evening news, on cereal box labels, in popular magazines, and by government agencies applies to them. They will become learned consumers of nutrients and nutrition information, realizing that nutrition knowledge allows them to personalize the information rather than follow every guideline issued to a population—which by definition actually consists of separate individuals with separate genetic backgrounds and responses to diet.

In addition we cover important questions that students often raise concerning vegetarianism, diets for athletes, the safety of our food supply, and fad diets. We emphasize the importance of behavior in terms of understanding one's food choices and changing one's diet. We discuss food behaviors in Chapter 1, focus on behaviors that lead to obesity in Chapter 9, and discuss in detail how to change behavior in Chapter 18.

AUDIENCE

This book has been designed for a diverse audience. It is most useful for students majoring in nutrition, the health sciences, home economics, nursing, physical education, and other health-related areas, and for pre-medical and pre-dental students. However, due to the flexibility of chapter organization and content and outstanding student appeal, it can be adapted to students of diverse background. While not absolutely necessary, most students will find having studied a course in biology, whether at the high school or college level, or having an understanding of basic biological concepts will provide a helpful background for taking the introductory nutrition course.

While the book is most suitable for a semester-length course, it can also be used in a quarter-length course by omitting chapters. A unique feature of this text is that it is presented in six segments:

Part I: Nutrition Basics
Part II: The Energy-Yielding Nutrients
Part III: Energy Production and Energy Balance
Part IV: The Vitamins and Minerals
Part V: Nutrition Applications in the Life Cycle
Part VI: Putting Nutrition Knowledge into Practice

This organization facilitates the ease of tailoring the text to your specific course needs.

FEATURES

Content

We have organized this text to make up for weaknesses seen in many current textbooks:

Early introduction to chemistry. An explanation of chemistry principles is presented early in the book to help students with weak chemistry backgrounds to more fully comprehend the nature of nutrient metabolism. Chemical structures are found primarily in the margins and can be used at your option.

Emphasis on nutrient density. Discussions of nutrients are based on the most nutrient-dense sources of foods. Leading food sources in the U.S. diet are identified for each nutrient when those data are available.

Emphasis on the exchange system. An outline of the exchange system is presented in Chapter 2 and can be used or not used at your option. The use of the exchange system is reinforced in Chapters 4 through 6, in the Student Study Guide and in the Mosby Diet Simple Software that accompanies this book.

Summary tables. Some chapters contain large detailed summary tables that include the major points made in the chapter. These tables provide convenient capsules for reference.

Content and controversial topics are well-referenced. Approximately 90 percent of the referenced material is from sources published since 1985; 60 percent is from sources published since 1987. As instructors, we demand the latest information to present to our students. Providing this up-to-date research will not only give students the most accurate picture of nutrition today but will also point them to current materials for further study.

Early introduction of digestion and absorption. These topics are discussed before the energy-yielding nutrients. This enables students to obtain a good background in the basic entry of nutrients into the body before they learn how nutrients function in the body.

Separate chapters on energy balance, weight control, and anorexia nervosa and bulimia. The student receives a thorough discussion on these very controversial and current topics.

Emphasis on changing behaviors. Chapter 18 both encourages the student to plan his or her own diet to enhance health maintenance and then outlines how to do so. This chapter allows the student to take the foundations of the course and apply them to daily life, allowing the student to put all of the concepts into perspective, set nutritional goals, and then change his or her own diet accordingly.

Career paths in the field of nutrition are developed. Chapter 20 informs the nutrition student of many possible avenues to pursue when looking for a job and eventual career. It is also very eye-opening to non-nutrition majors and spurs interest in possibly selecting a career in nutrition or working with nutrition professionals.

Design

Organizing the illustration program for this textbook has been quite exciting. We have drawn heavily from the biology and physiology expertise of Times Mirror/Mosby, and especially the illustrators under the direction of William Ober, M.D. This textbook is far ahead of any in the field in depicting important biological and physiological phenomenon, such as cell membranes, emulsification, glucose regulation, digestion and absorption, the progression of cancer, and fetal development. The extensive, 3-dimensional graphic presentations in this book will make nutrition and relevant physiological principles come alive for students.

In addition, we have drawn on many sources to provide what we consider the best photographic program in any nutrition text. The numerous 4-color photos for this text were researched and selected to reflect a modern view of food consumption and food presentation. This visually provides for the student the most outstanding and up-to-date view of the nutrition arena today.

Pedagogy

The following extensive pedagogical features were designed not only to interest the student but also to constantly reinforce the learning process:

Nutrition awareness inventory. This set of 15 true/false questions with answers at the end of each chapter serves to heighten awareness of chapter content. This feature also provides students with a gauge of how much they learned by repeating the quiz and comparing their scores.

Exploring issues and actions. These brief questions and comments throughout the margins of each chapter personalize the material by asking students to apply nutritional information to their own lives.

Margin notes. A liberal use of margin notes appear throughout the book. These notes provide clinical examples, references to other chapters, clarification of ideas, and further details for important concepts.

Margin definitions. Important key terms are boldfaced at first mention. More difficult terms include a definition in the text's margin. All boldfaced terms are included in the glossary at the back of the text.

Use of italics. Periodically, important points are italicized throughout the text. These are concepts that the student would usually highlight while studying.

Concept checks. This material summarizes recent chapter content every few pages, providing the student with the opportunity to monitor his or her understanding of the material presented.

Take action. This activity at the end of each chapter provides the student with an opportunity to put theory into practice. The suggested assignments are usually proactive and at times involve the student in an activity in which a registered dietitian or nutritionist may perform.

Summary points. Chapter content is summarized by highlighting 7 to 10 major points. This feature, together with the Concept Checks, should help students to study for examinations.

Suggested readings. This feature helps students find interesting and timely articles.

Up-to-date references. Each chapter contains approximately 30 current references, most published since 1987.

Nutrition Perspectives. These essays at the end of each chapter extend the chapter content by adding more detailed and often controversial material. Milestones in nutrition history and research are also discussed, including a look at pellagra, rickets, and the development of nutrition thought and nutrition careers since 1900.

Expert Opinion boxes. Each chapter contains an "Expert Opinion" written by a noted researcher. In most cases, the expert has received recognition from the American Dietetic Association.

Glossary. A comprehensive glossary of more than 500 words is included for the student's reference. The glossary contains a list of common medical terms and their root definitions, as well as pronunciation inclusions for many unfamiliar terms.

SUPPLEMENTARY MATERIALS

Both the student and the instructor are provided with the latest materials to make better use of the text and the concepts of the course:

Instructor's manual and test bank. Prepared by Mary C. Mitchell, Ph.D., R.D., this comprehensive teaching aid includes chapter summaries with suggestions for teaching difficult material; activities; suggested readings; nutrition assessments; conversion notes; source lists of supplementary materials; and a unique "Survival" chapter addressed to the novice instructor that discusses class organization, scheduling, and problem areas such as cheating.

Extensively reviewed for clarity and accuracy, the Test Bank features more than 2000 test items (multiple-choice, short-answer, and matching) coded for level of difficulty, the kind of knowledge being tested, topic, and text page reference. Test items in each chapter follow the sequence of chapter discussions to make selection easy. The resource manual also includes 75 transparency masters of key illustrations selected from the text.

Diploma II computerized test bank. Qualified adopters of the text receive a computerized Test Bank package compatible with the IBM, Macintosh, Apple IIc, or Apple IIe microcomputers. This software provides a unique combination of user-friendly aids and enables the instructor to select, edit, delete, or add questions, and construct and print tests and answer keys. The Gradebook segment features computerized record-keeping, and class, test, or individual grade analysis displayed as bar charts. The Proctor segment allows instructors to set up student tutorials, using items from the Test Bank or specially written tests.

Study guide. Prepared by Gordon M. Wardlaw, this student aid has been thoroughly reviewed by experienced instructors and developed in consultation with a learning theory expert. This comprehensive guide reinforces concepts presented in the text and integrates them with study activities, such as the use of flash cards to reinforce key concepts. It features vocabulary review and sample exams structured to reflect the actual exams students will face in the classroom. An ongoing dietary analysis highlights the content of each chapter.

Mosby Diet Simple nutrient analysis software. This interactive software includes a unique food list with more than 1500 items, selected activities, and food exchange lists. The disk allows students to input food intake and physical activities to determine total kcalories consumed and expended in a 24-hour period.

Transparency acetates. Seventy-eight full-color transparency acetates feature key illustrations from the text with large, easy-to-read labels.

ACKNOWLEDGMENTS

Reviewers

As our goal throughout this project has been to provide the most accurate, up-to-date, and useful introductory nutrition text available, we have constantly called on the expert assistance of many noted colleagues in nutrition research and instruction.

We would like to thank those people whose insight and direction guided us in the proposal stages in order to develop a game plan for an outstanding text:

Carol Byrd-Bredbenner, Ph.D., R.D.
Montclair State College

Susan Crockett, Ph.D.
North Dakota State University

Barbara Gilpin, M.S.
Mesa Community College

Robert Hackman, Ph.D.
University of Oregon

Wendy Hunt, M.S., R.D.
American River College

Nelda Loper, M.S., R.D.
Seminole Community College

Janice Peach, M.S.
Western Washington University

Diana Spillman, Ph.D., R.D.
Miami University

Special gratitude must go to those people who reviewed the entire text. They will find their "fingerprints" throughout the text, because their valuable reviews shaped its outcome:

Richard Ahrens, Ph.D., R.D.
University of Maryland

Kathy Beerman, Ph.D.
Washington State University

Wen Chiu, Ph.D.
Shoreline Community College

Sylvia Gartung, B.S.
Michigan State University

Catherine Justice, Ph.D., R.D.
Purdue University

Michael Keenan, Ph.D.
Louisiana State University

RoseAnn Kutschke, Ph.D.
University of Texas—Austin

Joseph Leichter, Ph.D.
University of British Columbia

Ricki Lewis, Ph.D.
State University of New York—Albany

Sandra Mitchell, Ph.D., R.D.
California State University—Chico

Jean Peters, M.S.
Oregon State University

Harry Sitren, Ph.D.
University of Florida

Joanne Slavin, Ph.D., R.D.
University of Minnesota

Anne Smith, Ph.D., R.D.
The Ohio State University

Linda Vaughan, Ph.D., R.D.
Arizona State University

We would like to thank the following people whose field of expertise was requested on specific chapters or sections of the book:

Stephen Barrett, M.D.
Psychiatrist and Consumer Advocate
Index, Chapters 1–20

Sue Bolze, Ph.D., R.D.
The Ohio State University (formerly)
Chapters 14–17

Linda Boyne, M.S., R.D.
The Ohio State University
Chapters 15 and 16

C. Russell Hille, Ph.D.
The Ohio State University
Chapter 7

Carol Johnston, Ph.D.
Arizona State University
Appendices

Murray Kaplan, Ph.D.
Iowa State University
Chapter 8

Donald McCormick, Ph.D.
Emory University
Chapters 11–14

Edward Naber, Ph.D.
The Ohio State University
Chapter 6

James Olson, Ph.D.
Iowa State University
Chapter 11

Karla Roehring, Ph.D.
The Ohio State University
Chapter 4

Walton T. Roth, M.D.
Stanford University
Chapters 1, 17, and 18

Rosita Schiller, Ph.D., R.D.
The Ohio State University
Chapter 20

Ann Voss, Ph.D., R.D.
The Ohio State University
Chapter 5

A unique feature of this book is the "Expert Opinion" boxes. We would like to thank the following experts whose outstanding and insightful articles are a highlight of this text:

Bruce Arnow, Ph.D.
Stanford University

Kelly Brownell, Ph.D.
University of Pennsylvania

James Ferguson, M.D.
University of Utah

Helen Guthrie, Ph.D., R.D.
The Pennsylvania State University

Al Harper, Ph.D.
University of Wisconsin

John Hathcock, Ph.D.
Food and Drug Administration

Victor Herbert, M.D., J.D.
Mount Sinai School of Medicine

Jules Hirsch, M.D.
Rockefeller University

Janet King, Ph.D., R.D.
University of California–Berkeley

David Klurfeld, Ph.D.
Wistar Institute of Anatomy and Biology

David Kritchevsky, Ph.D.
Wistar Institute of Anatomy and Biology

David Lamb, Ph.D.
The Ohio State University

Velimir Matkovic, M.D., Ph.D.
The Ohio State University

James Olson, Ph.D.
Iowa State University

Ellyn Satter, M.S., R.D.
Family Therapy Center, Madison, WI

Rosita Schiller, Ph.D., R.D.
The Ohio State University

Robert Stokstad, Ph.D.
University of California–Berkeley

Jean Weininger, Ph.D.
University of California–Berkeley

Jackie Wood, Ph.D.
The Ohio State University

Bonnie Worthington-Roberts, Ph.D., R.D.
University of Washington

Jack Yetiv, M.D., Ph.D.
Sequoia Hospital, Menlo Park, CA

Frank Young, M.D., Ph.D.
Food and Drug Administration

Special acknowledgements

We would like to thank our developmental editor, Vicki Van Ry, who nurtured and assisted us every step of the tortuous journey, and also Kathy Sedovic, the developmental editor who originally launched this project. Pat Coryell, Acquisitions Editor, and Ed Murphy, Vice President and Publisher, facilitated the difficult decisions that frequently arose. Francine Kohnen researched most of the outstanding photographs, Gina Chan provided excellent and careful copyediting and production work, and Mark Spann managed the text through a whirlwind production schedule.

This book would never have been completed without the help of our two wives. Marcia Insel provided excellent technical advice in developing and writing the manuscript, as well as adding a considerable flair to the prose. Much of the daily task of reforming the manuscript through many drafts also fell on her shoulders. Lorie Wardlaw typed the first draft of the manuscript and also contributed much assistance in refining the second and eventually the third draft. While this book was taking every free minute for the last two years, our children William and Elizabeth Wardlaw and Claire and Philip Insel had to sometimes wait for their parents to finish the book in order to have their bedtime stories, go to the swimming pool, or walk the dog. The book began with a dream, was fostered by the excitement that each element brought, and has ended in the establishment of an innovative and exciting textbook which we feel sets a new standard for introductory nutrition textbooks.

Gordon M. Wardlaw
Paul M. Insel

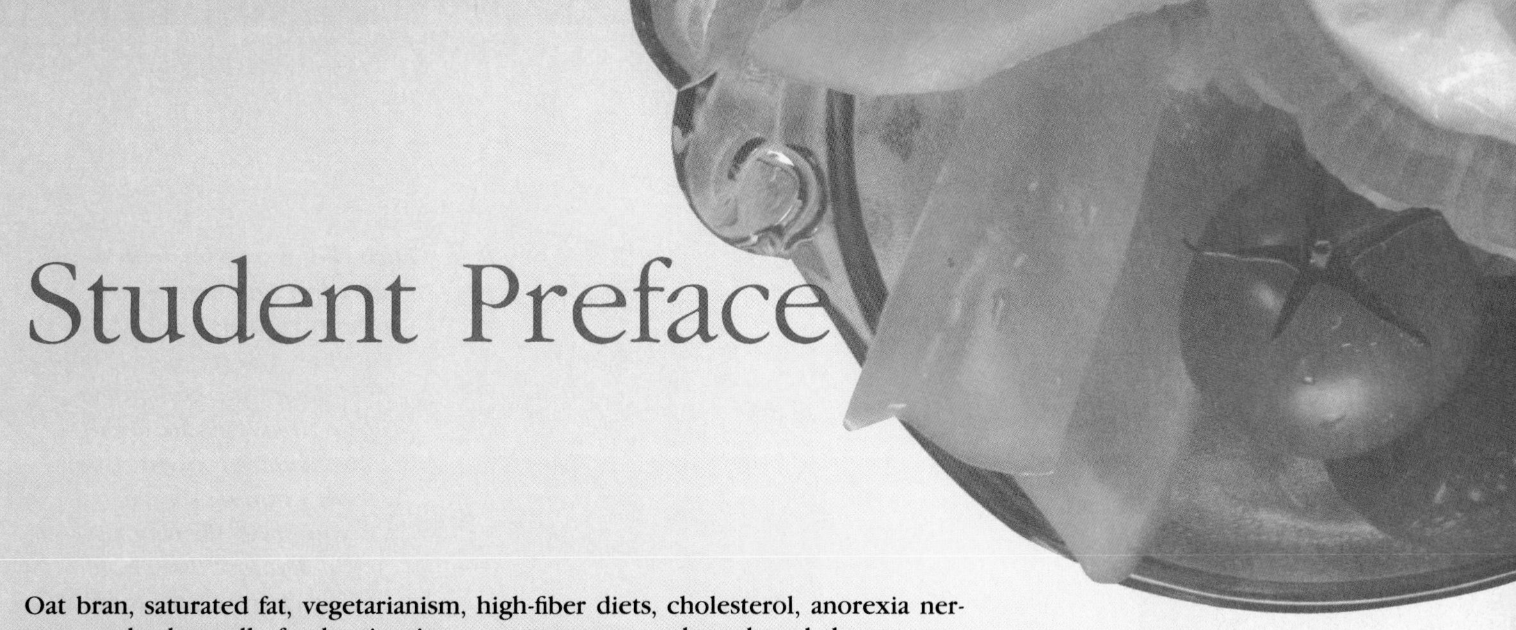

Student Preface

Oat bran, saturated fat, vegetarianism, high-fiber diets, cholesterol, anorexia nervosa, and salmonella food poisoning—we suspect you have heard these terms. Which are important enough to be a consideration in your life?

North Americans pride themselves on being individuals. Nutritional advice should be given in that manner. Not all of us have high blood cholesterol levels, and so don't face a risk for heart disease. The need to tailor dietary advice to the individual nature of each of us is the basic philosophy behind this book. We first carefully define terms and explain the relationship between nutrition and health. Then we encourage you to discover more about your own health status and apply nutrition concepts in this book that specifically pertain to you.

We think you will find that the study of nutrition is fascinating. This text combines some of the most interesting and important elements of biology, physiology, nutrition, and food composition to help you understand both how your body works and how what you eat affects your health.

FEATURES

We have included some features in this book that you should find especially interesting and valuable to your study of nutrition:

Chemistry review. In Chapter 2 we discuss the critical concepts you need to understand chemistry in the context of nutrition. Mixing a bit of chemistry knowledge with a lot of nutrition knowledge gives you a better understanding of how nutrients work and how nutrition information applies to you.

Planning a new way of eating. By Chapter 18 you will know more about how nutrients affect health, and should know a great deal about your own health and nutrient status. It is then time to change your diet where needed to reflect any weaknesses in your overall health. Chapter 18 begins with exploring your problems and ends with designing a plan to deal with those problems.

Careers in nutrition. At this time you are probably looking at many career options. Chapter 20 outlines the major roles, responsibilities and opportunities that various careers in nutrition hold. Even if you do not plan to pursue a career in a nutrition-related field, this chapter will help you understand more about what dietetic and nutrition professionals know and can do.

Pedagogy

Perspectives in Nutrition incorporates some important tools (called pedagogy) to help you learn nutrition. The next few pages graphically point out how to use these study aids to your best advantage.

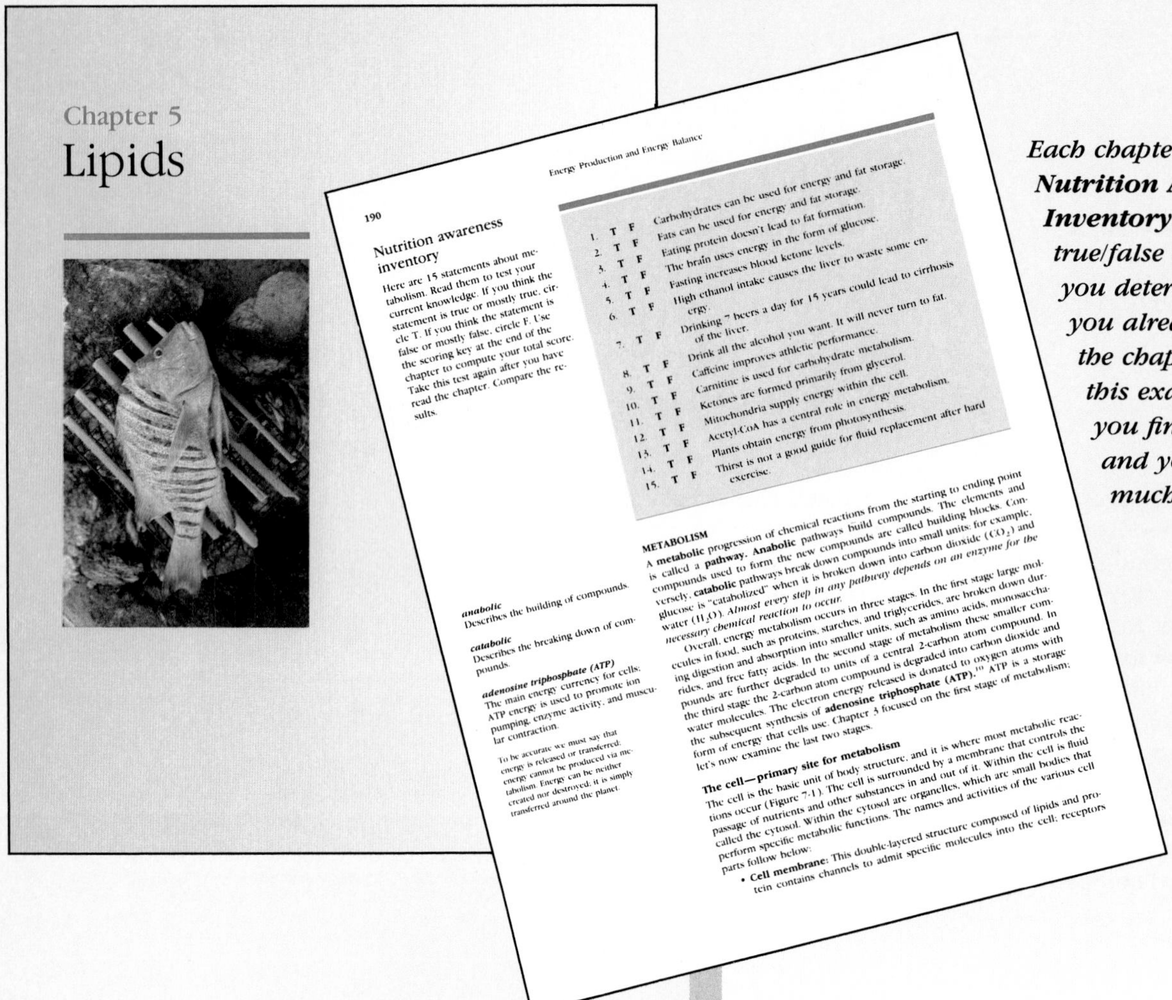
Chapter 5

Lipids

190 Energy Production and Energy Balance

Nutrition awareness inventory

Here are 15 statements about metabolism. Read them to test your current knowledge. If you think the statement is true or mostly true, circle T. If you think the statement is false or mostly false, circle F. Use the scoring key at the end of the chapter to compute your total score. Take this test again after you have read the chapter. Compare the results.

1. T F Carbohydrates can be used for energy and fat storage.
2. T F Fats can be used for energy and fat storage.
3. T F Eating protein doesn't lead to fat formation.
4. T F The brain uses energy in the form of glucose.
5. T F Fasting increases blood ketone levels.
6. T F High ethanol intake causes the liver to waste some energy.
7. T F Drinking 7 beers a day for 15 years could lead to cirrhosis of the liver.
8. T F Drink all the alcohol you want. It will never turn to fat.
9. T F Caffeine improves athletic performance.
10. T F Carnitine is used for carbohydrate metabolism.
11. T F Ketones are formed primarily from glycerol.
12. T F Mitochondria supply energy within the cell.
13. T F Acetyl-CoA has a central role in energy metabolism.
14. T F Plants obtain energy from photosynthesis.
15. T F Thirst is not a good guide for fluid replacement after hard exercise.

METABOLISM

A **metabolic** progression of chemical reactions from the starting to ending point is called a **pathway**. **Anabolic** pathways build compounds. The elements and compounds used to form the new compounds are called building blocks. Conversely, **catabolic** pathways break down compounds into small units; for example, glucose is "catabolized" when it is broken down into carbon dioxide (CO_2) and water (H_2O). *Almost every step in any pathway depends on an enzyme for the necessary chemical reaction to occur.*

Overall, energy metabolism occurs in three stages. In the first stage large molecules in food, such as proteins, starches, and triglycerides, are broken down during digestion and absorption into smaller units, such as amino acids, monosaccharides, and free fatty acids. In the second stage of metabolism these smaller compounds are further degraded to units of a central 2-carbon atom compound. In the third stage the 2-carbon atom compound is degraded into carbon dioxide and water molecules. The electron energy released is donated to oxygen atoms with the subsequent synthesis of **adenosine triphosphate (ATP)**.[10] ATP is a storage form of energy that cells use. Chapter 3 focused on the first stage of metabolism; let's now examine the last two stages.

anabolic Describes the building of compounds.

catabolic Describes the breaking down of compounds.

adenosine triphosphate (ATP) The main energy currency for cells; ATP energy is used to promote ion pumping, enzyme activity, and muscular contraction.

To be accurate we must say that energy is released or transferred; energy cannot be produced via metabolism. Energy can be neither created nor destroyed; it is simply transferred around the planet.

The cell—primary site for metabolism

The cell is the basic unit of body structure, and it is where most metabolic reactions occur (Figure 7-1). The cell is surrounded by a membrane that controls the passage of nutrients and other substances in and out of it. Within the cell is fluid called the cytosol. Within the cytosol are organelles, which are small bodies that perform specific metabolic functions. The names and activities of the various cell parts follow below:

- **Cell membrane:** This double-layered structure composed of lipids and protein contains channels to admit specific molecules into the cell; receptors

Each chapter begins with a ***Nutrition Awareness Inventory.*** *This group of 15 true/false questions helps you determine how much you already know about the chapter content. Take this exam again when you finish the chapter and you will see how much you have learned.*

Throughout each chapter are ***boldfaced key terms.*** *These are terms you will need to be familiar with throughout your study. The more difficult terms will include a definition in the text's margins. All boldfaced terms will appear with their definitions and pronunciations in the* ***glossary*** *at the end of the text.*

biological value of a protein
A measurement of the body's ability to retain protein absorbed from a food.

EVALUATION OF P

Protein quality refer
maintenance. Metho
will discuss the mor

Biological value

The **biological valu**
tein can be turned
amino acids, it shou
into body proteins.
its amino acid patt
ter the match, the n

BV = nitrogen r / nitrogen a

We actually measur
itself is easier to me

Table 6-3

Comparative protein quality of selected foods

Food	Chemical (amino acid) score	BV*	NPU†	PER‡
Egg	100	100	94	3.92
Cow's milk	95	93	82	3.09
Fish	71	76	—	3.55
Beef	69	74	67	2.30
Unpolished rice	67	86	59	—
Peanuts	65	55	55	1.65
Oats	57	65	—	2.19
Polished rice	57	64	57	2.18
Whole wheat	53	65	49	1.53
Corn	49	72	36	—
Soybeans	47	73	61	[illegible]
Sesame seeds	42	62	53	[illegible]
Peas	37	64	55	[illegible]

*Biological value
†Net protein utilization
‡Protein efficiency ratio

The numerous ***tables*** *throughout the text provide convenient capsules of information for reference.*

You'll find that the numerous 4-color, 3-dimensional ***illustrations*** *almost jump off the page. No other nutrition textbook provides you with effective, detailed anatomical drawings that virtually "come alive."*

8 Energy Balance 249

Take Action

Do you know your numbers? Complete the following table.

Height ______ centimeters ______ meters ______ inches
Weight ______ kilograms ______ pounds
Frame size (Table 8-6) (circle one): small medium large
Desirable body weight (Table 8-5): ______ pounds
(shortcut method, page 236): ______ pounds *

Percentage of desirable weight:

$$\frac{(\text{current weight} - \text{desirable weight})}{\text{desirable weight}} \times 100 = \underline{\qquad}$$

$$\text{Body mass index:} \frac{\text{weight (kilograms)}}{\text{height}^2\text{ (meters)}} = \underline{\qquad}$$

Waist circumference: ______ centimeters ______ inches
Hip circumference: ______ centimeters ______ inches
Waist to hip ratio: ______
Shape (circle if appropriate): android gynecoid
Resting energy needs (Harris-Benedict equation, Appendix M)
(Oliver formula, Appendix M)
H-B ______ kcalories; Oliver ______ kcalories
Total energy needs: RDA ______ kcalories
based on weight (see page 232) ______ kcalories
Percentage of total energy needs due to resting metabolic rate:

$$\frac{\text{resting energy needs}}{\text{total energy needs}} \times 100 = \underline{\qquad}\ \%$$

Thermic effect of food in 24 hours:

total energy needs × either .06 or .10 = ______—______ kcalories

REFERENCES

1. Anderson GH: Metabolic regulation of food intake. In Shils ME and Young VR, eds: Modern nutrition in health and disease, Philadelphia, 1988, Lea & Febiger.
2. Anonymous: Genetic differences in mitochondrial ATPase. Nutrition Reviews 45:248, 1987.
3. Anonymous: Role of fat and fatty acids in the modulation of energy exchange. Nutrition Reviews 46:382, 1988.
4. Atkinson RL: Opioid regulation of food intake and body weight in humans. Federation Proceedings 46:178, 1987.
5. Beutler B: Cachexia: a fundamental mechanism. Nutrition Reviews 46:369, 1988.
6. Blair D and Buskirk ER: Habitual daily energy expenditure and activity levels of lean and adult-onset and child-onset obese women. The American Journal of Clinical Nutrition 45:540, 1987.
7. Bray GA: Complications of obesity. Annals of Internal Medicine 103:1052, 1985.
8. Bray GA: Nutrient balance and obesity: classification and evaluation of the obesities. Medical clinics of North America 73:29, 1989.
9. Brownell KD: The psychology and physiology of obesity: implications for screening and treatment. The Journal of the American Dietetic Association 84:406, 1984.
10. Daily JM and others: Human energy requirements: overestimation by widely used prediction equation. The American Journal of Clinical Nutrition 42:1170, 1985.
11. Donahue RP and others: Central obesity and coronary heart disease in men. Lancet, p 11, April 11, 1987.
12. Fernstrom JD: Tryptophan, serotonin, and carbohydrate appetite: will the real carbohydrate craver please stand up. Journal of Nutrition 118:1417, 1988.
13. Garn SM: Family-line and socioeconomic factors in fatness and obesity. Nutrition Reviews 44:381, 1986.
14. Haffner SM and others: Do upper-body and centralized adiposity measure different as-

At the end of each chapter is a ***Take Action*** *that will help you put a major concept in each chapter into focus for your own life. The activity may include looking more carefully at your diet, examining your family history, or applying information you learned to others.*

14 Nutrition Basics

How do we rate our diets?
Judging from the responses given by well over half the people in several large surveys, we are extremely concerned about good nutrition and are well aware of possible health hazards from fat, salt, and sugar.[21] Still, the unwillingness of many people to examine their nutritional practices is probably the major impediment to improving their diet—concern does not necessarily translate into change.
Over half of the people in a USDA survey[22] described their nutritional intake as excellent or above average, 42% said it was average, and only 4% felt it was below average. They were not convinced they needed to know more about nutrition, in spite of scoring low on nutrition-knowledge questions. Only 7% of people surveyed said they were not very well informed. Most viewed food and cooking as a pleasure, not as a science. We hope you will think of it as both. One third agreed that "the impression I get is that nobody really knows the answers on the best foods to eat for a balanced diet." Almost one half agreed that "learning the basic ideas in nutrition will probably alter my personal eating habits very little." We hope we can convince you otherwise.

WHAT SHAPES OUR FOOD TASTES?
The basic purpose of food is nourishment, but to us it means far more than that, and that is fine. *Food symbolizes much of what we think about ourselves.*[11] We bond relationships and express friendships around the dinner table. We enhance and maintain our social status by entertaining creatively or lavishly. We cope with stress and tension by eating or not eating. We influence other's behaviors through our food practices. Some of us express religious beliefs and display our creative talents through food preparation and ceremonies. Since people eat 80,000 to 100,000 times in a lifetime (this takes 13 to 15 years of our waking hours), eating becomes an important key to the way we define ourselves politically, religiously, and socially. See Table 1-5 to review many factors that affect food consumption in the United States, and Figure 1-3 for a model illustrating the effects of behavior and environment on food habits.
Food likes and dislikes are probably the most important determinants of what we eat. Respondents to a USDA survey[22] rated taste as the chief consideration in selecting foods to serve their families; budget came in second. Respondents were much more likely to serve a meal based on taste, compared with one they knew would be more nutritious.

Early experiences
Food preferences are learned early as social and cultural preferences.[23] They are refined through interactions with parents and friends, our social class, and the need for status. Unfortunately for young children, adult caregivers may severely limit the child's experience with food. Adults may purchase only a small subset of foods available, and may consider even many of these foods inappropriate for children. For example, at what age were you first introduced to okra, lentils, spinach salad, or salmon?
Mere exposure to a variety of foods can help reduce the resistance to trying new foods. Young children seem to prefer foods that are sweet or familiar, but preschoolers are often quite willing to try new things. Caregivers need to provide that opportunity. It may take as many as fifteen introductions, but the odds are in favor of final acceptance (see Chapter 16).
Our innate preferences are important, including universal enjoyment of sweet foods and dislike of bitter and sometimes spicy, burning ones. Bitter tastes often portend poisonous substances. However, innate responses can be modified through exposure and **conditioning** (learning, that is). This allows some people—even whole cultures—to learn to enjoy very sour or hot, spicy foods, such as jalapeno peppers and fiery curries.

Vegetables are a good source of dietary fiber.

Exploring Issues and Actions
After eating dinner, your active 4-year-old cousin is still hungry and asks for a bowl of cold cereal for dessert. What do you think about this?

conditioning
The process where an originally neutral stimulus repeatedly paired with a reinforcing agent elicits a predictable response.

The Exploring Issues and Actions questions enable you to apply chapter information to your own experiences.

The full-color ***photos*** *reflect a modern view of food consumption and food presentation.*

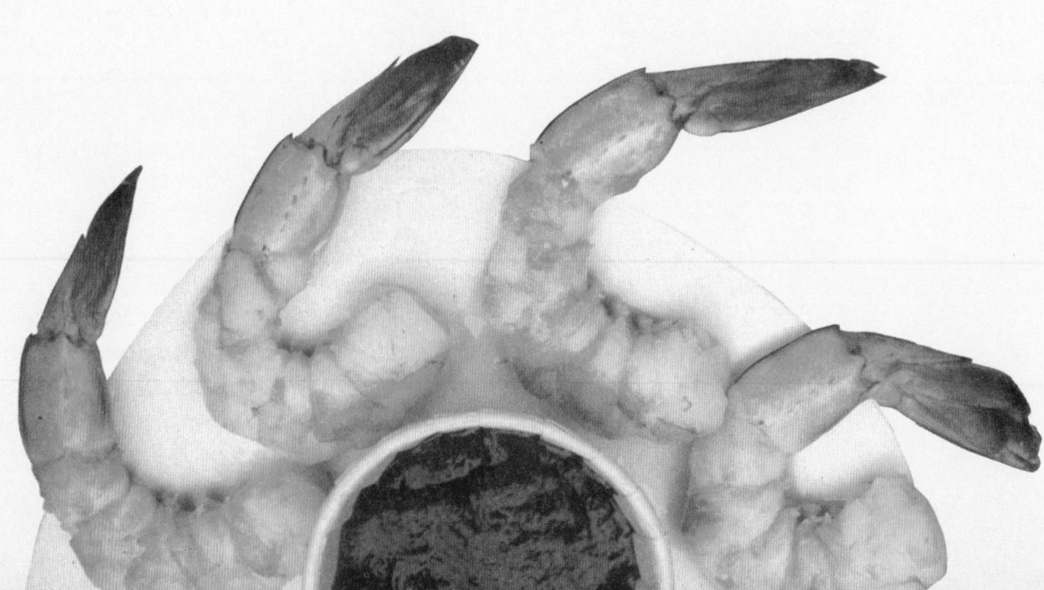

olecystokinin (CCK) to signal a natural satiety response, while giving the retch receptors in the stomach time to signal fullness. People who tend to eat *ything available* can stop purchasing foods they cannot resist.

Dieters must analyze their own particular shortcomings; they should sensi-ze themselves to facets of their life-style that make dieting difficult. Is snack-g, compulsive eating, or overeating at each meal a constant problem? Then spe-fic problems must be addressed. Table 9-3 provides many options for changing opping and eating behaviors. Table 9-5 shows step-by-step how to set goals and w to develop specific activities to meet these goals. It is usually best to develop written plan and show it to a friend or spouse. Social support is important. A

On almost every other page of the chapter are ***italicized sentences.*** *These are key ideas that you will probably want to highlight as you read, and will certainly want to reread before exams. These sentences summarize the major points that the chapter has been developing.*

The ***Concept Checks*** *list the major points made in a chapter section. If you don't understand what the Concept Check says, you should go back and reread that preceding section in the textbook.*

Ask your professor about new findings on the importance of fish oils to health. You may want to search the scientific literature yourself. A reference librarian can help you start.

The fish oil story unfolds daily. Increasing fish oil in the diet reduces both blood pressure and inflammation in certain diseases, such as psoriasis and asthma.[25,30] It will be exciting to follow this new area of research. (See the suggested readings on page 144.)

Concept Check

When cells use omega-3 fatty acids to synthesize hormone-like compounds called *eicosanoids*, the synthesized products differ markedly from those using omega-6 fatty acids. In general, products made from omega-3 fatty acids tend to lower blood clotting, blood pressure, and inflammatory responses in the body. In the future, there may be more specific recommendations for the deliberate inclusion of omega-3 fatty acids in diet planning. Presently the recommendation to eat fish about twice a week is our best guide.

Chain length—another factor to consider with fatty acids

Fats in foods that contain primarily saturated fatty acids are solid at room temperature, expecially if the fatty acids have a **long chain** (greater than 12 carbon atoms). **Medium-chain** saturated fatty acids (8 to 12 carbon atoms), such as those found in coconut oil, produce liquid oils at room temperature. The shorter chain length overrides the effect of saturation. **Short-chain** fatty acids (4 to 8 carbons) also form liquid oils at room temperature.[8] Food sources of short-chain fatty acids include dairy fats (see Appendix 1). *Fats containing primarily polyunsaturated or monounsaturated fatty acids are usually liquid at room temperature. Chain length is not an issue.*[8]

The capability of some saturated fatty acids of short- or medium-chain lengths to form oils at room temperature is significant. Non-dairy creamers initially appear to be a healthful substitute for cream because of cream's high content of saturated fats. However, many coffee creamers contain coconut oil, which is also high in saturated fatty acids. Manufacturers use coconut oil because it allows the product a long shelf life without turning rancid. You will see why in the following section. Low-fat milk is a much healthier choice than non-dairy creamers.

Hydrogenation of fatty acids

To solidify vegetable oils into margarines and shortenings the polyunsaturated fatty acids in plant oils must become more saturated. Hydrogen atoms are added across the double bonds in the fatty acids. *This process, called* ***hydrogenation,*** *turns many double bonds into single bonds and produces some trans fatty acids.*[16] Both changes increase hardness. Generally, the harder the product—stick margarine compared with tub margarine—the more hydrogenation has occurred. Hydrogenated fats are easier to use in some techniques of food production, such as in making pastries and cakes.

Recall from Chapter 2 that monounsaturated and polyunsaturated fatty acids can exist in two isomer forms—cis and trans. The cis form has the hydrogen atoms on the same side of the double bond. The trans form has the hydrogen atoms on opposite sides of the double bond (Figure 2-2). Plant fatty acids are in the cis form. A few trans fatty acids are in milk because the bacteria in a cow's multiple stomachs (rumen) rearrange the fatty acids from the cis form into the trans form. However, margarine has the highest concentration of trans fatty acids. *Presently the many studies done show that trans fatty acids are not linked to significantly increased risk for any disease, notably heart disease and cancer.*[16] Margarine—the major source of such fatty acids in our food—has been used increasingly for the last 20 years while heart disease rates have declined and cancer

UNSATURATED

ADDING HYDROGEN

HYDROGENATED

How liquid fatty acids become solid. (A) Unsaturated fatty acids in liquid form. (B) Hydrogen atoms are added (hydrogenation), changing double bonds to single bonds and producing *trans fatty acids.* (C) The hydrogenated product.

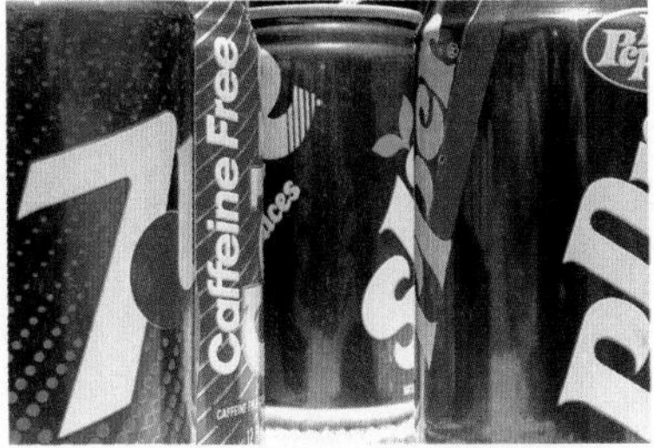

Soft drinks are today more popular than milk, although not as beneficial to the diet.

these trends are not fully known, but deaths from heart disease and strokes have dropped dramatically since the late 1960s. Better medical care and diets also deserve some credit. Still, affluence, when it leads to sedentary life-styles and high intakes of alcohol, can be a villain. *Because of better technology and greater choices, we have a much better diet today than ever before—if we know what to do with the choices. Overall, we are doing well, but many of us can do better. The goal here is to help you find your best path to good nutrition.*

Summary

1. Nutrition is the study of the food substances vital for health and how the body uses these substances to promote and support growth, maintenance, and reproduction of cells.
2. Nutrients in foods fall into six classes: carbohydrates, lipids (fats and oils), proteins, vitamins, minerals, and water. The first three, along with alcohol, provide energy for the body to use.
3. As nutritional health diminishes, nutrient stores in the body are depleted, then biochemical reactions in the body slow down and finally, clinical evidence (signs and symptoms) can be seen.
4. Overnutrition is a focus today in North America. This condition includes overconsumption of energy and certain vitamins and minerals.
5. The focus for nutrition planning should be food, not supplements. Using foods to supply nutrient needs essentially eliminates the possibility of severe nutrient imbalances.
6. Results from large nutrition surveys in North America suggest that on the whole the food supply is quite safe, but some North Americans need to concentrate on consuming foods that supply more vitamin A, vitamin C, vitamin B-6, calcium, magnesium, iron, zinc, and dietary fiber.
7. Our food choices are greatly affected by our culture, our family, our upbringing, our self-image, and the image we want to present to others.

If you can explain what the ***Concept Checks*** *represent and apply the information, as well as explain and apply the information listed in the* ***Summary,*** *you should be confident you understand the major points of the chapter and, therefore, are well-prepared to take an examination.*

Each chapter ends with a list of ***Summary Points.*** *These points constitute the major ideas in the chapter. These provide an ideal review for studying for exams.*

Expert Opinion

There's No Such Thing as "Junk Food" But There Are Junk *Diets*

HELEN A. GUTHRIE, PH.D., R.D.

During the past 15 years, the phrase "junk food" has invaded America's everyday vocabulary. As a nutritionist, I contend that this term is meaningless and should be discarded. There is no totally worthless food, any more than there is a perfect food that meets *all* our nutritional needs.

Obviously, some foods contribute more nutrients than do others. But almost any food has *some* redeeming value *under the right circumstances*. The problem arises when foods that contribute more calories than nutrients become so important in our diet that foods of higher nutritional value are excluded. It is equally possible to make an unbalanced selection of our most sacred nutritious foods and wind up with a diet overabundant in some nuturients yet deficient in others. In both cases, the result is a junk *diet*.

SOME FOODS GO HAND-IN-HAND

Foods of low nutrient density don't carry much nutritional weight by themselves. For example, in some cakes and cookies, most of the calories come from ingredients such as fat and sugar, and relatively few from milk, flour, and eggs. However, if eating a cookie means that a child also drinks milk or fruit juice, we should look at cookie-and-milk or cookie-and-juice as a unit and judge them together rather than condemn one and applaud the other. For an 8-year-old, milk and one or two cookies makes a nutritious combination. Milk and five cookies, though, may create an imbalance between calories and nutrients—and thus be considered lower in nutrition.

Potato chips are another example of a food that can be valuable in the right context. Eaten alone, potato chips add vitamin C, vitamin B_6, and copper to our diet. Eaten with a sandwich, potato chips become part of a balanced meal. But if we stuff ourselves with so many potato chips that we're too full to eat dinner, we are misusing them. What about the salt, you ask? One ounce of potato chips provides about one quarter gram of sodium—less than the amount in the bread in a sandwich and considerably less than the amount in two slices of bread with salted butter. Just because we see and taste the salt on potato chips doesn't mean they contain too much.

For another example, consider pizza. Some people see it as a junk food because it is high in calories, cholesterol, and fat. But pizza has nutritional merits comparable to a meat-and-cheese sandwich served with tomato.

TOO MUCH OF A GOOD THING?

How about the classically "healthful" foods like milk, eggs, orange juice, and oatmeal? Are they always desirable? Surprisingly, no. Milk, especially nonfat milk, has one of the most impressive nutrient profiles of any food. But it isn't perfect. Although high in calcium, protein, and riboflavin, it is low in iron and vitamin C. In contrast, oranges are high in iron and vitamin C, but low in calcium, protein, and riboflavin.

What does all this have to do with junk food? When a food doesn't meet an immediate nutritional need, its nutritional value is limited. After an adult has had two or three glasses of milk (which meet many nutritional needs), additional milk becomes less and less useful. If this additional milk (which does not provide vitamin C) displaces a fruit juice that does have vitamin C, that milk becomes worthless except as a source of calories. In this context, the extra milk would be a "junk" food. The key point to remember is that foods should not be judged in isolation but in relation to the total diet and the individual's needs.

If all our daily nutrient needs are met except for calories, we can obtain the rest of our calorie requirements from any food.

Of course, moderation is a virtue. And so is avoidance of excess amounts of saturated fats, sodium, calories, and cholesterol. Getting a maximum of 10% to 15% of our total daily calories from foods of limited nutritional value is reasonable.

COST PER NUTRIENT

In choosing nutritious foods, we might also consider cost per nutrient. Many parents feel good about giving their children buttered toast and honey for breakfast but feel guilty if they serve a doughnut. Since both bread and doughnuts are made with enriched flour—and often with whole-wheat flour—there is no appreciable difference in their nutrient content. Considering cost, however, the doughnut is not as good a buy. Similar considerations hold for french-fried and baked potatoes. Nutritionally, a serving of french fries cooked in oil compares favorably with a baked potato served with a fat such as sour cream or butter. However, the cost per nutrient of commercially prepared french fries can be considerably higher than that of home-prepared baked potatoes. Frequent eating of sticky sweets, especially between meals, should also be questioned because of its possible contribution to tooth decay. Nutritionists want people to eat the right amounts and combinations of nutrients to promote health, but they also want everyone to eat in a rational way, without feeling guilty about including a favorite food merely for the pleasure it provides. Special medical considerations aside, a healthful diet can include at least small amounts of any food you enjoy—as long as your overall diet is moderate in calories and properly balanced.

Dr. Guthrie is Professor of Nutrition at The Pennsylvania State University.

In the ***Expert Opinion*** *boxes, an expert in the field of nutrition and health outlines what he or she considers important information you need to understand nutrition issues of our day. Consider these boxed discussions like "visiting speakers" coming into your classroom to inform you of their latest research findings and information.*

4 Carbohydrates 117

REFERENCES

1. American Dietetic Association Reports: Position of The American Dietetic Association: appropriate use of nutritive and non-nutritive sweeteners. Journal of The American Dietetic Association 87:1689, 1987.
2. Anderson, JW: Fiber and health: an overview. Nutrition Today Nov Dec 1986.
3. Block, G and others: Nutrient sources in the American diet: quantitative data from the NHANES II. American Journal of Epidemiology 122:13, 1985.
4. Briggs, GM and Calloway DH: Nutrition and Physical Fitness, 11th edition, New York, 1984, Holt, Rinehart & Winston.
5. Bright-See, E: Dietary fiber and cancer. Nutrition Today July Aug 1988.
6. Burkitt, DP: Dietary fiber and cancer. Journal of Nutrition 118:531, 1988.
7. Castle, SC: Constipation. Archives of Internal Medicine 147:1702, 1987.
8. Costill, DL: Carbohydrates for exercise: dietary demands for optional performance. International Journal of Sports Medicine. 9:1, 1988.
9. Council on Scientific Affairs: Aspartame. Journal of the American Medical Association 254:400, 1985.
10. Cronin, FJ and Shaw, AM: Summary of dietary recommendations for healthy americans. Nutrition Today Nov Dec 1988.
11. Deutsch, RM: The New Nuts Among the Berries. Palo Alto, Calif, 1977, Bull Publishing Company.
12. Evans, WJ and Hughes, VA: Dietary carbohydrates and endurance exercise. The American Journal of Clinical Nutrition 41:1146, 1985.
13. U.S. Food and Drug Administration: New sweetener approved. FDA Consumer 22:4, 1988.
14. Filer, LJ: Modified food starch. Journal of the American Dietetic Association 88:342, 1988.
15. Hallfrisch, J and others: Acceptability of a 7-day higher-carbohydrate, lower-fat menu: the Beltsville diet study. Journal of The American Dietetic Association 88:163, 1988.
16. Hallfrisch, J and others: Mineral balance of men and women consuming high fiber diets with complex or simple carbohydrate. Journal of Nutrition 117:48, 1987.
17. Jenkins, DJA and others: Metabolic effects of a low-glycemic-index diet. American Journal of Clinical Nutrition 46:968, 1987.
18. Klurfeld, DM: The role of dietary fiber in gastrointestinal disease. The Journal of the American Dietetic Association 87:1172, 1987.
19. Kritchevsky, D: Dietary fiber. Annual Reviews of Nutrition 8:301, 1988.
20. Lanza, E and others: Dietary fiber intake in the U.S. population. American Journal of Clinical Nutrition 46:790, 1987.
21. Lanza, E and Butrum, RR: A critical review of food fiber analysis and data. Journal of The American Dietetic Association 86:732, 1986.
22. MacDonald, I: Carbohydrates. Schills, ME and Young, VR, editors: Modern Nutrition in Health and Disease. Philadelphia, Pa, 1988, Lea & Febiger.
23. Mayes, PA: Regulation of carbohydrate metabolism. Murray, RK and others, editors: Harper's Biochemistry. East Norwalk, Conn, 1988, Appleton & Lange.
24. Nelson, RL: Hypoglycemia: fact or fiction. Mayo Clinic Proceedings 60:844, 1985.
25. O'Neil, FT and others: Research and application of current topics in sports nutrition. Journal of The American Dietetic Association 86:1007, 1986.
26. Schiffman, SS and others: Aspartame and susceptibility to headache. New England Journal of Medicine 317:1181, 1987.
27. Slavin, JL: Dietary fiber: classification, chemical analyses, and food sources. Journal of The American Dietetic Association 87:1164, 1987.
28. Stegink, LD: The aspartame story: a model for the clinical testing of a food additive. American Journal of Clinical Nutrition 46:204, 1987.
29. Stevens, J and others: Comparison of the effects of psyllium and wheat bran on gastrointestinal transit time and stool characteristics. Journal of The American Dietetic Association 88:323, 1988.
30. Wolever, T and Jenkins, DJA: The use of glycemic index in predicting the blood glucose response to mixed meals. American Journal of Clinical Nutrition 43:167, 1986.

SUGGESTED READINGS

To learn more about aspartame read the article by Stegink, which provides a summary of the major research surrounding this popular low-calorie sweetener. For more information about dietary fiber study the article by Anderson. Although quite detailed, it is in a very readable and understandable format. We recommend that you read the journal it is published in, *Nutrition Today*, regularly if you want to learn more about nutrition. For more information about carbohydrate-loading, read the article by Costill. It summarizes the effects of dietary carbohydrates on sports performance in various sports and covers carbohydrate intake immediately before and during exercise.

CHAPTER 4
Answers to Nutrition Awareness Inventory

1. *True.* Glucose combined with fructose forms sucrose, or table sugar.
2. *True.* Few carbohydrates are present in animals foods.
3. *False.* Fat contains more kcalories per gram than carbohydrates (9 versus 4 kcalories per gram).
4. *True.* Carbohydrates are important energy-supplying nutrients.
5. *True.* Fiber is referred to as *bulk*, but *dietary fiber* is the preferred term.
6. *False.* Although there is no RDA for carbohydrates 50 to 100 grams per day is considered an adequate intake.
7. *False.* The body uses fiber to increase stool mass, which eases elimination.
8. *True.* In the exchange system milk yields 12 grams of carbohydrate per exchange.
9. *True.* When eaten in excess of energy needs carbohydrates are stored as glycogen and fat.
10. *False.* Honey, like table sugar, is a simple carbohydrate.
11. *True.* The average North American consumes about 125 pounds of simple sugars annually. Many nutritionists believe that this is too high. A diet including less than 50 pounds per year allows for more healthful foods in the diet.
12. *True.* Honey may contain bacteria spores that may grow and become fatal to infants because their stomachs have yet to develop the strong acidic environment that adult stomachs have. Acid reduces the bacterium's growth.
13. *False.* Diabetes mellitus is a disorder of high blood glucose levels.
14. *True.* Researchers have found that if an athlete eats greatly increased amounts of carbohydrates—about 70% of total kcalories—each day for 3 days before an event, he can greatly enhance carbohydrate storage in the muscles. This enhances "aerobic" athletic endurance.
15. *True.* This was observed by Dr. Denis Burkitt, who attributes this phenomenon to the high dietary fiber intakes of Africans as compared with North Americans.

We make a point of providing you with a detailed ***reference list*** *to back up material presented in the chapter. The research cited is from the latest available publications: more than two thirds of the references are from sources published in the last half of the 1980's.*

If you are preparing a research paper for your class, or would just like to read further into specific topics, consult the ***suggested readings*** *section at the end of each chapter for interesting and informative articles.*

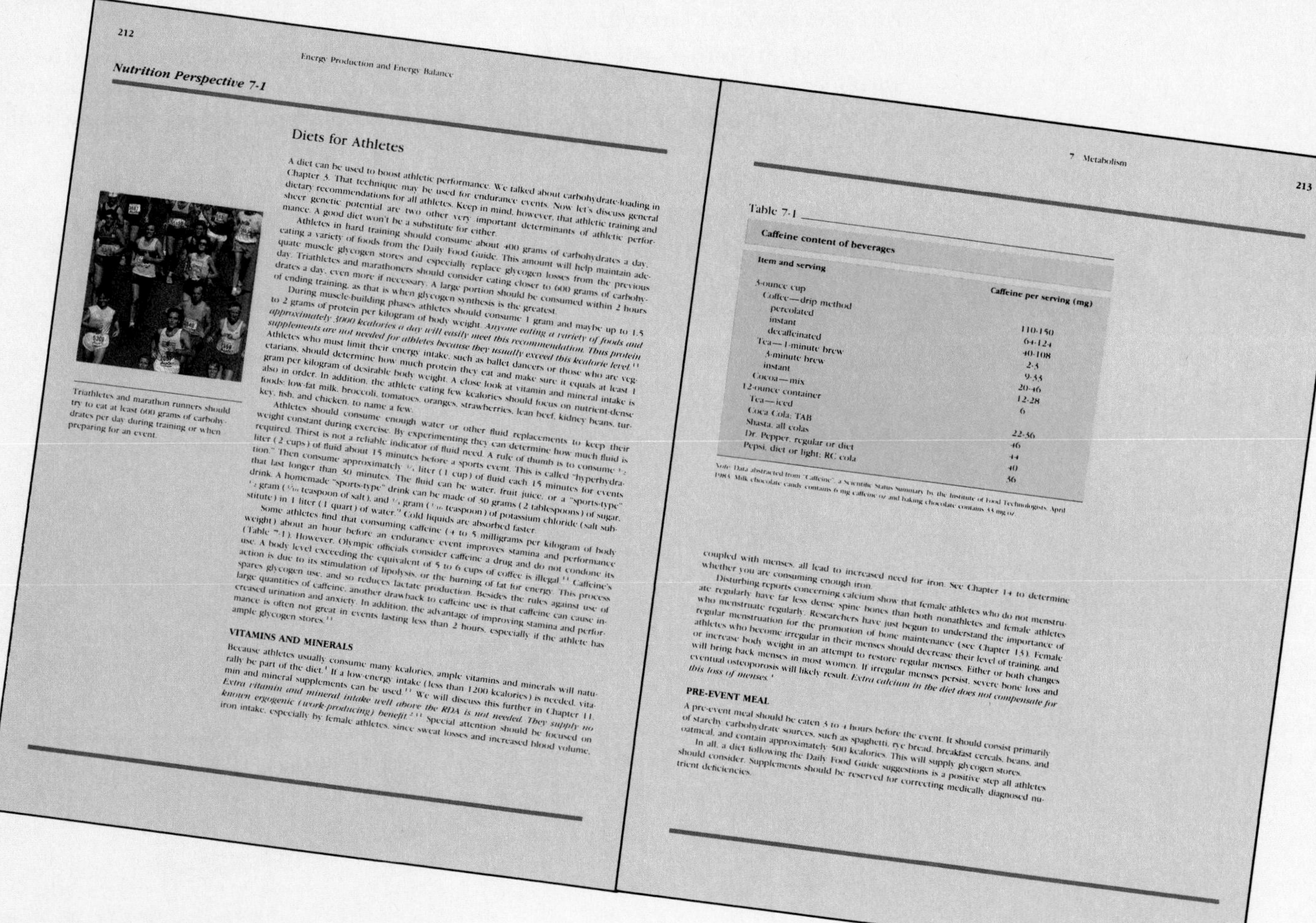

212 Energy Production and Energy Balance

Nutrition Perspective 7-1

Diets for Athletes

A diet can be used to boost athletic performance. We talked about carbohydrate-loading in Chapter 3. That technique may be used for endurance events. Now let's discuss general dietary recommendations for all athletes. Keep in mind, however, that athletic training and sheer genetic potential are two other very important determinants of athletic performance. A good diet won't be a substitute for either.

Athletes in hard training should consume about 400 grams of carbohydrates a day, eating a variety of foods from the Daily Food Guide. This amount will help maintain adequate muscle glycogen stores and especially replace glycogen losses from the previous day. Triathletes and marathoners should consider eating closer to 600 grams of carbohydrates a day, even more if necessary. A large portion should be consumed within 2 hours of ending training, as that is when glycogen synthesis is the greatest.

During muscle-building phases athletes should consume 1 gram and maybe up to 1.5 to 2 grams of protein per kilogram of body weight. *Anyone eating a variety of foods and approximately 3000 kcalories a day will easily meet this recommendation. Thus protein supplements are not needed for athletes because they usually exceed this kcalorie level.*[11] Athletes who must limit their energy intake, such as ballet dancers or those who are vegetarians, should determine how much protein they eat and make sure it equals at least 1 gram per kilogram of desirable body weight. A close look at vitamin and mineral intake is also in order. In addition, the athlete eating few kcalories should focus on nutrient-dense foods: low-fat milk, broccoli, tomatoes, oranges, strawberries, lean beef, kidney beans, turkey, fish, and chicken, to name a few.

Athletes should consume enough water or other fluid replacements to keep their weight constant during exercise. By experimenting they can determine how much fluid is required. Thirst is not a reliable indicator of fluid need. A rule of thumb is to consume 1/2 liter (2 cups) of fluid about 15 minutes before a sports event. This is called "hyperhydration." Then consume approximately 1/4 liter (1 cup) of fluid each 15 minutes for events that last longer than 30 minutes. The fluid can be water, fruit juice, or a "sports-type" drink. A homemade "sports-type" drink can be made of 30 grams (2 tablespoons) of sugar, 1/2 gram (1/10 teaspoon of salt), and 1/3 gram (1/16 teaspoon) of potassium chloride (salt substitute) in 1 liter (1 quart) of water.[2] Cold liquids are absorbed faster.

Some athletes find that consuming caffeine (4 to 5 milligrams per kilogram of body weight) about an hour before an endurance event improves stamina and performance (Table 7-1). However, Olympic officials consider caffeine a drug and do not condone its use. A body level exceeding the equivalent of 5 to 6 cups of coffee is illegal.[11] Caffeine's action is due to its stimulation of lipolysis, or the burning of fat for energy. This process spares glycogen use, and so reduces lactate production. Besides the rules against use of large quantities of caffeine, another drawback to caffeine use is that caffeine can cause increased urination and anxiety. In addition, the advantage of improving stamina and performance is often not great in events lasting less than 2 hours, especially if the athlete has ample glycogen stores.[11]

Triathletes and marathon runners should try to eat at least 600 grams of carbohydrates per day during training or when preparing for an event.

VITAMINS AND MINERALS

Because athletes usually consume many kcalories, ample vitamins and minerals will naturally be part of the diet.[1] If a low-energy intake (less than 1200 kcalories) is needed, vitamin and mineral supplements can be used.[11] We will discuss this further in Chapter 11. *Extra vitamin and mineral intake well above the RDA is not needed. They supply no known ergogenic (work-producing) benefit.*[2,11] Special attention should be focused on iron intake, especially by female athletes, since sweat losses and increased blood volume,

7 Metabolism 213

Table 7-1

Caffeine content of beverages

Item and serving	Caffeine per serving (mg)
5-ounce cup	
Coffee—drip method	110-150
percolated	64-124
instant	40-108
decaffeinated	2-5
Tea—1-minute brew	9-33
3-minute brew	20-46
instant	12-28
Cocoa—mix	6
12-ounce container	
Tea—iced	22-36
Coca Cola; TAB	46
Shasta, all colas	44
Dr. Pepper, regular or diet	40
Pepsi, diet or light; RC cola	36

Note: Data abstracted from "Caffeine", a Scientific Status Summary by the Institute of Food Technologists, April 1983. Milk chocolate candy contains 6 mg caffeine/oz and baking chocolate contains 35 mg/oz.

coupled with menses, all lead to increased need for iron. See Chapter 14 to determine whether you are consuming enough iron.

Disturbing reports concerning calcium show that female athletes who do not menstruate regularly have far less dense spine bones than both nonathletes and female athletes who menstruate regularly. Researchers have just begun to understand the importance of regular menstruation for the promotion of bone maintenance (see Chapter 13). Female athletes who become irregular in their menses should decrease their level of training, and or increase body weight in an attempt to restore regular menses. Either or both changes will bring back menses in most women. If irregular menses persist, severe bone loss and eventual osteoporosis will likely result. *Extra calcium in the diet does not compensate for this loss of menses.*[1]

PRE-EVENT MEAL

A pre-event meal should be eaten 3 to 4 hours before the event. It should consist primarily of starchy carbohydrate sources, such as spaghetti, rye bread, breakfast cereals, beans, and oatmeal, and contain approximately 500 kcalories. This will supply glycogen stores.

In all, a diet following the Daily Food Guide suggestions is a positive step all athletes should consider. Supplements should be reserved for correcting medically diagnosed nutrient deficiencies.

***Nutrition Perspectives** are essays at the end of chapters that develop current topics in nutrition in greater detail than the chapter can. Topics include heart disease, cancer, quackery, dietary advice for athletes, nutrition labeling, vegetarianism, and lactose intolerance.*

ACCElerate Your Growth!

A Student Study Guide and Mosby Diet Simple software are avilable with *Perspectives In Nutrition.* These instructional aids are designed to help you practice the major concepts developed in each chapter and prepare for classroom exams.

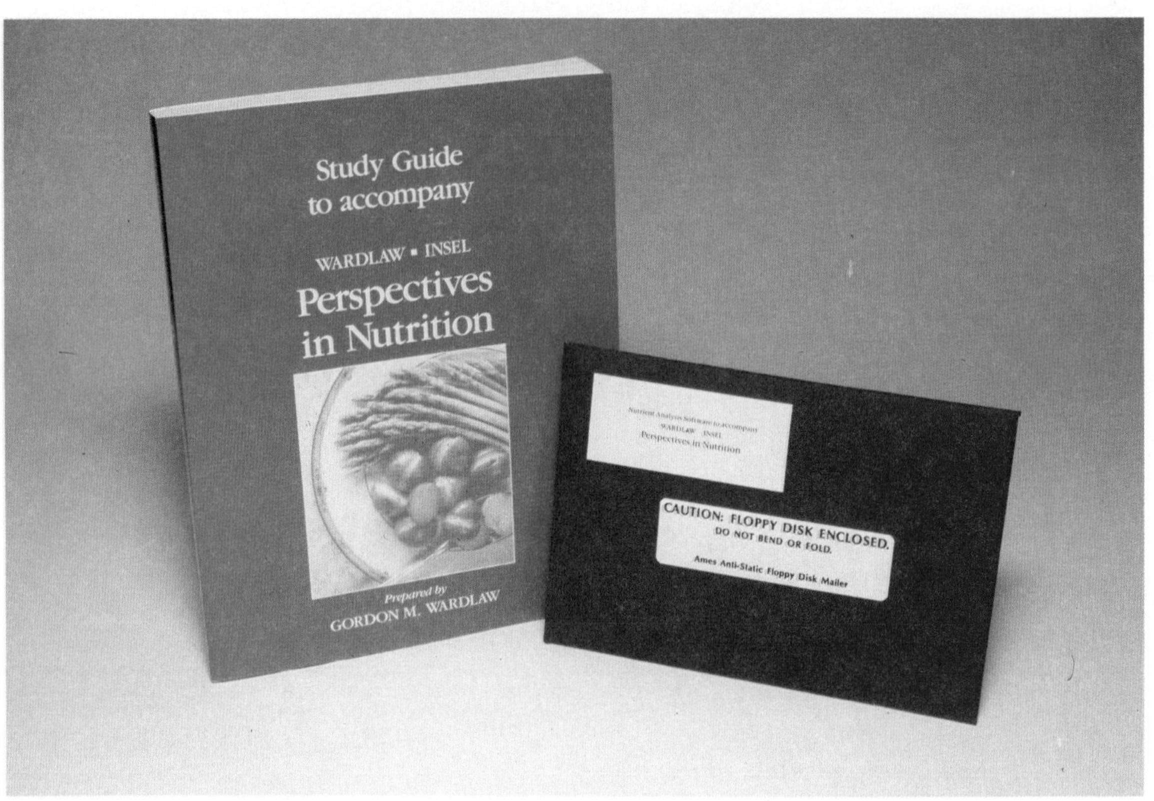

Study Guide

Reviewed by instructors and developed in consultation with a learning theory expert, this valuable Study Guide by Gordon Wardlaw reinforces concepts presented in the text and integrates them with activities to facilitate learning.

- Sample exams reflect the actual exams you will face in the classroom.
- Vocubulary review exercises increase your knowledge of terminology.
- Flash cards help you practice explaining the major concepts in the chapter to yourself, and in turn test your understanding of these important concepts.
- Activities include fill-in tables, labeling, and matching terms. These activities follow the text discussion and are anchored with quotations and page citations from the text. An ongoing dietary analysis highlights the content of many chapters.

Mosby Diet Simple Software

Created by N-Squared Computing, the nutrient analysis computer software is designed to help you quickly calculate the nutrient content of your diet, learn more about the Exchange System, and calculate how many kcalories you use each day. You will find that learning to run this software will make your study of nutrition more interesting, and certainly analysis of a diet much more efficient.

Perspectives in Nutrition

Part I

Nutrition Basics

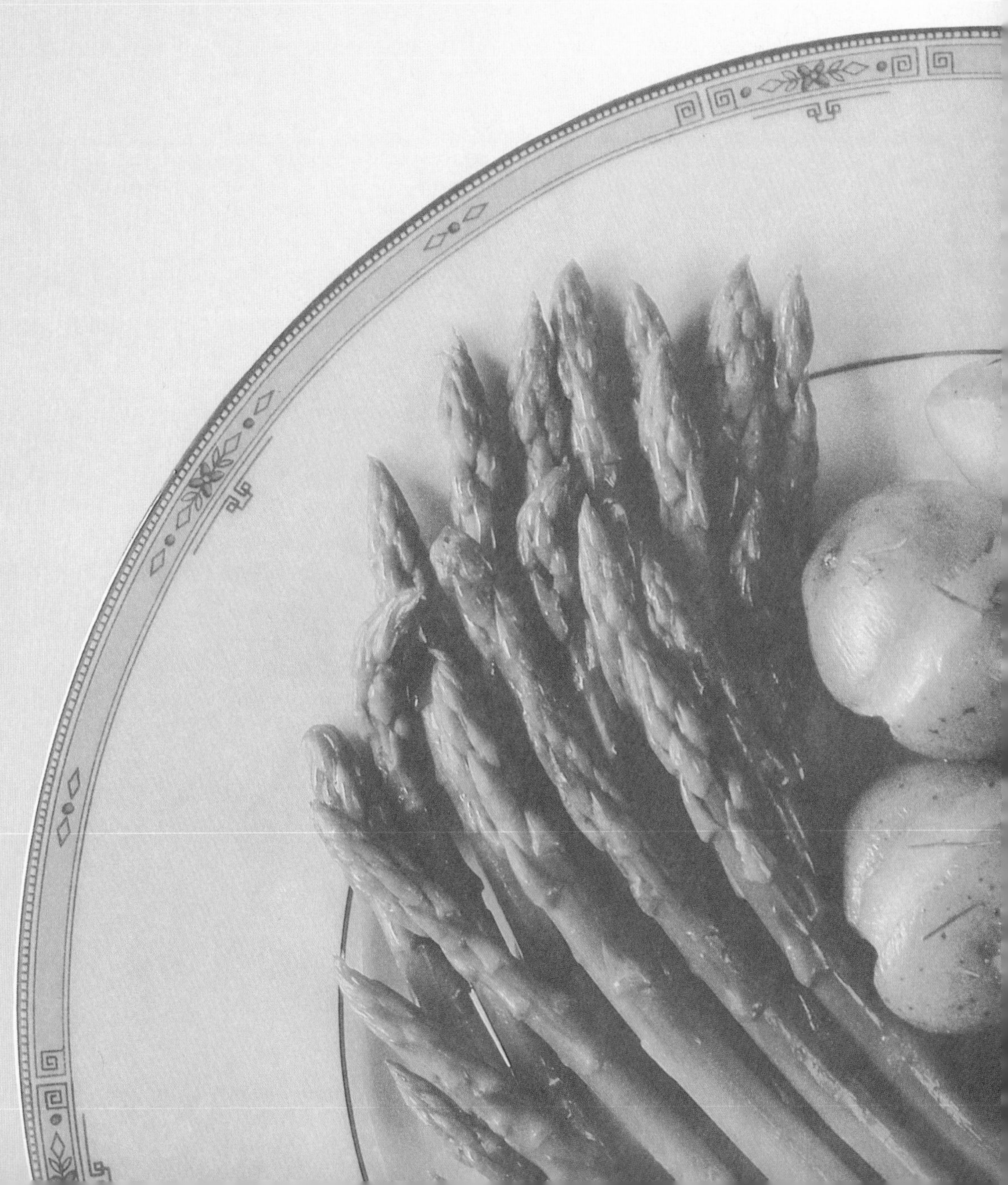

Chapter 1

What Nourishes You?

Overview

We are continually bombarded with information about nutrition and health. Almost daily, the news media report new studies showing how diet affects our well-being. The best-seller list usually contains at least one book about diet and health. Bookstores display rows and rows of books telling us what to eat and what to avoid. We're constantly getting mixed messages, which are confusing. Worse, diet "experts" encourage us to follow unbalanced and gimmicky diets. They try to exploit a concerned public seeking information on diet with their shortcuts to health and beauty.

Turning to a more knowledgeable source, the 1988 Surgeon General's Report on Nutrition and Health reminds us that "for the two out of three adult Americans who do not smoke and do not drink excessively, one personal choice seems to influence long-term health prospects more than any other: what we eat."[21] Some of us have nutritional life-styles that are out of balance with our physiology. And since we live longer than our ancestors did, we have to focus more on preventing nutrition-related diseases. By changing our food habits as necessary, we can strive to bring the goal of optimum health within reach.[23] This is a goal, not only for this chapter, but for this book as well.

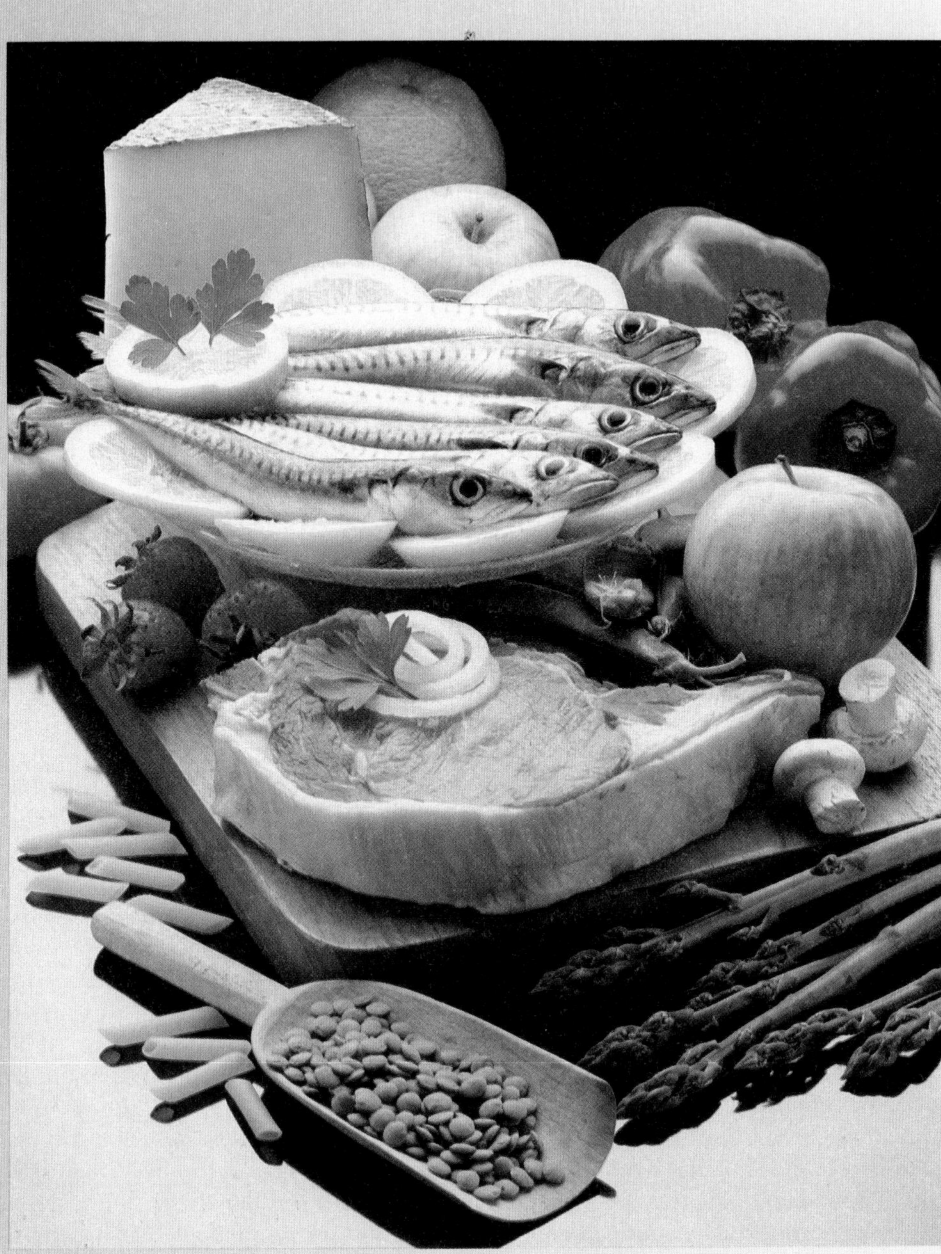

Food provides both the energy and materials needed to build and maintain all body cells.

Nutrition awareness inventory

Here are 15 statements about nutrition and food habits. Answer them to test your current knowledge. If you think the answer is true or mostly true, circle T. If you think the answer is false or mostly false, circle F. Use the scoring key at the end of this chapter to compute your total score. Take this test again after you have read this chapter. Compare the results.

1.	**T**	**F**	Your body's cells are mostly water.
2.	**T**	**F**	Minerals can be broken down into vitamins.
3.	**T**	**F**	The terms *kcalories* and *calories* can be used interchangeably; both are correct.
4.	**T**	**F**	Fats yield more energy per gram than do carbohydrates.
5.	**T**	**F**	Vitamins yield no energy.
6.	**T**	**F**	*Nutritional stores* refer to nutrients your body can call upon when needed.
7.	**T**	**F**	The body requires greater amounts of vitamins than minerals.
8.	**T**	**F**	The term *organic* is similar to the term *organic gardening*.
9.	**T**	**F**	When referring to nutritional states of health, the terms *signs* and *symptoms* can be used interchangeably.
10.	**T**	**F**	Fatigue and poor temperature control can be signs of an advanced iron deficiency.
11.	**T**	**F**	Increased weight is a sign of overnutrition.
12.	**T**	**F**	It is necessary to use vitamin and mineral supplements to maintain your nutritional health.
13.	**T**	**F**	Alcohol provides a large source of energy for some people.
14.	**T**	**F**	Many people who have poor diets are aware of it, but are unable to change their eating behavior.
15.	**T**	**F**	There is no such thing as "junk food."

THE IMPORTANCE OF EXPLORING YOUR OWN FOOD HABITS

In this opening chapter, you will be encouraged to explore your own food habits and discover the underlying reasons for them. This is an important first step as you study nutrition. *Ironically, people have good intuitions about healthy food choices, but all too often fail to act on them.* Yet, even small changes in behavior toward food can make big differences in achieving a long and vigorous life. The more you know about nutrition and about your health risks, the better you can plan a diet to meet your nutritional needs.

Recent evidence suggests that a poor diet is a **risk factor** for the major **chronic** diseases that are the leading causes of death: **heart disease, stroke, hypertension, diabetes mellitus,** and some types of **cancer.** Together, these disorders account for two thirds of all deaths in the United States and Canada. In addition, **cirrhosis** of the liver, accidents and suicides are associated with excessive alcohol consumption. These consequences of modern living are partly an "affliction of affluence" (Table 1-1). Knowing now about nutrition can help to minimize your risk for these diseases.

To begin your study of nutrition, we present some terms to describe the **nutrients** you need. Then we outline what those nutrients do in the body. Later we outline how to assess a person's nutritional health and describe the current "health" of the North American diet. Finally, we discuss why people eat the things they do.

risk factor
A characteristic or a behavior that contributes to the chances of developing an illness.

nutrients
Chemical substances in food that nourish the body by providing energy, building materials, and factors to regulate needed chemical reactions in the body. The body either can't make these nutrients, or can't make them fast enough for its needs.

Table 1-1

10 Leading Causes of Death: United States, 1987

Rank	Cause of death	Number	Percent of total deaths
1*	Heart diseases	759,400	35.7
	(Coronary heart disease)	(511,700)	(24.1)
	(Other heart disease)	(247,700)	(11.6)
2*	Cancers	476,700	22.4
3*	Strokes	148,700	7.0
4†	Unintentional injuries	92,500	4.4
	(Motor vehicle)	(46,800)	(2.2)
	(All others)	(45,700)	(2.2)
5	Chronic obstructive lung diseases	78,000	3.7
6	Pneumonia and influenza	68,600	3.2
7*	Diabetes mellitus	37,800	1.8
8†	Suicide	29,600	1.4
9†	Chronic liver disease and cirrhosis	26,000	1.2
10*	Atherosclerosis	23,100	1.1
	All causes	2,125,100	

*Causes of death in which diet plays a part.
†Causes of death in which excessive alcohol consumption plays a part.
From Estimates from the National Center for Health Statistics, Monthly Vital Statistics Report, 37:1, April 25, 1988.

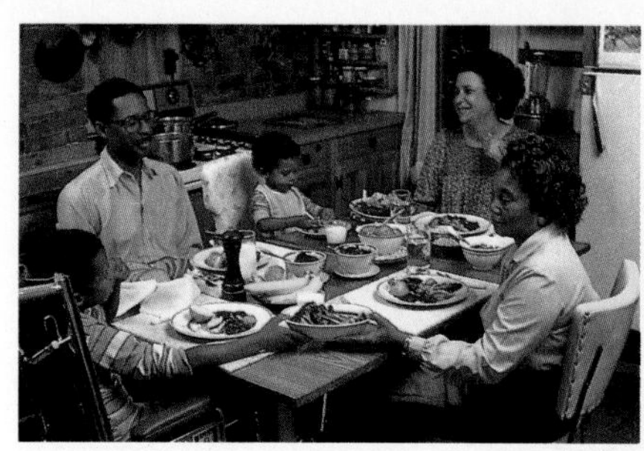

The need for nutrients is a uniting factor.

FOOD PROVIDES NUTRIENTS

Food, water, and oxygen are life-giving and life-sustaining substances. Food provides you with both the energy and materials needed to build and maintain all your body cells. It is important to distinguish between food and nutrients. Food is the source of nutrients. Nutrients are the nourishing substances in food: they are vital for the growth of the infant, the development that leads to adulthood, and the maintenance of body functions throughout life.

Nutrition is the study of these nutrients: what they consist of, how the body **metabolizes** them, and what they finally do in your body to support health.

metabolism Chemical reactions in the body that allow for life.

Classes of nutrients

The nutrients in food can be organized into six classes (Table 1-2). First, there are the energy-yielding nutrients, which constitute the major portion of most foods:

1. **Carbohydrates** are a mixture of mainly carbon, hydrogen, and oxygen **atoms.** Carbohydrates are known as sugars and **starches.** Starches are a storage form of the simple sugar called **glucose.** Chapter 4 focuses on this category.
2. **Lipids** (fats and oils) are a mixture of mainly carbon and hydrogen atoms. There are fewer oxygen atoms in lipids than in carbohydrates. The main form of lipid in food is a **triglyceride.** Chapter 5 focuses on this category. In most cases we will use the more familiar term *fat,* rather than lipid, in this book.
3. **Proteins** are a mixture of carbon, hydrogen, nitrogen, oxygen, and sometimes sulfur atoms. The building blocks of protein are **amino acids.** Chapter 6 focuses on this category.

The Council on Food and Nutrition of the American Medical Association defines nutrition as; "the science of food, the nutrients and the substances therein, their action, interaction, and balance in relation to health and disease, and the process by which the organism ingests, digests, absorbs, transports, utilizes, and excretes food substances."

Chapter 2 reviews many basic chemistry concepts. If you are unfamiliar with chemistry terms, you will find that review quite helpful.

Table 1-2

Essential Nutrients* in the Human Diet and Their Categories

Energy nutrients					
Carbohydrate	**Fat (lipid)†**	**Protein (amino acid)**	**Vitamins**	**Minerals**	**Water**
Glucose‡ (or a carbohydrate that yields glucose)	Linoleic acid (omega-6)	Histidine	A	Arsenic¶	Water
	α-Linolenic acid (omega-3)	Isoleucine	D§	Boron¶	
		Leucine	E	Calcium	
		Lysine	K	Chloride	
		Methionine	Thiamin	Chromium	
		Phenylalanine	Riboflavin	Copper	
		Threonine	Niacin	Cobalt	
		Tryptophan	Pantothenic acid	Fluoride‖	
		Valine	Biotin	Iodide	
			B-6	Iron	
			B-12	Magnesium	
			Folate	Manganese	
			C	Molybdenum	
				Nickel¶	
				Phosphorus	
				Potassium	
				Selenium	
				Silicon¶	
				Sodium	
				Sulfur	
				Zinc	

This table includes nutrients that the current RDA publication lists for humans. Some debate over other minerals not listed does exist.

*Dietary fiber could be added to the list of essential substances, but it is not a nutrient (see Chapter 4).

†The lipids listed are needed in only slight amounts, about 2% of total kcalorie needs (see Chapter 5).

‡In order to prevent ketosis and thus the muscle loss that would occur as protein was used to synthesize carbohydrate (see Chapter 4).

§Sunshine on the skin also allows the body to make vitamin D for itself. (see Chapter 11).

‖Primarily for dental health.

¶Based only on animal studies.

vitamins
Compounds needed in very small amounts in the diet to help regulate and support chemical reactions in the body.

minerals
Elements used in the body to promote chemical reactions and form body structures.

elements
Substances which cannot be broken down further using ordinary chemical procedures.

Again, aside from water, food is mostly a mixture of carbohydrates, fats, and proteins. Two other classes of nutrients are also vital but needed only in small amounts:

4. **Vitamins** are compounds that enable many biochemical reactions to occur, some of which unlock the energy potential of carbohydrates, fats, proteins, and alcohol. Vitamins are the focus of Chapters 11 and 12.
5. **Minerals** also play important parts in metabolic reactions. In addition, they form an integral part of the body's structure. Minerals are **elements**—groups of one or more of the same atoms (see Chapter 2). Minerals are the focus of Chapters 13 and 14.

Water is in a class by itself:

6. **Water** nourishes in many ways. It is vital in the body as a **solvent** and lubricant and as a medium for transporting nutrients and waste. The body even makes some water as a by-product of metabolism. Water is examined in detail in Chapter 13.

The 50 or so elements that make up these life-sustaining nutrients are some of the 105 elements found in nature.

Because minerals and water do not contain carbon atoms bonded to hydrogen atoms, they are called **inorganic** compounds. The other nutrients that contain carbon atoms bonded to hydrogen atoms are called **organic.** These terms have nothing to do with organic gardening, but instead are based on simple chemistry concepts that we describe in Chapter 2.

inorganic
Free of carbon atoms bonded to hydrogen atoms.
organic
Contains carbon atoms bonded to hydrogen atoms.

Concept Check

Food contains vital nutrients: carbohydrates, lipids (fats and oils), proteins, vitamins, minerals, and water. The first three yield energy. Vitamins and minerals aid in energy production, among other functions. Water is the solvent of life—the medium of transport of the body's substances.

Energy supplies for body functions

We get the energy necessary to perform body functions and to do work from carbohydrates, fats, and proteins (and **alcohol** for some of us). Energy is held in the chemical **bonds** of these compounds. In Chapter 7 we discuss how that energy is released and used by cells. The energy in food is often measured in terms of calories. A calorie is the amount of heat it takes to raise one **gram** of water one degree **Celsius** (1° C, centigrade scale). Because a calorie is such a tiny unit of heat measurement—like a penny in relation to dollars and cents—we can more efficiently express food energy in terms of kilocalories, which are 1000-calorie units. A kilocalorie (**kcalorie** or kcal) is the amount of heat it takes to raise 1000 grams (1 liter) of water 1° C. The abbreviation kcalorie (or kcal) is used throughout this book.

kcalories
The heat needed to raise 1,000 grams (1 liter) of water 1° Celsius.

A **bomb calorimeter** is used to determine the number of kcalories in a food portion (Figure 1-1). The food is burned inside a chamber that is surrounded by water. As the food burns, it gives off heat. This raises the temperature of water surrounding the chamber. The increase in water temperature seen after the food has burned indicates the amount of kcalories the food contained. Any food can be burned in the calorimeter but some foods must be dried first.

Today scientific journals often require the use of the term ***kilojoule*** (kjoule) instead of kcalorie to express the energy content of a food. One kjoule equals 4.18 kcalories. A kjoule is a measure of work, not heat. It is the amount of work involved in moving 1 kilogram for 1 meter with the force of 1 newton. Heat and work are just two forms of energy. Energy expressions in the form of either heat or work can be exchanged for each other. In kjoule units, 1 gram of carbohydrate equals 17 kjoules, 1 gram of protein equals 17 kjoules, 1 gram of fat equals 38 kjoules, and 1 gram of alcohol equals 29 kjoules.

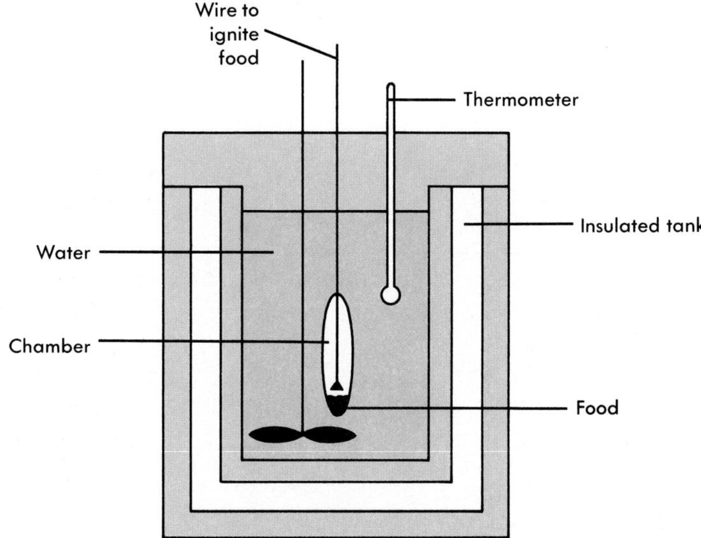

Figure 1-1
The bomb calorimeter. A food sample is put in the inner chamber, which is then charged with oxygen and tightly sealed. The heat produced by burning the food is measured as an increase in temperature in the surrounding water.

Chapter 2 reviews the metric system. If you are not familiar with the metric system, you will find that review quite helpful.

In Chapter 2 you will learn an easy way to estimate the grams of carbohydrate, lipid, and protein in foods—the *exchange system.* Once you know the gram quantities of these substances in a food, you can estimate the total kcalories in that food using the kcalorie values. For example, if a banana-rum drink had 10 grams of carbohydrate, 1 gram of protein, 1 gram of fat, and 15 grams of alcohol, it would contain 158 kcalories ($10 \times 4 + 1 \times 4 + 1 \times 9 + 15 \times 7 = 158$).

Exploring Issues and Actions

You are organizing a food relief program for victims of a tornado in a local town. You are looking for high-kcalorie foods. As you walk down the aisles of your local supermarket, what foods might you place on your high-kcalorie list? Why?

Information from the bomb calorimeter gives the energy equivalents of 1 gram of carbohydrate, fat, protein, and alcohol. Specifically, carbohydrates yield 4 kcalories per gram, proteins yield 4 kcalories per gram, fats yield 9 kcalories per gram, and alcohol yields 7 kcalories per gram. These kcalorie figures have been adjusted for (1) **digestibility** and (2) those substances in food that will burn in the bomb calorimeter but that the human body cannot use for energy, such as waxes and some parts of plants (see Appendix B).[16]

Are you what you eat?

The quantities of nutrients that a human needs vary widely from one nutrient to another. Nutrient quantities found in food also vary a great deal. Aside from water, the bulk of food we eat daily—and our daily food needs as well—consists of the energy-yielding substances, which amount to about 500 grams (~1 pound). Vitamins are needed daily in very small amounts, 100 milligrams or less. Although each day we require nearly a gram of some minerals like calcium and phosphorus, many minerals are also needed in quantities of only milligrams or less. For example, you need about 15 milligrams of zinc per day, which is just a few specks of zinc oxide. Figure 1-2 contrasts the relative concentration of all of these nutrients in a human body with the composition of both a cooked steak and a cooked stalk of broccoli. Note how your nutrient composition differs from the nutritional profiles of foods you eat.

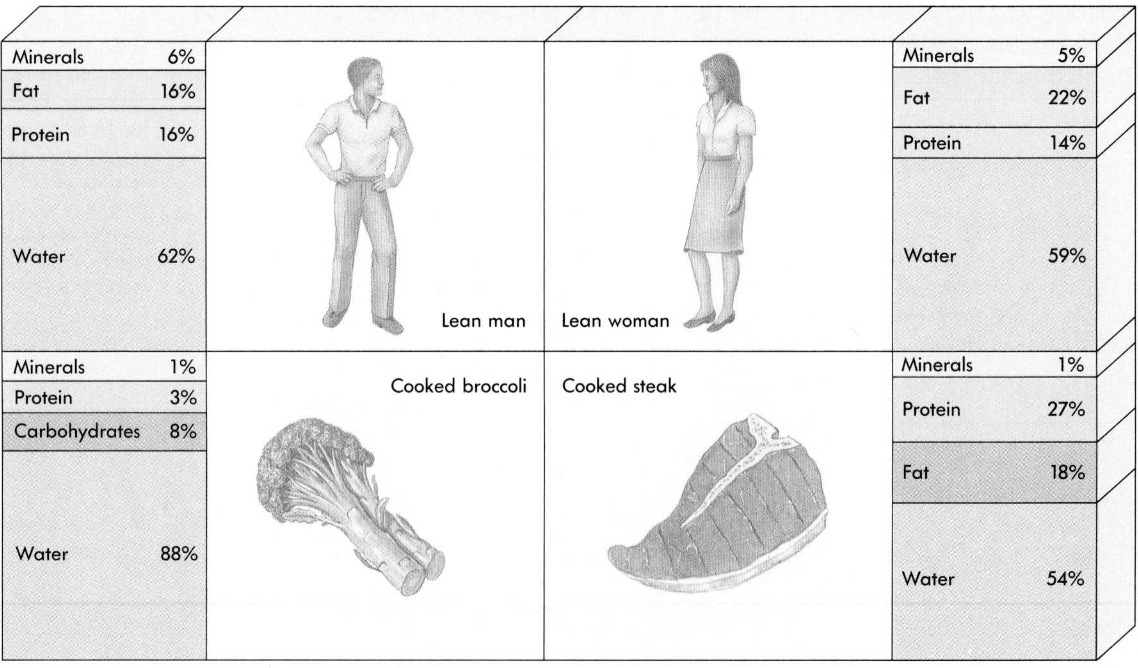

Figure 1-2

You aren't what you eat! Body cells primarily dictate their own composition; the form of the nutrients you consume has only a minor effect.

STATES OF NUTRITIONAL HEALTH

Theoretically, the body's **nutritional status** varies for each individual nutrient it needs (Table 1-3). The optimal nutritional status for a nutrient is achieved when body tissues have enough of a nutrient for both (1) metabolic functions and (2) surplus stores of it, which can be mobilized during times of increased need. When nutrient intake does not regularly meet the nutrient needs dictated by cell activities and body maintenance, stores of nutrients soon become depleted, some sooner than others. Although body stores briefly may be sufficient to compensate for an inadequate diet, over time serious problems can arise. Some women in North America, for example, do not consume sufficient iron and eventually deplete their iron stores (see Chapter 14).

A sign, such as flaky skin, is a result of a disease that is visible upon examination, while a symptom is a change in body function that is not necessarily apparent to an examiner, such as stomach pains.

Biochemical lesions

Once nutrient stores are depleted, a continuing nutrition deficit drains body tissues further. When tissue levels fall far enough, the body's metabolic processes eventually slow down, or even stop. A **biochemical lesion** then develops. This deficiency is termed **subclinical,** because there are no outward **signs** or **symptoms.** At the subclinical stage for poor iron status, low levels of the red blood cell protein, *hemoglobin,* are found in the bloodstream. Synthesizing hemoglobin requires iron.

biochemical lesion
Nutritional deficiency symptoms observed in the blood or urine, such as low levels of nutrient by-products or low enzyme activities, indicating reduced biochemical function.

nutritional status
The nutritional health of a person as determined by anthropometric measures (height, weight, circumferences, and so on), biochemical measures of nutrients or their by-products in blood and urine, a clinical (physical) examination, and a dietary analysis.

Clinical lesions

If a biochemical deficit becomes very severe, **clinical lesions** eventually develop and become outwardly apparent. It is now possible to actually note changes in the body, perhaps in the skin, hair, nails, tongue, and eyes (see Appendix C for common clinical signs and symptoms of nutritional deficiencies). The person also

subclinical
Not seen on a clinical (physical) examination.

sign
Seen on a physical examination.

symptom
A change in health status noted by the person with the problem, such as a stomach pain.

clinical lesion
Nutritional deficiency sign seen on physical examination.

Table 1-3

Levels of Nutritional Status with Respect to Iron

General condition	Condition with respect to iron
Overnutrition	Toxic damage to liver cells
Optimal nutrition: nutrients to support body functions and stores of nutrients for times of increased need	Adequate liver stores of iron, adequate blood values for iron-related compounds
Stores depleted: tissue levels fall	Serum ferritin*, an iron-containing protein in the blood, drops below 12 nanograms per 100 milliliters
Reduced biochemical function (biochemical lesion)	Hemoglobin, an iron-containing pigment in the red blood cell, drops below 11 grams per 100 milliliters of blood
Clinical signs and symptoms (clinical lesion)	Pale complexion, greatly increased heart rate during activity, "spooning" of the nails in a severe deficiency, poor body temperature regulation

*Serum is the liquid portion of blood present after it clots.

overnutrition
A state where nutritional intake exceeds the body's needs.

lacks that vigorous glow that good health conveys. In the case of an iron deficiency, the person may become very pale, and his or her heart rate will increase greatly during even moderate activity. In a severe deficiency, one's fingernails begin to curl up in a spoon shape.

Overnutrition

One nutritional state that is reaching epidemic proportions in North America today is **overnutrition,** especially from overloading the body with too many kcalories and nutrients. In the short run, for instance, a week or two, overnutrition may cause no sign or symptom. But keep it up and eventually body weight, or blood levels of some nutrients, will increase. In the long run, then overnutrition can then lead to serious diseases, such as the **obesity**-related diseases diabetes and hypertension, or even vitamin A toxicity. *One form of overnutrition, excessive energy intake, has been possible for many people. In recent times, with the introduction of vitamin and mineral supplements, overnutrition of many other nutrients has also become a concern.*

obesity
A condition characterized by excess body fat, usually defined as 20% above desirable body weight (see Chapter 8).

For most nutrients the gap between an optimal intake and overnutrition is wide. Therefore even if people take a typical multiple vitamin and mineral supplement daily, they probably won't receive a harmful amount of any nutrient. Some possible exceptions are vitamin A, vitamin D, and iron (see Chapters 11 and 14). Recent studies indicate that very high doses of vitamin B-6 and niacin can also cause health problems (see Chapter 12). Usually supplements need to be taken on a regular basis to build up toxic levels in the body. As a rule of thumb: the dose determines the poison. For some vitamins and minerals high doses are poisonous.

For vitamins A and D, a potentially harmful dose is only 5 to 10 times greater than recommended amounts for children or pregnant women who take these nutrients (usually as supplements) on a regular basis (see Chapter 11).

Concept Check

People should focus on foods for their nutrient sources rather than on supplements. Foods promote a balanced nutrient intake and possess very little likelihood of harmful intake of nutrients, provided good nutritional habits have been developed.

At the beginning of the twentieth century *undernutrition* was the battle cry for nutrition science. Today attention is needed for both undernutrition and overnutrition. In fact, the major nutritional problems in North America today are the result of overnutrition, principally caused by excess intakes of energy compared with energy needs and overconsumption of sodium and certain types of fat.[21] Some of us are susceptible to ill health when we consume too many of these nutrients. This is a problem we will focus on throughout the book.

In the United States more than 40% of elderly women take vitamin and mineral supplements.[13] Although this practice usually causes no harm, some people have overdone it and ended up sick or hospitalized. If you take nutrient supplements, keep a close eye on your total vitamin and mineral intake both from food and from supplements (see Nutrition Perspective 11-1 in Chapter 11 for further details on choosing nutrient supplements).

A Warning

Often a long time elapses between the development of a poor nutritional condition and the first clinical evidence of a problem. For example, a diet high in animal fat often increases one's blood **cholesterol** level without showing any clinical signs or symptoms for years. But when the blood vessels become sufficiently blocked by cholesterol and other materials, chest pain during physical activity may develop. This buildup of fatty substances also may eventually provoke a

cholesterol
A waxy lipid; it has a structure containing multiple chemical rings (see Chapter 5).

heart attack (see Chapter 5 for further details). Thus a person may be on the road to developing a serious disease but because it progresses so slowly the effects won't be obvious until quite late—perhaps too late.

Furthermore, clinical signs and symptoms of nutritional deficiencies are often not very specific. Typical signs to look for—diarrhea, an irregular walk, facial sores—can be caused by many different problems. It's often hard to decide if the problem is caused by faulty nutrition or by some other medical disorder. *Long lag times and vague signs and symptoms make it difficult to establish a link between an individual's current diet and nutritional state.*

anthropometric
The measurement of weight, lengths, circumferences, and thicknesses of the body.

Evaluating your nutritional state

To look at your nutritional status carefully requires an expensive procedure, most of which can be done only in specialized laboratories. **Anthropometric** evaluation of height, weight, and body circumference are simple compared with a biochemical evaluation using the activity of certain blood **enzymes** and measurements of blood levels of nutrients and their by-products. A thorough clinical (physical) examination and a detailed assessment of your last day's dietary intake also are required. For some nutrients it might take a year to obtain an accurate assessment of intake.[3] Together, these activities form the *ABCD* of nutrition assessment. Later in the book, we will describe in detail how these assessments are made.

enzyme
A compound that speeds the rate of a chemical reaction but is not altered by the chemical reaction. Almost all enzymes are proteins (see Chapters 3 and 5).

Does your nutritional intake make any difference?

As you study nutrition and learn the importance of nutrients in foods, you may notice people who, in spite of very poor diets, show no outward clinical signs or symptoms of poor health. Such cases primarily reflect our need for more research in nutrition. Better methods for early detection of nutritional disease are needed. Often it is not possible to separate the best nutritional state from one that is slightly jeopardized. *We can usually distinguish between* ***malnutrition*** *and good nutrition, but the gray area—the gradual slide from a "good" to a poor nutritional state—is hard to detect.* This is why it is important to strive to meet your nutrient needs each day. Otherwise, a subtle decline in health and performance may begin, but you will probably not know why.[4]

malnutrition
Failing health that results from a longstanding dietary intake that fails to meet nutritional needs.

Table 1-4

Components of a Nutrition Assessment

Component	Example
Background histories	Medical history including current diseases and past surgeries Medications history Social history; married, cooking facilities Economic status
Nutrition parameters	Anthropometric assessment; height, weight, skinfold thickness, arm muscle circumference, and other parameters Biochemical (laboratory) assessment of blood and urine; enzyme activities, levels of nutrients or their by-products Clinical assessment (physical examination); general appearance of skin, eyes, and tongue, rapid hair loss, sense of touch, ability to walk
Diet history	Usual intake or record of previous day's meals

THE NORTH AMERICAN DIET: HOW GOOD IS IT?

As we said, the major energy sources in the North American diet are carbohydrates, fats, and proteins. Alcoholic beverages provide a large source of energy for some people; in fact, alcoholic beverages are the third leading contributor to kcalorie intakes and supply 11% of all kcalories consumed in the United States.[6] Currently adults in the United States consume about 14% to 16% of kcalories as proteins, 44% to 47% as carbohydrates, and 35% to 38% as fats. Canadian diets are a bit higher in fat, about 42% of kcalories. These percentages are estimates and change slightly from year to year. Individual diets also vary widely.

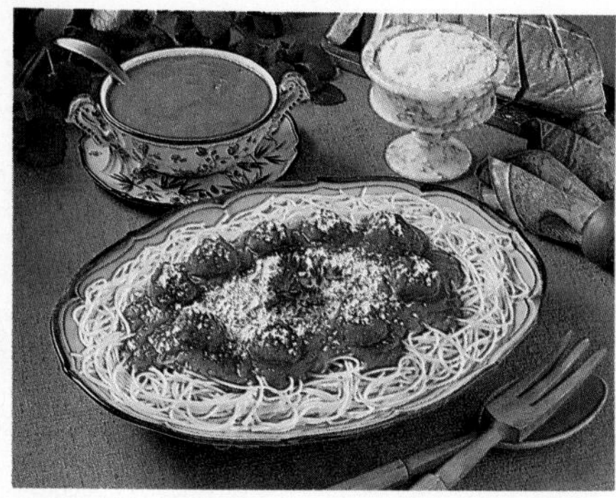

Pasta contributes carbohydrates to the diet.

In the North American diet most protein comes from animal sources; vegetable sources supply only about one third of our protein. In many other parts of the world, it is just the opposite: vegetable proteins—those found in rice, beans, corn, and other vegetables—dominate diets. About half of carbohydrates in the diets of North Americans come from simple sugars; the other half come from starches (such as peas, pastas, bread, grains, potatoes, and beans). About 60% of fats come from animal sources and 40% from vegetable sources.

United States and Canadian Nutrition Surveys

Federal governments perform large surveys to estimate the actual levels of nutrients in our food supply, as well as our nutrient intakes. The first such survey in the United States was the Ten State Survey done in the late 1960s. In Canada the first survey, called Nutrition Canada, began in the early 1970s. Because the Ten State Survey focused on poorer states, it did not accurately assess the average U.S. nutrient intake. Soon after, in the United States the first National Health and Nutrition Examination Survey (NHANES I 1971-74) was conducted, followed by NHANES II (1976-80).[26] The NHANES surveys included a cross section of about 20,000 Americans. This survey collected interviews about food intakes, assessed heights, weights, and blood pressures, measured vitamin and mineral levels in the blood, and examined other health parameters. Each time the NHANES survey is performed more and more parameters are added. NHANES III, already in process, will include 40,000 people.[24] Results should be available between 1992-1995. The U.S. Department of Agriculture (USDA) also conducts, as it has since the beginning of this century, various surveys that document the types of foods people eat.[18] Agriculture Canada performs the same type of food consumption surveys.

A North American nutrition profile

Results from the NHANES, Nutrition Canada, various food consumption surveys, and other studies show quite a diversity in our diets. Many people are meeting their nutrient needs; others are not. The studies suggest that some North Americans should try to choose more foods that are rich in iron, calcium, vitamin A, vitamin B-6, vitamin C, magnesium, zinc, and dietary fiber.[10,19] In addition, we generally should look for the possibility of having an excessive kcalorie and alcohol intake, and some black persons may especially need to limit their **salt** intake more because they have a much greater chance of developing hypertension than do whites. We also can be confident about the safety of our food supply (see Chapter 19).

Although the nutrients just listed are the most problematic, other nutrients can also be low in individual diets. Overall, many of us need to make better food choices.

Concept Check

Surveys show that we have plenty of food available to us in North America and that, overall, it is very safe to consume. Food availability and safety are major reasons why overall we enjoy such good health. Still *some* of us could *improve our diets* by focusing on good food sources of iron, calcium, vitamin A, vitamin B-6, vitamin C, magnesium, zinc and dietary fiber.

Expert Opinion

There's No Such Thing as "Junk Food," But There Are Junk *Diets*

HELEN A. GUTHRIE, PH.D., R.D.

During the past 15 years, the phrase "junk food" has invaded America's everyday vocabulary. As a nutritionist, I contend that this term is meaningless and should be discarded. There is no totally worthless food, any more than there is a perfect food that meets *all* our nutritional needs.

Obviously, some foods contribute more nutrients than do others. But almost any food has *some* redeeming value *under the right circumstances.* The problem arises when foods that contribute more calories than nutrients become so important in our diet that foods of higher nutritional value are excluded. It is equally possible to make an unbalanced selection of our most sacred nutritious foods and wind up with a diet overabundant in some nutrients yet deficient in others. In both cases, the result is a junk *diet.*

SOME FOODS GO HAND-IN-HAND

Foods of low nutrient density don't carry much nutritional weight by themselves. For example, in some cakes and cookies, most of the calories come from ingredients such as fat and sugar, and relatively few from milk, flour, and eggs. However, if eating a cookie means that a child also drinks milk or fruit juice, we should look at cookie-and-milk or cookie-and-juice as a unit and judge them together rather than condemn one and applaud the other. For an 8-year-old, milk and one or two cookies makes a nutritious combination. Milk and five cookies, though, may create an imbalance between calories and nutrients—and thus be considered lower in nutrition.

Potato chips are another example of a food that can be valuable in the right context. Eaten alone, potato chips add vitamin C, vitamin B-6, and copper to our diet. Eaten with a sandwich, potato chips become part of a balanced meal. But if we stuff ourselves with so many potato chips that we're too full to eat dinner, we are misusing them. What about the salt, you ask? One ounce of potato chips provides about one quarter gram of sodium—less than the amount in the bread in a sandwich and considerably less than the amount in two slices of bread with salted butter. Just because we see and taste the salt on potato chips doesn't mean they contain too much.

For another example, consider pizza. Some people see it as a junk food because it is high in calories, cholesterol, and fat. But pizza has nutritional merits comparable to a meat-and-cheese sandwich served with tomato.

TOO MUCH OF A GOOD THING?

How about the classically "healthful" foods like milk, eggs, orange juice, and oatmeal? Are they always desirable? Surprisingly, no. Milk, especially nonfat milk, has one of the most impressive nutrient profiles of any food. But it isn't perfect. Although high in calcium, protein, and riboflavin, it is low in iron and vitamin C. In contrast, oranges are high in iron and vitamin C, but low in calcium, protein, and riboflavin.

What does all this have to do with junk food? When a food doesn't meet an immediate nutritional need, its nutritional value is limited. After an adult has had two or three glasses of milk (which meet many nutritional needs), additional milk becomes less and less useful. If this additional milk (which does not provide vitamin C) displaces a fruit juice that does have vitamin C, that milk becomes worthless except as a source of calories. In this context, the extra milk would be a "junk" food. The key point to remember is that foods should not be judged in isolation but in relation to the total diet and the individual's needs.

If all our daily nutrient needs are met except for calories, we can obtain the rest of our calorie requirements from any food.

Of course, moderation is a virtue. And so is avoidance of excess amounts of saturated fats, sodium, calories, and cholesterol. Getting a maximum of 10% to 15% of our total daily calories from foods of limited nutritional value is reasonable.

COST PER NUTRIENT

In choosing nutritious foods, we might also consider cost per nutrient. Many parents feel good about giving their children buttered toast and honey for breakfast but feel guilty if they serve a doughnut. Since both bread and doughnuts are made with enriched flour—and often with whole-wheat flour—there is no appreciable difference in their nutrient content. Considering cost, however, the doughnut is not as good a buy. Similar considerations hold for french-fried and baked potatoes. Nutritionally, a serving of french fries cooked in oil compares favorably with a baked potato served with a fat such as sour cream or butter. However, the cost per nutrient of commercially prepared french fries can be considerably higher than that of home-prepared baked potatoes. Frequent eating of sticky sweets, especially between meals, should also be questioned because of its possible contribution to tooth decay. Nutritionists want people to eat the right amounts and combinations of nutrients to promote health, but they also want everyone to eat in a rational way, without feeling guilty about including a favorite food merely for the pleasure it provides. Special medical considerations aside, a healthful diet can include at least small amounts of any food you enjoy—as long as your overall diet is moderate in calories and properly balanced.

Dr. Guthrie is Professor of Nutrition at The Pennsylvania State University.

How do we rate our diets?

Judging from the responses given by well over half the people in several large surveys, we are extremely concerned about good nutrition and are well aware of possible health hazards from fat, salt, and sugar.[21] Still, the unwillingness of many people to examine their nutritional practices is probably the major impediment to improving their diet—concern does not necessarily translate into change.

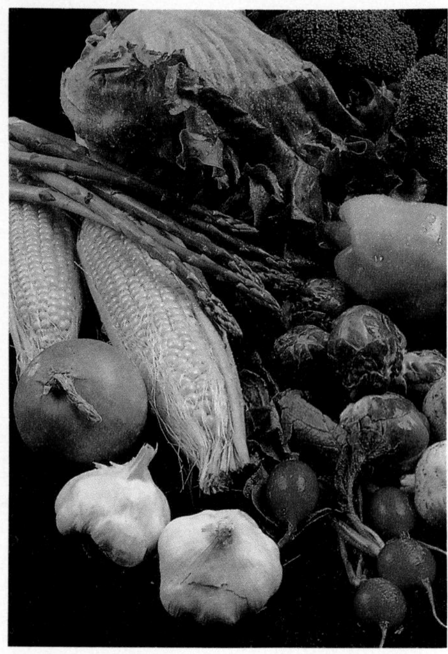

Vegetables are a good source of dietary fiber.

Over half of the people in a USDA survey[22] described their nutritional intake as excellent or above average, 42% said it was average, and only 4% felt it was below average. They were not convinced they needed to know more about nutrition, in spite of scoring low on nutrition-knowledge questions. Only 7% of people surveyed said they were not very well informed. Most viewed food and cooking as a pleasure, not as a science. We hope you will think of it as both. One third agreed that "the impression I get is that nobody really knows the answers on the best foods to eat for a balanced diet." Almost one half agreed that "learning the basic ideas in nutrition will probably alter my personal eating habits very little." We hope we can convince you otherwise.

WHAT SHAPES OUR FOOD TASTES?

The basic purpose of food is nourishment, but to us it means far more than that, and that is fine. *Food symbolizes much of what we think about ourselves.*[14] We bond relationships and express friendships around the dinner table. We enhance and maintain our social status by entertaining creatively or lavishly. We cope with stress and tension by eating or not eating. We influence other's behaviors through our food practices. Some of us express religious beliefs and display our creative talents through food preparation and ceremonies. Since people eat 80,000 to 100,000 times in a lifetime (this takes 13 to 15 years of our waking hours), eating becomes an important key to the way we define ourselves politically, religiously, and socially. See Table 1-5 to review many factors that affect food consumption in the United States, and Figure 1-3 for a model illustrating the effects of behavior and environment on food habits.

Food likes and dislikes are probably the most important determinants of what we eat. Respondents to a USDA survey[22] rated taste as the chief consideration in selecting foods to serve their families; budget came in second. Respondents were much more likely to serve a meal based on taste, compared with one they knew would be more nutritious.

Early experiences

Food preferences are learned early as social and cultural preferences.[2,5] They are refined through interactions with parents and friends, our social class, and the need for status. Unfortunately for young children, adult caregivers may severely limit the child's experience with food. Adults may purchase only a small subset of foods available, and may consider even many of these foods inappropriate for children. For example, at what age were you first introduced to okra, lentils, spinach salad, or salmon?

Exploring Issues and Actions

After eating dinner, your active 4-year-old cousin is still hungry and asks for a bowl of cold cereal for dessert. What do you think about this?

Mere exposure to a variety of foods can help reduce the resistance to trying new foods. Young children seem to prefer foods that are sweet or familiar, but preschoolers are often quite willing to try new things. Caregivers need to provide that opportunity. It may take as many as fifteen introductions, but the odds are in favor of final acceptance (see Chapter 16).

Our innate preferences are important, including universal enjoyment of sweet foods and dislike of bitter and sometimes spicy, burning ones. Bitter tastes often portend poisonous substances. However, innate responses can be modified through exposure and **conditioning** (learning, that is). This allows some people—even whole cultures—to learn to enjoy very sour or hot, spicy foods, such as jalapeno peppers and fiery curries.

conditioning
The process where an originally neutral stimulus repeatedly paired with a reinforcing agent elicits a predictable response.

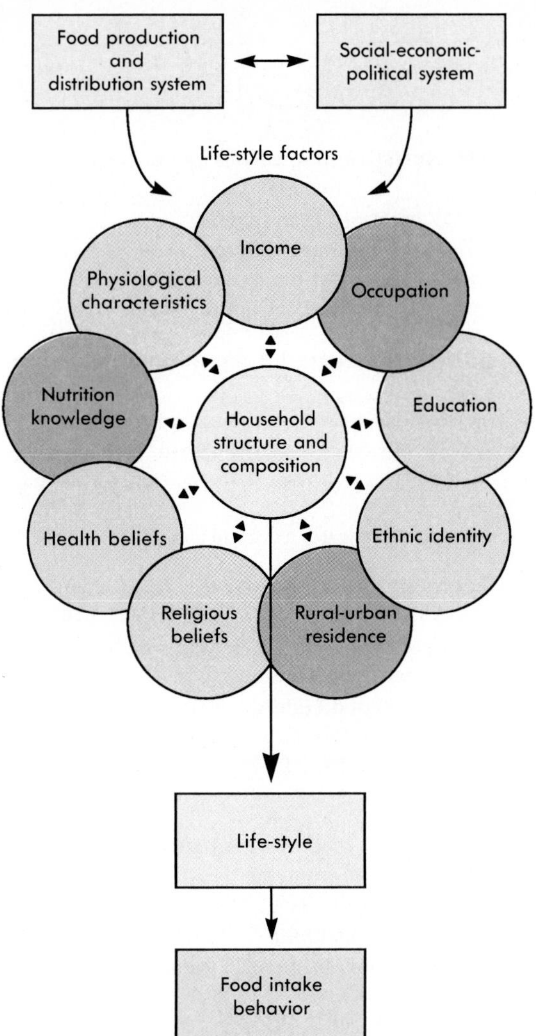

Figure 1-3

Food behavior can be influenced by many sources. Which are important in your life?

Habit

Most of us eat only from a core group of foods. One study estimated that only about 100 basic items account for 75% of the total amount of food we consume.[14] We may think we buy foods mainly based on their sensory appearance, freshness, safety, nutritional quality, healthfulness, convenience, and price. Those factors do figure in, but we still work within very narrow constraints, *primarily dictated by routine and habit in selecting foods.* Many of us could use cooking classes to expand our nutritional horizons. Of the respondents in a USDA survey of women,[22] 51% agreed that their cooking habits were very similar to their mothers'. Did your mother teach you healthy food habits?

Taboos further limit cuisine: Hindus would no more eat beef than they would eat a cat. And Swedes, who regard corn in general as food for hogs, do not enjoy a good ear of sweet corn. Adults even limit the time of day foods can be eaten. When did you last have nourishing vegetable noodle soup for breakfast, even though it can be highly comforting on a cold morning? Many Japanese prefer it at that time of day.

Table 1-5

Determinants of Food Consumption in The U.S. Household

1. Demographic characteristics affect food consumption: sex, age, income, marital status.

- Males, for example, may eat more than females
- Older people and infants usually have different food tolerances
- Those with lower incomes may not be able to afford costly foods
- Family members may eat more meals at home, sitting down, than singles

2. Food tastes and preferences may be the greatest determinant of what we eat.

- Cultural influences: caviar, for example, is an acquired taste
- Innate traits: almost everyone likes ice cream from the first taste
- Personality traits: for example, willingness to try new foods may broaden the menu
- Willingness of food preparer to cater to family tastes

3. Household management constraints of the food shopper and preparer limit menus.

- Skills and time allowance may limit choices
- Interest in experimenting with food
- Willingness to entertain, to expend energy, time, ideas
- Willingness to use convenience foods
- Planning skills: use of shopping list, leftovers, menus
- Budget

4. Beliefs about nutrition and nutrition information sources.

- What is believed to be the relationship between diet and health
- What does a nutrient do for you
- What foods are believed to be healthful
- How to apply nutrition information in menu planning

5. Attitudes toward nutrition and food color diet choices.

- Buys food because it is nutritious
- Buys food because of its emotional or other significance

6. Life change events and health and weight concerns may cause diet variation.

- Deaths, divorce, traumas
- Pregnancy, lactation, family size change, finance change
- Weight concerns: obesity, high blood pressure, cholesterol levels

7. Life-style and food routines affect what is eaten.

- Some households skip certain meals altogether
- Some eat away from home frequently
- Some permit extensive snacking; rarely sit down together
- Some eat a particular way because they consume cigarettes and alcohol

USDA, *Determinants of Food Consumption in American Households.* December 1982. Marketing Science Institute, Cambridge, Massachusetts, in conjunction with Community Nutrition Institute, Washington, D.C., 1982.

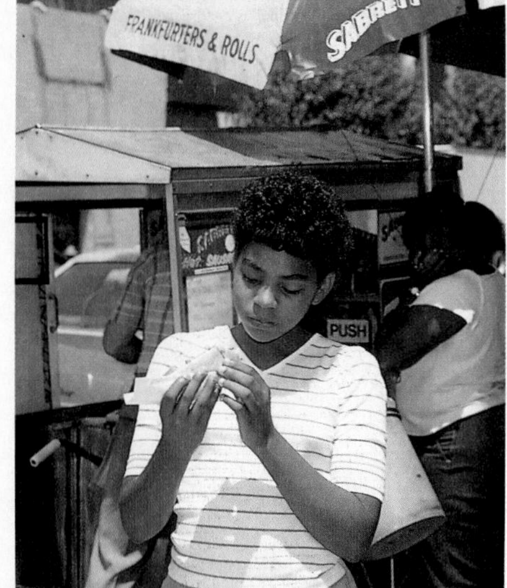

Food preferences are often culturally acquired.

Health

Several surveys have revealed that about half of the population considers nutrition, or what they think is good nutrition, is an important factor in influencing their food purchases.[21] Only about one fourth of people reported price as more important than nutrition. The North Americans who focus on better nutrition are mainly the well-educated professionals of the middle-class, the health-oriented and active life-style segment whose tastes can set a trend.

Some of the most successful products introduced in recent years to the U.S. markets are those with a healthy image, whether or not they actually contain healthful ingredients. Popular products of the 1980s have included fruit rolls and bars, bottled mineral water, granola bars, fruit juices, bulk frozen vegetables without sauce, and Oriental meals.

The recent movement toward better nutrition was sparked in the late 1960s when the American Heart Association labeled the fat- and cholesterol-rich diets in the United States as a major cause of heart disease. More recently, research shows diet may be linked to 10% to 35% of all cancers.[8] Some of us are responding to these health risks by attempting to change our diets. Nevertheless, as we said earlier, taste and habit still profoundly dictate choice. Recently, when people were asked why they did not include foods they knew were healthy in their diets—for instance, yellow vegetables, low-fat milk, margarine, and whole-wheat bread—they said they didn't like them. The response to why they didn't give up foods they thought they should decrease, such as whole milk, cheese, and fatty meat, was that they liked them too much.[25]

Weight concerns appear to be another important factor in influencing food choices. In a recent U.S. survey 59% of people said they have changed their diet because of concern over their body weight.

The food industry is responding to our health concerns. A modern supermarket provides extensive choices among fresh, frozen, international, gourmet, ethnic, vegetarian, and even not-so-healthy foods. Salad bars in supermarkets are a big hit, especially where single people shop. Stores are moving toward foods lower in fat, salt, and sugar. They are carrying dry-roasted and unsalted nuts, pure fruit juices, high-fiber cereals, whole-grain breads, fruits canned in natural juices, low-sodium soups and sauces, low-fat turkey and chicken franks, and many kinds of fish. Bulk foods sold in bins include beans, rice, flours, dried fruits, nuts, and grains. Some shelf tags in markets provide information on the nutritional content of foods, such as kcalories, vitamins and minerals, sodium, and cholesterol. The road to good nutrition is paved with the appropriate options.

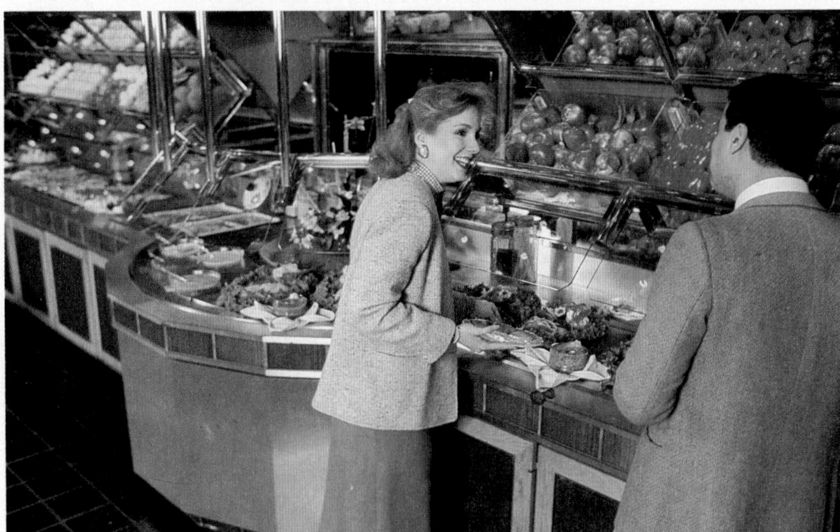

Salad bars are an increasingly popular feature of today's supermarkets.

Advertising

To capture consumers' interest, the food industry spends annually well over $6 billion on advertising and another $26 billion on packaging (another form of advertising)—a total of more than $32 billion. Some of this advertising is helpful—when it promotes the importance of calcium and dietary fiber in our diets and encourages us to consume more lowfat milk products, fruits, vegetables, and lean meats. The food industry, however, does not promote all foods equally: sellers tend to emphasize brand-name foods because they bring higher returns, especially highly sweetened cereals, cookies, cakes, and pastries. Food manufacturers

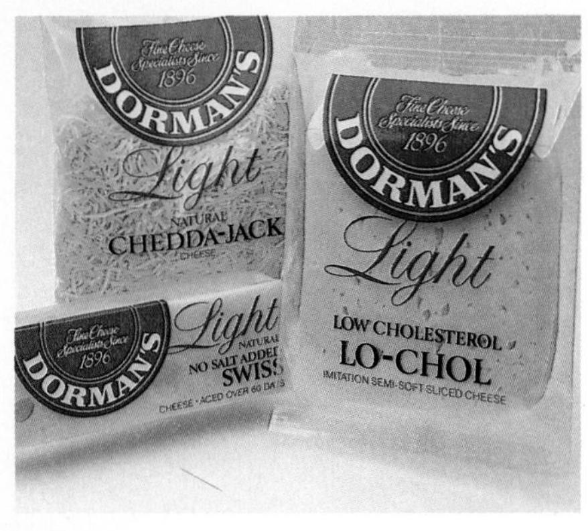

Eye-catching packaging indicating dietary benefits.

often pay for the best place in the supermarkets: at the end of the aisle and, depending on the product, at the child's or adult's eye level.[21]

Restaurants are a big growth industry in North America. Fast-food restaurants are especially zealous in advertising their fare. Many fast-food restaurants now offer healthy alternatives to their high-kcalorie and salty foods. Still, the temptation to consume the latter is often too hard to resist. Restaurant food is generally poorer in nutritional quality than food eaten at home.[20] The reality is that a hamburger, french fries, and a milkshake often have a greater appeal than a well-stocked salad bar.

Social factors

Many social changes in recent years have strongly affected the food marketplace. The increase in the number of working mothers and single parents, both young and old, means that less time is available for preparing meals. This limitation enhances the appeal of microwave ovens and frozen foods. Quick to meet the need, food producers have increased the number of foods that require little or no preparation. One third to one half of people state in surveys that to save time, those are the foods they eat most consistently. Households headed by men are particularly likely to use convenience items.[17]

As the age of our population has increased, so has the consumption of certain foods: for example, shellfish, fresh vegetables, and alcoholic beverages. For the elderly, new health and nutrition problems often arise and compel changes in food habits. We focus on these changes in Chapter 17.

As education levels rise, diet quality tends to improve as well, and families eat more meals together.[7] Today, it's relatively common to eat away from home and to skip meals. In one study, over one half of college students reported that they ate only two meals a day, eating many snacks to make up the difference.[15] For families, approximately 30% of adults skip breakfast. Breakfast is the time to replace carbohydrate stores used during the night's sleep (see Chapter 4). Skipping breakfast can interfere with proper nutrition.

Economics

The amount of money available for food influences eating habits. As income increases, so do meals eaten away from home. More affluent people also tend to consume more vegetables, fruits, cheeses, meats, fish, poultry, and fat, but they eat less dried beans, rice, and eggs. However, the relationship between income and overall food consumption is not as strong as you might expect, probably because food is relatively inexpensive in North America. Nevertheless, high meat prices have led to the use of beef as an ingredient rather than as a centerpiece in some households, encouraging the use of chicken and turkey as alternatives.

Concept Check

Our food choices are influenced mainly by taste and habit. Good food habits developed and strengthened now will benefit you in years to come.

GIVEN OUR FOOD CHOICES, WE CAN DO BETTER

Our cultural diversity, varied cuisines, and high nutritional status are points of pride for North Americans. In 1990, we have available a tremendous variety of food choices. Many recent diet changes are advantageous; some are not. Soft drinks now are more popular than milk, but frozen vegetable consumption is also on the rise. We live longer than ever before and enjoy better general health. Some of us also have more money, more overwhelming food and life-style choices to consider, and more time to relax and enjoy life. The end results of

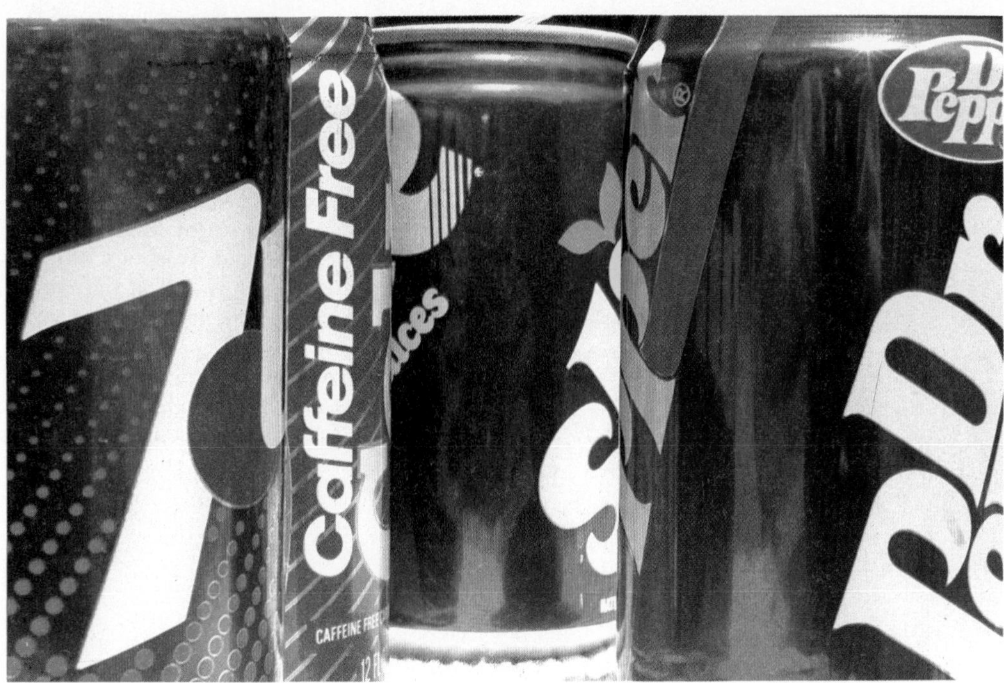

Soft drinks are today more popular than milk, although not as beneficial to the diet.

these trends are not fully known, but deaths from heart disease and strokes have dropped dramatically since the late 1960s. Better medical care and diets also deserve some credit. Still, affluence, when it leads to sedentary life-styles and high intakes of alcohol, can be a villain. *Because of better technology and greater choices, we have a much better diet today than ever before—if we know what to do with the choices. Overall, we are doing well, but many of us can do better. The goal here is to help you find your best path to good nutrition.*

Summary

1. Nutrition is the study of the food substances vital for health and how the body uses these substances to promote and support growth, maintenance, and reproduction of cells.
2. Nutrients in foods fall into six classes: carbohydrates, lipids (fats and oils), proteins, vitamins, minerals, and water. The first three, along with alcohol, provide energy for the body to use.
3. As nutritional health diminishes, nutrient stores in the body are depleted, then biochemical reactions in the body slow down and finally, clinical evidence (signs and symptoms) can be seen.
4. Overnutrition is a focus today in North America. This condition includes overconsumption of energy and certain vitamins and minerals.
5. The focus for nutrition planning should be food, not supplements. Using foods to supply nutrient needs essentially eliminates the possibility of severe nutrient imbalances.
6. Results from large nutrition surveys in North America suggest that on the whole the food supply is quite safe, but some North Americans need to concentrate on consuming foods that supply more vitamin A, vitamin C, vitamin B-6, calcium, magnesium, iron, zinc, and dietary fiber.
7. Our food choices are greatly affected by our culture, our family, our upbringing, our self-image, and the image we want to present to others.

Take Action

Where do your food preferences come from? What are your favorite foods? What foods do you particularly dislike? All of us have our own associations and idiosyncracies about food. However, it is not always easy to identify the origins of our food preferences and aversions. See if you can identify yours. Fill in the chart with your food preferences and dislikes. Do the same for your parents. Any surprises? What were/are the three most important reasons for food choices in your household? (Consider income, ages, cultural origins, advertising, etc.)

Foods I Like	Foods I Dislike
1. ____________	1. ____________
2. ____________	2. ____________
3. ____________	3. ____________
Foods My Mother Likes	**Foods My Mother Dislikes**
1. ____________	1. ____________
2. ____________	2. ____________
3. ____________	3. ____________
Foods My Father Likes	**Foods My Father Dislikes**
1. ____________	1. ____________
2. ____________	2. ____________
3. ____________	3. ____________

Most important reasons for food choices:

1. ____________
2. ____________
3. ____________
4. ____________
5. ____________

REFERENCES

1. Apparent nutrient content of the Canadian food supply 1960-1983 (per capita per day). Agriculture Canada Nutrient Assessment Program, July 1985 (revised).
2. Axelson ML: The impact of culture on food-related behavior, Annual Reviews of Nutrition 6:345, 1986.
3. Basiotis PP and others: Number of days of food intake records required to estimate individual and group nutrient intakes with defined confidence, Journal of Nutrition 117:1638, 1987.
4. Beaton GH: Towards harmonization of dietary, biochemical, and clinical assessments: the meaning of nutritional status and requirements, Nutrition Review 44:349, 1986.
5. Birch LL: The acquisition of food acceptance patterns in children. In eating habits: food, physiology, and learned behavior, Boakes RA and others, editors. John Wiley & Sons Inc, London, 1987.
6. Block G and others: Nutrient sources in the American diet. American Journal of Epidemiology 122:13, 1985.
7. Boakes R, Piopplewell D and Burton M: Eating habits: food, physiology and learned behavior, New York, John Wiley & Sons Inc., 1987.
8. Butrum RR and others: NCI dietary guidelines: rationale, American Journal of Clinical Nutrition 48:88, 1988.
9. Fuller E: Who is malnourished? Patient Care p. 143, June 15, 1986.
10. Gibson RS and others: Dietary fibre and selected nutrient intakes of some Canadian children, adolescents, and women. Journal of the Canadian Dietetic Association 48:82, 1987.
11. Harper AE: Nutrition: from myth and magic to science, Nutrition Today, p 8, Jan/Feb 1988.
12. Kim WW and others: Evaluation of long-term dietary intakes of adults consuming self-selected diets, American Journal of Clinical Nutrition 40:327, 1984.
13. Koplan JP and others: Nutrient intake and supplementation in the United States (NHANES II). American Journal of Public Health 76:287, 1986.
14. Logue AW: The psychology of eating and drinking, New York, WH Freeman & Co Publishers, 1986.
15. Marrale JC and others: What some college students eat, Nutrition Today, p 16, Jan/Feb 1986.
16. Miles CW: Metabolizable energy of human mixed diets, Human Nutrition. Applied Nutrition 40A:333, 1986.
17. Pearson JM and others: Convenience food use in households with male food preparers. Journal of the American Dietetic Association 86:339, 1986.
18. Peterkin BB and others: Nationwide food consumption survey, 1986, Nutrition Today, p 18, Jan/Feb 1988.
19. Posner BEM and others: Dietary characteristics and nutrient intake in an urban homebound population, Journal of the American Dietetic Association 87:452, 1987.
20. Reese CP and others: Impact of commercial eating on nutrient adequacy, Journal of the American Dietetic Association 87:463, 1987.
21. Surgeon General's report on nutrition and health, Nutrition Today, p 22, Sept/Oct 1988.
22. USDA, Determinants of Food Consumption of American Households, Marketing Science Research Institute, Cambridge, 1982.
23. White PL: Setting new diet and health directions, Nutrition Today, p 4, July/Aug 1986.
24. Woteki CE and others: National Health and Nutrition Examination Survey—NHANES, Nutrition Today, p 25, Jan/Feb 1988.
25. Yetiv JZ: Popular nutritional practices: a scientific appraisal, Toledo, 1986, Popular Medicine Press.
26. Yetley E and Johnson C: Nutritional applications of the Health and Nutrition Examination Surveys (HANES), Annual Review of Nutrition 7:441, 1987.

SUGGESTED READINGS

We want to call your particular attention to the article by Beaton that describes the many theoretical problems surrounding the establishment of nutrient needs. This article reminds us that we should not attribute extravagant values to nutrients, but instead have foods as our major focus. The article edited by Fuller describes for practicing physicians the major signs and symptoms of malnutrition seen in North Americans. Articles published in Patient Care are very practical and include numerous tables and figures that can be copied and distributed by physicians to their clients. Axelson looks in detail at various social influences on our food behavior, including income, education, gender, race, and attitude. Articles like this one published in *Annual Reviews of Nutrition* are generally quite detailed and provide numerous references. Finally, the article by Harper is an interesting look at the science of nutrition and emphasizes the importance of maintaining a skeptical mind when evaluating nutritional claims. He reminds us that nutrition-related diseases, such as diabetes and heart disease, are common not only because of our food habits, but also because of the increased life span that all of us have the potential to enjoy. As we age, these diseases have a longer time to develop.

CHAPTER 1

Answers to nutrition awareness inventory

1. *True.* Water is the medium in which most of the body's substances are dissolved; a lean human body is about 70% water.
2. *False.* Minerals are elements and cannot be further broken down by ordinary chemical means.
3. *False.* Kcalories (kilocalories) are 1000-calorie units. Although most people talk about energy units as calories, what they really mean is kilocalories. As a nutrition student, you need to be aware of the proper term.
4. *True.* One gram of protein yields 4 kcalories, 1 gram of carbohydrate 4 kcalories, 1 gram of fat 9 kcalories, and 1 gram of alcohol 7 kcalories.
5. *True.* Although vitamins, like carbohydrates, fats, and proteins, contain carbon atoms, vitamins yield no energy directly to the body.
6. *True.* When nutrient intake does not meet nutrient needs, your nutrient stores can be used. However, once these stores are depleted, serious health problems may result.
7. *False.* Some minerals such as calcium are required in larger amounts than vitamins.
8. *False.* Organic refers to carbon atoms bonded to hydrogen atoms and has nothing to do with organic gardening.
9. *False.* A sign is a visible result of disease, such as flaky skin; a symptom is a change in body function that you would complain of, such as a stomach pain.
10. *True.* If you are deficient in iron, you often become pale and your heart rate increases. If you are severely deficient, temperature control may be altered and you will feel cold.
11. *True.* If you overeat continually, you are likely to gain weight. This overnutrition may have long-term consequences, such as high blood pressure or diabetes.
12. *False.* People should get their nutrients from foods rather than from supplements. Vitamins A and D and minerals such as iron and selenium can even be harmful if taken in large amounts for long periods of time.
13. *True.* Alcoholic beverages are the third leading contributor to energy intakes in the United States.
14. *True.* Recent studies have shown that although people express concern about their nutritional intake, they are often unable to change their diets.
15. *True.* No food is totally worthless. Diets, however, that are unbalanced in needed nutrients can be described as "junk diets."

Nutrition Perspective 1-1

Establishing Nutrient Needs by Scientific Research

hypothesis
An "educated guess" by a scientist to explain a phenomenon.

theory
An explanation for a phenomenon that has numerous lines of evidence to support it.

The study of nutrient needs and nutrient metabolism derives information using the scientific method, a method designed to detect and eliminate error. Scientists begin by observing physical phenomena. They conjecture and speculate about the causes of the phenomena, and then suggest possible explanations or **hypotheses** about them. They critically examine these possibilities using rigorous experimental tests that may either support or refute them. If many lines of evidence support an hypothesis, it gains the status of a **theory.**

Science obliges us to view hypotheses and theories skeptically, to avoid hasty acceptance of them based on meager evidence and to discard those that fail to pass critical analyses (see Figure 1-4). Nutrition science requires skeptical minds that impose a critical evaluation of all current ideas.[14]

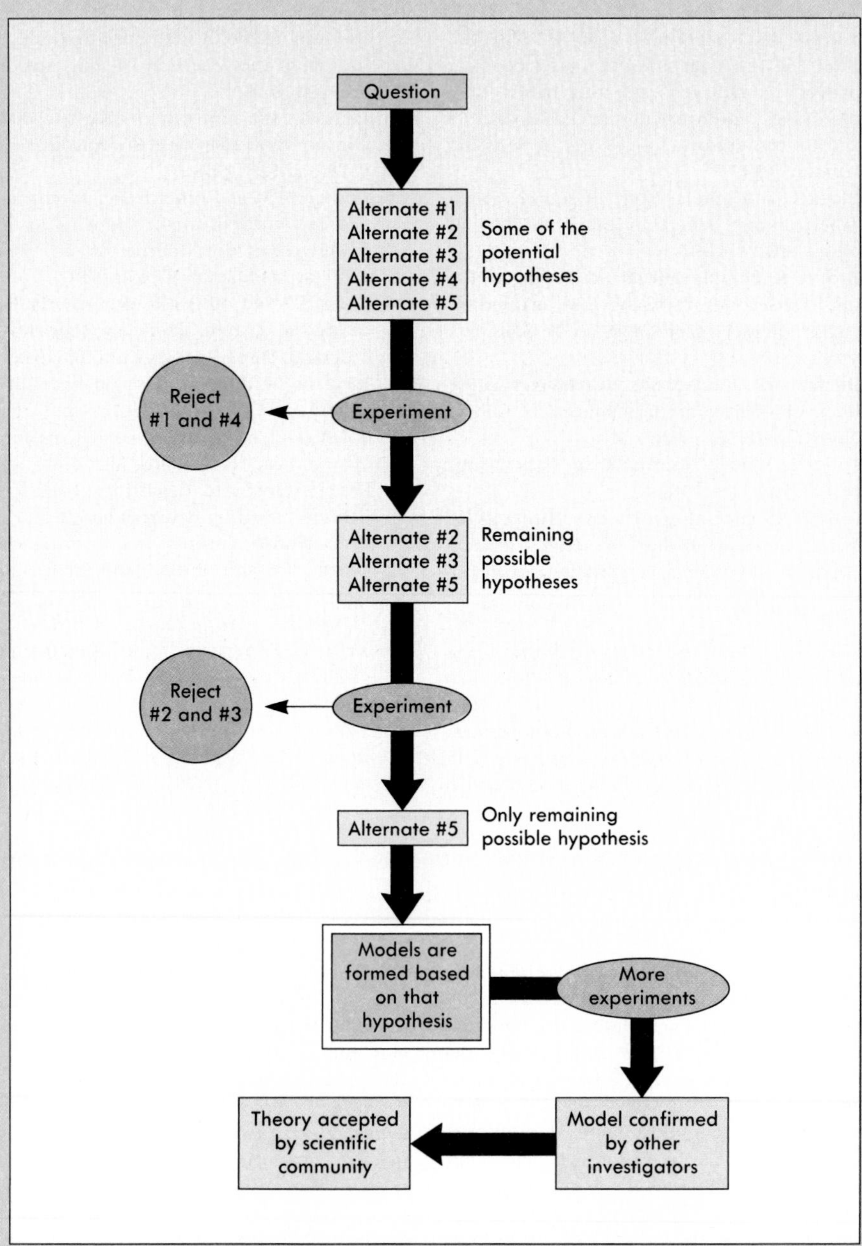

Figure 1-4

From question to theory—the process of science. Hypotheses are first suggested to answer a question. Then, experiments are done in an attempt to eliminate one or more hypotheses. Thus the most likely hypothesis is selected. If it is supported by experiments done by other investigators and stands the test of time, the hypothesis may eventually become theory.

Nutrition Perspective 1-1—cont'd

GENERATING HYPOTHESES

Historical events often give us clues to important relationships in nutritional science. For example, in the 15th and 16th centuries, when European explorers left Europe to come to the Americas, the disease **scurvy** developed during their voyages. This vitamin deficiency developed because the sailors ate few fruits and vegetables, and thus consumed very little vitamin C. Eventually British scientists discovered that lime juice cured the scurvy. About 300 years later vitamin C was discovered. Meanwhile the British Navy, run by "Limeys," had a healthy work force, and dominated the seas worldwide.

scurvy
The deficiency disease that results after a few months of consuming a diet free of vitamin C (see Chapter 12).

During World War II, the German army blockaded the Russian city Leningrad, causing widespread malnutrition there. Noting that this malnutrition was associated with increased infant **mortality,** scientists in North America evaluated the effect of food supplements on infant mortality. That work showed that food supplements given to poor women improved their chances of having a healthy baby.

mortality
This represents a population's death rate. The term *morbidity* refers to the rate/amount of sickness present.

EPIDEMIOLOGY

Another approach scientists pursue to establish nutritional hypotheses is to study the different dietary and disease patterns among various populations in the world. If one group tends to develop a certain disease while another group does not, speculation can occur about the role diet plays in this difference. The study of diseases in populations is called **epidemiology.**

epidemiology
The study of how disease rates vary between different population groups, such as the rate of stomach cancer in Japan compared with that in Germany.

In the 1920s epidemiological studies helped Dr. Joseph Goldberger determine that the disease **pellagra** was a dietary deficiency disease, rather than **infectious disease.** He noticed that prisoners in jail—but not their jailers—suffered from pellagra. If pellagra was an infectious disease, both populations would be expected to suffer from it.

In the 1970s, Dr. Denis Burkitt noted the low rate of intestinal problems in Africans compared with North Americans. Burkitt speculated that the large amount of dietary fiber Africans eat leads to greater intestinal health, and the low dietary fiber intakes seen in North America cause problems (see Chapter 4 for details).

CONFIRMING EPIDEMIOLOGICAL IMPRESSIONS

Epidemiological evidence, however, was not enough for either Goldberger or Burkitt to establish that a dietary problem caused the diseases they studied. Getting better evidence required **experimental** testing. In the 1920s various foods were fed to people in mental asylums who suffered from pellagra. The experiment showed that yeast and high-protein foods could cure pellagra (see Chapter 12 for a detailed discussion). Similarly, when typical North Americans diets were improved to contain more dietary fiber in the 1970s, intestinal health often improved. The research on pellagra is largely complete, but research on the importance of dietary fiber to health still continues.

pellagra
A disease characterized by inflammation of the skin, diarrhea, and eventual mental incapacity due to the lack of the vitamin niacin in the diet (see Chapter 12).

infectious disease
Any disease caused by an invasion of the body by microorganisms, such as bacteria, fungi, or viruses.

experiment
A test made to examine the validity of a hypothesis.

USING ANIMALS TO EXPLORE EPIDEMIOLOGICAL ASSOCIATIONS

When scientists cannot test their hypostheses on humans, they often use animals. Much of what we know about human nutritional needs and functions has been generated from animal experiments. Still, human experiments are the most convincing for scientists. In the 1930s scientists showed that a pellagra-like disease seen in dogs, called blacktongue, was cured by *nicotinic acid.* But only when nicotinic acid actually cured the disease in humans were scientists convinced that nicotinic acid, later called *niacin,* was the critical dietary factor.

Today we know that low doses of the mineral *fluoride* can stimulate growth in rats. However, we still do not know whether that is true for humans because no human experiment can be conducted. It is just not practical to control the fluoride intake of humans accurately enough. Thus there is speculation that fluoride might stimulate growth in humans, but real proof is lacking.

Nutrition Perspective 1-1—cont'd

In addition, some human experiments would not be ethical. You may think it is reasonable to feed rats a low copper diet to study copper's importance in the formation of blood vessels. (Some people argue that performing animal experiments is unethical.) Almost universally, however, people would find it unethical to study how copper affects the formation of blood vessels in infants.

Unfortunately, scientists often cannot advance their findings beyond the point of epidemiology. For example, perhaps no disease exists in animals that is comparable with a particular human disease, so no **animal model** can be used to answer the question. Or perhaps ethical questions or insufficient funds block experimentation in humans.

animal model
A disease in animals that duplicates human disease and thus can be used to understand more about the human disease.

Concept Check

Throughout this book we will point out areas where more research is needed to answer important nutritional questions. Many of these questions will have been raised by epidemiological studies or by other observations of scientists. They now await support from experiments done in the animal and, especially, the clinical laboratory. Until overwhelming evidence supports the hypothesis, it should not be considered a nutrition "fact."[11]

CONDUCTING EXPERIMENTS—THE DOUBLE-BLIND STUDY

An important type of experimental approach used to test hypotheses is the **double-blind study.** By definition, an experiment requires a group of **subjects** that follow a specific protocol, such as eating a certain food. An experiment also requires a **control group** with which the normal pattern of living is not altered. Scientists then observe the experimental group over time to see if there is any effect that is not found in the control group. Sometimes subjects are used as their own control: first, they are observed for a period of time, and then they are treated and their responses noted.

double-blind study
An experiment where the subjects and researchers are unaware of the outcome of the study until it is completed.

Bias (prejudice) can easily affect the outcome of an experiment. Researchers need to limit the amount of bias they and the subjects in the experiment contribute. The best way to do that is to "blind" the subjects and themselves so neither know which subjects are in the experimental group and which are in the control group. In addition, the effects of the experimental protocol are not disclosed until after the entire study is completed. This approach avoids the chance that the subjects may begin to feel better, for example, simply because they are part of an experiment. Also, it avoids the possibility that researchers may see the change they want to see in the subjects in order to prove a certain hypotheses, even though the change did not actually occur.

In a double-blind experiment, a **placebo** (fake medicine) is often given to the control group in order to camouflage who is in what group. Until the experiment is complete, a third party holds the code key that identifies each participant and his treatment. Sometimes only a single-blind protocol is possible, in which either the subjects *or* the researchers are kept in the dark.

placebo
A fake medicine used to disguise the roles of participants in an experiment; if fake surgery is performed, that is called a sham operation.

Drug studies lend themselves to a double-blind protocol because it is often easy to disguise the drug with a placebo. However, food studies often cannot be placebo-controlled. It is hard to disguise a diet high in fruits and vegetables from one devoid of them. However, in that case, the experimenters should try to ensure that the results from the blood assays or other samples are not revealed until the end of the study. In addition, the results should be kept from the subjects until the end of the study. In that way much potential bias can be eliminated. The more bias is controlled in the experiment, the more confidence we can have in the results.

When you read accounts of scientific experiments, ask yourself: "Was a double-blind study protocol used? If the use of a placebo was possible, was it used? Were the researchers 'blinded' as much as possible during the progress of the experiment to who received the experimental treatment and to the effects of that treatment?"

PEER-REVIEW OF EXPERIMENTAL RESULTS

Once an experiment is complete, scientists summarize the findings and publish the results in a scientific journal. At the ends of the chapters in this book, we list many citations for

Nutrition Perspective 1-1—cont'd

important experiments that have been published in scientific journals. Most of these journals are **peer-reviewed.** This means other scientists have judged the quality of the research, striving to allow only the highest quality research findings to be published. Research results published in the *American Journal of Clinical Nutrition,* the *New England Journal of Medicine,* or the *Journal of The American Dietetic Association* are much more reliable than those found in popular magazines or promoted on television talk shows. A major difference is that scientific journals are closely scrutinized by the scientific community to make sure the research results are of sufficient quality, deserving your attention.

peer-reviewed journal
A journal that publishes research only after two or three scientists, who were not part of the study, agree it was well conducted and the results are fairly represented. In this case, the research has been approved by peers of the research team.

THE NEED FOR FOLLOW-UP STUDIES

Finally, even if the study contains all the right factors and is accepted by the scientific community, one examination is not enough. Results from one laboratory must be confirmed by other laboratories. Only then can we really trust and use the results. We don't advise accepting new ideas as fact or incorporating them into your health habits until they are proven by several lines of evidence. Until then, the best goal is variety and moderation with any food.[11]

Chapter 2

Tools for Studying Nutrition

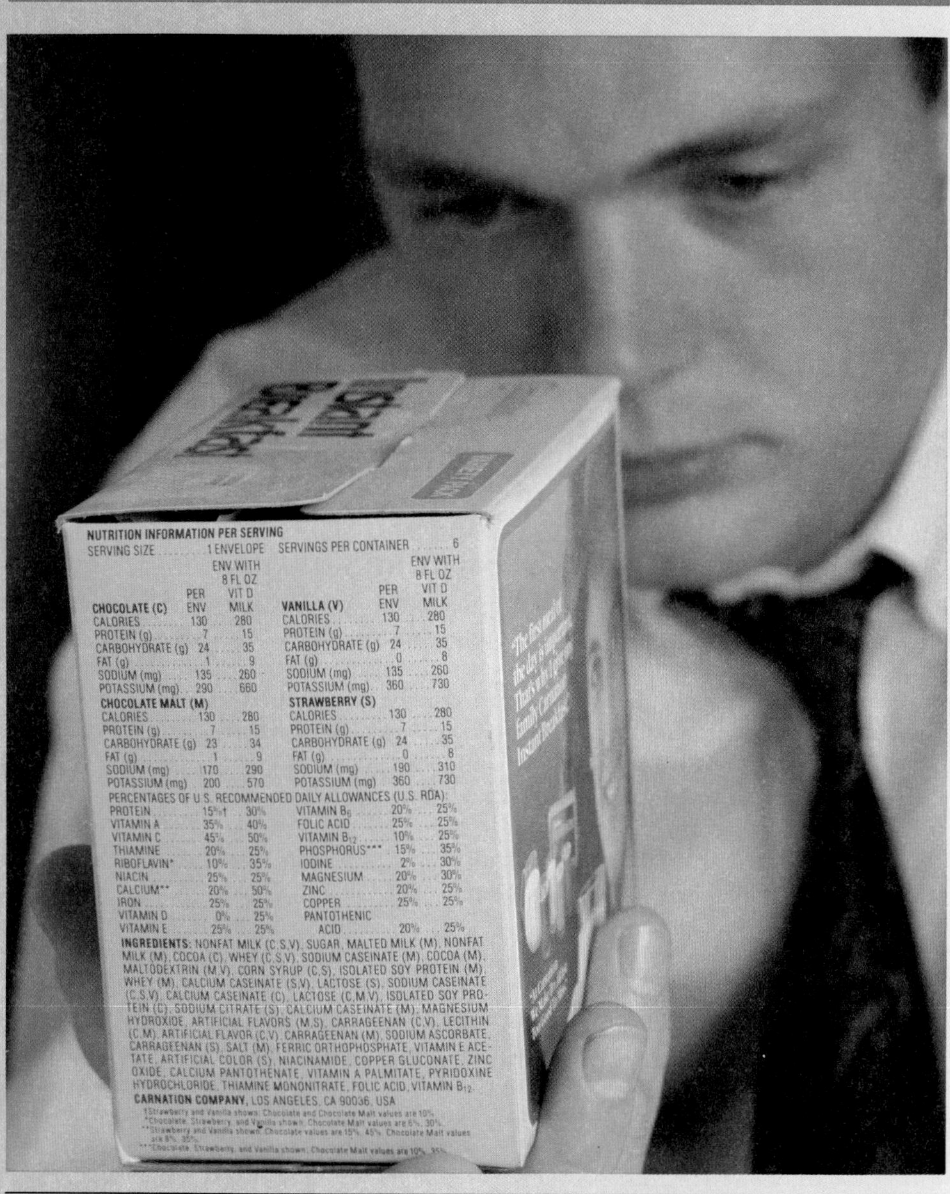

Use food labels to learn more about what you eat.

Overview

This chapter provides important tools for studying nutrition. Here we spell out critical terms and definitions to aid your understanding the rest of the book. The first three sections explain basic chemistry, discuss mathematical principles, and explain what the Recommended Dietary Allowances (RDA) represent. Last, we recommend basic good food choices by outlining the Daily Food Guide and discuss the Exchange System. This system is a method both for planning diets and tracking the amount of energy-yielding nutrients in a food plan.

If you are familiar with these basic concepts, briefly skim the sections. Some concepts may have been covered in previous coursework. We want to provide you with a firm understanding of basic chemistry, mathematics, and diet planning concepts now, before you study the nutrients in detail.

Nutrition awareness inventory

Here are 15 statements about the tools for studying nutrition. Answer them to test your current knowledge. If you think the statement is true or mostly true, circle T; if you think the statement is false or mostly false, circle F. Use the scoring key at the end of the chapter to compute your total score. Take this test again after you have read this chapter. Compare the results.

1. T F The basic chemical components of nutrition are carbohydrates, fats, proteins, vitamins, minerals, and water.
2. T F Atoms bonded together form a molecule.
3. T F The term *joule,* used in Britain, is similar to the use of the term calorie in the United States.
4. T F A cup of water equals a milliliter (ml) of water.
5. T F 100 grams equals about 1 pound.
6. T F RDA is the abbreviation for recommended daily allowance.
7. T F Most vitamins are needed daily to maintain good health.
8. T F Recommended nutrient intakes differ from country to country.
9. T F Establishing personal nutritional needs is the main purpose of the RDA.
10. T F An intake of 1500 kcalories per day is considered adequate for most people.
11. T F Although potatoes are vegetables, their nutrient content more closely resembles that of bread than of broccoli.
12. T F The Exchange System works on the premise that foods with similar fat, protein, and carbohydrate composition can be substituted for each other.
13. T F Nutrient density is one way to evaluate a food's quality.
14. T F A kcalorie is the amount of heat required to raise the temperature of 1 liter of water 1° C.
15. T F There is no perfect food.

CHEMISTRY: A TOOL FOR UNDERSTANDING NUTRITION

A basic understanding of chemistry can make the study of nutrition much easier and more exciting. It enables you to connect nutrient characteristics with a mental picture of their structures. At this course level memorizing complex chemical structures is unnecessary, since they are not the key to understanding the most important aspects of nutrition. However, a basic knowledge of chemical structures can help you visualize important concepts in nutrition. Let's briefly examine the chemistry of nutrition. If at first things are not clear to you, step back and read the section again. Again, our goal in this book is to use some chemistry concepts to help you learn a lot about nutrition. We hope this introduction will make it easier to see what nutrition is all about.

molecule
A group of like or unlike atoms chemically combined (see compound).

The basic units of chemistry

The body is composed of **molecules,** which are simply clusters of atoms. The term **compound** refers to a cluster of unlike chemicals grouped into molecules. If identical atoms "bond" together, the group is considered an element, as is a single atom. Thus pure sodium and pure gold are elements, and so are gold and sodium atoms. Atoms, however, usually combine with different types of atoms, thus compounds, not elements, are the rule in nature. The basic chemicals of nutrition—carbohydrates, fats, proteins, vitamins, minerals, and water—are either elements or compounds composed of atoms.

compound
A group of different types of atoms bonded together in definite proportion (see molecule).

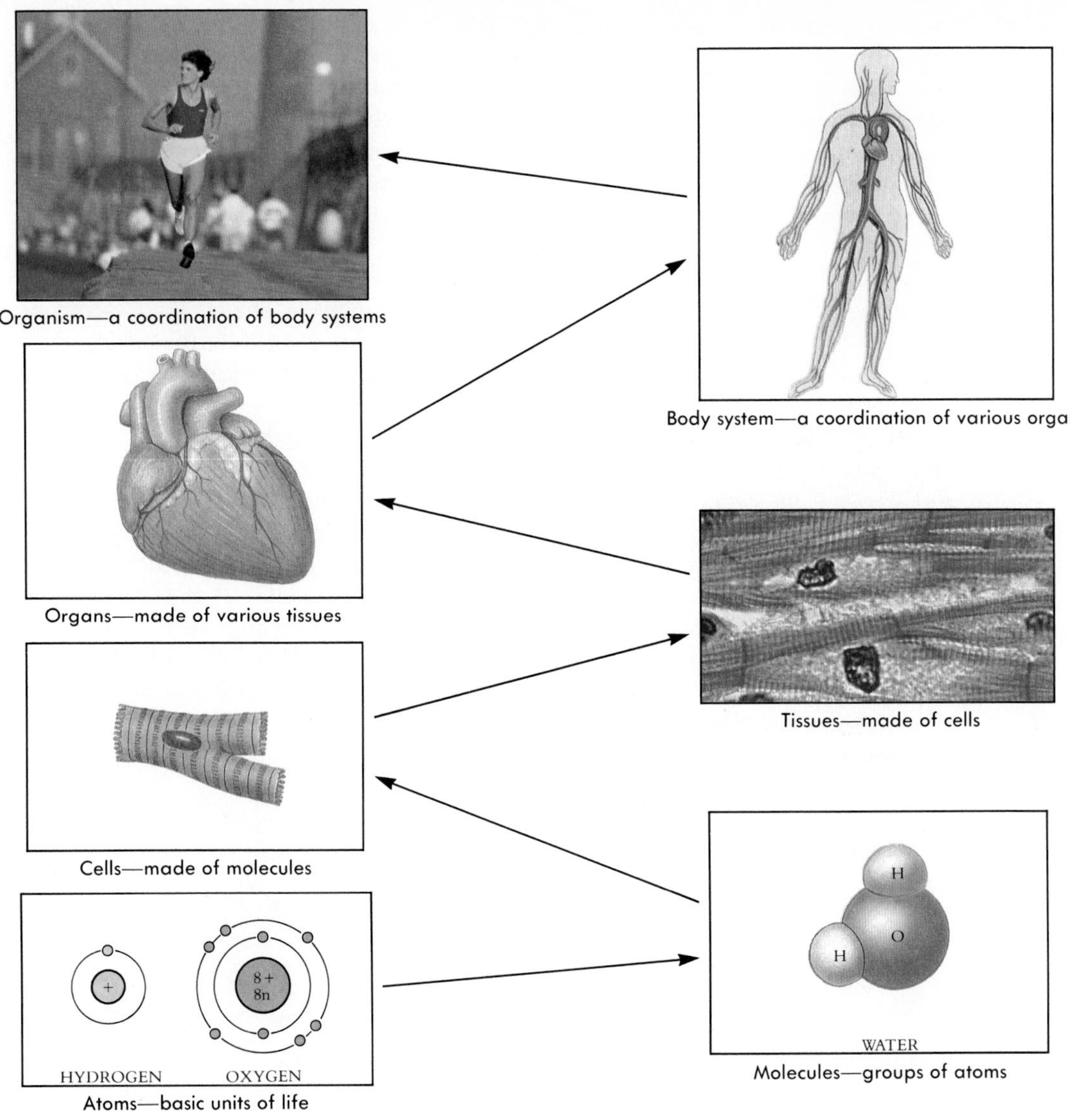

Organism—a coordination of body systems

Body system—a coordination of various organs

Organs—made of various tissues

Tissues—made of cells

Cells—made of molecules

Molecules—groups of atoms

Atoms—basic units of life

Figure 2-1

Levels of human biological organization. We are as simple as a collection of atoms and as complex as a single organism.

Beginning as tiny units, atoms combine millions of times to form living organisms. First molecules form, then many molecules combine to form **cells.** Cells combine and become **tissue,** which connects to form **organs.** The interaction of organs forms a coordinated system, called an **organism.** The human body is just such a coordinated unit of many organ systems (Figure 2-1).

A closer look at the atom. In its simplest form, an atom can be described as having a central core, or **nucleus,** composed of **protons** and **neutrons. Electrons** orbit the nucleus. These components are called subatomic particles. In a typical atom, the number of protons equals the number of neutrons, and together these determine molecular weight. If the number of neutrons differs from the number typically associated with a particular element, the atom exists in an **isotope** form. Examine the isotopes of hydrogen, called deuterium and tritium, that are drawn on page 30. Note that both possess extra neutrons.

nucleus
The core of an atom; it consists of ***protons*** (positively charged particles) and ***neutrons*** (uncharged particles). ***Electrons*** are negatively charged and orbit the nucleus.

When an atom holds fewer electrons than protons, it exists as a positive **ion,**

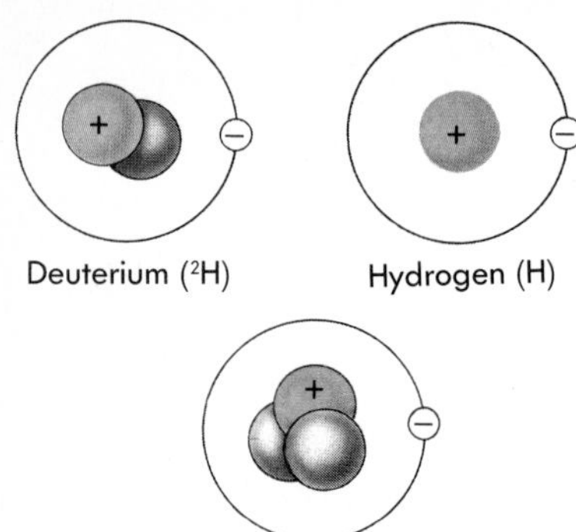

Isotopes of hydrogen

such as a sodium ion, (Na^+). (See the Periodic Table in Appendix D for abbreviations of elements.) When electrons outnumber protons, an atom exists as a negative ion, such as a chloride ion (Cl^-). In table salt, the negatively charged chloride ion is attracted to the positive sodium ion; this attraction forms a chemical **bond.** Since interacting ions actually form the bond, it is called an **ionic bond.** When salt dissolves in water, the ionic bond returns to the original ion forms. These sodium and chloride ions are called **electrolytes** (see Chapter 13).

Forming chemical bonds

Electrons orbit the nucleus in several different layers or shells. Two electrons form the first shell, and eight electrons form the second shell. Further shells contain varied numbers of electrons, but for our purposes the first two shells are most important.

Many atoms exist with incomplete electron shells. Hydrogen's first shell has only one electron, so it attracts electrons from other atoms to complete that shell and stabilize its structure. Carbon possesses a completed first shell of two electrons but has only four electrons in its second shell; it can accept four other electrons to fill spaces in its second shell. Thus four hydrogen atoms will react with one carbon atom to form methane (CH_4). In this molecule, all the atoms complete their electrons' shells, making it a very stable compound. The two atoms, then, share electrons: the same electrons fill spaces in the shells of both atoms. *Two atoms sharing electrons create a chemical bond called a* ***covalent bond.*** Note below how the carbon atom forms four separate covalent bonds with four individual hydrogen atoms.

covalent bond
A union of two atoms formed by the sharing of electrons.

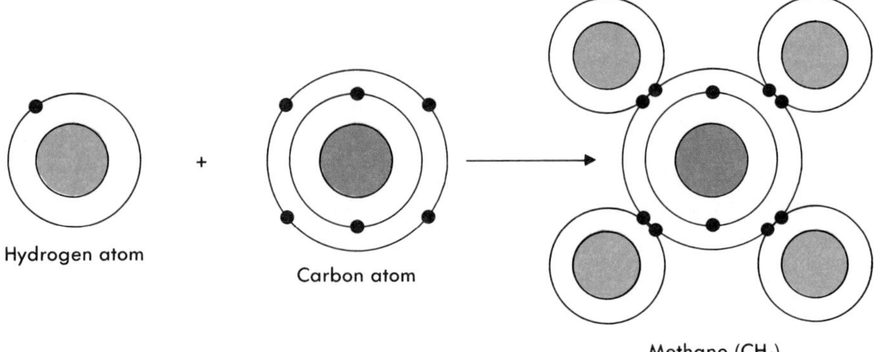

In nature, different atom types have different numbers of electrons in their various shells. Thus atoms need different numbers of covalent bonds to create a stable molecular structure. We see that hydrogen atoms need only one bond, while carbon atoms require four bonds. Other important atoms in nutrition include nitrogen, which needs three bonds; oxygen, which needs two bonds; sulfur, which needs two or more bonds; and phosphorus, which requires five bonds.

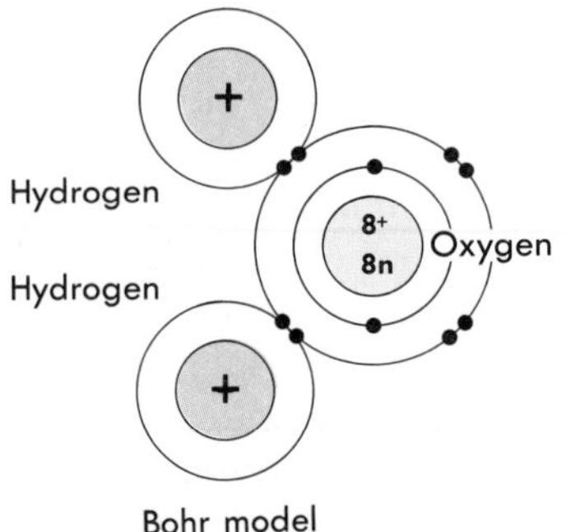

Bohr model

Note the structure of water at the bottom of page 30. It fulfills the need of both types of atoms: hydrogen now has two electrons in its only shell and oxygen has two electrons in its first shell and eight electrons in its second shell. We also depict what methane could look like in a molecular model and also in a ball and stick model. Both techniques for drawing molecules and their chemical bonds will be used throughout the next few chapters.

More about chemical bonds. Sharing electrons creates a powerful covalent bond; it takes a lot of energy to break one of these bonds. Below are drawings of structures for the simple sugar glucose, the amino acid alanine, and the fatty acid (part of a triglyceride) from butter, butyric acid. Note that various atoms are bonded to make each molecule.

Molecular model

104.5°

Ball and stick model

Glucose **Alanine** **Butyric acid**

When you see chemical bonds, think of electrons and energy. Electrons have a lot of energy and can power electric lights and motors. Even your body "runs on" electrons. Chapter 7 explains this process, but for now, keep in mind that the power to run your body resides in the bonds of many molecules.

Drawing chemical structures

To reduce the time required to draw all the atoms of a compound in its chemical structure, we will shortcut that procedure in the next chapters. Instead of drawing a carbon atom, we will depict it as a corner. Glucose becomes a hexagon with five carbon atoms and one oxygen atom in the hexagon. We represent all the carbon atoms as corners of the hexagon and only specifically indicate where the oxygen atom is located. We *draw* any group attached to a carbon atom only if it is *not* a hydrogen atom. It is unnecessary to draw all the hydrogen atoms because we know all carbon atoms must have four bonds. Assume that if a corner exists with nothing or only one group on it, enough hydrogen atoms are present to form four bonds.

Look below for the shortcut form we are using to redraw glucose, alanine, and butyric acid. Throughout your studies in biology, physiology, organic chemistry, biochemistry, and advanced nutrition science, this shortcut method of drawing chemicals will be used.

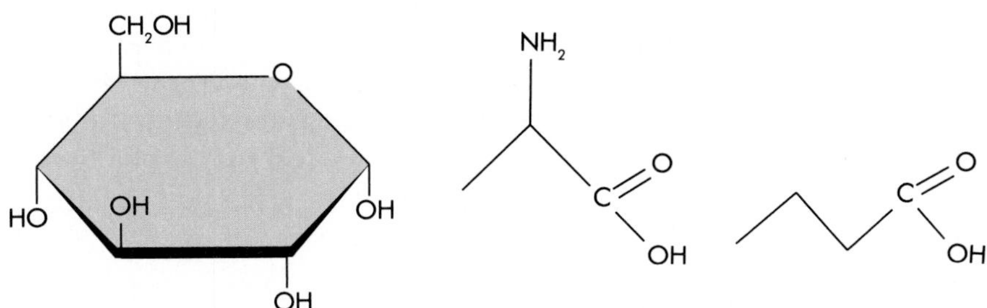

Exploring Issues and Actions

How can you approach mastering enough chemistry to reach your goals in studying nutrition? What strategies do you think might be helpful? The flash cards in the student study guide are one approach. Consider pairing up with another student and together developing other strategies for mastering these ideas.

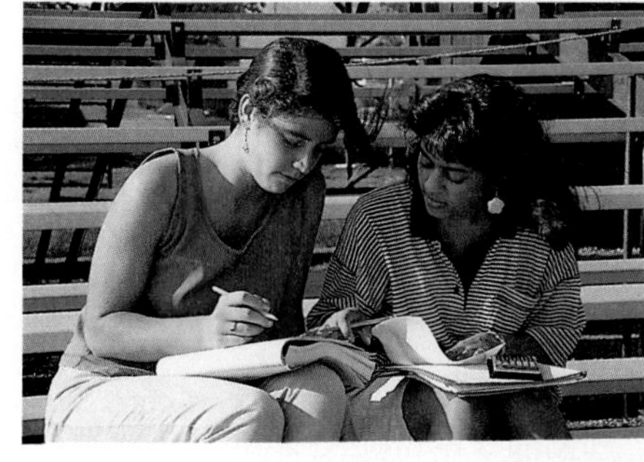

Common chemical groups

Certain groups of atoms appear repeatedly in the human body and in the foods we eat. Below are listed a few of the most common groups, for example, a hydroxyl group (—OH), an aldehyde group ($-\overset{\displaystyle O}{\overset{\|}{C}}-H$), a ketone group ($C-\overset{\displaystyle O}{\overset{\|}{C}}-C$), a carboxyl (acid) group ($-\overset{\displaystyle O}{\overset{\|}{C}}-OH$), a disulfide group (—S—S—), an amine group ($-NH_2$), and a phosphate group ($-O-\underset{\underset{\displaystyle OH}{|}}{\overset{\overset{\displaystyle O}{\|}}{P}}-O-$). Study the name and structure of these groups because you will see them throughout the next chapters.

An amine group is actually an ammonia group (NH_3) with one or more hydrogen atoms replaced by carbon atoms (or other types of atoms).

Condensation and hydrolysis reactions

chemical reaction
An interaction between two chemicals that changes both participants.

condensation reaction
A reaction that forms a bond between two compounds by removing a water molecule.

hydrolysis reaction
A reaction in which one compound is split into parts, releasing water in the process.

Various **chemical reactions** either create or break down compounds. By definition, a reaction results in changing the chemical participants. Body cells employ one basic type of reaction over and over again. When two compounds need to join, a hydroxyl group (−OH) from one compound is released, as is a hydrogen atom (−H) from the other compound. A bond is formed, and water is lost. This process makes a covalent bond and is called a **condensation reaction.**

Breaking a compound into smaller parts involves adding water to a covalent bond. A hydrogen atom from water transfers to one of the breakdown products, and the leftover hydroxyl group from water goes to the other breakdown product. The bond is now broken; this process is called a **hydrolysis reaction.** As compounds form, cells typically use condensation reactions. As compounds are broken down, cells typically employ hydrolysis reactions. When the body makes proteins for muscles, carbohydrates for storage in muscles, or fat to fuel muscles, it uses condensation reactions. When the body breaks down foods during digestion to absorb them, it uses hydrolysis reactions. See an example of these reactions in the margin.

Oxidation and reduction

oxidize
The process of losing an electron or gaining an oxygen atom.

reduce
The process of gaining an electron or losing a hydrogen atom.

When a compound is **oxidized,** it loses an electron; when it is **reduced,** it gains an electron. An easy way to differentiate oxidation from reduction is to imagine gaining a "negative" electron as actually subtracting something from the compound. Thus the compound is "reduced" by gaining a negatively charged electron.

For example, reducing iron as Fe^{+3} ion by an electron, changes it to an Fe^{+2} ion. Fe^{+2} then can oxidize back to Fe^{+3} by losing an electron. Adding the negative electron to iron (reduction) subtracts one of its positive charges. Removing the negative electron from the iron atom (oxidation), adds a positive charge.

Oxidizing a compound sometimes involves adding an oxygen atom or removing a hydrogen atom. To reduce a compound, add a hydrogen atom. *However, to include all examples of oxidation and reduction reactions in the body we must discuss the process in terms of electrons lost and electrons gained.*

Many oxidation and reduction reactions occur in cells, such as the example of changing the charge on iron. In addition, pyruvic acid (made from glucose) is reduced to form lactic acid by gaining two hydrogen atoms. This happens during intense exercise (see Chapter 7). Lactic acid is oxidized back to pyruvic acid by losing two hydrogen atoms. When you see the term oxidation or reduction, concentrate on electrons but also look for gains or losses of hydrogen or other atoms.

Isomers

Isomers are compounds that share the same chemical formula (have the same number of hydrogen atoms, carbon atoms, and so on) but have different chemical structures. A common isomer exists in nutrition when a carbon atom bonds to four different types of groups. In the margin is a drawing of alanine, an amino acid. At the center a carbon atom links with a hydrogen ($-H$), a methyl group ($-CH_3$), an amine group ($-NH_2$), and an acid group. A carbon with four different groups can always exist in two isomeric forms; in the case of alanine, they are called D and L. These two forms of alanine are much like a pair of gloves: each is different and functions differently, just as a right hand glove doesn't fit on a left hand.

The concept of isomers is important. Often the enzymes driving many chemical reactions in the body function with only one type of isomer. For example,

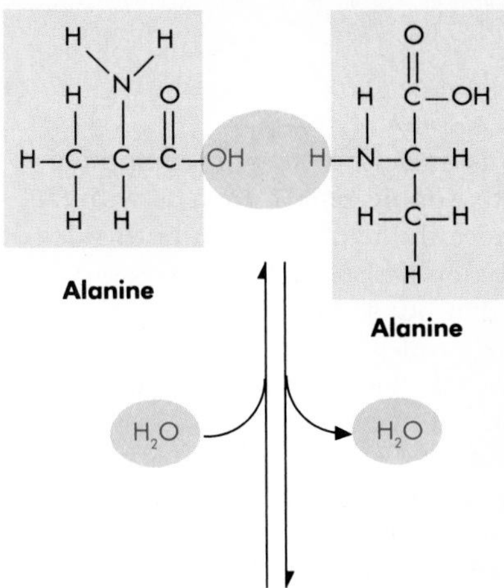

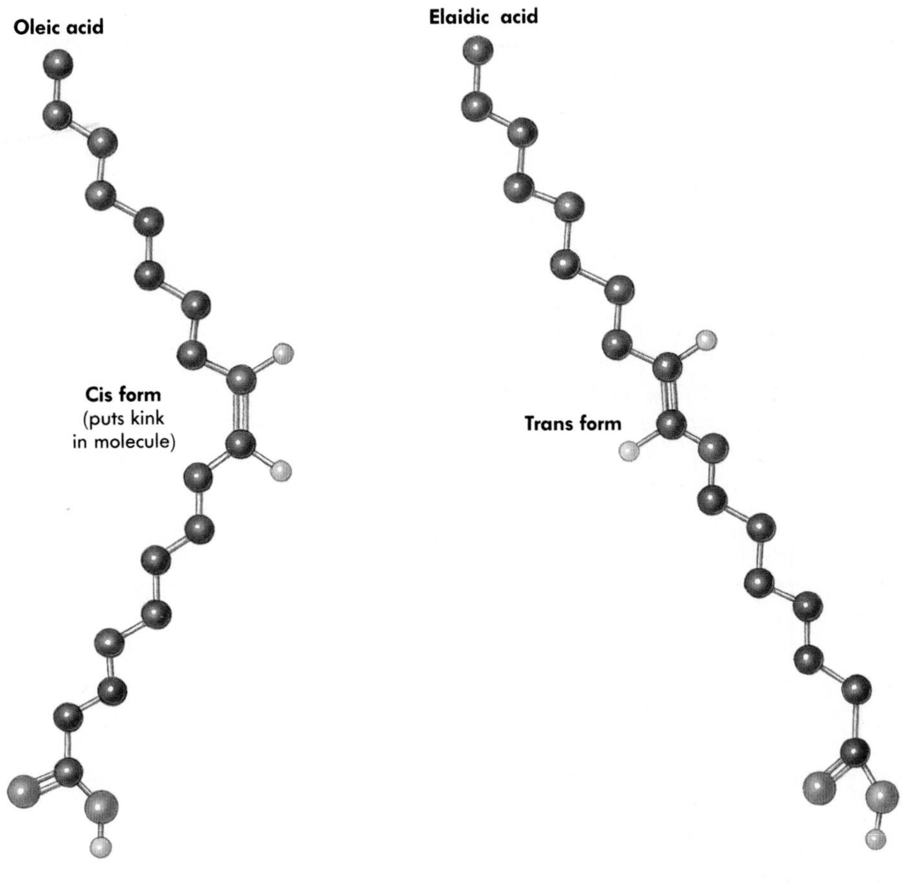

Figure 2-2
Cis and trans isomers of fatty acids. Cis forms are the most common forms in unprocessed foods.

isomer
Different chemical structures of compounds that share the same chemical formula.

An example of D and L isomers.

D-alanine

L-alanine

the body metabolizes only D-glucose, not L-glucose. Most amino acids are L-form; the body uses these and has a limited ability to metabolize some D forms.

cis isomer
An isomer form seen in compounds with double bonds, such as with fats, where the hydrogens on both sides of the double bond lie on the same side of that bond.

trans isomer
An isomer form found in compounds with double bonds, such as with fats, where the hydrogens on both sides of the double bond lie on opposite sides of that bond.

Another type of isomer is the **cis** and **trans** isomer. Figure 2-2 is a drawing of oleic acid, an important part of many fats. Notice the single bonds. When two carbon atoms possess only a single bond between them, they rotate separately around that single bond, almost like two pinwheels next to each other. In oleic acid, however, a double bond also exists. This bond forms a rigid part in the chemical structure. The two carbon atoms in the double bond are welded in space: one carbon atom cannot rotate without the other carbon atom also rotating. Those carbon atoms are attached to hydrogen atoms, which then also end up fixed into position. *If the hydrogen atoms lie on the same side of the double bond, the isomer is in the cis form. If hydrogen atoms lie across from each other, the isomer is in the trans form.*

Oleic acid is a cis isomer. In making margarine some trans oleic acid forms, which is called *elaidic acid* (see Chapter 5). We will use this cis and trans isomer terminology only when discussing fat compounds. The D and L isomer terminology will be used to describe proteins, carbohydrates, and other chemical structures in the body.

pH

pH
A measure of the hydrogen ion concentration in a solution.

The term ***pH*** describes the hydrogen ion (H^+) concentration of a solution. Specifically, pH is equal to the negative exponent of the hydrogen ion concentration. As the hydrogen ion concentration increases, the pH decreases. Because of the exponential relationship, a one unit change in pH represents a tenfold change in

Figure 2-3

The pH values of common substances. Note that "acid" tomatoes aren't really that acidic.

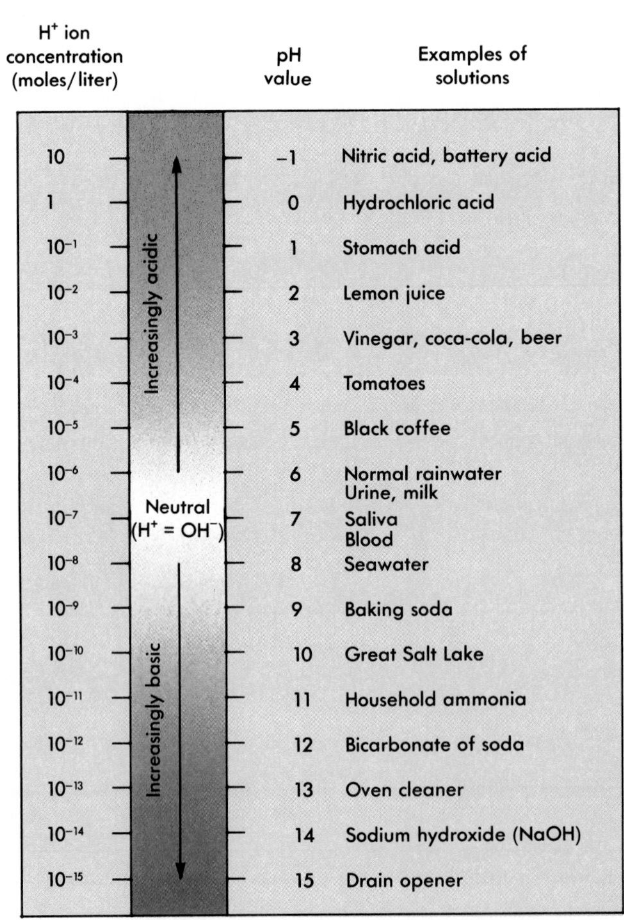

hydrogen ion concentration. Keep in mind that a neutral pH is 7, an **acid** pH lies between −1 and 7, and an **alkaline,** or basic, pH lies between 7 and 15. The blood has a pH between 7.35 and 7.45. Therefore it is slightly alkaline.

The stomach has a pH of 1 to 2 and so is very acidic. Since pH is based on an exponent, the stomach doesn't have merely seven times more hydrogen ions than the blood. *It actually has one million times more hydrogen ions than the blood.* Other acidic solutions include coffee at pH 5, orange juice at pH 4, and vinegar at pH 3 (Figure 2-3).

In a basic solution, hydroxyl ions (OH^-) are in a greater concentration than hydrogen ions. Basic solutions include household ammonia at pH 11 and concentrated lye (sodium hydroxide) at pH 14.

This brief look at chemistry should allow you to understand more about a compound's chemical structure. If you know the names of some compounds and develop a sense of chemical structure, you can understand much more about nutrition. You can tell simply by looking at their structures that glucose and amino acids are quite different in form, and thus probably perform different functions in the body. So, a little familiarity with chemistry makes it easier to learn and remember nutritional concepts.

acid pH
A pH less than 7. Lemon juice has an acid pH.

alkaline (basic) pH
A pH greater than 7. Baking soda in water yields an alkaline pH.

Concept Check

Atoms bond together to form molecules. These molecules combine to form cells, which combine to create body tissues, organs, and ultimately an entire human body. Atoms usually join using covalent bonds. These bonds represent a sharing of electrons and therefore represent storage forms of energy that the cell can later mobilize for its energy needs. The same types of atoms can group into various isomer forms. Different isomer forms possess different properties.

MATHEMATICAL TOOLS IN NUTRITION

The mathematical concepts you need for studying nutrition are few. Besides performing addition, subtraction, multiplication, and division, you need to calculate percentages and convert English units of measurement to metric units.

Percentages

The term *percent* (%) refers to a part of the total when the total represents 100 parts. For example, if you earn 80% on your first nutrition exam, you will have answered the equivalent of 80 out of 100 questions correctly, and the other 20 questions incorrectly. We have already discussed percentages when describing the North American diet (Chapter 1). The best way to master this concept is to calculate some percentages. We have included some problems below.

Question	Answer
What is 6% of 45?	0.06 × 45 = 2.7
What is 32% of 8?	0.32 × 8 = 2.6
What percent of 16 is 6?	6/16 = .375 or 37.5%
What percent of 99 is 3?	3/99 = 0.03 or 3%

Joe ate 15% of the adult RDA for vitamin C at lunch.
How many milligrams did he eat?
(RDA = 60 milligrams)

0.15 × 60 milligrams = 9 milligrams

It is difficult to succeed in a nutrition course unless you know what a percentage means and how to calculate one. We use the concept of percentages frequently in refering to diets and nutrient composition.

A millimeter is about the thickness of a dime.

The metric system

The basic units of the metric system are the **meter** for length, the gram for weight, and the **liter** for volume. The inside cover contains conversion factors for the English system units of pounds, feet, and cups to metric units. Here is a brief summary.

A meter is 39.4 inches long, or about 3 inches longer than 1 yard (3 feet). A meter is divided into 100 units called **centi**meters. A meter divided into 1000 units yields **milli**meters. There are 2.54 centimeters in 1 inch, and about 30 centimeters in 1 foot. A 6-foot tall person is 183 centimeters tall.

A gram is about 1/30 of an ounce. Five grams of sugar or salt is about 1 teaspoon. A **kilo**gram is 1,000 grams, a kilogram is equivalent to 2.2 pounds. A 156-pound man weighs 71 kilograms. A milligram breaks a gram into 1000 parts; a **micro**gram breaks 1 gram into 1,000,000 parts.

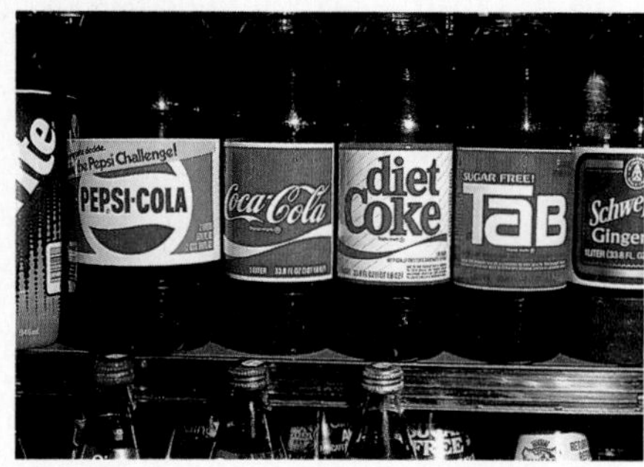

Liters are divided into 1000 units called milliliters. One teaspoon equals about 5 milliliters, 1 cup is about 240 milliliters, and 1 quart (4 cups) equals almost 1 liter (0.946 liters to be exact).

If you plan to work in any realm of science, you should study the metric system until you become quite comfortable with it. For now, remember that a kilogram equals 2.2 pounds, 2.54 centimeters equals 1 inch, and a liter is almost the same as a quart. In addition, know what the prefixes *micro-, milli-, centi-,* and *kilo-* represent. With that, you can get an approximation of any metric quantity into English units and approximate English units into the metric system.

Exploring Issues and Actions

Closely observe your environment to determine which familiar objects or measurements are already in metric units. Start by looking for 1 or 2 liter soft drink bottles in the supermarket.

RECOMMENDED DIETARY ALLOWANCES

Now that you have reviewed some basic chemistry and math skills, it is time to use them in developing some tools for studying nutrition. To begin, a major nutrition controversy arose when many men were rejected from military service during World War II because of the effects of poor nutrition on their health. In response, a group of 25 scientists met in 1941 and formed the first Food and Nutrition Board. They were given the responsibility to establish dietary standards both to evaluate the nutritional intakes of large population groups and to provide a guide for planning agriculture production.[7] This Board developed the first **Recommended Dietary Allowances (RDA).** Because their standards were based on insufficient scientific information, they realized the RDA they set needed alterations as new information became available.

Recommended Dietary Allowances (RDA)
Recommended intakes of nutrients that meet the needs of almost all healthy people of similar age and gender. These are established by the Food and Nutrition Board of the National Academy of Sciences.

Subsequently, the RDA was revised every four to five years. The Food and Nutrition Board uses the following plan to set the new levels[5]:

1. Estimate the average **requirement** of a population for a given nutrient and the **variability** for that requirement in a population. In other words, estimate how much of a nutrient each person requires to be healthy and how much those requirements vary among people.

2. Increase that average requirement by amounts sufficient to meet the needs of nearly all members of the population. This usually means increasing the average requirement by about 30% to 50%. Thus if the average requirement for a vitamin is 20 milligrams per day, the RDA may be approximately 28 milligrams per day, or 40% higher than the average figure.

3. Increase the RDA to account for inefficient use by the body of the nutrients when consumed. This inefficiency could be due to poor absorption, poor conversion of an inactive form to an active form, or other causes.

4. Use judgment to interpret and establish allowances when information about requirements is limited. In other words the members of the Food and Nutrition Board needed to use their scientific judgment in lieu of specific scientific data in certain cases.

Using this process, the Board set the RDA for males and females according to various age groups (see the inside cover for the specific recommendations).

The RDA serves as a guide to help you meet your nutritional needs with food rather than with vitamin and mineral supplements. This aim is important because only 19 of approximately 40 necessary nutrients—not counting essential amino acids—have an RDA. Not enough is known about many nutrients for the Food and Nutrition Board to establish an RDA.

One common misconception about the term *RDA* is that the "D" stands for "daily." It does not; it stands for "dietary." It is not necessary to consume the RDA for each nutrient every day. Think instead of *averaging the RDA for vitamins and minerals over a week's time.* No nutrient (even water) is absolutely needed every day. You can survive for a few days on a diet without water, and about 1 year on a diet without vitamin A.[6,7,12]

Because the RDA is based on our average needs and increased to account for variability in the population, it is by definition a generous allowance. The Food and Nutrition Board expects that the allowances are high enough so that for healthy people no improvement in health results from consuming more than RDA levels.[7,12] The Board believes the RDA generally covers any possible benefit that may be achieved from the nutrients obtainable in a typical diet.[6] The goal is to protect Americans from receiving either too much or too little of the needed nutrients; the RDA guideline provides good protection against both possibilities.

Thus the RDA is an estimate of the amount of nutrient that should be consumed by healthy people to meet their nutritional need. The word **healthy** needs emphasis. The RDA guideline also assumes that people are not taking medications that increase nutrient needs.

A close look at one RDA: Protein

The RDA of 0.8 grams of protein per kilogram of body weight per day for an adult aims for a state of protein **equilibrium:** where protein intake balances daily losses. The recommendation includes an extra amount to keep protein stores full in the body (Figure 2-4). Thus the overall economy of protein in the body should remain stable.

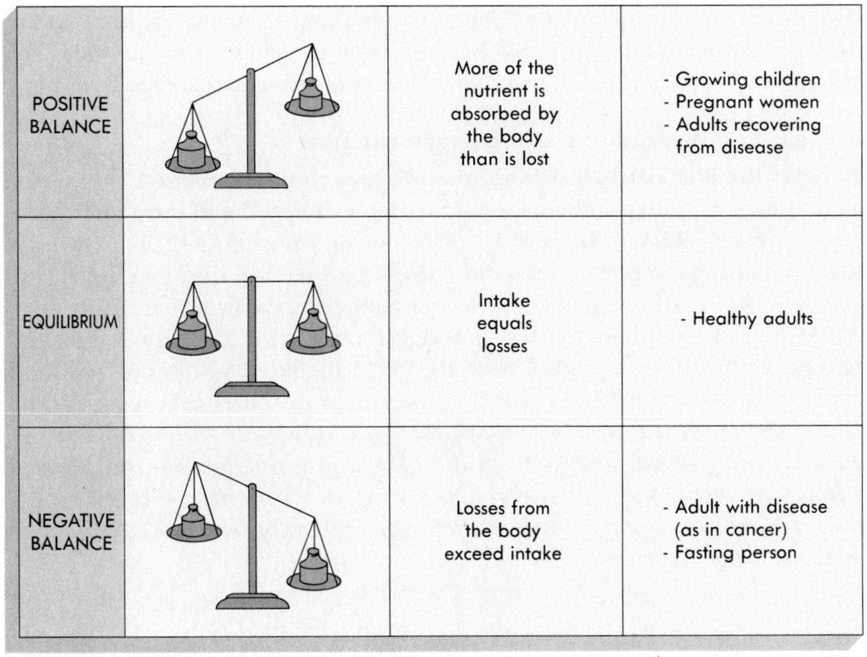

POSITIVE BALANCE		More of the nutrient is absorbed by the body than is lost	- Growing children - Pregnant women - Adults recovering from disease
EQUILIBRIUM		Intake equals losses	- Healthy adults
NEGATIVE BALANCE		Losses from the body exceed intake	- Adult with disease (as in cancer) - Fasting person

Figure 2-4

Nutrient balance using protein as an example. This balance concept can be applied to all nutrients.

In setting the RDA for children, scientists include enough protein to meet daily losses and maintain stores, plus some extra to accommodate growth and storage in new tissue that is built each day. The RDA for children then must attempt to promote a **positive protein balance.** Equilibrium is not good enough because children need to gain new protein tissue. Children, then, should regularly consume a greater amount of protein than they lose. The same is true for pregnant women and people recovering from weight loss due to disease.

Whether we need to be in equilibrium or positive balance, none of us knows exactly how much protein we need each day. From examining the adult RDA for protein we know that if we each consume 0.8 grams of protein per kilogram of body weight per day (56 grams for a 70 kilogram person), probably all of us will meet our needs. However, the RDA does not indicate that if you eat only 0.6 grams per kilogram instead, you will necessarily not get enough protein. Because allowances are generous, many of us get enough protein when we eat less than the RDA. This is an example of why the RDA does not actually apply to individuals.

positive balance
A state where a nutrient intake exceeds losses. This causes a net gain of the nutrient in the body, such as when tissue protein is gained during growth. The opposite of this would be negative balance, where losses exceed intake, as in cases of starvation.

If you calculate the amount of protein you eat in a week, divide by 7, compare it with the RDA, and find that your intake is close to the RDA, fine. You are most likely consuming enough protein. However, if you take in less protein than the RDA suggests, you do not know whether you are eating enough protein. You could need less than the RDA. *Overall, the further you stray from the RDA, the greater your risk of a nutritional deficiency.* Based on statistical theory, when you are eating less than half of the RDA, it is likely that you are not eating enough of that nutrient.[2]

Signs and symptoms of nutritional deficiencies may be subtle and develop slowly. Decreased effectiveness of the immune system, reduced enzyme functions, or an impaired ability to carry oxygen in the bloodstream may not become apparent for a long period of time. You may become ill more often and not know the cause. Though your diet may be inadequate, you still may show no tell tale signs. No "smoke detector" will sound the alarm. Thus it is best to eat a diet that meets your RDA for all the recommended nutrients. These recommendations form the basis for the dietary advice in this book.

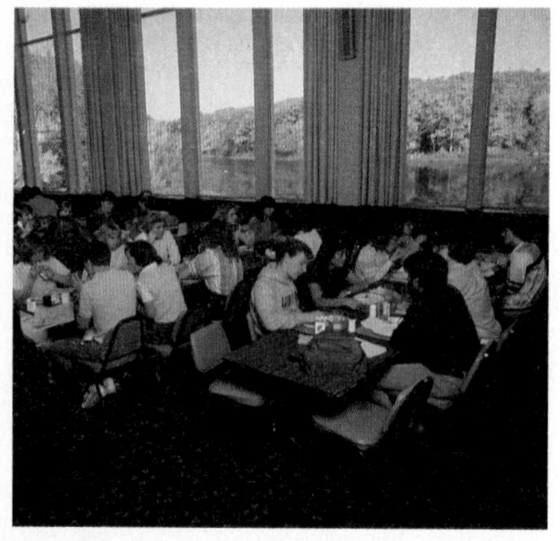

The RDA applies to groups—not individuals.

Correctly applying the RDA to groups

The RDA is not designed for individuals. It is designed for groups and should be used primarily to plan and evaluate what groups eat. Recall one original purpose of the RDA when established in the 1940s: to plan and evaluate soldiers' diets. That is still the basic function of the RDA, except its scope now includes all healthy groups of Americans, such as college students eating on campus.

Estimated Safe and Adequate Daily Dietary Intakes

As noted above, the Food and Nutrition Board revises the RDA every 4 to 6 years in response to new scientific information. In 1980, **estimated safe and adequate daily dietary intakes (ESADDI)** were listed for several nutrients that previously had no RDA, including copper, biotin, and chromium (see the inside cover). The Food and Nutrition Board felt that there were insufficient data on these nutrients to set an RDA, but enough data existed to suggest a range for a reasonable intake for groups. In 1989, the 10th edition of the RDA included minimum requirements for sodium, potassium, and chloride rather than ESADDIs that were in the 9th edition. *Even including the estimated safe and adequate daily dietary intakes and minimum requirements with the RDA, some nutrients—like carbohydrates and fats—still are not covered. Meeting all nutrient needs stated by the Food and Nutrition Board through diet, not with supplements, should account for those other nutrients.*

Estimated Safe and Adequate Daily Dietary Intake (ESADDI)
Nutrient intake recommendations first made in 1980 by the Food and Nutrition Board, where a range for intake of some nutrients was given because not enough information was available to set an RDA.

RDA for energy needs

The Food and Nutrition Board sets the RDA for energy at the average energy needs for various age groups and also provides a wide range for the allowance (see the inside cover for recommendations). The Board warns that the energy RDA is only a rough estimate. Energy intake should depend more on energy use. For most adults, weight maintenance is the best yardstick.

The tenth edition of the RDA

The tenth edition of the RDA, published in 1989, was due by 1985. During its development, a controversy arose concerning the suggestions for vitamins A and C.[6,8,16,17,18] These were lower than the 1980 values, and reviewers at the National Academy of Sciences, the overseeing organization of the Food and Nutrition Board, believed the lower values were unwise. The reviewers thought the evidence was insufficient to justify lowering the RDA for these nutrients, especially when some health agencies were emphasizing them to reduce cancer risk. The controversy grew to include other aspects of the way the tenth edition of the RDA was determined. Finally, the National Academy of Sciences stopped the publication and formed a new Food and Nutrition Board.

In 1987, some recommendations of the first Food and Nutrition Board for the tenth edition of the RDA were published in the *American Journal of Clinical Nutrition* (see Appendix F). These included the nutrients iron, folate, and vitamins A, C, B-12, and K. Many of the recommendations appear in the final tenth edition of the RDA published in 1989. However, vitamins A and C were left at 1980 levels.

World nutrient guides

Canada has its own version of RDA, called **Recommended Nutrient Intakes (RNI)**, set by the Department of National Health and Welfare (Appendix G). Great Britain also has its own guideline as do other countries. The World Health Organization, together with the Food and Agriculture Organization (FAO/WHO) of the United Nations publishes a counterpart to the RDA to apply worldwide. All

Recommended Nutrient Intakes (RNI)
The Canadian version of the RDA.

Table 2-1

Comparison of United States (1989), United Kingdom (1980), Canadian (1990), and WHO (1974) dietary standards for the adult male and adult female

Classification	Kcal	Protein (grams)	Calcium (mg)	Iron (mg)	Vitamin A (RE)	Thiamin (mg)	Riboflavin (mg)	Vitamin C (mg)
United States								
Female (63 kg, 1.63 m)	2200	50	800	15	800	1.1	1.3	60
Male (79 kg, 1.76 m)	2900	63	800	10	1000	1.5	1.7	60
United Kingdom								
Female	2150-2500	54-62	500	12	750	0.9-1.0	1.3	30
Male	2500-3350	63-84	500	10	750	1.0-1.3	1.6	30
Canada								
Female (59 kg)	2000	44	700	13	800	0.8	1.0	30
Male (74 kg)	2700	61	800	9	1000	1.1	1.4	40
FAO/WHO								
Female	2300	39	400-500	18	750	0.9	1.3	30
Male	3200	46	400-500	10	750	1.2	1.8	30

Shils ME and Young UR: Modern Nutrition in Health and Disease, ed 7, Philadelphia, 1988, Lea & Febiger.

these nutrient recommendations are set by separate groups of scientists. The groups do not always agree, so the recommended nutrient levels may differ from country to country, although they are usually close. If they are not close, a good explanation for the difference often exists. For example, different countries consume different amounts of protein. This can lead to varying vitamin and mineral needs (see Table 2-1).

Concept Check

Recommended Dietary Allowances represent the nutrient needs of groups, not of individuals. RDA are established for specific age and gender categories. No one knows his own personal nutritional requirements. The best general rule is that the further you stray from your RDA for your age and gender, the greater the chance of experiencing a nutritional deficiency.

U.S. RDA

U.S. Recommended Daily Allowances (U.S. RDA)
Standards established by the FDA for use on nutrition labels. Generally the four existing versions use the highest nutrient recommendation in the appropriate age and gender category from the 1968 publication of the RDA. The version that includes children over 4 years of age and adults is most commonly seen on nutrition labels.

One practical application of the RDA is the **U.S. Recommended Daily Allowances (U.S. RDA).** The U.S. RDA, set in 1974 by the Food and Drug Administration (FDA), is used on **nutrition labels** on foods (Figure 2-5). It replaced the minimum daily requirements (MDR). The U.S. RDA for adults basically represents a compilation from the 1968 publication of the RDA and primarily uses the highest RDA values within specific age categories. For example, consider iron: the RDA for adult men was 10 milligrams per day; for adult women it was 18 milligrams per day. The U.S. RDA for adults used the higher value of 18 milligrams per day. Table 2-2 lists U.S. RDA values. Note that certain nutrients do not quite follow the rule. The highest adult RDA in 1968 was 1200 milligrams for calcium, but the U.S. RDA is 1000 milligrams. The FDA believed that 1000 milligrams was high enough. The reason for not updating the U.S. RDA when each new RDA is published is mostly economic.

See Nutrition Perspective 2-1 to learn more about regulations that apply to nutrition labeling of foods.

Four versions of the U.S. RDA exist: (1) for children over 4 years and adults, (2) for infants less than 1 year, (3) for toddlers 1 to 4 years, and (4) for pregnant and lactating (breast-feeding) women. Most nutrition labels that list the U.S. RDA use the "adult" version. Infant formulas will use the infant U.S. RDA, "junior" baby foods use the "toddler" U.S. RDA, and vitamin supplements designed for pregnant women use the U.S. RDA designed for pregnancy and lactation.

Figure 2-5 shows a typical nutrition label and how the U.S. RDA for children over 4 years of age and adults are depicted as percentages. The label states that one serving of this food contains 20% of the U.S. RDA for iron. Since the U.S. RDA for iron is 18 milligrams and 0.2 × 18 is 3.6 milligrams, this product contains

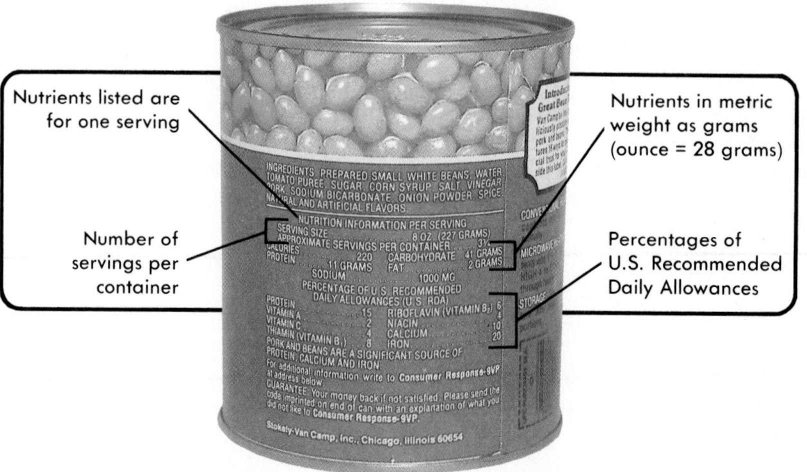

Figure 2-5
A nutrition label. This label is a source of detailed nutrient information.

Table 2-2

U.S. Recommended Daily Allowances (U.S. RDA)

Vitamins and minerals	Unit of measurement	Adults and children 4 or more years of age*	Infants	Children under 4 years of age	Pregnant or lactating women
Protein	Grams	65†	25†	28	‡
Vitamin A	International Units	5000	1500	2500	8000
Vitamin D	"	400	400	400	400
Vitamin E	"	30	5.0	10	30
Vitamin C	Milligrams	60	35	40	60
Folic Acid	"	0.4	0.1	0.2	0.8
Thiamin	"	1.5	0.5	0.7	1.7
Riboflavin	"	1.7	0.6	0.8	2.0
Niacin	"	20	8.0	9.0	20
Vitamin B-6	"	2.0	0.4	0.7	2.5
Vitamin B-12	Micrograms	6.0	2.0	3.0	8.0
Biotin	Milligrams	0.3	0.05	0.15	0.3
Pantothenic Acid	"	10	3.0	5.0	10
Calcium	Grams	1.0	0.6	0.8	1.3
Phosphorus	"	1.0	0.5	0.8	1.3
Iodine	Micrograms	150	45	70	150
Iron	Milligrams	18	15	10	18
Magnesium	"	400	70	200	450
Copper	"	2.0	0.6	1.0	2.0
Zinc	"	15	5.0	8.0	15

*These U.S. RDA values are on most nutrition labels.
†If protein efficiency ratio of protein is equal to or better than that of casein. U.S. RDA is 45 g for adults, 20 g for children under 4 yrs, and 18 g for infants (see Chapter 6).
‡Not specified because this U.S. RDA is used only in vitamin and mineral supplements for pregnant or lactating females.

about 3.6 milligrams of iron per serving. For the vitamin niacin, the label states a content of 4% of the U.S. RDA. With a U.S. RDA of 20 milligrams, the niacin content is 0.04 × 20, or 0.8 milligrams.

Nutrient density

The RDA is used to evaluate the diets of groups, but what is used to evaluate the nutritional quality of an individual food? **Nutrient density** is a concept that has gained acceptance in the last few years. To calculate nutrient density, simply compare the vitamin or mineral content of the food with the number of kcalories it provides. For any nutrient, the higher the nutrient density in the food, the better the food source is for that nutrient.

A way of quantifying nutrient density for a food is to determine its **Index of Nutritional Quality (INQ).**[21] The INQ is calculated by dividing the amount of nutrient in 100 grams of the food by the U.S. RDA for that nutrient. That becomes the numerator for the INQ. The denominator is the number of kcalories in that 100 grams of food divided by an RDA for energy. Then, divide the numerator by the denominator to calculate the INQ.

$$\text{INQ} = \frac{\text{amount of nutrient in 100 grams of the food} \,/\, \text{U.S. RDA for that nutrient}}{\text{kcalories in 100 grams of the food} \,/\, \text{U.S. RDA for energy (2700 kcalories is often used)}}$$

nutrient density
The ratio formed by dividing a food's contribution to nutrient needs by its contribution to kcalorie needs. When the contribution to nutrient needs exceeds that of kcalorie needs, the food is considered to have a favorable nutrient density.

Index of Nutritional Quality (INQ)
The numerical value for nutrient density.

Table 2-3

Index of Nutrient Quality of Selected Foods*

Food	Protein	Calcium	Iron	Vitamin A	Thiamin	Riboflavin	Vitamin C
Milk							
whole	3.0	5.2	0.1	2.3	1.3	4.3	0.9
nonfat	6.2	9.2	0	4.6	1.6	6.2	1.5
Bread							
white	1.8	1.3	1.6	0	3.1	1.8	0
whole wheat	2.2	0.6	1.8	0	2.2	1.1	0
Vanilla ice cream	1.1	1.7	0.1	1.3	0.4	2	0.1
Hamburger (10% fat; cooked)	5.5	0.1	1.2	0	0.3	1.2	0
Orange juice	0	0.7	0	1.2	3.5	1.2	141
Green beans	3	5	5	5	3	4	14
Honey	0	0.1	0.3	0	0	0.2	0.1

*Calculations based on 2700 kcalories for an adult male. See text for details on how the quality ratings are determined.

An INQ of 1 indicates that the food contributes as much toward meeting the day's need for a specific nutrient as it does for meeting the day's need for kcalories. If the INQ is greater than 1, then the food is considered an adequate source for that nutrient. When the INQ reaches 2 or above, the food is considered a good source of the nutrient. An INQ of 6 indicates the food is an excellent source for that nutrient. An INQ of less than 1 indicates that the food is not a very good source for that nutrient.

No food has INQ values greater than 1 for all nutrients. *There is just no perfect food.* Every food has a weakness in one or more INQ values. For example, whole milk has a very low INQ value for iron (0.1).

The INQ can be used to find the best foods for supplying any particular nutrient at the least kcalorie cost (Table 2-3). However, it is difficult to apply when designing an overall diet. To juggle numerous INQ values for the 20 to 30 foods you eat each day is just not practical.

Concept Check

The U.S. RDA, designed in 1974 by the FDA, is used as a benchmark for representing the nutrient content of foods on nutrition labels. Nutrient content is expressed as a percentage of the U.S. RDA. The values used to set the U.S. RDA are taken primarily from the 1968 publication of the RDA. The concept of nutrient density uses the U.S. RDA to evaluate the nutrient contributions made by each food in a diet in comparison with its contribution to total kcalorie needs.

DIET PLANNING TOOLS

Food plans

In the 1940s nutritionists began translating the RDA into more practical terms so that people with no special training could estimate whether their nutritional needs were being met. A seven-food-group plan was designed first, and daily food choices had to include some from each group. This later was simplified to five food groups. By the mid-1950s a four-food-group plan was established that included a milk group, a meat group, a fruit and vegetable group, and a breads and cereals group. In 1979 the names of the groups were revised, and a fifth group containing fats, sweets, and alcoholic beverages was added as part of the "Hassle-Free Daily Food Guide." Caution was urged in consuming this last group, though some foods in it can supply needed vitamin E. This is the Daily Food Guide we use today (Figure 2-6). It is designed to provide a minimum foundation for a complete diet and represents about 1200 to 1400 kcalories. Canada has a similar food guide (Figure 2-7).

Using the Daily Food Guide

The number of servings and portion sizes to eat from each food group in the Daily Food Guide depends on a person's age. Table 2-4 lists serving sizes and amounts for various ages. The traditional adult plan basically consists of two servings from the milk and cheese group; two servings from the meat, poultry, fish, and beans group (2 to 3 ounces each, with emphasis on poultry and fish); four servings from fruits and vegetables (emphasis on citrus fruits and dark green vegetables); and four servings from breads and cereals (emphasis on whole grains). Again, use caution when choosing from the fats, sweets, and alcoholic beverages group. Table 2-4 lists the major nutrients each food group supplies. Note the similarities and differences for various nutrients between the groups.

Table 2-4

The daily food guide: a summary

Nutritional group	Serving	Major nutrients	Foods and nutritional service sizes*
Milk and cheese group	2 (adult‖) 2-3 (child) 3-4 (teens, young adults, and pregnant or lactating women)	Calcium Riboflavin Protein Potassium Zinc	1 cup milk 1-⅓ oz cheese 1 cup yogurt 2 cups cottage cheese 1 cup custard/pudding 1-½ cups ice cream
Meat, poultry, fish, and beans group	2 (adult) 3 (pregnant or lactating women)	Protein Niacin Iron Vitamin B-6 Zinc Thiamin Vitamin B-12†	2-3 oz cooked meat, poultry, fish 1-1½ cup cooked dry beans 4 T peanut butter 2 eggs ½ - 1 cup nuts
Fruits and vegetables	4	Vitamin A Vitamin C Folate Fiber	½ cup cooked fruit or vegetable ½ cup juice 1 whole fruit 1 small salad
Bread and cereal	4	Thiamin Riboflavin§ Iron Niacin Magnesium‡ Fiber‡ Zinc‡	1 slice bread 1 oz ready-to-eat cereal ½ - ¾ cup cooked cereal, rice, or pasta
Fats, sweets, and alcohol		Foods from this group should not replace any from the four groups. Amounts consumed should be determined by individual energy needs.	

*May be reduced for child servings
†Only in animal food choices
‡Whole grains
§If enriched
‖≥ 25 years of age

Figure 2-6
The Hassle-free Daily Food Guide.

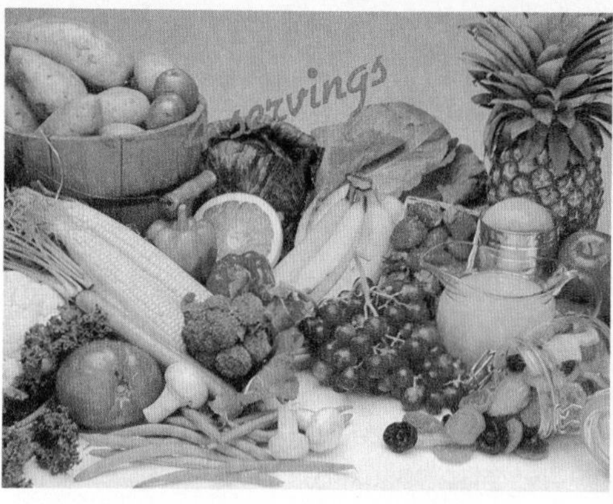

VEGETABLE AND FRUIT GROUP

1 serving is:

½ cup	an orange
a small salad	½ cantaloupe
a medium-sized potato	½ grapefruit

Have citrus fruit, melon, berries, or tomatoes daily and a dark-green or dark-yellow vegetable frequently. For a good source of fiber, eat unpeeled fruits and vegetables and fruits with edible seeds—such as berries or grapes.

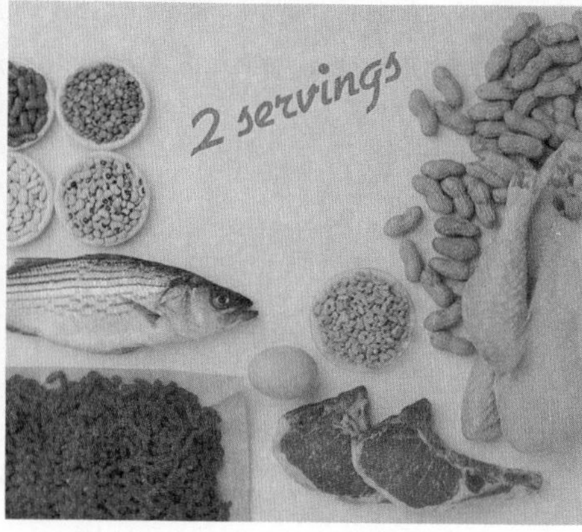

MEAT, POULTRY, FISH, AND BEANS GROUP

½ serving is:
1 to 1½ ounces lean, boneless, cooked meat, poultry, or fish
1 egg
½ to ¾ cup cooked dry beans, peas, lentils, or soybeans
2 tablespoons peanut butter
¼ to ½ cup nuts, sesame or sunflower seeds

Poultry and fish have less fat content than red meats.

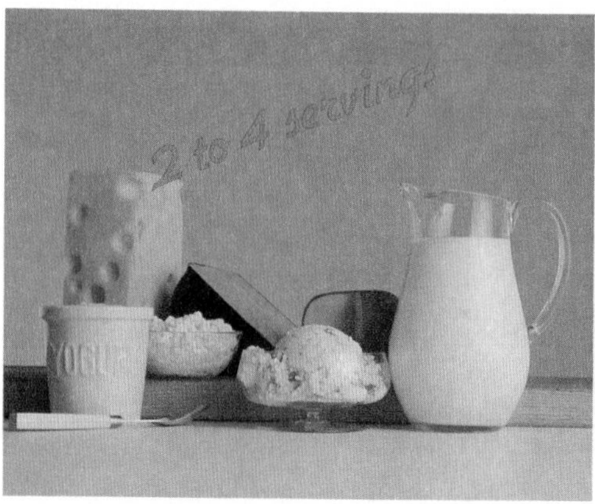

MILK AND CHEESE GROUP

Servings:	
Adults	2
Children under 9 years old	2-3
Children 9 to 12 years old and pregnant women	3
Teens and nursing mothers	4

1 serving is:
1 cup milk or yogurt
1 1/3 ounces cheddar or swiss cheese
2 ounces processed cheese food
1½ cups ice cream or ice milk
2 cups cottage cheese

Skim, nonfat, and low-fat milk and milk products provide calcium and keep fat intake down.

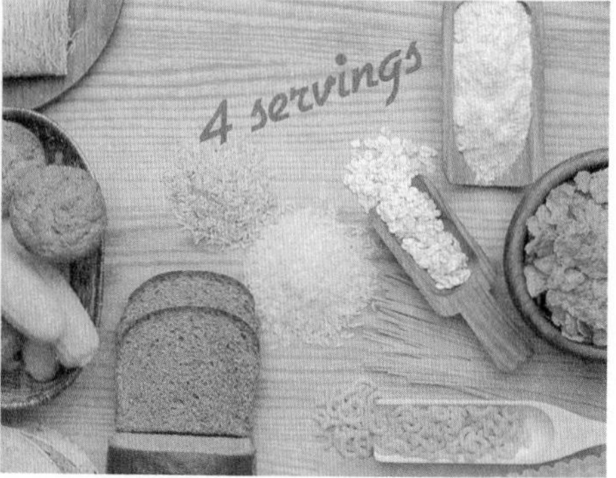

BREAD AND CEREAL GROUP

1 serving is:
1 slice bread
½ to ¾ cup cooked cereal or pasta
1 ounce ready-to-eat cereal

Choose whole-grain products often.

CAUTION

FATS, SWEETS, AND ALCOHOL GROUP

These foods provide kcalories but few nutrients.

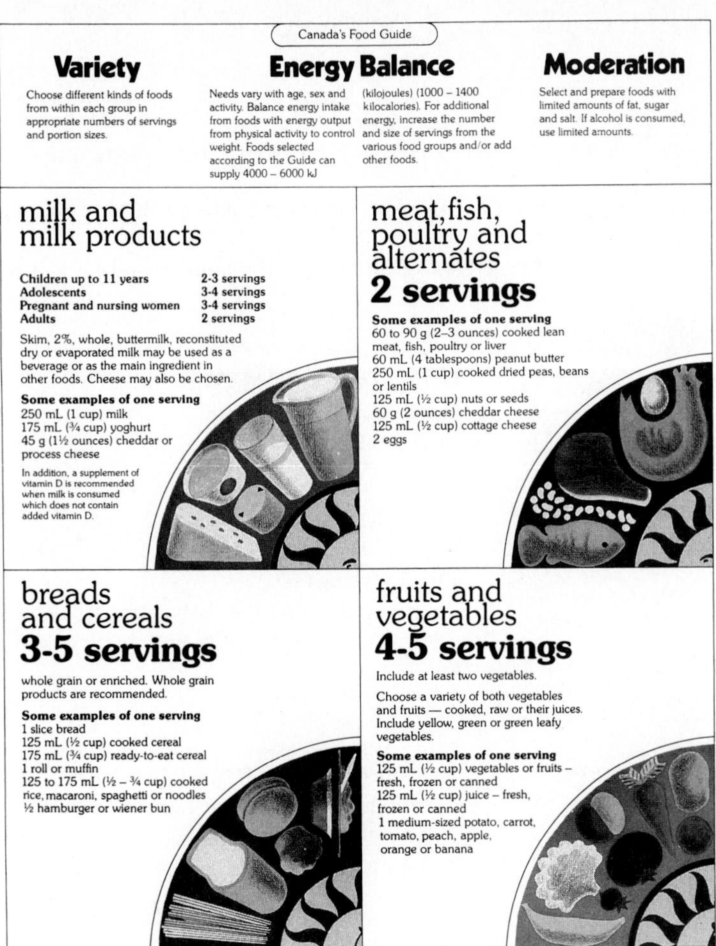

Figure 2-7
The Canadian food guide.

Another pattern of servings was recently published by the U.S. Department of Agriculture (USDA). Following the Daily Food Guide framework, this represents a total diet plan rather than just a foundation for a diet plan (Figure 2-8), and so includes more servings to account for the greater energy needs that many people will have.

Here are several important points to keep in mind when you use the Daily Food Guide:

1. The guide does not deal with infant feeding.
2. No one food is absolutely essential to good nutrition. Each food is low in at least one essential nutrient.
3. No one food group alone provides all essential nutrients in adequate amounts. Each food group makes an important, distinct contribution to nutritional intake.
4. Variety is the key to the Daily Food Guide. Variety is first guaranteed by using all the groups. Furthermore, one should consume a variety of foods within each group.

The foundations of balanced nutrition are variety and moderation.[14] The Daily Food Guide and variations of it specifically speak to both of these parameters. Choosing from every group and varying choices within groups allows a healthy variety of foods. The nutritional adequacy of the Daily Food Guide is compromised unless variety of choices is practiced.

Following the Daily Food Guide makes it easy to create daily diets that contain as little as 1200 to 1400 kcalories. The diets usually meet the adult RDA for

A Pattern for Daily Food Choices

When shopping, planning, and preparing meals for yourself and others, use this guide for a varied and nutritious diet . . .

- Choose foods daily from each of the first five major groups shown below.
- Include different foods from within the groups. As a guide, you can use the subgroups listed below the major food group heading.
- Have at least the smaller number of servings suggested from each group. Limit total amount of food eaten to maintain desirable body weight.
- Most people should choose foods that are low in fat and sugars more often. (See the bulletins on fat and sugar in this series.)
- Go easy on fats, sweets, and alcoholic beverages.

FOOD GROUP	SUGGESTED DAILY SERVINGS*
Breads, cereals, and other grain products ▪ Whole-grain ▪ Enriched	6 to 11 (Include several servings a day of whole-grain products.)
Fruits ▪ Citrus, melon, berries ▪ Other fruits	2 to 4
Vegetables ▪ Dark-green leafy ▪ Deep-yellow ▪ Dry beans and peas (legumes) ▪ Starchy ▪ Other vegetables	3 to 5 servings (Include all types regularly; use dark-green leafy vegetables and dry beans and peas several times a week.)
Meat, poultry, fish, and alternatives (eggs, dry beans and peas, nuts and seeds)	2 to 3 servings—total 5 to 7 ounces lean. Include dry beans and peas several times a week
Milk, cheese and yogurt	2 servings (3 servings for teens and women who are pregnant or breastfeeding; 4 servings for teens who are pregnant or breastfeeding)
Fats, sweets, and alcoholic beverages	Avoid too many fats and sweets. If you drink alcoholic beverages, do so in moderation.

WHAT COUNTS AS A SERVING?

- **Breads, cereals, and other grain products:** 1 slice of bread; 1/2 hamburger bun or english muffin; a small roll, biscuit, or muffin; 3 to 4 small or 2 large crackers, 1/2 cup cooked cereal, rice, or pasta; or 1 ounce of ready-to-eat breakfast cereal.
- **Fruits:** A piece of whole fruit such as an apple, banana, orange; a grapefruit half; a melon wedge; 3/4 cup of juice; 1/2 cup berries, or 1/2 cup cooked or canned fruit; or 1/4 cup dried fruit.
- **Vegetables:** 1/2 cup of cooked or chopped raw vegetables or 1 cup of leafy raw vegetables, such as lettuce or spinach.
- **Meat, poultry, fish, and alternates:** Serving sizes will differ. Amounts should total 5 to 7 ounces of lean meat, fish, or poultry a day. A serving of meat the size and thickness of the palm of a woman's hand is about 3 to 5 ounces and a man's, 5 to 7 ounces. Count 1 egg, 1/2 cup cooked dry beans, or 2 tablespoons of peanut butter as 1 ounce of lean meat.
- **Milk, cheese, and yogurt:** 1 cup of milk, 8 ounces of yogurt, 1-1/2 ounces natural cheese, or 2 ounces of process cheese.

***WHAT ABOUT THE NUMBER OF SERVINGS?**

The amount of food you need depends on your age, sex, physical condition, and how active you are. Almost everyone should have at least the minimum number of servings from each food group daily. Many women, older children, and most teenagers and men need more. The top of the range is about right for an active man or teenage boy. Young children may not need as much food. They can have smaller servings from all groups except milk, which should total 2 servings per day.

Note: The pattern for daily food choices described here was developed for Americans who regularly eat foods from all the major food groups listed. Some people, such as vegetarians and others, may not eat one or more of these types of foods. These people may wish to contact a nutritionist in their community for help in planning food choices.

Source: USDA Home and Garden Bulletin Number 232-1, 1986.

Figure 2-8

A pattern for daily food choices. This pattern helps you follow the Dietary Guidelines. This is a complete diet plan, whereas the Daily Food Guide is a foundation diet.

protein, thiamin, niacin, riboflavin, calcium, and other important nutrients. Unfortunately, the diets may be low in vitamin E, vitamin B-6, magnesium, iron, and zinc. Most people also need to eat more foods than those in the Daily Food Guide, both to meet energy needs and to turn the food choices into meals. The extra foods needed can be selected to supply any nutrients lacking from those in the Guide. Following the expanded pattern in Figure 2-8 is a good place to start.

However, if an adult does not need many more kcalories—as could be the case for small, inactive, and elderly people—he or she may just want to follow the Daily Food Guide. Thus that person may not meet the RDA for the nutrients needed within the amount of kcalories consumed. In this case, he or she should tailor the Daily Food Guide as needed, since choices within a food group are not nutrient equivalent.

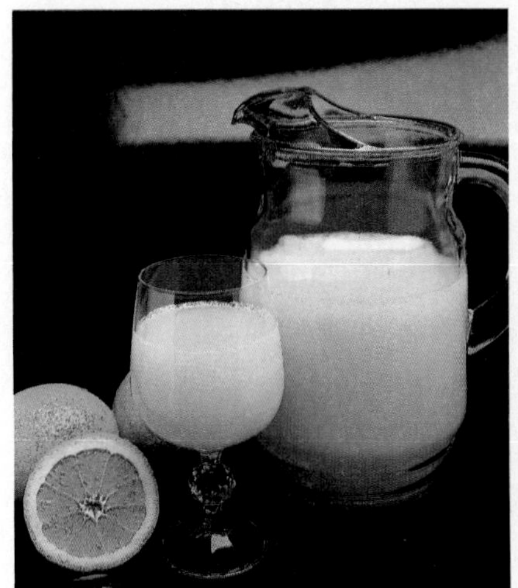

Orange juice is an excellent source of the vitamins C and folate.

We recommend some changes, based on an article published in 1978.[13] These recommendations essentially follow those of the "Hassle-Free Food Guide":

1. Use low-fat and nonfat choices for the milk and cheese group.
2. Add one or two servings from vegetable proteins to the two from animal sources.
3. For fruits and vegetables include a vitamin C source and a dark green vegetable each day.
4. For breads and cereals all servings should be made with whole grains.
5. Finally, include one serving of fat, preferably vegetable oil.

Table 2-5 lists the totals for important nutrients in two diets side-by-side. One diet follows the Daily Food Guide, and the other diet conforms to the above suggestions. As predicted, a typical day's Daily Food Guide menu can be low in vitamin E, vitamin B-6, magnesium, and zinc. Following our suggestions, the revised plan adds significant amounts of vitamin E, vitamin B-6, and magnesium, as well as more zinc. At the same time, the protein level adds up to twice a woman's RDA. This extra protein is not necessary. However, this is approximately the amount of

Table 2-5

Comparison of one day nutrient intakes from the daily food guide plans— traditional and improved.

	Daily Food Guide*	Improved Daily Food Guide†
kcalories	1400	1600
Protein	162%‡	240%
Vitamin B-6	72%	138%
Vitamin E	42%	123%
Iron§	100%	95%
Magnesium	73%	157%
Zinc	90%	110%

*The diet follows the Hassle-Free Daily Food Guide: 1 cup whole milk, 1 ounce cheddar cheese, 2 ounces bologna, 3 ounces ground beef, 1/2 cup carrots, 1 cup orange juice, 1 apple, 3/4 cup mashed potatoes, 2 slices enriched bread, 1/2 cup egg noodles, 3/4 cup ready-to-eat cereal.

†With an emphasis on lowfat dairy products, inclusion of vegetable proteins, some dark green leafy vegetables, whole grains, and vegetable oil. The actual diet was: 2 cups 1% fat milk, 2 ounces turkey, 3 ounces roast beef, 1/2 cup pork and beans, 3 tablespoons peanut butter, 1/2 cup carrots, 1/2 cup broccoli, 1 orange, 1 apple, 1/2 cup brown rice, 2 slices whole wheat bread, 1/2 cup oatmeal, and 1 teaspoon margarine.

‡Percentage of RDA for 25-year-old women.

§The drop in iron on the improved food guide was due to the substitution of oatmeal for an iron-fortified breakfast cereal.

protein most men and women in North America already eat. The protein adds a little more expense, but aside from that, it causes no harm. The addition of the vegetable proteins is needed to supply extra vitamin B-6, magnesium, iron, zinc, and other nutrients. Thus the vegetable proteins are useful additions to the food plan.

Our diet suggestions yield a total of only 1600 kcalories. This level of kcalories does not meet the needs of an active adult, but it will probably meet the needs of a sedentary adult or an elderly person. If 1600 kcalories are too many kcalories for you, first try to become more active. *It is very difficult to obtain enough nutrients from a food plan that supplies less than about 1600 kcalories total.* You probably don't need to meet the RDA for all nutrients, but you may never know for which ones those are. If you can't increase your energy output, you may need to include some nutrient-fortified foods, like ready-to-eat breakfast cereals. In addition, if your diet does not include meat or other animal products, see Nutrition Perspective 6-1 on vegetarianism in Chapter 6.

Dietary guidelines

The Daily Food Guide was designed to help meet nutritional needs for protein, vitamins, and minerals. However, most of the major chronic "killer" diseases in North America, such as heart disease, cancer, and cirrhosis of the liver, are not associated with deficiencies in protein, vitamins, or minerals. Deficiency diseases such as rickets (vitamin D deficiency) and pellagra (niacin deficiency) are no longer common. It appears the real problems in the North American diet for many of us are excess kcalories, saturated fat, cholesterol, alcohol, and sodium (salt).[15,19] You can also include insufficient calcium, iron, zinc, and dietary fiber for some people in that list.

Dietary Goals
Specific goals for nutrient intakes set in 1977 by a Committee of the U.S. Senate.

In response to concerns regarding disease patterns in the United States, a Senate Select Committee developed **dietary goals** for the United States. The first dietary goals were published and then quickly revised in 1977 (Table 2-6).

In response to criticisms that the Dietary Goals lacked sufficient scientific data to support such strict recommendations, the USDA and Department of Health and Human Services (DHHS) published more general *Dietary Guidelines* in 1980, and a slight revision in 1985. They are as follows:

Chapter 5 defines saturated fat and polyunsaturated fat and discusses these concepts in detail.

1. Eat a variety of foods.
2. Maintain desirable body weight.
3. Avoid too much fat, saturated fat, and cholesterol.
4. Eat foods with adequate starch and fiber.
5. Avoid too much sugar.
6. Avoid too much sodium.
7. If you drink alcoholic beverages, do so in moderation.

This plan, published in a pamphlet called *Nutrition and Your Health—Dietary Guidelines for Americans,* tries to ensure adequate vitamin and mineral intake with the first guideline: eat a variety of foods. Then the guidelines try to create changes that will reduce risk for obesity, hypertension, heart disease, diabetes, and alcoholism. We will discuss diet recommendations of other scientific groups in Chapter 17.

The dietary goals for Canadians proposed in 1977 include:[3]

1. The consumption of a nutritionally adequate diet as outlined in Canada's food guide;
2. A reduction in kcalories from fat to 35% of total calories, while including a source of polyunsaturated fatty acids (linoleic acid) in the diet;
3. The consumption of a diet that emphasizes whole grain products, fruits, and vegetables, and minimizes alcohol, salt, and refined sugars.

Table 2-6

U.S. dietary goals 2nd edition, 1977
1. To avoid overweight, consume only as much energy (calories) as is expended; if overweight, decrease energy intake and increase energy expenditure. 2. Increase the consumption of complex carbohydrates and "naturally occurring" sugars from about 28% of energy intake to about 48% of energy intake. 3. Reduce the consumption of refined and processed sugars by about 45% to account for about 10% of total energy intake. 4. Reduce overall fat consumption from approximately 40% to about 30% of energy intake. 5. Reduce saturated fat consumption to account for about 10% of total energy intake; and balance that with polyunsaturated and monounsaturated fats, which should account for about 10% of energy intake each. 6. Reduce cholesterol consumption to about 300 mg a day. 7. Limit the intake of sodium by reducing the intake of salt to about 5 g a day.
The Goals Suggest the Following Changes in Food Selection and Preparation: 1. Increase consumption of fruits and vegetables and whole grains. 2. Decrease consumption of refined and other processed sugars and foods high in such sugars. 3. Decrease consumption of foods high in total fat, and partially replace saturated fats, whether obtained from animal or vegetable sources, with polyunsaturated fats. 4. Decrease consumption of animal fat, and choose meats, poultry and fish which will reduce saturated fat intake. 5. Except for young children, substitute low-fat and non-fat milk for whole milk, and low-fat dairy products for high fat dairy products. 6. Decrease consumption of butterfat, eggs and other high cholesterol sources. Some consideration should be given to easing the cholesterol goal for pre-menopausal women, young children and the elderly in order to obtain the nutritional benefits of eggs in the diet. 7. Decrease consumption of salt and foods high in salt content.

US Senate Select Committee on Nutrition and Human Needs: Dietary Goals for the United States, ed 2, 1977.

Combining the major food plans

Ideally, we should combine concepts from the Daily Food Guide and the various dietary guidelines. Good eating habits can yield life-long dividends.

Some nutritionists are uneasy about the "Nutrition and Your Health" Plan. They think it is too general because it does not acknowledge that individual people may need to follow different dietary objectives. As we show in later chapters, some people are bothered by cholesterol in foods, while others are not; some are bothered by sodium in foods, while others are not; and controversy rages over the detriments of sugar. For now, keep in mind these two plans, the Daily Food Guide and the Dietary Guidelines. If what you are currently eating is far from what these plans recommend, try to make some appropriate changes.

In your study of the next few chapters, you may find it exciting to design a more personal set of plans for yourself. This is the power of studying nutrition: You no longer must follow general recommendations. You can learn more about your body and find ways to stay healthy, even from plans that vary from those we have just reviewed.

Concept Check

Dietary guidelines have been set by a variety of private and government organizations. These guidelines are designed to minimize the risk of developing obesity, hypertension, heart disease, and alcoholism. To do so, they first encourage us to eat a variety of foods, ideally, by following the Daily Food Guide. Then they encourage us to limit consumption of kcalories to match energy output and to limit saturated fat, salt, sugar, and alcohol intake while focusing more on starches and dietary fiber.

THE EXCHANGE SYSTEM

exchange system
A grouping of foods in six lists. When the serving size for any food in a list is consumed, all foods within the list yield a similar amount of carbohydrate, fat, protein, and energy.

The **Exchange System** is a valuable tool for quickly estimating the energy, protein, carbohydrate, and fat content of a food or meal. Using it also creates greater understanding about what one eats. Rather than memorizing the tables of composition of all foods, your work is greatly simplified by using the exchange system because it generalizes those details into a manageable framework.

The exchange system arranges food into six different categories: milk, fruit, vegetables, starch/bread, meat, and fat. These categories are designed so that after noting the proper serving size, each food within a category provides about the same amount of carbohydrate, protein, fat, and kcalories. This equality allows the exchange of foods within a category. Hence the term *exchange system.*

The exchange system arranges foods based on nutrient composition, not origin.

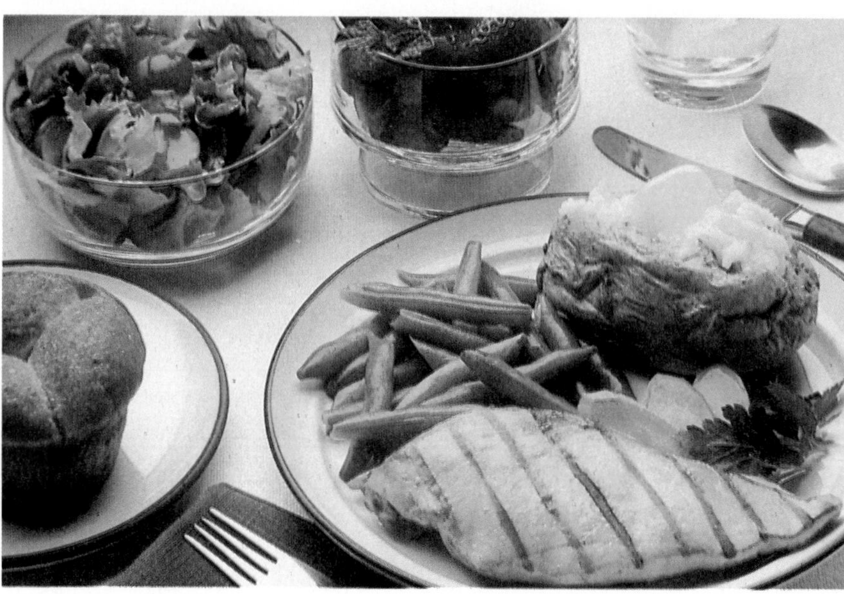

The exchange system was revised in 1976 and again in 1986. Each time it has changed slightly. When using the exchange system listed in any book, it is important to note which version you are consulting.

The exchange system was developed in the 1950s for planning diabetic diets. Diabetes is easier to control if the person's diet has about the same composition day after day. If a certain number of "exchanges" from each of the six categories is eaten each day, that regularity is easier to achieve. However, the utility of this system goes beyond that, since it yields a quick way for anyone to estimate energy and carbohydrate, protein, and fat content in a food or meal. Learning it is a bit tedious. As in learning a foreign language, you will need some practice before you feel comfortable with the exchange system.

Using the exchange system

Using the exchange system requires knowing which foods are in each group and knowing the serving sizes for each food. We have listed the entire U.S. exchange system in Appendix H. You will need to consult this Appendix many times before you can apply the system.

Table 2-7

The exchange lists composition (1986 edition)

Exchange list	Household measures*	Carbohydrate (grams)	Protein (grams)	Fat (grams)	Kcalories
Starch/Bread	1 slice, ¾ cup raw, or ½ cup cooked	15	3	trace†	80
Meat	1 ounce				
Lean		—	7	3	55
Medium-Fat		—	7	5	75
High-Fat		—	7	8	100
Vegetable	½ cup cooked	5	2	—	25
Fruit	1 small piece	15	—	—	60
Milk	1 cup				
Skim		12	8	trace	90
Low-fat		12	8	5	120
Whole		12	8	8	150
Fat	1 teaspoon	—	—	5	45

The American Diabetes Association and American Dietetic Association, Exchange Lists for Meal Planning, 1986.
*Just an estimate. See exchange lists for actual amounts.
†Calculated as 1 gram for purposes of energy contribution

Table 2-7 shows the carbohydrate, protein, fat, and energy composition of each of the six exchange groups. The starch/bread group has 15 grams of carbohydrate, 3 grams of protein, and a trace of fat per **exchange.** The trace of fat is calculated as 1 gram of fat when the total energy contribution of an exchange is determined. The meat group is divided into three subclasses: lean, medium fat, and high fat. Each exchange has 7 grams of protein. Lean meats contain 3 grams of fat per exchange, medium fat meats have 5 grams of fat per exchange, and high fat meats have 8 grams of fat per exchange. Meats have essentially no carbohydrate. The vegetable group contains 5 grams of carbohydrate, 2 grams of protein, and no fat per exchange. The fruit group has 15 grams of carbohydrate per exchange. Fruit has no appreciable fat or protein.

exchange
The serving size of a food within a specific exchange group.

The milk group is divided into three subclasses: nonfat, low-fat, and whole. Each exchange has 12 grams of carbohydrate and 8 grams of protein. Nonfat milk has a trace of fat (calculated as 1 gram when energy content is expressed) per exchange. Low-fat milk has 5 grams of fat per exchange, and whole milk has 8 grams of fat per exchange. Finally, the fat group contains 5 grams of fat per exchange. Fats contain no appreciable amount of carbohydrate or protein.

An exchange from the starch/bread group contains 80 kcalories. Lean meats have 55 kcalories per exchange, medium fat meats have 75 kcalories per exchange, and high fat meats have 100 kcalories per exchange. Vegetables have 25 kcalories per exchange. Fruits have 60 kcalories per exchange. Skim milk has 90 kcalories per exchange; low-fat milk has 120 kcalories per exchange; and whole milk has 150 kcalories per exchange. Finally, fat has 45 kcalories per exchange.

To fully use the exchange system requires memorizing Table 2-7. Doing so will take time, but if you plan to use this system regularly, there is no alternative.

Taking a closer look at the exchange groups

Before you can turn a group of exchanges into a meal plan for one day, you first have to see what each exchange group contains (see Appendix H). The starch/

bread group contains dry cereal, cooked cereal, rice, pasta, baked beans, corn on the cob, potatoes, bread, and tortillas. This list is not the same as that used for the Daily Food Guide groups. *The exchange system is not concerned about the origin of the food, animal or vegetable. It is primarily concerned with the nutrient composition in terms of carbohydrate, protein, and fat of each food in a group.* For example, the carbohydrate composition of potatoes resembles that of bread more than of broccoli, although bread is not a vegetable.

The lean meat list contains round steak, lean ham, veal, chicken (without skin), fish, cottage cheese, and 95% fat-free luncheon meat. The medium-fat meat list contains T-bone steak, pork roast, lamb chops, well-drained duck and goose, salmon, mozzarella cheese, and eggs. The high-fat meat list contains prime cuts of beef (marbled), ribs, sausage, fried fish, cheddar cheese, salami, and peanut butter.

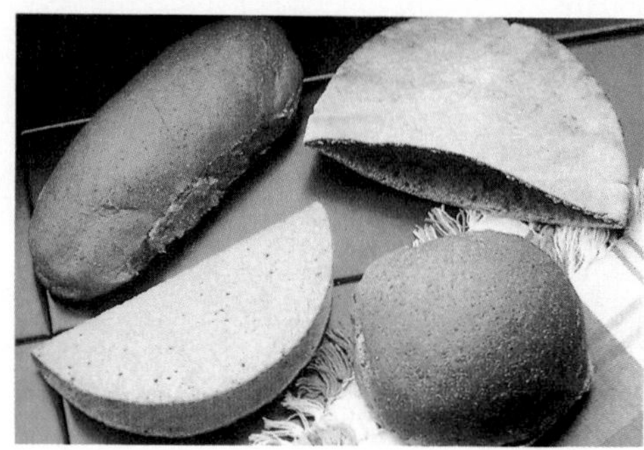

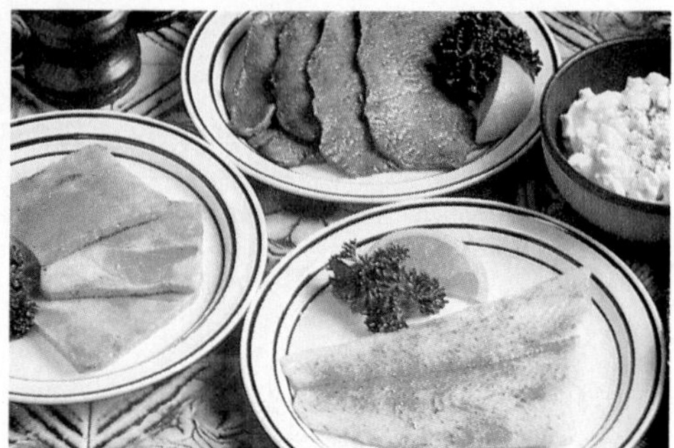

The starch/bread exchange group (left).

The meat exchange group (right).

The vegetable list contains most vegetables. Some starchy vegetables were listed above in the starch/bread group. Some vegetables, such as cabbage, celery, mushrooms, lettuce, and zucchini, are "free foods": their minimal energy contribution does not count in the calculations. The fruit list contains fruits and fruit juices.

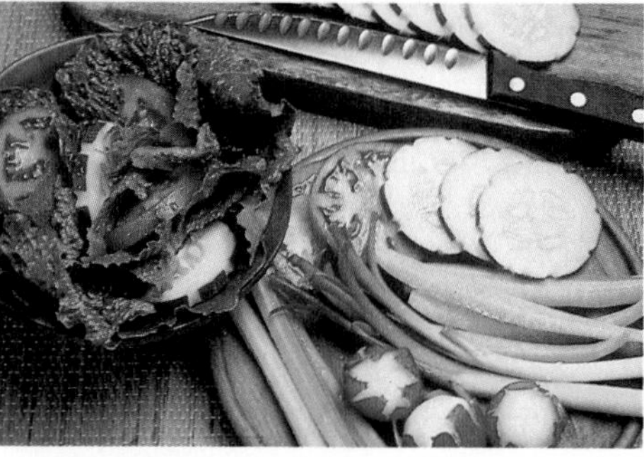

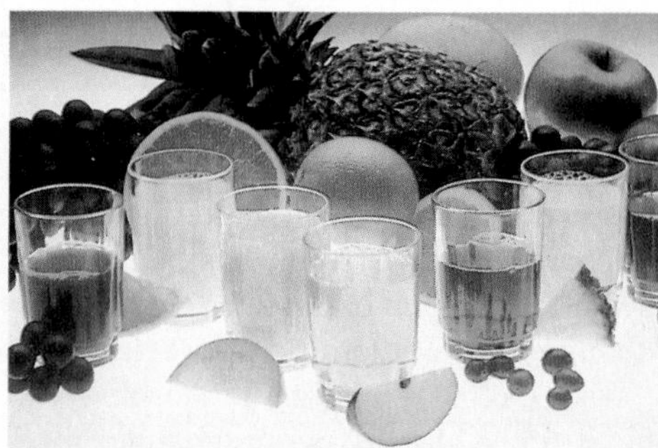

The vegetable exchange group (left).

The fruit exchange group (right).

The milk exchange list contains milk, plain yogurt, and buttermilk. The amount of fat in a product determines whether the serving is nonfat, low-fat, or whole.

The fat list contains margarine, mayonnaise, nuts and seeds, salad oils, olives, sour cream, and cream cheese. Bacon is considered a fat, rather than a high-fat meat.

Free foods, other than the vegetables already mentioned, include bouillon, diet soda, coffee, tea, dill pickles, and vinegar, as well as herbs and spices.

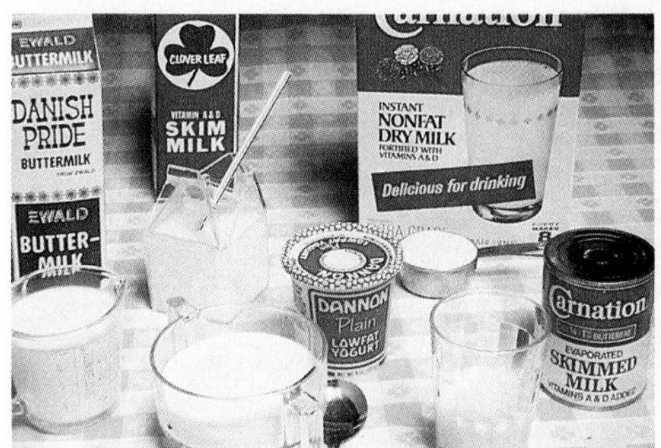

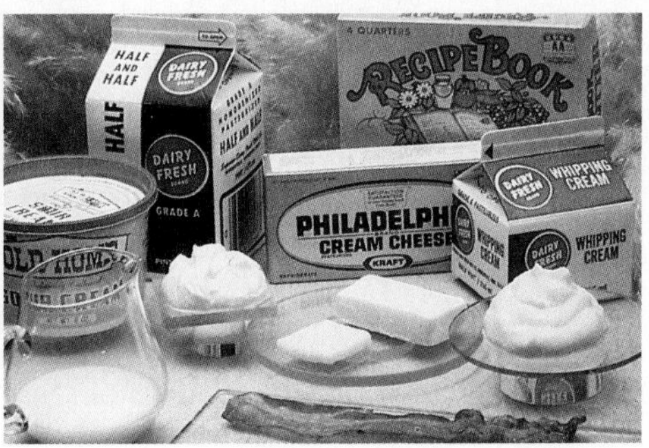

The milk exchange group (left).

The fat exchange group (right).

Let's now turn an exchange food plan into 1 day's menu. We want 2000 kcalories, consisting of 55% energy from carbohydrates, 15% energy from protein, and 30% energy from fat. This can be translated into 2 low-fat milk exchanges, 3 vegetable exchanges, 5 fruit exchanges, 11 bread exchanges, 3 medium-fat meat exchanges, and 8 fat exchanges (Table 2-8). Note this is only one of many possible combinations; the exchange system offers great flexibility.

Table 2-9 arbitrarily separates these exchanges into breakfast, lunch, dinner, and a snack. Breakfast includes 1 low-fat milk exchange, 2 fruit exchanges, 3 starch/bread exchanges, and 2 fat exchanges. This total corresponds to ¾ cup cold cereal eaten with 1 cup of 2% milk, 2 slices of bread with 2 teaspoons margarine, and 1 cup of orange juice.

Table 2-8

Turning a diet prescription into a plan of servings from each Exchange Group

Prescription: 2000 kcalories, 55% carbohydrate, 30% fat, and 15% protein
55% carbohydrate 0.55 × 2000 = 1100;
1100 kcalories ÷ 4 kcalories/gram = 275 grams carbohydrate
30% fat 0.30 × 2000 = 600 kcalories;
600 kcalories ÷ 9 kcalories/gram = 67 grams fat
15% protein 0.15 × 2000 = 300;
300 kcalories ÷ 4 kcalories/gram = 75 grams protein

Prescription	Carbohydrate	Protein	Fat
	275	75	67
2 low-fat milk exchanges	24	16	10
SUBTOTAL	251	59	57
3 vegetable exchanges	15	6	—
SUBTOTAL	236	53	57
5 fruit exchanges	75	—	—
SUBTOTAL	161	53	57
11 starch/bread exchanges	165	33	—
SUBTOTAL	—	20	57
3 medium-fat meat exchanges	—	21	15
SUBTOTAL	—	—	42
8 fat exchanges	—	—	40
SUBTOTAL	—	—	—

Table 2-8—cont.

To convert a diet prescription in grams into the number of exchanges from each group, list across the top of a page the total grams of carbohydrate, protein, and fat. In this case you have 275 grams of carbohydrate, 75 grams of protein, and 67 grams of fat. Then decide how many exchanges from the milk group you want. We have chosen two low-fat exchanges. This choice yields 24 grams of carbohydrate, 16 grams of protein, and 10 grams of fat. Subtract those values from the total amounts with which you started; what remains is 251 grams of carbohydrate, 59 grams of protein, and 57 grams of fat.

Now choose the number of exchanges of vegetables you want. We have chosen 3, which give 15 grams of carbohydrate and 6 grams of protein. Subtract those figures from our subtotals; this leaves 236 grams of carbohydrate, 53 grams of protein, and 57 grams of fat.

Now choose the exchanges of fruit. We have chosen 5, which provide 75 grams of carbohydrate. Again, subtract those 75 grams of carbohydrate from the subtotals. The plan now has 161 grams of carbohydrate, 53 grams of protein, and 57 grams of fat remaining for distribution.

The only exchange group left with any carbohydrate in it is the starch/bread group. Each serving contains 15 grams of carbohydrate. Now divide by 15 the number of grams of carbohydrate left—in this case, 161 grams divided by 15. This division yields 11 exchanges (rounded off) from the starch/bread group. Those 11 exchanges of starch/bread also provide 33 grams of protein. After subtracting the carbohydrate and protein contributions from the subtotals, 20 grams of protein and 57 grams of fat remain.

Now determine the number of meat exchanges. This is the only group left that contains protein. Divide the grams of protein by 7, which is the grams of protein from each exchange from the meat group. This division yields 3 exchanges of meat. We chose medium-fat meat, which also gives 15 grams of fat. Subtract those values from the subtotals. The plan now has only 42 grams of fat left unassigned. Since each exchange contains 5 grams of fat, divide 42 by 5. This yields 8 servings (rounded off) of fat exchanges.

We started with a prescription of 2000 kcalories: 55% from carbohydrate, 15% from protein, and 30% from fat. We have turned that into various exchanges from the exchange groups; namely, 2 low-fat milk exchanges, 3 vegetable exchanges, 5 fruit exchanges, 11 bread exchanges, 3 medium-fat meat exchanges, and 8 fat exchanges. We could have designed this plan with other relative numbers of exchanges. We could have chosen to exclude meat, to double the number of fruit exchanges, or to use lean meat, thereby increasing the number of fat exchanges available. This is the beauty of the exchange system. You start with a nebulous diet prescription of percentages and kcalories and end up with a pattern of servings from food groups that is tailored to an individual's likes and dislikes, while also adhering—if necessary—to the type of diet pattern the person needs to follow.

Lunch consists of 3 fat exchanges, 4 starch/bread exchanges, 1 vegetable exchange, and 2 fruit exchanges. This translates into 2 slices of bacon with 1 teaspoon mayonnaise, two slices of bread, and tomato. In other words, a bacon and tomato sandwich. Add to this a 9-inch banana (1 exchange = ½ banana), and 16 animal cookies.

Dinner consists of 3 medium-fat meat exchanges, 1 low-fat milk exchange, 1 fruit exchange, 2 vegetable exchanges, 1 fat exchange, and 2 starch/bread exchanges. This total corresponds to a 3-ounce broiled T-bone steak, 1 large baked potato (1 exchange = 1 small baked potato) with 1 teaspoon of margarine, 1 cup broccoli, 1 cup of 2% milk, and 1 kiwi fruit.

Finally, we have a snack containing two starch/bread exchanges and two fat exchanges. This translates into 1 bagel with 2 tablespoons of cream cheese.

We have listed only one of many possibilities for a day's food plan. Orange juice could be exchanged for apple juice. The banana could be an apple. The T-bone steak could be 3 ounces of chicken breast with the skin. The choices are endless. Notice that an exchange diet is much easier to plan if you use individual foods, as we have; however, the exchange system tables list some combination foods to help you (see Appendix H). Using combination foods, such as pizza or lasagna, however, makes it more difficult to calculate the number of exchanges in a serving. For instance, lasagna has meat exchanges, vegetable exchanges, and starch/bread exchanges. With experience, you will be able to tackle such complex foods. For now, using individual foods makes learning the exchange system much easier. Finally, you might want to prove to yourself that our food choices

Table 2-9

Turning an exchange system plan into a menu for one day

Breakfast	
1 low-fat milk exchange	1 cup 2% milk (put some on cereal)
2 fruit exchange	1 cup orange juice
3 bread exchanges	¾ cup cold cereal, 2 pieces whole-wheat toast
2 fat exchanges	2 teaspoons margarine on toast
Lunch	
4 bread exchanges	2 slices whole-wheat bread, 16 animal cookies
3 fat exchanges	2 slices bacon 1 teaspoon mayonnaise
1 vegetable exchange	1 sliced tomato
2 fruit exchanges	1 banana (9 inches)
Dinner	
3 medium-fat meat exchanges	3 ounces broiled T-bone steak
2 bread exchanges	1 large baked potato
1 fat exchange	1 teaspoon margarine
2 vegetable exchange	1 cup broccoli
1 fruit exchange	1 kiwi fruit
1 low-fat milk exchange	1 cup 2% milk
Snack	
2 bread exchanges	1 bagel
2 fat exchanges	2 tablespoon cream cheese

Values calculated using a computer and nutrient analysis software		Prescription
kcalories	2037	2000
Carbohydrate	55%	55%
Protein	16%	15%
Fat	29%	30%

Table 2-10

Exchange patterns to get you started

kcalories/day	1200	1600	2000	2400	2800	3200	3600
Exchange Group							
Milk (lowfat)	2	2	2	2	2	2	2
Vegetables	2	2	2	3	3	3	3
Fruit	5	4	6	8	8	10	10
Bread	4	8	10	11	15	17	20
Meat (medium fat)	2	2	4	5	5	7	8
Fat	4	7	7	9	12	12	14

These are just one set of options. More meat could be included if less milk is used, for example. The breakdown is: 55% kcalories as carbohydrate, 30% kcalories as fat, 15% kcalories as protein.

really meet the exchange plan. This demonstration will give you practice turning exchanges into actual food servings.

To recap, Table 2-9 lists the original prescription for carbohydrate, protein, fat, and energy intake. The actual percentages of carbohydrate, protein, fat, and kcalories in the diet have also been calculated using a nutrient software package and a computer. Note that the exchange system values closely match the computer analysis shown in Table 2-9. The exchange system is a very useful tool for diet planning. If used correctly, there is no easier way to plan a precise menu pattern. Table 2-10 gives you a head start in planning diets.

Concept Check

The Exchange System enables us to design and follow a precise diet that balances ratios of carbohydrate, fat, and protein, while watching total energy intake. Within each of the six exchange lists, when serving sizes are considered, all foods yield similar contributions of carbohydrate, fat, protein, and kcalories. Their similar nutrient profiles allow the foods in each group to be "exchanged" for each other.

The need for tools in the study of nutrition

When you have a personal or professional goal that requires skills, the tools you need to master those skills are especially valuable. Tools are mastered only when they are frequently used. As you will discover, the tools reviewed in this chapter are the stock and trade of the student of nutrition.

Summary

1. Individual atoms form molecules, which can combine to form cells. Cells form tissue, which can build into organ systems. The combined systems can then be organized into an entire human body.
2. Atoms attach to each other primarily by sharing electrons, forming covalent bonds. Molecules frequently join together by forming a water molecule together and then separating from it. Each molecule contributes part of the water molecule. This is called a condensation reaction. Large molecules are frequently broken down by adding a water molecule to a covalent bond, with each part of the molecule accepting part of the water molecule. This is called a hydrolysis reaction.
3. The metric system is used throughout science. Lengths are expressed in meters, weights are expressed in grams, and volumes are expressed in liters. A

meter equals about 39 inches, a kilogram is about 2.2 pounds, and a liter is about 1 quart.

4. Recommended Dietary Allowances are set for many nutrients. These levels represent the amount of each nutrient that people on the whole should consume regularly to meet their needs for that nutrient. Different RDA guidelines have been set for different genders and ages.
5. The four versions of the U.S. RDA are based primarily on the highest RDA levels found in the 1968 publication. The U.S. RDA is used as a basis for expressing the nutrient levels in foods on a nutrition label.
6. The "Hassle-free Food Guide" is designed to convert nutrient recommendations from the RDA into a food plan. The guide focuses on using low-fat (or nonfat milk) products, some vegetable proteins in addition to animal protein foods, citrus fruits, and dark green vegetables, and emphasizes whole grain breads and cereals.
7. Dietary guidelines have been issued to help reduce the amount of chronic "killer" diseases. The guidelines emphasize eating a variety of foods, maintaining desirable body weight, and watching consumption of fats, cholesterol, sugar, salt, and alcohol while focusing on starches and fiber.
8. The exchange system provides a powerful tool for estimating the carbohydrate, fat, protein, and kcalorie content of a food or meal and for planning a diet to correspond to specific goals for carbohydrate, fat, protein, and kcalorie consumption.

Take Action

PRODUCT: ______________________________

INGREDIENTS:

1. ____________	11. ____________
2. ____________	12. ____________
3. ____________	13. ____________
4. ____________	14. ____________
5. ____________	15. ____________
6. ____________	16. ____________
7. ____________	17. ____________
8. ____________	18. ____________
9. ____________	19. ____________
10. ____________	20. ____________

1. Become a label reader! This is one of the best ways to learn what foods contain. Start with a package of one of your favorite foods. Make a list of all the ingredients. On a separate sheet of paper, write a brief description of them using the glossary in the book and Appendix R. What nutrients is this product a good source of?

CHAPTER 2

Answers to nutrition awareness inventory

1. *True.* These are the substances provided by foods that are necessary for life.
2. *True.* Still, atoms bonded together retain their chemical identity when in the form of a molecule.
3. *True.* Joules are a measure of work energy, while calories are a measure of heat energy. Both are used as measures of food energy.
4. *False.* A cup of water equals about 250 milliliters, or ¼ liter.
5. *False.* One pound equals about 454 grams.
6. *False.* RDA is the abbreviation for recommended dietary allowances.
7. *False.* No nutrient is absolutely required daily. You can survive for about 4 days on a diet free of water and about 10 days on a diet free of the vitamin thiamin.
8. *True.* While nutrient recommendations are often similar, groups of scientists from different countries may disagree with each other. In addition, the type of diet consumed influences nutrient needs.
9. *False.* The RDA is a recommendation only for group needs. It does not provide personal nutrient requirements.
10. *False.* Active people are likely to require closer to 2200 to 2800 kcalories or more to meet energy needs.
11. *True.* Potatoes and bread have very similar carbohydrate : protein : fat ratios.
12. *True.* The exchange system relieves us of having to memorize the composition of all foods: rather, it is a powerful tool for quickly and conveniently estimating the energy, protein, carbohydrate, and fat of a food or meal.
13. *True.* Nutrient density is an important concept, especially for people on a low-kcalorie diet. It refers to the ratio of a food's nutrients to its kcalorie content.
14. *True.* The term *Kilocalories,* or *kcalories,* is used to measure food energy. Nutritionists often use the term *calories* when speaking, but the written word should use the term *kcalories.*
15. *True.* No one food contains all the nutrients needed to maintain good health. Milk, for example is low in iron, while eggs are low in calcium.

REFERENCES

1. American Dietetic Association: Nutrition information on food labels, Journal of the American Dietetic Association 89:266, 1989.
2. Beaton, GH: Toward harmonization of dietary, biochemical, and clinical assessments: the meanings of nutritional status and requirements, Nutrition Reviews 44:349, 1986.
3. Beare-Rogers, JL: Dietary goals and recommendations in Canada, Journal of the Canadian Dietetic Association 45:325, 1984.
4. Cooper, RM: Health claims of foods—reflections on the food/drug distinction and on the law of misbranding, American Journal of Clinical Nutrition 44:560, 1986.
5. Food and Nutrition Board, National Academy of Sciences—National Research Council: Recommended dietary allowances, revised 1989, Washington D.C.
6. Guthrie, HA: The 1985 recommended dietary allowance committee: an overview, Journal of The American Dietetic Association 85:1646, 1985.
7. Harper, AE: Scientific substantiation of health claims: how much is enough, Nutrition Today March/April 17, 1989.
8. Hegsted, DM: Dietary standards—guidelines for prevention of deficiency or prescription for total health, Journal of Nutrition 116:478, 1986.
9. Herbert, V: Recommended dietary intakes (RDI) of folate in humans, The American Journal of Clinical Nutrition 45:661, 1987.
10. Herbert, V: Health claims in food labeling and advertising, Nutrition Today 25, May/June 1987.
11. Jeejeebhoy, KN: Nutritional balance studies: indicators of human requirements or adaptive mechanisms, Journal of Nutrition 116:2061, 1986.
12. Kamin, H: Additional thoughts on the RDA, Nutrition Forum, 4:69, 1987.
13. King, JC and others: Evaluation and modification of the basic four food guide, Journal of Nutrition Education 10:27, 1978.
14. Krebs-Smith, SM and others: The effects of variety in food choices on dietary quality, Journal of The American Dietetic Association 87:897, 1987.
15. Miller, SA and Stephenson, MG: The 1990 national nutrition objectives: lessons for the future, Journal of The American Dietetic Association 87:1665, 1987.
16. Olson, JA: Should RDA values be tailored to meet the needs of their users? Journal of Nutrition 117:220, 1987.
17. Olson, JA: Recommended nutrient intakes: guidelines for the prevention of deficiency or prescription for total health, Journal of Nutrition 116:1581, 1986.
18. Press, F: Postponement of the 10th edition of the RDAs, Journal of the American Dietetic Association. 85:1644, 1985.
19. Surgeon General's report on Nutrition and Health, Nutrition Today 22, September/October 1988.
20. USDA: Eat a variety of foods, Home and Garden Bulletin Number 232-1, April 1986.
21. Wittwer, AJ and others: Nutrient density—evaluation of nutritional attributes of foods, Journal of Nutrition Education 9:26, 1977.

SUGGESTED READINGS

The articles by The American Dietetic Association, Harper, and Herbert provide an excellent background for understanding the issues surrounding health claims on food labels. The article by Guthrie will help you understand how the Food and Nutrition Board thinks about the RDA and how, as scientists, they must work together to form a consensus using the information available at one time. Finally, the articles by Olson will add further insights to setting the RDA. Reading these articles, along with the RDA book itself, will help you develop a deep understanding of this concept and the ramifications inherent in setting a specific RDA.

Expert Opinion

Deceptive Health Claims in Food Labeling and Advertising

VICTOR HERBERT, M.D., J.D.

"Giving Americans more facts on diet and health" appears to be a specious catch phrase for "Misleading Americans into making unwise food choices based on misinformation." It borders on health fraud to give a message that a product delivers more health efficacy and safety than there is general scientific agreement that it does. "Telling the truth" on labels is specious, deceptive, and misleading when it is not the *whole* truth. Too frequently, it is deception by omission of adverse facts, which nearly always includes omission of the fact that too much of anything can be harmful. The consumer is deprived of informed choice when adverse facts are withheld. When industry works with nutrition politicians who suppress disagreement with their "killer fat," "miracle fiber," and "miracle vitamin" claims—claims based largely on inference instead of evidence—the deception is deepened that good nutrition comes from certain products, rather than as a function of the total diet.

An example is the promotion of wheat bran as a "preventative health tip" to "reduce your risk of some kinds of cancer." The adverse facts omitted are as follows: (1) that there are no data showing the Americans who eat wheat bran cereals have less cancer than Americans who do not; (2) that there are many kinds of fiber; (3) that rat research shows *more* colon cancer with intakes of too much wheat bran; (3) that too much bran can produce deficiencies of iron, zinc, calcium and even intestinal obstruction; and (4) that in 1989 the National Academy of Sciences noted that benefits against cancer may relate to substances coincidentally present in some high-fiber foods and may have nothing to do with the fiber itself.

Deception by omission is the core of "snake-oil" nutrition. To not be deceptive and misleading, claims must relate to the entire diet and must be generic rather than relate to individual products. That is, consumers ought to be advised not to "eat more fiber" or "eat more bran" but to "eat adequate fiber" and "eat not less than 15 grams or more than 35 grams daily of assorted fibers taken from a variety of grains, fruits, and vegetables." Health claims for specific foods or food supplements are by definition distortions and misrepresentations because they are not generic and do not focus on the entire diet, and they are irresponsible because they do not warn of the dangers of excess intakes of the specific foods or supplements.

Honest health claims relate to the total daily diet and not to any one product. To "give Americans more facts on diet and health," industry must tell *all* the relevant facts, both favorable and unfavorable, and should position products generically as part of the total daily diet if they indeed are appropriately a part (supplements are not, according to the 1989 National Academy of Sciences report "Diet and Health." It is confusing, deceptive,and misleading to provide facts not relevant to making informedfood choices, to withhold relevant ones, and to claim special health properties for any one product. Moderate amounts of vitamin C, carotene, and fiber may inhibit cancer. Excessive amounts may promote it.

WHO ARE THE GOOD GUYS?

"There is a basic conflict between the public health scientists or "activists" (the "good guys?") and the academic scientists or "traditionalists" ("the bad guys?") concerning health claims on food labels. The conflict is misrepresented as one in which academic scientists believe that the existence of *any* doubt in the relationship between diet and disease is sufficient to withhold accepting the relationship.

This type of statement falsely represents the position of the academic community as a rigid straw man, and many media writers have been deceived by it. It is the old "health foods" scam argument in a new form. We academic scientists are not "traditionalists"—inquiry and skepticism are our lifeblood. Many of us are activists. We believe in responsibly informing the public regarding total daily diet and health, both qualitatively and quantitatively; speaking in terms of appropriate and adequate total dietary quantities—and always in terms of efficacy and safety; and giving the public both the upside and the downside. We oppose overaggressive product promotion that falsely represents unresolved scientific issues as facts. Some public health epidemiology enthusiasts, who misrepresent themselves as "*the* activists" and "*the* good guys" irresponsibly give the public only the upside, promote specific products rather than the total daily diet, and talk in terms of "eat more of this and less of that," which is bad advice for many people who already are eating more than enough of this and less than they should of that.

Some would argue that it is fair for the public to know what we think the best information is today, just as a doctor would give advice in a clinical situation. I say, "Amen"—but we should give the public the *whole* truth, as a doctor does, instead of just the upside. We must say that the daily dietary fiber intake should be from a *variety* of grain, fruit, and vegetable sources and should be not less than 15 grams or more than 35 grams daily. We must always warn that just as too little fiber is bad for you, so is too much.

I believe the current petitions to the FDA to legalize "truthful health claims on labels," which are "not false or misleading" and are "adequately substantiated," are not in the public interest. The reason for this belief is that every health claim that is not for total dietary intake but rather for a specific food is, by definition, deceptive and misleading. Such

Continued.

Expert Opinion—cont'd

claims cause the consumer to inappropriately choose too much of specific products rather than make appropriate choices from all foods. The deception is primarily by presentation of ***irrelevant positive truths and irresponsible omission of relevant negative facts.*** The claims state literal truths but send false messages. The consumer is deprived of informed choice when relevant information is withheld, whether it is withheld by intent or by ignorance.

Let us look at the ads for a product promoted as a good source of dietary fiber as an illustration of the type of soft-core nutrition deception the FDA is being asked to follow. Note the literally truthful statement "The National Cancer Institute believes eating the right foods *may* reduce your risk of some kinds of cancer." Note the false message: "Product X protects against cancer." If the industry promotes eating wheat bran as a means to reduce the frequency of cancer, there is a duty to warn that it has been shown in rats that too much wheat bran promotes, rather than inhibits, colon cancer. Similarly, according to a recent Australian study, eating too much cereal fiber may increase colon cancer in female humans.

I hope now you can see that the current argument is not between "activitists" and "traditionalists" but between enthusiasts, who give advice using epidemiologic *inference,* and responsible nutrition scientists, who give advice using laboratory and clinical *evidence* and whose watch words are efficacy and safety. We do not demand absolute proof—all we ask is evidence from studies clearly applicable to the American public that the message is valid. When that evidence is not provided with the message in any ads, we are deceived by not being told it is missing.

In the example of brand X cereal, it would have been just as easy to place a responsible message on the label, such as: "The National Cancer Institute suggests Americans should eat not less than 15 and not more than 35 grams daily of a variety of fibers from an assortment of grains, fruits, and vegetables. One portion of this product contains 9 grams of one form of fiber: wheat bran fiber."

THE RIGHT MESSAGE

Three basic words, four basic food groups, and seven dietary guidelines constitute the message of good nutrition, a message that food processors should be spreading to the public. The three basic words are moderation, variety, and balance. The four basic food groups are fruits and vegetables; grains and grain products; meat and alternates (including fish, poultry, eggs, nuts, and legumes); and milk and milk products. Moderation means to not eat too much and too little of each. Variety means the variety of the four food groups and variety *within* each group.

Note also that the HHS-USDA Dietary Guidelines for Americans say "avoid too much," which is good advice for everyone, and not "eat less," which is bad advice for some. Note as well that they say "eat adequate amounts," which is good advice for everyone, not "eat more," which is bad advice for some."

A responsible health message would be: "eat *appropriate* amounts of fiber (15 grams to 35 grams daily)," not "eat *more* fiber." To the many complete and partial vegetarians already eating more than 35 grams of fiber daily, the advice to "eat more fiber" can bring only harm. Because of their heavy intake of fiber and poorly absorbed vegetable minerals, vegetarians have twice the frequency of iron deficiency as nonvegetarians, and more zinc deficiency and vegetarian rickets among their children. Why increase the casualties?

The next time you look at a "food supplement" ad, ask yourself the following: (1) will this product favorably affect *my* health? (2) Is the product effective for me? (3) Is it safe for *me* (4) Why doesn't it contain a disclaimer? Why doesn't it mention adverse effects? (6) Why doesn't it mention what the U.S. government says about supplements? (7) What does the local FDA office say about it? and (8) What has *Consumer Reports* said about it? Always remember: under U.S. law, it is legal to lie about the benefits of a product everywhere but on the label. If the benefit is not on the label (or in a package insert, which is legally part of the label), it probably is not true.

Dr. Herbert is Professor of Medicine and Chairman of the Committee to Strengthen Nutrition, Mount Sinai School of Medicine and Chief, Hematology and Nutrition Research Laboratory, Bronx V.A. Medical Center.

Nutrition Perspective 2-1:

What's on the Label?

In the United States the FDA is responsible for most food labeling, except for meat and poultry products, which are regulated by the USDA, and alcoholic beverages, which are regulated by the Bureau of Alcohol, Tobacco and Firearms. The Federal Trade Commission (FTC) regulates the advertising of food products and has authority to take action against unsubstantiated claims. In doing so, it uses the FDA as the lead agency.

Foods packaged and sold in any United States supermarket usually are labeled with the product name, the name and address of the manufacturer, the amount of product in the package, and the ingredients in descending order of weight. With the exceptions of fresh fruits, vegetables, and meats, almost all other foods are so labeled.

Another exception to this amount of labeling is given to foods with a **standard of identity.** Products with a standard of identity must follow a certain recipe on file with the FDA. In those cases, the manufacturer does not have to list ingredients. These foods include catsup, ice cream, mustard, and mayonnaise. Notice, however, that many manufacturers now list the ingredients on labels for these foods, though they do not have to by law. This trend is due to consumer demand. Most of us want to see what ingredients are in our foods, now more than ever.

Standard of Identity
If a food is produced according to a specific recipe on file with the FDA, the label does not have to list its ingredients. In that case the manufacturer is using its Standard of Identity to avoid disclosing its ingredients.

If a manufacturer adds a nutrient to the food product or makes a nutritional claim about the product, then a "nutrition label" must also be provided. An example of such a label is shown in Figure 2-5. The label lists the serving size of the product, servings per package, and kcalories, protein, carbohydrate, fat, and sodium per serving. If the product contains more than 2% of the U.S. RDA for certain vitamins and minerals, those percentages of the U.S. RDA must be listed. These nutrients include protein, vitamin A, vitamin C, thiamin, riboflavin, niacin, calcium, and iron. Additional information may be provided on dietary fiber, the amount of sugars and cholesterol, and other information the manufacturer believes the consumer wants. The Surgeon General of the United States has encouraged manufacturers to make full use of this opportunity to educate the public.

LABELING PITFALLS

Some pitfalls accompany label reading. The meanings of terms on labels are not always apparent. Here are some legal definitions for terms you are likely to see on food labels. Note that these definitions may change in the future as food labeling laws change.

Diet or dietetic: Usually the product contains no more than 40 kcalories per serving (also called low-calorie), or has at least one-third fewer kcalories than the regular product (also called reduced-calorie).

Imitation: The product does not follow the usual recipe for that type of product. For instance, more water may have been added to margarines to make it lower in kcalories. Note that such products may also be lower in nutrients, such as protein, vitamins, or minerals.

Natural: This term is usually meaningless. It simply states that the product occurs in nature. When applied to meats, it means the meat contains no added artificial flavors, colors, preservatives, or synthetic ingredients.

Sugar-free: The product cannot contain sucrose (table sugar), honey, fruit juice, molasses, or other simple sugars (see Chapter 3).

Light (lite): There are no laws concerning the use of this term with beer or other foods. It may or may not be lower in kcalories than the standard product (read the label).

Low-calorie: The product contains no more than 40 kcalories per serving and no more than 0.4 kcalories per gram.

Sodium-free: The product contains less than 5 milligrams of sodium per serving.

Very-low-sodium: The product contains no more than 35 milligrams of sodium per serving.

Low-sodium: The product contains no more than 140 milligrams of sodium per serving.

Nutrition Perspective 2-1—cont'd

What's on the Label?

Reduced sodium: The product contains 75% less sodium than the product it replaces.
No artificial flavors: The product contains no flavors other than those from naturally occurring products.
No artificial coloring: The product contains only colors from naturally occurring products, such as beet juice, grape skin, or carrot oil.
May contain one or more of the following: The product can contain any of the ingredients listed after this phrase. Usually the ingredient(s) will be the one(s) found to be least expensive at the time of production.
No cholesterol: The product contains no cholesterol.
Cholesterol-free: The product contains less than 2 milligrams of cholesterol per serving.
Low-fat: Milk described as such can contain 0.5% to 2% milk fat. Low-fat meat can contain no more than 10% fat by weight.
New: The product is either brand new or has been substantially changed within the last 6 months.
Organic: This term has no legal meaning as far as the U.S. federal law is concerned.
Wheat: The product contains wheat but not necessarily whole wheat. The label will say whole wheat if the product uses only whole-wheat flour.
Enriched: The vitamins thiamin, riboflavin, and niacin and the mineral iron have been added to the product to replace (and in some cases augment) that lost in processing.
Fortified: Vitamins and/or minerals that were not originally present have been added to the product.

There are other fine points to labeling laws. These definitions represent the most important ones to keep in mind.

HEALTH CLAIMS ON LABELS

A debate exists concerning the extent to which a manufacturer can make health claims on a food product label.[1,4,7,10] It is permissible to state that a food contains certain nutrients: this simply requires a nutrition label to back up the claim. The debate concerns whether a manufacturer can state that these nutrients will provide specific health benefits, such as the claim that dietary fiber in food helps prevent some types of cancer. The current trend is for manufacturers to want to make health claims. The Kellogg Company markets its high-fiber cereals as a possible preventive measure against certain forms of cancer. Whether this should be allowed is far from settled. Government agencies are not sure how far they should let manufacturers go. Many nutritionists think this particular claim lacks scientific merit and that claims in general are a bad idea.[1,10]

The American Dietetic Association feels health claims are permissible as part of a labeling or marketing system, as long as they are presented in the context of a total diet and are generally supported by the scientific community. Those claims supporting the messages in "Dietary Guidelines for Americans" are especially appropriate. The Association supports both positive and negative health claims on food labels to prevent the public from being misled. For example, a high-fiber claim on a food must also state if the food is high in fat. Such an approach would protect the consumer against deception by omission.

The danger with health claims is that not *all* the facts may be presented.[10] For example, with dietary fibers, some adverse facts are omitted: No studies show that Americans who eat wheat bran cereals have less cancer than Americans who do not; many kinds of fiber exist; animal research shows *more* colon cancer occurs with too much wheat bran in the diet; too much bran can lead to poor absorption of iron, zinc, and calcium, as well as intestinal problems such as gas. The warning should be that too little—as well as too much—dietary fiber can be harmful (see Chapter 3 for details).

The bottom line for health claims on food packages comes down to honesty. The whole story needs to be told. How the federal agencies in the United States will ensure that such is the case remains unanswered. For you, the best tactic will continue to be defensive shopping: read the small print and be skeptical.

Chapter 3

Digestion and Absorption

Overview

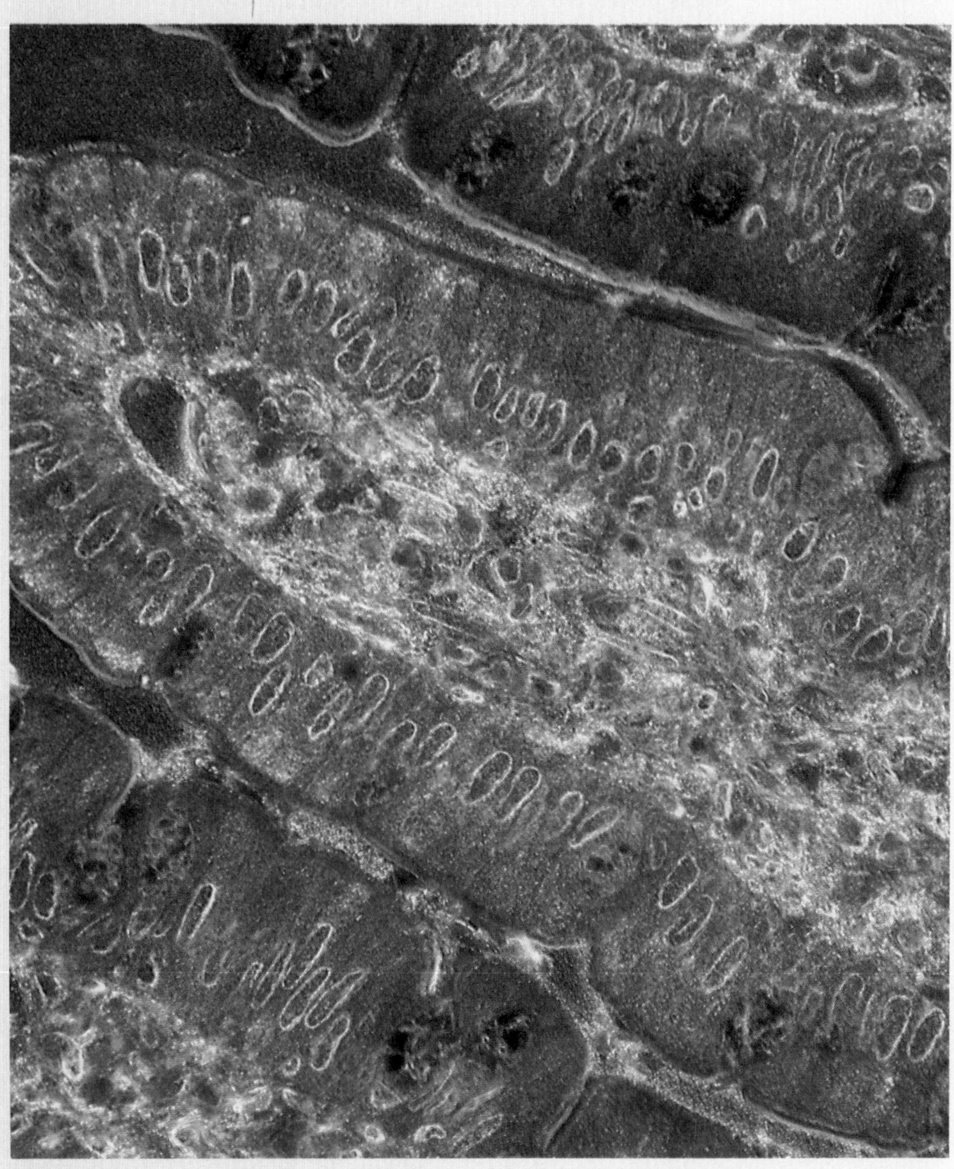

Intestinal villi—gatekeepers of the GI tract.

Merely ingesting the foods we have discussed doesn't nourish you. In many cases you must first break down the nutrients contained in the foods, and in all cases you must absorb them. Only then can nutrients be taken up by the bloodstream and distributed to all of your body's cells. The major parts of the body involved in this process are the gastrointestinal tract, pancreas, liver, and gallbladder.

We take digestion and absorption for granted because most of the processes involved are autonomic; that is, they control themselves. We don't decide when the pancreas will secrete digestive enzymes into the small intestine, what the liver will do with absorbed glucose, or how quickly foodstuffs will be propelled down the intestinal tract. Hormones, hormone-like compounds, and nerves control these functions.[5] We have two choices: how well to chew food and when to eliminate the stool. Those are voluntary responses. Thus while you go about your daily routine—playing the piano, working in a laboratory session, walking home from classes, and eating lunch—many reactions and functions occur in your intestinal tract. Let's examine these processes.

Nutrition awareness inventory

Here are 15 statements about digestion and absorption. Answer them to test your current knowledge. If you think the answer is true or mostly true, circle T. If you think the answer is false or mostly false, circle F. Use the scoring key at the end of this chapter to compute your total score. Take the test again after you have read this chapter. Compare the results.

1. **T F** Digestion primarily begins in the mouth.
2. **T F** Nutrients absorbed directly into the bloodstream from the digestive tract first go to the liver.
3. **T F** The small intestine is longer than 8 feet.
4. **T F** Mucus kills most bacteria that enter the stomach.
5. **T F** The colon is another name for the large intestine.
6. **T F** Fruit and meat should not be eaten together.
7. **T F** Many stomach enzymes work less efficiently in the small intestine.
8. **T F** Hormones and nerves coordinate all digestive processes.
9. **T F** As we age, our ability to digest lactose, a carbohydrate found in milk, often declines.
10. **T F** Stress interferes with the absorption of nutrients.
11. **T F** Total parenteral nutrition bypasses the intestines.
12. **T F** Glucose requires energy to be absorbed, whereas fat does not.
13. **T F** Peristalsis utilizes a coordinated muscle action.
14. **T F** Malabsorption of some foods results in the production of gas in the colon.
15. **T F** The gastrointestinal tract, except the colon, is essentially free of bacteria.

THE PHYSIOLOGY OF DIGESTION

The **gastrointestinal (GI) tract** is a long tube stretching from the mouth to the anus (Figure 3-1). This tube, also known as the **alimentary canal,** is in one sense "outside" the body. *It is partitioned from the body in such a way that nutrients must pass through the walls of the tube for absorption into the bloodstream.* Just eating a food is not enough—the nutrients must also be absorbed. As we will describe, certain diseases may hamper absorption, in turn denying the body some of the consumed nutrients.

The GI tract is a very complex system that performs a variety of physiological functions: movement (motility), secretion, digestion, absorption, elimination, and nutrient production.[5] Nutrient production refers to the synthesis of vitamins by bacteria that live in the intestine. In this chapter we discuss the most important aspects of GI physiology from a nutritional viewpoint. You can find a more detailed discussion in a physiology textbook.

gastrointestinal (GI) tract
The main sites in the body used in digestion and absorption of nutrients. It consists of the mouth, esophagus, stomach, small intestine, large intestine, rectum, and anus.

alimentary canal
Another name for the GI tract.

saliva
A watery fluid produced by the salivary glands in the mouth; it contains lubricants, enzymes, and other substances.

mucus
A thick fluid secreted by glands throughout the body. It contains a compound that has both a carbohydrate and protein nature (glycoprotein). This acts as both a lubricant and a means of protection for cells.

lysozyme
A substance produced by a variety of cells in the body that can destroy bacteria.

The flow of digestion

Let's begin by reviewing the major parts of the body used in digestion (Figure 3-1). In the mouth, glands produce **saliva.** Saliva contains enzymes that break down carbohydrates, as well as **mucus** that lubricates the foods. Chewing also breaks up solid food into smaller, more manageable pieces. This increases the surface area of the food, thus allowing more efficient and greater digestive action by enzymes. In addition, saliva contains **lysozyme,** which kills bacteria.

The tongue contains taste receptors for sweet, salt, sour, and bitter.[15] The sweet and salt receptors are near the tip of the tongue, and the sour and bitter

Figure 3-1

The organization of the gastro-intestinal (GI) tract.

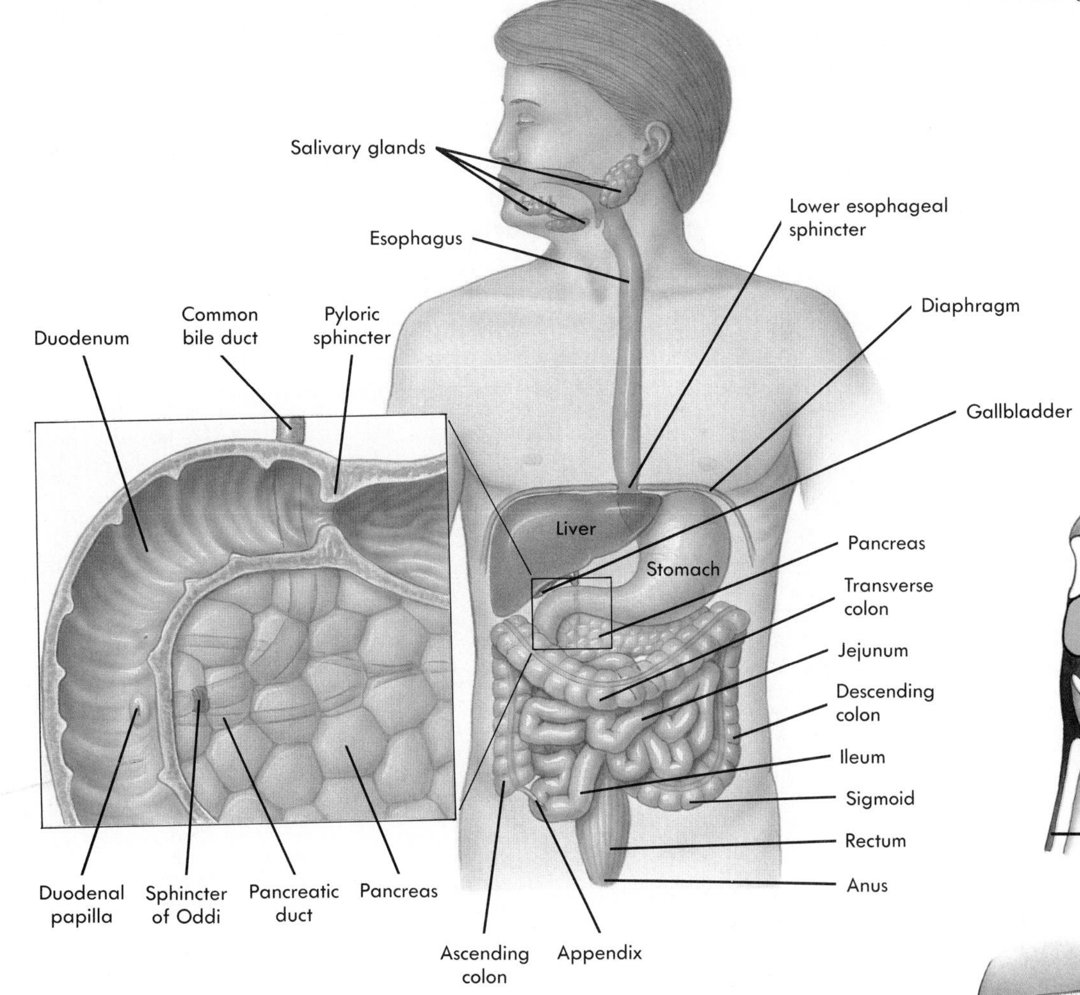

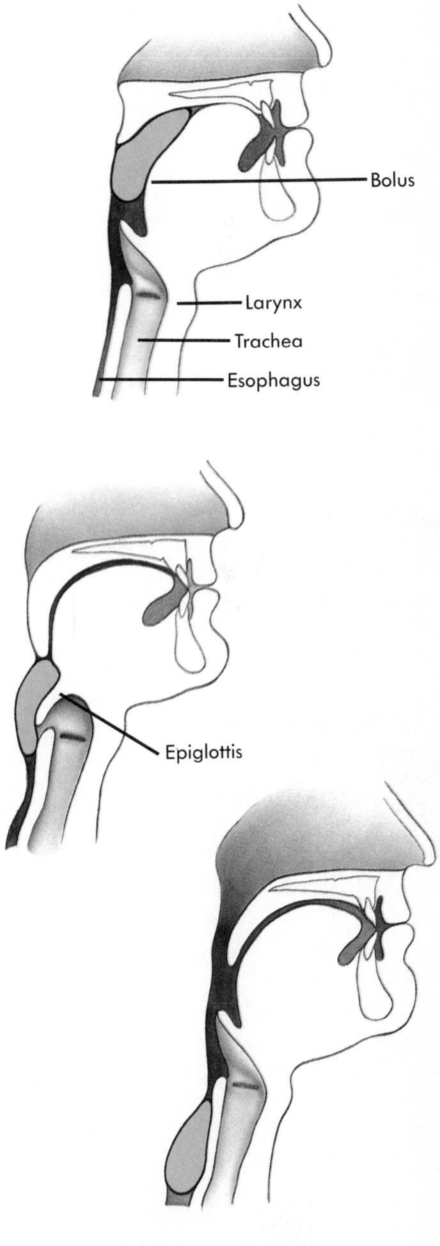

receptors are near the base. A variety of diseases and drugs can alter the sense of taste; adding more spices and flavorings to foods can help in these cases.

The mouth and stomach are connected by a "food tube," the esophagus. At its top is a valve-like epiglottis, a flap of tissue that prevents food from being swallowed into the trachea (wind pipe). In the margin, diagrams show that during swallowing, food lands on the epiglottis. When that happens the epiglottis covers the larynx, the opening of the trachea. Breathing also automatically stops. These involuntary responses ensure that swallowed food will travel only down the esophagus, helped along by its muscular contractions and gravity.

Food now enters the stomach, a holding tank with about a 1 liter (4 cup) capacity. The stomach continues the digestive process by secreting acid and enzymes, and then slowly churning them into the food. A meal usually leaves the stomach within 2 to 3 hours of eating. Solids take longer than liquids to leave the stomach, and a fatty meal usually leaves later than a meal containing mostly protein or carbohydrate.

The stomach is connected to the small intestine, which is coiled in the abdomen. The small intestine is divided into three sections: the **duodenum** is the first

At autopsy, the small intestine muscles relax, allowing the jejunum and the ileum to both lengthen to about 11 feet each. The small intestine then ends up about 23 feet long, a figure often cited in textbooks.

foot; the **jejunum** is the next 4 feet; the last 5 feet are called the **ileum.**[17] *Due to this total length, the small intestine can only be considered small because of its narrow diameter.* Most digestion is completed in the jejunum with the help of enzymes made by intestinal cells and the pancreas. The intestinal enzymes are often found on hair-like projections called the *glycocalyx* (Figure 3-2), which are attached to the intestinal walls.

Muscular contractions in the small intestine constantly mix the food, enhancing digestive action. A meal remains in the small intestine about 3 to 10 hours.

The small intestine connects with the large intestine, or colon. This organ measures about 3½ feet and is separated into five sections: the cecum, ascending colon, transverse colon, descending colon, and sigmoid colon. Bacteria in the colon digest some leftover plant fibers; otherwise little digestion occurs. However, there is no need for it—*about 95% of a total meal is digested in the small intestine.* In addition, much of the remaining 5% is indigestible. A meal remains in the colon for about 24 to 72 hours before elimination from the body.

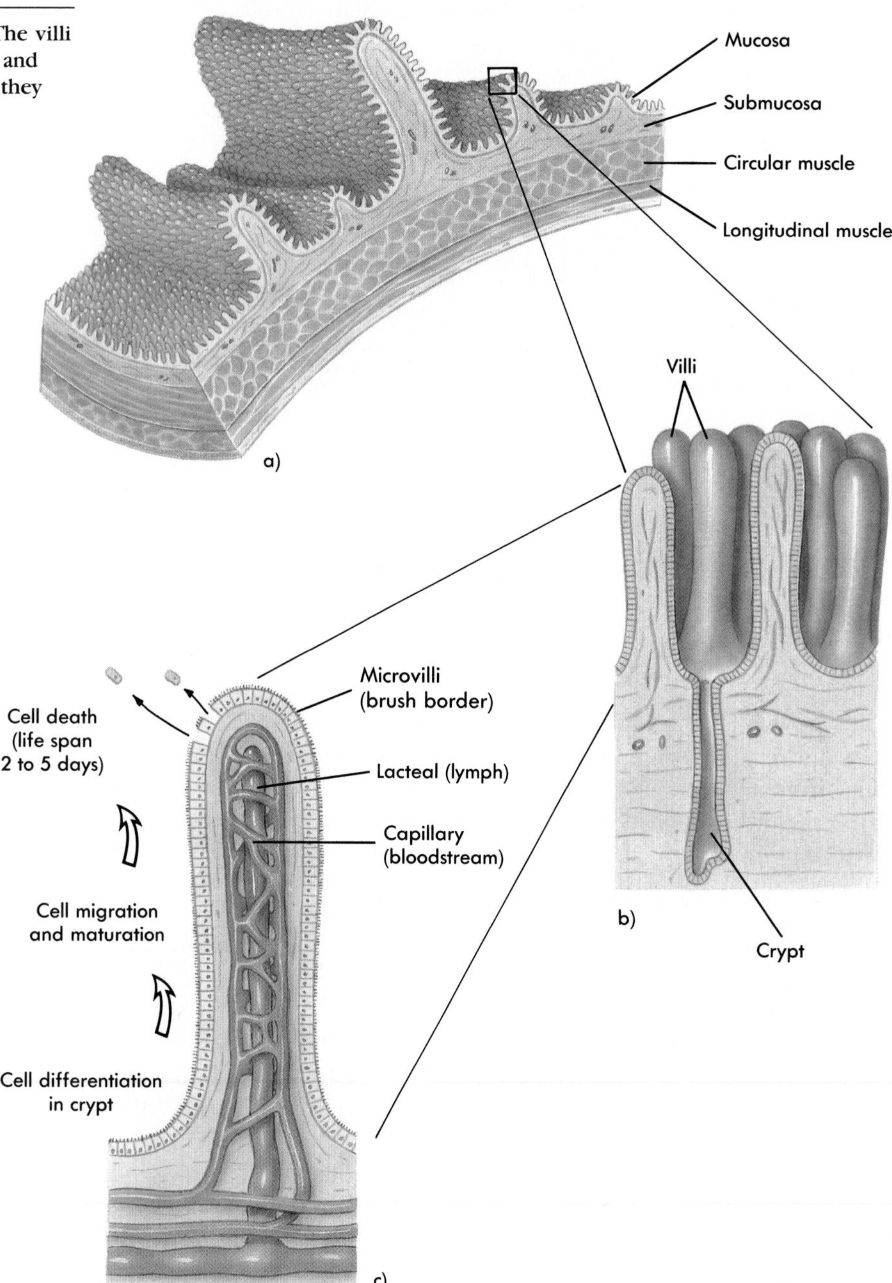

Figure 3-2

The villi in the small intestine. The villi are critical participants in digestion and absorption. The harsh environment they face limits their life span.

The end of the colon is connected to the rectum, which is connected to the anus. These final sections work with the colon to prepare the feces for elimination.

The liver, which provides **bile** to aid fat digestion and absorption, is connected to the gallbladder; the gallbladder stores this bile until it is needed for digestion. A duct leading from the gallbladder connects with a duct from the pancreas. This organ provides critical enzymes as well as other products for use in digestion. This output from the pancreas merges with that of the gallbladder before all of it enters the duodenum for digestive purposes. *Thus the liver, pancreas, and gallbladder work with the GI tract but are not part of it.*

GI control valves: sphincters

A variety of valves **(sphincters)** are located throughout the intestinal tract.[5] These sphincters respond to stimuli from nerves, **hormones,** hormone-like compounds, and the amount of pressure that builds up around them (Tables 3-1 and 3-2). The flow of food through the esophagus is controlled by the upper and lower esophageal sphincters. The lower esophageal sphincter is important for preventing backflow (reflux) of stomach contents up into the esophagus. The stomach contents are highly acidic, and if these come in contact with the esophagus, they can cause pain known as **heartburn.** Coffee, alcohol, and nicotine can weaken the tension of the lower esophageal sphincter and thus are likely to cause heartburn in some people (see Nutrition Perspective 3-1).

The pyloric sphincter, which is located at the base of the stomach, controls the movement of acidic stomach contents into the small intestine. *The pyloric*

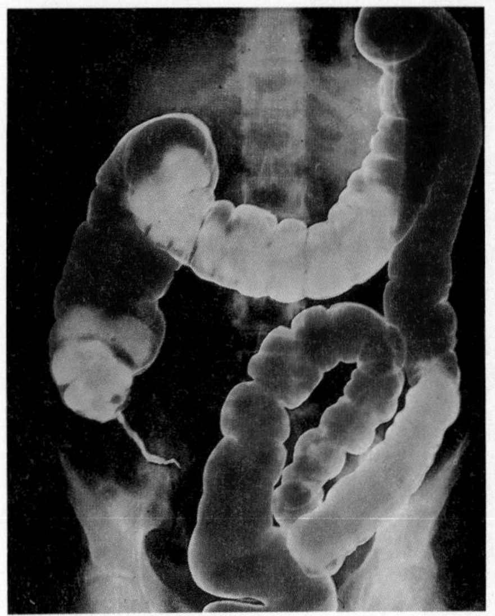

The colon has a large diameter and no villi.

bile
A substance that is made in the liver and stored in the gallbladder; it is released into the small intestine to aid fat absorption (see Chapter 5).

sphincter
A muscular valve that controls flow of foodstuffs in the GI tract.

hormone
A compound secreted into the bloodstream that acts to control the function of distant cells. Hormones can be either protein-like (such as insulin) or fat-like (such as estrogen).

heartburn
A pain emanating from the esophagus due to stomach acid backing up into the esophagus and irritating the tissue in that organ.

Table 3-1

Hormones that regulate the digestive tract[17]

Hormone	Origin	Stimulus to secretion	Action
Gastrin	Pyloric region	Food and other substances in the stomach, especially proteins, caffeine, spices, alcohol; nerve input	Stimulates flow of stomach enzymes and acid
Gastric inhibitory peptide	Duodenum, jejunum	Fats, protein	Inhibits secretion of stomach acid and enzymes; reduces stomach motility
Cholecystokinin (CCK)	Duodenum, jejunum	Food, especially fat and protein in duodenum	Causes contraction of gallbladder and flow of bile to duodenum; causes secretion of enzyme-rich pancreatic juice and bicarbonate-rich pancreatic juice
Secretin	Duodenum, jejunum	Acid chyme; peptones	Causes secretion of thin bicarbonate-rich pancreatic juice and reduces gastric motility

Table 3-2

Hormone-like compounds that help regulate the digestive process[17]

Compound	Main location	Proposed main actions
Motilin	Upper small intestine	Stimulates intestinal motility
Pancreatic polypeptide	Pancreas	Inhibits pancreatic secretion, relaxes gallbladder
Somatostatin	Widespread	Inhibits glandular secretions and nerve transmissions in intestinal muscles
Neurotensin	Ileum	Inhibits stomach acid release and stomach emptying; stimulates pancreatic bicarbonate release
Enteroglucagon	Ileum, colon	Slows intestinal transit; stimulates intestinal mucosa
Vasoactive intestinal peptide (VIP)	Widespread	Dilates blood vessels; relaxes GI muscles; stimulates pancreatic, gallbladder, and intestinal secretion; inhibits stomach acid secretion
Substance P	Widespread	Dilates blood vessels; contracts GI muscles, stimulates pancreatic and salivary secretions
Enkephalins	Widespread	Inhibits nerve transmission in GI muscles

sphincter allows the stomach contents to squirt only a few milliliters at a time into the small intestine. This slow rate allows bicarbonate ions (HCO_3^-) from the pancreas to efficiently neutralize the hydrogen ions (H^+) in the stomach contents. This neutralization reduces the risk of acid erosion of the small intestine, and in turn possible production of an **ulcer** (see Nutrition Perspective 3-1).

ulcer
Erosion of the tissue lining in either the stomach or upper small intestine, generally referred to as a peptic ulcer.

At the end of the gallbladder duct is the sphincter of Oddi. When the hormone cholecystokinin (CCK) stimulates the gallbladder to contract during digestion, the sphincter of Oddi relaxes and allows the contents of the gallbladder to enter the duodenum (Table 3-1).

The ileocecal valve forms the end of the small intestine. This sphincter prevents the contents of the large intestine from backing up into the small intestine. Thus bacteria from the large intestine are prevented from invading and colonizing the small intestine. It is important for the small intestine to have a relatively low concentration of bacteria because these can compete for nutrients, in turn absorbing nutrients before the body can. These bacteria also tend to break down the bile supplied by the gallbladder; in this case the bile can then neither help in

People who have had surgery involving the small intestine fare much better if their ileocecal valve is left intact to control the bacteria count in the small intestine.

the digestion of dietary fat nor be reabsorbed and used again. Unreabsorbed bile enters the colon and acts as a powerful **laxative,** often producing diarrhea.

laxative
A medication or other substance that stimulates evacuation of the intestinal tract.

At the end of the colon are two anal sphincters, both under voluntary control. Once a child is toilet-trained he can fairly well determine when these sphincters will relax and when they will stay rigid.

Thus sphincters along the intestinal tract perform important functions. Without them we would suffer more heartburn, ulcers, and diarrhea.

GI propulsion: peristalsis

Food is propelled down the GI tract partly by a process called **peristalsis.** One group of muscles forms a circular pattern around the GI tract (Figure 3-3). They constrict behind and relax in front of the ingested food, thus moving it down the intestinal tract. At the same time muscles lying lengthwise down the tract contract to make it shorter. After swallowing, this coordinated squeezing and shortening occurs in the esophagus in the form of two waves closely following each other. In the stomach, peristaltic waves create a mixing and grinding action as often as 3 times per minute during digestion. The most prominent peristalsis occurs in the small intestine where contractions occur about every 4 to 5 seconds. The colon has very sluggish peristalsis, employing occasional **mass movements** to help eliminate the feces.

peristalsis
A coordinated muscular contraction that is used to propel food down the GI tract.

mass movements
A peristaltic wave that simultaneously coordinates contraction over a large area of the colon. These move material from one portion of the colon to another, and from the colon into the rectum.

Laxatives stimulate peristalsis. They do this either by irritating the nerve junctions in the intestine to stimulate the peristaltic muscles or by drawing water into the intestine to enlarge the stool. A larger stool stretches the peristaltic muscles, making them rebound and then constrict. Chronic laxative use, especially the ir-

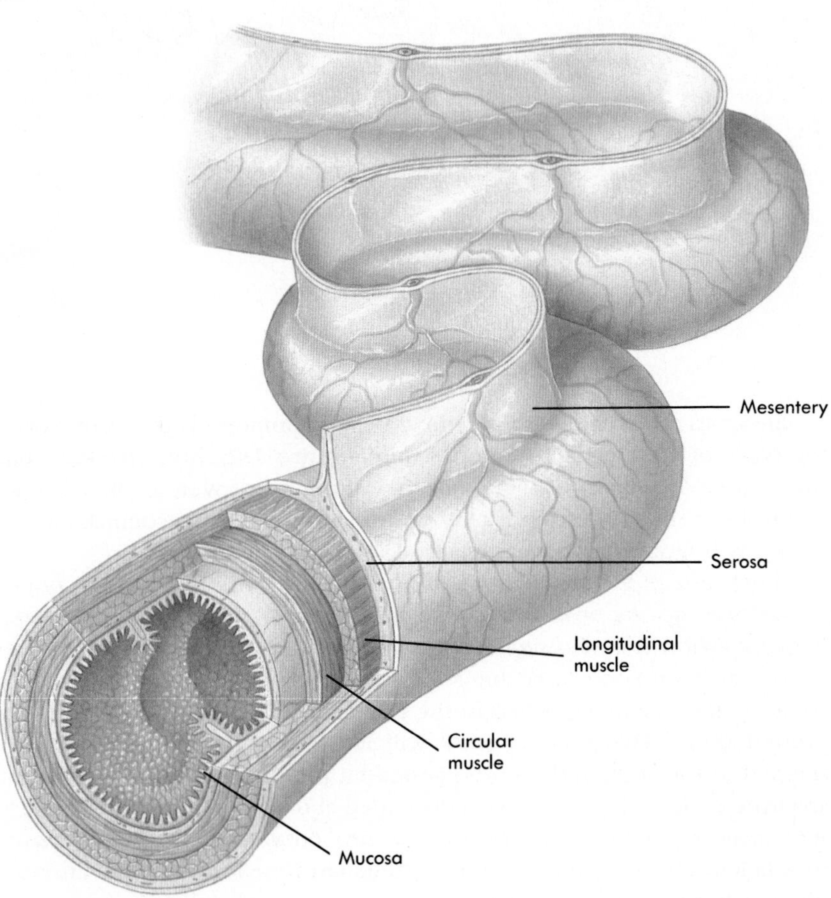

Figure 3-3
The small intestine. This diagram shows the muscle layers, circular folds, and blood supply for this organ.

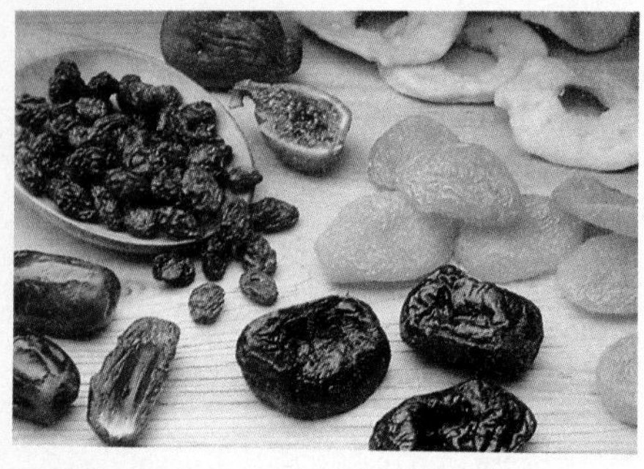

Eating dried fruit is another excellent way to increase your dietary fiber.

ritating varieties, can decrease muscle tone in the colon, causing more constipation.

A better alternative is the use of dietary fibers, such as those in whole grain breads and cereals. These also stimulate peristalsis by helping form a bulky stool but do so in a much safer manner. Thus the person with constipation should first increase fluid and fiber intake (see Chapter 4 for a detailed discussion). Eating dried fruits may also help. In addition, the person may need to develop more regular bowel habits; allowing the same time each day for a bowel movement can help train the colon to respond routinely. Finally, relaxation contributes to regular bowel movements, as does regular exercise.

Enzymes in digestion

The names of enzymes often end in "ase," like lipase, the enzyme that digests certain lipids.

Enzymes speed up digestion by facilitating chemical reactions (making them more likely to happen). Recall that most enzymes are proteins and work by bringing certain molecules in close proximity and then creating an environment favorable for the intended chemical reaction. This environment primarily consists of lowering the amount of energy needed to allow the reaction to proceed (Figure 3-4). *Almost every reaction in the body requires an enzyme to hasten its occurrence. This is especially true for digestion.* Most digestive enzymes are made by the pancreas and small intestine. A few are made by the mouth and stomach (Table 3-3).

Figure 3-4

A model of enzyme action. With some enzymes, the reaction can go both ways.

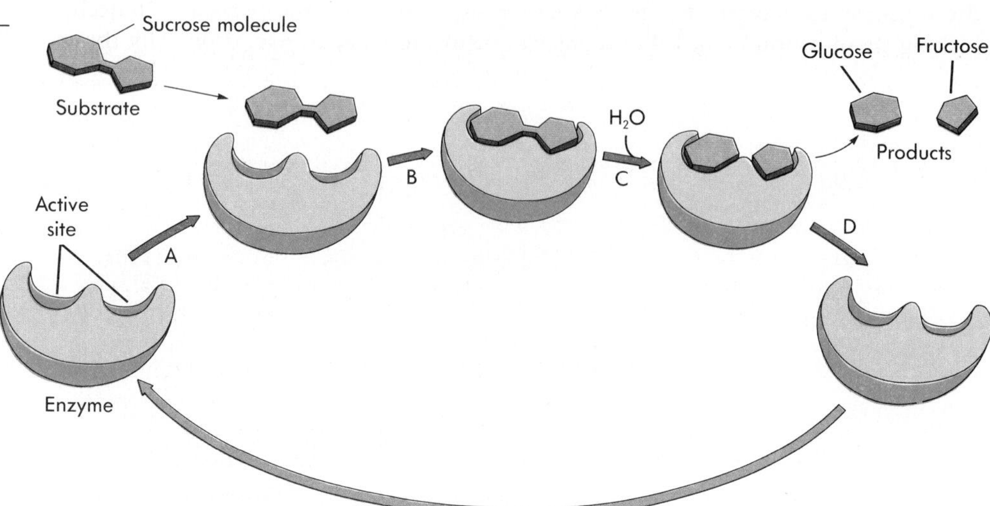

Enzymes are sensitive to pH, the types of compounds they can work with, and the types of vitamins and minerals they require. Digestive enzymes that work in the acid environment of the stomach will not work well in the alkaline environment of the small intestine. Furthermore, enzymes that recognize table sugar (sucrose) will ignore milk sugar (lactose).

People who have pancreatic disease, which is often found in people with **cystic fibrosis,** may not produce sufficient enzymes for digestion. In cystic fibrosis excess mucus production may block the release of the enzymes from the pancreas. This results in malabsorption of nutrients and associated discomfort. Such a person can consume replacement enzymes with their meals. Some forms are coated to protect against destruction by stomach acid.

When either the small intestine or the pancreas is diseased, important enzymes may not be produced in adequate quantities. This scarcity can result in poor digestion and, consequently, very poor absorption. In such cases the foodstuffs travel into the large intestine instead of being absorbed into the bloodstream. They are metabolized in the large intestine into acids and gas by bacteria present there. The person's stool will look foamy and greasy due to the gases trapped in the stool and the undigested fat present. A person with intestinal malabsorption also will often have a distended abdomen due to intestinal gas present. *Whenever digestion and absorption are hampered, the body pays a price.* Insufficient enzyme production or insufficient time for complete enzyme action is often at the root of these problems.[11]

Table 3-3

Summary of digestive enzymes

Secretion origin	Enzyme	Substrate	Major end products
Salivary glands	Salivary amylase	Starch, glycogen	Maltose
Lingual glands	Lingual lipase	Short-chain triglycerides, medium-chain triglycerides	Fatty acids, monoglycerides
Stomach glands	Pepsin	Protein	Peptides, peptones
	Gastric lipase	Short-chain triglycerides, medium-chain triglycerides	Fatty acids, monoglycerides
Pancreas	Trypsin	Protein, peptides	Polypeptides, smaller peptides
	Chymotrypsin	Protein, peptides	Same as trypsin, more coagulating power for milk
	Carboxypeptidase	Polypeptides	Smaller peptides, free amino acids
	Pancreatic amylase	Starch, glycogen	Maltose
	Lipase	Triglycerides	Monoglycerides, free fatty acids
Intestinal wall	Aminopeptidase	Peptides	Amino acids, smaller peptides
	Maltase	Maltose	Glucose
	Sucrase	Sucrose	Glucose, fructose
	Lactase	Lactose	Glucose, galactose
	Enterokinase	Trypsinogen	Trypsin

Concept Check

The gastrointestinal (GI) tract includes the mouth, esophagus, stomach, small intestine, large intestine (colon), rectum, and anus. Associated with the GI tract are the liver, gallbladder, and pancreas. Together these organs perform the digestion and absorption needed to both extract nutrients from food and funnel them into the bloodstream. In the GI tract, a coordinated muscular activity, called *peristalsis,* propels food from the esophagus to the anus. During this journey, enzymes produced by the mouth, stomach, pancreas, and small intestinal cells digest the food so that the nutrients present can be absorbed. The lag time from ingesting food to the eventual elimination of the remains from the body is usually about 1 to 3 days.

Exploring Issues and Actions

In 1981 products called *Starch Blockers* were placed on the market. The manufacturer suggested that starch blockers inhibit starch digestion. It is true that in the laboratory starch blockers do work, but they were never shown to be effective in the body.[3] If they were effective, in what manner, if any, would they affect the eating of a starch-rich meal?

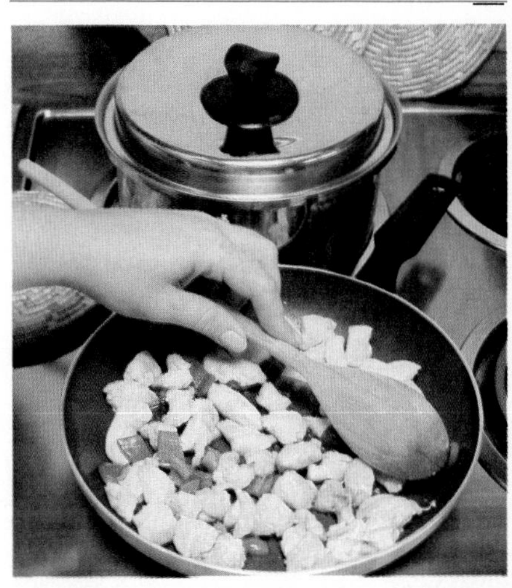

Cooking makes many foods safer to eat.

DIGESTION

A good way to study digestion of food is to track a single food from the time it enters the mouth until it is either absorbed into the bloodstream or eliminated in the feces. We have done that for banana bread in Figure 3-5.

Digestion actually begins before we start eating. Cooking food can be viewed as a first step in digestion. When starches are heated, the starch granules swell as they soak up water, making them much more easily digested and absorbed. Cooking also unfolds proteins and softens tough connective tissues in meats as well as in the fibrous tissue of plants, such as broccoli stalks. All these effects of cooking make the food easier to chew, swallow, and break down during later digestion and absorption. As you will see in Chapter 19, *cooking also makes many foods, such as meats, fish, and poultry, much safer to eat.*

Protein digestion

Protein digestion begins in the stomach. The stomach secretes **pepsin,** a major enzyme used for this process. Pepsin attacks all proteins and breaks them down

Figure 3-5

Digestion in practical terms. Many enzymes contribute to the digestion of foods.

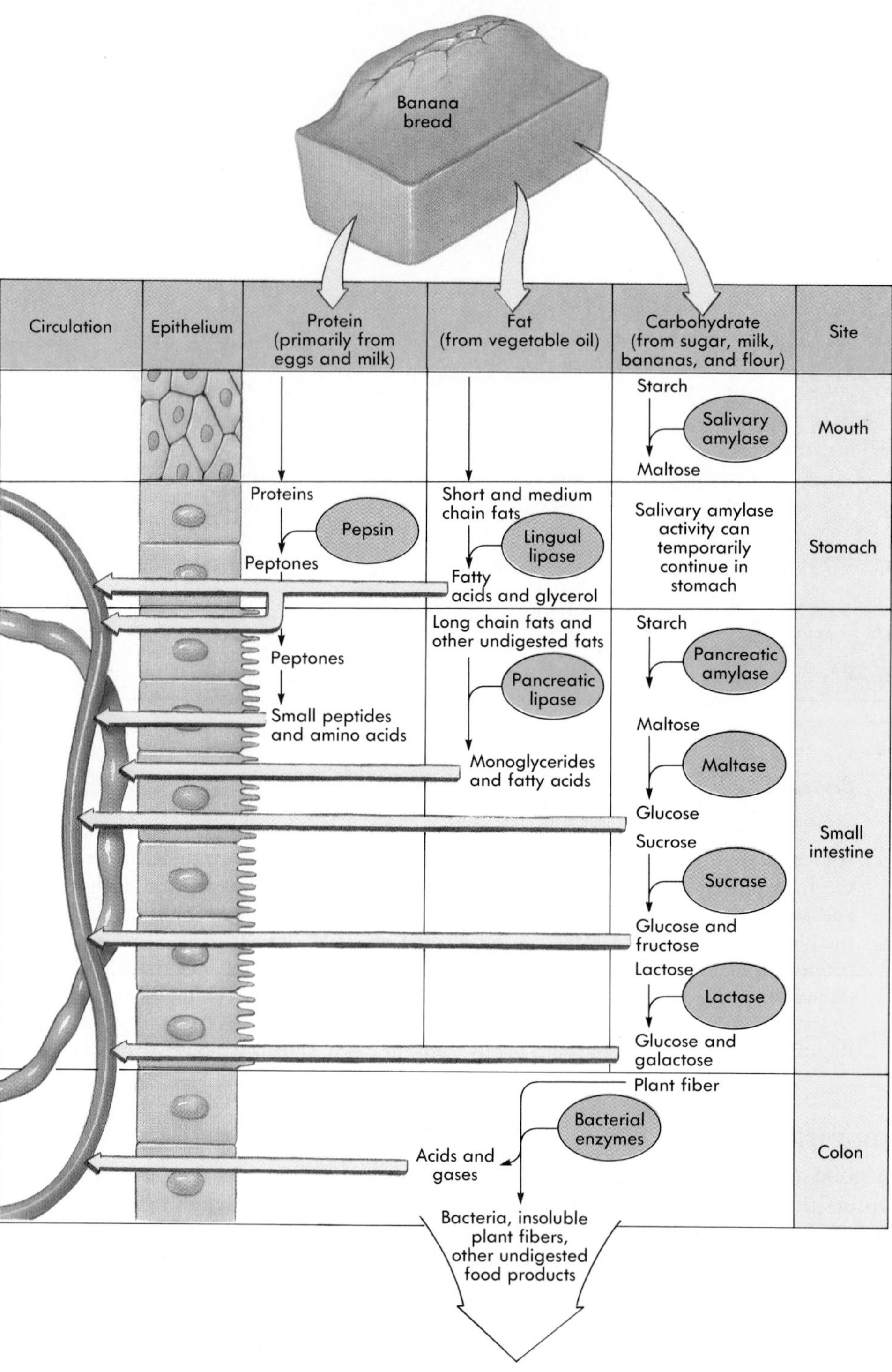

peptones
A partial breakdown product of proteins.

into shorter units, called **peptones.** Pepsin does not completely separate the protein into amino acids (the building blocks of protein) because it can break only a few of many types of bonds found in protein molecules. Thus it has limited activity.

Pepsin is stored in the chief cells of the stomach as *pepsinogen,* its inactive form. These cells, along with parietal (acid-forming) cells and mucus-forming cells, lie in gastric pits in the stomach. If pepsin were not stored as an inactive enzyme, it would digest the stomach glands while waiting to be secreted. Once pepsinogen enters the stomach's acidic environment, part of the enzyme is broken off, thus forming the active enzyme, pepsin. This storage of the inactive form of pepsin is just one way the stomach prevents **autodigestion** (digesting itself).

The release of pepsin is controlled by the hormone **gastrin** (Table 3-1). Just thinking about food or chewing food stimulates nerves in the brain that control special gastrin-producing cells in the base of the stomach (Figure 3-6). Gastrin then signals the chief cells in the stomach to begin producing pepsinogen. This is another means by which the stomach prevents autodigestion. Pepsin is present only when food enters or is about to reach the stomach because gastrin is released only at those times.

Gastrin also strongly stimulates the stomach's parietal cells to produce acid. The parietal cells are likewise stimulated by a breakdown product of proteins, called **histamine,** as well as by stomach distention (Figure 3-7). The parietal cells then produce hydrochloric acid (HCL);[19] the starting reactants are water, carbon dioxide, and chloride ions. *Hydrochloric acid activates pepsin and also improves the absorption of iron and calcium, keeps the stomach essentially bacteria-free, and inactivates plant and animal hormones that might otherwise act in the body* (see Nutrition Perspective 3-1). The parietal cells also produce intrinsic factor, a compound needed for vitamin B-12 absorption (see Chapter 12).

Since gastrin is released only when we eat or think about eating, acid production follows this same pattern. Furthermore, as the stomach's pH approaches 1.5 to 2, gastrin release stops. These are two other ways the stomach is protected

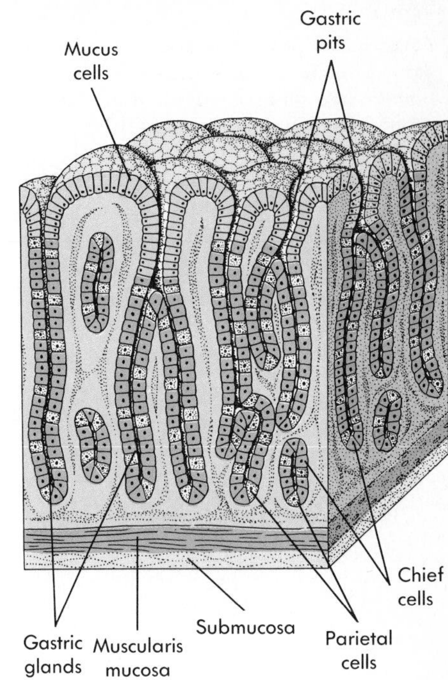

autodigestion
Literally, "self digestion." The stomach limits autodigestion by covering itself with a thick layer of mucus and producing enzymes and acid only when needed for digestion of foodstuffs.

gastrin
A hormone that stimulates enzyme and acid secretion by the stomach.

histamine
A breakdown product of the amino acid histidine that stimulates acid secretion by the stomach.

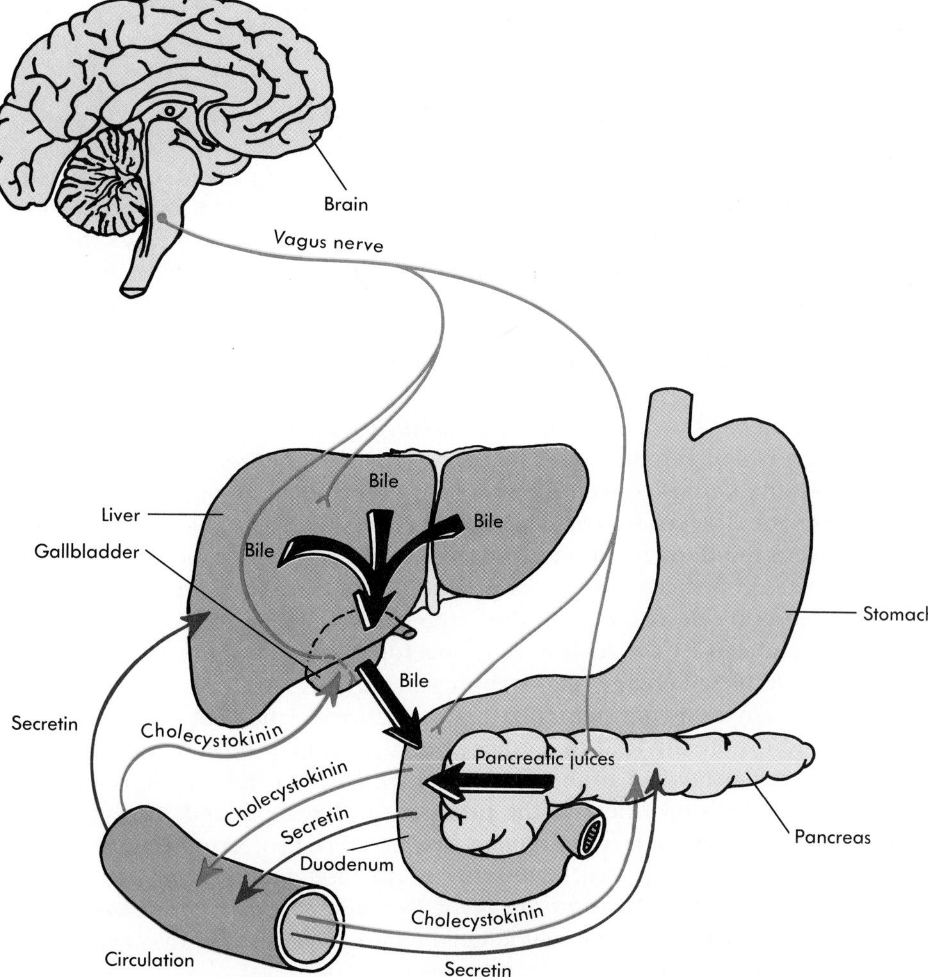

Figure 3-6
The mind-GI tract connection. Nerve input from the brain interacts with hormones and other factors to help regulate digestion.

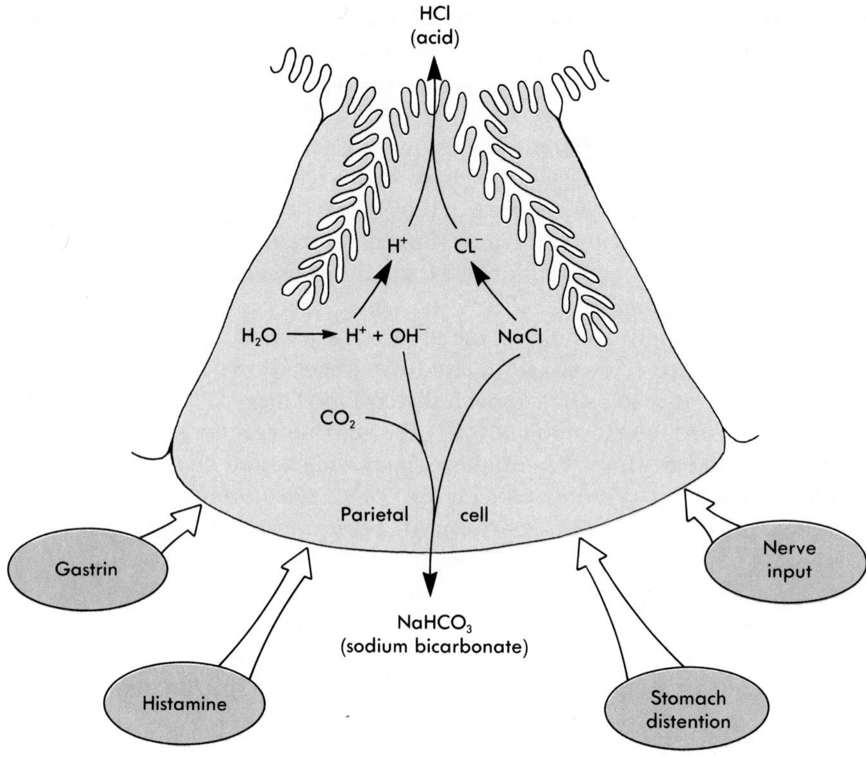

Figure 3-7
Factors that stimulate acid secretion in the stomach. The reactants are water, carbon dioxide, and sodium chloride. The product is hydrochloric acid (HCl).

from autodigestion. The first involves acid production: acid is produced only when food is present, and only enough is made to digest the food that is present. The second barrier against autodigestion is the thick layer of mucus the stomach secretes. The mucus lines the inside of the stomach, insulating it from the acid and pepsin produced for digestion.

Protein digestion continues in the small intestine

The peptones now move with the rest of the meal from the stomach into the small intestine. As we mentioned, the mixture actually squirts through the pyloric sphincter, which separates the stomach from the upper small intestine (duodenum). All the liquids consumed, plus the acid produced by the stomach, have together created a very watery food mixture, called **chyme.** As soon as the chyme squirts into the duodenum, bicarbonate ions made in the pancreas neutralize the acid. This is coordinated by the hormone **secretin.** Acid entering the duodenum causes secretin release. Secretin then stimulates the pancreas to release bicarbonate ions, and causes a reduction in stomach peristalsis (motility).

chyme
A mixture of stomach secretions and partially digested food.

secretin
A hormone that causes bicarbonate ion release from the pancreas.

The neutralized chyme is now approximately pH 5 to 7, rather than pH 2 to 3. If the acid chyme is not neutralized, it will corrode the wall of the duodenum.[7] This could eventually lead to an ulcer because, unlike the stomach, the small intestine is not protected from acid by a thick layer of mucus. Because the small intestine must absorb most of the products of digestion, and absorption cannot occur through a thick layer of mucus, that mode of protection is unavailable. *The stomach absorbs only small amounts of alcohol and certain fats; therefore a thick layer of mucus poses no problem. The duodenum is protected instead by quick neutralization of the acidic chyme and the constant shedding of its cell lining.*

Once in the small intestine, the peptones mix with the protein-digesting enzymes **trypsin,** chymotrypsin, and carboxypeptidase, which are secreted by the pancreas. These enzymes divide the peptones into short **peptides** and amino acids. All three enzymes exist in inactive forms in the pancreas and become active enzymes only when a protein tail from each is removed. The enzyme that cuts off this protein tail is called *enterokinase.* It is produced by cells in the wall of the small intestine. As we will cover in a later section, eventual digestion of all the peptides into amino acids then occurs inside the villi cells of the small intestine.

trypsin
A protein-digesting enzyme secreted by the pancreas to act in the small intestine.

peptides
A few amino acids bonded together (often two to four).

Fat digestion

The tongue produces lingual **lipase,** an enzyme that digests fat.[10] (*Lingual* refers to the tongue.) This enzyme acts primarily on short- and medium-chain fats, such as those found in butter fat (see Chapter 5). The actual digestion occurs while the fats are in the stomach because lingual lipase can function in an acid environment. The stomach produces a similar gastric lipase (*gastric* refers to the stomach). The action of both of these enzymes, however, is usually dwarfed by pancreatic lipase action in the small intestine. Long-chain fats, such as those found in common vegetable oils, must wait for this intestinal digestion.

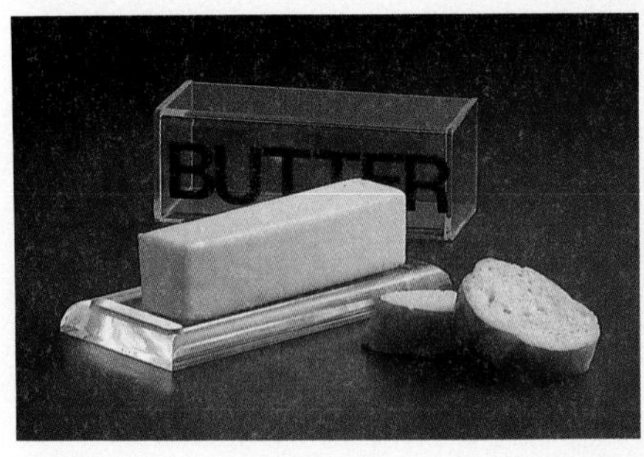

Digesting fats, such as those found in butter, requires pancreatic lipase.

Pancreatic lipase digests fats into smaller breakdown products, called **monoglycerides** and fatty acids. Pancreatic lipase enters the small intestine in a concentration 1000 times greater than needed. This "overkill" makes fat digestion very rapid and thorough given the right circumstances. "Right" circumstances include the presence of bile from the gallbladder. This helps **emulsify** the digestive products produced by lipase action. This improves digestion and absorption because large fat globules break down into smaller ones. This increases the total surface area for lipase action.

The hormone **cholecystokinin (CCK)** controls the release of enzymes, including lipase, from the pancreas as well as bile from the gallbladder. When food enters the small intestine, CCK is released from the wall of the duodenum into the bloodstream. This hormone then travels to the pancreas and gallbladder and causes these organs to release their products.

Fats and proteins in the chyme also stimulate the release of the hormone **gastric inhibitory peptide (GIP).** Stomach motility is reduced by GIP. Both the hormones secretin and GIP then keep the stomach from overwhelming the intestine with chyme. *This helps explains why fats in a meal cause a feeling of fullness: the chyme remains in the stomach longer, and so we feel full longer.* [5] On the other hand, hunger returns quickly after a low-fat meal—a common occurrence after eating a low-fat meal (see Chapter 5).

lipase
Fat-digesting enzymes; linguinal lipase is produced by the tongue, gastric lipase by the stomach, and pancreatic lipase by the pancreas.

monoglycerides
A breakdown product of a triglyceride consisting of one fatty acid bonded to the carbohydrate glycerol.

emulsify
To suspend fat in water by isolating individual fat drops using sheets of water molecules to prevent the fat from coalescing.

Carbohydrate digestion

Carbohydrate digestion begins as carbohydrates mix with saliva during the chewing of food. Saliva contains the enzyme salivary **amylase.** This enzyme converts starch into sugars, specifically maltose, which is glucose bonded to glucose. You can observe this conversion while chewing a saltine cracker. Prolonged chewing of the cracker causes it to taste sweeter as some starch is converted into the sweeter sugars.

Salivary amylase does not work in an acidic environment. Once food moves down the esophagus into the stomach, the stomach's acidity halts further salivary amylase action and consequently starch digestion. However, salivary amylase is not that important because pancreatic amylase will finish in the small intestine what salivary amylase does not finish in the mouth.

When the carbohydrates are in the intestine, the pancreas releases its amylase to continue the digestion of the starches into maltose. The original carbohydrates from the original meal are now present in their more simple sugar forms: Glucose, fructose, maltose, lactose, sucrose, and others. *The sugars are then digested*

cholecystokinin (CCK)
A hormone that stimulates enzyme release from the pancreas and bile release from the gallbladder.

gastric inhibitory peptide
A hormone that slows gastric motility and stimulates insulin release from the pancreas.

amylase
Starch-digesting enzymes from the salivary glands or pancreas.

to their single sugar forms by specialized enzymes that are synthesized by and attached to the cells of the small intestine. The maltose is acted on by maltase to produce two glucose molecules. Sucrose (table sugar) is acted on by sucrase to produce glucose and fructose. Lactose (milk sugar) is acted on by lactase to produce glucose and galactose. The single sugars are then absorbed (see Chapter 4).

When considering carbohydrate digestion, *it is important to remember that the needed digestive enzymes come from both the pancreas and cells of the intestinal wall.* Intestinal diseases can interfere with the production of the intestinal wall enzymes. Such conditions may interfere with the efficient digestion of the sugars maltose, lactose, and sucrose. If these carbohydrates are not fully digested, they will not be absorbed. When they end up in the colon, the bacteria present will use the sugars to produce acid and gas, causing abdominal discomfort. People recovering from intestinal disorders such as diarrhea or bacterial infections need to especially avoid lactose for a few weeks in case of possible temporary lactose intolerance. Two weeks will give time for the small intestine to again begin producing enough lactase enzyme to allow for lactose digestion (see Nutrition Perspective 3-2).

Hormones—helping to orchestrate the process

We have now seen the four true hormones of the GI tract: Gastrin, secretin, cholecystokinin, and gastric inhibitory peptide.[16] Many other hormone-like compounds also control important aspects of GI function. These compounds diffuse from cells or nerve endings to nearby cells, rather than traveling through the bloodstream. To be a true hormone a compound must enter the bloodstream; however, while some of the compounds that regulate GI tract function are not true hormones, they are important nevertheless (Table 3-2). Many are found in both the intestine and brain. When a person thinks about eating or prepares to eat, his or her whole GI tract begins to prime itself for action. Hormone-like substances participate in this "priming." The cells that make all these hormones and hormone-like compounds are scattered throughout the GI tract.[9]

Concept Check

Digestion begins with cooking; heat and moisture unfold proteins, swell starch granules, and soften tough fibrous tissues in plants. Enzymes produced in the mouth begin to digest starch. The stomach primarily digests protein, producing breakdown products called peptones. The small intestine is the major site of all digestion. There, peptones separate into small peptides and amino acids, carbohydrates yield single sugars, and fats form monoglycerides and free fatty acids. Peristaltic muscle contractions in the stomach and small intestine constantly mix the food, enhancing the digestive process. Enzymes used for digestion in the small intestine come from the pancreas and the cells lining the intestinal wall. Fat digestion is aided by bile, which is produced by the liver and later released by the gallbladder.

SMALL INTESTINE: SITE FOR MOST NUTRIENT ABSORPTION

Most nutrient absorption occurs in the small intestine and colon. The small intestine can absorb about 95% of the kcalories it receives in the form of protein, carbohydrate, fat, and alcohol. Only water, small amounts of alcohol, certain types of fats, and glucose are absorbed by the mouth and/or stomach. Some minerals, water, and short-chain fats (produced by bacterial action) are absorbed in the colon.

One cancer treatment is the use of medications (chemotherapy) to prevent rapid cell growth. This can stop tumor cells from growing. However, chemotherapy also affects body cells that normally have a rapid turnover such as villi cells. Because the cells of the villi are affected, people on these medications usually develop diarrhea as a side effect from such cancer treatments.

The incredible surface area of the small intestine greatly contributes to efficient absorption. The wall of the small intestine is folded. Within the folds are finger-like *villi* projections (see Figure 3-2). The "fingers" trap foodstuffs between each other to enhance absorption. Each villi "finger" is made up of numerous **absorptive cells,** and each of these cells has a brush border, or microvilli, cap. *All these folds, fingers, and indentations in the small intestine increase surface area 600 times beyond that of a simple tube.*

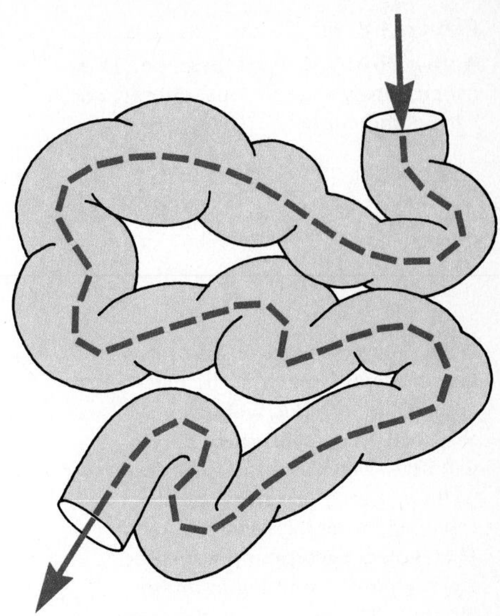

Absorptive cells

The absorptive cells are produced in crypts buried deep in the wall of the small intestine (see Figure 3-2). They migrate up from the crypts to the tip of the villi. As the cells migrate, they mature, and their absorption efficiency increases. By the time they reach the top of the villi, however, they are partially degraded by digestive enzymes that have been acting on them. They are then ready to be sloughed off. Newly formed absorptive cells are constantly produced, and these march up from the crypts to replace the dying ones.

The journey from the crypt to the top of the villi takes 2 to 5 days for each absorptive cell. Thus these cells have a very short life span. This short life span probably serves as an important adaptive mechanism because absorptive cells face a harsh environment due to contact with the enzymes, bacteria, and various toxins found in the small intestine. Contact with alcohol also reduces the integrity of the intestinal lining.[1] In essence, constantly making a new intestinal lining is probably a biological necessity.

When a cell has a short life span, it has a high need for nutrients, since cell production requires many nutrients. With the same logic one can predict that the small intestine will rapidly deteriorate during a nutrient deficiency or in starvation. Researchers have shown that the products of digestion and the hormones associated with digestion have a direct growth-promoting (trophic) action on the cells of the small intestine.[4] The absorptive cells in the small intestine are healthier when GI tract hormones and digestive products are present.

If a disease flattens the villi, the surface area in the small intestine decreases and so malabsorption often results. This is what happens in **celiac disease** (gluten-induced enteropathy). A person having this disease shows an allergic response to a protein found in wheat, rye, oats, and barley. To prevent attacks the person must avoid eating those grains.

lumen
The inside cavity of the GI tract.

passive absorption
Absorption that requires permeability for the substance through the wall of the small intestine, as well as a concentration gradient higher in the lumen of the small intestine than in the absorptive cell.

facilitated absorption
Absorption using a carrier to shuttle substances into the absorptive cell but not expending energy. A concentration gradient higher in the intestinal lumen than in the absorptive cell drives the absorption.

active absorption
Absorption using a carrier and expending ATP energy. In this way the absorptive cell can absorb nutrients, such as glucose, against a concentration gradient.

Types of absorption

The small intestine uses four basic types of absorption processes: **Passive, facilitative, active,** and **phagocytosis/pinocytosis.** Passive absorption occurs when nutrients enter the absorptive cells without any need for a carrier or energy expenditure. To allow for this the wall of the intestine must be permeable to the nutrient and the nutrient must be present in a higher concentration in the intestinal **lumen** than in the absorptive cells. *The difference in concentration drives passive absorption.* Water and some minerals are passively absorbed.

Facilitative absorption involves a carrier molecule to shuttle the nutrients from the lumen of the small intestine into the absorptive cells, but no energy is expended. Again, a concentration difference drives the reaction. Facilitative absorption takes place for the simple sugar fructose, which mostly arises from the digestion of table sugar (sucrose).

Active absorption uses a carrier and expends energy in the process. The single sugars glucose and galactose, amino acids, and other nutrients are actively absorbed (Figure 3-8). Adenosine triphosphate (ATP) is the energy source (see Chapter 7). Using this energy, an absorptive cell can take up even a low concentration of a substance from the intestinal lumen because *energy can be used to actively pump the compound, such as glucose, into the villi.* This is important since glucose is always in a high concentration in the absorptive cells, as these cells are bathed by the bloodstream, which also has a high concentration of glu-

Because fructose follows facilitated absorption, a large amount of fructose in a meal can easily overwhelm the intestine's capacity to absorb it. Eating more than 100 grams (400 kcalories) of fructose at one time then can lead to diarrhea; fructose pulls water upon entering the large intestine.

Figure 3-8

Active absorption of glucose. This process uses sodium ions, energy, and a carrier molecule.

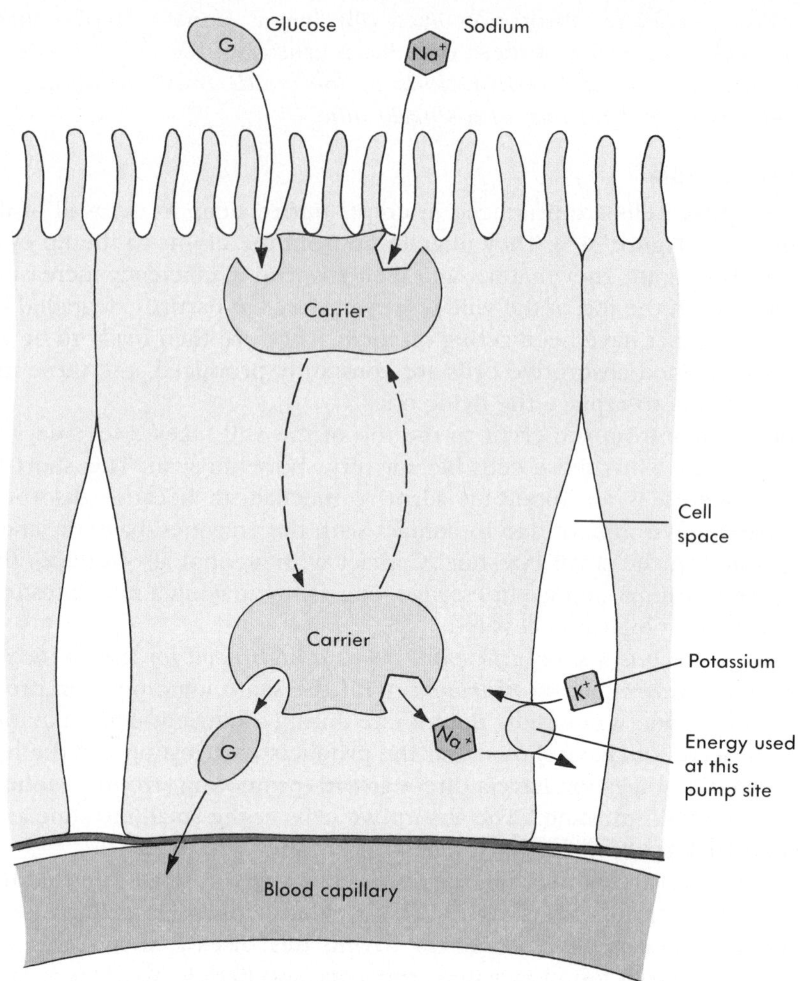

If the pump for glucose absorption does not work, much of the glucose in the intestine will not be absorbed. The unabsorbed glucose will draw water into the small intestine, causing diarrhea. This is essentially what happens in cholera. The cholera bacterium poisons the glucose pump, resulting in massive diarrhea. If a person with cholera is not given adequate fluid support while infected, he or she will quickly become dehydrated and die.

cose. Then there is no alternative to active absorption because a concentration gradient favoring glucose absorption from the intestinal lumen does not exist.

A second type of active absorption by villi cells involves phagocytosis/pinocytosis. This process involves the absorptive cells literally engulfing compounds or liquids. A cell can indent itself such that when particles or fluids move into the indentation, the cell surrounds and engulfs them. This process is used when an infant absorbs antibodies from the mother's milk.[8]

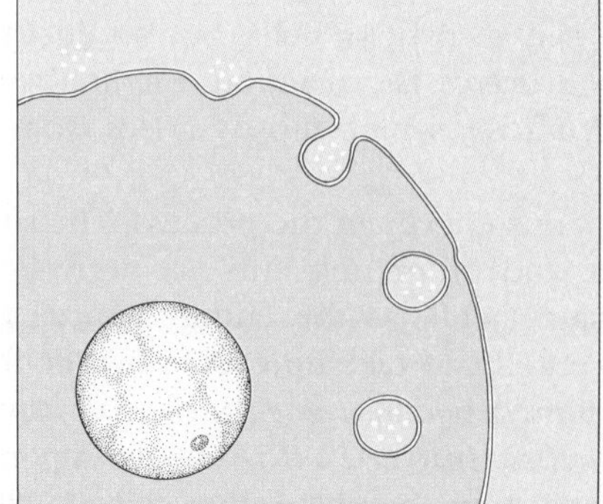
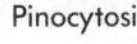
Pinocytosis

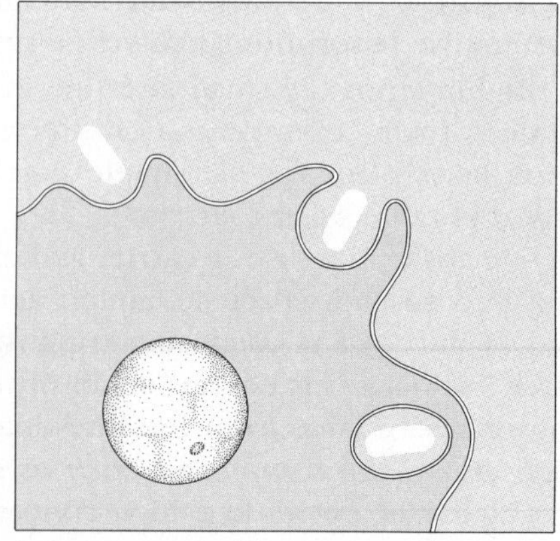
Phagocytosis

phagocytosis/pinocytosis
A form of active absorption in which the absorptive cell forms an indentation and particles entering the indentation are then engulfed by the cell.

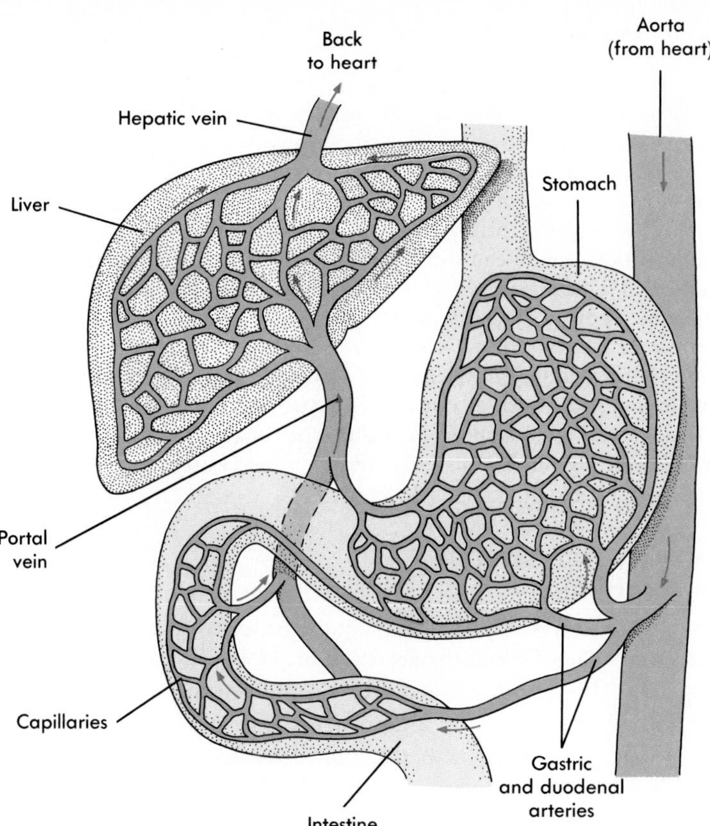

Figure 3-9

Hepatic-portal circulation. Blood from the stomach and small intestine collects in the portal vein and is carried to the liver. After flowing through the liver, the blood enters the general venous bloodstream.

portal vein
Capillaries from the intestine drain into a large portal vein that leads to the liver.

lymphatic system
System of vessels that can accept large particles, such as chylomicrons, and eventually pass them into the bloodstream.

Some cancer cells also travel through the lymph. When cancer is found in the body during surgery, the surgeon will examine the lymph nodes closest to the site of the cancer to see if it has traveled from the original site to other sites in the body. If cancer cells are found in the lymph nodes, they have probably already spread to other organs in the body.

Portal and lymphatic circulation

The villi in the intestine are drained by two different circulation systems. One is the bloodstream. Blood flow during digestion uses 30% of the heart's total output. This blood, laden with oxygen and nutrients, leaves the heart through arteries, travels to the intestine, and ends up in capillary beds inside the villi (Figure 3-9). The blood then passes through veins leaving the capillary beds and collects into a large vein called the **portal vein.** This vein leads directly to the liver. Most veins in the body double back directly to the heart. *However, by going directly to the liver the portal vein enables the liver to process absorbed nutrients before they enter the general circulation of the bloodstream.* Water-soluble products of digestion use the portal vein to enter the bloodstream.

The other circulatory system that drains the villi is the **lymphatic** system. The lymphatic vessels carry particles that are too large to pass through the capillaries into the bloodstream. Large proteins that escape from the bloodstream and **chylomicrons** formed after the absorption of fat are just two of many substances that travel through the lymphatic system. After substances enter the lymphatic system, they are squeezed through the sponge-like vessels by muscular activity. The lymphatic vessels from the intestine drain into the thoracic duct, which stretches from the abdomen to the neck. This duct connects into the bloodstream via the subclavian vein near the neck.

enterohepatic circulation
A continual recycling of compounds between the small intestine circulation and the liver; bile acids are a recycled compound.

Enterohepatic circulation

During meals, bile circulates about twice through the liver, then to the gallbladder, the small intestine, into the portal vein, and then back to the liver. This cycling is called **enterohepatic circulation.** Approximately 98% of the bile is recycled. Only 1% to 2% of the bile ends up in the colon and is eliminated in the feces. Enterohepatic circulation also occurs during the digestion of some vitamins and minerals.

Concept Check

The small intestine is the major site for nutrient absorption. Numerous folds and finger-like projections increase the surface area 600 times that of a simple tube. This provides a large area for nutrient absorption. Absorptive cells have a life span of 2 to 5 days, and so the lining of the small intestine is constantly being renewed. These cells can perform passive absorption, promoted by a concentration gradient; facilitative absorption, promoted by a concentration gradient plus a carrier; and active absorption, which can work against a concentration gradient because energy is expended. This method requires a carrier as well. Absorptive cells can also engulf compounds (phagocytosis/pinocytosis). The products of absorption, if water-soluble, pass into the portal vein and enter the liver. The products of fat digestion are mostly formed into chylomicrons and enter the lymphatic system. Some participants in digestion, such as bile, are reabsorbed after use in the small intestine and returned to the liver, only to be again sent back to the small intestine during another bout of digestion. This circulation is called enterohepatic circulation.

A common way to control very high blood cholesterol levels is to consume resins that bind bile and draw its constituents into the feces. This treatment reduces enterohepatic circulation. The liver is then forced to make new bile, rather than use recycled bile. The building block for bile synthesis is cholesterol. The liver must take this cholesterol out of the bloodstream to make new bile, thus lowering the blood cholesterol level.

ABSORPTION: STEP BY STEP

Protein absorption

Peptides and amino acids are actively absorbed into the absorptive cells of the small intestine. These products are then broken down into individual amino acids (Figure 3-10). The amino acids travel via the portal vein to the liver. From there the liver either combines the amino acids into protein, converts them into glucose or fat, or puts them into the bloodstream. The liver can break down all amino acids and gets help from the muscles in breaking down certain amino acid varieties (see Chapter 6).

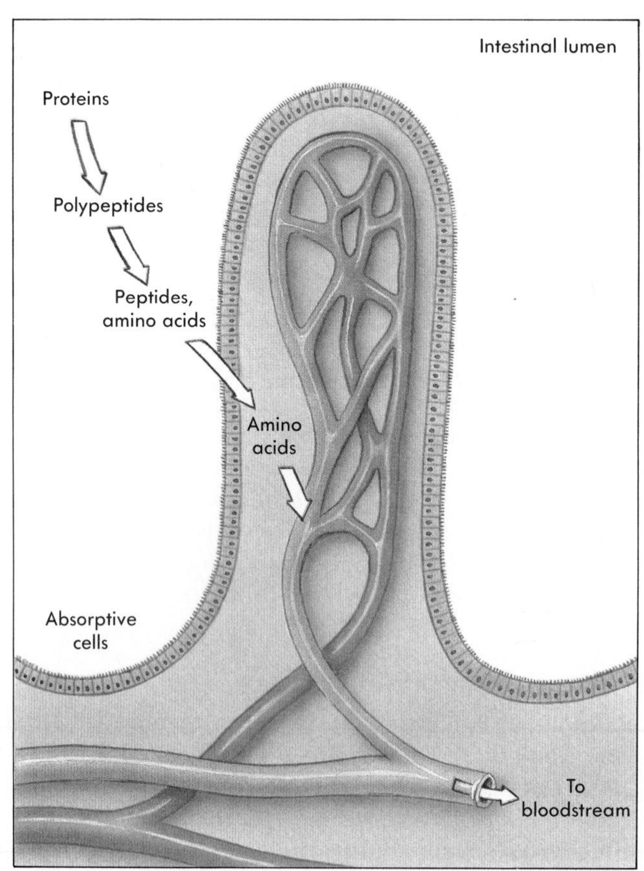

Figure 3-10

Final protein digestion. This takes place in the absorptive cells of the small intestine.

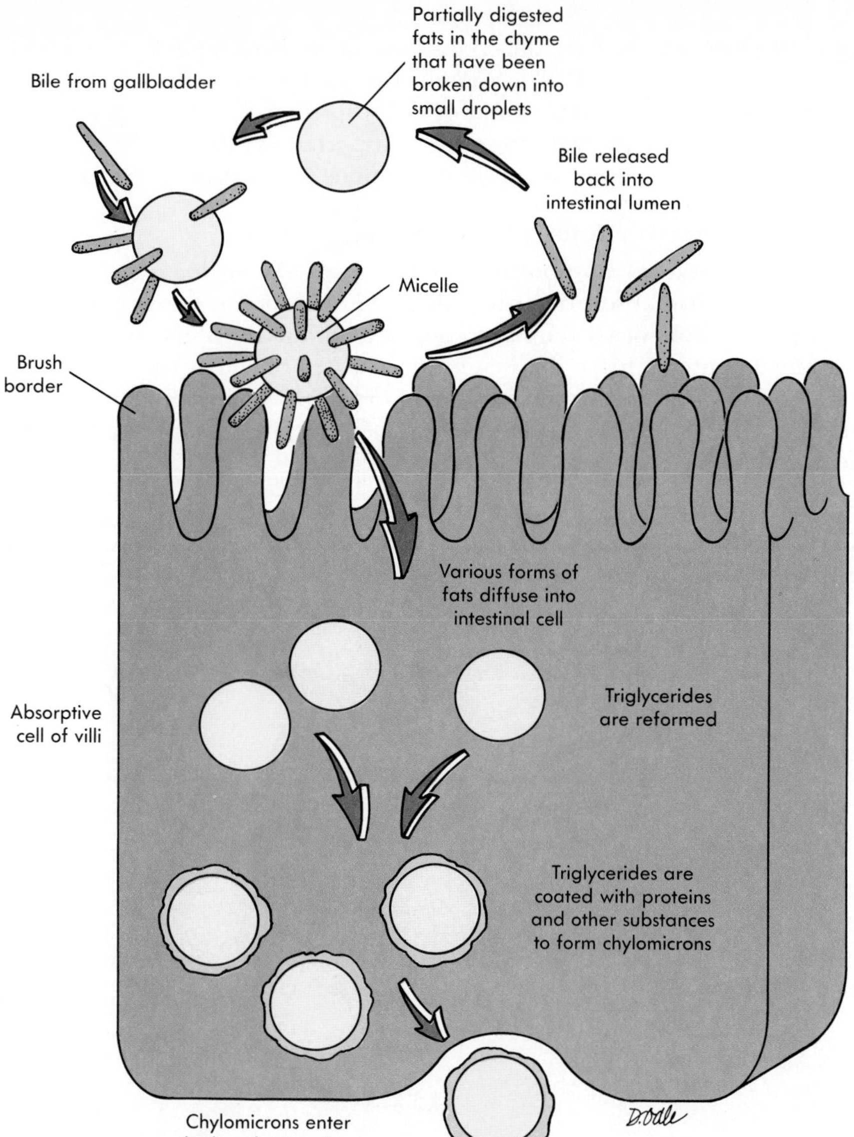

Figure 3-11

A simplified look at fat absorption. Triglycerides form primarily monoglycerides. These are absorbed using bile, and then reformed into triglycerides in the absorptive cells. Triglycerides are then formed into chylomicrons, and enter the lymphatic system.

Fat absorption

The products of fat digestion are passively absorbed into the absorptive cells. Two characteristics of fats affect the manner of their absorption. If the chain length of a fatty acid is less than 12 carbon atoms (a short- or medium-chain variety), it is water-soluble and so will probably travel as such through the portal vein to the liver. If the fatty acid is a long-chain variety (16 or more carbon atoms), then it must eventually be reformed into a triglyceride molecule and go via the lymphatic system as part of a chylomicron (Figure 3-11).

The major by-products of lipid digestion are long-chain free fatty acids and monoglycerides. These are resynthesized into triglycerides in the villi. The triglycerides are then combined with cholesterol and other substances and covered with a protein coat. This chylomicron enters the lymphatic system and eventually the bloodstream (see Chapter 5 for more details).

Carbohydrate absorption

Finally, we come to the single sugars. Fructose follows facilitative absorption as it is taken up by the villi cells. A carrier is involved, but no energy is used. Glucose

Exploring Issues and Actions

While you and your friend are discussing the benefits of eating good food, he suggests that eating fruit and meat together is bad for digestion. He claims each stops the digestion of the other. The authority for this statement is a popular book he has read. How do you respond to this common misconception, now that you have learned about the digestive process?

and galactose are actively absorbed. Sodium is cotransported during active absorption (see Figure 3-8). The ATP energy used in the process is actually needed to pump the sodium ion back out of the absorptive cell. Once glucose, galactose, and fructose enter the villi, they are transported via the portal vein to the liver. The liver then exercises its metabolic options (see Chapters 4 and 7).

The large intestine finishes absorption

The small intestine is responsible for 85% to 90% of the water absorbed from the GI tract. This absorption can reduce the 9 liters it receives (2 liters of dietary fluid plus 7 liters of GI tract secretions) to about 1.5 liters. Nevertheless, as the intestinal contents leave the ileum, some water remains. The remnants of digestion entering the colon consist mostly of water, along with some minerals and undigested food fibers. Again, only a minor amount (5%) of carbohydrate, protein, and fat have escaped absorption.

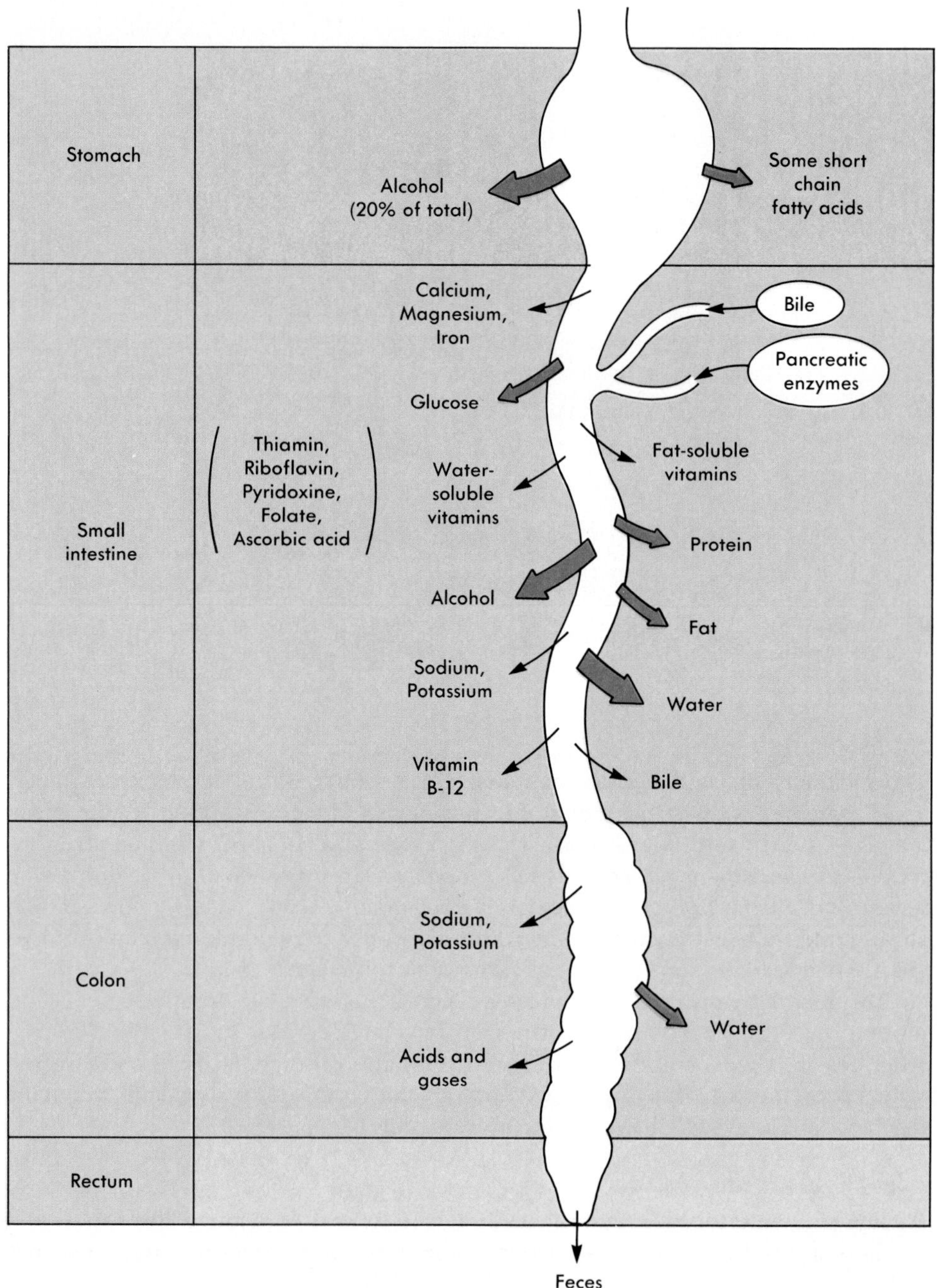

Figure 3-12
Major sites of absorption along the GI tract.

The colon absorbs primarily the minerals sodium and potassium, along with some water (Figure 3-12). This occurs mostly in the first half of the colon. The unabsorbed water now amounts to only about 200 milliliters. Short-chain fatty acids produced from the metabolism of some plant fibers and undigested starches are also absorbed in the colon,[6] along with some vitamins synthesized by bacteria, such as vitamin K and biotin (see Chapters 11 and 12). By the time the contents of the colon have passed through the first two-thirds of its length, they are semisolid. The stool remains in the colon until peristaltic waves and mass movements push it into the rectum for eventual elimination.

The presence of feces in the rectum powerfully stimulates defecation. This process involves powerful muscular reflexes in the sigmoid colon and rectum, as well as relaxation of the anal sphincters. What remains in the feces are undigestible plant fibers, tough connective tissues from animal foods, and bacteria from the colon.

Concept Check

In protein absorption peptides and amino acids are actively absorbed into the villi and broken down into amino acid forms. These enter the portal vein enroute to the liver. During fat absorption, the breakdown products are passively absorbed into the villi. These products are mostly resynthesized into triglycerides and combined with cholesterol, protein, and other substances to yield a chylomicron. Chylomicrons enter the lymphatic system and eventually the bloodstream. In carbohydrate absorption the single sugars glucose and galactose are actively absorbed into the villi; however, fructose requires facilitated absorption, a process in which a carrier is used but no energy is expended. These single sugars then travel via the portal vein to the liver. In the colon further water and mineral absorption occurs. The remaining fecal material contains primarily undigestible plant fibers and bacteria.

Summary

1. The gastrointestinal (GI) tract consists of the mouth, esophagus, stomach, small intestine, large intestine (colon), rectum, and anus. Most absorption of nutrients occurs in the small intestine.
2. The liver, gallbladder, and pancreas participate in digestion and absorption. Products from these organs enter the small intestine. The enzymes and bile supplied play important roles in digesting protein, fat, and carbohydrates.
3. Along the GI tract are valves (sphincters) that control the flow of foodstuffs. Muscular contractions, called peristalsis, propel the foodstuffs down the GI tract. A variety of nerves, hormones, and hormone-like compounds control the activity of sphincters and peristaltic motions.
4. In digestion the mouth chews food to break it into smaller parts, thereby increasing surface area. Enzyme activity is enhanced when the surface area of the food is increased. Some starch digestion also occurs in the mouth. Much protein digestion occurs in the stomach. In the small intestine carbohydrate and protein digestion is finished and fat digestion begins in earnest. Some plant fibers are digested by the bacteria present in the colon; undigested plant fibers end up in the feces.
5. Digestive enzymes are secreted by the pancreas, mouth, stomach, and wall of the small intestine. Pancreatic enzyme release is controlled by the hormone cholecystokinin (CCK). The presence of food in the small intestine stimulates the release of this hormone. Bile needed for fat digestion is synthesized by the liver, stored in the gallbladder, and released in digestion due to the action of CCK.
6. The major absorptive sites consist of finger-like villi projections in the small

intestine. The cells that cover the villi have a life span of 2 to 5 days. Thus the intestinal lining continually renews itself. Absorptive cells can perform passive, facilitated, and active absorption, and phagocytosis/pinocytosis, a second type of active absorption.

7. The products of protein digestion—amino acids and peptides—are actively absorbed into the villi. Most of the end products of fat digestion are passively absorbed into the intestinal villi and rebuilt into triglycerides. Single sugars from carbohydrate digestion are actively absorbed in the cases of glucose and galactose; facilitated absorption is used for fructose.
8. Water-soluble compounds in villi enter the portal vein and travel to the liver. Fat-soluble compounds are incorporated into chylomicrons and enter the lymphatic system, which eventually connects to the bloodstream. Some factors used in digestion, such as bile, are reabsorbed by the small intestine, sent back to the liver and returned to the small intestine to act in further digestion of foodstuffs. This recycling is called enterohepatic circulation.
9. In the colon final water and mineral absorption takes place, as well as absorption of products from bacterial breakdown of some plant fibers. Once the feces enter the rectum, the impetus for eventual elimination is strong.

Take Action

First read Nutrition Perspective 3-2. Then find a person who thinks he or she has lactose intolerance. Discover what diet changes have been made or should be made to adjust to the problem. Consider helping the person learn more about the options for treatment that you have learned in this chapter.

SYMPTOMS: ____________________

____

____

____

CURRENT DIET CHANGES: ____________________

____

____

____

OTHER CHANGES TO CONSIDER: ____________________

____

____

____

____

____

____

Expert Opinion

The GI Tract Has a Mind of Its Own

JACKIE D. WOOD, Ph.D

Every time we eat a meal or a snack our digestive machinery goes into high gear. Remarkable events take place in the gastrointestinal (GI) tract, especially in the stomach and the small and large intestines. Muscles provide automation and digestive juices, which have special enzymes, flow from glands. When the digestive intent—the absorption of as many nutrients as possible—has been met, the end of the GI tract sends the debris from the body. Overall, this is a complex process. Yet, even when we abuse the GI tract (and it usually lets us know about that) by overindulging or eating foods that upset it, it valiantly tries to return to an even keel and, more often than not, succeeds.

The intricate, specialized events that occur in the GI tract are orchestrated differently from those of the rest of the body. The digestive tract has, in a sense, a mind of its own.

PRIVATE PROGRAMS

Does the GI tract actually have its own brain? Probably not. The brain has memory banks and can learn. It's unlikely that the enteric nervous system (ENS)—the nervous system of the GI tract—stores information it can later use. I sometimes refer to the "little brain" in the GI tract primarily to point out that the classical idea of the control of the GI tract lying *entirely* in the brain and spinal cord—the central nervous system (CNS)—is indefensible and should be discarded.

Most of the nerve circuits determining the behavior of the GI tract are located within its walls. These circuits contain the programmed directions that guide the GI tract to make the proper motor and secretory responses to the commands of the CNS. Intriguingly, these responses are different from those occurring elsewhere in the body.

Typically, when the spinal cord communicates with a skeletal muscle, it excites nerve cells, or neurons, which are called motor neurons. A motor neuron, by definition, terminates on a skeletal muscle and stimulates it to contract. But when the spinal cord communicates with the GI tract, something different happens: processing of the nervous input from the CNS takes place within the GI tract itself, forming a decision-making point for action. Your arm muscles or leg muscles can't decide how to interpret input from motor neurons. However, the GI tract can by using its own nervous system, the ENS. In essence, the ENS constitutes a semiautonomous control system that, like an intelligent computer terminal, contains its own programs. The CNS, or "mainframe computer," then acts to select the ENS "programs" needed for a particular digestive state.

But that's not the only difference between skeletal motor neurons and motor neurons in the GI tract. Unlike the spinal cord, the ENS has both inhibitory and excititory motor neurons. Whereas spinal motor neurons can only excite relaxed skeletal muscle fibers to contract, the ENS can suppress the activity of certain GI tract muscles and enhance the activity of others. A further distinction involves neurotransmitters, which are chemical messengers from the brain that transmit nerve impulses that either excite or inhibit target cells. Spinal motor neurons release one excititory neurotransmitter, namely acetylcholine, to fire muscle fibers at the nerve-muscle junction. ENS motor neurons release four or perhaps more neurotransmitters from motor neurons, including acetylcholine, substance P, and vasoactive intestinal peptide (VIP). (See Chapter 8 to review the link between these neurotransmitters and hunger regulation.) In addition, unlike spinal motor neurons, which release acetylcholine at highly structured end plates (the sites where motor nerve fibers join skeletal muscle fibers), ENS motor neurons release neurotransmitters from sites called varicosities, which are strung like beads along the length of the nerve terminal. From all this you can see that the ENS does indeed have properties that are much similar to those of the brain.

TRACT TROUBLES

Considering the intricacies of the ENS motor neuron setup, it's not surprising that sometimes it goes haywire. For instance, Hirschsprung's disease is a classical condition in which at birth the lower parts of the large intestine lack specific nerve cells—especially inhibitory motor neurons—to allow for the peristaltic motions (wormlike waves of contraction) that produce bowel movements. There is contraction of the muscles—but because there is nothing to inhibit this motion, it is continuous and hyperactive, causing abnormal distention of the colon, obstruction, and severe constipation.

This type of obstruction, which is due to lack of neurons rather than to a physical bottleneck, is called intestinal pseudo-obstruction. It can be seen anywhere along the intestine where hereditary factors, the effects of aging, or disease lead to decreased action of inhibitory motor neurons. The result is often a medical emergency requiring surgery and intravenous feeding.

Continued.

Expert Opinion—cont'd

Paralytic ileus, or paralysis of the intestines, is the opposite of the spasticity associated with the absence of inhibitory motor function. Here, unremitting release of inhibitory neurotransmitters (due to the inability to "switch off" inhibitory neurons) causes the muscles to be inactive for abnormally long periods so that, again, peristalsis can proceed. Paralytic ileus often results from an abdominal insult, such as handling the GI tract during surgery. In reaction to such an insult, the ENS does something perfectly normal: it programs the GI tract for muscle quiescence. Unfortunately, of course, the upshot is a lack of peristalsis, which, in turn, causes gas to accumulate and distend the large intestine. The surgery patient can't eat again until this unhappy situation remits and normal bowel function resumes.

THE PACING OF PERISTALSIS

No commands from motor neurons are needed to initiate the contractions in the GI muscular system. The circular muscles contain a built-in pacemaker system designed for self-excitability. Release of neurotransmitters from *excititory* motor neurons increases the responsiveness of the muscles to the pacemaker system and, in some instances, may even be organized to override the pacemaker in initiating muscle contraction. Release of neurotransmitters from *inhibitory* motor neurons can suppress the muscles' responsiveness to the pacemaker system.

The muscle fibers of the GI tract are coupled in such a way that the force that triggers contractions can spread from cell to cell. This force is summoned by the pacemaker and generated by action potentials (the electrical activity developed in a muscle or nerve fiber when it is stimulated). Contractions are initiated simultaneously around the circumference of the bowel by these action potentials. Propagation then occurs more slowly in the longitudinal direction. Overall, inhibitory motor neurons determine not only when it's time for the ever-ready pacemaker system to initiate a contraction but also what the distance and direction of propgagation should be once contraction has begun. In contrast, skeletal muscle fibers are "slaves" to their individual motor neurons and contract only on command.

The peristaltic reflex occurs in response to activation of stretch receptors, which are located on muscles that are stimulated by a stretch or pull. When the GI tract distends, it triggers a pattern of motor behavior that causes contraction of the circular muscle that is in the direction of the mouth (oral to the stimulus), while shortening of the longitudinal muscle and inhibition of the circular muscle occur at the end opposite to the stimulus (in the direction of the anus). This behavior is produced by a fundamental neural circuit that is expressed repeatedly along the length of the intestine. The overall action results in a one-way propulsion of intestinal contents by linking basic persistaltic reflex circuits that are repeated over and over until the end of the bowel is reached.

THE ENS AND THE FUTURE OF GASTROENTEROLOGY

Our understanding of the ENS suggests that malfunctions may be the cause of certain disorders that are thought of today as functional disorders—diseases that we can describe but whose cause we can't explain in terms of a structural defect. Irritable bowel syndrome, which commonly affects college students and leads to pain and alternate bouts of diarrhea and constipation, is one such functional disorder. The present state of clinical gastroenterology—the study of the stomach and intestine and their diseases—is reminiscent of neurology in the early part of this century. Many brain disorders were originally referred to as functional because too little was known about their neurophysiological basis. For example, Parkinson's disease was considered a functional disorder until we discovered in the late 1950s that depletion of the neurotransmitter dopamine in the midbrain was the culprit. This is an example of how unraveling the mechanism of chemical neurotransmission in the "big brain" has pushed a CNS disorder from the shadows of a functional classification into the enlightened domain of basic scientific understanding.

Successful application of basic neuroscientific advances to the treatment of CNS disorders is already one of the brightest chapters in the history of medicine. Soon we might write a similar chapter in gastroenterology as we learn more about how the little brain in the gut controls the behavior of the digestive tract.

Dr. Wood is professor and chairman of the Department of Physiology of The Ohio State University College of Medicine, Columbus. He received his Ph.D. in physiology and biophysics from the University of Illinois and was awarded the Hoffmann LaRoche Prize for Gastrointestinal Research in 1986.

REFERENCES

1. Anonymous: The leaky gut of alcoholism, Nutrition Reviews 43:72, 1985.
2. Anonymous: Prevalence of lactose maldigestion, American Journal of Clinical Nutrition 48:1086, 1988.
3. Anonymous: Starch-blockers do not block starch digestion, Nutrition Reviews 43:46, 1985.
4. Bienenstock, J: Mucosal barrier functions, Nutrition Reviews 42:105, 1984.
5. Cashman, MD: Principles of digestive physiology for clinical nutrition, Nutrition in Clinical Practice 1:241, 1986.
6. Cummings, JH and others: The role of carbohydrates in lower gut function, Nutrition Reviews 44:50, 1986.
7. Feldman, M: Bicarbonate, acid, and duodenal ulcer, New England Journal of Medicine 316:408, 1987.
8. Gardner, MLG: Gastrointestinal absorption of intact proteins, Annual Reviews of Nutrition 8:329, 1988.
9. Giduck, SA and others: Cephalic reflexes: their role in digestion and possible roles in absorption and metabolism, Journal of Nutrition 117:1191, 1987.
10. Hamosh, M: Lingual lipase, Gastroenterology 90:1290, 1986.
11. Hermann-Zaidins, MG: Malabsorption in adults: etiology, evaluation, and management, Journal of The American Dietetic Association 86:1711, 1986.
12. Leiber, CS: Biochemical and molecular basis of alcohol-induced injury to liver and other tissues, New England Journal of Medicine 319:1639, 1988.
13. Kamath, SK: Taste acuity and aging, American Journal of Clinical Nutrition 36:766, 1982.
14. Kumar, N and others: Effect of milk on patients with duodenal ulcers, British Medical Journal 293:666, 1986.
15. Martini, MC and Savaiano, DA: Reduced intolerance symptoms from lactose consumed during a meal, American Journal of Clinical Nutrition 47:57, 1988.
16. Mattes, RD and Mela, DJ: The chemical senses and nutrition, Nutrition Today May/June, 1988.
17. Mayes, PA: Nutrition, digestion, and absorption. In Murray, RK and others, editors: Harper's Biochemistry, East Norwalk, Conn, 1988, Appleton & Lange.
18. Nicholl, CG and others: The hormonal regulation of food intake, digestion, and absorption, Annual Reviews of Nutrition 5:213, 1985.
19. Quimby, GF and others: Active smoking depresses prostaglandin synthesis in human gastric mucosa, Annals of Internal Medicine 104:616, 1986.
20. Strum, MB: Prevention of duodenal ulcer recurrence, Annals of Internal Medicine 105:757, 1986.
21. Wolf, MM and Soll, AH: The physiology of gastric acid secretion, New England Journal of Medicine 319:1707, 1988.

SUGGESTED READINGS

The article by Cashman is a clearly represented description of digestion and absorption designed for the practicing clinician. Thus it is detailed but also quite practical. The article by Leiber, a world authority on alcohol metabolism, is very technical but contains drawings that clearly depict the manner in which alcohol affects many cells in the body including those in the GI tract. The chapter by Mayes in Harper's *Biochemistry* is a step-by-step review of digestion and absorption that includes many tables, figures, and chemical structures of the most important participants. This is one of many books by Appleton & Lange. Finally, the artical by Hermann-Zaidens provides a comprehensive look at malabsorption—which is the result when this fine system we have discussed goes awry.

CHAPTER 3

Answers to nutrition awareness inventory

1. *True.* However, for many foods some digestion actually begins during cooking when protein structures unfold, starch granules swell, and tough vegetable fibers are softened.
2. *True.* A special portal vein connects the intestinal tract to the liver. Many nutrients can enter the bloodstream only after passing through the liver.
3. *True.* A living person's small intestine is approximately 15 feet; at autopsy it is approximately 23 feet.
4. *False.* Acid produced by the stomach is responsible for killing most of the bacteria that enter the stomach.
5. *True.* The term *colon* also refers to the large intestine.
6. *False.* The digestive enzymes work efficiently no matter what combination of foods is eaten.
7. *True.* Stomach enzymes require an acid pH for maximum activity, whereas the small intestine has a more neutral pH.
8. *False.* Hormone-like factors made by cells scattered throughout the GI tract also contribute to the coordination of digestive processes.
9. *True.* For about 70% of people worldwide, the ability to digest the milk carbohydrate, *lactose,* declines in adulthood.
10. *False.* Unless stress leads to significant diarrhea, it is unlikely to greatly affect the absorption of nutrients. Under almost all circumstances a healthy person digests and absorbs about 95% of the protein, carbohydrates, and fat consumed.
11. *True.* In total parenteral nutrition a tube is inserted into a vein close to the heart. Nutrients are infused into the bloodstream, bypassing the small intestine and liver.
12. *True.* The sugar *glucose* is absorbed from the small intestine into the bloodstream against a concentration gradient. Much glucose from the bloodstream is present in the cells of the intestine. So energy must be expended if more glucose in the intestinal tract is to enter the intestinal cells. Conversely, the concentration of fat in the intestinal cells is low, allowing fat to be passively absorbed into them.
13. *True.* The peristaltic waves that propel food down the intestinal tract requires a coordination of both longitudinal muscles, which lie lengthwise down the intestinal tract, and circular muscles, which surround the intestinal tract.
14. *True.* Many undigested foods that enter the colon are nutrient sources for bacteria there. The bacteria then make a variety of products, including hydrogen gas.
15. *True.* Bacterial growth is most prominent in the colon. Growth is hampered in the stomach by acid and in the small intestine by the muscular action of peristalsis.

Nutrition Perspective 3-1

Acid Autodigestion: Ulcers and Heartburn

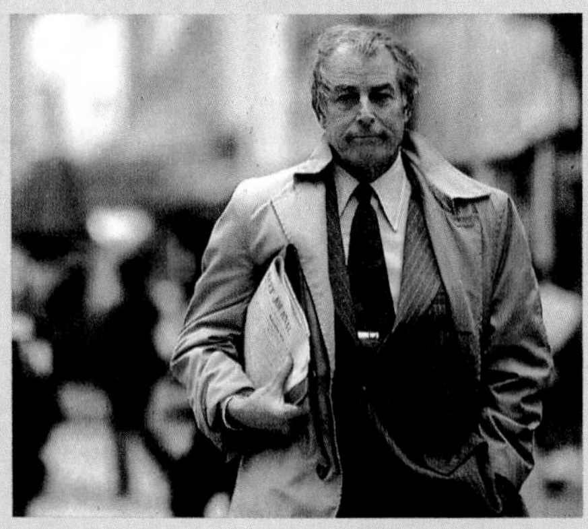

All of us need to take time to care for our bodies.

ULCERS

An unfortunate sign of success can be an ulcer. For some people stress and tension greatly excite the nerves that control the stomach. This in turn increases acid secretion by the stomach's parietal cells. More tension means more acid, and eventually the acid erodes through the mucus layer in the stomach into the stomach tissue or into the tissue of the duodenum. A peptic ulcer results in such cases. Some people are more susceptible to ulcers than others because of a decreased ability of their stomach and intestinal cells to protect themselves from the acid. Recent research suggests that an infection by Campylobacter bacteria may also be an important provoker of ulcers.

Most ulcers in young people occur in the duodenum; in older people they occur mostly in the stomach.[7] The typical symptom of an ulcer is pain about 2 hours after eating. Digestive acids that were working on a meal irritate the ulcer after most of the meal has moved to the small intestine.

The primary risk in having an ulcer concerns the possibility of it eating entirely through the stomach or intestinal wall. The GI contents could then spill into the body cavities causing a massive infection. In addition, an ulcer may erode a blood vessel, leading to massive blood loss (hemorrhage). In the past milk and cream therapy—the Sippy diet—was used to help cure ulcers. *Today we know that milk and cream are two of the worst foods for an ulcer.*[13] The calcium in these foods stimulates gastrin, the hormone that increases stomach acid secretion. Thus this therapy actually inhibits ulcer healing.[14]

Antacid medications are the first line of medical treatment for ulcers. Added to these is a class of medicines called **H_2 blockers,** for example, cimetidine, ranitidine, and famotidine. They prevent histamine-related acid secretion in the stomach (see Figure 3-7). The stomach cells produce histamine, and the diet supplies histamine from the decarboxylation (removal of $-\overset{\overset{\large O}{\|}}{C}-OH$) of the amino acid histidine. By preventing histamine from increasing acid secretion, the H_2 blockers greatly speed up ulcer healing, and so have greatly reduced the need for surgical treatment.

H_2 blockers
Medications, such as cimetidine, that block the increase of stomach acid production caused by histamine.

The person should also stop smoking, if practiced, and minimize the use of aspirin and other aspirin-like compounds.[17,18] These reduce stomach mucus secretion. This combination of therapies along with the use of antacids as needed has so revolutionalized ulcer therapy that changing one's diet is of secondary importance today (see Table 3-4).

Table 3-4

Recommendations to prevent ulcers and heartburn from recurring

Ulcers

1. *Stop smoking, if you are now a smoker.*
2. Avoid aspirin, ibuprofen, and other aspirin-like compounds.
3. Avoid coffee, tea, and alcohol (especially wine).
4. Limit pepper, chili powder, and other strong spices, if this helps.
5. Eat nutritious meals on a regular schedule.
6. Chew foods well.
7. Lose weight if you are now overweight.

Heartburn

1. Wait about 3 hours after a meal before lying down.
2. Don't overeat at mealtime.
3. Observe the recommendations for ulcer prevention.

Is stomach acid also an enemy for those not prone to ulcers? The answer is no. The hydrochloric acid in the stomach enhances the ability to absorb iron, calcium, and vitamin B-12. Acid also minimizes bacterial growth in the stomach; the stomach is essentially bacteria-free because of its acid content. Bacteria in food are quickly destroyed by hydrochloric acid. This reduces the risk of these bacteria either forming cancer-causing agents or leading to food poisoning (see Chapter 19). Thus acid production by the stomach is an important part of the physiology of digestion and absorption. Ideally one should not take a medication that hampers it.[20]

HEARTBURN

Some people are very susceptible to heartburn. This gnawing pain in the upper chest is caused by the backflow (reflux) of acid from the stomach into the esophagus. Unlike the stomach, the esophagus has no mucus lining to protect it. The acid quickly erodes the esophageal tissue, causing pain. *An important dietary measure for avoiding heartburn is to eat smaller meals low in fat.* Large meals containing much fat remain in the stomach longer than lower fat meals. The large volume of chyme then creates pressure in the stomach, which can force the stomach contents up into the esophagus. One should also stop smoking if practiced, not lie down after eating, and avoid foods and other substances that can specifically contribute to heartburn, such as chili powder, onions, garlic, caffeine, alcohol, and chocolate. Each person must discover what bothers him or her and tailor the diet accordingly.

Certain physical conditions can lead to heartburn. For example, both pregnancy and obesity result in increased production of estrogen and progesterone. These hormones relax the lower esophageal sphincter, making backflow more likely. A pregnant woman may find it helpful to eat more frequently but consume smaller meals until she delivers her child. The obese person should slim down to a more normal weight so that blood levels of these hormones decrease. *Adipose,* or fatty, tissue turns circulating hormones into estrogen. Thus the more adipose tissue one has, the more estrogen is produced.

Heartburn that recurs several times a week for a month should be investigated by a physician. Long-standing heartburn may require aggressive medical therapy because it can lead to alteration in the cells of the esophagus, which increases the risk of a rare form of cancer.

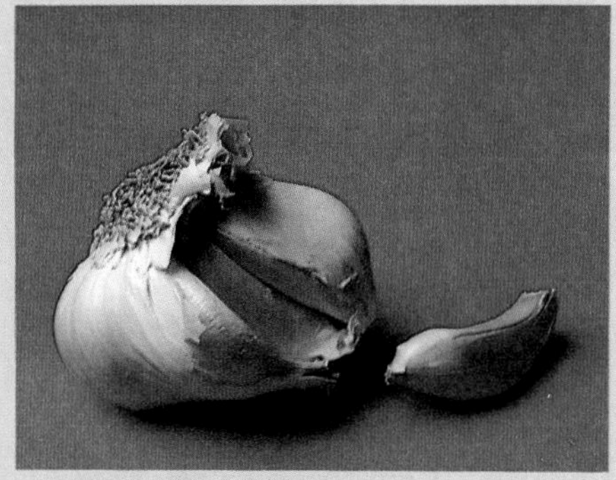

Garlic may contribute to heartburn.

Nutrition Perspective 3-2

Lactose Intolerance

A common carbohydrate disorder is lactose intolerance. If lactose is not digested by lactase in the small intestine, it then travels into the colon. Bacteria in the colon metabolize the lactose into acids and gas. About 2 hours after consuming milk products, the person with lactose intolerance then experiences abdominal distention and gas symptoms associated with drinking milk.

primary and secondary lactose intolerance
Primary lactose intolerance occurs when lactase production declines for no apparent reason. Secondary lactose intolerance occurs when a specific cause, such as long-standing diarrhea, results in reduced lactase production.

Primary lactose intolerance is common in Asians, Hispanics, people of Mediterranean descent, and blacks. However, though lactose intolerance is more prevalent in some races than in others, almost anyone is susceptible. As people age, probably 70% of adults worldwide experience a large decrease in their abilities to synthesize lactase.[2] Although when younger they could digest lactose, as they age lactose from milk products tends to remain undigested. This loss of lactase activity is not due to disease; it happens naturally. If another disease, such as an intestinal bacterial infection, is the source of the intolerance, then that is called **secondary lactose intolerance,** since it is secondary to having another disease.

In the clinic lactose intolerance can be diagnosed from a history of gas and bloating after milk consumption. This history can then be confirmed by having the person consume 50 grams of lactose, which is equal to 1 liter (4 cups) of milk. If the blood glucose level does not rise much after consuming the lactose, poor digestion is the likely cause. Some clinicians prefer using 12.5 grams of lactose, which they consider a much more reasonable (realistic) dose. Other tests can also be performed.

If one has lactose intolerance, *it is not a good idea to relinquish all milk and milk products because these are very good sources of calcium, riboflavin, potassium, and magnesium.* All four of these nutrients are present in other foods in the North American diet, but there are always groups of people who underconsume them. Diet planning for these nutrients is much easier if one uses milk and milk products.

Several options are available to lactose-intolerant people who prefer to continue using milk products. First, they should consume smaller serving sizes of milk products and take them with other foods; this often works,[14] probably because their digestive systems can digest some lactose, but not large loads. Secondly, they can eat cheese. Much lactose is lost when milk is made into cheese. Finally, they can consume yogurt. The bacteria that make yogurt can provide their own lactase activity, so the lactose in yogurt essentially digests itself. However, sweetened yogurt may have as many as 240 kcalories per serving, approximately three times more kcalories than a glass of skim milk—making it a high-kcalorie option.

In the last few years, manufacturers have been producing low-lactose milk. They treat regular milk with lactase that has been isolated from yeast. After a day of treatment, 70% of the lactose is digested into glucose and galactose. This milk tastes a bit sweeter, since glucose is much sweeter than lactose (see Chapter 4).

One can also reduce the lactose content of milk at home by putting drops of lactase into a gallon of milk and waiting 24 hours before consuming it. Lactase can be bought at drug or grocery stores; it works at refrigerator temperatures. Lactase pills can also be purchased for consumption with milk products. Although these procedures increase the cost of using dairy products, the nutritional benefits can be worth it. Thus several options are available to lactose intolerant people, only one of which is abandoning milk products.

Part II

The Energy-Yielding Nutrients

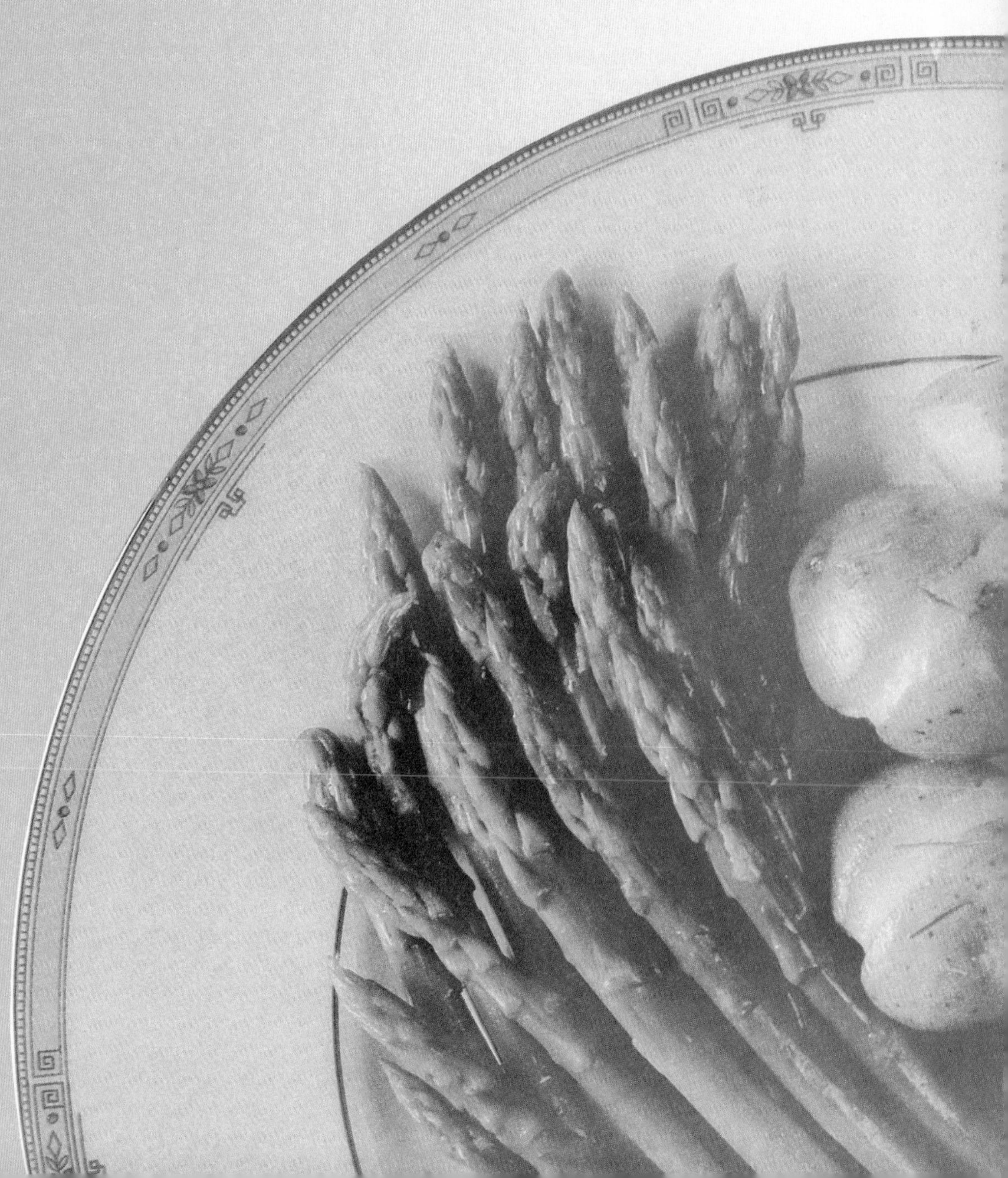

Chapter 4
Carbohydrates

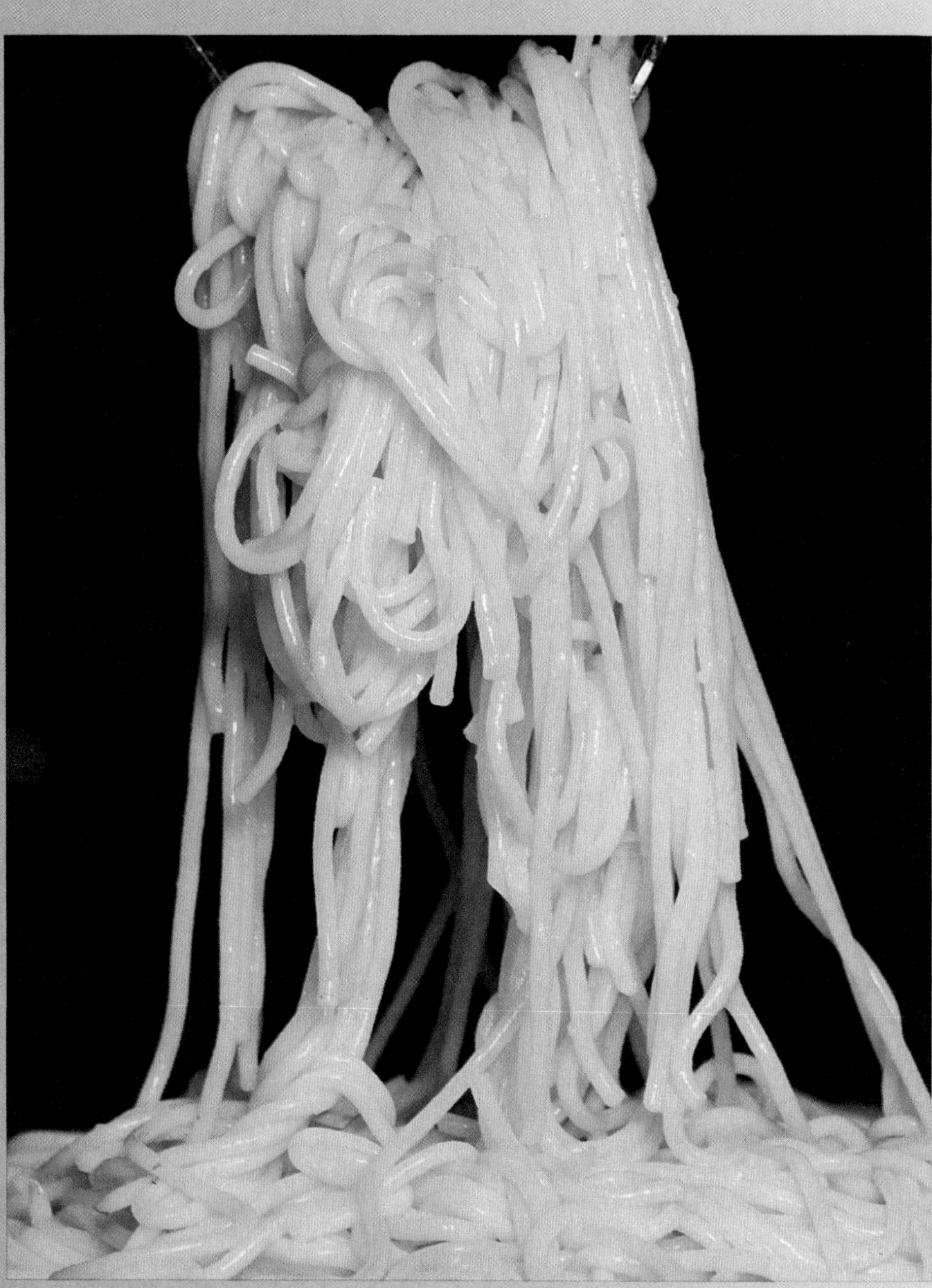

Carbohydrates are the nutrient most promoted by diet recommendations.

Overview

You have now studied why we eat and what we eat, basic tools used to plan a diet, and digestion and absorption of some major nutrients. The next three chapters examine the energy-yielding nutrients—carbohydrates, proteins, and fats. Knowing about them will give you an advantage over the average consumer. Most people know that potatoes have carbohydrates and steak has fat and protein, but few people know what those terms actually signify. These chapters give you the opportunity to learn that, and much more.

It is important to study carbohydrates in detail because these compounds are often misunderstood. Many people think carbohydrates are necessarily fattening—they are not. People also think carbohydrates cause diabetes—they don't. Some people think carbohydrates can make them hyperactive—again, this is unlikely. *In fact, carbohydrates, especially starches, have been the nutrient most promoted by diet recommendations in the last 10 years.*[10] The link between fat—especially animal fat—and heart disease has prompted many nutrition scientists to urge North Americans to switch their focus from high-fat foods to more high-carbohydrate foods.

Nutrition awareness inventory

Here are 15 statements about carbohydrates. Answer them to test your current knowledge of carbohydrates. If you think the statement is true or mostly true, circle T. If you think the statement is false or mostly false, circle F. Take this test again after you have read this chapter. Compare the results.

1. **T F** Common table sugar is called *sucrose.*
2. **T F** Carbohydrates are obtained mostly from plants.
3. **T F** Carbohydrates are necessarily fattening.
4. **T F** The primary role of carbohydrates is to supply energy.
5. **T F** Fiber and "roughage" are the same thing.
6. **T F** There is an RDA for carbohydrate.
7. **T F** The human body uses dietary fiber mainly for energy.
8. **T F** Milk is a source of carbohydrates.
9. **T F** Excess dietary carbohydrate is converted into fat in the body.
10. **T F** Honey is a complex carbohydrate.
11. **T F** No desirable level of sugar intake has been established but current levels may be too high.
12. **T F** Honey is not safe to feed to infants.
13. **T F** Diabetes mellitus is a disorder of low blood glucose levels.
14. **T F** Carbohydrate-loading can help long-distance runners run farther.
15. **T F** Africans have fewer intestinal disorders than North Americans.

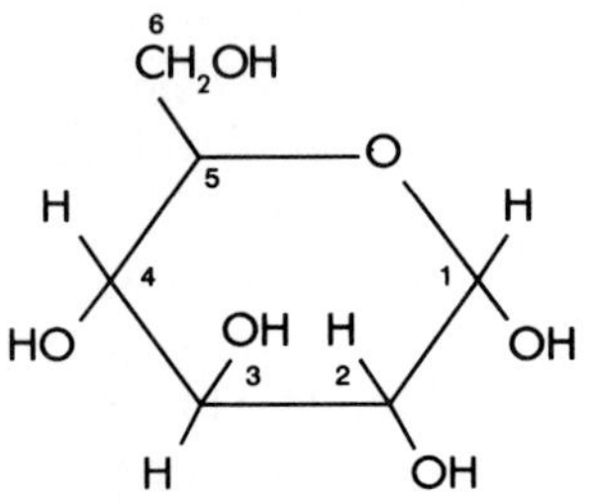

FORMS AND FUNCTIONS OF SIMPLE CARBOHYDRATES

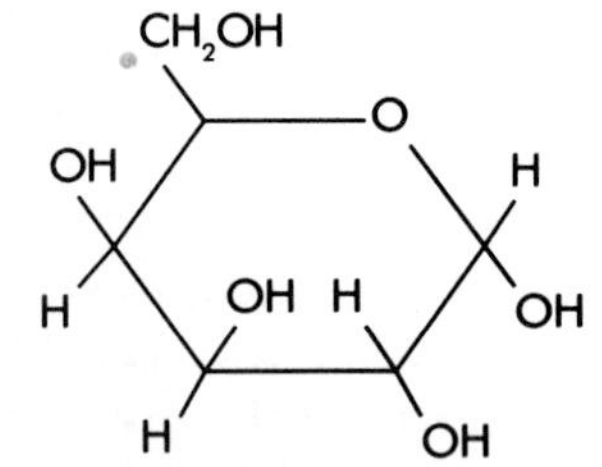

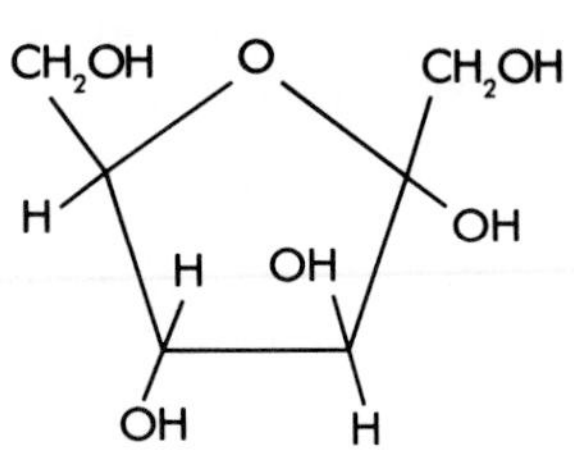

Most forms of carbohydrates are composed of just carbon, hydrogen, and oxygen atoms. These atoms bond together according to the rules we discussed in chapter 2. The simpler forms of carbohydrates are called *sugars,* and the more complex forms are either *starches* or *dietary fibers.*

D-glucose

D-galactose

D-fructose

Monosaccharides

Monosaccharides are single sugars. Glucose is the major monosaccharide. Other names for glucose are dextrose and blood sugar. In the margin, glucose is drawn in the D isomer form; note the oxygen in the ring. Your body can metabolize only this D form. This may make it possible to use the L isomer form in the future as a low-kcalorie sweetener. Glucose is called a **hexose** because it has six carbon atoms. *Hex* means six, and *-ose* is the standard ending used to indicate carbohydrate.

Fructose—also called levulose and fruit sugar—is another hexose, but it forms a five-membered ring containing an oxygen atom. **Galactose** is the last single sugar we will consider. Galactose has the same structure as glucose, except that the hydrogen atom (−H) and the hydroxyl groups (−OH) are reversed on carbon no. 4. Galactose does not exist free in nature in large quantities. Instead, it usually forms part of the double sugar lactose, which is found in milk and other dairy products. The other monosaccharides found in nature, such as **ribose,** (a five-carbon sugar present in a cell's genetic material), are not so plentiful in our diets.

Once you are familiar with the chemical forms of the simple sugars, it is much easier to see how they are interrelated. Glucose is the major sugar found in the bloodstream. Fructose, after absorption by the small intestine and transport to the liver, is quickly metabolized—mainly into glucose, with some into **lactic acid.** After absorption galactose is transformed into either glucose or a storage form of glucose in the liver, called **glycogen.**[23] Chapter 6 discusses a disease that results in the inability to metabolize galactose, and the consequences of this inability.

Disaccharides

Disaccharides are formed when two monosaccharides combine (*di* means two). A condensation reaction occurs: the two monosaccharides are joined, and a water molecule is split off (Figure 4-1).

This reaction forms a **glycosidic bond** (C − O − C). Two forms of this bond exist and are labeled alpha (α) and beta (β). An **alpha bond** is drawn as └O┘, and a **beta bond** looks like ⌜O┘. The corners do not represent carbon atoms; this notation is simply used to represent the two types of bonds. When glucose molecules bond together, we can digest the compound if it has alpha—but not beta—bonds. This will be discussed in detail later.

Glucose bonded to fructose forms **sucrose,** which is the form of *table sugar.* Sucrose is found in sugar cane, sugar beets, honey, and maple syrup. Glucose bonded to galactose forms lactose. Again, our major food source for lactose is milk products. Some people lose their ability to digest lactose as they age and show lactose intolerance. This can cause intestinal gas and bloating as the unabsorbed lactose is metabolized by bacteria in the large intestine, as we discussed in Chapter 3.

Maltose is formed when two glucose molecules combine using an alpha bond. Our major source is germinating grains. As the starch in grains breaks down during germination, maltose is formed. This is done before grains are used to make beer. In the process of beer making, yeast metabolizes this "malt," which is easier for the yeast to metabolize than the original starch in the grain. We have few other sources of maltose in our diets.

Monosaccharides and disaccharides are often referred to as "simple" sugars. Food labels sometimes lump all these sugars under that one category, listing them as "sucrose and other sugars."

Maltose

Sucrose

Lactose

Single-sugar alcohols

A few single-sugar alcohols appear in foods. Today the major ones are **sorbitol** and **mannitol** (see Appendix E for their chemical structures). Another one, **xyli-**

H_2O

1. alpha (α) 1,4 bond (Maltose)

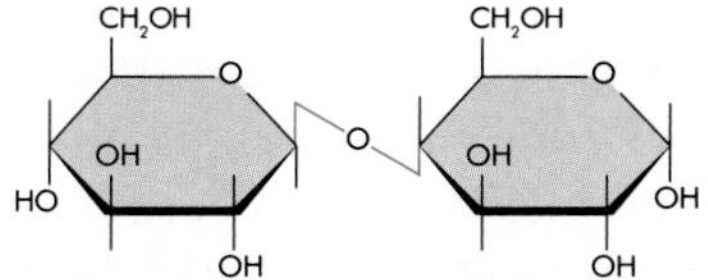

2. beta (β) 1,4 bond (found in cellulose)

Figure 4-1

Maltose is formed using a condensation reaction. Water is a by-product.

Figure 4-2

A dental carie. Bacteria can collect in various areas on a tooth. Using simple sugars, it creates acid that can dissolve tooth enamel, leading to a carie. The bacteria also produce plaque to adhere themselves to the tooth surface.

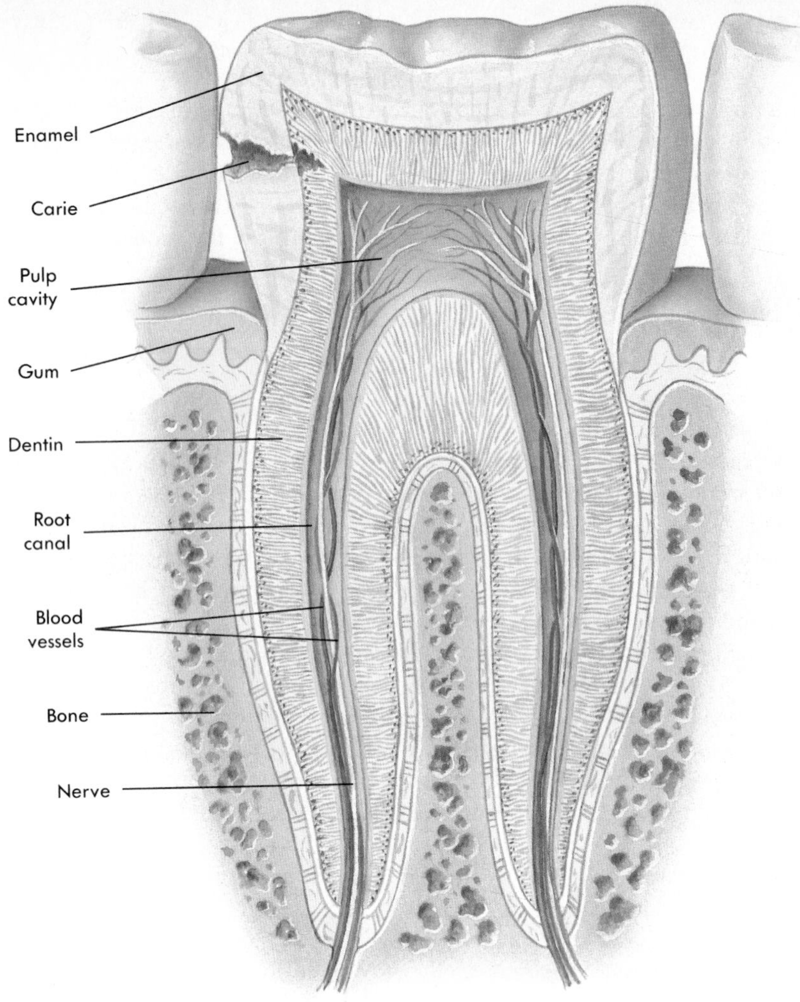

tol, is no longer used widely in the United States, partly because of past safety concerns, although its use is still legal in the United States, and it is used in Canada.[1] Sorbitol is used in sugarless gum. It yields kcalories but is not readily metabolized by the bacteria in the mouth. Thus sorbitol does not promote **dental caries** (cavities) nearly so readily as other simple sugars, like sucrose.

Dental caries are formed when sugars are metabolized to acid by bacteria that live on the teeth (Figure 4-2). The acid then dissolves the tooth enamel and underlying structure. Sticky or gummy foods high in sugars, such as caramels and raisins, are the worst types. These foods are **cariogenic;** *cario* means cavity. Liquid sugar sources—for example, fruit juices—are not nearly as potent for causing dental caries. Snacking regularly on sugary foods is also likely to cause caries since it allows the bacteria on the teeth to continually make acid. Thus the frequency of sugar consumption also affects dental health, in the absence of good dental hygiene.

In the last 15 years, simple-sugar consumption has remained about constant in the United States, but dental-caries rates have decreased by 30%.[1] This decline is primarily due to the addition of fluoride to water. When teeth develop in the presence of the mineral fluoride, they become much more resistant to acid (see Chapter 14).

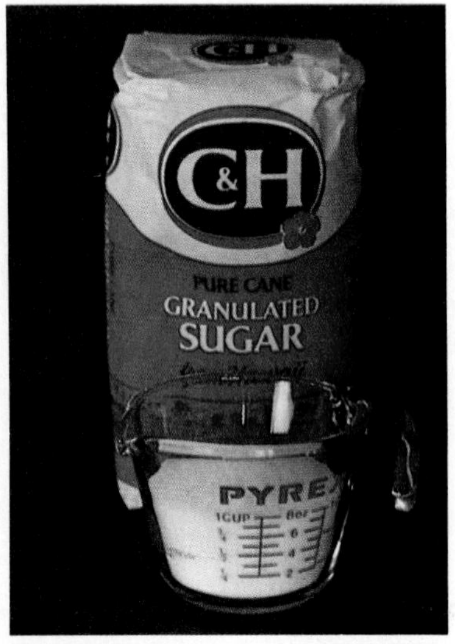

If you can afford the kcalories, sugar in moderation can be included in your diet.

Besides affecting teeth, are the simple sugars bad for us?

Many people think it is not healthy to consume sugars. True, simple sugars by themselves have very low nutrient densities. In other words, sugary foods may supply few, if any, vitamins, minerals, or proteins compared with the number of kcalories they supply. However, if one can afford to consume some extra kcalories, there is probably nothing wrong with eating sugar. Scientists estimate that sugar is mostly a problem when substituted for more nutritious foods. In that case, a person could become deficient in vitamins and other important nutrients.

Some people claim sugar causes heart disease, diabetes, hyperactivity, obesity, and other problems. Little or no credible research supports these allegations. Many major scientific groups have examined the research surrounding sugar and basically given it a clean bill of health, except for its tendency to cause dental caries.[1] (See Chapter 16 for a full discussion of whether sugar causes hyperactivity in children.)

In the final analysis, use of sugar should follow the safe advice given for many other food products—moderation. By regularly visiting the dentist and keeping blood sugar levels and weight under control, sugar can be enjoyed in "moderation," meaning a limit of about 10% of total kcalorie intake.

A common misconception is that honey contains vitamins and minerals. We showed this is not true in Table 2-3. You can prove to yourself that honey is also no more nutrient dense than sucrose by using Appendix A. Only the sweetener molasses, a by-product of sugar production, contains any appreciable amount of minerals. However, our consumption of molasses in foods is very low.

Concept Check

Monosaccharides are single sugars. Important monosaccharides in the diet are glucose, fructose, and galactose. *Disaccharides* are double sugars. Important disaccharides in the diet are sucrose (glucose bonded to fructose), maltose (glucose bonded to glucose), and lactose (glucose bonded to galactose). Once absorbed, the majority of these carbohydrates are ultimately transformed into glucose by the liver.

PUTTING CARBOHYDRATES TO WORK IN THE BODY

Energy production

The main functions of the simple sugar glucose (and so carbohydrates in general, since most can yield glucose) is to supply energy for the body. *Certain tissues in the body derive energy only from glucose, such as the red blood cells and most parts of the brain.* In fact, except when the diet contains almost no carbohydrates, the brain and nervous system use mostly carbohydrates for fuel. Carbohydrates can also fuel muscle cells and other body cells, but many of these cells can usually use fat for energy needs.

Carbohydrates supply about 44% to 47% of dietary energy needs in the United States. About half that comes from sugars and half from starches. Worldwide, however, carbohydrates account for about 70% of all kcalories consumed. In some countries, carbohydrates account for up to 80% of kcalories consumed. In North America and in many other industrialized areas where fat intake is high, carbohydrates supply a lower percentage of total kcalories.

Regulating this energy source in the bloodstream. Under normal circumstances, blood glucose usually varies between about 70 and 120 milligrams per 100 milliliters of blood.[23] If blood glucose rises above 170 milligrams per 100 milliliters of blood, it begins to spill over into the urine. If blood glucose falls below 40 to 50 milligrams per 100 milliliters of blood, a person begins to feel nervous, irritable, and hungry and may develop a headache. Having high levels of blood glucose is called **hyperglycemia.** Having low levels of blood glucose is called **hypoglycemia.**[24]

hyperglycemia
High blood glucose levels above 140 milligrams per 100 milliliters of blood.

hypoglycemia
Low blood glucose levels below 40 to 50 milligrams per 100 milliliters of blood.

Recall that carbohydrates are primarily digested in the small intestine. The resulting monosaccharides—glucose, fructose, and galactose—are absorbed via cells of the intestinal villi into the portal vein. The portal vein empties into the liver, where much of the galactose and fructose is turned into glucose.[23] The liver is the body's main organ for controlling the amount of glucose that eventually enters the bloodstream. Since it is the first organ to screen the absorbed sugars, the liver appropriately serves as guard, preventing excess glucose from entering the bloodstream after a meal (Figure 4-3).

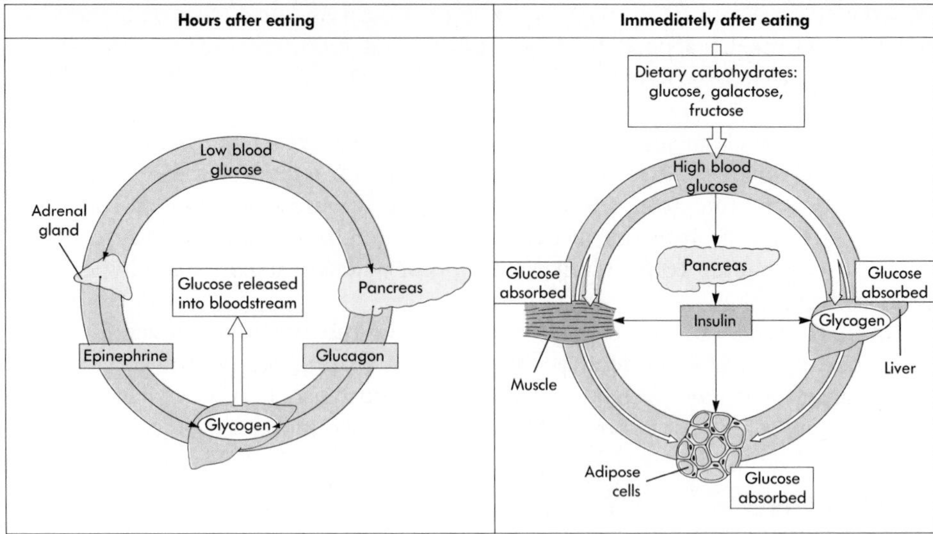

Figure 4-3

The regulation of blood glucose. (A) When blood sugar levels are low, cells in the pancreas release the hormone glucagon into the bloodstream. Cells in the adrenal gland (situated on top of the kidneys) release another hormone, epinephrine, into the bloodstream. When these hormones reach the liver, they increase liver breakdown of glycogen to glucose, in turn raising the blood glucose level. (B) When blood glucose levels are high, other cells within the pancreas produce the hormone insulin. This stimulates the liver and muscles to convert blood glucose into glycogen and initiate other processes that lower the blood glucose level.

Although insulin has a profound effect on carbohydrate metabolism in the liver, glucose uptake in that organ does not require insulin.

Small amounts of the hormone **insulin** are released by the pancreas as soon as a person begins eating. Once glucose has entered the bloodstream, the pancreas releases large amounts of insulin. Insulin affects the body in a variety of ways. It promotes increased glycogen synthesis in the liver to stimulate glucose storage, as well as increased glucose uptake by the muscle cells, **adipose (fat) cells,** and many other cells. By this means, *insulin triggers both glucose storage in the liver and glucose movement out of the bloodstream into cells.* This dual action of insulin is one key of keeping blood glucose levels within a narrow normal range.[22]

Hormones that counteract the effects of insulin. When a person has not eaten carbohydrates for a few hours, the blood glucose level begins to fall. As the level of blood glucose falls the pancreas releases the hormone **glucagon.** This hormone prompts the breakdown of glycogen in the liver, and the resulting glucose is released into the bloodstream. In this way glucagon helps restore blood glucose levels to a normal level.

At the same time, the hormone **epinephrine (adrenaline)** triggers a breakdown of glycogen in the liver and so a release of glucose into the bloodstream. Other hormones, such as **cortisol,** growth hormone, and thyroid hormone also help regulate the blood glucose level.

In essence, the actions of insulin in the body are balanced by the actions of glucagon, epinephrine, cortisol, and other hormones. [23] If hormonal balance is not maintained, such as when insulin or glucagon are either overproduced or underproduced, major changes in blood glucose levels occur. See Nutrition Perspective 4-1 for examples of this phenomenon.

Epinephrine is responsible for the "flight or fight" reaction. This is how the body responds to a threat, such as suddenly seeing a car approaching head-on. Epinephrine is released in large amounts from the adrenal gland and various nerve endings. The resulting rapid flood of glucose into the bloodstream helps promote a quick reaction.

Concept Check

Blood glucose levels are maintained within a very narrow range, between about 70 and 120 milligrams per 100 milliliters of blood. When blood glucose rises after a meal, the hormone insulin attempts to restore normal levels by increasing glucose uptake by muscles and adipose tissues. If blood glucose levels fall during fasting, then glucagon, epinephrine, and other hormones increase the liver's release of glucose into the bloodstream to restore normal levels. Whether a person has eaten or fasted overnight, hormone activity attempts to maintain blood glucose levels within a very narrow range.

Table 4-1

The sweetness of sugars and artificial sweeteners

Type of sweetener	Relative sweetness* (sucrose = 1.0)	Typical sources
Sugars		
Fructose	1.7	Fruit, honey, some soft drinks
Invert sugar†	1.3	Some candies, honey
Sucrose	1.0	Table sugar, most sweets
Glucose	0.7	Corn syrup
Maltose	0.4	Sprouted seeds
Lactose	0.2	Dairy products
Sugar alcohols		
Mannitol	0.7	Dietetic candies
Sorbitol	0.6	Dietetic candies, sugarless gum
Xylitol	0.9	Sugarless gum
Artificial sweeteners		
Saccharin (sodium salt)	500	Diet soft drinks
Aspartame	200	Diet soft drinks, diet fruit drinks, sugarless gum, powdered diet sweetener
Acesulfame	200	Sugarless gum, diet drink mixes, powdered diet sweetener

*On a per gram basis
†Sucrose broken down into glucose and fructose

Flavoring and sweetening foods

From birth humans respond to sugars with a smile. On the tip of the tongue are receptors for tasting sweetness. These recognize a variety of sugars, and even some noncarbohydrate substances. The sugars are not equally sweet; per gram fructose is almost twice as sweet as sucrose under either acid or cold conditions; sucrose is 30% sweeter than glucose; lactose is less than half as sweet as sucrose[4] (Table 4-1).

Sparing protein

Sugars and starches that form sugars are *protein sparing.* This term means that dietary protein can be used to make tissues and perform other vital processes only when carbohydrate intake is sufficient. As mentioned before, red blood cells and the brain require glucose for fuel under normal circumstances. *Therefore if you do not eat enough carbohydrates to yield that glucose, your body is forced to make it from other nutrients, such as proteins.* The process is termed **gluconeogenesis,** which means "production of new glucose". The hormone cortisol stimulates this process, and the liver and kidney perform most gluconeogenesis in the body.

gluconeogenesis
The production of new glucose molecules by metabolic pathways in the cell. Amino acids usually provide carbon atoms for these new glucose molecules.

The source of most of this new glucose must be protein, because fat generally cannot be synthesized into glucose. Amino acids from the proteins in muscles, heart, liver, kidneys, and other vital organs supply the carbon atoms needed to make this glucose.[23] If the process occurs over weeks at a time, these organs can become partially weakened. (See Chapter 6 for a discussion of the specific effects of starvation.)

Preventing ketosis

Sugars and starches that form glucose are necessary for complete fat metabolism. Insufficient carbohydrate intake (intake not meeting glucose needs) leads to an incomplete breakdown of fats in the metabolic pathways. In essence, *"fats burn in a fire of carbohydrate."* Without sufficient dietary carbohydrates, carbon dioxide (CO_2) and water (H_2O) molecules are not formed during fat metabolism. Instead, fats are turned into **ketones**—acetoacetic acid and its derivatives (see Appendix E for their structures). The compounds are called ketones because their structure includes a ketone group $\left(-\mathrm{C}-\overset{\overset{\mathrm{O}}{\|}}{\mathrm{C}}-\mathrm{C}-\right)$. The liver is the major organ producing these ketones.[23]

ketone
Incomplete breakdown products of fat containing three or four carbon atoms. These contain a ketone group, hence, the name. An example is acetoacetic acid.

The metabolic reason for this response by the liver is discussed in Chapter 7. For now, remember that you need to eat at least 50 to 100 grams of carbohydrates per day to ensure complete fat metabolism and so avoid **ketosis.** This prevents the body weakness that usually results from an insufficient carbohydrate intake.

In starvation conditions people do not eat enough carbohydrate, and ketones soon appear in their bloodstreams. Again, this is the normal metabolic response. Part of the brain and other tissues can use these ketones for fuel. In fact, the use of ketones by the brain and other organs, such as the heart, is an important adaptation measure for survival during starvation; it reduces protein breakdown by one third. If part of the brain could not use ketones, the body would be forced to produce much more glucose from protein to support the brain's extra needs. The resulting self-cannibalization would rapidly break down muscle, heart, and other organs, severely limiting the body's ability to tolerate starvation. Thus a person could not exist nearly as long in starvation if the brain could not use ketones for energy.[23]

In untreated diabetes mellitus, ketones are also formed, partly because there is not enough insulin to push glucose into the cells to be metabolized. Diabetic people may have a full load of glucose in the bloodstream but unless that glucose can get into the muscle and adipose cells, it cannot be of much use. The body then acts as if it lacks glucose, and the liver responds by producing ketones. However, in this case the ketone level rises excessively in the bloodstream, eventually spilling ketones into the urine, pulling sodium and potassium ions with them. This ion loss can contribute to a chain reaction that can lead to coma and even death in people with uncontrolled insulin-dependent diabetes mellitus.

Concept Check

The major reason for consuming carbohydrates is to provide glucose for the energy needs of red blood cells and parts of the brain. Eating less than 50 to 100 grams of carbohydrates per day forces the liver and kidneys to make glucose (gluconeogenesis), primarily using amino acids from proteins in vital organs. This change in metabolism inhibits efficient fat metabolism by the liver and can lead to ketosis.

FORMS AND FUNCTIONS OF COMPLEX CARBOHYDRATES

Oligosaccharides

Oligosaccharides contain 3 to 10 single sugar units (*oligo* means scant). Two oligosaccharides of nutritional importance are **raffinose** and **stachyose.** Our bodies don't make the enzymes for digesting raffinose and stachyose, thus when we eat these carbohydrates in beans and other legumes, the raffinose and stachyose molecules remain undigested upon reaching the large intestine. Bacteria in the large intestine then metabolize them, producing gas and other by-products. Plant breeders have been trying to produce "gasless" beans—those without a great amount of oligosaccharides.

Polysaccharides

Polysaccharides for the most part contain many glucose units. Some have 3000 or more. The major digestible polysaccharides are called either *starch* or *complex carbohydrates.* These forms include **amylose** and **amylopectin** in plants and *glycogen* in animal tissues. Most vegetables turn glucose into starch as they age, so peas and corn are sweetest when they are young. On the other hand, fruits, such as bananas and peaches, turn starches into sugar as they age.

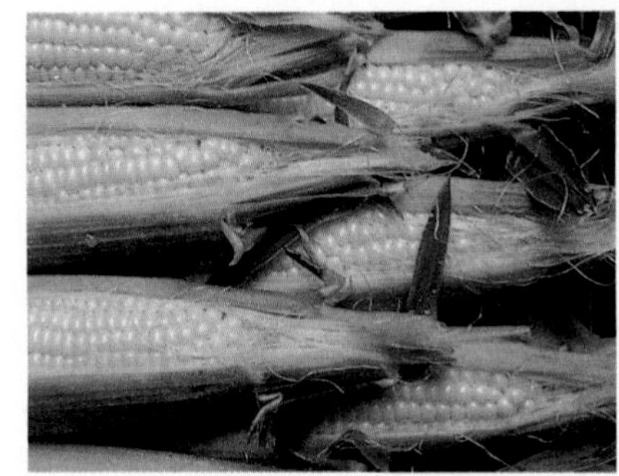

Amylose is a long, straight chain of glucose with alpha bonds. Recall that these alpha bonds can be broken during digestion. Amylopectin has a "backbone" of glucose molecules with alpha bonds, and many branches from the backbone that also use alpha bonds. These starches can be found in potatoes, beans, breads, pasta, rice, and other food products.

The branches in amylopectin allow it to form a very stable starch gel, enabling it to retain water and resist water seepage. Food manufacturers commonly use amylopectin in sauces and gravies for frozen foods for this reason. Manufacturers may also use processes to bond the starch molecules to each other, further increasing their stability. These products are listed as **modified food starch** on food labels.[14]

Another polysaccharide, **cellulose,** has beta bonds. Beta bonds are indigestible, thus cellulose is a part of dietary fiber, not a starch. Otherwise its structure is identical to amylose. The next section discusses this and other dietary fibers in detail.

Glycogen, an animal starch, is made of glucose molecules with alpha bonds and has many branches. Enzymes that digest starches can start digestion only at the ends of the molecule. The more numerous the branches of a starch molecule, the more sites (ends) are available for enzyme action. Because it is highly branched, glycogen is quickly broken down. Therefore it is an ideal form for carbohydrate storage in the body.[25]

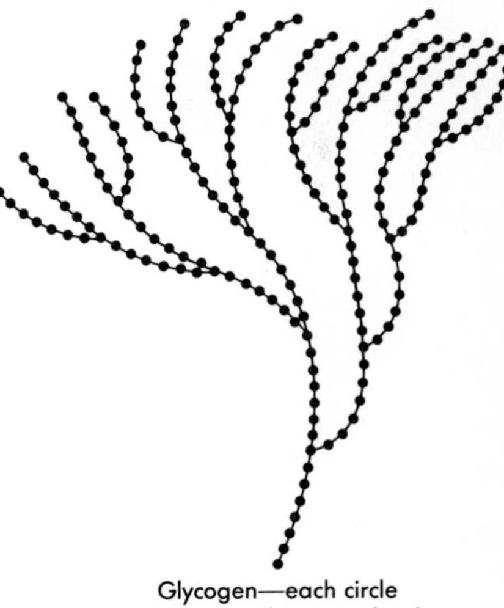

Glycogen—each circle represents a glucose molecule.

The liver and muscles are the major storage sites for glycogen. Liver glycogen can be turned into blood glucose but muscle glycogen cannot.[23] Still, the glycogen in muscles can supply glucose for muscle use, especially during high-intensity and endurance exercise. (See Nutritional Perspective 4-2 for a discussion of carbohydrate use in exercise).

Dietary fiber

Dietary fibers are primarily polysaccharides that are not digested in the small intestine. These consist of the carbohydrates cellulose, **hemicelluloses, pectins, gums,** and **mucilages,** as well as the only noncarbohydrate class **lignins** (an alcohol derivative).[19,27]

Cellulose, hemicellulose, and lignin form the structural part of the plant. A cotton ball is pure cellulose. Bran fiber is rich in hemicelluloses. The woody fibers in broccoli are partly lignins. These compounds generally will not dissolve in water, and so are called **insoluble fibers.** Pectins, gums, and mucilages are contained around and inside plant cells. These compounds either dissolve or swell when put into water, and so are called **soluble fibers.** They exist as gum arabic,

The term *fiber* almost defies definition. Fiber differs from other nutrients, such as the B vitamins, because there is really no common thread among fibers. Rather, fibers are a group of diverse and complex compounds whose single common property is their ability to resist digestion in the small intestine. Even the definitions of insoluble fiber and soluble fiber are debatable. Besides the ones listed, insoluble fibers could also be described as those that are not metabolized *(nonfermentable)* in the colon, while soluble fibers are those that are metabolized *(fermentable)* in the colon.

guar gum, locust bean gum, and various pectin forms in foods, especially in salad dressings, inexpensive ice creams, jams, and jellies.

One workable definition of dietary fiber is: the foodstuffs that remain undigested as they enter the large intestine.[19] Since some fibers—especially the soluble fibers—are digested by bacteria in the large intestine, it is not accurate to say that dietary fiber is the carbohydrate found in the feces.

Bacteria in the large intestine metabolize soluble dietary fibers into products such as acids (such as acetic acid and propionic acid) and gas. Both can then be absorbed, in turn yielding about 3 kcalories per gram. The actual value is still in question.[27] Some gases produced by the bacteria, such as methane (CH_4) and hydrogen gas, increase in the breath when dietary fiber intake increases but this is not harmful.

Another term used for dietary fiber is **crude fiber.** This term developed in the early 1900s to reflect the amount of indigestible foodstuff present in animal feed. The animal feed was boiled for 1 hour in acid, then for another hour in an alkaline solution. The remains of that chemical digestion was called crude fiber; it consisted mostly of cellulose and lignins. All other types of fibers were destroyed by the chemicals.

Many food composition tables still report dietary fiber values in terms of crude fiber. These values often bear little resemblance to dietary fiber values because crude fiber no longer contains many fiber components. This point is important. *When nutrition scientists talk about fiber, they refer to dietary fiber. Crude fiber is just another outmoded term.* Other outmoded terms for dietary fiber include roughage and bulk (Table 4-2).

Table 4-2

Classification of dietary fiber[2]

Type	Component	Physiological effects	Major food sources
Insoluble			
Noncarbohydrate	Lignins	Uncertain	All plants
Carbohydrate	Cellulose	Increases fecal bulk	All plants
	Hemicelluloses	Decreases transit time	Wheat, rye, vegetables
Soluble			
Carbohydrate	Pectins, gums, mucilage	Delays gastric emptying; slows glucose absorption; lowers serum cholesterol	Citrus fruits, oat products, beans

We still need much more data concerning the dietary fiber content of foods. In fact, researchers still disagree on the manner of determining dietary fiber content of foods.[21] All procedures used today lose some dietary fiber in the analysis. This explains why food tables and food labels often disagree on how much dietary fiber is in a given food.

Why do we need dietary fiber? Dietary fiber supplies mass to the feces, making this much easier to eliminate.When enough fiber is consumed, the stool will be large and soft because many types of plant fibers can attract water. The larger size stimulates the intestinal muscles, which aids peristalsis (see Chapter 3). Consequently, less pressure is necessary to expel the larger stool. This link between dietary fiber and the large intestine's function has interested people for hundreds of years (see The History of Fiber in America in this chapter for details).

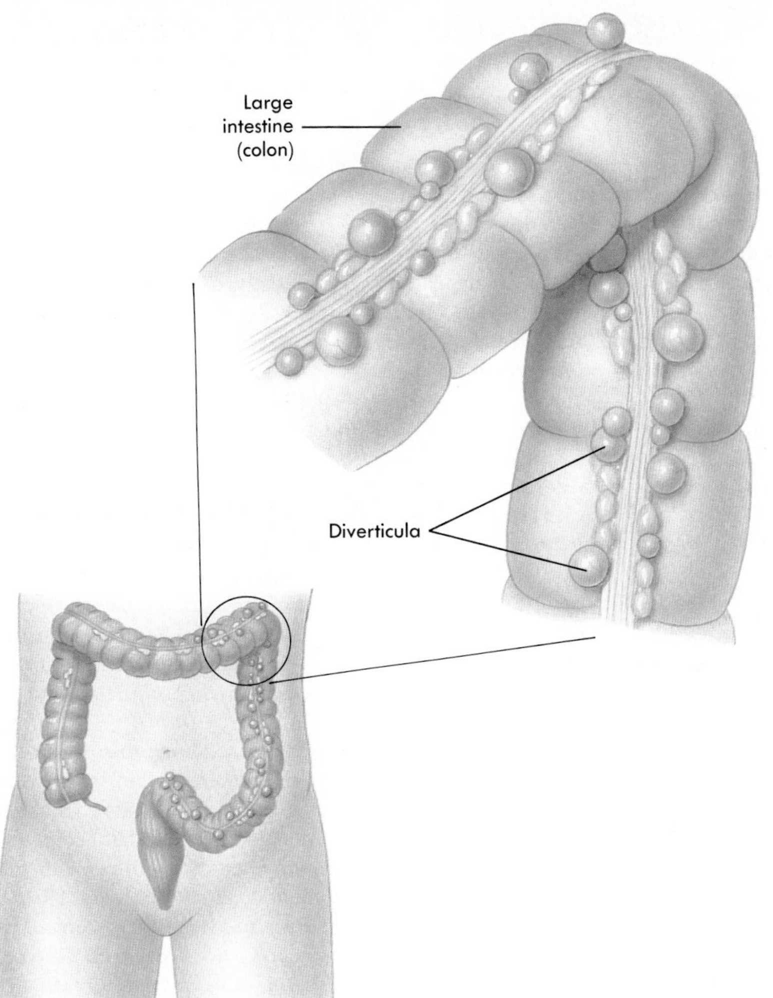

Figure 4-4

Diverticula in the colon. A low-fiber diet increases the risk for their development.

When eating too little dietary fiber, the opposite can occur: the stool may be small and hard. Constipation may result, which may force one to exert high pressures in the large intestine during defecation.[7,18] These high pressures can force parts of the large intestine wall to pop out from between the surrounding bands of muscle, forming small pouches. A person can have many of these pouches, called **diverticula.** About 50% of elderly people have diverticula (Figure 4-4). **Hemorrhoids** may also result from excessive straining during defecation.

diverticula
Pouches that protrude through the outside wall of the large intestine.

hemorrhoid
A pronounced swelling in a large vein, particularly those found in the anal region.

Diverticula are normally asymptomatic; that is, they are not noticeable. The asymptomatic form of this disease is called **diverticulosis.** If the diverticula become filled with food particles, such as hulls or seeds, bacteria can metabolize these food particles into acids and gases. The acids and gases irritate the diverticula and may eventually cause them to become inflamed. This condition is known as **diverticulitis.** Antibiotics then may be needed to counter the bacterial action, and dietary fiber intake will be reduced to limit further bacterial activity. Once the inflammation subsides, a high dietary fiber intake (but free of seeds) is begun to ease stool elimination and reduce the risk of a future attack. In the past low-fiber diets were recommended after an attack but research has shown high-fiber diets work much better.[18]

diverticulitis
An inflammation of the diverticula caused by acids produced by bacterial metabolism inside the diverticula.

As noted above, diverticula commonly occur in the lower large intestine of elderly people in Western countries. These rarely occur in people in Third World countries. The low dietary fiber intake in Western countries, in contrast to that of the the Third World, is probably the major reason for the difference.[6]

History of Fiber in America

Folklore surrounding dietary fiber has been a part of American culture since the 1800s.[11] Sylvester Graham, a minister, traveled up and down the East Coast extolling the virtues of fiber in the 1820s and 1830s. He left us a legacy—the Graham cracker. However, today's graham cracker bears little resemblance to the whole-grain product he promoted.

The next wave of fiber frenzy crested in the mid-1870s. Dr. John Harvey Kellogg was hired by the Seventh Day Adventist Church to manage their health sanitarium in Battle Creek, Michigan. He believed fiber would cure the ills that existed in his time. People came from throughout the United States, including many famous people, to "take the cure" at the sanitarium. Fiber was an important part of that cure. Dr. Kellogg became the first person to earn a million dollars from "health foods."

One gentlemen who came for a cure in 1891 was Charles W. Post. Post saw what Dr. Kellogg was doing and decided he could do the same. He created the Post Toasted Cornflakes Company and started producing Postum Cereal Food Coffee and Grape Nuts Cereal. Not to be outdone, William Kellogg, John Harvey Kellogg's brother, revived the Kellogg Toasted Corn Flake Company in 1906. Today both companies are active in the breakfast cereal market. True to form, the Kellogg Company is still "promoting" fiber to Americans.

Fiber finally received its scientific letters in the early 1970s. Dr. Denis Burkitt, a noted British physician, observed that in Africa many "western" diseases did not exist.[6] These included diverticulosis, colon cancer, appendicitis, hemorrhoids, constipation, and other intestinal disorders. He also noted that heart disease was rare in Africa. Burkitt surmised that the high-fiber intake of Africans was an important reason these diseases did not occur. He noticed that Africans had very large stools, almost twice the weight of stools from Westerners.

Many researchers followed Burkitt's lead. Soon studies showed that high-fiber intakes decreased transit time. That is, by eating more fiber less time is needed for the undigested part to pass through the intestinal tract and be eliminated. Researchers suggested that if stool stayed in the colon for only a short time, less bacterial metabolism of the stool would occur, thus probably fewer toxins and perhaps fewer carcinogens would form.[5] This faster transit time is especially true for insoluble fibers. Researchers also found that soluble fibers can bind cholesterol-containing substances in the intestine. That strengthened the link between a high-fiber diet and low levels of coronary heart disease (see Chapter 5).

As we discussed in Chapter 2, the fiber argument sharpened in the mid-1980s when the Kellogg Company began promoting high-fiber cereals in the war against colon cancer. Actually, the company was following the lead of the National Cancer Institute. Scientists at the National Cancer Institute believed that a verifiable link existed between low fiber diets and colon cancer and thought the public needed to be alerted.

The bold move by the Kellogg Company to promote fiber to Americans has been criticized as premature by many scientists (see Chapter 2). They believe that if fiber intake is related to colon cancer, it is not that strong. Many scientists are still not convinced that a high-fiber diet will prevent enough colon cancer to justify giving fiber much publicity. Fiber is important for regular bowel habits and it can help control hyperglycemia in diabetes mellitus and lower blood cholesterol levels. However, scientific research does not support the promotion of fiber much beyond that.

How much dietary fiber do we need? A reasonable goal for dietary fiber intake is 20 to 35 grams per day (10 to 13 grams per 1000 kcalories).[19] The average North American intake is closer to 10 to 13 grams per day.[20] *Thus most of us should probably increase our dietary fiber intake.* A goal of 20 to 35 grams should prevent much of the diverticulosis that typically develops in Western countries and is not hard to attain, as we will show later.

To help control blood glucose levels in persons with diabetes mellitus, some researchers recommend consuming up to 60 grams of dietary fiber per day, emphasizing soluble fibers.[2] A carefully planned diet is necessary to meet this much fiber recommendation. This also carries the risk of producing a stool too large for comfortable elimination and other problems we will discuss below.

More about soluble and insoluble fiber. *All dietary fibers do not have the same effect on the body* (Table 4-2). Insoluble fibers, particularly certain types of hemicelluloses, are the best fiber source for increasing stool size.[29] Bran, the fibrous covering of grain kernels, is rich in hemicelluloses. Bran adds mass to stool

Dietary Fiber: Different Types, Different Effects

DAVID KRITCHEVSKY, Ph.D.

One of the most enduring dietary interests of the 1980s worldwide has been dietary fiber. One probable reason is that, for once, physicians and other health professionals have been asking us to add something to the diet instead of declaring another taboo. Another reason may be that any substance that is touted to help prevent or cure a large number of maladies—from obesity, constipation, and ulcers to cancer, diabetes mellitus, and heart disease—is bound to garner considerable attention.

What is fiber? Grandmother called it "roughage" and it is presently defined as a plant substance that resists breakdown by the body's digestive processes in the stomach and small intestine. Whenever we eat vegetables, fruits, legumes, grains, or seeds, we're ingesting fiber.

In general, fiber is classified as insoluble or soluble. Insoluble fiber doesn't dissolve in water and is made of cellulose (such as in wheat bran, apples, and carrots), hemicelluloses (such as in wheat bran and whole grains), and lignins (such as in wheat bran, whole wheat, pears, and asparagus). It exerts a "push" effect, reducing transit time and increasing fecal bulk. Soluble fiber dissolves in water and is composed of pectins (such as in apples, citrus fruits, and carrots), gums (such as in oat bran, oatmeal, barley, dried beans), and mucilages (such as in seeds). It doesn't influence stomach emptying but does seems to slow absorption of the products of digestion, such as sugars and cholesterol. This effect is most likely due to its gelling properties.

Except for lignins, which act as binders for cellulose fibers and add strength to the cell walls of plants, all the fibrous substances are carbohydrate in nature and are broken down to some extent (some are broken down completely) by the bacteria in the large intestine. This process produces water, methane, carbon dioxide, hydrogen, and volatile fatty acids.

There is no universally accepted method for analyzing dietary fiber. The method used to provide data found in older tables was inadequate: it crudely measured what was called "crude fiber" (a meaningless term still found on some labels)—completely missing the soluble fibers—while also giving poor recovery of the insoluble ones. Most modern methods are based on enzymatic breakdown of the carbohydrate materials followed by anaylsis of individual sugars. Protein, mineral ash and lignins are determined separately. Although the variations in methodology are complex, all are coming up with similar answers. Accurate tables of fiber content of various foodstuffs are now becoming available.

Whereas people generally think of wheat bran as pure fiber, it is actually as you have seen, a mixture of a number of types of fiber. It even contains some protein, fat, and trace minerals. Soy and rice brans differ from wheat bran in their makeup of nutrients. The age of a vegetable may also influence its fiber composition; thus young carrots contain very little lignin, whereas old carrots may contain 10% to 20% of this material. And the form in which fruit is eaten affects the fiber content. For example, an apple (with skin) has far more fiber than applesauce, and apple juice has virtually no fiber at all.

Not all soluble fibers are alike, either. Pectin, for example, consists of a uronic acid (a carbohydrate) backbone with natural carbohydrate side chains. Oat gum, on the other hand, is primarily a beta glucan, which is a mixture of three or four linked glucose units. Whether one type of structure is more effective than others, regarding physical or metabolic properties, remains to be seen.

In almost every case, insoluble fibers, such as wheat bran and corn bran, have no effect on serum cholesterol levels. Doses of wheat bran as high as 60 grams per day have been ineffective in lowering these levels. On the other hand, 60 grams of oat bran per day does have a cholesterol-lowering action, probably because it contains a soluble fiber, oat gum. Likewise, when 6 grams to 36 grams per day (an average of 19 grams) of pectin is ingested for 2 to 12 weeks (an average of 7 weeks), cholesterol levels decrease by 5% to 18% (an average of 8%). Guar gum has similar effects at similar dosages.

Why do fibers, such as pectin and oat gum, have cholesterol-lowering effects? The existence of several competing hypotheses suggests that none is totally satisfactory. According to one hypothesis, some fibers tend to bind bile acids, which are needed for the absorption of cholesterol. But scientific data are not consistent enough to validate this idea. Another hypothesis involves the roles of volatile fatty acids. The intestinal bacteria degrade soluble fibers to a greater extent then they do insoluble fibers. The acids produced (acetic, propionic, butyric) are absorbed from the colon and enter the circulation. The result is an increase in serum concentrations of acetate and propionate, which have been shown to inhibit cholesterol synthesis.

Are there risks from eating too much fiber? In countries whose populations ingest low-kcalorie, high-fiber diets, there is evidence of growth retardation primarily due to negative zinc balance—since virtually all fibers bind positive ions, such as zinc, calcium, and magnesium. There is always the danger that a diet too high in fiber will lead to a mineral imbalance and, indeed, such cases have been reported. It is easy to overshoot fiber in the diets of certain groups such as elderly people, whose energy intake is normally low. In addition, some people can tolerate more fiber than others. In any case, if you want to increase fiber consumption, do so gradually because your body needs time to learn to deal with the added bulk and to let you know when enough's enough; if the change is made too fast, your body will complain by producing gas and bloating. Expert panels convened in Canada and the United States have arrived independently at similar suggestions for fiber intake. They propose that it be geared to energy intake, and recommend 10 grams to 13 grams of fiber per 1000 kcalories. This amount would provide 20 grams to 35 grams of dietary fiber for the average healthy North American adult. The ratio of insoluble to soluble fiber should be about 3:1, as it is in nature. The same panels suggest that the fiber we do eat come from the grocery and not the pharmacy.

Dr. Kritchevsky is Associate Director and Institute Professor at the Wistar Institute of Anatomy and Biology in Philadephia.

Table 4-3

Dietary fiber values for fiber-containing foods[21]

Food group	Serving	kcalories	Grams of dietary fiber
Breads and cereals			
100% Bran	½ cup	75	8.4
Air-popped popcorn	1 cup	25	2.5
All Bran	⅓ cup	70	8.5
Bran Buds	⅓ cup	75	7.9
Bran Chex	⅔ cup	90	4.6
Corn Bran	⅔ cup	100	5.4
Cracklin' Oat Bran	⅓ cup	110	4.3
Bran Flakes	¾ cup	90	4.0
Grapenuts	¼ cup	100	1.4
Oatmeal (cooked)	1 cup	144	2.2
Whole-wheat bread	1 slice	60	1.4
Legumes, cooked			
Kidney beans	½ cup	110	7.3
Lima beans	½ cup	130	4.5
Vegetables, cooked			
Beans, green	½ cup	15	1.6
Broccoli	½ cup	20	2.2
Brussels sprouts	½ cup	30	2.3
Cabbage, red & white	½ cup	15	1.4
Carrots	½ cup	25	2.3
Cauliflower	½ cup	15	1.1
Corn	½ cup	70	2.9
Green pepper	½ cup	12	0.8
Green peas	½ cup	55	3.6
Kale	½ cup	20	1.4
Lettuce	1 cup	7	0.8
Parsnip	½ cup	50	2.7
Potato, with skin	1 medium	95	2.5
Tomato, chopped	½ cup	17	1.5
Fruits			
Apple	1 medium	80	3.5
Apricot, fresh	3 medium	50	1.8
Apricot, dried	5 halves	40	1.4
Banana	1 medium	105	2.4
Blueberries	½ cup	40	2.0
Cantaloupe	¼ melon	50	1.0
Cherries	10	50	1.2
Dates, dried	3	70	1.9
Grapefruit	½ cup	40	1.6
Orange	1 medium	60	2.6
Peach	1 medium	35	1.9
Pineapple	½ cup	40	1.1
Prunes, dried	3	60	3.0
Raisins	¼ cup	110	3.1
Strawberries	1 cup	45	3.0

most effectively if it is coarsely ground. Finely ground bran does not significantly increase stool size or frequency. *Since bran layers form the outer covering of all grains, whole grains are good sources of insoluble fiber.*

Soluble fibers are the best fiber source for inhibiting cholesterol absorption from the small intestine and for slowing down glucose absorption from the small intestine.[2] Rich sources of soluble fibers include fruits, vegetables, legumes, soybean fiber, **psyllium** seeds (found in many commercial fiber laxatives), dried beans, and oat bran.

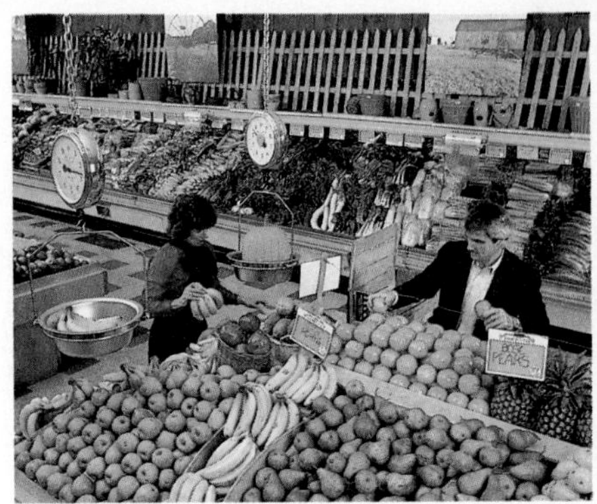

The first step in increasing fiber intake should be towards whole foods, not supplements.

Increasing your dietary fiber intake. Before increasing your dietary fiber intake, first calculate the amount of fiber you are already eating. If it is less than 20 to 35 grams per day, find some higher-fiber foods to substitute for foods you already eat, or add some new ones (Table 4-3). Eating a high-fiber cereal for breakfast is one possibility. *We suggest whole food sources over bran supplement sources because foods can provide a broader variety of nutrients.* This is especially true for many natural high-fiber foods.

Table 4-4 lists a diet containing about 35 grams of dietary fiber but only 1600 calories. We think you will agree that this would be an easy diet to follow if you like fruits and beans. *By eating whole-grain breads, beans, high-fiber cereals, and fruits and vegetables, it is easy to eat enough dietary fiber.* However, some people may need to minimize their intake of foods made with refined flour, such as doughnuts, sweet rolls, coffee cakes, and white bread, to control kcalorie intake. Table 4-5 lists tips on increasing dietary fiber intake.

Read the label. We have already mentioned that a good place to look for dietary fiber is in whole-grain breads and cereals. The way you check for whole grains is to read the label. Manufacturers are now listing enriched white flour as wheat flour on food labels. Most people think that if "wheat bread" is on the label, they are getting a whole-wheat product. *Not so; the label must say whole-wheat flour in the ingredient list.* If it does not say whole-wheat flour, it is not whole-wheat bread, and so probably will not contain as much dietary fiber as it could.

Problems with high-fiber diets

Very high dietary fiber intakes—for example, 60 grams per day—may pose some health risks. *A high dietary fiber intake requires a high water intake.* Not consuming enough water with the dietary fiber can leave the stool very hard and make it difficult and painful to eliminate. Large amounts of dietary fiber may also bind important minerals, especially those with a positive charge, like calcium, zinc, and iron.[16] More studies are needed concerning the long-term effects of high-fiber diets on mineral status.

High-fiber diets also often contribute to intestinal gas. In addition, high fiber intakes may lead to the production of fiber balls, called **phytobezoars,** in the stomach. These have been found in diabetic people who consume large amounts of dietary fiber. *Finally, great amounts of dietary fiber may add such an excess of bulk to a child's diet that energy consumption would suffer;* dietary fiber would fill the child before food intake could meet kcalorie needs.

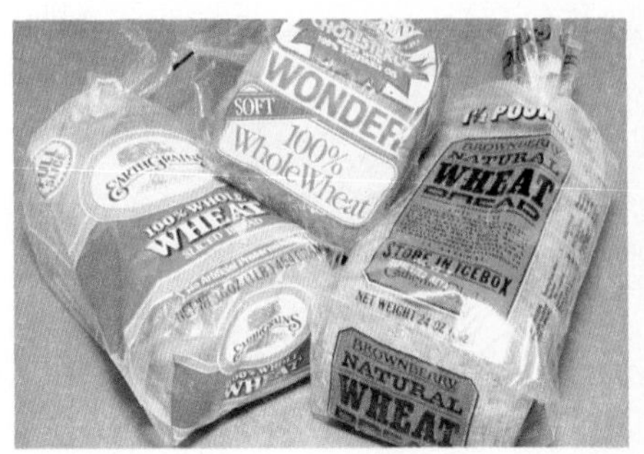

If you want whole-wheat bread, you need to read the fine print.

Concept Check

Dietary fiber has been the focus of human attention for centuries. Fiber forms a vital part of the diet by providing mass to the stool, which helps ease elimination. It is also useful for controlling blood glucose levels in people with diabetes and in lowering high blood cholesterol levels. Some types of fiber yield energy after they are metabolized by bacteria in the large intestine. Whole grains, vegetables and fruits are excellent sources of dietary fiber.

Table 4-4

A 35-gram fiber diet

1600 kcalories:
250 grams of carbohydrate (61% of kcalories)
76 grams of protein (19% of kcalories)
36 grams of fat (20% of kcalories)

Menu	**Fiber†**	**Exchanges**	**Carbohydrate content based on the exchange system**
Breakfast			
1 orange	2.6	1 fruit	15
¾ cup Corn Bran	6.0	1 starch/bread	15
½ cup 1% milk	—	½ low-fat milk	6
2 slices whole-wheat toast	2.4	2 starch/bread	30
1 t margarine	—	1 fat	0
coffee	—	free	0
Lunch			
1 oz lean ham	—	1 lean meat	0
2 slices whole-wheat bread	2.8	2 starch/bread	30
½ cup cooked white beans	7.1	1-½ starch/bread	23
2 t mayonnaise	—	2 fat	0
¼ cup lettuce	.2	free	0
1 pear (with skin)	6.2	1 fruit	15
Dinner			
3 oz broiled chicken (no skin)	—	3 lean meat	0
1 baked potato (medium)	2.5	2 starch/bread	30
1-½ t margarine	—	1-½ fat	0
½ cup green beans	1.6	1 vegetable	5
½ t margarine	—	½ fat	0
1 cup 1% milk	—	1 lowfat milk	12
1 apple (with peel)	3.5	1 fruit	15
Snack			
¼ cup raisins	3.1	2 fruit	30
TOTAL:	39 grams		TOTAL: 226

See Reference 21.

Table 4-5

Increasing dietary fiber

Try this:	Instead of this:
Whole-wheat bread	White bread
Brown rice	White rice
Baked potato in the skin	Mashed potatoes
Unpeeled apple (or applesauce made with unpeeled apples)	Regular applesauce
Orange segments	Orange juice
Whole-grain cereals (hot or ready-to-eat)	Sweetened cereals
Popcorn (lightly seasoned with butter or salt, if at all)	Potato chips
Bean dip	Sour cream dip
Kidney beans on salad	bacon bits on salad

A glycemic index for carbohydrates

Research concerning the body's response to various dietary fibers has led to the development of a clinical tool known as the **glycemic index.**[17,30] This index compares the total amount of glucose appearing in the bloodstream after eating a food with the total amount of glucose appearing in the bloodstream after eating the same amount of carbohydrate in the form of white bread. (Some researchers use glucose itself.)

glycemic index
A ratio that compares the relative ability of a carbohydrate to raise blood glucose levels to the ability of white bread to raise blood glucose levels.

$$\text{Glycemic index} = \frac{\text{Total amount of glucose appearing in the bloodstream within a specified time period (often 2 hours) after eating a food}}{\text{Total amount of glucose appearing in the bloodstream in that same time period after eating the same amount of carbohydrate in the form of white bread (or glucose)}}$$

Predictions concerning the glycemic index of a food often cannot be based on its simple or complex carbohydrate composition. Several factors must be considered, including the food's amount of dietary fiber, the food's digestion rate, and its total fat content. Some foods, such as oatmeal, contain much soluble fiber. Soluble fiber causes the food to gel in the intestine, yielding a slow increase in blood glucose after eating. In contrast, foods such as potatoes are quickly digested, in turn producing a rapid increase in blood glucose after eating. Table 4-6 lists glycemic index values for many foods.

Noting these differences of blood glucose levels after eating has a practical use. In treating diabetes mellitus, the main goal is to keep blood glucose within the normal range (see Nutrition Perspective 4-1). One way to do that is to eat foods that cause a gradual rise in blood glucose levels rather than a rapid rise. Foods with low glycemic indexes provide this. If a diabetic person eats many foods having low glycemic indexes, then each meal in the entire diet will encourage normal glucose levels. A low-glycemic—index diet can then help reduce high blood glucose levels in diabetes, thus leading to better blood glucose control.

There is a danger, however, in relying too much on glycemic index values for the treatment of diabetes mellitus. Ice cream has a very low glycemic index (52 versus white bread at 100) because it is high in fat. Fat reduces the rate of stom-

Table 4-6

Glycemic index values of foods

Food	Glycemic Index
Grain and Cereal Products	
White bread	100
Whole-wheat bread	99
Brown rice	96
White rice	83
White spaghetti	66
Breakfast Cereals	
Cornflakes	119
Shredded Wheat	97
All Bran	73
Oatmeal	85
Fruits	
Raisins	93
Banana	79
Orange juice	67
Orange	66
Grapes	62
Apple	53
Pear	47
Peach	40
Grapefruit	36
Plum	34
Vegetables	
Baked potato	135
Instant potatoes	116
New potatoes	81
Yams	74
Frozen peas	74
Sweet potato	70
Dried legumes	
Canned baked beans	60
Kidney beans	54
Butter beans	52
Chickpeas	49
Lentils	43
Soybeans	20
Dairy products	
Ice cream	52
Yogurt	52
Whole milk	49
Skim milk	46
Sweeteners	
Maltose	152
Glucose	138
Honey	126
Sucrose	86
Fructose	30

Modified from Jenkins DA and others: The glycemic response to carbohydrate foods, Lancet 2:388, 1984.

ach emptying. Assuming that diabetic persons should consume foods with a low glycemic index, you may conclude that ice cream is a good food for a diabetic person to eat. But it isn't. Diabetics must also monitor their butter fat intake. Butter fats tend to raise cholesterol levels in the bloodstream, which can increase the risk of heart disease. Diabetic people are already at high risk for heart disease, so they should not add to that risk. Instead, foods consumed by diabetic people should be low in fat and have a low glycemic index. Thus the diet should emphasize beans, oats, pasta, bran cereals, and apples rather than ice cream and whole milk.

RECOMMENDATIONS FOR CARBOHYDRATE INTAKE

No RDA for carbohydrates has been established. As discussed before, it is important to consume about 50 to 100 grams of carbohydrates per day to prevent ketosis. This amount assumes the diet also contains enough total kcalories to meet energy needs.

It is easy to consume 50 grams of carbohydrate. Just 3 pieces of fruit or 3 slices of bread or a little more than 3 cups of milk will suffice. In fact, it is difficult to follow a diet that *will* produce ketosis. Using the exchange system, estimate the amount of carbohydrates you eat each day. Table 4-4 will help you practice.

The average North American eats more than 200 grams of carbohydrates per day. The top five contributors of carbohydrates to the U.S. diet are white breads, sugared soft drinks, baked goods, sugar itself, and milk.[3]

Table 4-7

Suggestions for reducing sugar intake

At the Supermarket

- Read ingredient labels. Identify all the added sugars in a product. Select items lower in total sugar when possible.
- Buy fresh fruits or fruits packed in water, juice, or light syrup rather than those in heavy syrup.
- Buy fewer foods that are high in sugar such as prepared baked goods, candies, sweet desserts, soft drinks, and fruit-flavored punches and soft drinks.

In the Kitchen

- Reduce the sugar in foods prepared at home. Try new recipes or adjust your own. Start by reducing the sugar gradually until you've decreased it by one third or more.
- Experiment with spices such as cinnamon, cardamom, coriander, nutmeg, ginger, and mace to enhance the flavor of foods.
- Use home-prepared items (with less sugar) instead of commercially prepared ones that are higher in sugar, when possible.

At the Table

- Use less of all sugars. This includes white and brown sugar, honey, molasses, and syrups.
- Choose fewer foods high in sugar such as prepared baked goods, candies, and sweet desserts.
- Reach for fresh fruit instead of a sweet for dessert or when you want a snack.
- Add less sugar to foods—coffee, tea, cereal, or fruit. Get used to using half as much; then see if you can cut back even more.
- Cut back on the number of sugared soft drinks and punches, you drink.

Modified from USDA Home and Garden Bulletin No 232-5, 1986.

In *Nutrition and Your Health—Dietary Guidelines for Americans* an emphasis is placed on starch and fiber in the diet. We suggest you aim for a goal of at least 35% to 45% of kcalorie intake as starches is reasonable. As carbohydrate intake increases, fat intake should decrease.[15]

The average North American eats about 125 pounds of simple sugars per year.[1] Three quarters of this comes from sucrose and one quarter from corn sweeteners. Most of these sugars (two thirds) are added to foods and beverages in manufacturing. The rest is accounted for in what occurs naturally in foods and what is added from the sugar bowl. Overall consumption of sucrose has dropped in the last 10 years but consumption of corn sweeteners has increased. Corn sweeteners are cheaper than the other forms of sugar food manufacturers use.

Exploring Issues and Actions

Do you have a bad impression of sugar? If so, why? If not, why not? Is it a valid position? Can you defend your position?

A goal to avoid too much sugar also is included in the *Dietary Guidelines for Americans.* A desirable level of intake has not been established, but less than 10% of total kcalorie intake is considered a reasonable level.[1] This corresponds to about 44 pounds of simple sugars per year or about 35% of our current intake. Table 4-7 provides ideas to help us reduce our sugar intake.

CARBOHYDRATES IN FOODS

In the Exchange System the milk group yields 12 grams of carbohydrates per exchange. The starch/bread group and the fruit group both yield 15 grams of carbohydrates per exchange and the vegetable group yields 5 grams of carbohydrates per exchange (Table 2-7).

For foods in general, the greatest nutrient densities for carbohydrates are found in sugar, honey, jams and jellies, fruit, and a plain baked potato. They are essentially pure carbohydrate (Figure 4-5). Corn flakes, rice, bread, and noodles all contain at least 75% of kcalories as carbohydrates. Foods with moderate amounts of carbohydrates are peas, broccoli, oatmeal, pork and beans, cream pies, french fries, and skim milk. In these foods the carbohydrate content is diluted either by protein, as in the case of skim milk, or by fat, as in the case of a cream pie.

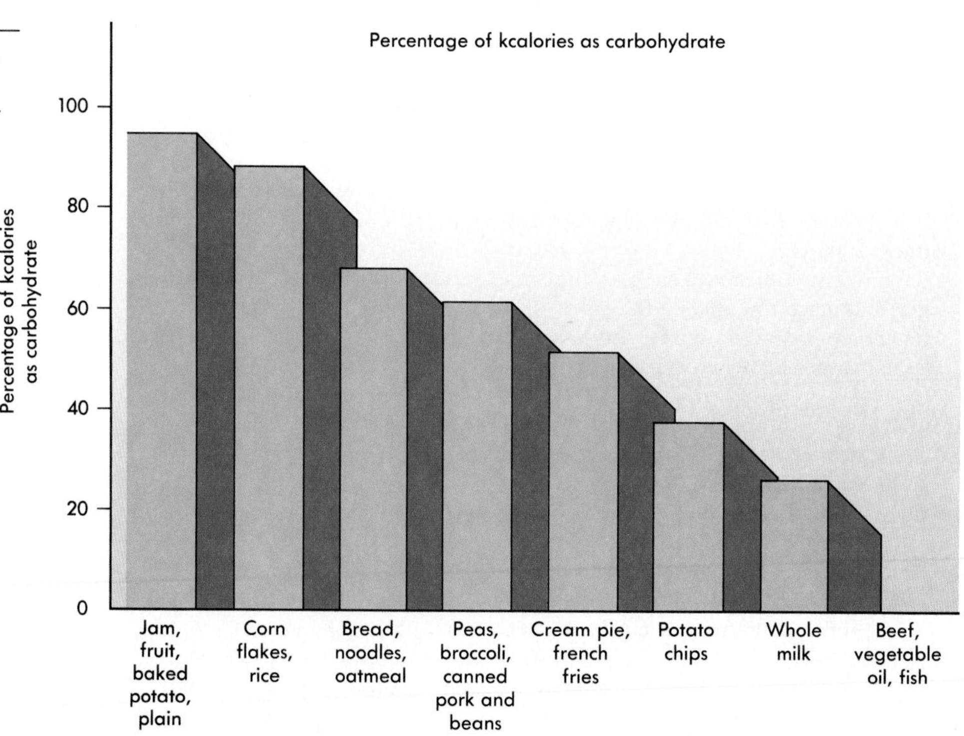

Figure 4-5

Percent of kcalories as carbohydrates in foods. Jams, fruits, rice, and many breakfast cereals provide almost all kcalories as carbohydrates.

Chocolate, potato chips, and whole milk contain 30% to 40% of kcalories as carbohydrates. Again, the carbohydrate content of these foods is overwhelmed by either their fat or protein content. Foods with essentially no carbohydrates include beef, chicken, fish, vegetable oils, butter, and margarine.

Recall that the recommendation for a high-carbohydrate diet primarily means one high in complex carbohydrates.[15] *Figure 4-5 shows that the emphasis for a high-carbohydrate diet needs to be on potatoes, grains, pasta, and vegetables.* A person cannot form a high-carbohydrate diet from chocolate, potato chips, and french fries because these foods contain too much fat.

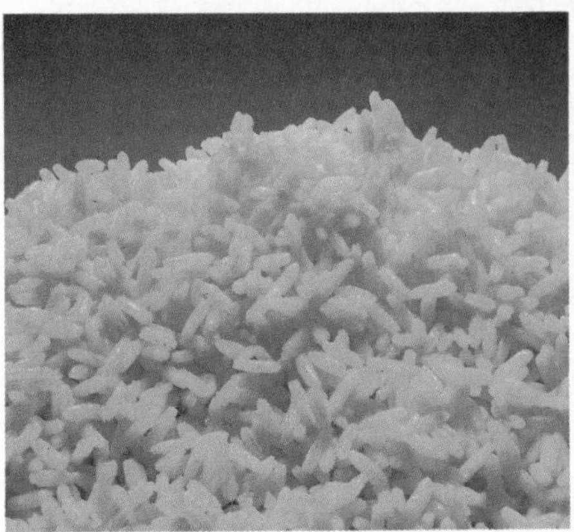

The carbohydrates in rice supply much of the fuel in the Asian diet.

Sweeteners in foods

Sucrose is the tried-and-true sweetener. A relatively new sweetener in food is **high-fructose corn syrup,** which contains 40% to 90% fructose. [1] To make this, cornstarch is first treated with acid and enzymes. Much of the starch is broken down into glucose, then some or all of the glucose is changed by enzymes into fructose. The syrup is usually as sweet as sugar. Its major advantage is that it is cheaper than sugar. Also, it doesn't form crystals and it has better freezing properties. High-fructose corn syrups are used in soft drinks, candies, jams, jellies, other fruit products, and desserts.

In addition to sucrose and high-fructose corn syrup, brown sugar, turbinado sugar, honey, maple syrup, and other sugars are also added to foods. (Table 4-8.) No raw (unrefined) sugar can be sold in the United States because the U.S. Food and Drug Administration (FDA) considers raw sugar unfit for human consumption. Turbinado sugar, a partially refined version of raw sugar, can be sold and has a slight molasses flavor. Brown sugar is basically white sugar containing some molasses; either the molasses is not totally removed from the sugar during processing or it is added back to the sucrose crystals.

high-fructose corn syrup A corn syrup containing between 40% and 90% fructose.

Maple syrup is made by boiling down and concentrating the sap that runs in the spring and autumn in sugar maple trees. Most pancake syrup sold in supermarkets is not maple syrup. Pure maple syrup is available in specialty food shops and from catalogs.

Honey is a product of plant nectar that has been altered by bee enzymes. The enzymes break down much of the nectar's sucrose into fructose and glucose. Honey basically offers the same nutritional value as other simple sugar sources—a source of energy and little else (Table 2-3). However, honey is not safe to use with infants because it can contain spores of the bacterium *Clostridium botulinum.* These spores can become the bacteria that cause fatal food poisoning. Honey does not pose a problem for adults because the acidic environment of an adult's stomach inhibits the growth of the bacteria. An infant's stomach, however,

Table 4-8

Names of sugars used in foods

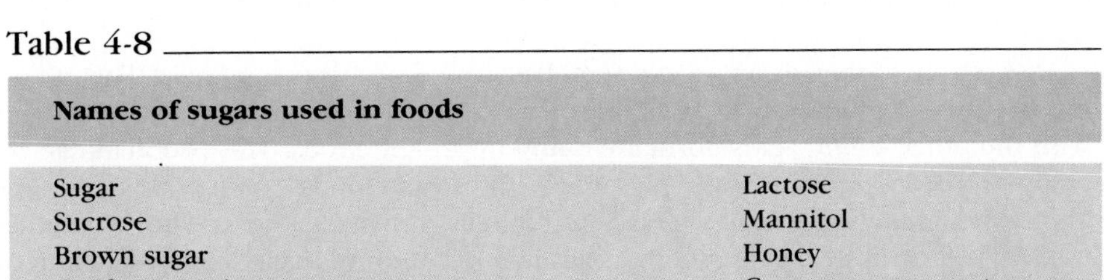

Sugar	Lactose
Sucrose	Mannitol
Brown sugar	Honey
Confectioners' sugar (powdered sugar)	Corn syrup or sweeteners
	High-fructose corn syrup
Turbinado sugar	Molasses
Invert sugar	Maple syrup
Glucose	Dextrose
Sorbitol	Fructose
Levulose	Maltose

does not have a very acidic environment, making infants susceptible to the risks this bacterium poses.

The artificial sweetener cyclamate was banned in 1970 by the FDA due to a link with cancer and birth defects. Some officials at the FDA now believe, after considering new research, that a ban may be unwarranted. Thus you could see it back on grocery shelves soon.

ARTIFICIAL SWEETENERS

Three major artificial sweeteners are available in the United States today—**saccharin, aspartame,** and **acesulfame** (see Appendix E for their structures).

Saccharin

Saccharin, first produced in 1879, has been recently linked with cancer. Laboratory animals suffer from bladder cancer when given high doses of saccharin, especially animals in the second generation after exposure.[1] Arguments continue concerning the amount of cancer actually resulting from saccharin intake. We will further discuss this issue in Chapter 19.

In 1977 the FDA attempted to ban saccharin because of this link to cancer. Many users protested because it left them with no low-kcalorie sweetener (the others mentioned above were not yet available). Although knowing of the association between saccharin and cancer, some people still wanted to use saccharin. Due to this public pressure, Congress prevented the FDA from banning saccharin. Until 1992, when the current moratorium set by Congress expires, the FDA cannot act.

Aspartame

In 1981 a new artificial sweetener, aspartame, became available. Its trade name is NutraSweet when added to foods and Equal when sold as powder. Aspartame is composed of the amino acids phenylalanine and aspartic acid, with the addition of methanol. Recall that amino acids are the building blocks of proteins. *Thus aspartame belongs more in the protein class than in the carbohydrate class.* Aspartame yields energy—4 kcalories per gram—but is 180 to 200 times sweeter than sucrose. This means much less aspartame yields the same sweetening potency as sucrose. Today aspartame is used in beverages, gelatin desserts, chewing gum, and other food items.[28]

Aspartame never has been linked with cancer, but approximately 4000 complaints have been filed with the FDA (as of October 1987) by individuals claiming adverse reactions to aspartame. These individuals complain of headaches, dizziness, seizures, nausea, allergic reactions, and other side effects.

It is important for people who are sensitive to aspartame to avoid it. But the percentage of sensitive people is extremely small—4000 potentially sensitive users compared with 258 million Americans, of whom at least 50% are consuming aspartame. Considering its wide use in food products, the relatively small number of complaints made against aspartame means that most people can use it. In addition, careful double-blind research casts doubt on whether it causes headaches.[26]

Aspartame's phenylalanine content has concerned some people. The blood levels of this amino acid may increase too much if aspartame is not consumed with the other amino acids normally found in protein foods. This problem can be easily avoided by consuming aspartame with protein foods. Some people also are concerned about aspartame's methanol content. However, the amount of methanol in a soft drink sweetened with aspartame is not more than is found in a cup of fruit or vegetable juice.

Overall, the scientific community does not agree that aspartame itself is harmful. In fact numerous scientific and medical groups support its use.[1,9,28] The acceptable daily intake set by the FDA is 50 milligrams per kilogram of body weight per day. This is equivalent to about 14 cans of diet soft drinks a day for an adult. Aspartame appears to be safe for pregnant women and children, but some scientists suggest cautious use by these groups. As more and more foods incorporate aspartame, there is a possibility that more adverse reactions may occur. For now its use is quite limited, therefore so is our consumption of it.

One final note about aspartame. A rare disease called **phenylketonuria (PKU)** prevents a person from metabolizing phenylalanine. (We discuss PKU further in Chapter 6.) Labels on products containing aspartame warn people with PKU to not use the product. Individuals carrying only one PKU *gene* do not have the disease and can consume aspartame. Only someone with two PKU genes has inherited the disease and should not use aspartame.[28]

CALCIUM AND IRON.
CONTAINS: CARBONATED WATER, ORANGE JUICE, CITRIC ACID, NUTRASWEET* BRAND OF ASPARTAME**, POTASSIUM BENZOATE (A PRESERVATIVE), CITRUS PECTIN, POTASSIUM CITRATE, CAFFEINE, MALTODEXTRIN, GUM ARABIC, NATURAL FLAVORS, BROMINATED VEGETABLE OIL, YELLOW #5 AND ERYTHORBIC ACID (TO PROTECT FLAVOR).
*NUTRASWEET® AND THE NUTRASWEET SYMBOL ARE REGISTERED TRADEMARKS OF THE NUTRASWEET COMPANY.
PHENYLKETONURICS: CONTAINS PHENYLALANINE.

Note the warning for people with PKU to not consume aspartame.

Acesulfame

The newest artificial sweetener in the United States, acesulfame (Sunette), was approved by the FDA in July 1988.[13] Acesulfame is 200 times sweeter than sucrose. For the present it can be used in chewing gum, powdered drink mixes, gelatins, puddings, and nondairy creamers. It contributes no kcalories to the diet because it is not broken down by the body.

Some studies show that laboratory animals develop cancer after exposure to acesulfame. However, the FDA's analysis of these studies suggests that the tumors were not due to acesulfame consumption because they could be routinely expected in these animal species studied. Therefore acesulfame has FDA approval. It is already used as a sweetener in foods and beverages in at least 20 countries. Acesulfame can be used in baking, whereas aspartame cannot because it breaks down when heated. So acesulfame may have wider uses. Currently little information has been published about acesulfame. Ask your professor if new information is available.

Concept Check

North Americans consume about 125 pounds of simple sugars a year. About two thirds of these sugars are added to foods and beverages in manufacturing. The rest occurs naturally in foods or is added from the sugar bowl. To reduce simple sugar consumption one must reduce consumption of items that have had sugar added, such as some baked goods, beverages and breakfast cereals.

Take Action

How much dietary fiber are you eating? Write down your estimate of your daily intake of dietary fiber. Then keep a one-day record of foods that have dietary fiber (ignore meats, fish, poultry, dairy products, and liquids—except juices) and determine how close your estimate is to your actual intake.

Food	Amount	Dietary Fiber

TOTAL _____

Summary

1. The monosaccharides in our diet include glucose, fructose, and galactose. Once absorbed via the small intestine into the liver, much of the fructose and galactose is turned into glucose.
2. The major disaccharides are sucrose (glucose plus fructose), maltose (glucose plus glucose), and lactose (glucose plus galactose). When digested, these yield the monosaccharides forms. The ability to digest lactose can diminish as we age. This is especially true for some ethnic groups.
3. The major polysaccharides contain multiple glucose units linked together with alpha bonds. These bonds allow for the digestion of straight-chained amylose and branched-chain amylopectin starches in the upper GI tract. Glycogen is animal starch and acts as a storage form of carbohydrate in the liver.
4. Carbohydrates provide energy, protect against needless metabolism of protein (to supply glucose for the body's needs), prevent ketosis, and provide flavor and sweetness to foods.
5. Dietary fibers include the carbohydrates cellulose, hemicelluloses, pectins, gums, and mucilages, as well as the noncarbohydrate lignins. Dietary fiber provides mass to the stool, thus easing elimination. In therapeutic doses it helps control blood glucose levels in diabetic people and lowers high blood cholesterol levels.
6. There is no RDA for carbohydrates. An intake of 50 to 100 grams should prevent ketosis. If carbohydrate consumption is inadequate, the body can make what it needs to support energy production. However, the price is a loss of body protein, ketosis, and thus a general weakening of the body if a low-carbohydrate diet is continued for weeks at a time.
7. Diets high in complex carbohydrates are encouraged as a replacement for high-fat diets. A goal of at least 35% to 45% of kcalories as starches is a good one. Foods to emphasize are potatoes, grains, pastas, and vegetables.

REFERENCES

1. American Dietetic Association Reports: Position of The American Dietetic Association: appropriate use of nutritive and non-nutritive sweeteners, Journal of The American Dietetic Association 87:1689, 1987.
2. Anderson, JW: Fiber and health: an overview, Nutrition Today Nov/Dec 1986.
3. Block, G and others: Nutrient sources in the American diet: quantitative data from the NHANES II, American Journal of Epidemiology 122:13, 1985.
4. Briggs, GM and Calloway DH: Nutrition and Physical Fitness, 11th edition, New York, 1984, Holt, Rinehart & Winston.
5. Bright-See, E: Dietary fiber and cancer, Nutrition Today July/Aug 1988.
6. Burkitt, DP: Dietary fiber and cancer, Journal of Nutrition 118:531, 1988.
7. Castle, SC: Constipation, Archives of Internal Medicine 147:1702, 1987.
8. Costill, DL: Carbohydrates for exercise: dietary demands for optional performance, Internation Journal of Sports Medicine. 9:1, 1988.
9. Council on Scientific Affairs: Aspartame, Journal of the American Medical Association 254:400, 1985.
10. Cronin, FJ and Shaw, AM: Summary of dietary recommendations for healthy americans, Nutrition Today Nov/Dec 1988.
11. Deutsch, RM: The New Nuts Among the Berries, Palo Alto, Calif, 1977, Bull Publishing Company.
12. Evans, WJ and Hughes, VA: Dietary carbohydrates and endurance exercise, The American Journal of Clinical Nutrition 41:1146, 1985.
13. U.S. Food and Drug Administration: New sweetener approved, FDA Consumer 22:4, 1988.
14. Filer, LJ: Modified food starch, Journal of the American Dietetic Association 88:342, 1988.
15. Hallfrisch, J and others: Acceptability of a 7-day higher-carbohydrate, lower-fat menu: the Beltsville diet study, Journal of The American Dietetic Association 88:163, 1988.
16. Hallfrisch, J and others: Mineral balance of men and women consuming high fiber diets with complex or simple carbohydrate, Journal of Nutrition 117:48, 1987.
17. Jenkins, DJA and others: Metabolic effects of a low-glycemic-index diet, American Journal of Clinical Nutrition 46:968, 1987.
18. Klurfeld, DM: The role of dietary fiber in gastrointestinal disease, The Journal of the American Dietetic Association 87:1172, 1987.
19. Kritchevsky, D: Dietary fiber, Annual Reviews of Nutrition. 8:301, 1988.
20. Lanza, E and others: Dietary fiber intake in the U.S. population, American Journal of Clinical Nutrition 46:790, 1987.
21. Lanza, E and Butrum, RR: A critical review of food fiber analysis and data, Journal of The American Dietetic Association 86:732, 1986.
22. MacDonald, I: Carbohydrates, Schills, ME and Young, VR, editors: Modern Nutrition in Health and Disease, Philadelphia, Pa, 1988, Lea & Febiger.
23. Mayes, PA: Regulation of carbohydrate metabolism, Murray, RK and others, editors: Harper's Biochemistry, East Norwalk, Conn, 1988, Appleton & Lange.
24. Nelson, RL: Hypoglycemia: fact or fiction, Mayo Clinic Proceedings 60:844, 1985.
25. O'Neil, FT and others: Research and application of current topics in sports nutrition, Journal of The American Dietetic Association 86:1007, 1986.
26. Schiffman, SS and others: Aspartame and susceptibility to headache, New England Journal of Medicine 317:1181, 1987.
27. Slavin, JL: Dietary fiber: classification, chemical analyses, and food sources, Journal of The American Dietetic Association 87:1164, 1987.
28. Stegink, LD: The aspartame story: a model for the clinical testing of a food additive, American Journal of Clinical Nutrition 46:204, 1987.
29. Stevens, J and others: Comparison of the effects of psyllium and wheat bran on gastrointestinal transit time and stool characteristics, Journal of The American Dietetic Association 88:323, 1988.
30. Wolever, T and Jenkins, DJA: The use of glycemic index in predicting the blood glucose response to mixed meals, American Journal of Clinical Nutrition 43:167, 1986.

CHAPTER 4

Answers to Nutrition Awareness Inventory

1. *True.* Glucose combined with fructose forms sucrose, or table sugar.
2. *True.* Few carbohydrates are present in animals foods.
3. *False.* Fat contains more kcalories per gram than carbohydrates (9 versus 4 kcalories per gram).
4. *True.* Carbohydrates are important energy-supplying nutrients.
5. *True.* Fiber is referred to as ***bulk,*** but ***dietary fiber*** is the preferred term.
6. *False.* Although there is no RDA for carbohydrates 50 to 100 grams per day is considered an adequate intake.
7. *False.* The body uses fiber to increase stool mass, which eases elimination.
8. *True.* In the exchange system milk yields 12 grams of carbohydrate per exchange.
9. *True.* When eaten in excess of energy needs carbohydrates are stored as glycogen and fat.
10. *False.* Honey, like table sugar, is a simple carbohydrate.
11. *True.* The average North American consumes about 125 pounds of simple sugars annually. Many nutritionists believe that this is too high. A diet including less than 50 pounds per year allows for more healthful foods in the diet.
12. *True.* Honey may contain bacteria spores that may grow and become fatal to infants because their stomachs have yet to develop the strong acidic environment that adult stomachs have. Acid reduces the bacterium's growth.
13. *False.* Diabetes mellitus is a disorder of high blood glucose levels.
14. *True.* Researchers have found that if an athlete eats greatly increased amounts of carbohydrates—about 70% of total kcalories—each day for 3 days before an event, he can greatly enhance carbohydrate storage in the muscles. This enhances "aerobic" athletic endurance.
15. *True.* This was observed by Dr. Denis Burkitt, who attributes this phenomenon to the high dietary fiber intakes of Africans as compared with North Americans.

SUGGESTED READINGS

To learn more about aspartame read the article by Stegink, which provides a summary of the major research surrounding this popular low-calorie sweetener. For more information about dietary fiber study the article by Anderson. Although quite detailed, it is in a very readable and understandable format. We recommend that you read the journal it is published in, *Nutrition Today,* regularly if you want to learn more about nutrition. For more information about carbohydrate-loading, read the article by Costill. It summarizes the effects of dietary carbohydrates on sports performance in various sports and covers carbohydrate intake immediately before and during exercise.

Nutrition Perspective 4-1

When Blood Glucose Regulation Fails

Two problems arise with blood glucose regulation; the major one concerns diabetes mellitus. There are two forms of diabetes mellitus—insulin dependent and noninsulin dependent. The **insulin-dependent form** often begins in late childhood, around the age of 8 to 12 years, but can strike at any age. The hallmark of the disease is the tendency to develop ketosis. A viral infection may play an important part in the development of insulin-dependent diabetes by triggering an immune response that attacks the pancreas, especially the pancreatic beta cells. These cells make insulin. The pancreas then gradually loses its ability to make insulin. When about 90% of the beta cells are lost, blood glucose levels are apt to rise very high after eating because not enough insulin is produced. Excess glucose spills over into the urine. Figure 4-7 shows a typical glucose tolerance curve seen in diabetes mellitus.

The disease is treated by having the person eat regular meals and snacks of a precise carbohydrate:protein:fat ratio and by replacing the missing insulin, either with injections 1 to 6 times a day or with an insulin pump. The pump dispenses insulin on a regular basis into the body and higher amounts after each meal. Regular meals are especially important for people with diabetes mellitus who use insulin because insulin requires glucose in the bloodstream on which to act. This adds much regulation and possible inconvenience to a person's life. However, if the person with diabetes doesn't eat, the injected insulin can cause severe hypoglycemia as it acts on whatever little glucose is available.

Figure 4-6

Glucose tolerance test. These are typical responses seen after eating 50 grams of glucose in a healthy person and in a person with uncontrolled diabetes mellitus.

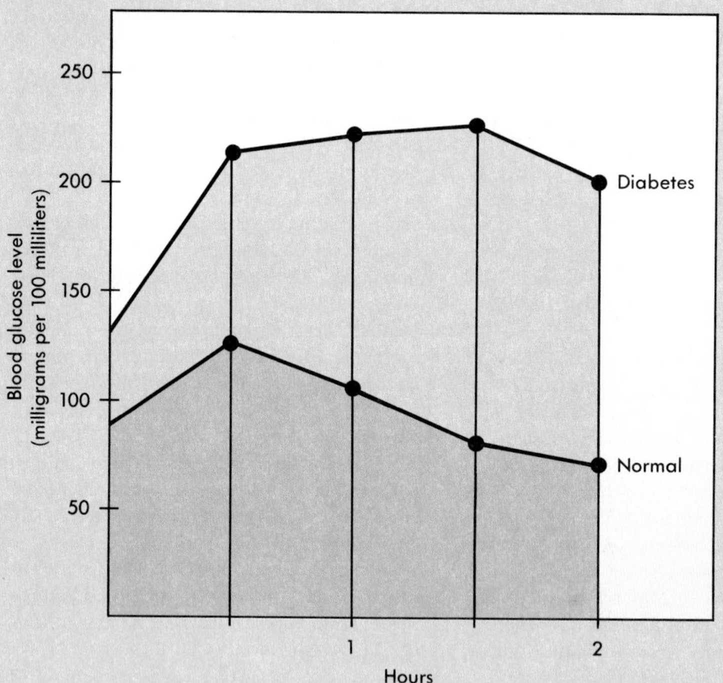

Typical responses seen after eating 50 grams of glucose in normal and uncontrolled diabetic states.

The *noninsulin-dependent form* usually begins in adulthood. Ketosis is not usually seen in this group. This is the most common type of diabetes mellitus, accounting for 90% of cases. *Most of these cases are due to obesity.* Obesity, with its large fat cells, causes an insulin resistance. The pancreas still makes some insulin but body cells, especially the adipose cells, resist insulin action. Therefore blood glucose is not transferred into adipose cells and the person develops hyperglycemia.

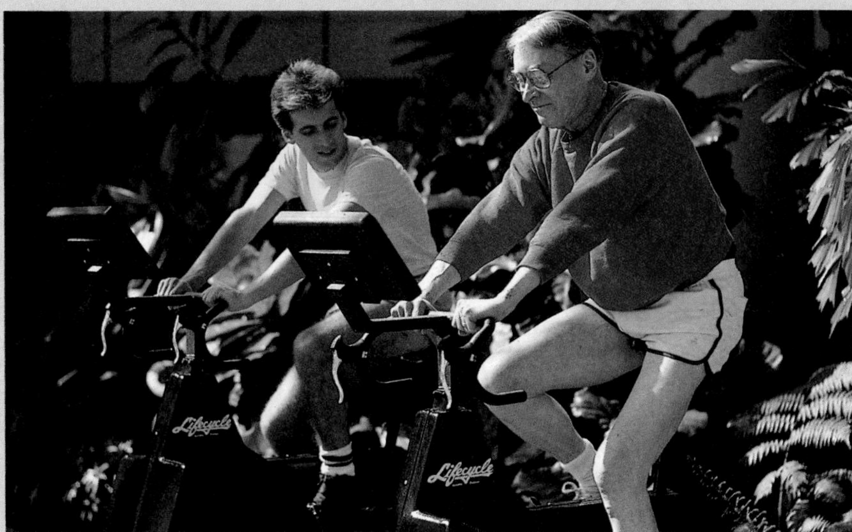

Regular exercise is an important part of the therapy for people who have diabetes mellitus.

If obesity is corrected, often the diabetes mellitus also disappears. People with this noninsulin-dependent form sometimes take oral medications that increase the ability of the pancreas to produce insulin. Regular exercise also helps because the muscles will absorb more glucose, and regular meal patterns help by spreading carbohydrates throughout the day. This helps minimize the high and low swing in blood glucose levels. Sometimes even insulin injections are used.

Although many cases of the noninsulin-dependent form can be relieved by losing excess fat stores, many people are not able to lose weight. They remain diabetics and suffer the consequences of both forms of this disease—blindness, loss of fingers and toes, kidney failure, and heart disease. These problems are due to nerve deterioration caused by high blood glucose levels and to a rapid progression of fatty buildup in blood vessels, which eventually chokes off the blood supply to nearby organs. See Chapter 5 for details on this latter process, called **atherosclerosis.**

HYPOGLYCEMIA

The second carbohydrate disorder is hypoglycemia. This problem comes in two forms—reactive and fasting.[24] **Reactive hypoglycemia** is characterized by irritability, nervousness, headache, sweating, and confusion 2 or 4 hours after eating a meal, especially one high in simple sugars. It is not clear what causes the reactive hypoglycemia. It may be due to an overproduction of insulin by the pancreas in response to rising blood glucose levels.

The second type, **fasting hypoglycemia,** is usually caused by cancer in the pancreas, which may lead to excessive insulin secretion. Blood glucose levels fall to low levels after fasting for about a day. This form of hypoglycemia is rare.

Exploring Issues and Actions

Your best friend eats a sugar donut and has a soft drink for breakfast almost every morning. She also later complains that she has a headache and can't sit still in class. Any clues to her problem? What do you say to her?

To diagnose hypoglycemia a physician needs to observe the usual symptoms and a low blood glucose level at the same time. This level of blood glucose is about 40 to 50 milligrams per 100 milliliters of blood. Some of us have bouts of hypoglycemia and never know it. Just having a low blood glucose level after eating, however, is not enough evidence to make the diagnosis of hypoglycemia. Both a low blood glucose level and the typical symptoms must appear together to make up the whole pattern.[24]

Many people think they have hypoglycemia but few actually do. Nevertheless, *if you sometimes feel you do develop hypoglycemia, the nutrition therapy is one we all could follow. You need to eat regular meals, make sure you have some protein and fat in each meal, and eat complex carbohydrates with ample soluble fiber.* Fat, protein, and soluble fiber in the diet tend to moderate swings in blood glucose.

Nutrition Perspective 4-2

Carbohydrate-Loading

Fat is the main fuel for muscles at rest (how this fuel is used to power muscle and other cells is discussed in Chapter 7). During endurance exercise, such as in long distance running, muscles continue to metabolize fat for energy. However, as a muscle works harder and harder, and constricts faster and faster, eventually it can no longer metabolize enough fat to receive the energy it needs. There is a limit to how much fat can be pushed through the metabolic cycles to yield enough energy. At this point carbohydrate metabolism plays a major role with fat in supplying the energy needed.[8]

WHEN DOES THIS CARBOHYDRATE ENERGY KICK IN?

In endurance exercise, the switch from using primarily fat for fuel to using fat plus a lot of carbohydrate occurs when a person's total oxygen consumption exceeds approximately 40 to 60% of the **maximum volume of oxygen consumption (VO_2 max,** measured in milliliters of oxygen per kilogram of body weight per minute). Little carbohydrate is used by muscles at workloads of 20% to 30% VO_2 max, as found in brisk walking.[8]

VO_2 max is calculated from oxygen intake while running on a treadmill. The technician will increase treadmill speed and raise the incline during the test. Both these changes make the person work harder. The object is to work harder and harder until it is not possible to work any harder. The point right before total exhaustion is VO_2 max. That is the most oxygen one can use (Figure 4-7).

At 70% VO_2 max typical of endurance exercise, fat/carbohydrate use by the muscles is 75% / 25%. By the time one reaches 90 to 100% of VO_2 max, carbohydrate is the dominant energy source for muscles. *If one wants to perform workloads at or above 70% of VO_2 max for more than an hour (a 3 hour marathon is run at 60% to 70% VO_2 max), a lot of carbohydrate must be stored in the muscles.* Endurance at this level of exertion for

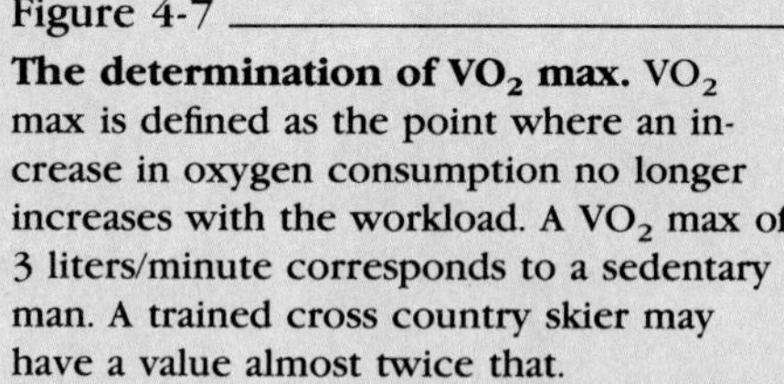

Figure 4-7

The determination of VO_2 max. VO_2 max is defined as the point where an increase in oxygen consumption no longer increases with the workload. A VO_2 max of 3 liters/minute corresponds to a sedentary man. A trained cross country skier may have a value almost twice that.

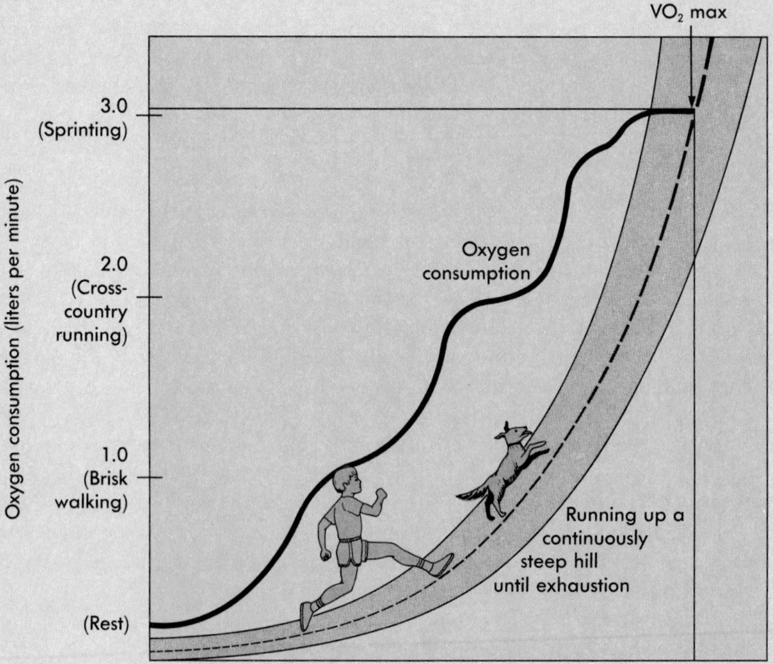

VO_2 max is where oxygen consumption no longer increases with a further increase in workload. A VO_2 max of 3 liters per minute corresponds to a sedentary man. A trained cross country skier may have a value almost twice that high.

Table 4-9

A 600-gram carbohydrate diet

4000 kcalories:

623 grams of carbohydrates	(61% of kcalories)
139 grams of protein	(14% of kcalories)
118 grams of fat	(26% of kcalories)

Menu	Carbohydrate (grams)
Breakfast	
1 orange	14
2 cups oatmeal	50
1 cup skim milk	12
2 bran muffins	48
Snack	
¾ cup chopped dates	98
Lunch	
Lettuce salad:	
1 cup romaine lettuce	2
1 cup garbanzo beans	45
½ cup alfalfa sprouts	5.5
2 Tablespoon French dressing	2
3 cups macaroni and cheese	80
1 cup apple juice	28
Snack	
2 slices whole-wheat toast	26
1 teaspoon margarine	—
2 Tablespoon jam	14
Dinner	
2 ounce turkey breast (no skin)	—
2 cups mashed potatoes	74
1 cup peas and onions	23
1 banana	27
1 cup skim milk	12
Snack	
1 cup pasta with	33
2 teaspoon margarine and	—
2 Tablespoon parmesan cheese	—
1 cup cranberry juice	36
TOTAL	628 grams

Continued.

Nutrition Perspective 4-2, cont'd

Carbohydrate-Loading

more than an hour is closely tied to the amount of glycogen stored in the muscles.[8] When carbohydrate fuel is gone, it is not possible to maintain the high initial workload. Athletes call this "hitting the wall."

CARBOHYDRATE-LOADING

If a person works at levels of exertion greater than 70% of VO_2 max for more than an hour, it may be wise to increase the amount of carbohydrate stored in muscles. This is called **carbohydrate-loading.** Carbohydrate-loading can double the usual storage of muscle glycogen.[8,12]

carbohydrate-loading
A process where a 600-gram carbohydrate intake (or an intake of 70% of total energy as carbohydrate, whichever is larger) is consumed for 7 days before an athletic event in an attempt to increase muscle glycogen stores.

Carbohydrate-loading requires some complicated procedures involving about 7 days of alternating hard and light workouts while alternating high- and low-carbohydrate diets. This process becomes is very time-consuming. In addition, training is difficult during the low-carbohydrate phase because of the limited glycogen stores produced. *Researchers have found recently that a simpler procedure is to eat 70% of total kcalories, or 600 grams (whichever is greater) of carbohydrates each day for 7 days before an event while gradually decreasing activity. Carbohydrate (glycogen) storage in muscles will then be greatly enhanced.* (See Table 4-9 provides for an example of a 600-gram carbohydrate diet.) Most of the carbohydrate should be eaten within 2 hours of ending training because the rate of glycogen synthesis is greatest then. To maximize these stores for the event, the person should also rest for the 24 hours immediately before the event.

A 600-gram carbohydrate diet is necessary only for endurance events (those lasting an hour or longer) or during intensive training for endurance events. A 350-gram intake will keep muscle glycogen at a sufficient level for most sports events.

One disadvantage to carbohydrate loading is that 2.6 grams of water are stored with every gram of glycogen stored in the muscles. This water adds weight and may cause muscle stiffness. Some people choose to not practice carbohydrate-loading because of this extra weight and stiffness.

Sports nutritionists emphasize the need to distinguish between a high-carbohydrate meal and a high-carbohydrate/high-fat meal.[25] Before endurance events, such as marathons or triathalons, some athletes attempt carbohydrate-loading by eating potato chips, french fries, banana cream pie, and pastries. These foods do contain carbohydrate but they also contain a lot of fat. *Better foods for carbohydrate-loading are those high mostly in starches, such as spaghetti and other noodles, rice, mashed potatoes, and oatmeal.*

People considering carbohydrate-loading should try it once before an important event to experience its effects on performance. In this way they can determine if it is worth the effort. They should also realize that for extremely long endurance events, such as ultramarathons, even carbohydrate-loading will not suffice. Carbohydrate must be consumed during such events to keep glucose continuously available for muscle energy production.

Chapter 5
Lipids

Overview

Lipids (fats and oils) in our diets are the nutrients that probably concern us most. Lipids contain more than twice the kcalories per gram (9 instead of just 4) compared with proteins and carbohydrates. Dietary saturated fats are closely linked to high serum cholesterol levels and consequently to the risk of developing heart disease. Some concern about lipids is warranted, but lipids also play several very important roles in the body and in foods. Their presence in the diet is vital to health. Let's look at the lipids in detail—their functions, metabolism, food sources, and links to the major "killer" diseases, heart disease and cancer.

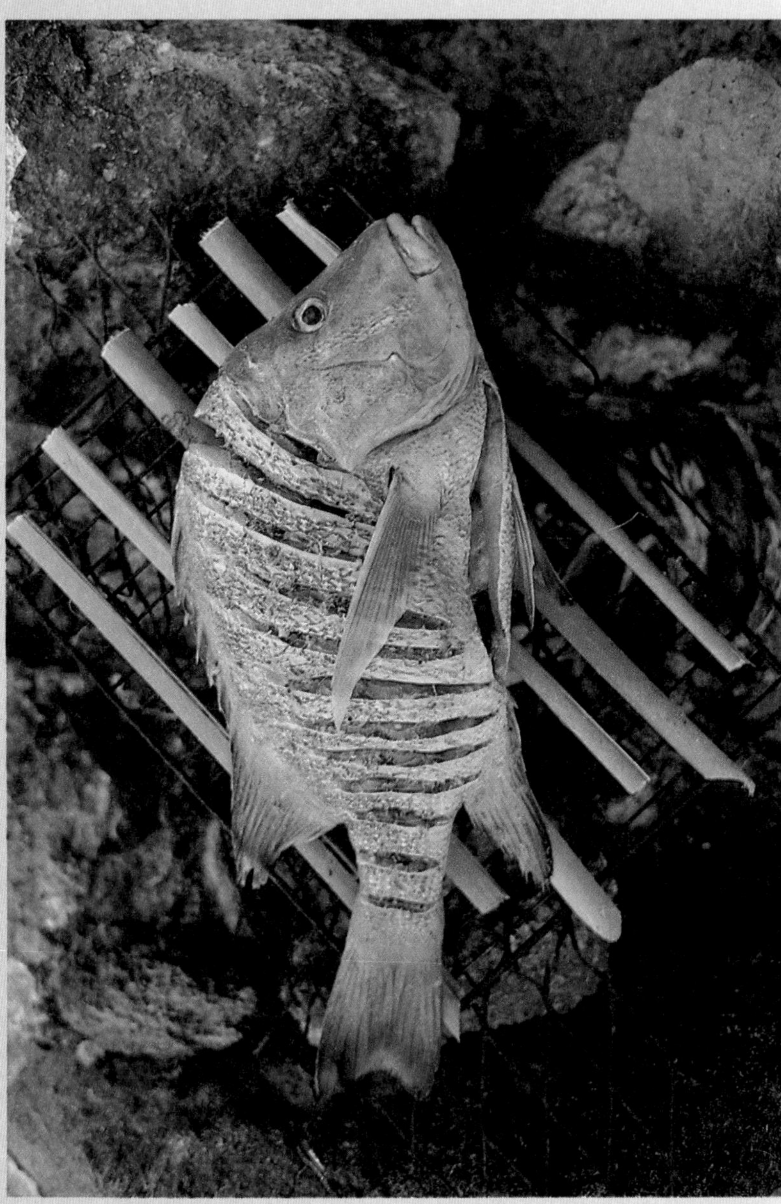

Fish oils have received much publicity lately; many health authorities encourage weekly fish consumption.

Nutrition awareness inventory

Here are 15 statements about carbohydrates. Answer them to test your current knowledge of carbohydrates. If you think the statement is true or mostly true, circle T. If you think the statement is false or mostly false, circle F. Take this test again after you have read this chapter. Compare the results.

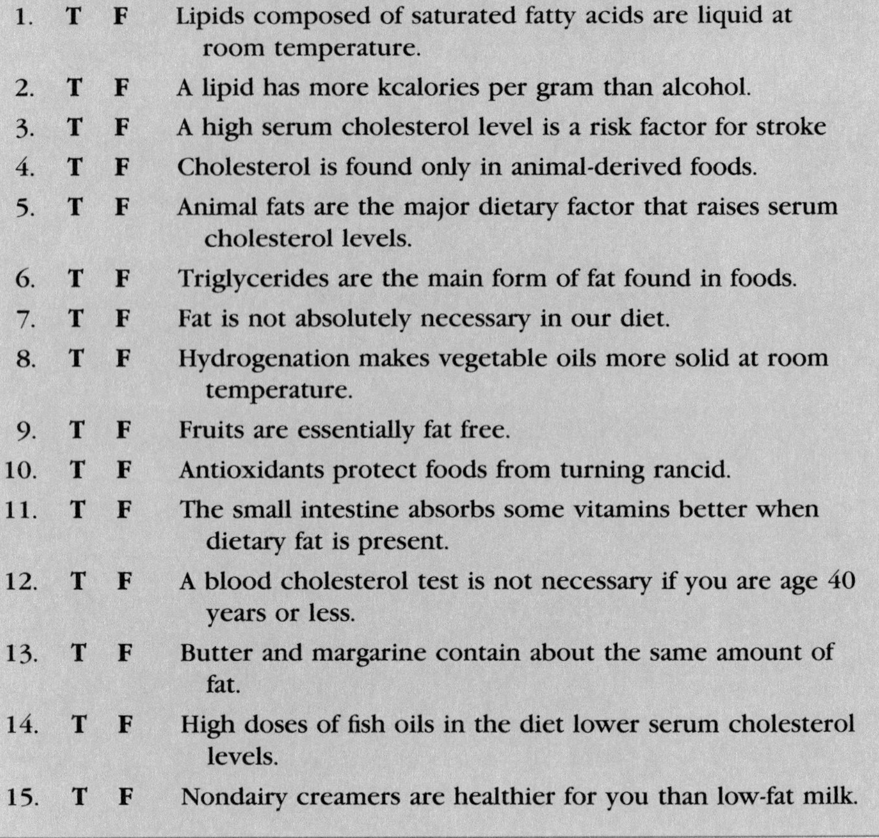

1. **T F** Lipids composed of saturated fatty acids are liquid at room temperature.
2. **T F** A lipid has more kcalories per gram than alcohol.
3. **T F** A high serum cholesterol level is a risk factor for stroke
4. **T F** Cholesterol is found only in animal-derived foods.
5. **T F** Animal fats are the major dietary factor that raises serum cholesterol levels.
6. **T F** Triglycerides are the main form of fat found in foods.
7. **T F** Fat is not absolutely necessary in our diet.
8. **T F** Hydrogenation makes vegetable oils more solid at room temperature.
9. **T F** Fruits are essentially fat free.
10. **T F** Antioxidants protect foods from turning rancid.
11. **T F** The small intestine absorbs some vitamins better when dietary fat is present.
12. **T F** A blood cholesterol test is not necessary if you are age 40 years or less.
13. **T F** Butter and margarine contain about the same amount of fat.
14. **T F** High doses of fish oils in the diet lower serum cholesterol levels.
15. **T F** Nondairy creamers are healthier for you than low-fat milk.

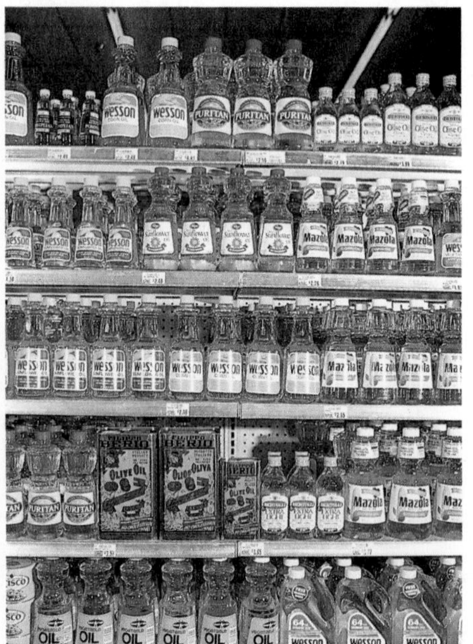

A small amount of vegetable oil in a diet makes a healthful contribution.

You probably know lipids as fats and oils. At room temperature, fats are solid and oils are liquid. Referring to them both as lipids simplifies the terminology, and considering a food's temperature is now irrelevant. Otherwise, butter can be an oil on a hot day and a fat on a cold day.

Lipids are a diverse group, but they share one main characteristic: they all dissolve in chloroform, benzene, and ether. They also contain fewer oxygen atoms per carbon atom than do carbohydrates, protein, or alcohol.[8] Little else relates some types of lipid to others. Compare the structures of lecithin and cholesterol as these are discussed in the following pages for an example.

When we discuss lipid chemistry or metabolism, we will use the term *lipid* or the actual name of the compound, such as serum triglycerides. When we discuss lipids in foods, we will use the terms *fats,* or *fats and oils.* This usage is common today in health care settings.

FREE FATTY ACIDS

The **fatty acid** is common to most lipids in the body and in foods. Its basic structure is a long chain of carbon atoms bonded to hydrogen atoms. At the end of the molecule is an acid group $(\text{—}\overset{\text{O}}{\overset{\|}{\text{C}}}\text{—OH})$ (Figure 5-1).

If all bonds between carbon atoms are single bonds, a fatty acid is called **saturated.** Animal fats are often high in saturated fatty acids. If a fatty acid has one double bond, it is **monounsaturated.** Olive and canola oils have a high percentage of these. If two or more bonds between carbon atoms are double

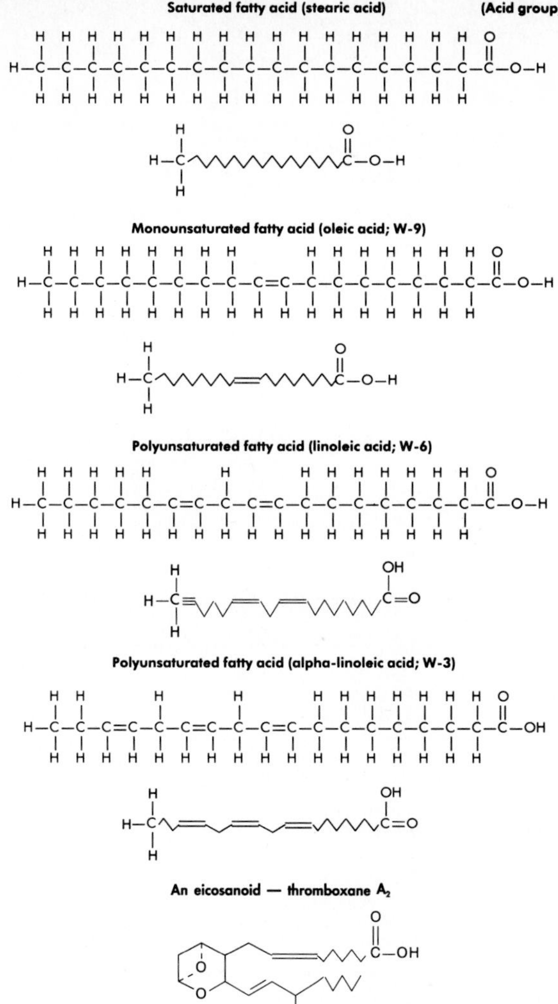

Figure 5-1

The family of fatty acids found in foods.

bonds, the fatty acid is **polyunsaturated.** Corn, soybeans, and safflower oils are good sources of polyunsaturated fatty acids (Table 5-1).

The point at which the double bonds begin in the fatty acid can make a big difference in how the body metabolizes it. If the double bonds start after the third carbon atom from the methyl end ($-CH_3$), it is an **omega-3 (w-3) fatty acid.** If the double bonds start after the sixth carbonator from the methyl end, it is an **omega-6 (w-6) fatty acid,** and so on (Figure 5-1). ***Alpha-linolenic acid** is the major omega-3 fatty acid in food; **linoleic acid** is the major omega-6 fatty acid; oleic acid is the major omega-9 fatty acid.*

Humans can obtain omega-3 and omega-6 fatty acids only by ingesting them.[8] When a human cell builds a fatty acid, it can't create double bonds in these sites. A human cell can only produce double bonds after the ninth carbon atom. Nevertheless, omega-3 and omega-6 fatty acids only form parts of vital structures in the body—they perform roles in immune system activity and vision, help form cell membranes, and produce hormone-like compounds called **eicosanoids.** So we must eat these fatty acids to maintain health

Another terminology used in place of omega-3 (w-3) and omega-6 (w-6) is *n-3* and *n-6.* Both n and omega represent the same thing: the number of the carbon atom where the double bonds begin, counting from the methyl end.

Essential fatty acids

Because some polyunsaturated fatty acids—linoleic acid and alpha-linolenic acid—are available to us only by ingestion, they are called **essential fatty acids.** The RDA states that people need to consume about 1% to 2% of their total kcalories from linoleic acid; current consumption is 7%. Up to 10% of kcalories from polyunsaturated fatty acids is generally recommended as a safe upper level. Since many plant oils—corn, soybean, sunflower, and safflower oils—contain over

Table 5-1

Comparison of Dietary Fats

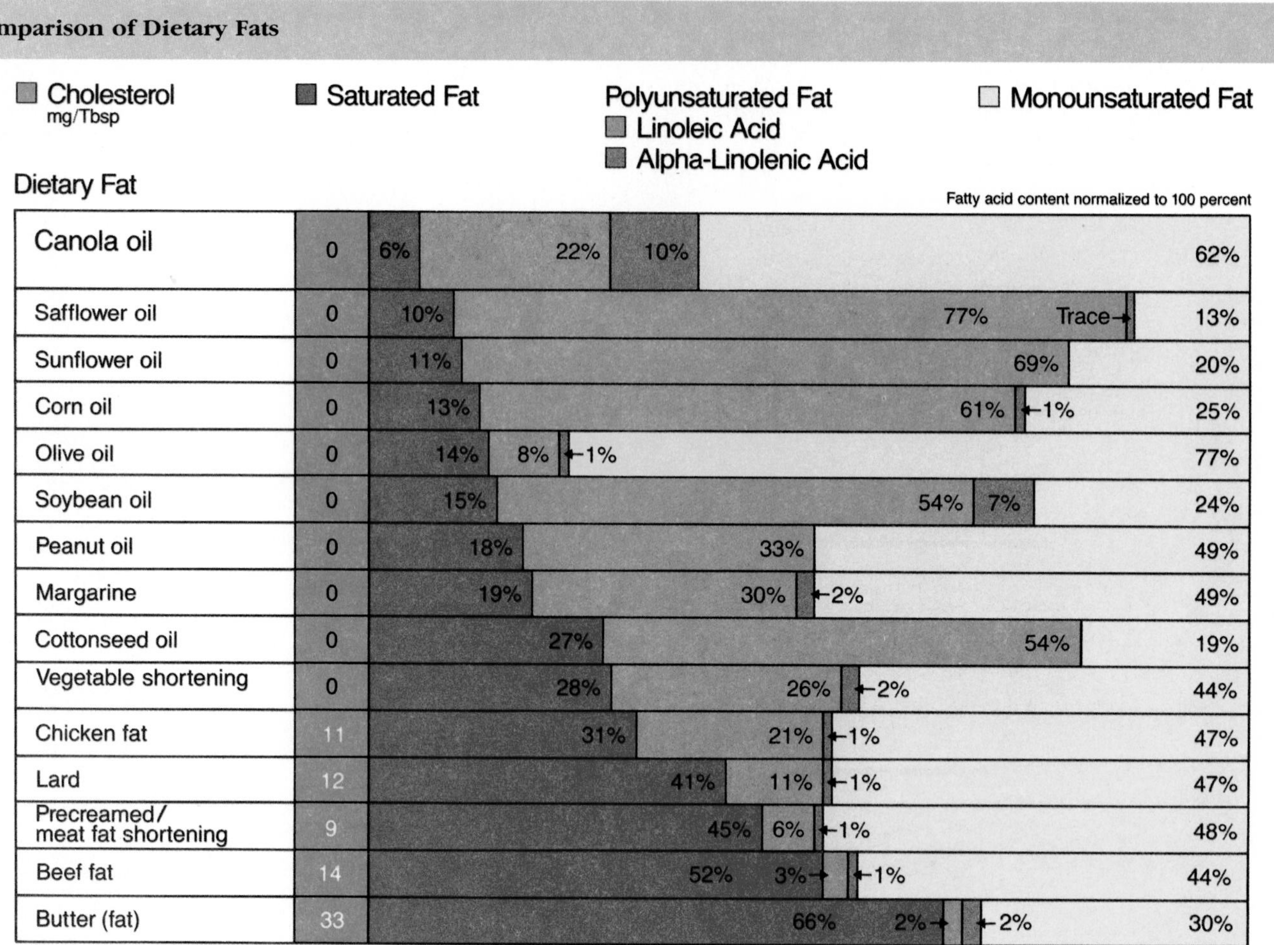

50% of fatty acids as linoleic acid, they should supply about 4% of our total kcalorie intake. *On a 2500 kcalorie diet this corresponds to 1 tablespoon of plant oil per day.*

The RDA also states that in the future an allowance for omega-3 fatty acids should be considered. Leading researchers support that statement.[23] They think that diet planning should include a regular supply of alpha-linolenic acid or its related omega-3 form **eicosapentenoic acid (EPA).** This would essentially require weekly consumption of fatty fish, such as salmon, tuna, and sardines, or canola or soybean oil. All are good sources of omega-3 fatty acids. It is too early to know who is right. This is a vital research area that we will explain further in the next few pages.

eicosapentenoic acid (EPA)
An omega-3 fatty acid with 20 carbon atoms and 5 double bonds; present in fish oils.

Essential fatty acid deficiency

Unless enough essential fatty acids are consumed, skin becomes flaky and itchy and diarrhea and other symptoms often develop. Today these signs of deficiency appear in people fed **intravenous** solutions for long periods that contain no lipid. However, since we need only about 1 tablespoon of polyunsaturated plant oil a day to meet essential fatty acid needs, even a low-fat diet, if it follows the Daily Food Guide, is likely to provide enough.

intravenous
Introduced directly into the bloodstream.

Concept Check

Lipids are a group of compounds that have few oxygen atoms in their structures and dissolve in chloroform, benzene, or ether. Fatty acids form one class of lipids. Saturated fatty acids contain no double bonds, monounsaturated fatty acids contain one double bond, and polyunsaturated fatty acids contain two or more double bonds. If the double bonds begin at the third carbon atom from the methyl end ($-CH_3$), the fatty acid is an omega-3 fatty acid. If the double bonds begin at the sixth carbon atom, it is an omega-6 fatty acid. Both omega-3 and omega-6 fatty acids are essential parts of a diet.

Putting fatty acids to work: forming eicosanoids

Once linoleic acid is in a cell, it can be lengthened to 20 carbon atoms and have two more double bonds added to yield **arachidonic acid.** Alpha-linolenic acid can be elongated to 20 carbon atoms and have two double bonds added to form EPA. The rate at which EPA is formed in humans is still debatable.[23]

Arachidonic acid and EPA form the group of compounds called eicosanoids: prostaglandins, prostacyclins, thromboxanes, and leukotrienes (Figure 5-1). As mentioned, these eicosanoids are important regulators of vital body functions, such as blood pressure, childbirth, blood clotting, immune responses, and stomach secretions.[9]

Aspirin has such diverse effects on the body—from lowering body temperature to easing muscle pain—because it blocks the synthesis of prostaglandins and thromboxanes.

The w-3 fatty acid EPA is especially concentrated in some fish oils. Research has shown that Greenland Eskimos have one-tenth the risk of heart attacks compared with Danish people.[30] These Eskimos eat primarily fish and about 40% of their kcalories comes from fish oils. Studies have also shown that people with very high serum lipid levels markedly reduce those levels (primarily the level of serum triglycerides) by consuming about 20% to 25% of their daily kcalories from fish oils (about 50 grams).[20] Scientists now wonder whether the ability of EPA to lower the risk of heart attack suggests that it should also be considered essential to the diet, particularly since converting alpha-linolenic acid—another omega-3 fatty acid—to EPA appears to be inefficient.[23] To increase EPA content in cells we probably need to eat fish regularly

W-3 fatty acids reduce blood clotting

Another line of evidence supports the recommendation to regularly eat fish. *Studies from Scandinavia show that people who eat fish about 2 times a week (240 grams or 8 ounces of total weekly intake) run lower risks for heart disease than people who rarely eat fish.*[30] In these cases the fish oil probably affects blood clotting. We will soon discuss how blood clots are linked to heart attacks. Decreasing the tendency for blood to clot reduces the risk of heart attack, especially for people at high risk.

Fish oils reduce the tendency for blood to clot by changing the nature of eicosanoid synthesis in the body.[20,30] An important class of prostaglandins and thromboxanes are usually made from arachidonic acid, an omega-6 fatty acid. Since fish oils contain a lot of the omega-3 fatty acid, EPA (plus a related compound, docosahexaenoic acid [DHA]), cells of people who eat a lot of fish have a greater tendency to synthesize eicosanoids with EPA and DHA. In effect, EPA and DHA compete with arachidonic acid for the same metabolic pathways. When they are highly concentrated in a cell, EPA and DHA win.

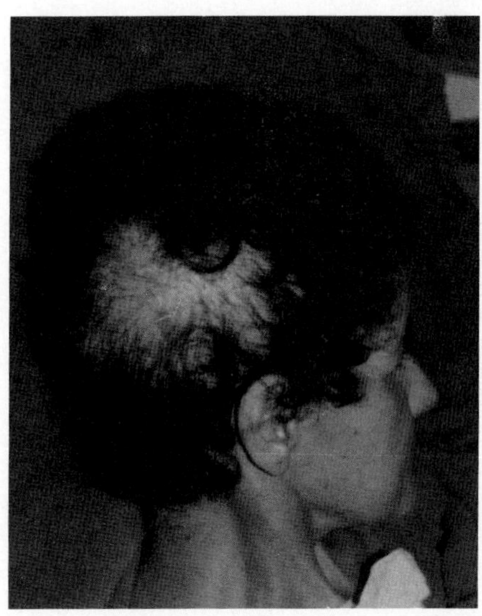

About 1 tablespoon of plant oils per day protects against essential fatty acid deficiency.

When cells use these different starting compounds, they synthesize different types of eicosanoids. Arachidonic acid yields **Prostaglandin I_2** and **Thromboxane A_2.** From EPA and DHA the cells make *prostaglandin I_3* and *thromboxane A_3*. The subtle differences in eicosanoid structure between these compounds (2-class vs 3-class) yield profound differences in function, particularly concerning blood clotting (Table 5-2). Overall, the 2-class products from arachidonic acid

Table 5-2

Effects of products made from omega-3 (w-3) and omega-6 (w-6) fatty acids in man

Site of synthesis	w-6 (linoleic acid)	w-3 (EPA, DHA)
Cells lining blood vessels	Form prostaglandin I_2, which inhibits blood clotting	Form prostaglandin I_3, which inhibits blood clotting
Platelets* in the blood	Form thromboxane A_2, which is a strong promoter of blood clotting	Form thromboxane A_3, which is a very weak promoter of blood clotting

The net result is that omega-3 fatty acids reduce the tendency for blood to clot.
*Plate-like fragments in the bloodstream that contribute to blood clotting.

(omega-6) increase blood clotting and the 3-class products from EPA and DHA (omega-3) decrease it.[10]

Does this mean we should eat "Eskimo" diets?

Blood clotting is a normal physiological process. Eskimos who eat a lot of fish have a higher risk for strokes than Danish people, maybe because their blood does not readily clot. This is not the case in Japan, however, where fish consumption is also high.[23] Still, significantly altering blood clotting *may* be a two-edged sword.[30] Because of this possibility we recommend eating fish about twice a week. Atlantic and Pacific herring, sardines, Atlantic halibut and salmon, lake trout, coho, pink and king salmon, blue fish, albacore tuna, and Atlantic mackerel are among those fish with the greatest omega-3 fatty acid contents (see Appendix I). New research may soon add more types of fish to this list.

We do not recommend consuming fish oil capsules without a physician's advice. Besides the potential for seriously altering blood clotting, fish oil capsules often contain high amounts of cholesterol, vitamins A and D, and rare fatty acids, such as cateoleic and gadoleic acids.[30] Any of these substances taken in high amounts can lead to health problems. However, some of them may be removed during processing; check the label on any fish oil supplement to see if they have been removed. Simply not listing the substances on the label is not enough; the label should state that the substances have been removed.

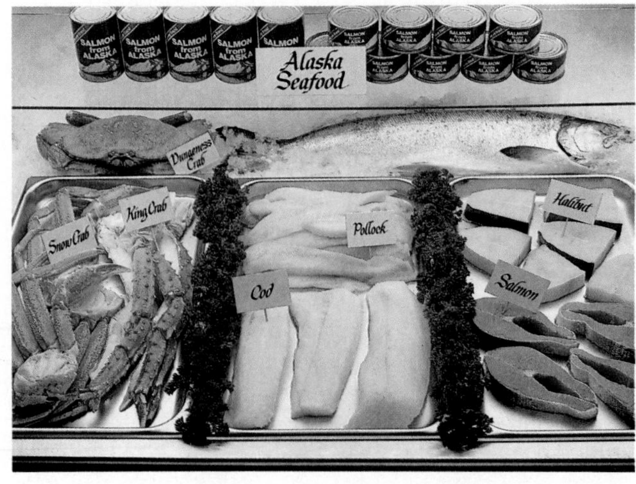

Fish is a good source of omega-3 fatty acids.

Expert Opinion

Fishing for Cardiovascular Health

JACK Z. YETIV, M.D., Ph.D.

When you were a child, your folks probably told you that fish and codliver oil were good for you. And, unlike some other things you may have been told (such as "finish *everything* on your plate"), the fish recommendation may have some basis in fact.

Dutch researchers recently reported that fish eaters had half the mortality from heart disease as people who don't eat fish! The really remarkable fact was that the fish eaters had to eat only 1 ounce of fish per day to achieve this heart-protective effect.

Why the sudden interest in fish and fish oil? Well, scientists sought an explanation for the observation that Greenland Eskimos have a very low rate of heart disease, even though their diet is as high in fat as other North Americans. This seeming paradox may be due to the fact that much of their fat intake comes from marine sources (such as fish, whale, seal, and walrus). Marine fat is especially rich in a group of fats called *omega-3 fatty acids.* These omega-3 fatty acids decrease the "stickiness" of platelets, the blood cells that are responsible for blood clotting. Excessively "sticky"platelets are believed to play a major role in blocking arteries, and this sudden arterial blockage causes strokes and heart attacks.

Another report in the same journal suggested a possible reason for the improved longevity in fish eaters—fish and fish oil intake can lower blood cholesterol levels—although large quantities must be ingested to do this. The fish-rich diet contained the equivalent of over a pound of fish per day.

Although these studies are the best publicized, they certainly do not stand alone. Many other articles support the improved mortality experience of fish eaters, although some studies do not show such a benefit.

In addition to decreasing the formation of blood clots and lowering cholesterol levels, omega-3 fatty acids have other potential beneficial effects: they lower blood pressure and decrease blood viscosity. The latter effect enables blood to flow more easily. These beneficial effects of fish fats seem to occur at different dose levels. It appears that only high doses of fish (or fish oil supplements) decrease CHOL and blood pressure. Such doses are in the range of a pound of marine foods per day (the amount that Greenland Eskimos eat) or about 10 to 30 fish oil supplements per day. A much lower dose (in the range of two to three 4-ounce fish servings per week or three to six supplement pills per day) may decrease platelet stickiness and affect blood viscosity.

This assessment represents an educated guess, and much more data must be gathered before scientifically solid recommendations can be made. For instance, the Dutch study quoted earlier found that men who ate lean fish containing 1% fish fat had as low a mortality as men eating fattier fishes (which contain up to 10% fish fat). This suggests that *something else in fish—not only or necessarily the omega-3 fatty acids may be beneficial to the heart.* This is one reason some researchers recommend eating fish rather than taking fish oil supplements. Finally, if fish intake replaces a meat meal, this would confer additional advantages.

But supposing you absolutely refuse to eat fish. Is taking a fish oil supplement reasonable? Several factors may be considered in answering this question:

First, children, adolescents, pregnant women, people taking anticoagulants (blood thinners), or those with bleeding or bruising problems should not take fish oil supplements. Little is known about fish oil use in these individuals and some fish oils (primarily cod-liver oil) contain large amounts of vitamin A, which can cause birth defects, among other problems. The last two groups are predisposed to bleeding, and adding fish oil supplements to their blood thinners could lead to serious—perhaps fatal—bleeding.

Second, patients under a doctor's care for a serious medical disorder should discuss plans for fish oil supplementation with their physician. If he or she is not receptive to even discussing the issue, the patient may wish to search for a genuine fish oil researcher in their geographic area. Finding such an individual may take some effort—but a literature search in the local medical library may turn up a local researcher. Alternatively, the chief dietitian at a local medical center may be able to direct the patient to an appropriate research facility. *Your local health food store does not qualify as a bone fide research facility.*

Third, patients with very high CHOL levels (over 300 to 350) and/or very high TG levels (over 500) are reasonably treated with fish oil, *under medical supervision.* None of the drugs currently used to treat such high CHOL and TG levels are very satisfactory and, although current experience with fish oil supplements is limited, sufficient evidence allows at least a trial of fish oil supplementation. Such trials are presently considered experimental. Other experts in this field may legitimately disagree with this view and may prefer to prescribe other drugs. And of course these suggestions are subject to modification as further research accumulates.

Fourth, it seems reasonable to increase fish intake to the levels noted to be beneficial in the Dutch study—two or three fish dishes per week.

Dr. Yetiv, a physician and pharamacologist is the author of Popular Nutritional Practices: A Scientific Appraisal. He has published widely in the scientific literature.

Ask your professor about new findings on the importance of fish oils to health. You may want to search the scientific literature yourself. A reference librarian can help you start.

The fish oil story unfolds daily. Increasing fish oil in the diet reduces both blood pressure and inflammation in certain diseases, such as psoriasis and asthma.[23,30] It will be exciting to follow this new area of research. (See the suggested readings on page 145.)

Concept Check

When cells use omega-3 fatty acids to synthesize hormone-like compounds called *eicosanoids,* the synthesized products differ markedly from those using omega-6 fatty acids. In general, products made from omega-3 fatty acids tend to lower blood clotting, blood pressure, and inflammatory responses in the body. In the future, there may be more specific recommendations for the deliberate inclusion of omega-3 fatty acids in diet planning. Presently the recommendation to eat fish about twice a week is our best guide.

Chain length—another factor to consider with fatty acids

Fats in foods that contain primarily saturated fatty acids are solid at room temperature, expecially if the fatty acids have a **long chain** (greater than 12 carbon atoms). **Medium-chain** saturated fatty acids (8 to 12 carbon atoms), such as those found in coconut oil, produce liquid oils at room temperature. The shorter chain length overrides the effect of saturation. **Short-chain** fatty acids (2 to 6 carbons) also form liquid oils at room temperature.[8] Food sources of short-chain fatty acids include dairy fats (see Appendix I). *Fats containing primarily polyunsaturated or monounsaturated fatty acids are usually liquid at room temperature. Chain length is not an issue.*[8]

The capability of some saturated fatty acids of short- or medium-chain lengths to form oils at room temperature is significant. Non-dairy creamers initially appear to be a healthful substitute for cream because of cream's high content of saturated fats. However, many coffee creamers contain coconut oil, which is also high in saturated fatty acids. Manufacturers use coconut oil because it allows the product a long shelf life without turning rancid. You will see why in the following section. Low-fat milk is a much healthier choice than non-dairy creamers.

A

B

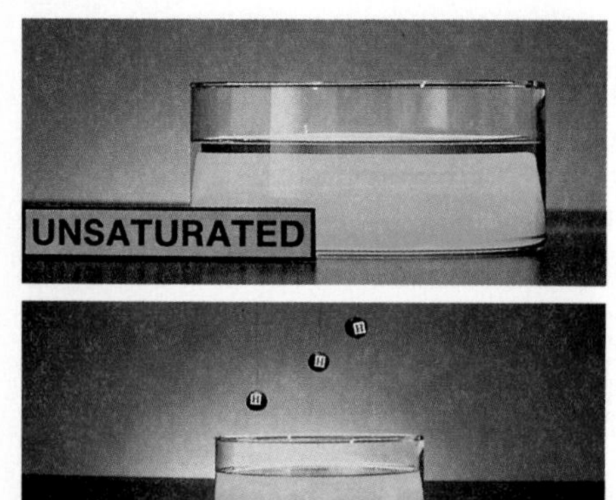

C

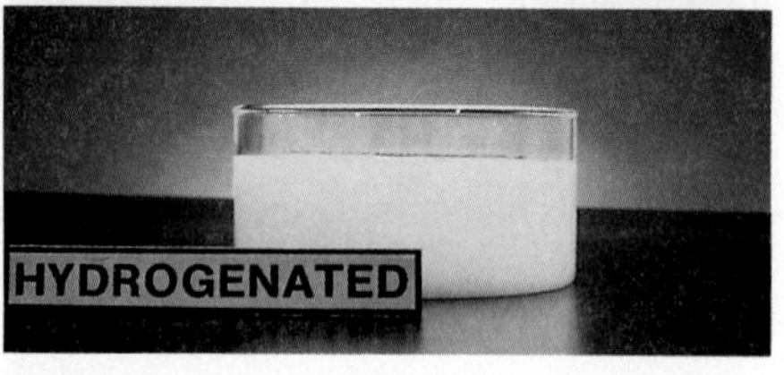

How liquid fatty acids become solid. (A) Unsaturated fatty acids in liquid form. (B) Hydrogen atoms are added (hydrogenation), changing double bonds to single bonds and producing *trans fatty acids.* (C) The hydrogenated product.

Hydrogenation of fatty acids

To solidify vegetable oils into margarines and shortenings the polyunsaturated fatty acids in plant oils must become more saturated. Hydrogen atoms are added across the double bonds in the fatty acids. *This process, called* ***hydrogenation,*** *turns many double bonds into single bonds and produces some trans fatty acids.*[16] Both changes increase hardness. Generally, the harder the product—stick margarine compared with tub margarine—the more hydrogenation has occurred. Hydrogenated fats are easier to use in some techniques of food production, such as in making pastries and cakes.

Recall from Chapter 2 that monounsaturated and polyunsaturated fatty acids can exist in two isomer forms—cis and trans. The cis form has the hydrogen atoms on the same side of the double bond. The trans form has the hydrogen atoms on opposite sides of the double bond (Figure 2-2). Plant fatty acids are in the cis form. A few trans fatty acids are in milk because the bacteria in a cow's multiple stomachs (rumen) rearrange the fatty acids from the cis form into the trans form. However, margarine has the highest concentration of trans fatty acids. *Presently the many studies done show that trans fatty acids are not linked to significantly increased risk for any disease, notably heart disease and cancer.*[16] Margarine—the major source of such fatty acids in our food—has been used increasingly for the last 20 years while heart disease rates have declined and cancer rates, except for lung cancer, have remained steady. For now it appears that trans fatty acids produced by hydrogenation are a problem mainly because they act like saturated fatty acids in affecting serum cholesterol level—both tend to raise it.

Rancidity

Another reason manufacturers hydrogenate plant oils is to reduce their deterioration, which forms **rancid** products. The double bonds in polyunsaturated fatty acids easily break down. Ultraviolet light and various chemicals attack the double bonds, break them, destroying the structure of the polyunsaturated fatty acids. You may have recognized the disagreeable odor and sour, stale taste of decomposing oils. There appears to be no health threat from these, as long as enough essential fatty acids remain in the diet. Even though rancid oils are potentially toxic, their unappealing taste and odor normally discourage people from eating enough to pose a threat. However, rancidity reduces a product's shelf life and is therefore costly to the manufacturer.

*Nature provides polyunsaturated fatty acids some natural protection against rancidity. Vitamin E is an **antioxidant** found in plant oils.* Antioxidants, such as vitamin E, stop **oxidizing agents** from breaking the double bonds in fatty acids. Oxidizing agents are usually seeking electrons to capture. Vitamin E and antioxidants in general donate electrons to oxidizing agents. This keeps the electrons in the double bonds of fatty acids, and the bonds they form, safe from attack. When food manufacturers want to prevent rancidity in polyunsaturated fats, they often add the antioxidants **BHA** and **BHT.** Look for these food additives in salad dressings, cake mixes, and other products that contain fat. Manufacturers also tightly seal their products from the atmosphere and use other methods to reduce the presence of oxygen inside packages.

antioxidant
A compound that can donate electrons to electro-seeking compounds.

BHA and BHT
Butylated hydroxyanisole and butylated hydroxytoluene—two common synthetic antioxidants added to foods.

Concept Check

At room temperature saturated fatty acids tend to form solid fats, and polyunsaturated and monounsaturated fatty acids tend to form liquid oils. *Hydrogenation* is the process of turning double bonds of fatty acids into a single bond by adding hydrogen atoms. This solidifies the fat and reduces the breakdown of fatty acids commonly found in polyunsaturated varieties, in turn reducing rancidity. The presence of antioxidants in oils, such as vitamin E, naturally protects unsaturated fatty acids against rancidity.

TRIGLYCERIDES

Fatty acids usually do not exist in a free form in the body. Some free fatty acids are bound to albumin proteins in the bloodstream while they are transferred from storage in the adipose cells to the liver, muscles, and other sites. *However, most fatty acids in the body, as in food, are in the form of triglycerides.*

Triglyceride molecules contain a backbone of a three-carbon carbohydrate, **glycerol.** On the three hydroxyl groups (−OH) of the glycerol are atttached three fatty acids (Figure 5-2).

To form a triglyceride, three fatty acids attach their acid ends ($-\overset{\overset{\displaystyle O}{\|}}{C}-OH$) to the hydroxyl ends of the glycerol molecule. The bond between an acid group and a hydroxyl group is formed as a water molecule is removed. *Because water is a by-product, this is a condensation reaction.* The net result is that glycerol and three fatty acids form a triglyceride and three water molecules. Most triglycerides are in mixed forms, meaning they contain different types of fatty acids on each glycerol molecule.

The term **triacylglyceride** is the more formal name for a triglyceride. The addition of *acyl* to the word signifies that the three compounds on the glycerol molecule are long chains of carbons with hydroxyl groups missing from the acid groups at one end.

Figure 5-2

Forming a triglyceride. This uses a condensation reaction, yielding water as a byproduct while creating ester bonds.

Ester bond

Glycerol + 3 Fatty acids → Fat (triglyceride) + 3 H_2O (water)

The bonds formed in a triglyceride are ester bonds $(-C-O-\overset{O}{\overset{\|}{C}}-C-)$. So the process of putting fatty acids on the glycerol molecule is called **esterification.** Taking the fatty acids off the glycerol molecule is called *deesterification.* Removing the fatty acids from the glycerol molecule and then putting them back on is called *reesterification.* Surprisingly, the body reesterifies triglycerides over and over again. Every time a triglyceride crosses a cell membrane it must be broken down, or *deesterified.* Then, when the fatty acids enter the cell, they often must be *reesterified* into a triglyceride.

esterification
The process of attaching fatty acids to a glycerol molecule, creating an ester bond. Removing a fatty acid is called deesterification, reattaching a fatty acid is called reesterification.

A glycerol containing only one fatty acid forms a *monoglyceride.* A glycerol that contains two fatty acids forms a *diglyceride.* Recall that during digestion most fatty acids must be removed from the triglyceride molecules. This aids fat absorption because triglycerides can't easily cross through the intestinal cells into the bloodstream. What occurs is that many triglycerides are turned into monoglycerides. When the free fatty acids, monoglycerides, and any free glycerol molecules are absorbed into the intestinal cells, the parts are mostly rebuilt into triglycerides.

Monoglyceride

Putting triglycerides to work

Energy storage. Triglycerides are the main form of energy storage in the body. The ability to store lipid is essentially limitless. The storage sites, adipose cells, can increase about 50 times in weight. If the amount of lipid to be stored exceeds the ability of the cells to expand, the body can form new adipose cells. We will discuss that further in Chapter 8.

Chapter 8 discusses how to determine the amount of fat stored in the body.

When we store lipids in adipose cells, we store little else. *Adipose cells are about 80% lipid and only 20% water and protein.* In contrast, if we stored energy as muscle tissue, we would need to store much water, since muscle is about 73% water. The same is true for energy stored as glycogen. About 2.6 grams of water are stored for every gram of glycogen. Think of the consequences if we stored energy as muscle tissue or glycogen—for most of us body weight would greatly increase due to the excess water we would need to carry. Another advantage to storing triglycerides for energy is that they are energy-dense. Recall that triglycerides yield over twice the kcalories per gram as proteins and carbohydrates do.

Providing energy for the body. The free fatty acids on triglycerides are the main fuel for muscles at rest and during light activity. In endurance exercises the muscles burn a lot of carbohydrate in addition to fatty acids. We discussed that in Nutrition Perspective 4-2 on carbohydrate-loading. Mostly, however, muscles derive energy from fatty acids. Other body tissues also use fatty acids for energy—about 40% of the energy used by the entire body at rest and during light activity comes from fatty acids. This amount, perhaps coincidentally, is about the same as the percentage of total kcalories in our food that comes from fat.

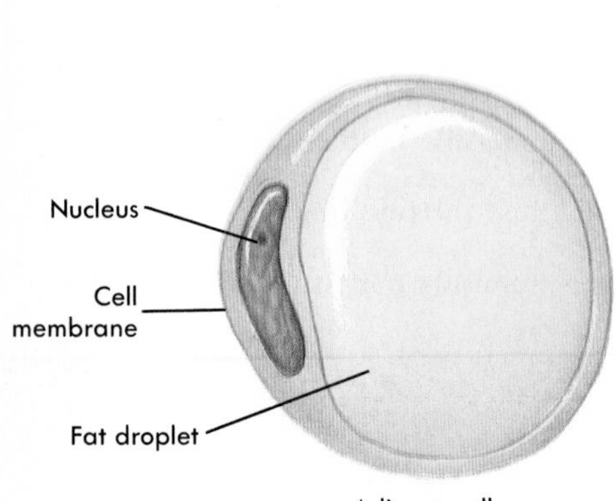

Adipose cell

Providing satiety. Triglycerides in foods are very important for **satiety,** that is, feeling satisfied after eating. The composition of what is eaten helps determine the rate of stomach clearance, due to hormonal responses (see Chapter 3). Slower emptying allows food to remain in the stomach longer while acidic juices complete this important phase of digestion. Since eating fat in food causes the stomach to empty slower than eating carbohydrate or protein, a high-fat meal makes us feel full longer.

Many people who want to reduce weight know that fats are high in kcalories and they find it easiest to cut kcalories by cutting out much of the fat they eat. *However, if dieters lower fat intake too much, they lose its satiety value and get hungry quicker. Thus lowering fat intake too much when dieting can actually be self-defeating.* (See Chapter 9 for further discussion.)

Exploring Issues and Actions

Which of your favorite foods do you suspect are satisfying because of their fat content? Does understanding this relationship make you want to change your eating habits?

Insulating and protecting the body. A layer of adipose tissue made mostly of triglycerides insulates and protects the body, especially the breasts and kidneys. We usually don't notice the important insulating function of adipose tissue because we wear clothes but it is quite apparent in animals. Polar bears, whales, and other animals that live in cold climates build a thick layer of adipose tissue around themselves to insulate against their cold-weather environment. It also represents stored energy for winter.

People with the disease **anorexia nervosa** often lose 25% or more of body weight, ending up almost fat-free. We can never be totally fat-free, because fat is an essential part of all cells. However with anorexia nervosa a person may get as lean as its biologically possible. The person then often develops downy hair all over the body, called **lanugo.** These hairs stand up, trapping air around them. The air acts as insulation and represents an attempt to substitute for the missing layer of adipose tissue usually present under the skin. Lanugo also insulates a growing **fetus** before its layer of adipose tissue is laid down late in pregnancy.

anorexia nervosa
An eating disorder involving a psychological loss of appetite and self-starvation, due in part to a distorted body image and various social pressures associated with puberty (see Chapter 10).

fetus
A developing infant in utero from 8 weeks until birth.

Transporting fat-soluble vitamins. Triglycerides and other lipids carry fat-soluble vitamins to the small intestine and aid their absorption. If the small intestine is diseased, however, dietary fat may not be properly digested and absorbed. Rather, the fat bypasses the small intestine and ends up in the colon. When this happens, the fat-soluble vitamins—A, D, E, and K—are bound by the unabsorbed fat and carried into the colon, bypassing their absorption sites in the small intestine. People who absorb fat poorly, such as those with cystic fibrosis, are at risk for deficiencies of fat-soluble vitamins, especially vitamin K. So are people who use mineral oil as a laxative during meal times, since we cannot digest or absorb mineral oil. The undigested mineral oil carries fat-soluble vitamins into the colon where they are eliminated in the stool. This can make mineral oil a poor choice for a laxative.

Unabsorbed fatty acid can also bind minerals, such as calcium and magnesium, and pull them into the stool for elimination. This can harm mineral status (see Chapter 13).

Providing flavor and texture to foods. Triglycerides and other fats in foods provide important texture and carry flavors. Many flavors are fat soluble; their essences dissolve in fat, and the fat carries them to the sensory cells in the mouth that discriminate taste and smell. Thus we quickly associate flavorful foods with fatty foods.

If you have ever eaten a high-fat cheese or cream cheese, you will probably agree that fat melting on the tongue feels good. This love of fat is universal. Western diets, Eskimo diets, and Mediterranean diets are all high in fat. Immigrants to Western cultures quickly embrace the high-fat diet found here.

Concept Check

Triglyceride is the major form of fat in food and in the body. Triglycerides in the body provides energy, energy storage, insulation and protection, transportation for fat-soluble vitamins, and satiety after eating. In foods, triglycerides provide flavor and texture.

H–C–O–C(=O)–fatty acid chain
H–C–O–C(=O)–fatty acid chain
H–C–O–P(=O)(O⁻)–O–CH₂–CH₂–N⁺(CH₃)₃

2 Fatty acids

Choline

Glycerol

Phosphate

Lecithin

PHOSPHOLIPIDS

Lipids sometimes contain only one or two fatty acids. Structures other than fatty acids bond to other sites on the glycerol backbone. For example, an important participant in fat digestion in the intestine, **lecithin,** is called a *phospholipid.* Egg yolks contain it in abundance. On the bottom carbon of the glycerol molecule in lecithin is a phosphate group $\left(-\text{O}-\underset{\underset{\text{O}-}{|}}{\overset{\overset{\text{O}}{\|}}{\text{P}}}-\text{O}-\right)$ bonded to a choline molecule. This phosphate group is what makes lecithin a phospholipid. Many other phospholipids exist in the body, such as *sphingomyelins* and *cerebrosides* found in the brain.

Phospholipids form important parts of cell membranes. A cell membrane looks much like a sea of phospholipids with protein islands (Figure 5-3). The protein island form receptors for hormones and function as enzymes, and act as transporters, among other functions.

Health food literature promotes choline as a vitamin. However, because the human body can make choline from the amino acid methionine, choline is not a vitamin for humans (see Chapter 12).

Phospholipids also function as *emulsifiers,* compounds that can break fat globules into small droplets. In doing so emulsifiers have the ability to suspend fat in water. Look at Figure 5-4. The charged end of a lecithin molecule attracts lipids while the other end attracts water. The lipid-attracting end is made of fatty acids. These long chains of carbon atoms and attached hydrogen atoms show no positive or negative charges, so they have no polarity. They are **nonpolar.** Triglycerides are also nonpolar and so are attracted to fatty acids.

Water, in contrast, is **polar.** the slightly negatively charged oxygen atom and the two slightly positive hydrogen atoms create poles similar to magnetic poles. The phosphate group and nitrogen at the bottom of the lecithin molecule are charged—so this area is also polar. The polar water is attracted to the charges on lecithin. This part of lecithin is called **hydrophilic,** which means "liking water." In contrast, the parts with fatty acids are **hydrophobic,** since they don't attract (fear) water.

When many emulsifier molecules are mixed together with oil and water, the emulsifiers organize into ***micelles*** *by orienting their hydrophobic parts to the inside and their hydrophilic parts to the outside.* Oil is attracted to the hydro-

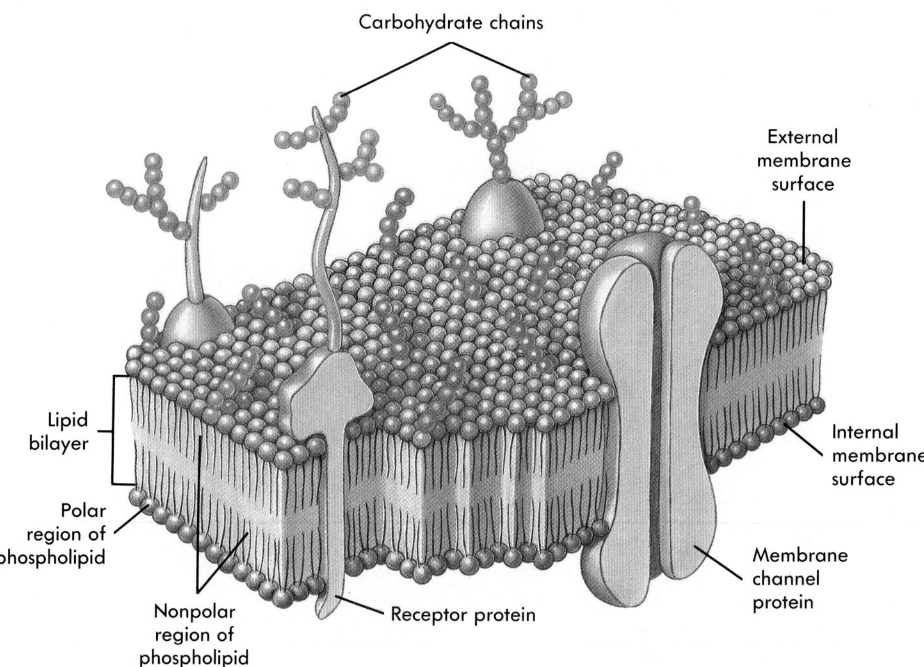

Figure 5-3

A cell membrane. This membrane is composed of protein islands within a sea of lipids. The lipids are mostly phospholipids.

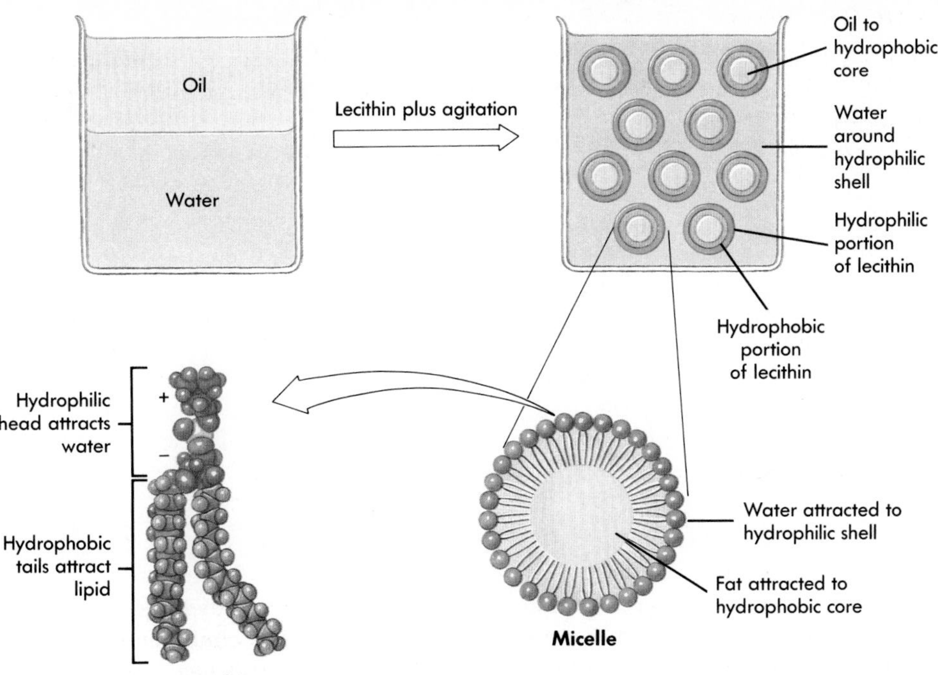

Figure 5-4

Emulsification and emulsifiers. Emulsifiers can organize oil and water into micelles—droplets of oil surrounded by shells of water. Forming micelles is a key step in fat digestion.

Cholesterol

Cholesterol

Testosterone

Cortisol

phobic core of the micelles, and water is attracted to the hydrophilic shells. The mixture produced then has tiny oil droplets surrounded by thin shells of water.

In an emulsified solution there are millions of these tiny oil droplets, all separated from each other by shells of water (Figure 5-4). Commercial salad dressings are examples of emulsification put to practical use—emulsifiers, such as Polysorbate 60 and lecithin, are added to salad dressings to keep the vegetable oil suspended in the water. Eggs used in cake recipes likewise emulsify the fat with the water in the milk used.

Complete digestion and absorption of fat requires emulsification of dietary fats in the small intestine. Recall that digestion requires a large surface area for the fat-digesting enzymes to act. Breaking the fats in foods into tiny oil droplets by emulsification (and by the warming action of the body) greatly increases their surface areas, and so improves enzyme action.

Lecithin and **bile acids** are produced by the liver and secreted into the small intestine via the gallbladder to emulsify dietary fats. These two substances are the body's main emulsifiers. The breakdown products of fat digestion, monoglycerides and diglycerides, are also good emulsifiers and are sometimes used in cake mixes and salad dressings for that reason.

STEROLS

Sterols show how diverse lipids can be. These compounds have a multi-ringed (steroid) structure. An important sterol is the waxy substance cholesterol. The hydroxyl group (−OH) on the cholesterol molecule makes it a sterol. Cholesterol doesn't look like a triglyceride but since it dissolves in ether, it is a lipid. It shares another characteristic with fatty acids, triglycerides, and phospholipids–synthesis of most parts of these molecules uses a derivative of the smallest fatty acid, acetic acid.

Cholesterol forms part of some important hormones, such as the estrogens, testosterone, and the active vitamin D hormone **calcitriol.** Cholesterol also forms the bile acids needed for fat digestion and is incorporated into cell membranes.

Cholesterol is found only in animal foods (Table 5-3). However, humans can make all they need when dietary cholesterol is inadequate.[8] Some plants have related sterols, such as *ergosterol,* that can form a type of vitamin D. How-

Table 5-3

Cholesterol content of common measures of selected foods (in ascending order)

Food	Amount	Cholesterol in milligrams	Food	Amount	Cholesterol in milligrams
Milk, skim	1 cup	4	Clams, halibut, tuna	3 oz	55
Mayonnaise	1 T	10	Chicken, turkey, light meat	3 oz	70
Butter	1 pat	11	Beef*, pork*, lobster	3 oz	75
Lard	1 T	12	Lamb, crab	3 oz	85
Cottage cheese	1/2 cup	15	Shrimp	3 oz	125
Milk, low fat, 2%	1 cup	22	Heart, beef	3 oz	164
Half and half	1/4 cup	23	Egg, (egg yolk)*	1 each	220-275†
Hot dog*	1	29	Liver, beef	3 oz	410
Ice cream, ≈ 10% fat	1/2 cup	30	Kidney	3 oz	587
Cheese, cheddar	1 oz	30	Brains	3 oz	2637
Milk, whole*	1 cup	34			
Oysters, salmon	3 oz	40			

†New evidence suggests the lower value (200 to 220 milligrams).
*Leading contributors of cholesterol to the U.S. diet.

ever, plants do not contain cholesterol. Manufacturers who advertise peanut butter, vegetable shortening, margarines, and vegetable oils as containing no cholesterol are taking advantage of consumer naivete. *Of course peanut butter and margarine have no cholesterol—no purely plant food has!*

Concept check

Phospholipids are derivatives of triglycerides. They can have both polar and nonpolar parts. If polarities are present, they make the phospholipids effective emulsifiers—compounds that can suspend fat in water. Phospholipids also form important parts of cell membranes and other body molecules. The compound *cholesterol* forms compounds vital to the body, such as hormones, parts of cell membranes, and bile acids. Cholesterol is so essential to the body that if sufficient amounts are not available from the diet, the body synthesizes cholesterol for its needs.

CARRYING LIPIDS IN THE BLOODSTREAM

By their natures, lipids and water don't mix. Overcoming this incompatibility challenges the ingenuity of the body.

Carrying lipids from dietary sources

Once dietary fat is digested and absorbed into the small intestine cells, triglycerides are reformed. They combine with phospholipids and cholesterol to turn into a chylomicron, which is a large droplet of lipid surrounded by a thin shell of protein, cholesterol, and phospholipid. This combination of lipid and protein is called a **lipoprotein** (Figure 5-5). The shell around the chylomicron allows the lipid inside to float freely in the water-based bloodstream (Figure 5-6). Some of the proteins, **apolipoproteins,** also help other cells identify this particle as a chylomicron.[13]

lipoprotein A compound found in the bloodstream containing a core of lipids with a shell of protein, phospholipid, and cholesterol.

The chylomicron structure, in essence, emulsufies dietary fats before they enter the bloodstream. This process resembles the action of lecithin and bile acids in the small intestine when they emulsify dietary fats during digestion. The difference is that in digestion a layer of water—rather than of protein, cholesterol, and phospholipid—surrounds the droplets.

Chylomicrons enter the lymphatic system and travel to the thoracic duct, which is located along the spinal column and opens into a large vein in the neck. In this way chylomicrons enter the bloodstream.

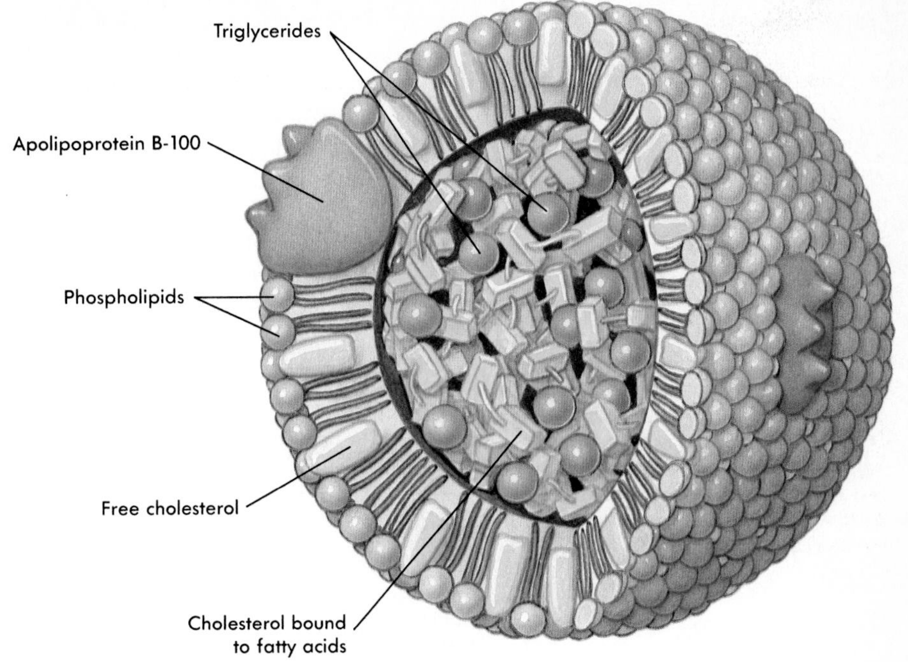

Figure 5-5

The structure of lipoprotein. This structure allows fats to circulate in the water-based bloodstream.

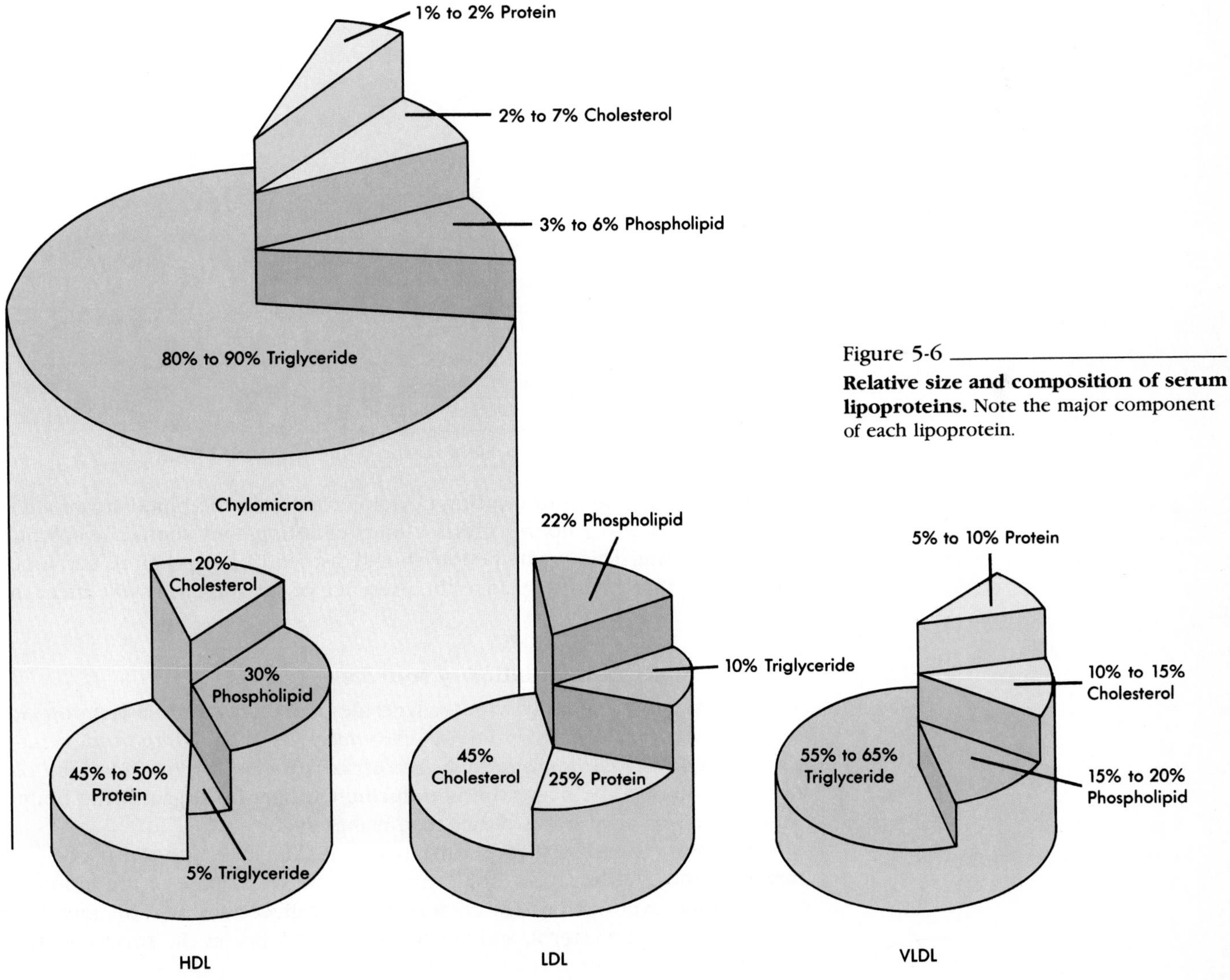

Figure 5-6

Relative size and composition of serum lipoproteins. Note the major component of each lipoprotein.

1% to 2% Protein
2% to 7% Cholesterol
3% to 6% Phospholipid
80% to 90% Triglyceride
Chylomicron

20% Cholesterol
30% Phospholipid
45% to 50% Protein
5% Triglyceride
HDL

22% Phospholipid
10% Triglyceride
45% Cholesterol
25% Protein
LDL

5% to 10% Protein
10% to 15% Cholesterol
55% to 65% Triglyceride
15% to 20% Phospholipid
VLDL

Chylomicrons in the bloodstream are acted on by **lipoprotein lipase.** This enzyme is attached to the outside surface of blood vessel and other cells. Lipoprotein lipase *deesterifies* (breaks down) the triglycerides in the chylomicrons into free fatty acids and glycerol (Figure 5-7). Muscle, adipose, and other cells in the vicinity then absorb most of the fatty acids. Absorbed fatty acids can immediately be either used for fuel or *reesterified* (reformed) into triglycerides. Muscle cells tend to perform deesterification and then metabolize the fatty acids, while adipose cells tend to perform reesterification. Once lipoprotein lipase has removed most of the triglycerides from a chylomicron, the remnant, which contains mostly cholesterol and protein, is taken up by the liver and metabolized (Figure 5-7).

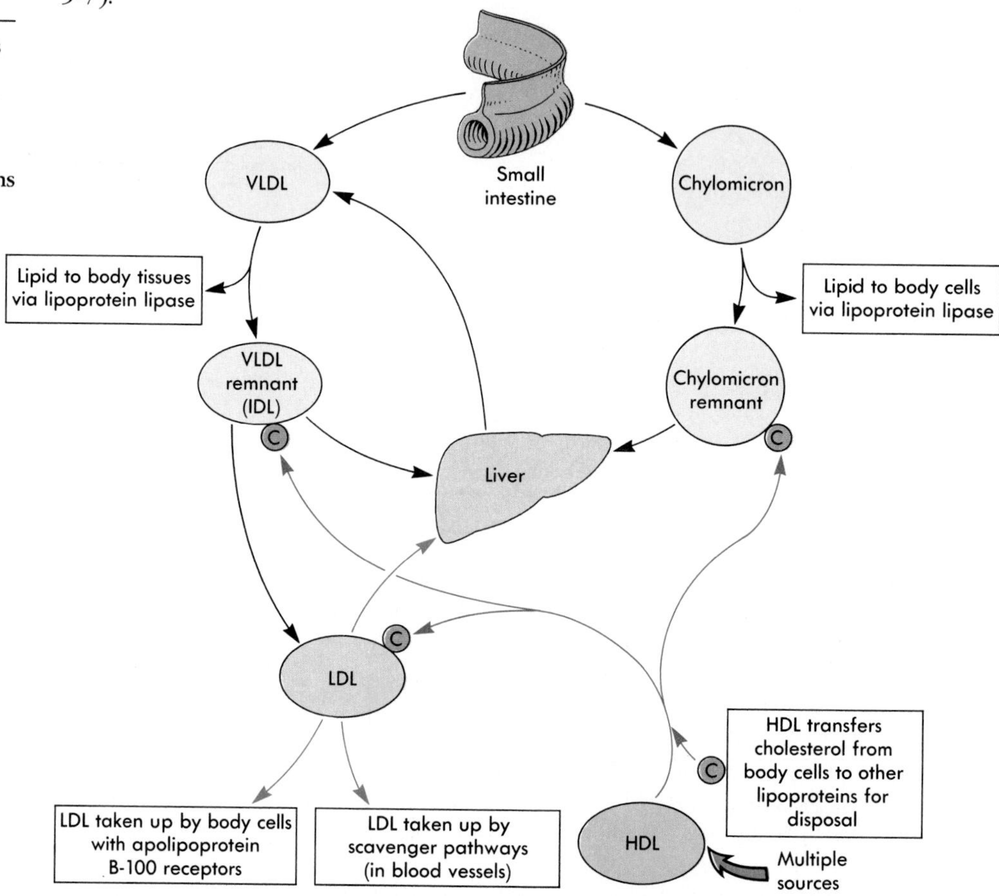

Figure 5-7

Lipoprotein interactions. Chylomicrons carry absorbed fat to body cells. VLDLs carry fats synthesized in the liver to body cells. LDLs arise from VLDLs and carry mostly cholesterol *to* cells. HDLs carry cholesterol *from* cells to other lipoproteins for excretion.

Most of the process of clearing chylomicrons from the bloodstream after eating takes about 1 to 2 hours. After 14 hours of fasting, they should be absent from the bloodstream. This is why people should fast for 14 hours before certain blood tests—then there is little chance the presence of chylomicrons will affect the results.

Carrying lipids from nondietary sources

The liver supplies the body with triglycerides and cholesterol. *When you eat too much protein or carbohydrate, the liver degrades these compounds, and then uses the resulting carbon and hydrogen atoms to make triglycerides and cholesterol.* The liver is the major lipid-producing **(lipogenic)** organ in the body. Adipose tissue primarily stores rather than makes lipid.

The liver must resolve the same problem the small intestine faced—equip newly synthesized lipids so they can float in the water base of the bloodstream. So when the liver synthesizes cholesterol or triglycerides, it too coats the lipid with a protein, cholesterol, and phospholipid shell, just as the small intestine did for chylomicrons.[8] The liver's version of a chylomicron is a **very low density lipoprotein (VLDL).**

When the VLDLs leave the liver, lipoprotein lipase again deesterifies the triglyceride in the VLDLs. With less triglyceride in the VLDL it becomes much heavier because lipids are less dense than water. The remnant of the VLDL then becomes an **intermediate density lipoprotein (IDL)**—called intermediate density due to the lipid it has lost. Half the IDLs are taken up by the liver and the rest are converted to **low density lipoprotein (LDL).** An LDL is composed primarily of cholesterol because most triglyceride was removed from the original VLDL. It is even lower in lipid than an IDL, an so even heavier. For a cell to absorb an LDL, it needs a receptor to bind it.

To measure the amount of chylomicrons, VLDLs, LDLs, HDLs in a serum sample, the serum can be centrifuged at high speeds for approximately 24 hours. These lipoproteins are named for their relative densities because this is a common method of separation. An alternate method for separating lipoproteins is to apply an electrical current to the sample by a specialized instrument.

To review, VLDL has most of its triglyceride removed upon leaving the liver, changing it to an IDL, then to an LDL. The LDL particle in the bloodstream still contains cholesterol that originally left the liver. Cells with LDL receptors pick up the LDL particles in a process called the **receptor pathway.** When the LDL particles are received by a cell, they are broken down and parts of the LDL—the cholesterol and protein—are transported throughout the cell. In this way the cell absorbs the building blocks it needs to make sex hormones and other compounds.

Research has demonstrated the importance of the LDL receptor. About 1 in 500 people have a genetic defect; they make only about half the LDL receptors needed to latch onto and remove circulating LDLs from the bloodstream. Recall that LDLs are high in cholesterol. When scavenger cells buried in the blood vessels detect the extra circulating LDL particles, they engulf and digest them. This process is called the **scavenger pathway** for LDL uptake. A key part of this process appears to be alteration of the LDL molecule (oxidation) by the scavenger cells so that it cannot reenter the bloodstream.[25] Cholesterol then inundates the scavenger cells.

When this process recurs over many years, cholesterol builds up on the vessel wall, and **plaque** develops. This plaque is eventually mixed with protein and then covered with a cap of muscle cells and calcium. Atherosclerosis develops as plaque grows in the vessel. *The actual key to atherosclerosis may lie in the liver. Because it contains about 50% to 75% of the LDL receptors in the body, the liver is the main regulator of blood cholesterol levels.* Recently, a child born essentially without LDL receptors in her liver received a liver transplant. Before the operation the patient's cholesterol level was 1100 milligrams per 100 milliliters of serum. After the operation her serum cholesterol dropped to 270 milligrams per 100 milliliters. A desirable serum cholesterol level is below 200 milligrams per 100 milliliters.[2] This demonstrates the importance of the liver in controlling serum cholesterol levels.

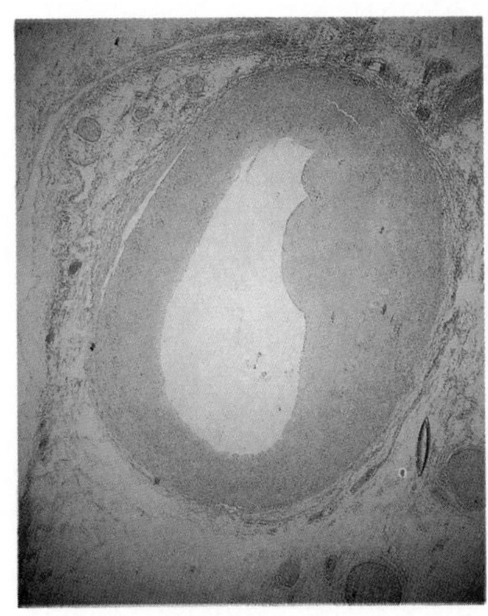

Over time, cholesterol and other substances can build up in a blood vessel, in turn retarding blood flow.

A final critical participant in this whole process of lipid transport is the **high-density lipoprotein (HDL).** The liver and intestine produce HDLs that roam the bloodstream, picking up cholesterol from dying cells and other sources. HDLs donate the cholesterol primarily to other lipoproteins for transport back to the liver for excretion (Figure 5-7). Some HDLs may interact directly with the liver as well. This process is called **reverse transport of cholesterol.**

Large-scale studies clearly show that a person's HDL cholesterol level is very predictive of the risk for heart disease. If the serum HDL level is greater than 60 milligrams per 100 milliliters, the risk of heart disease is likely to be low. If the HDL cholesterol level is less than 40, the risk of developing heart disease is increased.[1] Men often have HDL cholesterol levels in the high 30s and to high 40s. Women often have HDL cholesterol levels in the low 50s to low 60s. This is one reason why women, at least before **menopause,** have a lower risk for atherosclerosis, and therefore for heart attacks, than men. The estrogen produced by women in their child-bearing years appears to help keep serum HDL cholesterol levels high. For men, regular exercise may raise their serum HDL cholesterol levels a bit—about 5 milligrams per 100 milliliters. The more exercise, the better result.

Since a high HDL cholesterol level is associated with a lower chance of developing heart disease, the HDL form of cholesterol has been considered "good" cholesterol. If so, the LDL form would be the "bad" cholesterol because a high serum LDL cholesterol level increases the risk for heart disease. However, LDLs are not all bad; they carry needed cholesterol to cells and take cholesterol from the HDLs back to the liver for excretion. *Probably only when serum LDL cholesterol level is high—greater than 130 to 160 milligrams per 100 milliliters—are LDLs really "bad" for the body.*

Concept Check

The bloodstream carries absorbed dietary fat as chylomicrons. Lipid synthesized by the liver is carried in the bloodstream as *very low density lipoproteins (VLDL).* Once a VLDL has most of its triglycerides removed, it eventually turns into a *low density lipoprotein (LDL).* This lipoprotein is high in cholesterol. The LDLs are picked up by body cells, especially liver cells. A final lipoprotein is the *high density form, HDL.* It picks up cholesterol from cells and transports it primarily to other lipoproteins for eventual transport back to the liver. An elevated serum LDL cholesterol level is associated with high risk for heart disease as in a low serum HDL cholesterol level.

RECOMMENDATIONS FOR FAT INTAKE

There is no RDA for fat. A good goal, as suggested earlier, is to consume about 4% of energy from plant oils to get the essential fatty acids. Recall that this percentage amounts to about 1 tablespoon of oil per day.

The U.S. diet contains about 38% of total kcalories as fat. In Canada the diet is about 42% of total kcalories as fat. Vegetable sources supply about half this fat and animal sources supply the other half. Major sources of fat in the U.S. diet include animal flesh, whole milk, and pastries.

The ratio of saturated to monounsaturated to polyunsaturated fatty acids in the U.S. diet is about 42:40:18. Sometimes the ratio of polyunsaturated fatty acids to saturated fatty acids (P:S ratio) is calculated for a diet. The P:S ratio for the U.S. diet is 18:42, or about 0.43. A ratio of 1 is generally recommended to reduce the risk of heart disease. *Registered dietitians worry less today about a diet's P:S ratio and focus instead on the saturated fat content.* It is saturated fat that most affects blood cholesterol levels (see Nutrition Perspective 5-1).

The American Heart Association (AHA) recommends a fat intake of no more than 30% of total kcalories, with a ratio of about 10:10:10 for saturated to monounsaturated to polyunsaturated fatty acids (Table 5-4). (Note that the P:S ratio would be 1.) The AHA further recommends lowering fat intake to 20% of total kcalories in cases where elevated serum cholesterol level does not respond to this moderate recommendation. The National Cholesterol Education Program, established in 1985 in the United States, recommends reducing saturated fatty acids to 7% of total kcalories if a high serum cholesterol level does not respond to reducing it to 10%. By encouraging a reduction in total fat and saturated fat intake, all these suggestions are in line with the Dietary Guidelines for Americans.

FATS IN FOODS

The Exchange System provides an easy method for estimating the amount of fat in food (Table 5-5). Exchanges from both vegetables and fruit groups are fat-free. In the milk group the amount of fat varies with food choice—skim milk has a trace (sometimes calculated as 1 gram), low-fat has 5 grams, and whole has 8

Table 5-4

Dietary guidelines for healthy american adults
A statement for physicians and health professionals by the nutrition committee, American Heart Association

1. Total fat intake should be less than 30% of kcalories.
2. Saturated fat intake should be less than 10% of calories.
3. Polyunsaturated fat intake should not exceed 10% of calories.
4. Cholesterol intake should not exceed 300 mg/day.
5. Carbohydrate intake should constitute 50% or more of calories, with emphasis on complex carbohydrates.
6. Protein intake should provide the remainder of the calories.
7. Sodium intake should not exceed 3 g/day.
8. Alcoholic consumption should not exceed 1 to 2 oz of ethanol per day. Two ounces of 100 proof whisky, 8 oz of wine, or 24 oz of beer each contain 1 oz of ethanol.
9. Total kcalories should be sufficient to maintain the individual's recommended body weight.
10. A wide variety of foods should be consumed.

Source: Circulation 77:721A, 1988.

Monounsaturated fatty acids can lower serum cholesterol levels when they replace saturated fatty acids in the diet. The P:S ratio ignores this effect. Furthermore, not all saturated fatty acids raise serum cholesterol levels. Stearic acid, which has 18 carbon atoms, doesn't, while many saturated fatty acids with chain lengths of 16 carbons or less do. This gives further evidence for questioning the importance of the P:S ratio; this concept is too simplistic.

grams per exchange. The starch/bread group has a trace of fat (sometimes calculated as 1 gram) per exchange. Again, in the meat group, fat values vary with food choice—lean has 3 grams, medium-fat has 5 grams, and high-fat has 8 grams per exchange. The fat group has 5 grams of fat per exchange.

For foods in general the highest nutrient density for fat is found in salad oils, butter, margarine, and mayonnaise. All contain about 100% of kcalories as fat (Figure 5-8). Walnuts, bologna, avocados, and bacon have about 80%. Peanut butter and cheddar cheese have about 75% of their kcalories as fat. Steak and ham-

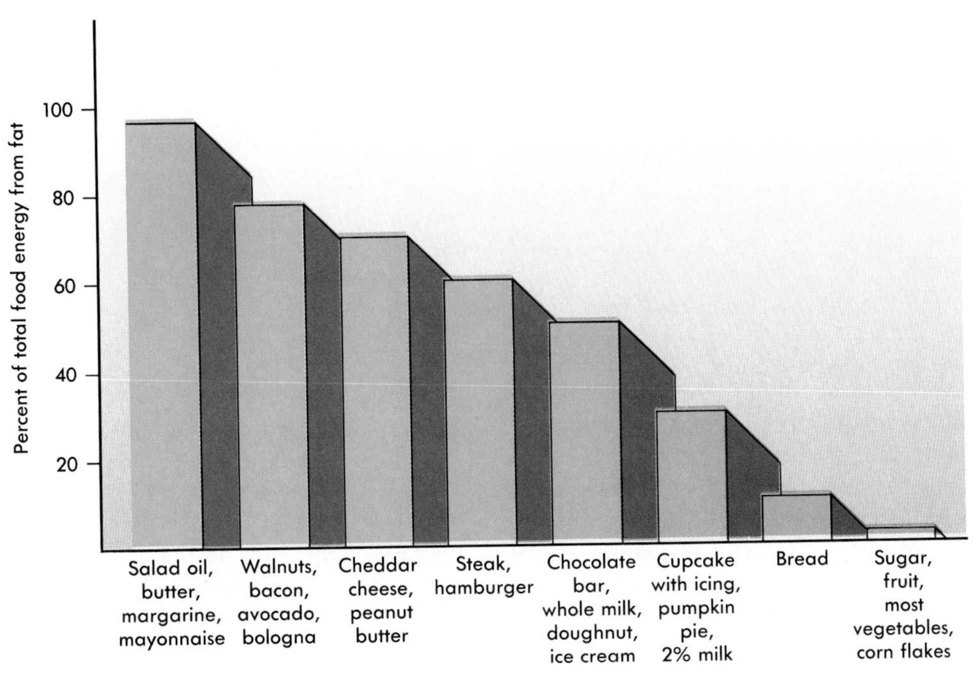

Figure 5-8
Percent of kcalories as fats in foods. Vegetable oils, butter, margarine, and mayonnaise provide almost all kcalories as fats.

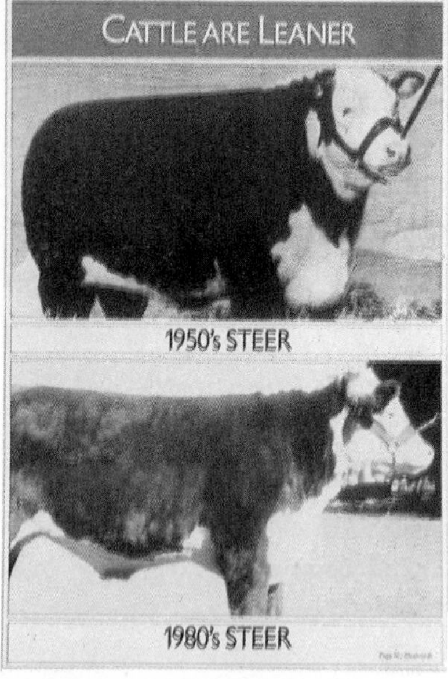

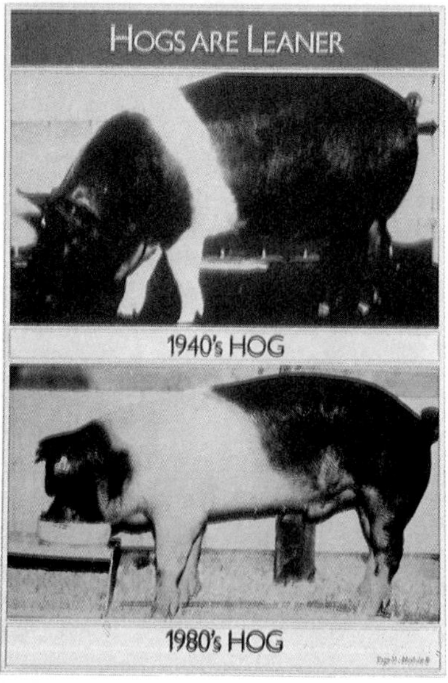

Table 5-5

Exchanges	30% of kcalories as fat	25% of kcalories as fat	20% of kcalories as fat
Milk	2 low-fat	2 low-fat	2 non-fat
Fruit	4	5	7
Vegetable	2	3	2
Starch/bread	11	11	11
Meat	4 medium-fat	4 medium-fat	4 lean
Fat	7	5	4
Menu			
Breakfast			
	1 cup orange juice	same	same
	3/4 cup shredded wheat	same	same
	1 toasted bagel	same	same
	2 t margarine	1 t margarine	1 t margarine
	1 cup 2% milk	same	1 cup nonfat milk
Lunch			
	2 slices whole wheat bread	same	same
	1 oz roast beef	same	1 oz boiled ham
	2 t mayonnaise	1 t mayonnaise	1 t mayonnaise
	lettuce	same	same
	1 sliced tomato	same	same
	8 animal crackers	same	same
Snack			
	1 apple	same	same
Dinner			
	3 oz broiled lamb chop	same	3 oz broiled halibut
	1-1/2 cup pasta	same	same
	2 t margarine	same	1 t margarine
	1/2 cup broccoli	1 cup	1/2 cup
	1 cup 2% milk	same	1 cup nonfat milk
			1 banana
Snack			
	2 T raisins	1/4 cup	1/4 cup
	6 cups air-popped popcorn	same	same
	with 1 t margarine	same	same

burgers have about 60%, and chocolate bars, ice cream, doughnuts, and whole milk have about 50% of kcalories as fat. Pumpkin pie and cupcakes have 35%. Bread contains about 15% of its kcalories as fat. Cornflakes, sugar, and most fruits and vegetables have essentially no fat.

Animal fats contain about 40% to 60% saturated fatty acids and are the chief contributor of saturated fatty acids to the U.S. diet. Recent evidence suggests that only saturated fatty acids with 16 or less carbons tend to raise serum cholesterol levels.[3] These problem saturated fatty acids constitute about 25% to 50% of animal fats. Some plant products also contain significant amounts of problem saturated fatty acids; for example, cottonseed oil (27%), palm oil (46%), palm kernel oil (79%), and coconut oil (89%). Researchers suggest that the 18-carbon saturated stearic acid does not raise serum cholesterol levels because it quickly has a double bond added to it, transforming it into the monounsaturated fatty acid, oleic acid.[3]

Plant fats contain mostly unsaturated fatty acids, ranging from 73% to 94%, excluding palm and coconut oils. Plant oils supply the majority of the linoleic and linolenic acid in the U.S. food supply. Olive oil, canola oil, and peanut oil contain a moderate to high amount of monounsaturated fatty acids (49% to 77%). Some animal fats are also good sources (30% to 47%; Table 5-1). Corn, cottonseed, sunflower, soybean, and safflower oils contain mostly polyunsaturated fat (54% to 77%). Note that plant oils vary in their amounts of polyunsaturated fat. While many oils are similar in composition, significant variations are common. "Vegetable oil" is too general a term to list on a label. The specific oil used, for example, corn or palm oil, should be known. Unfortunately, the label may list a variety of oils, and any one could have been used. That makes it difficult for people trying to limit their intake of saturated fat.

Concept Check

There is no recommended dietary allowance for fat. We need about 4% of total energy intake from plant oils to get the needed essential fatty acids. Many health-related agencies recommend a diet containing no more than 30% of energy as fat, and no more than one third of that as saturated fat. The current North American diet contains about 38% to 42% of energy as fat, with two fifths of that from saturated fat. Foods high in fat (over 60% of total kcalories) include plant oils, butter, margarine, mayonnaise, walnuts, bacon, avocados, peanut butter, cheddar cheese, steak and hamburger.

Exploring Issues and Actions

Your best friend eats heavily buttered popcorn at home every night. What reasons might you suggest for switching to a small amount of margarine?

FAT REPLACEMENTS

Recently there has been much public and scientific interest in two fat substitutes—sucrose polyester (Olestra) and Simplesse. Only Simplesse is approved for use in foods yet. Sucrose polyester is made by adding fatty acids to the hydroxyl groups (−OH) on a sucrose (table sugar) molecule.[15] Usually eight fatty acids are added to each sucrose molecule. The manufacturer can change the characteristics of the product by adding greater or fewer numbers of fatty acids. Sucrose polyester with many fatty acids attached cannot be digested by either human digestive enzymes or bacteria that live in the intestine. Therefore it yields no kcalories to the body. As it leaves the body, it can even pull cholesterol-containing substances found in the intestine with it, thereby lowering the person's serum cholesterol level. The product is quite versatile as an ingredient. The manufacturer feels it can replace up to 35% of the fat is salad dressings and cakes made in the home, and it can be used for frying in food manufacturing.

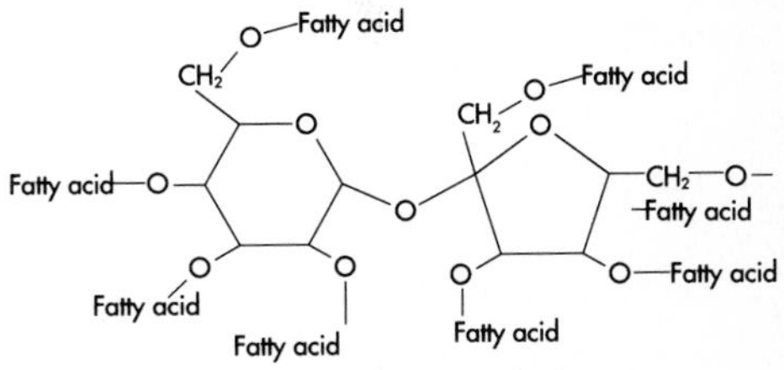

Fatty acid
CH_2
O
Fatty acid
CH_2
O
Fatty acid—O
O
CH_2—O—Fatty acid
O—Fatty acid
Fatty acid
Fatty acid
Fatty acid

Sucrose polyester (with the maximum number of fatty acids attached)

There are still some problems with sucrose polyester. It tends to bind the fat-soluble vitamin E, reducing its absorption. The manufacturer has proposed adding vitamin E to it to compensate. Some years ago the Food and Drug Administration (FDA) would not permit the use of mineral oil in foods as a no-kcalorie fat because it bound up fat-soluble vitamins. Because of that and other questions, it is unclear when this product will be available. If approved by the FDA, it would reduce the fat content of many foods and permit us to eat some rich desserts and fried foods and better control fat intake.

Little has been published about Simplesse. The manufacturer has developed a technique in which egg and milk proteins are mixed together with heat in such a way that microscopic, mist-like protein globules are produced. The globules feel like fat in the mouth. While it yields energy, Simplesse has only about 1.3 kcalories per gram, which is much less than regular fat's 9 kcalories per gram.

Simplesse is most useful for replacing fat in mayonnaise, salad dressings, ice cream, and other dairy products. Because high heat alters Simplesse'structure so much that it no longer resembles fat, it cannot be used for cooking or frying. The manufacturer petitioned the FDA for approval of the product in early 1988. It may reach the market in 1990.

Ask your professor about the latest information on these fat substitutes. Research is moving rapidly in this area. There is much scientific and economic interest in producing flavorful snack and dessert foods that yield less fat.

See Nutrition Perspectives 5-1 on heart disease to do the Take Action activity.

Summary

1. Lipids are a group of relatively oxygen-poor compounds that dissolve in chloroform, benzene, or ether. Saturated fatty acids contain no double bonds, monounsaturated fatty acids contain one double bond, and polyunsaturated fatty acids contain two or more double bonds.
2. If the double bonds in the fatty acid begin at the third carbon atom from the methyl end ($-CH_3$), then the fatty acid is an *omega-3 fatty acid.* If the double bonds begin at the sixth carbon atom, it is an *omega-6 fatty acid.* Both omega-3 and omega-6 fatty acids are essential parts of a diet.
3. When cells use omega-3 fatty acids to synthesize hormone-like compounds called *eicosanoids,* the products tend to reduce blood clotting, blood pressure, and inflammatory responses in the body.
4. Lipids composed of saturated fatty acids tend to be solid at room temperature and those with polyunsaturated fatty acids are usually liquid at room temperature. *Hydrogenation* is the process of turning double bonds in fatty acids into single bonds by adding hydrogen atoms. This solidifies vegetable oils and reduces the rancid breakdown of fatty acids.
5. The triglyceride is the major form of fat in food and in the body. Phospholipids are derivatives of the triglycerides. Phospholipids are important parts of cell membranes, and some act as efficient emulsifiers.
6. Cholesterol forms vital compounds, such as hormones, parts of cell membranes, and bile acids. We eat cholesterol, and cells in the body make it.
7. Lipids are carried in the bloodstream by various lipoproteins: chylomicrons, very low density lipoproteins (VLDL), low density lipoproteins (LDL), and high density lipoproteins (HDL).
8. An elevated serum LDL cholesterol level is associated with a high risk of developing heart disease, as in a low serum HDL cholesterol level.
9. There is no RDA for fat. We need about 4% of total energy intake from plant oils to get the needed essential fatty acids.

REFERENCES

1. Anderson JW and Gustafson NJ: Hypocholesterolemic effects of oat bran and bean products, American Journal of Clinical Nutrition 48:749, 1988.
2. Anonymous: Heart-liver transplantation in a child with homozygous familial hypercholesterolemia, Nutrition Reviews 43:274, 1985.
3. Bonanome A and Grundy SM: Effect of dietary stearic acid on plasma cholesterol and lipoprotein levels, New England Journal of Medicine 318:1244, 1988.
4. Butrum RR and others: NCI dietary guidelines: rationale, American Journal of Clinical Nutrition, 48:888, 1988.
5. Canadian Dietetic Association: Diet and cancer prevention, Journal of the Canadian Dietetic Association 48:144, 1987.
6. Carroll KK: Dietary fat and cancer: specific action or caloric effect? Journal of Nutrition 116:1130, 1986.
7. Cleveland LE and Pfeffer AB: Planning diets to meet the National Research Council's

guidelines for reducing cancer risk, Journal of the American Dietetic Association 87:162, 1987.
8. Council for Agricultural Science and Technology: Diet and coronary disease, Nutrition Today March/April:26, 1986.
9. Das UN and others: Clinical significance of essential fatty acids, Nutrition 4:337, 1988.
10. Dyerberg J: Linolenate-derived polyunsaturated fatty acids in prevention of atherosclerosis, Nutrition Reviews 44:125, 1986.
11. Garfinkel L: Overweight and cancer, Annals of Internal Medicine 103:1034, 1985.
12. Greenwald P and others: Dietary fiber in the reduction of colon cancer risk, Journal of the American Dietetic Association 87:1178, 1987.
13. Grundy SM: Monounsaturated fatty acids, plasma cholesterol, and coronary heart disease, American Journal of Clinical Nutrition 45:1168, 1987.
14. Grundy SM: Comparison of monounsaturated fatty acids and carbohydrates for lowering plasma cholesterol, The New England Journal of Medicine 314:745, 1986.
15. Haumann BF: Getting the fat out, Journal of the American Oil Chemists Society 63:278, 1986.
16. Hunter JE and Applewhite TH: Isomenic fatty acids in the U.S. diet, The American Journal of Clinical Nutrition 44:707, 1986.
17. Kris-Etherton PM and others: The effect of diet on plasma lipids, lipoproteins, and coronary heart disease, Journal of the American Dietetic Association 88:1373, 1988.
18. Lane HW and Carpenter JT: Breast cancer: incidence, nutritional concerns and treatment approaches, The Journal of the American Dietetic Association 87:765, 1987.
19. Lands WEM: Renewed questions about polyunsaturated fatty acids, Nutrition Reviews 44:189, 1986.
20. Leaf A and Weber PC: Cardiovascular effects of n-3 fatty acid, The New England Journal of Medicine 318:549, 1988.
21. Mensink RP and Katan MB: Effect of monounsaturated fatty acids versus complex carbohydrates on high-density lipoprotein in healthy men and women, Lancet 1:122, 1987.
22. Pariza MW: Dietary fat and cancer risk: evidence and research needs, Annual Reviews of Nutrition 8:167, 1988.
23. Simopoulos AP: W-3 fatty acids in growth and development and in health and disease, Nutrition Today, March/April: 10 and May/June: 12, 1988.
24. Snetselaar L: Update on nutrition and cardiovascular disease, Topics in Clinical Nutrition 4:31, 1989.
25. Steinberg D and others: Beyond cholesterol: modifications of low-density lipoprotein that increase its atherogenicity, New England Journal of Medicine 320:915, 1989.
26. Thompson PD and others: Modest changes in high-density lipoprotein concentration and metabolism with prolonged exercise training, Circulation, 78:25, 1988.
27. Wardlaw GM: Assessing the cancer risk from foods, Journal of the American Dietetic Association 85:1122, 1985.
28. Watson RR and Leonard PK: Selenium and vitamins A, E, and C: nutrients with cancer prevention properties, Journal of the American Dietetic Association 86:505, 1986.
29. Willit WC and others: Dietary fat and the risk of breast cancer, The New England Journal of Medicine 316:22, 1987.
30. Yetiv JZ: Clinical Applications of fish oils, Journal of the American Medical Association 260:665, 1988.
31. Ziegler RE: A review of epidemiological evidence that carotenoids reduce the risk of cancer, Journal of Nutrition 119:116, 1989.

CHAPTER 5

Answers to the Nutrition Awareness Inventory

1. *False.* Saturated fats are solid at room temperature.
2. *True.* Alcohol yields 7 kcalories per gram and lipid yields 9 kcalories per gram.
3. *True.* People who suffer from strokes have elevated serum cholesterol levels.
4. *True.* But don't be misled by advertisers who state certain products are "cholesterol-free." The product may still contain saturated fat, which is a more important determinant of blood cholesterol level.
5. *True.* Animal fats are often rich in saturated fat.
6. *True.* Triglyceride is the primary form of lipid in both foods and the body.
7. *False.* Fat is absolutely necessary for life because it supplies essential fatty acids used to make vital body compounds.
8. *True.* In some cases this process makes food production easier; hydrogenation prevents the oils in peanut butter from separating during storage.
9. *True.* Most fruits contain only a trace amount of fat.
10. *True.* BHA and BHT are examples of antioxidants found in salad dressings.
11. *True.* Because vitamins A, E, D, and K are fat soluble their absorption is enhanced by dietary fat.
12. *False.* Everyone age 20 years or more should monitor and track his or her blood cholesterol levels. (Some groups recommend that anyone over 2 years old who has a family history of early heart disease should do the same.) Elevated blood cholesterol is a risk factor for cardiovascular disease. Early action to reduce elevated cholesterol levels is the best plan.
13. *True.* Butter, however, contains more saturated fats than margarine.
14. *True.* Studies with both animals and humans have shown high doses of fish oil can moderately lower serum cholesterol levels. However, high fish oil doses mainly affect serum triglyceride levels.
15. *False.* Nondairy creamers often contain coconut oil, which is very high in saturated fat.

SUGGESTED READINGS

To learn more about interactions between diet and lipoproteins see both articles by Grundy, and that by Kris-Etherton. All three focus strongly on the effects of diet. For a review of how cancer develops in a cell and how to evaluate the potential for a food to cause cancer consult the article by Wardlaw. The article by Greenwald to explore in detail the relationship between dietary fiber and cancer. Finally, for a detailed discussion of omega-3 fatty acids see both articles by Simopoulos. After reading those articles consider reading the more technical reports by Leaf and Yetiv. These four articles will give you a strong background in this developing area of nutrition research.

Nutrition Perspective 5-1

Heart Disease

Heart disease is the major killer of North Americans. About 600,000 people die of heart disease each year in the United States. The figure rises to almost 1 million if we include strokes and other circulatory diseases. Heart disease is a chronic disease—it takes years to develop symptoms. There is no single cause of heart disease but many factors increase the risk for its development.

Heart disease and strokes are associated with poor blood circulation. When the flow of blood through arteries supplying the heart muscle with oxygen and nutrients is interrupted, part of the heart muscle can be affected. A heart attack, or **myocardial infarction,** may ensue (Figure 5-9). This may cause the heart to beat irregularly or not at all, leading to little or no heart function. If blood flow to part of the brain stops, that part of the brain may die. This event is called a **cerebrovascular accident (CVA),** or stroke. When it causes loss of muscle control, death may result.

myocardial infarction Death of part of the heart muscle.

cerebrovascular accident (CVA) Death of part of the brain tissue due to a blood clot.

Blood clots are the agents that stop the blood flow to the heart or brain. These clots have a greater tendency to form when cholesterol plaque has built up in the arteries that lead to the heart or brain. The plaque is probably first deposited to repair injuries in the vessel lining. The plaque thickens as layers of cholesterol and other factors in the bloodstream are laid down. The rate of plaque deposition partly depends on the amount of cholesterol in the bloodstream.

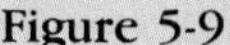

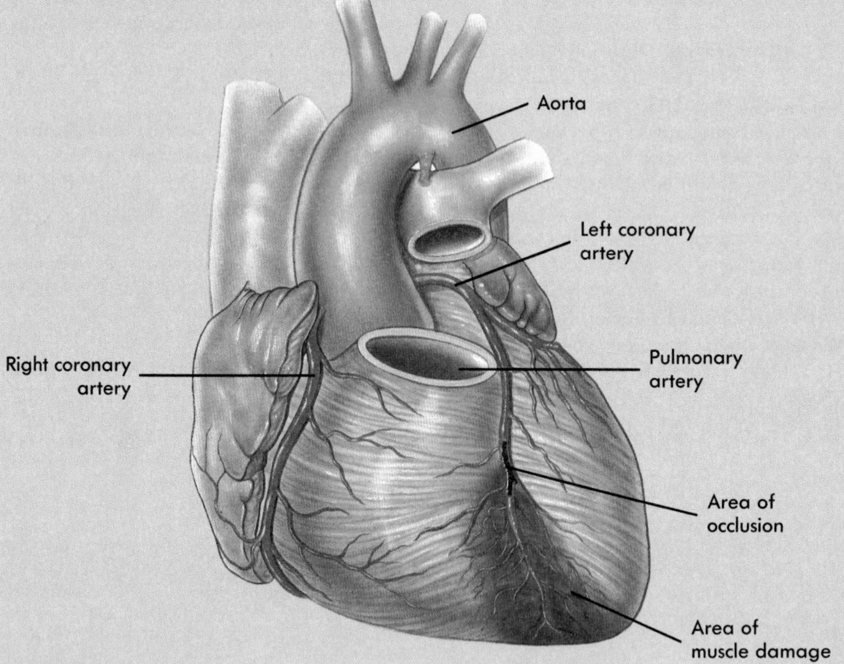

Figure 5-9

A heart attack. This heart attack resulted from blockage of the left coronary artery. The heart muscle serviced by the portion of the coronary artery beyond the point of blockage is damaged, and may die. This can lead to a significant drop in heart function.

WHAT IS YOUR RISK FOR HEART DISEASE?

The three most important risk factors for heart disease are smoking, hypertension (high blood pressure), and high serum cholesterol levels. Family history is also important, particularly if a parent suffers a heart attack or stroke before age 60. So is a low serum HDL cholesterol level. These factors should signal us to take aggressive early steps for prevention. Still significant but less important risk factors are diet, stress, inactivity, diabetes, and obesity. All these factors can contribute to heart disease. However, the most important contributors—smoking, hypertension, and high serum cholesterol levels—are the ones we should focus on first to prevent early heart disease.[8]

Do you smoke? Do you have hypertension? Specifically, is your **systolic blood pressure** about 140 millimeters of mercury or your **diastolic blood pressure** about 90 millimeters of mercury? Is your serum cholesterol over 200 milligrams per 100 milliliters? In addition, what is your serum HDL cholesterol level? If it is below 35 milligrams per 100 milliliters, you have an increased risk for coronary heart disease. Finally, what is your LDL cholesterol level? If it is greater than 160 milligrams per 100 milliliters of serum, you have a greater risk of heart disease. (Have yourself tested at least two more times if you show high values the first time because all the levels can vary day to day.) Add your family history and you can put heart disease into perspective for yourself.

Early heart disease, before age 70, should be the focus. Eventually we all die. The key is to prevent premature death. Heart attacks at age 40 through 60 are closely linked to these risk factors. Preventing heart attacks at these ages is an important goal. See Chapter 17 for a further discussion of this concept of premature disease and how to strive to prevent it.

Serum LDL and HDL cholesterol levels—rather than the total cholesterol level—are really the most important levels to focus on, especially for women. If total serum cholesterol level greater than 200 milligrams per 100 milliliters is primarily due to a high HDL cholesterol level, which is sometimes the case for women, the risk of heart disease is still low. Unfortunately, when men have elevated total cholesterol levels, it is usually due to an elevated LDL cholesterol level.

The National Institutes of Health in the United States encourage all people over age 20 to have their total serum cholesterol level checked. We recommend having your serum HDL cholesterol and triglyceride levels checked also. That way the serum LDL cholesterol can be calculated. If you don't know your cholesterol levels, you don't know your risk of developing heart disease.

LOWERING AN ELEVATED SERUM CHOLESTEROL LEVEL

When discovering that someone has a high serum cholesterol level, the first step for the person should be to consult a physician. Some diseases raise serum cholesterol levels. By treating the disease, the levels will naturally fall. If disease isn't present, diet change is the next step.

To change a diet to lower an elevated serum cholesterol level, first reduce the amount of saturated fat eaten.[17,24] (Even if the serum cholesterol level is normal, it is still wise to lower saturated fat intake.) Lowering serum saturated fat intake is more important for most people than reducing dietary cholesterol. Only about 10% to 25% of people find that they lower their serum cholesterol level when they eat less cholesterol. Most people show only a minimal effect or no effect. However, almost everyone who lowers saturated fat intake can lower an elevated serum cholesterol level about 10% to 20%, especially if he or she is already eating many foods high in saturated fats. Table 5-6 contains tips for lowering saturated fat intake.

Saturated fats in the diet probably affect serum cholesterol levels by changing the number of receptors for LDL cholesterol in the liver.[13] When saturated fat intake is low, the number of LDL receptors in the liver increases. Recall that the liver is the major organ for clearing LDL cholesterol from the bloodstream. Serum cholesterol levels fall as more cholesterol is cleared from the bloodstream and pulled into the liver for excretion as bile acids into the small intestine.

A reasonable goal is to eat no more than 10% of kcalories as saturated fats. A reduction to only 7% is better. *To do this one must watch the intake of fatty animal products, butter, coconut oil, palm oil, shortening, and other hydrogenated (solid) fats.* Reading labels is important. Saturated fats are often hidden in foods. In addition, broil, bake, or boil meats; don't fry them. Limit use of gravies and fatty desserts. Use only low-fat—and preferably nonfat—dairy products. Thus important foods to avoid should be processed meats (like sausage), butter, ice cream, cheese (except maybe mozzarella and other low-fat cheeses), whole milk, stick margarine (tub margarine is generally less hydrogenated, and so has fewer saturated fatty acids), sour cream, nondairy coffee creamers, granola bars, crackers, biscuits, and all visible animal fat (Table 5-6).

New analyses show an egg containing closer to 200 to 220 milligrams of cholesterol, rather than the earlier figure of 275 milligrams. Nevertheless, the focus should be on reducing saturated fat intake.

Continued

Nutrition Perspective 5-1, cont'd

Table 5-6

Tips for avoiding too much fat and saturated fat

1. Steam, boil, or bake vegetables. For a change, stirfry in a small amount of vegetable oil.
2. Season vegetables with herbs and spices rather than with sauces, butter, or margarine.
3. Try lemon juice on salad or use limited amounts of oil-based salad dressing.
4. To reduce saturated fat use tub margarine instead of butter or stick margarine in baked products and when possible, use vegetable oil instead of these solid fats.
5. Try whole-grain flours to enhance flavors when making baked goods with less fat and cholesterol-containing ingredients.
6. Replace whole milk with skim or low-fat milk in puddings, soups, and baked products.
7. Substitute plain low-fat yogurt, blender-whipped low-fat cottage cheese, or buttermilk in recipes that call for sour cream or mayonnaise.
8. Choose lean cuts of meat.
9. Trim fat from meat before and after cooking.
10. Roast, bake, or broil meat, poultry, or fish so fat drains away as the food cooks.
11. Remove skin from poultry before cooking.
12. Use a nonstick pan for cooking so added fat will be unnecessary; use a vegetable spray for frying.
13. Chill meat or poultry broth until the fat becomes solid. Spoon off the fat before using the broth.
14. Eat a vegetarian main dish at least once a week. Include fish (cooked without much added fat) in the diet every week.
15. Limit high-fat cheese intake.

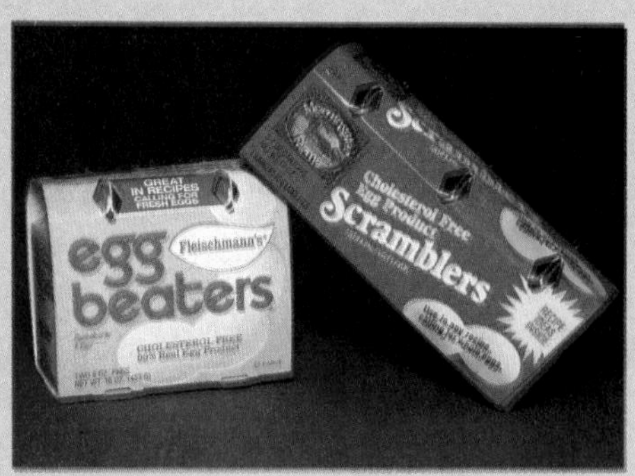

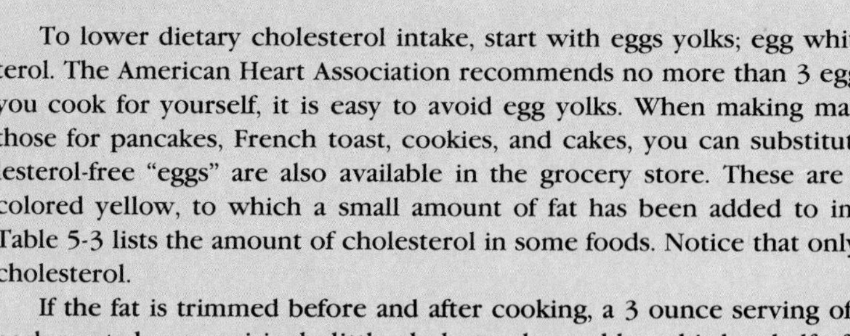

To lower dietary cholesterol intake, start with eggs yolks; egg whites have no cholesterol. The American Heart Association recommends no more than 3 egg yolks per week. If you cook for yourself, it is easy to avoid egg yolks. When making many recipes, such as those for pancakes, French toast, cookies, and cakes, you can substitute egg whites. Cholesterol-free "eggs" are also available in the grocery store. These are usually egg whites colored yellow, to which a small amount of fat has been added to improve their flavor. Table 5-3 lists the amount of cholesterol in some foods. Notice that only animal foods have cholesterol.

If the fat is trimmed before and after cooking, a 3 ounce serving of chicken, beef, and pork meats has surprisingly little cholesterol, roughly a third to half of that in an egg. *For North Americans it is the portion size that causes them trouble with meat and cholesterol intake.* A 10 ounce serving of meat can contain 260 milligrams of cholesterol, more than is in one egg. Meats have a reputation for being high in cholesterol. However, this mainly is due to the amount of meat we eat rather than to the amount of cholesterol in an ounce of meat.

MONOUNSATURATED VERSUS POLYUNSATURATED FATS

There are some encouraging new observations on the ability of monounsaturated fatty acids in diet to lower serum cholesterol levels.[13,14,21] Recall that these have only one double bond. In the past saturated fatty acids were thought to contribute to high serum cholesterol levels, and polyunsaturated fatty acids were believed to lower serum cholesterol levels.[19] Polyunsaturated fatty acids were then recommended to replace saturated fatty acids. However, recent studies show that when foods high in monounsaturated fatty acids replaced those high in saturated fatty acids, serum cholesterol levels also went down. So both are now considered good replacements for saturated fatty acids.

FIBER AND REDUCED HEART DISEASE

Another recent development in lowering serum cholesterol levels is increasing the intake of soluble fiber, which is found in oatmeal, oat bran, beans, vegetables, and fruits. Some laxatives—those with psyllium fiber—are also food sources. Diets very high in overall fiber (50 to 60 grams per day), especially those that emphasize soluble fibers, can lower serum cholesterol levels.[1] The fiber probably binds cholesterol and bile acids in the small intestine and carries them into the colon for elimination. This action resembles that of some medications in lowering serum cholesterol levels; removing bile acids from the body forces the liver to pull more cholesterol out of the bloodstream to make new bile acids. Other mechanisms to account for the effects of soluble fibers have also been suggested.

One may have to considerably change diet to follow a diet high in soluble fiber, but the change is possible (see Chapter 4). Currently researchers caution against eating more than 35 grams of dietary fiber a day, so it is best to consult a physician before embarking on a very high-fiber diet. We think that eating a diet low in saturated fats may be an easier and safer alternative to raising fiber intake so dramatically.

RAISING THE SERUM HDL CHOLESTEROL LEVEL

An important first step in lowering a serum total cholesterol level is not to lower the serum HDL cholesterol level. Only the serum LDL cholesterol level should fall. If the serum HDL cholesterol level does fall, an emphasis on monounsaturated fat, rather than polyunsaturated fat, is a good idea. Exercising at least 45 minutes 4 times a week will also protect the serum HDL cholesterol level, and maybe will even raise it by about 5 milligrams per 100 milliliters.[26] In addition, regular eating habits (three balanced meals per day), an energy intake matched to energy output, and a lower total fat intake often help by lowering serum triglyceride levels. Lowering serum triglyceride levels often results in increased serum HDL cholesterol levels. Why this is so is not clear. Nevertheless, the goal is to have fasting serum triglyceride levels below 150 milligrams per 100 milliliters. Certain medications also act to lower serum triglyceride levels. When this happens, serum HDL cholesterol levels also often increase. It is unfortunate that raising HDL cholesterol levels is usually difficult. Lowering LDL cholesterol levels is usually much easier.

WHAT SHOULD ONE DO?

To lower a high serum LDL cholesterol level:

• Reduce saturated fat intake	This is the best method and should be the major focus
• Reduce cholesterol intake	This helps some people and is not harmful to anyone
• Perform regular exercise	This may protect serum HDL cholesterol levels
• Lose weight to attain a desirable body weight	This helps reduce serum triglyceride levels (if elevated)
• Increase intake of soluble fiber	This binds cholesterol and bile acids in the small intestine to encourage their elimination via the colon rather than absorption into the bloodstream; there also may be other causes for the drop
• Reduce total fat intake	This may help achieve the other goals

National Cholesterol Education Program for Adults—Dietary Advice

GOAL: Total blood cholesterol <200 mg/dl*
LDL cholesterol <160 mg/dl or <130 mg/dl with 2 or more risk factors

If total blood cholesterol is >200 mg/dl and an individual has two or more of the following risk factors:

- Family history of coronary heart disease
- Smokes cigarettes
- Diabetes
- Obesity
- Hypertension
- Low HDL cholesterol
- Male

Test for LDL cholesterol

If LDL cholesterol >130 mg/dl:

- Reduce saturated fat intake to 10% of total kilocalories
- Reduce total fat intake to 30% of total kilocalories
- Reduce cholesterol intake to 300 mg/day

For 6 months

If unsuccessful (that is, LDL cholesterol >130 mg/dl)

- Reduce saturated fat intake to 7% of total kilocalories
- Reduce cholesterol intake to 200 mg/day

For 6 months

*mg/dl represents milligrams per 100 milliliters of serum.

New analyses show an egg containing closer to 200 to 220 milligrams of cholesterol, rather than the earlier figure of 275 milligrams. Nevertheless, the focus should be on reducing saturated fat intake. This correction in egg composition is of trivial importance.

Continued

Nutrition Perspective 5-1—cont'd

Everyone needs to find what works for himself. The plan should be to make some changes and recheck the serum total cholesterol and HDL cholesterol level in a couple of weeks to compare results. Steady progress toward these goals often reaps the benefit of a lower risk for developing heart disease.

MEDICATIONS TO LOWER SERUM CHOLESTEROL LEVELS

Medications are a last resort for treating high serum cholesterol levels because of their expense and side effects. Nevertheless, the effects of diet changes are sometimes insufficient to control high serum cholesterol levels, especially in people with strong genetic tendencies toward that problem. Current medications work in one of two ways. One group decreases lipoprotein synthesis by the liver and includes nicotinic acid, lovastatin, probucol, and gemfibrozil. The other group—which includes cholestyramine and cholestipol—binds bile acids in the small intestine and prevents their reabsorption. This forces the liver to synthesize new bile acids. The liver pulls cholesterol out of the bloodstream to do this, which lowers the serum cholesterol level. All these medications work better when a proper diet is followed—they do not substitute for diet changes.

Take Action

Do you have . . .	*yes*	*no*
a history of smoking?	☐	☐
high blood pressure?	☐	☐
a high serum cholesterol level, especially LDL cholesterol?	☐	☐
a low serum HDL cholesterol level?	☐	☐
diabetes mellitus?	☐	☐
a history of inactivity?	☐	☐
a history of early heart disease?	☐	☐
a history of obesity?	☐	☐

Other factors also could be considered. This will be a good start, however.

1. Do you know your HDL and total cholesterol levels? If not, discover where you can have them checked and make an appointment this week.
2. Write a one-page assessment of your risk for having a heart attack. Describe how you could modify your diet and life-style to reduce your risk.

Nutrition Perspective 5-2

Nutrition and Cancer

Cancer is the second leading cause of death for adults in the United States. Cancer is actually many diseases; different types of cells are affected, and many different causes contribute to cancer. What causes skin cancer differs from what causes breast cancer, and their treatments also differ. We each need to look seriously at cancer in general and at the risk we have of getting it. Cancer tends to occur in some families more than in others; genetic background plays a role in the risk for cancer, especially colon cancer. However, life-style is also a critical factor. We know this because rates of cancer differ around the world. The Japanese, for example, have higher rates of stomach cancer and Americans tend to have a higher rate of colon cancer. When Japanese people immigrate to the United States, their rates for stomach cancer decrease but their rates for colon cancer increase. *In addition, one third of all cancer cases in North America is due to smoking tobacco.*

MECHANISMS

To understand how to prevent cancer we first need to examine how cancer develops in the body. The process begins with an alteration in *DNA,* the genetic material in the cells. The DNA is altered so that the cell no longer responds to normal physiological controls. The cell can now dictate its own rate of growth and is not inhibited from growing at the expense of the cells around it. There are many ways to alter DNA. A substance or phenomenon capable of altering DNA and in turn causing cancer is known as a **genotoxic carcinogen,** or **initiator** (Figure 5-10).[27] The alteration requires from only minutes to days to occur.

Radiation from the sun can cause DNA to bind to itself or break into pieces. This is how skin cancer begins. The altered skin cells may then begin to grow out of control and cancer results.

DNA can be altered by chemicals, especially multi-ringed chemicals, such as aflatoxin and benzo(a)pyrene (see the structure of cholesterol on page 135 for an example of a multi-ringed structure). Aflatoxin is formed when mold is present in peanuts and peanut butter. The FDA regulates how much aflatoxin can be present in peanut butter (see Chapter 19). Rejecting moldy foods is another way to avoid possible carcinogens. Benzo(a)pyrene is found in charcoal-broiled foods. All these ringed compounds can insert themselves into DNA and cause breaks and other changes. A third agent that alters DNA is viruses. Viruses can insert their **genes** into human cells. If the genes promote growth (so-called **oncogenes**), then the cell may begin to grow out of control.

Human cells contain their own growth-promoting oncogenes. These are called **proto-oncogenes.** Scientists think that viruses have previously infected humans and taken proto-oncogenes from the human cells. The viruses then can multiply and reinfect other humans. When a growth-promoting gene from one human is placed in another human by a virus and later turned on, the newly infected cell grows autonomously.

Thus the three basic means of altering DNA are through radiation, chemicals, and viruses. However, having a cell with altered DNA does not guarantee cancer. Special enzymes travel up and down the DNA to repair breaks and changes in it. The repair enzymes may find alterations caused by chemicals or radiation and fix them before the cell begins to grow out of control.

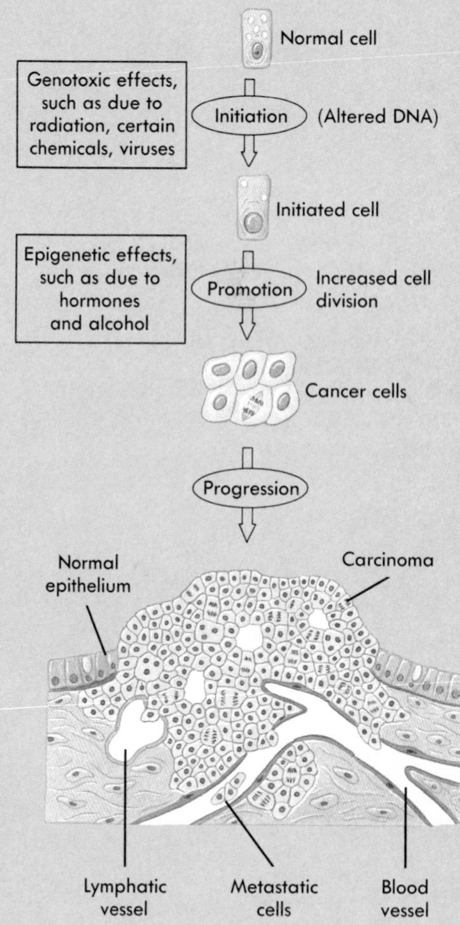

Figure 5-10

Progression from a normal cell to a tumor. The ball of cells is a developing tumor. As the mass of cells grows, it can invade surrounding tissues, eventually penetrating into lymphatic vessels and blood vessels. These vessels carry metastatic cancer cells throughout the body, where they can form new tumors.

EPIGENETIC CARCINOGENS

Anything that increases the rate of cell division decreases the chance that the repair enzymes will find the altered part of the DNA. Once a cell multiplies and incorporates its newly altered DNA into its genetic instructions, the cell no longer realizes that the DNA is altered.

Compounds that increase cell division are called **promoters,** or **epigenetic carcino-**

Nutrition Perspective 5-2, cont'd

gens. They are thought to promote cancer by either decreasing the time available for repair enzymes to act or by encouraging cells with altered DNA to develop and grow (Figure 5-10). Development and growth of these altered cells may take up to 20 years. Common promoters are estrogen, alcohol, and probably high levels of dietary fat.

Once an altered cell has multiplied, there is still no guarantee that cancer will result. First, a stage of progression must occur where the cell mass increases to an extent that it can significantly affect body metabolism. During this initial stage of growth, the immune system may find the altered cells and destroy them. In addition, the cancer cells also may be so defective that their own DNA limits their ability to grow, and they die anyway.

DIET AND CANCER

Besides a generally nutritious diet, other factors related to diet and life-style can reduce your risk of cancer initiation and promotion. For example, maintain a desirable body weight and practice regular physical activity. *Both obesity and physical inactivity are linked to an increased risk for many types of cancer.*[6]

endometrium
A layer of cells lining the wall of the uterus.

prostate
A gland located near the urinary tract in males that produces a fluid used for the discharge of semen.

Obesity is related to all major forms of cancer except lung cancer, including breast cancer, colon cancer, **endometrial** cancer, and **prostate** cancer.[11,12,18] The link probably occurs because adipose tissue can synthesize estrogen from other hormones in the bloodstream, and high levels of estrogen in the bloodstream promote cancer. A long-standing excess energy intake may also promote cancer. When animals are fed diets high in fat or total kcalories, they tend to experience more cancer, especially in the colon and breast. The effect is most apparent when a carcinogen is fed first and then a high-fat or high-kcalorie diet is used to promote cancer.[22] Thus fat and kcalories usually are not considered initiators of cancer.

The National Cancer Institute believes there is a sufficient link between dietary fat and cancer, especially breast cancer, to warrant encouraging Americans to eat less fat. It recommends decreasing dietary fat consumption to about 20% to 30% of total kcalories.[4,29] Some nutritionists, however, believe that this agency has overreacted to the fat and cancer issue. Epidemiological evidence relates fat to cancer but the evidence is not strong. The question of how much fat can be eaten while minimizing the risk of cancer is not settled.[22]

A stronger link between diet and cancer concerns total kcalories in the diet.[22] If a rat is treated with a carcinogen for either breast cancer or colon cancer and then is allowed a typical kcalorie intake versus a reduced kcalorie intake, the rat with a low kcalorie intake will have about a 40% reduction in tumor yield compared with the rat consuming a typical intake. The amount of fat in the diet is not important, as long as the low kcalorie diet is about 70% of the animal's usual kcalorie intake.[6]

The mechanism behind this effect of total kcalorie intake is probably hormonal. The kcalorie-restricted animals have higher levels of the hormone *cortisol* and lower levels of the hormone *prolactin* than the animals allowed to feed at will. This hormonal state inhibits tumor growth, while higher prolactin levels and lower cortisol levels increase tumor growth. The restricted diet may also lower serum estrogen levels. As noted, this hormone can promote cancer.

Can we use this evidence from animals? We North Americans don't want to suffer from cancer, but very few of us want to eat only 70% of our usual kcalorie intake. While there is a strong link between some types of cancer and obesity, this evidence has been insufficient to convince many of us to slim down to ideal body weights. It is a much bigger task to reduce kcalories to 70% of usual intake. So while the animal data are interesting, nutritionists do not know how to use these data to help us. In addition, once cancer is present, kcalorie restriction is no longer helpful.

ANTIOXIDANTS MAY BE ANTICARCINOGENS

Many single nutrients are promoted as keys to preventing cancer. They are called *anticarcinogens* (Table 5-7). The most important ones are beta-carotene (a plant form of vitamin A), vitamin E, vitamin C and selenium.[28,31] All four of these nutrients function as or contribute to antioxidant systems in the body. These antioxidant systems help prevent the alteration of DNA by electron-seeking substances. Note that the antioxidant vitamin E also protects unsaturated fatty acids from electron-seeking compounds. *A diet that follows the Daily Food Guide, so that fruits, vegetables, and plant oils are eaten daily, should provide enough of these nutrients to gain any possible benefit.*[5,7]

Table 5-7

Possible anticarcinogens in foods

Nutrient	Source	Action
Vitamin A	Liver, fortified milk, fruits and vegetables*	Encourages normal cell division and development
Vitamin E	Whole grains, vegetable oil, and green leafy vegetables	Antioxidant
Vitamin C	Fruits and vegetables	Antioxidant
Selenium	Meats and whole grains	Part of an antioxidant system (glutathione peroxidase system) (Chapters 11 and 14)
Carotenes	Fruits and vegetables	Bind free atoms of oxygen
Indoles, phenols	Vegetables, especially cabbage, cauliflower, and brussels sprouts	May reduce carcinogen activation
Dietary fibers	Whole grains, fruits, vegetables, and beans	May bind carcinogens in stool, decrease stool transit time
Calcium	Dairy products	Slows cell division in the colon, binds bile acids and free fatty acids

*Fruits and vegetables contain caratenes, many of which are converted to vitamin A (see Chapter 11).

IS DIETARY FIBER AN ANTICANCER AGENT?

In Chapters 3 and 4 we mentioned the possible role of fiber in preventing colon cancer. Fiber may do this by decreasing transit time so that the stool is in contact with the colon for a shorter period of time.[12] This would reduce the contact of carcinogens with the colon wall. In addition, soluble fibers bind bile acids. Bile acids are thought to contribute to cancer risk by irritating the colon cells, increasing cell division. However, the evidence

Continued

Nutrition Perspective 5-2—cont'd

regarding the importance of fiber in preventing colon cancer is still inconclusive. *For now the recommendation to eat 20 to 35 grams a day is probably best. Liberal use of whole grains, fruits, and vegetables should suffice to yield this amount.*

Calcium is also linked to a decreased risk for developing colon cancer. As with fiber the evidence is weak. Some studies show that calcium decreases the growth of cells in the colon; therefore it probably decreases the risk of an altered cell developing into a cancer. Calcium may also bind free fatty acids and bile acids in the colon so they are less apt to interact with cells there and cause cancer. We need more research before calcium can be promoted as a cancer-preventing agent. Nevertheless, there are many important reasons for consuming the RDA for calcium. We will discuss those in Chapter 13.

A BOTTOM LINE?

Table 5-8 lists a variety of changes you can make in your diet to possibly reduce the risk of cancer. Start by controlling energy and total fat intake (if necessary), and by increasing intake of fruits, vegetables, whole grains, beans, and low-fat dairy products. In other words, follow the Daily Food Guide. In addition, moderate the use of alcohol, if you drink alcohol. We remind you again that 35% of all cancer cases are due to cigarette smoking. Therefore a priority in avoiding cancer is not smoking tobacco—not even using smokeless varieties (chewing tobacco).

Table 5-8

General dietary recommendations to reduce the risk of cancer*
1. Avoid obesity.
2. Reduce fat intake to 30% of total kcalories.
3. Eat more high-fiber foods, such as fruits, vegetables, and whole-grain cereals.
4. Include foods rich in vitamins A and C in the daily diet.
5. If alcohol is consumed, do not drink excessively.
6. Use moderation when consuming salt-cured, smoked, and nitrite-cured foods.

*The National Cancer Institute (U.S.) endorses all the above but warns not to exceed 35 grams of dietary fiber intake.

The American Cancer Society endorses all the above, but sets no percentage for fat intake, and adds a recommendation to include cruciferous vegetables in the diet (cabbage, broccoli, and brussels sprouts). These may decrease carcinogen activation.

The Canadian Dietetic Association generally endorses all of the above, but the specific language differs.

Chapter 6
Proteins

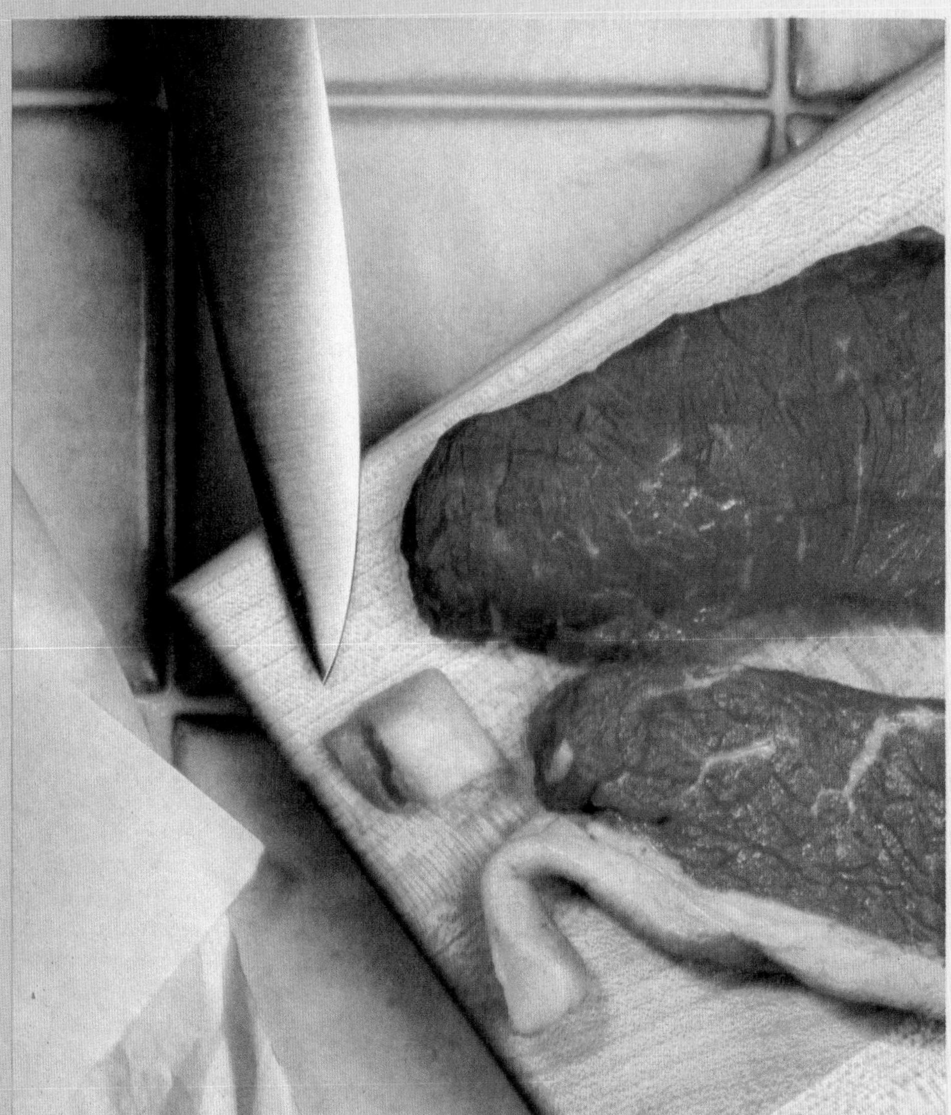

Trim meats before cooking to help reduce your fat intake.

Overview

A regular dietary intake of protein is vital for maintaining health. According to studies by anthropologists using fossilized teeth, our Stone Age ancestors obtained most of their protein from vegetables. Not until the emergence of our immediate ancestors, *Homo erectus,* about 1.5 million years ago, was there evidence of much meat in a primarily vegetarian diet. Food gathering, rather than hunting, was the primary means of obtaining dietary protein.[4]

Today, animal products hold a central position in the North American diet—roast turkey, grilled hamburgers, ice cream, and T-bone steak are just a few of the animal protein foods that most of us hold in high regard. Animal products contribute considerably to the total nutrient intake of North Americans, but plant proteins should also play a valuable role in our diets. Few of us would wish to exchange our comfortable modern life-styles with those of our Stone Age ancestors. However, it is possible to incorporate the best of both worlds nutritionally, enjoying the benefits of both animal and plant protein. In this chapter we will discuss why this nutrition message is important.

Nutrition awareness inventory

Here are 15 statements about proteins. Answer them to test your current knowledge. If you think a statement is true or mostly true, circle T; if you think the statement is false or mostly false, circle F. Use the scoring key at the end of the chapter to compute your total score. Compare the results.

1. **T F** Most people have trouble eating a diet containing all the essential amino acids.
2. **T F** An insufficient protein intake can stunt a child's growth.
3. **T F** Most enzymes are proteins.
4. **T F** The hormone insulin is a protein.
5. **T F** The quality of protein can be measured by its biological value—nitrogen retention divided by nitrogen absorption.
6. **T F** Milk provides higher quality proteins than most other foods.
7. **T F** The greatest need for protein occurs in the elderly years.
8. **T F** Athletes usually need at least double the protein intake of nonathletes. Supplements are the preferred source.
9. **T F** Animal protein sources often contain high amounts of saturated fat.
10. **T F** Lack of energy can be a symptom of severe protein deficiency.
11. **T F** Gelatin supplements can strengthen the protein in fingernails.
12. **T F** Marasmus is a disease caused by starvation and can be seen in large cities of impoverished countries.
13. **T F** There is little difference in nutrient content between animal and vegetable protein sources.
14. **T F** Water-packed tuna is almost pure protein.
15. **T F** Fruits contain very little protein.

Other than water, proteins compose the major part of a lean body, about 16% of body weight. Virtually all the building blocks for these proteins—amino acids—were originally made by plants. Plants combine nitrogen from the soil and air with carbon and other atoms to form amino acids. Humans must consume nitrogen in the amino acid form via proteins: directly using simple forms of nitrogen is, for the most part, impossible for humans.

The day-to-day and minute-to-minute regulation and maintenance of the body requires a variety of proteins. They contribute to key body functions, such as blood-clotting, fluid balance, production of hormones and enzymes, vision, and cell repair. Many of these proteins are very large: their molecular weights can exceed 1 million. In contrast, glucose has a molecular weight of only 180. Furthermore, the thousands of different varieties of proteins in the body greatly exceed the variety of types found among either carbohydrates or fats. Thus proteins deserve their name, which means "to come first."

If a person regularly fails to eat enough protein, major metabolic changes occur. An important change is a decrease in immune function. *Whether this is a child suffering in a famine or an adult hospitalized with a severe body burn, a poor protein intake can increase the risk of infections, disease, and possibly death.*[20,21]

AMINO ACIDS

Amino acids contain carbon, hydrogen, oxygen, nitrogen, and sometimes sulfur atoms. All 20 types of amino acids from the diet used to make protein have similar backbones, each composed of a carbon atom bonded to an amine group ($-NH_2$) (sometimes called an amino group); an acid group ($-\overset{O}{\overset{\|}{C}}-OH$); a hydrogen atom ($-H$), and another group, often signified by R. In the margin we show a basic model of an amino acid and the actual structures of glycine and alanine.

NH$_2$ O
R—C—C—OH
H

"Generic" amino acid

NH$_2$ O
H—C—C—OH
H

Glycine

NH$_2$ O
CH$_3$—C—C—OH
H

L-alanine

Form determines function

The form that the R portion assumes determines the type and name of the amino acid. If the R is a hydrogen, the amino acid is glycine. If the R is a methyl group ($-CH_3$), the amino acid is alanine, and so on (see Appendix E). Some amino acids have chemically similar R portions. These related amino acids form special classes, such as acidic amino acids, basic amino acids, or branched-chain amino acids (Table 6-1).

The key part of the amino acid is the amine group. This is the distinguishing feature of amino acids: all amino acids contain this nitrogen group. Cells can produce carbon skeletons and then add amine groups from other amino acids to synthesize 11 of the 20 different types of amino acids the body needs.

In the case of the other nine animo acids the body needs, body cells either cannot make the needed carbon skeleton, cannot put an amine group on the carbon skeleton, or just cannot do the whole process fast enough. The amino acids that body cells cannot make are called **essential (indispensable) amino acids** (Table 6-1). The 11 amino acids the body can make are then called **nonessential**

essential amino acids
The amino acids that cannot be synthesized by humans and must therefore be included in the diet; there are nine essential amino acids.

nonessential amino acids
Amino acids that can be synthesized by the body; there are 11 nonessential amino acids in the diet.

If the R portion on the amino acid is anything other than a hydrogen, the amino acid will have four different groups attached to it. Recall from Chapter 2 that a carbon atom with four different groups attached to it can exist as two isomer forms, in this case D and L. In nature almost all amino acids are the L form. However, we can metabolize some D isomer forms.

Table 6-1

Classification of amino acids

Classification	Essential amino acids	Nonessential amino acids
Neutral—one amine group ($-NH_2$) and one carboxyl group ($-\overset{O}{\overset{\|}{C}}-OH$)		
• Aliphatic (carbon-carbon chain)	Threonine Valine* Leucine* Isoleucine*	Glycine Alanine Serine
• Aromatic—contains benzene ring (⌬)	Phenylalanine	Tyrosine†
• Heterocyclic (some are multiringed)	Tryptophan Histidine	Proline
• Sulfur-containing	Methionine	Cysteine† (Cystine)
Basic—two amine groups and one carboxyl group	Lysine	Arginine
Acidic—one amine group and two carboxyl groups		Aspartic acid Asparagine‡ Glutamic acid Glutamine‡

*Branched-chain amino acids.
†These amino acids are classed as semi-essential.
‡Asparagine and glutamine contain an amine group attached to the additional carboxyl group.

(dispensable) amino acids.[13] Note that both essential and nonessential amino acids are present in foods that contain protein.

semi-essential amino acids
Amino acids that, when consumed, spare the need to use an essential amino acid for their synthesis. Tyrosine, for example, spares the need to use phenylalanine for its synthesis.

When health is compromised, such as when a child is born prematurely, some amino acids normally nonessential in the adult diet may become an essential part of the diet of the compromised person such as arginine.

All amino acids are essential, considering their necessity for proper body function. However, only the essential amino acids must be derived from the diet. If we don't eat enough essential amino acids, the rate of protein synthesis slows progressively until protein breakdown exceeds protein synthesis. A state of poor health can then result.

Two amino acids are considered **semi-essential (conditionally indispensable).** They can spare the need for two essential amino acids. Methionine and cysteine are an essential-semi-essential amino acid team, as are phenylalanine and tyrosine. Both methionine and phenylalanine are essential amino acids. Cysteine and tyrosine, the semi-essential amino acids, must be made from their essential amino acid counterparts, unless they are consumed in the diet. If cysteine and tyrosine are indeed consumed, the body uses them—instead of their essential amino acid partners—to synthesize protein. In so doing, cysteine and tyrosine spare methionine and phenylalanine from being transformed into themselves, leaving more methionine and phenylalanine to be used for protein synthesis. About 50% of an adult's dietary methionine needs are spared if ample cysteine is in the diet.

A common metabolic process for synthesizing nonessential amino acids is called **transamination.** In Figure 6-1 pyruvic acid accepts the amine group ($-NH_2$) from glutamic acid and becomes the amino acid alanine. In the process, by losing its amine group, glutamic acid turns into a carbon skeleton, called alpha-ketoglutaric acid.

Some amino acids, such as glutamic acid, simply lose their amine group without transferring it to another carbon skeleton. This process is called **deamination.** The amine group is incorporated into urea in the liver, and the kidneys ex-

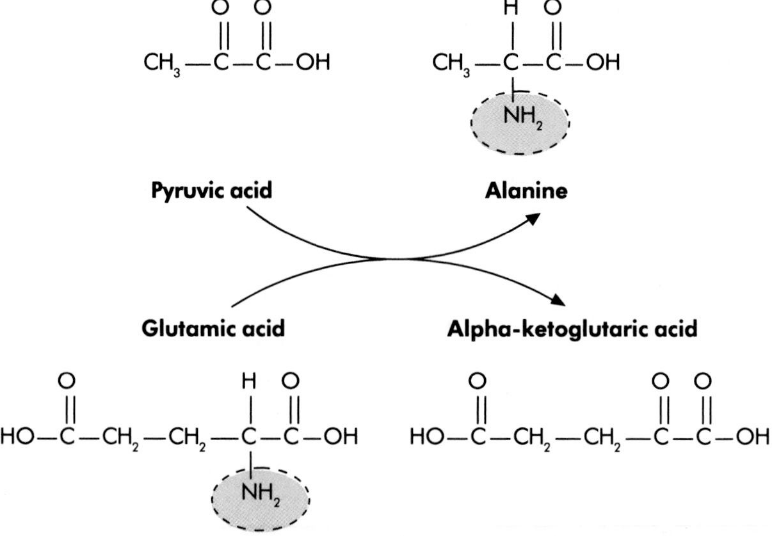

Figure 6-1
Transamination. This pathway allows cells to synthesize nonessential amino acids. In this example, pyruvic acid gains an amine group to form the amino acid alanine.

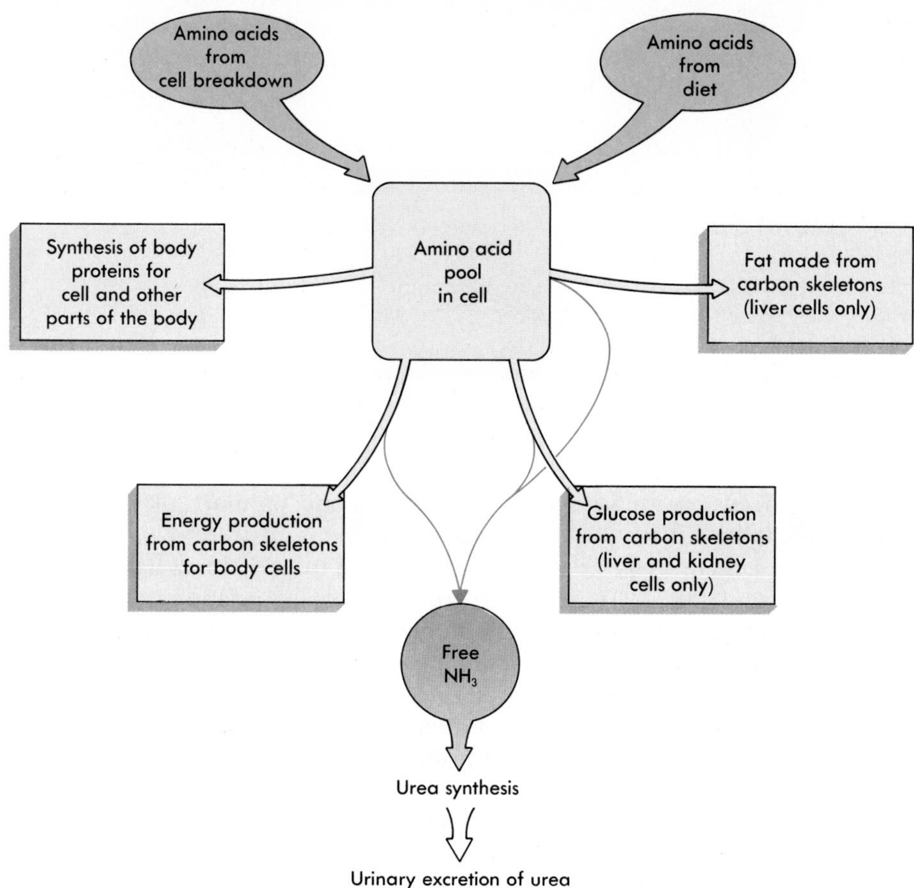

Figure 6-2

Amino acid metabolism. This yields a variety of products, from fat and glucose to urea.

crete the urea in urine (Figure 6-2). Once an amino acid breaks down to its carbon skeleton, the carbon skeleton can be burned for fuel or synthesized into other compounds, such as fatty acids (see Chapter 7).

Exploring Issues and Actions

What is generally meant by the word *essential?* What do nutritionists mean when referring to essential amino acids?

Putting essential amino acids into perspective

Physiological aspects. The disease phenylketonuria (PKU) illustrates the concept of essential and nonessential amino acids. Again, phenylalanine is an essential amino acid. Tyrosine is a nonessential amino acid because phenylalanine can be coverted into tyrosine. However, the liver of a person with PKU can lack sufficient enzyme activity to efficiently convert phenylalanine to tyrosine. This defect can vary from a mild to severe impairment of enzyme activity. Now both amino acids become essential amino acids because both now must come from food.

The diet of a person with PKU often must be carefully designed to contain enough phenylalanine for protein synthesis—because it is an essential amino acid—but no more than that. The inability to readily metabolize excess phenylalanine to tyrosine can lead to a buildup of abnormal products from alternate routes of phenylalanine metabolism. These products are thought to cause the severe mental retardation seen in untreated PKU cases.

Dietary considerations. Animal proteins and plant proteins can differ greatly in composition of essential and nonessential amino acids. Animal proteins, except gelatin, contain ample amounts of all essential amino acids. Gelatin, since it originates from the protein collagen, contains all essential amino acids, but heat and acid processing destroys the tryptophan present. Plant proteins, when compared

Table 6-2

Limiting amino acids in plant foods

Food	Limiting amino acid	Good plant source of limiting amino acid
Soybeans and other legumes	Methionine	Grains; nuts and seeds
Grains	Lysine, threonine	Legumes
Nuts and seeds	Lysine	Legumes
Vegetables	Methionine	Grains; nuts and seeds

with human needs, are always relatively low in one or more of the essential amino acids (Table 6-2).

complete proteins
Contain ample amounts of all nine essential amino acids.

incomplete proteins
Lack an ample amount of one or more essential amino acids for human protein needs.

limiting amino acid
The essential amino acid in lowest concentration in a food in proportion to body needs.

In essence, human tissue composition resembles that of animal tissue far more than it does plant tissue. Thus animal proteins, except gelatin, are considered **complete proteins.** They can support body growth and maintenance because they contain a balance of all essential amino acids. Plant proteins are either partially complete or **incomplete proteins.** Partially complete proteins only can support body maintenance. Incomplete proteins cannot support either growth or maintenance of the body because of an inadequate amount of one or more essential amino acids.

If you eat foods that do not contain a complete protein balance, you will not have all the essential amino acids needed for protein synthesis. *Protein synthesis stops when the supply of any one essential amino acid is depleted.* Considering body needs, the amino acid in shortest supply in a food or diet is called the **limiting amino acid.** This situation—when protein synthesis stops because one type of essential amino acid is used up—is said to follow the "all-or-none law": if all nine essential amino acids are not available to synthesize needed protein, the ones present cannot be used at that time, and protein synthesis stops.

Both the "all-or-none law" and the concept of the limiting amino acids may presently be overemphasized when typical North American eating patterns are considered.[14] *Most of us eat such a varied assortment of proteins that we would have to go far out of our way to eat a diet in which the combined amino acid contributions from each food did not yield enough of all nine essential amino acids—or, in essence, complete protein.* Furthermore, adults need only about 11% of their protein intake supplied by essential amino acids, while our diets average 50% essential amino acids.[24] Even most adults worldwide who eat sufficient protein will be supplied with enough essential amino acids to yield a complete protein intake. So there is little reason for the average adult to worry about balancing proteins that specifically complement deficiencies of other amino acids (see Nutrition Perspective 6-1 for more details on protein complementarity as we discuss vegetarianism).

Infants and preschool children, on the other hand, require that approximately 32% to 43% of their protein come from essential amino acids.[24] So food for young children must be more carefully planned to include enough of all the essential amino acids. If an infant consumes enough breastmilk or commercial formula to meet its protein needs, essential amino acid needs will be automatically met. A major health risk for children occurs in famine situations where only one type of grain is available, increasing the probability that some of the nine essential amino acids may be lacking in the total diet.

Concept Check

Twenty amino acids useful to the body exist in food. A healthy body synthesizes 11 of these (nonessential amino acids). The other nine must be in the diet (essential amino acids). Foods that contain all nine essential amino acids are called complete protein foods, while foods greatly lacking one or more of the essential amino acids are called incomplete protein foods. Two incomplete protein foods can be combined in a meal to complement each other's lack, providing a complete protein meal.

PROTEINS—AMINO ACIDS JOINED TOGETHER

Two amino acids bonded together form a dipeptide, and three amino acids bonded together form a tripeptide. A **polypeptide** has 50 to 100 amino acids, and a protein has at least 100 amino acids. Most foods contain just the large protein form. However, specialized feeding supplements used in hospitals often contain various sizes of peptides.

Amino acids are joined together by a **peptide bond.** Notice in the margin that the bond is formed by a condensation reaction. An amine group (-NH_2) reacts with a carboxyl group ($-\overset{O}{\overset{\|}{C}}-OH$) and a water molecule is split off. The process requires an enzyme to catalyze the reaction. In this peptide bond, electrons are shared (covalent), and so it is a difficult bond to break apart. The body can synthesize thousands of different proteins by joining the 20 different types of amino acids together with peptide bonds.

A peptide bond can be broken using a hydrolysis reaction. Water is added back to the molecule. Acids, enzymes, or other agents can lead to the hydrolysis of a peptide bond.

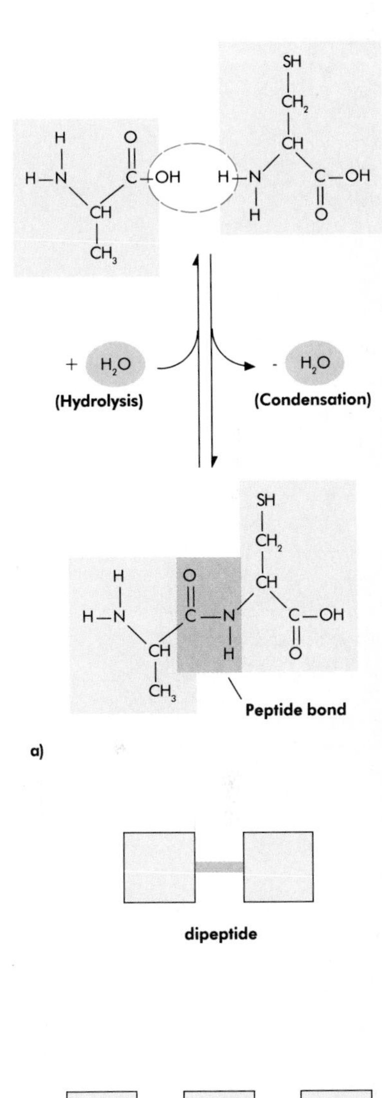

Levels of protein organization

The order of amino acids in a protein—in other words, the sequence created by amino acids bonded to each other—forms the **primary structure of the protein.** The primary structure sequence determines the function of the protein since it dictates the three-dimensional shape of the protein, called **tertiary structure.** The tertiary structure is then stabilized by hydrogen bonds and disulfide bonds (—S—S—), as well as by other forces. These bonds are referred to as **secondary structure** (Figure 6-3).

It may help to view secondary structure as stabilizing attractions formed between amino acids located close together in the primary structure, and tertiary structure as the complex folded form stabilized by attractions between amino acids located far apart in the primary structure. If two separate protein units then interact to form an even larger new protein form, they show quarternary structure.

Note that proteins have a specific sequence for their building blocks. The proper primary structure sequence of a protein ensures that each amino acid in the protein will end up in the right position in relationship to the other amino acids when the secondary and tertiary orientations form. Only appropriately positioned amino acids can bond properly so that the correct folded shape—whether coiled or globular—forms.

The disease **sickle-cell anemia** (also called sickle cell disease) illustrates the importance of having a protein with the correct primary structure. Blacks are especially prone to this genetic disease. The major problem is an altered formation of the protein chains in the red blood cell protein, hemoglobin. Only one incor-

Figure 6-3

Structural levels of protein. The amino acid sequence, called its primary structure, encourages the formation of hydrogen and disulfide bonds between nearby amino acids, producing secondary structure. The protein assumes a three-dimensional shape like a ball of string; this is called its tertiary structure. Many individual proteins associate in clusters to form quarternary structure.

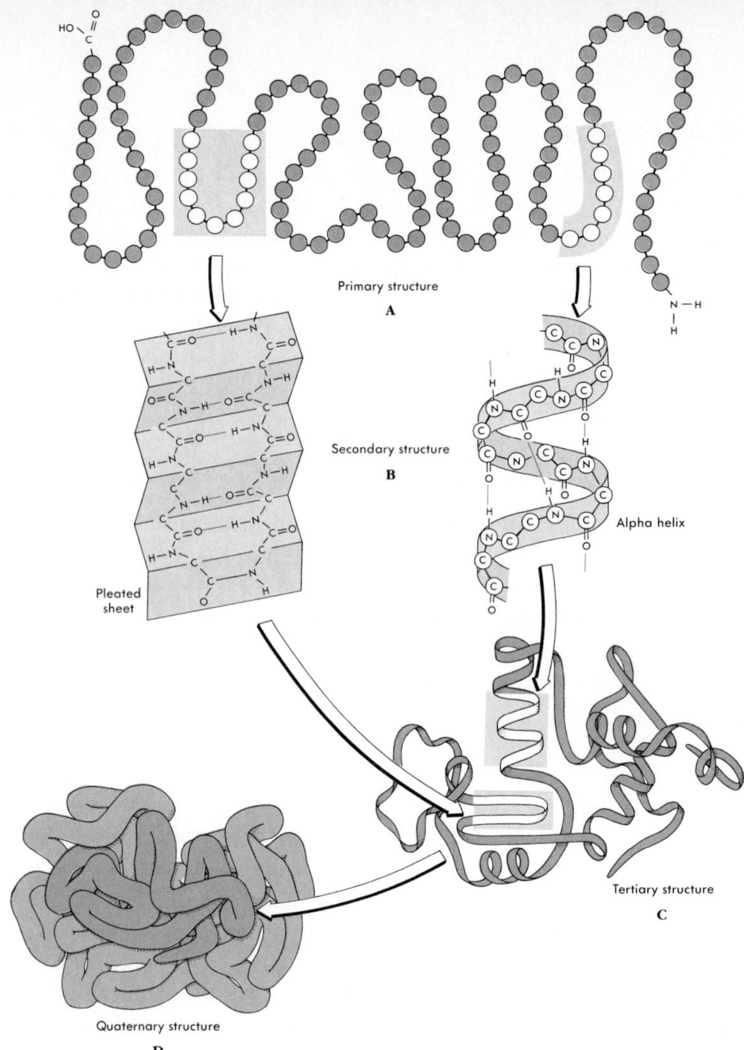

rect amino acid is present in two of the four protein chains. However, this small error produces a profound change in the structure of hemoglobin: it can no longer form the proper shape needed to carry oxygen efficiently inside the red blood cell. The red blood cells then form crescents rather than circles. Sickness results, which can lead to episodes of severe bone and joint pain, abdominal pain, headache, convulsions, and paralysis. This demonstrates how critical even a minor error in the primary structure can be. The template containing directions for this proper primary structure lies in the genetic material (the DNA, which forms genes on chromosomes) in the nucleus found in almost every cell in the body.

Normal blood cell.

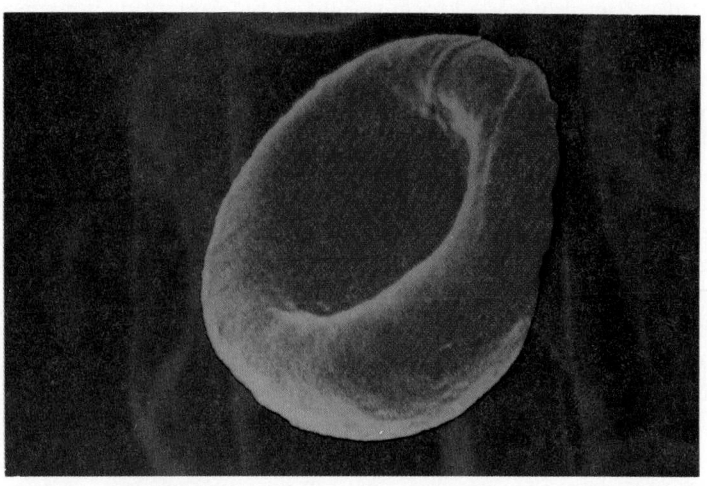

Denaturation of proteins

Treatment with acid or alkaline substances, heat, or agitation can severely alter the tertiary structure, leaving the protein in an unfolded, or **denatured,** state. Now the protein can no longer function as originally intended. For example, once an egg is cracked into a hot frying pan and solidifies, it can no longer produce a chicken. (The same is true for whipped egg whites.) Once the bacteria in yogurt have synthesized enough acid and enzymes to precipitate the milk protein casein, the protein can never be resuspended in the water base.

Destroying a protein's tertiary structure often effectively destroys its normal physiological function. The body uses this characteristic of protein to its advantage. When foods reach the stomach, stomach acid denatures some bacteria, plant hormones, many active enzymes, and other forms of proteins in the food. These processes render the foods safer to eat and contribute to the digestive process. Denaturing proteins in some foods can also reduce their tendencies to cause allergic reactions. Recall that we need proteins in the diet to supply essential amino acids—not the active proteins themselves. We can build the proteins we need.

FUNCTIONS OF PROTEINS

Proteins play myriad key roles in body metabolism and the formation of body structures. As discussed above, we rely on diet to supply this protein. However, to use dietary protein efficiently, we must also consume enough total kcalories to meet energy needs. Otherwise, the amino acids in proteins will be broken down and used for energy production, rather than for synthetic purposes.

Producing vital body constituents

Proteins form muscles, connective tissue, blood-clotting factors, blood transport proteins, lipoproteins, visual pigments, and the support structure (protein matrix) inside bones. Measurements of the amount of certain structural proteins in the body, such as the circumference of the upper arm muscle, are often used to estimate body protein levels in health and disease.[2,10]

Each cell membrane contains protein. In fact, as discussed in Chapter 5, a cell membrane is essentially composed of islands of protein in a sea of fats. Some cell membrane proteins act as receptors for absorption of nutrients into the cell. Others act as receptor sites for some hormones or as pumps to help maintain ion balance in a cell.

Most of these vital body proteins are in a constant state of breakdown, rebuilding, and repair, especially in the intestine and bone marrow. Most of the protein breakdown products, namely amino acids, can be reused, and so add to the pool of amino acids available for future protein synthesis (Figure 6-2). However, other protein breakdown products end up being lost to reuse. When a person continually does not eat enough protein to replace lost protein, the rebuilding and repairing process slows. Then the skeletal muscles, heart, liver, blood proteins, and other organs all decrease in size or amount. The exception is the brain. It is quite resistant to breakdown in this case. For health's sake, a person must eat enough protein to ensure the support of the growth and maintenance of the body's structures.

Maintaining fluid balance

The blood proteins—albumins and globulins—help maintain fluid balance in the body. Blood pressure in the arteries acts to force the blood fluid (serum) out of the blood vessels into the capillary beds. The fluid then spills out into the **extracellular spaces** to provide nutrients to cells (Figure 6-4). Proteins in the bloodstream can counteract this effect of blood pressure because they are too large to move out of the capillary beds into the tissues. Their presence in the blood vessels attracts fluid to them, counteracting the force of the blood pressure. This causes most of the fluid to remain in the blood vessels.

extracellular space
The space between cells.

Figure 6-4

Blood proteins are important for maintaining the body's fluid balance. Without sufficient protein in the bloodstream, edema develops.

Blood pressure

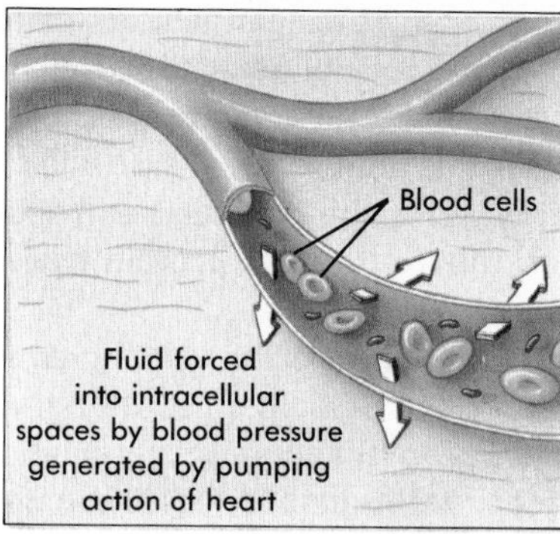

Osmotic pressure of blood proteins

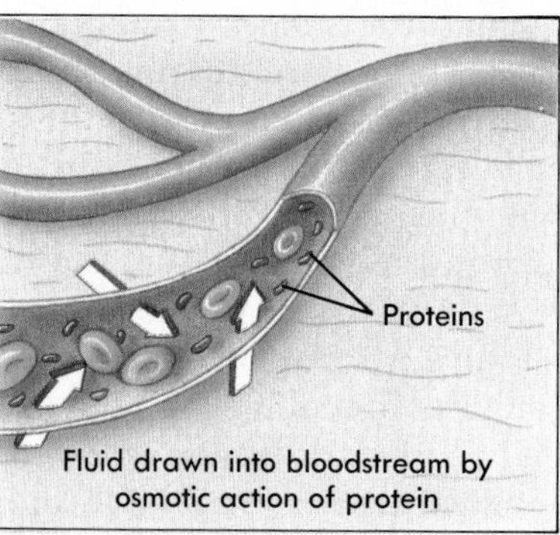

Blood pressure exceeds osmotic pressure

Blood pressure balanced by osmotic pressure

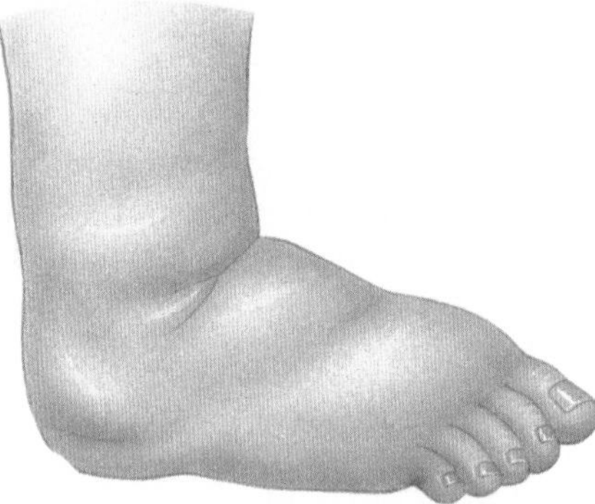

Swollen tissue (edema)

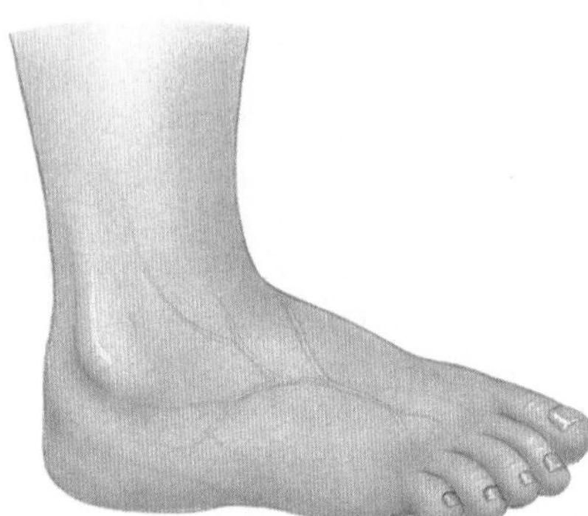

Normal tissue

edema
The buildup of excess fluid in extracellular spaces.

osmotic potential
The tendency to attract water across a semi-permeable membrane, usually to dilute some constituent in a fluid.

If a person's blood protein level falls below a certain level, and oncotic pressure falls, insufficient nutrient absorption from the small intestine will also result. Blood proteins attract fluid from the GI tract into the bloodstream. Thus when a hospitalized person shows malabsorption of food, it is important to determine if sufficient albumin and other blood proteins are present in the bloodstream to allow for proper nutrient absorption. If not, blood proteins can be infused intravenously to allow for a rapid improvement in intestinal absorption.

The ability of blood proteins, simply by their presence, to attract and retain fluid in the bloodstream is due to their **osmotic potential** (see Chapter 13 for a full discussion of osmosis). In essence, the blood proteins exert an attraction—also called **oncotic force**—on the fluid in the bloodstream that counters the force of blood pressure.

If a person doesn't eat enough protein, eventually the amount of protein in the bloodstream decreases. Blood pressure then can force excessive fluid out of the blood vessels and into the extracellular spaces because there is no strong counteracting force to oppose it. As more and more fluid pools in the extracellular spaces, clinical **edema** results. Other conditions, such as heart failure, kidney disease, liver disease, and pregnancy can also lead to edema. Because edema sometimes leads to serious medical problems, the cause needs to be investigated. A first step is to measure the blood protein concentration to see if it is adequate.

Children with protein malnutrition often show severe edema.[16,20] If they are fed protein along with the other nutrients needed for optimal health, their bodies can make more blood proteins. The fluid is then attracted back into bloodstream, and the edema disappears. We will discuss this in detail later in this chapter along with other effects of a protein deficiency.

Contributing to acid-base balance

The concentration of hydrogen ions in the bloodstream determines the acid-base balance (pH) of the blood. Proteins help regulate the amount of free hydrogen ions by readily accepting or donating hydrogen ions. This regulation helps to keep the blood pH fairly constant and slightly alkaline (pH 7.35 to 7.45). Compounds that act to keep pH within a narrow range are called **buffers.** Blood proteins are especially important buffers in the body.

Forming hormones and enzymes

Many hormones, such as the thyroid hormones T_3 and T_4, are derivatives of amino acids, while insulin is a polypeptide. These and other hormones that belong within the protein classification perform many important regulatory functions in the body, such as increasing glucose uptake from the bloodstream and controlling metabolic rate.

Neurotransmitter compounds, those made by nerve endings, are often derivatives of amino acids. This is true for dopamine, epinephrine, and serotonin. A current area of research is the study of how diet influences the synthesis of some of these neurotransmitters (see Chapter 8 for details).

Many hormone medicines from the protein class, such as insulin, must be injected. If taken orally, insulin would be destroyed: the stomach and small intestine would digest the hormone, dismantling it into amino acids, as they do with foods.

Almost all enzymes are proteins (a few are composed of nucleic acids). Enzymes are organic compounds than catalyze (speed) chemical reactions. Occasionally a cell lacks the correct DNA structure to instruct it how to make needed enzymes. An infant, for example, suffering from the disease **galactosemia,** cannot make the enzyme needed to metabolize the single sugar galactose. If the infant is not put on a galactose-free diet soon after birth, its growth and mental development will be depressed. This case demonstrates the crucial roles that enzymes, and thus proteins, play in cell function.

galactosemia
A disease characterized by the buildup of the monosaccharide, galactose, in the bloodstream due to the inability of the liver to metabolize it. If present at birth and left untreated, it results in severe growth and mental retardation.

Contributing to the immune function

Proteins compose key parts of the cells used by the immune system. Also, the **antibodies** produced by one type of immune cell (B-lymphocytes) are proteins. These antibodies can bind to foreign proteins in the body, an important step in ridding invaders from the body (see Chapter 14 for a description of how the immune system works). Without enough protein in the diet, the immune system will lack the cells and other tools needed to function properly (Figure 6-5). Thus immune incompetence—**anergy**—and a protein deficient diet often appear to-

antibody
Blood proteins that inactivate foreign proteins found in the body to prevent infections.

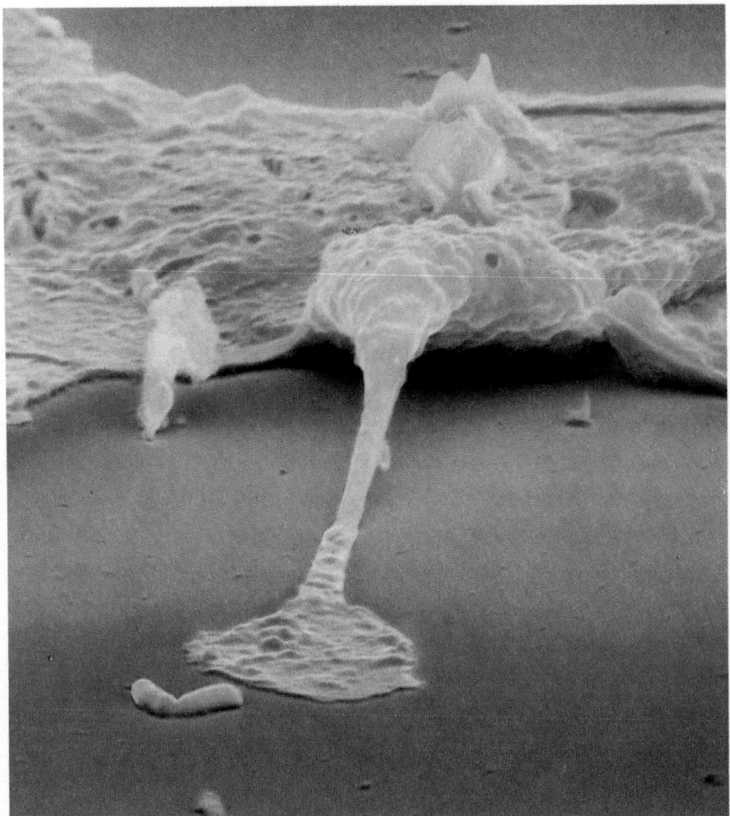

Figure 6-5

Going in for the kill. Ever vigilant, a patrolling white blood cell (macrophage) attacts a bacterium. Adequate protein in the diet aids immune system responses like this one.

gether. Anergy can turn measles into a fatal disease for a malnourished child.[16,20] It also can encourage unusual infections, such as widespread yeast *(Candida)* growth in the mouth and throat of hospitalized adults.[21] This yeast can more easily reproduce and spread when an immune system functions poorly.

Forming glucose

In Chapter 4 we noted that the body must maintain a fairly constant level of glucose in the bloodstream to supply energy for red blood cells and nervous tissue. The brain uses about 35% of the body's energy needs at rest, and it gets most of that energy from glucose. If a diet does not contain enough carbohydrate to supply the glucose, the liver and to a lesser extent the kidneys will be forced to metabolize amino acids to make the glucose (Figure 6-2). Many types of amino acids can be used for this purpose. Recall the metabolic process of turning amino acids into glucose is called gluconeogenesis.

Some gluconeogenesis is normal, for example, it occurs after skipping breakfast when you haven't eaten since a 7 PM dinner. Taken to the extreme, however, a constant need for gluconeogenesis causes much of the muscle wasting that occurs in starvation.

Providing energy

We have discussed how proteins can be used for energy. About 10% of body energy comes from this source. Still, most cells more readily use carbohydrates and lipids for energy. Proteins and carbohydrates contain the same amount of usable energy, 4 kcalories per gram. However, proteins are a very costly source of energy, in terms of both the amount of metabolism and handling required by the liver and kidneys and the original cost of protein foods.

Concept Check

Amino acids are bonded together in a specific order to form proteins. The order of the amino acids in a protein determines its primary structure. This primary structure dictates the three dimension, or tertiary, structure of the protein that is eventually formed. Destruction of the tertiary structure by acid or alkaline conditions, heat, or other factors unfolds—denatures—the protein, yielding an inactive form. Proteins form vital body constituents, such as muscles, connective tissues, blood transport proteins, enzymes, hormones, and immune bodies. Proteins can also provide fuel for the body and carbon atoms for the synthesis of glucose.

EVALUATION OF PROTEIN QUALITY

Protein quality refers to the ability of a food protein to support body growth and maintenance. Methods exist to both measure and estimate protein quality. We will discuss the more important approaches.

Biological value

biological value of a protein A measurement of the body's ability to retain protein absorbed from a food.

The **biological value (BV) of a protein** is a measure of how efficiently food protein can be turned into body tissues. If a food possesses enough of all essential amino acids, it should allow a person to efficiently incorporate the food protein into body proteins. *The biological value of a food then depends on how closely its amino acid pattern reflects the amino acid pattern in body tissues.* The better the match, the more completely food protein turns into body protein.

$$\text{BV} = \frac{\text{nitrogen retained}}{\text{nitrogen absorbed}} = \frac{\text{dietary nitrogen} - (\text{urinary nitrogen} + \text{fecal nitrogen})}{\text{dietary nitrogen} - \text{fecal nitrogen}}$$

We actually measure protein retention by measuring nitrogen retention. Nitrogen itself is easier to measure than protein, and all amino acids contain nitrogen. Both

Table 6-3

Comparative protein quality of selected foods

Food	Chemical (amino acid) score	BV*	NPU†	PER‡
Egg	100	100	94	3.92
Cow's milk	95	93	82	3.09
Fish	71	76	—	3.55
Beef	69	74	67	2.30
Unpolished rice	67	86	59	—
Peanuts	65	55	55	1.65
Oats	57	65	—	2.19
Polished rice	57	64	57	2.18
Whole wheat	53	65	49	1.53
Corn	49	72	36	—
Soybeans	47	73	61	2.32
Sesame seeds	42	62	53	1.77
Peas	37	64	55	1.57

*Biological value
†Net protein utilization
‡Protein efficiency ratio

humans and laboratory animals are used to generate data for biological value determinations (Table 6-3).

If the amino acid pattern in a food is quite unlike human tissue amino acid patterns, many amino acids in the food will not end up as body protein. They are simply leftovers. Their amine groups are removed and excreted in the urine as urea. The carbon skeleton that remains is turned into either glucose or fat or is burned for energy needs (Figure 6-2). Since the nitrogen is not retained, the ratio of retained nitrogen to absorbed nitrogen, and consequent biological value, is small.

Egg white protein has the highest biological value of any single protein source. (Recall that cholesterol is only in the yolk.) Milk and meat proteins also have high biological values. This makes sense because humans and other animals have similar amino acid compositions. Because plant amino acid patterns differ greatly from those of humans, corn has only a moderate biological value: it is high enough to support body maintenance, but not growth. Peanuts have a poor biological value.

As with essential amino acids, the importance of the biological value of a single food can be overemphasized. *It is the biological value of an entire meal that must be considered.* Rarely will a meal yield an overall low biological value, even if only plant foods are eaten. The amino acids in peanuts and bread combine to yield complete protein in a sandwich. Given a variety of foods in a meal, different amino acids usually combine to yield complete protein. This then gives a good overall amino acid balance, hence a high biological value for the meal.

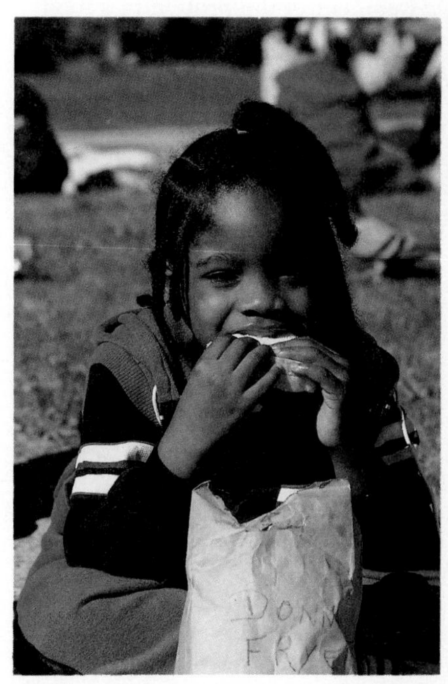

Plant proteins in a peanut butter sandwich combine to yield complete protein.

The concept of biological value is very important in treating some kidney and liver diseases. These organs must metabolize and dispose of extra amino acids, especially the amine groups ($-NH_2$). In treating these diseases it is desirable to have as much protein as possible synthesized into body tissues with as few amino acids as possible leftover to burden the already elevated blood urea or ammonia (NH_3) levels. Only egg protein or egg and milk proteins should be eaten: they provide the highest biological value possible from foods, allowing protein synthesis to occur without generating large amounts of unneeded amino acids.

Net protein utilization

The biological value of a food can be adjusted to account for its digestibility. This adjusted value is called **net protein utilization** (NPU). *Most proteins are almost entirely digested and absorbed.* Thus the biological value and the NPU for most proteins are similar (Table 6-3).

$$\text{NPU} = \text{BV} \times \text{digestibility}$$

Protein efficiency ratio

protein efficiency ratio
A measure of protein quality in a food determined by the ability of the protein to support growth in a young rat.

The **protein efficiency ratio (PER)** provides another means for measuring a food's protein quality. The FDA uses this method to set standards for food labeling. The PER compares the amount of weight gained by a growing rat after 10 or more days while eating a set amount of protein (9.09% of its kcalorie intake) from one food source to the total grams of protein eaten.

$$\text{PER} = \frac{\text{weight gained in a time period (grams)}}{\text{protein intake in that time period (grams)}}$$

The PER of a food reflects its biological value, since both basically measure protein retention by body tissues (Table 6-3). Plant proteins, due to their incomplete nature, yield low PER values. However, as with biological value, the low PER values for individual plant proteins are often of little consequence. Usually we eat many foods—not just one—at a meal. The PER of a peanut butter sandwich will be higher than that of either the bread or peanut butter alone. Why?

The PER also has a practical side. By definition the PER of the milk protein casein is 2.5. If the PER of a protein is less than 2.5, the US RDA used on a nutrition label for that food protein increases from the usual value of 45 grams to 65 grams.

Chemical score of proteins

chemical score
A ratio comparing the essential amino acid content of the protein in a food with the essential amino acid content in a reference protein, such as one established by the Food and Agriculture Organization of the United Nations; the lowest ratio for any essential amino acid becomes the chemical score.

Protein quality of a food can be estimated by its **chemical score.** To calculate a food's chemical score the amount of each essential amino acid provided by a gram of protein in the food is divided by an "ideal" amount for that essential amino acid per gram of food protein. The "ideal" protein pattern is based on the minimal amount (in milligrams) of each essential amino acid that is needed per gram of the food protein to provide a complete protein balance.

$$\text{chemical score} = \frac{\text{milligrams of amino acid per gram of test protein} \times 100}{\text{milligrams of amino acid per gram of the "ideal" protein}}$$

The lowest amino acid ratio calculated for any essential amino acid is the chemical score. Various "ideal" patterns are available. The pattern set by the Food and Agriculture Organization (FAO) of the United Nations for preschool children is often used. It is designed to represent the amino acid levels in human tissue proteins. Note that because children need a greater pecentage of protein as essential amino acids than do adults, applying the children's standard to adults underestimates the chemical score value for adults.

For an example of a chemical score calculation, assume the "ideal" lysine level in a diet is 5.5% or 5.5 milligrams per 100 milligrams of total protein. Wheat protein is most deficient in lysine, with a concentration of 2.4% of total protein. The chemical score for wheat would be:

$$\frac{2.4}{5.5} \times 100 = 44$$

The chemical score is quite similar in concept to biological value since both are based on meeting the body's need for the right balance of essential amino acids. The main advantage of the chemical score method is that it can easily be determined because of the availability of instruments that can measure the amino acid content of a food. *A disadvantage for using the chemical score for protein evaluation is that is does not consider whether toxic substances are also present in the protein. Feeding the protein to animals, as is done for a biological value or PER determination, would indicate that.*

Again, keep in mind that we usually eat meals, not single foods, as protein sources. The concepts of biological value, NPU, PER, and chemical score have important uses, such as in designing diets for sick people, evaluating individual proteins for famine relief, and determining the effects of food processing on food proteins. *However, if you eat enough protein from a variety of foods, you will meet your essential amino acid needs.* Remember also that protein quality is an issue only if the food you eat provides adequate kcalories. Otherwise, high quality or not, protein will be used for energy needs first, not protein needs.

Concept Check

Protein quality can be measured by determining a food's biological value. This essentially represents the body's ability to retain the food protein absorbed. Protein quality can also be measured by a food's capability to support weight gain in a young growing rat: this measurement is the protein efficiency ratio. To only estimate protein quality, the essential amino acid composition of the protein can be compared with a reference protein. A chemical score can then be calculated that indicates how well the food protein matches body tissue needs. The protein quality values of individual foods is important but the protein quality of a total meal is primarily what counts.

THE RECOMMENDED DIETARY ALLOWANCE FOR PROTEIN

How much protein (actually, how many amino acids) do we need to eat each day? If a person is not growing, he or she simply needs to eat enough protein to match daily losses from the urine, feces, skin, hair, nails, and so on. In short, the person needs to balance protein output with intake. Balancing output with intake allows for a state of protein equilibrium.

When either growing or recovering from an illness, the body needs to achieve a positive balance to supply the resources needed for producing new tissues. Consequently protein intake must exceed daily losses. This positive balance requires an appropriate hormonal state. The hormones insulin, growth hormone, and testosterone all stimulate positive protein balance. *Merely eating protein does not guarantee a positive balance: the body also needs the right hormonal condition to build extra tissues.*

During starvation or illness, protein losses often exceed intake, and the body falls into a negative protein balance. Hormones that encourage this state are cortisol and thyroid hormone (Table 6-4). They both can stimulate muscle tissue breakdown.

To measure protein balance we measure nitrogen balance; as we noted with foods, nitrogen intake and output are easier to measure than protein intake and output. Nitrogen makes up about 16% of the weight of a protein. So nitrogen intake or output divided by 0.16 yields a rough estimate of protein intake or output. We can also multiply by the reciprocal of 0.16, which is 6.25:

$$\text{Nitrogen (grams)} \times 6.25 = \text{protein (grams)}$$

In a healthy person the amount of dietary protein needed to yield nitrogen balance can be determined by increasing protein intake until nitrogen intake just equals nitrogen losses. Energy needs must be met so that the protein is not diverted for that use. Any nitrogen level above nitrogen equilibrium also will lead to an equal intake and output. However, what we actually need to determine is

Newer techniques use **stable isotopes** of nitrogen to measure protein synthesis and breakdown rates in the body as a person eats different amounts of various foods.[24]

Table 6-4

Nitrogen balance

N equilibrium: body protein constant
N intake = N excretion

Positive N balance: Increase in body protein
N intake > N excretion

Negative N balance: decrease in body protein
N excretion > N intake

Positive N balance	**Negative N balance**
Growth	Inadequate intake of protein (fasting, intestinal tract diseases)
Pregnancy	Inadequate energy intake
Recovery stage after illness	Illnesses, such as fevers, burns, and infections
Athletic training*	Immobilization
Increased secretion of insulin, growth hormone, and testosterone	Deficiency of essential amino acids
	Accelerated protein loss (as in some kidney diseases)
	Increased secretion of thyroid hormone and cortisol

*Only when additional lean body mass is being gained. Nevertheless, the athlete is probably already eating enough protein to support this extra protein synthesis; protein supplements are not needed.

the *least* amount of nitrogen intake that still allows for intake to equal output. An optimal protein intake should yield a balance in the rate of protein synthesis and breakdown. Too little protein in the diet will slow protein synthesis and may not allow synthesis to keep up with breakdown.

The best estimate for the amount of protein required to keep nearly all adults in nitrogen equilibrium—where intake equals output—is 0.6 grams of protein per kilogram of desirable body weight. (We will discuss values for infants and children in future chapters.) This figure needs to be increased by 25% to allow for individual variation. So we project that about 0.75 grams [0.6 + 0.25(0.6)] of protein is actually needed per kilogram of body weight.

This amount of protein would suffice if the body could absorb all protein eaten. But that is not the case. A reasonable estimate of absorption of dietary protein by North Americans is 94% of intake. So we must divide 0.75 by 0.94. *Using this formula, we have calculated the RDA for protein: 0.8 grams of protein per kilogram of desirable body weight* (Table 6-5). This works out to about 56 grams of protein per day for a 70-kilogram (154-pound) man, and about 44 grams of protein per day for a 55-kilogram (120-pound) woman.

Desirable body weight is based on height (see Chapter 8). Desirable body weight is preferred to actual body weight because extra fat storage does not increase protein needs. You may also see the term *ideal body weight.* Both terms—*ideal* and *desirable*—represent about the same thing.

Canadians use 0.82 grams of protein per kilogram of body weight for adult men and 0.74 grams of protein per kilogram of body weight for adult women

Table 6-5

Establishing the RDA for protein

1. Estimated amount of protein needed to keep the average adult in nitrogen equilibrium	0.6 grams/kilogram desirable body weight
2. 25% increase in protein needs to account for individual variation	0.15 grams/kilogram desirable body weight
TOTAL	0.75 grams/kilogram desirable body weight
3. 6% increase in protein needs to account for absorption efficiency	0.05 grams/kilogram desirable body weight
RDA	0.8 grams of protein/kilogram of desirable body weight

In Canada the RNI for protein is 0.82 grams per kilogram of desirable body weight per day for men and 0.74 grams per kilogram of body weight per day for women. Below are calculations that turn these recommendations into actual intakes of protein:

United States 0.8 grams of protein per kilogram of desirable body weight

Man 0.8 × 70 kg = 56 grams
Woman 0.8 × 60 kg = 48 grams

Canada 0.82 grams of protein per kilogram of body weight
For males 0.82 × 70 kg = 57 grams
0.74 grams of protein per kilogram of body weight
For females 0.74 × 60 kg = 44 grams

(Table 6-5). The World Health Organization currently recommends 0.75 grams of protein per kilogram of body weight for adults. The British use a protein recommendation of 10% of kcalories consumed. For a 2000-kcalorie diet, this intake totals about 50 grams of protein per day. The British recommendation deserves some caution. Low-kcalorie diets still need enough protein. Using a percentage will not guarantee enough protein when on a low-kcalorie diet. Table 6-5 shows recommended protein intakes using average weights for men and women from both the United States and Canadian guidelines.

Recall that an RDA is an allowance, not a requirement. Some people require less than this amount. Even so, the average man and woman in the United States consumes about 90 and 70 grams of protein, respectively, per day, a level in excess of the RDA.[11] Canadian values are similar. People just happen to eat many high protein foods in North America and can afford them. The excess protein cannot be stored as such. As noted before, the amine group is removed and the carbon skeleton is turned into glucose or fat and then either stored or burned for energy needs (Figure 6-2).

To consume the RDA for protein, adults must eat about 8% of their kcalories as protein. Registered dietitians in North America usually plan diets with 10% to 15% of total kcalories from protein to account for possible low kcalorie intakes, and to allow people to eat the amount of protein foods they are accustomed to.

Mental stress, physical labor, and sports activity do not require an increase in the RDA for protein. Elderly people might need 1 gram of protein per kilogram of body weight.[7,19] In addition, to support either substantial gains in muscle tissue from sports activities or a large muscle mass formerly acquired, increasing the allowance up to twice the RDA might be considered—but keep in mind that many

Expert Opinion

How Much Protein Do We Really Need?

A. E. HARPER, Ph.D.

In 1862, Dr. Edward Smith, a British physician who had studied energy and protein metabolism, concluded that to ensure the working capacity of the labor force during periods of food shortage a physically active man would need 80 grams of protein daily. During the next 40 years, other estimates of protein needs, which were based on records of the amounts of protein consumed by healthy working men, ranged up to 150 grams per day. But a controversy developed in the early 1900s after Russell Chittenden, an American chemist and educator, concluded from the results of studies on himself and his collegues and students at Yale that 35 to 45 grams of protein per day was sufficient for healthy adults.

This controversy has not been entirely resolved but the gap between the lower and higher estimates of protein needs of adults has narrowed. A practical recommendation of 0.8 grams per kilogram of body weight per day, or 56 grams per day for a 70-kilogram adult, is now widely accepted. Problems encountered in estimating protein needs have been discussed in detail in "Energy and Protein Requirements," a 1985 publication of the Food and Agriculture and World Health Organizations and United Nations University (FAO/WHO/UNU).

PROBLEMS IN ESTABLISHING PROTEIN NEEDS

Researchers face four problems in determining how much protein we need. First, there's the matter of measurement. Until the early 1900s, a measurement of the nitrogen content of a food was accepted as a reliable estimate of its value as a protein source ($N \times 6.25$ = protein). About that time, however, the amount of dietary protein required to prevent loss of body nitrogen was found to differ from one food source to another. The differences were explained when some of the amino acids in proteins were discovered to be essential nutrients and proteins were shown to differ in their content of these amino acids. This meant that the protein requirement was a dual one and that the ability of foods to supply certain indispensable amino acids could not be estimated from their nitrogen content alone. Some measure of this ability was also needed. What this measure should be is still being debated.

Second, clear signs of protein deficiency don't develop until protein depletion is severe. So it is not possible to reduce the protein intake of human subjects to the point where signs of severe depletion appear and then establish the requirement by determining how much is needed just to prevent their appearance. The initial effect of consuming a protein-deficient diet is loss of body protein. To gauge this loss requires accurate measurements of the amount of nitrogen consumed and the amounts lost in urine and feces. By feeding subjects a series of diets in which the protein content has been increased incrementally and determining the amount required merely to maintain nitrogen equilibrium, we can estimate the requirement. It tends to be an underestimate, however, because nitrogen lost in sweat, hair, and minor body secretions is rarely measured. An element of judgment is therefore involved in appropriately correcting for the loss.

Third, if protein intake is reduced, adaptation occurs and nitrogen equilibrium is achieved at the lower intake.

Fourth, amino acids, besides being essential nutrients, can also serve as sources of energy. If energy intake is low, a portion of the amino acids from dietary protein will be burned for fuel and additional protein will be required to compensate for this; hence protein requirements will be overestimated. If energy intake is high, amino acids are used quite efficiently so protein requirements may be underestimated. Differences in opinion over the significance of these effects have led to differences in estimates of protein needs.

DIGESTIBILITY AND AMINO ACID BALANCE

Estimates of protein requirements are based mainly on results of studies in which the diets have contained proteins of the highest quality. Such proteins are almost completely digestible and provide amino acids in proportions closely resembling those of the amino acid requirements. Because they have "well-balanced" amino acid patterns they are used very efficiently in synthesizing body proteins. Values for requirements established with such proteins are minimal.

Proteins in many plant products are only 80 to 90 percent digestible. To meet protein needs from such sources protein intake must be increased to compensate for the incomplete digestibility. Moreover, if the amino acid pattern of the dietary protein is "unbalanced"—that is, if one or more of the indispensable amino acids is present in disproportionately low amounts in relation to the requirements—the protein will be used inefficiently for synthesis of body proteins. That's true of cereal grain proteins, which are low in lysine. Young children therefore must consume a larger amount of unbalanced proteins, such as cereal grain proteins, than of well-balanced pro-

Expert Opinion—cont'd.

teins, such as milk proteins, to meet their amino acid requirements. With increasing age amino acid requirements per unit of body weight decline more rapidly than the need for total nitrogen; therefore the quantities of individual amino acids in the mixed diets of most adults are high enough when the requirements for total nitrogen is met. So a correction for protein quality isn't necessary.

In many poor countries where diets are composed largely of plant products, mixtures of cereal grains and legumes are traditionally used. Cereal grains are low in lysine; legumes are low in sulfur-containing amino acids. The amino acid patterns of the two thus complement each other, making the quality of the mixture of foods better than that of either one alone.

QUANTIFYING PROTEIN NEEDS

The FAO/WHO/UNU committee has estimated from the results of the best nitrogen-balance studies that the average need of adults for high quality proteins is 0.6 grams per kilogram of body weight per day. As half the population should have protein requirements below the average (and half above) public health recommendations for meeting protein needs must be high enough to cover the needs of those with the highest requirements. The FAO/WHO "safe" intake was therefore set at 0.75 grams of high quality protein per kilogram of body weight per day, and the RDA for adults at 0.8 grams.

Men and women don't differ in their protein requirements per unit of body weight but women, because they generally weigh less, need less total protein than men. Information about the needs of elderly adults is limited and not entirely consistent. There is little evidence to suggest that protein needs either decline or rise with increasing age.

PHYSICAL ACTIVITY AND DIETING

If you're doing heavy work in a hot, humid environment, the amount of nitrogen lost in sweat can increase substantially. Under most conditions, the loss appears to be small and transitory so no extra allowance for protein is recommended for physically active people. They usually eat enough extra food to meet their increased energy needs and ensure that their protein intake will also meet any increased needs.

The body's ability to use amino acids as energy sources has some implications for weight-loss regimens. To lose body fat, energy intake must be kept below the amount expended. Under these conditions the body will use some of the amino acids from food or mobilized from tissues as a source of energy. But to minimize the loss of body protein, protein intake must not be reduced. If, for example, the usual energy intake of an overweight person is 2500 kcalories, 9% of them as protein would provide 56 grams of protein. If he or she decides to slim down by cutting energy intake to 1500 kcalories a day, then 15% of them would have to come from protein to provide 56 grams daily.

APPROPRIATE INTAKES OF PROTEIN

Recommended intakes of protein for different age groups are listed on the inside cover of this textbook. These are sufficient to meet protein needs if there's adequate consumption of all other essential nutrients and energy. That these amounts of protein are a lot less than most people desire is evident from the average U.S. intake of nearly 100 grams per day. Considering the American penchant for high-protein food, for example, meat, poultry, fish, and dairy products, it's hardly surprising that protein consumption tends to be excessive. For example, since 1 ounce of meat, fish, or poultry supplies 7 grams of protein, a 55-kilogram woman can fulfill her entire daily protein requirement (44 grams) with a 5.6-ounce hamburger. High-protein foods are appetizing and flavorful and are excellent sources of many minerals and vitamins. So perhaps the question we should ask is "What is an appropriate dietary guideline for protein?" rather than "How much protein do we really need?"

The committee that established the Recommended Intakes of Nutrients for the United Kingdom proposed a guideline for protein of not less than 10% of kcalories. We might well recommend from 10 to 15% of kcalories as protein—not on the basis of meeting protein needs as such—but rather on the basis of evidence that diets rich in protein are ordinarily highly nutritious. There is no evidence of risk to health from such intakes. As caloric expenditure declines during aging, the appropriate guideline for the elderly should probably be toward the upper end of the range but, as kidney function also tends to decline with increasing age, it should probably not exceed 15% of total kcalories.

Dr. Harper is Professor of Nutritional Sciences at the University of Wisconsin at Madison.

North Americans eat that much protein already. *Extra protein intakes above usual adult intakes for athletes are usually not needed.* In addition, there is usually no reason for athletes to take either protein or individual amino acid supplements. All of us—athletes included—can meet our protein needs using basic foods.

Are the high-protein intakes of North Americans harmful?

It is unclear whether or not the high intake of protein by North Americans is harmful. The extra vitamin B-6, iron, and zinc that this provides is often a welcome addition. But research in the 1970s suggested that a high-protein diet might cause greater calcium loss in the urine. This worried researchers because they thought that protein caused calcium to leach out of the bones. In the long run this depletion can demineralize bones and lead to **osteoporosis,** a severe bone disease. However, follow-up studies show that if extra phosphorus is also consumed, urine calcium does not increase so much. Animal foods are excellent sources of both protein and phosphorus. So typical North American intakes probably don't threaten calcium balance as long as the RDA for calcium[22] is met (see Chapter 13 for further discussion).

osteoporosis
A bone disease characterized by decreased bone density that develops primarily after menopause in women.

Infants' diets must not contain excess protein since their kidneys have difficulty excreting the excess urea and minerals leftover after protein metabolism. Thus regular cow milk must not be used by itself for feeding young infants—it is too high in protein and other nutrients (see Chapter 16 for details).

There is some concern that high protein intakes may unduly burden the kidneys to excrete the resulting excess nitrogen (mostly as urea) into the urine. Animal studies show that protein intakes that just meet nutritional needs preserve kidney function over time better than high-protein diets. However, the same can be said for low-kcalorie diets. Thus the animal research has yet to determine which is more important for preserving kidney function—a conservative protein intake or a conservative energy intake.[18]

Exploring Issues and Actions

Your former high school gym teacher wants your advice on the amount of protein the field hockey team should eat. Is a poor protein intake likely contributing to their losing record?

Preserving kidney function is especially important for people with diabetes mellitus and for people who have only one functioning kidney. Presently many U.S. medical centers are studying whether a conservative protein intake preserves kidney function better in people with diabetes mellitus than does the typical North American very high-protein intake. For people without diabetes the risk of suffering kidney failure is very low and so the risk of a high-protein diet contributing to kidney disease in later life is probably also low.

The importance of plant proteins

Vegetable proteins deserve more attention from North Americans. These proteins, in proportion to the amount of energy they supply, provide much magne-

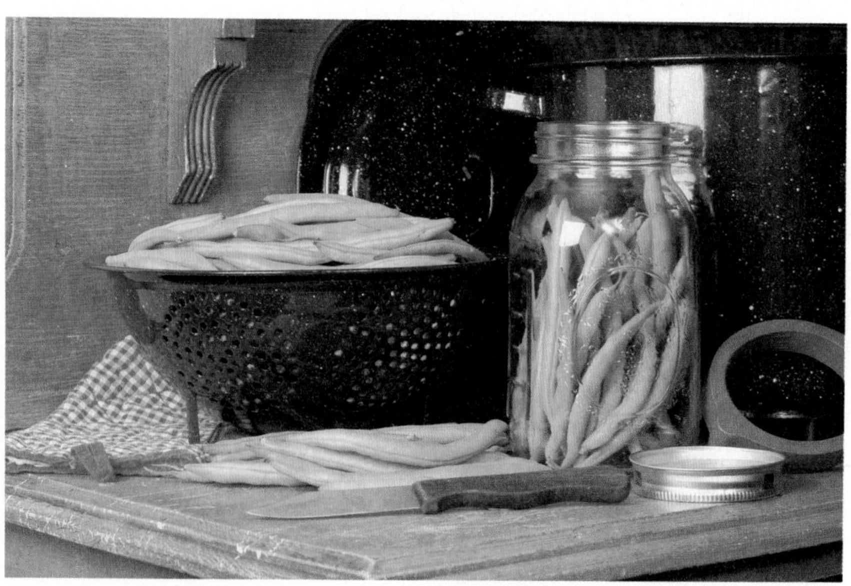

Legumes are a good sources of plant protein.

sium, soluble fiber, and other important benefits. Furthermore, vegetable proteins contain no cholesterol and are low in saturated fat, unless saturated fat is added during processing. As we discovered in Chapter 2, 1 to 2 servings of plant proteins per day make a valuable addition to the Daily Food Guide. Presently plant proteins are not very popular in North America, except for maybe peanut butter, pork and beans, and refried beans. Should you give them a second look?

Concept Check

The Recommended Dietary Allowance of protein for adults is 0.8 grams of protein per kilogram of desirable body weight. For a 70-kilogram (156-pound) person, this adds up to 56 grams of protein per day. The average North American man consumes about 90 grams of protein per day and the average woman consumes about 70 grams of protein per day. Thus typical protein intakes in North America are more than ample to meet protein needs.

PROTEIN IN FOODS

The exchange system provides easy means of estimating the protein content of a food. The fruit and fat groups contain no protein. The vegetable group yields 2 grams of protein; the starch/bread group yields 3 grams of protein; the meat group yields 7 grams of protein; and the milk group yields 8 grams of protein per exchange.

You will find that the actual amounts of protein in a diet and those predicted by the exchange system are very similar (Table 6-6). Note that Table 6-6 also shows that it is quite easy to obtain the RDA for protein by following the Daily Food Guide, even when consuming only 1200 kcalories a day.

The most nutrient-dense source of protein is water-packed tuna, which has over 80% of kcalories as protein (Figure 6-6). Notice that all the foods with more than 20% of kcalories as proteins are animal foods. They are also the major sources of protein in the North American diet: over two thirds come from animal sources. Worldwide, 54% of protein comes from animal sources. In Africa and East Asia less than 25% of the protein eaten comes from animals.[16]

In the United States in 1988, red meat and poultry consumption reached an all-time high of 253 pounds per person per year—nearly 58 pounds above the 1960 figures. Beef still leads with an annual per person consumption of 104 pounds, but chicken is gaining fast, with consumption increasing from 28 pounds in 1960 to 64 pounds in 1988.

The amino acids most likely to be low in a diet are lysine, methionine, threonine, and tryptophan. Table 6-2 lists plant foods that are characteristically low in these amino acids, although new strains of high-lysine and high-tryptophan corn are now available, as well as other improved grains. These strains yield better protein quality. The most toxic amino acids are methionine and tyrosine. The potential for amino acids imbalance and toxicities are too great to recommend any be taken individually as supplements. If a diet is low in an amino acid, we recommend finding a good food source to supply it.

PROTEIN DEFICIENCY CONDITIONS

In poorer areas of the world, people often eat diets low in kcalories and protein. Such diets stunt growth and increase susceptibility to disease. A person who eats too little protein and energy food can develop **protein-energy malnutrition (PEM),** also referred to as protein-calorie malnutrition (PCM). In its milder form it is difficult to tell if a person with PEM is suffering primarily from a poor intake of kcalories, protein, or both. But as the diet becomes more and more deficient, the signs and symptoms of primarily a kcalorie deficiency (clinical **marasmus**) differ from those of primarily a protein deficiency (clinical **kwashiorkor**), although similarities can still be seen (Figure 6-7).[16]

marasmus
A disease that results from not consuming sufficient protein and kcalories; thus it is the equivalent of protein-energy malnutrition. The infant or adult will have little or no fat stores, little muscle mass and poor strength. Death from infections is common.

kwashiorkor
A disease occurring primarily in young children when sufficient kcalories, but insufficient protein is consumed; the child suffers from edema, poor growth, weakness, and an increased susceptibility to infections.

Table 6-6

The protein content of a 1200 kcalorie diet

This table illustrates how few kcalories can be consumed while still meeting the RDA for protein.

Exchange	Food	Grams of protein based on exchange system
Breakfast		
1 skim milk	1 cup skim milk	8
1 starch/bread	¾ cup Cheerios	3
1 fruit	1 orange	—
Lunch		
2 starch/bread	2 slices whole-wheat bread	6
2 lean meat	2 oz chicken breast	14
1 fat	1 t mayonnaise	—
1 vegetable	1 cup carrot sticks	2
1 fruit	2 figs	—
	diet soda	—
Dinner		
2 lean meat	2 oz beef tenderloin	14
2 starch/bread with 1 fat	1 cup spinach pasta with 1 t garlic butter	6
1 vegetable with 1 fat	½ cup zuccini sauteed in 1 t oil	2
1 skim milk	1 cup skim milk	8
Snack		
1 starch/bread	½ toasted bagel	3
1 fat	1 t margarine	—
TOTAL		66 grams

Actual protein content based on Food Processor II software (ESHA Research, Salem, Oregon) 70 grams
RDA for 70-kilogram (156-pound) person in the United States 56 grams

General effects of semi-starvation

Detailed experiments studying the effects of human semi-starvation were performed by Dr. Ansel Keys in the 1940s. He maintained 32 men on a diet averaging about 1600 kcalories daily for 6 months. During this time the men lost an average of 24% body weight. After about 3 months, the subjects complained of tiredness, muscle soreness, irritability, and hunger pains. They showed a loss of ambition, poor self-discipline, and poor concentration. They were often moody and depressed. Their ability to laugh heartily or sneeze was reduced, and intolerance to heat appeared. Decreases in heart rate and muscle tone were also noted.[20]

These cumulative stresses of semi-starvation, then, eventually caused emotional instability and an overall apathetic frame of mind. Persistent hunger made it difficult for the subjects to pursue cultural interests, manual activities, and studies, in turn producing a frustrating discrepancy between the desire and the ability to pursue activities. After 12 weeks of rehabilitation, the desire for more food and

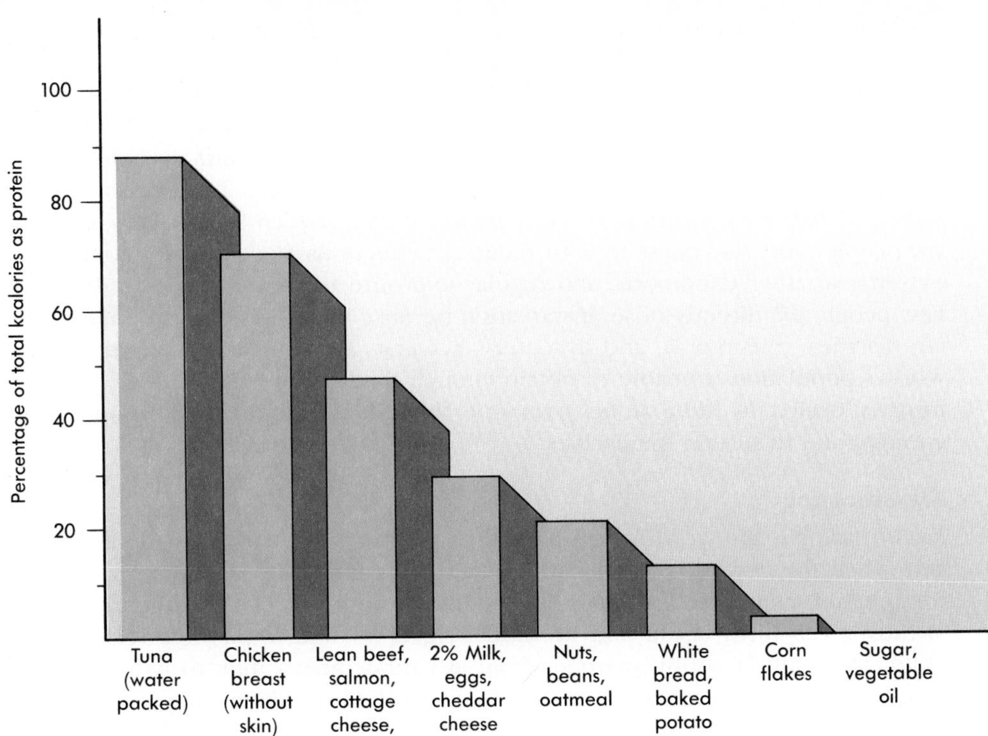

Figure 6-6

Percent of kcalories as proteins in foods. Water-packed tuna provides almost all kcalories as proteins.

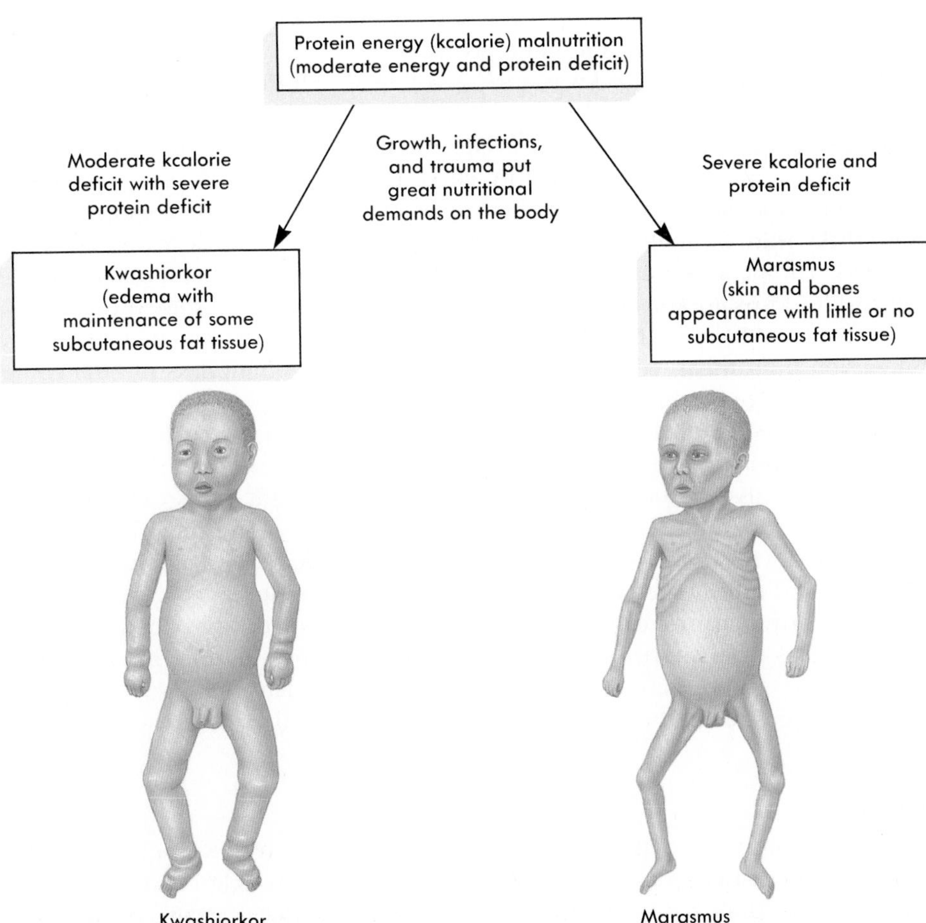

Figure 6-7

A schema for classifying malnutrition. The presence of subcutaneous fat (directly underneath the skin) is a diagnostic key.

a feeling of tiredness continued for the subjects. By 20 weeks they had largely, but not fully, recovered—full recovery required about 33 weeks.

These same responses can be expected in semi-starvation wherever it appears in the world. *Semi-starvation diminishes the ability of people, communities, and even whole countries to perform at peak levels of physical and mental capabilities, robbing people and nations of human resources.* The effects of semi-starvation in poor countries are even greater than that seen by Dr. Keys, because the people must also contend with recurrent infections, poor sanitary conditions, extreme weather conditions, and regular exposure to very **infectious diseases.** Few people die directly of semi-starvation because infectious diseases, in particular, diarrhea, pneumonia, and dysentery, act first. Today nearly a quarter of the world's population is unable to obtain enough food to support the level of activity they desire. In India alone, over one third of the population cannot afford enough food to sustain themselves.

infectious disease
Any disease caused by an invasion of the body by microorganisms, such as bacteria and fungi, or by viruses.

Kwashiorkor

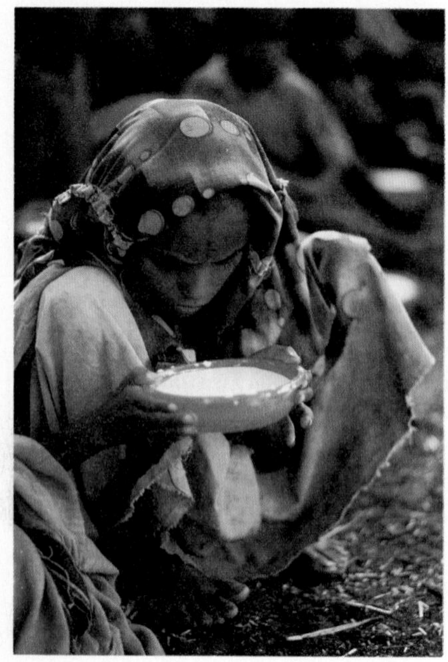

Kwashiorkor is the word from Ghana that means "the disease that the first child gets when the new child comes." From birth the child is probably breastfed. By the time the child reaches 1 to 1.5 years, the mother is probably pregnant or has already given birth again, and breastfeeding is no longer possible for the first child. This child abruptly switches from nutritious breast milk to native starchy roots and gruels. These foods have such low protein densities compared with total kcalories that they cannot meet the child's protein needs. The foods are also often so bulky and full of plant fibers that it is difficult for the child to eat much of them. So these children between ages 2 to 5 years have their energy needs met only marginally, but their protein needs, and probably many vitamin and mineral needs as well, are far from being met. Feeding famine victims starchy roots, such as casava (tapioca), sets up the same problem.

The major symptoms of kwashiorkor are apathy, listlessness, failure to grow and gain weight, withdrawal from the environment, and most importantly, an increased susceptibility to infections.[16] This can make conditions such as measles, a disease that normally makes a healthy child ill for only a week or so, a severely debilitating and fatal disease. Further signs of the disease are changes in hair color, flaky skin, fat infiltration in the liver, and massive edema in the abdomen and legs. The presence of edema with some subcutaneous fat still present is the hallmark of kwashiorkor (Figure 6-7). You would also notice something strange about these children—they hardly move. If you pick them up, they don't cry. When you hold them, you realize you are seeing the plumpness of edema, not muscle and fat tissue.

We can predict all these signs of kwashiorkor based on what we know about proteins. Proteins play important roles in fluid balance, immune function, and production of tissues such as skin and hair. We should not expect children with insufficient protein intakes to grow and mature normally. And they don't!

If a child with kwashiorkor is helped in time and fed a diet ample in protein, kcalories, and other essential nutrients, the disease symptoms reverse. The child begins to grow again and may even show no signs of the previous condition, aside perhaps from shortness of stature.[16] However, by the time many of these children reach a hospital or care center, they already have severe infections. In spite of the best care, they still die. Or, if they survive, they return home and repeat the cycle.

Marasmus

Marasmus is a disease that occurs when a child receives insufficient protein, kcalories, and other nutrients. The condition is also generally referred to as protein-energy malnutrition. The word *marasmus* means "to waste away." Children do just that. They have the "skin and bones" appearance that appears on posters from relief agencies (Figure 6-7). Little or no subcutaneous fat is present. The child is usually under age 2 and was either not breastfed or stopped breastfeeding in the early months. The weaning formula was then probably improperly prepared, partly because of poor water supplies and partly because the parents lacked money to afford sufficient formula for the child's needs. So the parents probably diluted the formula to provide more feedings. All this does is provide more water for the child, but the parents do not realize that.

Marasmus commonly occurs in the large cities of poverty-stricken countries. In the cities it is more fashionable to bottlefeed. When people are poor and sanitation is lacking, bottlefeeding often leads to marasmus (see Chapters 15 and 16 for further discussion). Even if a child with marasmus is helped in time and fed, he may never fully recover from the disease. Most brain growth takes place between conception and the first birthday. In fact, the brain is growing at its most rapid rate at birth. If the diet does not support brain growth during the first months of life, the brain may not grow to its full adult size. This reduced growth can lead to a decrease in intelligence.

Both kwashiorkor and marasmus wreak havoc on infant and childhood mortality rates: in poorer countries the rates are often 10 to 20 times higher than in the United States. Over 40,000 infants worldwide die of starvation each year. This high mortality rate in part encourages the high birthrate in poorer countries: if a mother wants four children, she had better have ten to make sure four survive. The overload makes infant mortality just that much more likely. The problem is further fueled by politics and war. In all, it often creates an intolerable environment for raising children (Figure 6-8). Better food availability and improved sanitation would greatly improve the health of many children worldwide.

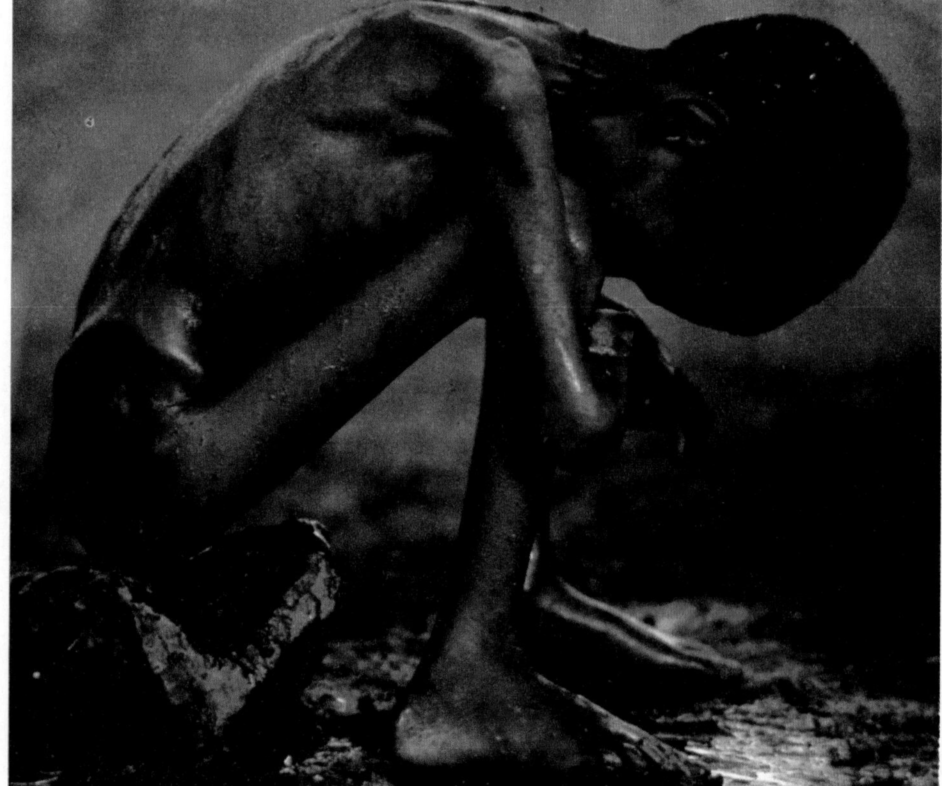

Figure 6-8
The tragedy of poverty and illness.

Protein malnutrition in the hospital

Kwashiorkor in the hospital results when a patient is fed primarily glucose intravenously. This may happen when a slow recovery from surgery prevents the use of a person's intestinal tract. In addition, a person may feel too sick to eat much. The intravenous feeding meets kcalorie needs to some extent but does not provide protein. The person develops edema, and often the immune function is diminished, leaving the patient at great risk for infections. One of the best markers for kwashiorkor is a person's serum albumin level. When it falls below 3.5 grams per 100 milliliters, the person is at risk. By the time the serum albumin level falls to 2.2 grams per 100 milliliters, the person is at a very high risk for infections and disease.

Studies have demonstrated that a hospital patient with a low body weight, a low serum albumin level, and a low white blood cell (especially lymphocyte) count is at a 4 to 6 times greater risk for complications and death than is a patient with normal levels for those three factors.[21] The lymphocyte count is a good monitor for immune function. In the last 10 years nutrition support teams have been formed in hospitals. One of their missions is to ensure that patients receive enough oral or intravenous nutrition support to enable them to meet their needs for proteins, carbohydrates, and other nutrients.

Marasmus occurs in a hospitalized patient when a person simply does not eat enough kcalories.[19] This can be the case in anorexia nervosa, in cancer, and in some intestinal disorders. The person either does not eat enough food or does not absorb enough nutrients from the intestinal tract to meet nutritional needs. Muscle, vital organ tissue, and fat stores waste away, and the person eventually looks like "skin and bones." Death from starvation or heart failure can then result. A hospitalized person may also have mixed kwashiorkor-marasmus. This is characterized by edema in a person with greatly diminished fat stores.

Concept Check

If a person regularly consumes sufficient energy but insufficient protein, a condition known as kwashiorkor develops. The person suffers decreased immune function, edema, weakness, and increased susceptibility to infections. Preschool children are especially susceptible to kwashiorkor, particularly in famine situations where only starchy root products are available for consumption. Marasmus is a condition in which neither protein nor kcalorie needs are met. Whether one is an adult suffering from cancer or an infant suffering from famine, the symptoms are muscle wasting, absence of fat stores, and weakness. Both protein deficiency conditions must be prevented if health is to be maintained.

Take Action

Using Table 6-5, calculate your own RDA for protein. Then record your food intake for a day and use the exchange system to estimate how much protein you ate. Are you surprised by the difference?

Your RDA for protein ______?

−

Your protein intake for one day ______?

DIFFERENCE ______?

Summary

1. Amino acids are the building blocks of protein. They contain nitrogen in the form of an amine ($-NH_2$) group. Of 20 types of amino acids found in food, 9 are essential in the diet and 11 can be synthesized by the body if amine groups from extra amino acids are available.
2. Complete protein foods contain an ample supply of all nine essential amino acids. This is typical of animal foods. Incomplete protein foods lack good supplies of one or more of the essential amino acids. This is typical of plant foods. Two plant foods can be combined to complement each other's amino acid deficiencies, in turn providing a complete protein meal.
3. Individual amino acids bond together to form proteins. The order of the amino acids is called the primary structure. This order determines the ultimate form and thus the function of the protein. The three-dimensional shape the protein eventually forms is called tertiary structure. This structure can be unfolded—denatured—by treatment with heat, acid or alkaline solutions, and other processes. Then the protein can no longer function as intended.
4. Proteins form essential body constituents, such as muscles, connective tissue, transport proteins, visual pigments, enzymes, hormones, and immune bodies. Proteins also provide a source of carbon atoms that can be synthesized into glucose.
5. Protein quality can be measured by determining the extent to which the body can retain the protein absorbed. This ratio of nitrogen retention to nitrogen absorption is called biological value. The ability of a food to support the growth of rats is also a measure of protein quality, known as the protein efficiency ratio. In addition, the balance of essential amino acids in a food can be compared to an ideal balance. The ability to match the ideal balance is referred to as a chemical store. It predicts the ability of the body to retain in tissues the food protein eaten.
6. The RDA for protein for adults is 0.8 grams per kilogram of desirable body weight. For a 70-kilogram (156 pound) person this corresponds to 56 grams of protein per day. The average North American man consumes about 90 grams of protein per day and women consume closer to 70 grams of protein per day. Thus the North American diet generally supplies ample protein.
7. Animal proteins are the most nutrient-dense sources of protein. Plant foods generally contain less than 20% of their kcalories as protein. Contrast that to water-packed tuna, which contains 85% of its kcalories as protein.
8. Protein deficiency conditions include kwashiorkor and marasmus. Kwashiorkor results primarily from a poor protein intake despite an ample kcalorie intake, while marasmus results primarily from a poor intake of both protein and kcalories. Marasmus commonly occurs in famine conditions, especially in infants. Kwashiorkor can result in that situation if children are fed starchy gruels that contain ample kcalories but insufficient protein. Variations of these diseases appear in hospitalized people in North America.

CHAPTER 6

Answers to Nutrition Awareness Inventory

1. *False.* Most of us eat such a varied assortment of food that if enough kcalories are consumed, it would be difficult not to have a complete protein diet that contains enough of all nine essential amino acids.
2. *True.* Protein is particularly important for building new tissue during periods of rapid growth.
3. *True.* Only a few enzymes are composed of other compounds.
4. *True.* It contains only amino acids.
5. *True.* Biological value represents the body's ability to retain the protein absorbed.
6. *True.* Milk proteins provide one of the highest possible biological values from foods. An egg white has the very best biological value.
7. *False.* People require more protein per weight when they are growing.
8. *False.* All of us, including athletes, can meet our protein needs with basic foods, and rarely is an intake greater than twice the RDA necessary.
9. *True.* For this reason trimming meats of fat and broiling them is a good idea.
10. *True.* Although lack of energy can be caused by other things, it is a symptom of severe protein deficiency.
11. *False.* Gelatin is an incomplete protein; it lacks the amino acid tryptophan.
12. *True.* Starvation in infancy leads to marasmus, which means "to waste away."
13. *False.* Plant proteins contain much fiber and magnesium; in comparison, animal proteins supply the most absorbable form of iron.
14. *True.* It is 85% protein.
15. *True.* These contain mostly carbohydrate and water.

REFERENCES

1. ADA Reports: Position of the American Dietetic Association: vegetarian diets, Journal of the American Dietetic Association 88:351-355, 1988.
2. Bishop CW and Ritchey SJ: Evaluating upper arm anthropometric measurements, Journal of The American Dietetic Association 84:330, 1984.
3. Dwyer JT: Health aspects of vegetarian diets, American Journal of Clinical Nutrition 48:712, 1988.
4. Eaton SB, Shostak M, and Konner M: The paleolithic Prescription, New York, 1988, Harper & Row.
5. Freeland-Graves JH: Mineral adequacy of vegetarian diets, American Journal of Clinical Nutrition 49:859, 1988.
6. Freeland-Graves JH and others: Health practices, attitudes, and beliefs of vegetarians and nonvegetarians, Journal of The American Dietetic Association 86:913, 1986.
7. Fukagawa NK and Young VR: Protein and amino acid metabolism and requirements in older persons, Clinics in Geriatric Medicine 3:329, 1987.
8. Grandjean AC: The vegetarian athlete, The Physician and Sports Medicine 15:191-194, 1987.
9. Herbert V: Vitamin B-12: plant sources, requirements, and assay, American Journal of Clinical Nutrition 46:852, 1988.
10. Kergoat M and others: Discriminant biochemical markers for evaluating the nutritional status of elderly patients in long-term care, American Journal of Clinical Nutrition 46:849, 1987.
11. Kim WW and others: Evaluation of long-term dietary intakes of adults consuming self-selected diets, American Journal of Clinical Nutrition 40:1327, 1984.
12. Kowalski R and others: Congress investigates vegetarian nutrition, Nutrition Today, p 30, July/August 1987.
13. Laidlaw SA and JD Kopple: Newer concepts of the indispensable amino acids, American Journal of Clinical Nutrition 46:593, 1987.
14. Lappe' FM: Diet For a Small Planet, New York, 1971, Ballantine/ Books.
15. Mudambi SR and Rajageopal MV: Is a vegetarian patient at risk? Nutrition 3:373, 1987.
16. Olson RE: World food production and problems in human nutrition, Nutrition Today p. 15, January/February 1989.
17. Robertson L and others: The New Laurel's Kitchen, Berkeley, Calif., 1986, Ten Speed Press.
18. Rudman D: Kidney senescence: a model for aging, Nutrition Reviews 46:209, 1988.
19. Russell RM: Nutritional Support of the long-term care patient, Nutrition Support Services 8:12, 1988.
20. Scrimshaw NS: The phenomenon of famine, Annual Reviews of Nutrition, 7:1-21, 1987.
21. Seltzer MH and others: Instant nutritional assessment, Journal of Parenteral and Enteral Nutrition 3:157, 1979.
22. Spencer H and others: Factors contributing to calcium loss in aging, American Journal of Clinical Nutrition 36:776, 1982.
23. Truesdell DD and Acosta PB: Feeding the vegan infant and child, Journal of The American Dietetic Association 85:837, 1985.
24. Young VR: Kinetics of amino acid metabolism: nutritional implications and some lessons, 1987 McCollum Award Lecture, American Journal of Clinical Nutrition 46:709, 1987.

SUGGESTED READINGS

For more details on amino acid metabolism and protein needs see the review by Young. His research on protein needs spans many years and has led to much of our understanding of this topic. To learn more about the reasons for famine and the effects on humans see the review by Scrimshaw. This article chronicles the major famines recorded in history and the effects they have had on the people involved. Finally, to learn more about the possible health benefits of vegetarianism see the review by Dwyer. This article covers essentially every possible effect of a vegetarian versus an omnivorous diet. An excellent vegetarian cookbook is that by Robertson and others. In addition, this book contains an easily understandable discussion of nutrition as it applies to vegetarianism.

Nutrition Perspective 6-1

Vegetarianism

Vegetarianism has sparked the interest of men and women for centuries. The practice of vegetarianism is as old as the human species, yet today it is new to many people. Throughout human history vegetarianism has changed from being a necessity to being a personal option. Historically vegetarians have been people particularly interested in philosophy, religion, or science. Today vegetarianism in this country usually appeals to a younger segment of people.

As nutrition science has grown, our ability to plan adequate vegetarian diets has improved. If you choose to be a vegetarian, you can be confident you can meet your nutritional needs by following a few basic rules.[8,12,23] Recent studies of all causes of death show that mortality rates are lower for vegetarians than for nonvegetarians. Diet, healthy life-styles (leanness, not smoking, abstinence from alcohol and drugs, and increased physical activity), and social class selection bias probably all account for these findings.

WHY DO PEOPLE PRACTICE VEGETARIANISM?

People choose vegetarianism for a variety of reasons. Some think it is more ethical not to kill animals for food. Religious orders, such as Hindus and Trappist monks, eat vegetarian meals as a practice of their religion. In the United States many Seventh Day Adventists base their practice of vegetarianism on Biblical texts and believe it is a healthier way to eat.

People might choose vegetarianism because they want to eat fewer pesticides. By eating plants animals concentrate the pesticides that plants take up. The greater variety of plants a person eats, the less chance of eating a food highly concentrated in pesticides. A person might also become a vegetarian after realizing that animals are not efficient protein factories. In fact, the reverse is true: animals use up much of the protein they eat for maintenance, rather than for synthesizing new muscle tissue. A cow eats 21 pounds of plant protein for every pound of meat protein it produces. The ratio for pigs is 8 to 1, and 5 to 1 for chickens. Food animals do sometimes eat grasses that humans cannot eat. However, they also eat grains fit for human consumption.

People might eat vegetarian because it encourages a high intake of carbohydrates, vitamin A, vitamin E, beta-carotene, vitamin C, magnesium, and fiber, while limiting cholesterol and saturated fat intake.[6] If this rationale sounds similar to the Dietary Guidelines covered in Chapter 2, it is. And some people might pursue vegetarianism because meat is expensive.

FOOD PLANNING

There are a variety of vegetarian styles. **Vegans** eat only plant foods. **Fruitarians** eat primarily fruits, nuts, honey, and vegetable oils. **Lacto-vegetarians** eat dairy products and plant foods. **Lacto-ovo-vegetarians** eat dairy products, eggs, and plant foods. **Lacto-ovo-pesco-vegetarians** eat dairy products, eggs, and fish, as well as plant foods. The wider the variety of foods eaten, the easier it is to meet nutritonal needs.[1]

The practice of eating no animal protein separates the vegans and fruitarians from all other vegetarian styles. *Including some animal protein in a diet makes diet planning much easier.* Most vegetarians consume at least dairy products, if not dairy products and eggs. A four-food-group plan has been developed for lacto-vegetarians (Table 6-7).[17] This plan has a protein group that includes nuts, grain, legumes, and seeds. There is also a vegetable group, a fruit group, and a milk and/or eggs group.

This plan differs a little from the typical Daily Food Guide pattern for **omnivores,** but it shares some similarities. The key to this plan is seeking protein sources in foods other than meats. It's not enough to just cut out meat and to eat everything else. One really needs to search for good quality protein sources to replace the meat in the diet. That is where the nuts, grain, legumes, and seed group comes in; they become the new "meat" group. By following the food plan, there should be no problem achieving an adequate diet.

omnivore
A person who consumes both plant and animal food sources.

Continued

Nutrition Perspective 6-1, cont'd

Table 6-7

A four-food-group plan for lacto-vegetarians[17]

Group*	Servings	Key nutrients supplied
Grains, legumes, nuts and seeds	6	Protein, thiamin, niacin, vitamin B-6, folate, vitamin E, zinc, magnesium, and fiber
Vegetables	3 or more (include one dark-green leafy)	Vitamin A, vitamin C, folate
Fruits	1 to 4	Vitamin A, vitamin C, folate
Milk	2 or more	Protein, riboflavin, vitamin D, vitamin B-12, and calcium

*Base serving size on those listed in the Daily Food Guide (see Chapter 2).

THE VEGAN

The vegan has to do some special diet planning.[3,5,15] First, it is a good idea to purchase some vegetarian cookbooks. These provide numerous ideas for nutritious ways to creatively use plant foods. A real effort must be made to eat grains and legumes to obtain good quality protein. Then if kcalorie needs are met, protein needs should also be met. *A wide variety of protein sources, including the excellent ones just mentioned, should provide* ***complementarity*** *of individual amino acids to yield a complete protein diet.* In other words, the deficiencies in essential amino acids in one food protein are made up for by the essential amino acid content of another food protein in the meal. Furthermore, the vegan diet needs some good sources for riboflavin, vitamin D, vitamin B-12, calcium, iron, and zinc (Table 6-8).

complementarity of proteins
A state in which two food protein sources make up for each other's lack in specific essential amino acids, such that together they yield complete protein.

Table 6-8

Nutrients likely to be low in the diet of a total vegetarian (vegan)

Nutrient	Plant sources
Vitamin D	Fortified margarines, fortified breakfast cereals
Riboflavin	Whole and enriched grains, leafy vegetables, mushrooms, beans, nuts, seeds
Vitamin B-12	Fortified breakfast cereals, fortified yeast, fortified soy milk
Iron	Whole grains, prune juice, dried fruits, beans, nuts, seeds, leafy vegetables
Calcium	Fortified soy milk*, tofu, almonds, dry beans, leafy vegetables, some fortified breakfast cereals, flours, and brands of orange juice*
Zinc	Whole grains, wheat germ, beans nuts, seeds

*Fortified soy milk and fortified orange juice are the best sources.

Riboflavin can be obtained by eating green leafy vegetables, whole grains, yeast, and legumes. Most vegans do eat these foods. Note that the major source of riboflavin in the North American diet is milk, which has been omitted from the diet. Vitamin D can be obtained by regular sun exposure. Otherwise, a supplement containing vitamin D should be considered. *Vitamin B-12 only naturally occurs in animal foods,* but plants may contain soil or microbial contamination that provide some vitamin B-12. However, the vegan should find a more reliable source of vitamin B-12, such as fortified soy bean milk or special yeast grown on media rich in vitamin B-12 (check the label).[9]

To obtain calcium, the vegan could consume fortified soy milk or fortified orange juice. Tofu, green leafy vegetables, and nuts also contain calcium, but it is either not well absorbed or not very plentiful. Calcium supplements are another possibility.

For iron the vegan can consume whole grains, dried fruits, and legumes. The iron in these foods is not as well absorbed as that found in animal foods, but a good source of vitamin C consumed with these foods can greatly enhance the iron absorption. Thus an excellent recommendation is to include a source of vitamin C in every meal that contains an adequate source of iron from plant foods (see Chapters 12 and 14).

The vegan can find zinc in whole grains and legumes. The phytic acid present in whole grains limits absorption; it is best if the grains are leavened, as in bread, to reduce the influence of phytic acid (see Chapter 14). Of all these nutrients sufficient calcium is the most difficult to consume (Table 6-8).[3]

Veganism in childhood deserves special attention. The sheer bulk of a plant-based diet may make it difficult for a child to consume sufficient kcalories to meet energy needs, to allow dietary protein to be used for synthetic, rather than energy, needs. Concentrated sources of kcalories should be included in the diet of a child vegan to avoid this problem. Examples include fortified soy milk, nuts, dried fruits, cookies made with vegetable oils, and fruit juices.

Anyone trying vegetarianism should realize that a healthful diet does not happen automatically. It takes some planning and common sense. We keep stressing the importance of eating a wide variety of foods. This is especially important for the vegetarian.

Part III

Energy Production and Energy Balance

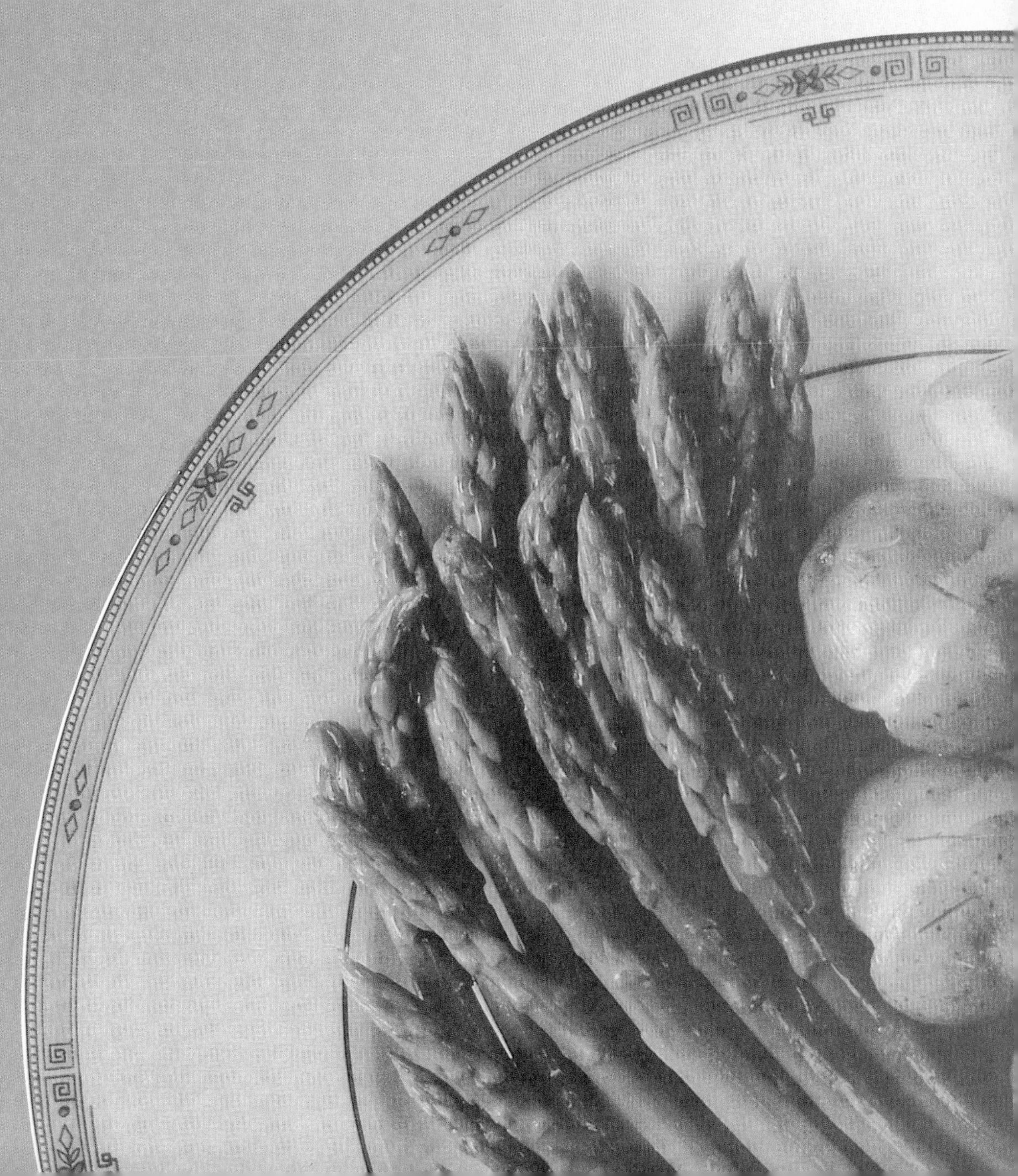

Chapter 7
Metabolism

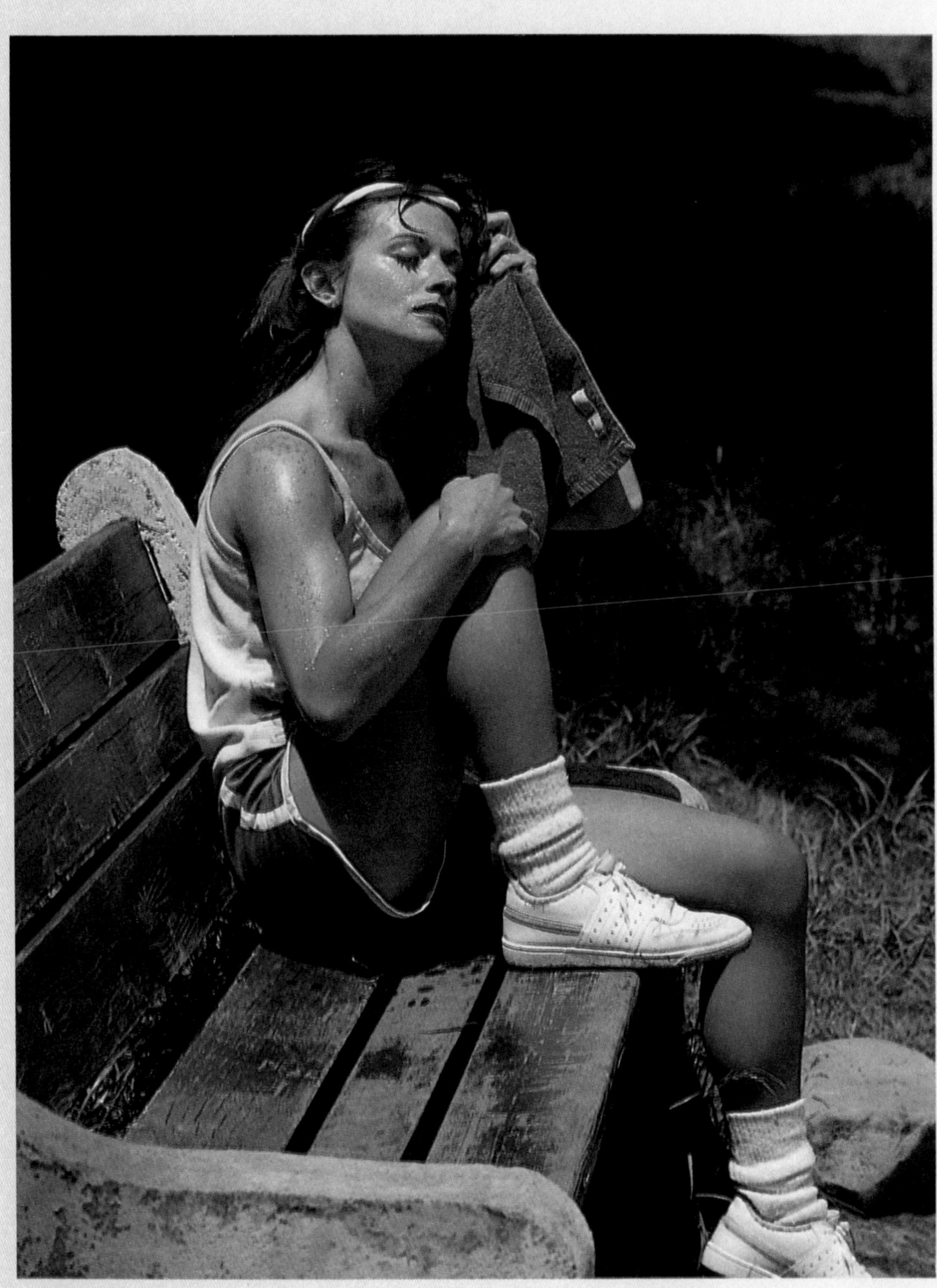

Exercise is an important part of a healthy life-style.

Overview

Metabolism refers to the entire network of physical and chemical processes involved in maintaining life. It encompasses all the sequences of chemical reactions that occur in the body. These reactions enable us to release and use energy from foods, convert one substance into another, and prepare the products for excretion. More than 1000 different kinds of chemical reactions take place in a simple single-cell bacterium.

Studying metabolism can help us understand other nutrition concepts. Understanding metabolism clarifies how proteins, carbohydrates, fats, and alcohol interrelate. It shows how carbon atoms in protein molecules become the carbon atoms of glucose and why carbon atoms of most fatty acids cannot become the carbon atoms of glucose. Second, studying metabolic pathways in the cell sets the stage for examining the roles of vitamins and minerals. Most vitamins function as coenzymes. Most minerals function as cofactors. By their natures, these compounds—coenzymes and cofactors—promote enzyme function and so contribute to important metabolic reactions in the cell. The functions of vitamins and minerals are easier to understand when you are familiar with the basic metabolic processes in the cell.

Nutrition awareness inventory

Here are 15 statements about metabolism. Read them to test your current knowledge. If you think the statement is true or mostly true, circle T. If you think the statement is false or mostly false, circle F. Use the scoring key at the end of the chapter to compute your total score. Take this test again after you have read the chapter. Compare the results.

1. **T F** Carbohydrates can be used for energy and fat storage.
2. **T F** Fats can be used for energy and fat storage.
3. **T F** Eating protein doesn't lead to fat formation.
4. **T F** The brain uses energy in the form of glucose.
5. **T F** Fasting increases blood ketone levels.
6. **T F** High ethanol intake causes the liver to waste some energy.
7. **T F** Drinking 7 beers a day for 15 years could lead to cirrhosis of the liver.
8. **T F** Drink all the alcohol you want. It will never turn to fat.
9. **T F** Caffeine improves athletic performance.
10. **T F** Carnitine is used for carbohydrate metabolism.
11. **T F** Ketones are formed primarily from glycerol.
12. **T F** Mitochondria supply energy within the cell.
13. **T F** Acetyl-CoA has a central role in energy metabolism.
14. **T F** Plants obtain energy from photosynthesis.
15. **T F** Thirst is not a good guide for fluid replacement after hard exercise.

anabolic
Describes the building of compounds.

catabolic
Describes the breaking down of compounds.

adenosine triphosphate (ATP)
The main energy currency for cells; ATP energy is used to promote ion pumping, enzyme activity, and muscular contraction.

To be accurate we must say that energy is released or transferred; energy cannot be produced via metabolism. Energy can be neither created nor destroyed; it is simply transferred around the planet.

METABOLISM

A **metabolic** progression of chemical reactions from the starting to ending point is called a **pathway. Anabolic** pathways build compounds. The elements and compounds used to form the new compounds are called building blocks. Conversely, **catabolic** pathways break down compounds into small units: for example, glucose is "catabolized" when it is broken down into carbon dioxide (CO_2) and water (H_2O). *Almost every step in any pathway depends on an enzyme for the necessary chemical reaction to occur.*

Overall, energy metabolism occurs in three stages. In the first stage large molecules in food, such as proteins, starches, and triglycerides, are broken down during digestion and absorption into smaller units, such as amino acids, monosaccharides, and free fatty acids. In the second stage of metabolism these smaller compounds are further degraded to units of a central 2-carbon atom compound. In the third stage the 2-carbon atom compound is degraded into carbon dioxide and water molecules. The electron energy released is donated to oxygen atoms with the subsequent synthesis of **adenosine triphosphate (ATP).**[10] ATP is a storage form of energy that cells use. Chapter 3 focused on the first stage of metabolism; let's now examine the last two stages.

The cell—primary site for metabolism

The cell is the basic unit of body structure, and it is where most metabolic reactions occur (Figure 7-1). The cell is surrounded by a membrane that controls the passage of nutrients and other substances in and out of it. Within the cell is fluid called the cytosol. Within the cytosol are organelles, which are small bodies that perform specific metabolic functions. The names and activities of the various cell parts follow below:

- **Cell membrane:** This double-layered structure composed of lipids and protein contains channels to admit specific molecules into the cell; receptors

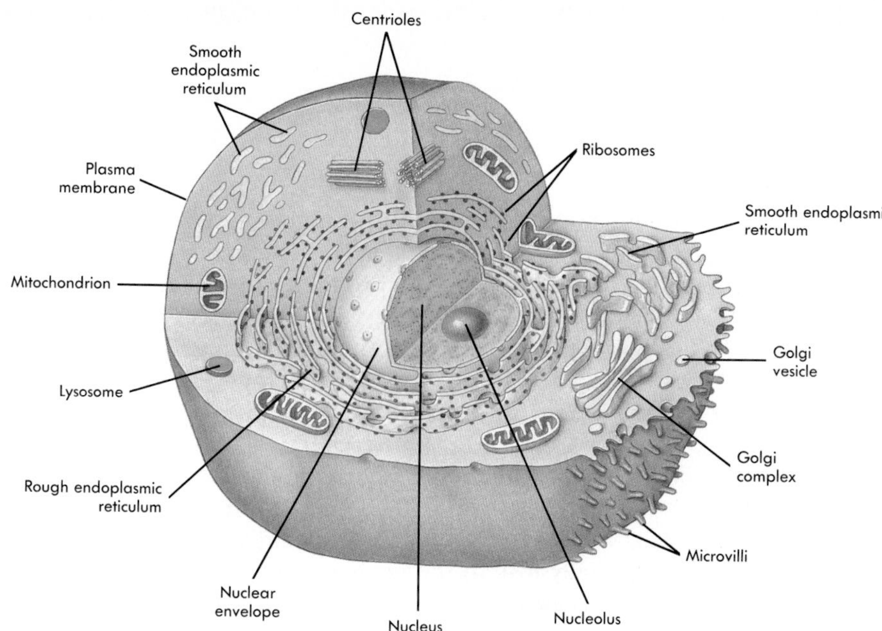

Figure 7-1

An animal cell. Almost all humans cells contain these various organelles.

that bind hormones and other compounds that send signals to the cell; and protein markers on the outside of the cell membrane that allow the immune system to recognize it as a human cell, as opposed to an invading bacterium (see Figure 5-3).

- **Nucleus:** This spherical structure is bounded by its own double membrane. Within the nucleus are chromosomes, which are long threads of DNA that contain hereditary information for directing cell protein synthesis and cell reproduction. Inside the nucleus is a nucleolus. Here a type of RNA (ribosomal RNA) is synthesized that eventually helps assemble ribosomes (see below).
- **Mitochondria:** These have their own outer membrane and an inner membrane that is highly folded. The mitochondria are the major sites of energy production in the cell. Mitochondria also synthesize important cell components, such as parts for nonessential amino acids.
- **Endoplasmic reticulum:** This network of internal membranes serves as a communication network within the cell. Small granules called ribosomes cover parts of the outside of the endoplasmic reticulum, known as the rough endoplasmic reticulum; protein is synthesized at these granules. Fat is synthesized in other areas of the endoplasmic reticulum, namely, the smooth endoplasmic reticulum.
- **Golgi complex:** This consists of stacks of flattened structures that both package proteins for export from the cell and help form other cell organelles. Budding off the golgi complex are golgi vesicles, which are fluid-filled sacs destined either for other parts of the cell or for excretion from the cell.
- **Lysosomes:** These small bodies contain digestive enzymes that break down worn-out cell parts and other cell debris. A lysosome is prevented from digesting the entire cell because each maintains a very low pH, which inhibits the digestive enzyme action. When a lysosome fuses with a particle that is to be digested, the pH in the lysosome then rises, promoting digestive enzyme activity.
- **Storage forms of energy:** These occur as glycogen granules and lipid droplets.

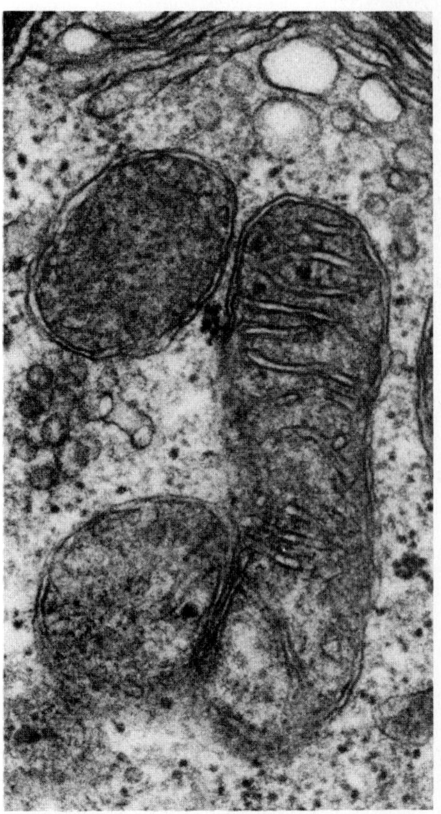

The mitochondrion is the major site of energy production in the cell.

- **Peroxisomes:** These carry enzymes, such as catalase, that can break down peroxides.

Let's begin by reviewing energy metabolism in general. Later we will identify the types of metabolism with their locations of occurrence in the cell.

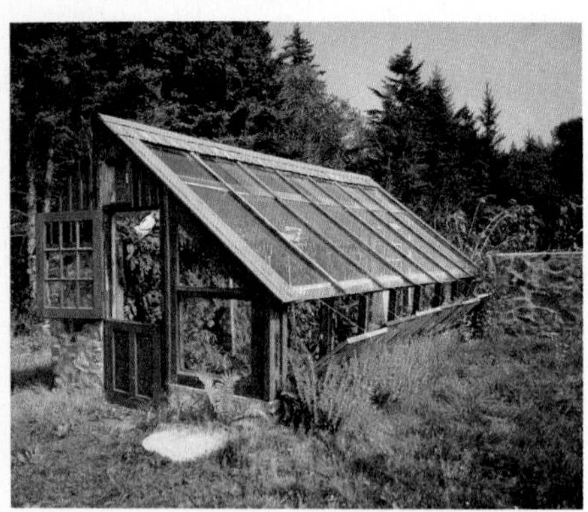

Unlike us, plants can use the direct energy of the sun to produce glucose and the organic compounds.

Energy for the cell

The energy that runs your body is captured in the chemical bonds of carbohydrate, protein, and fat molecules and in alcohol. This energy is a product of photosynthesis. Plants use energy from the sun to produce glucose and other organic compounds. In doing so they trap solar energy as electron energy in the compounds. The body then transforms the electron energy trapped in the carbohydrates, fats, and proteins *into* other forms: *chemical* energy to transform carbohydrates to fats; *mechanical* energy to propel muscular movements; *electrical* energy to drive nerve transmissions; and *osmotic* energy to maintain ion balance between cells. The flow of chemical energy from ingested foodstuffs throughout the body, in the final analysis, is then eventually and irretrievably dissipated to the environment as heat. Thus we rely on plants to convert solar energy into a form we can use, but eventually lose to the environment.

Each covalent bond between the atoms of molecules in foods (carbon atoms, hydrogen atoms, oxygen atoms, and so on) represents potential energy through the sharing of electrons. In every amino acid, glucose, and fatty acid molecule are many sites where solar energy is stored as chemical energy. One function of metabolism is to convert this chemical energy into a form human cells can use.

Many chemical reactions in the body could not occur without the addition of outside energy that food supplies. The outside energy permits compounds such as glucose to be transformed into end products such as glycogen. While glucose molecules themselves contain the energy needed, this form of food energy we consume neither provides us the right amount of energy for a chemical reaction nor provides a form our cells can use directly. *Human cells must always convert the chemical energy stored in the bonds of foodstuffs into a more appropriate form.* A glucose molecule contains over 100 times more energy than required to drive an individual chemical reaction in a cell. A triglyceride molecule contains about 500 times more energy than is needed. So a cell must have a means of breaking down the glucose and fatty acid molecules to both release and then convert the chemical energy trapped in them into usable and smaller energy packets.

Adenosine triphosphate (ATP)

The form of energy that cells generally use is ATP. Every body cell makes ATP to help meet energy needs. The active form of ATP is usually a complex of it with a magnesium or manganese ion. To release the energy in ATP, cells split it into adenosine diphosphate (ADP) plus Pi (Figure 7-2). The Pi stands for a free-phosphate group

$$\begin{array}{c} \mathrm{O} \\ \| \\ -\mathrm{O}-\mathrm{P}-\mathrm{O}- \\ | \\ \mathrm{O}- \end{array}$$

In other words, adenosine *tri*phosphate is split split into adenosine *di*phosphate plus a free-phosphate group. Splitting ADP into adenosine monophosphate (AMP) plus Pi also yields energy. Muscles do that during intense exercise in an attempt to maintain adequate ATP levels when the rate of ATP synthesis from ADP does not keep pace with energy needs.

Breaking the bond between either the first and second phosphate group or between the second and third phosphate group on ATP releases energy. This form of energy resembles the energy released when a bond is broken between a

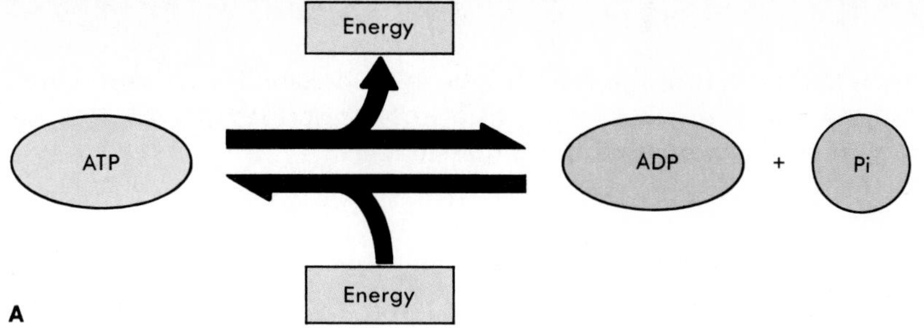

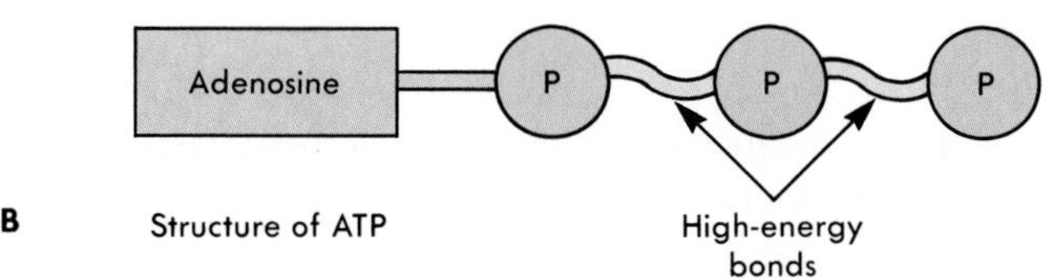

Figure 7-2

ATP stores and yields energy. ATP is the high-energy state, while ADP is the lower-energy state—some energy has been released to form the molecule.

carbon atom and a hydrogen atom in a glucose molecule. But unlike the energy released from breaking the bonds between carbon and hydrogen atoms, ATP energy can be used by cells. Energy released when breaking typical chemical bonds releases heat, but unless it also forms ATP, the energy cannot be used directly to promote enzyme action, ion pumping, or muscle contractions, the three processes human cells need energy for. *Only ATP energy or its derivatives can be used directly for energy by the cell.*

Pathways in every cell combine ADP and Pi to form ATP. This process captures chemical energy from food between the phosphate groups of ATP (Figure 7-2). An enzyme can then break that bond to release the energy for driving metabolic reactions. ATP itself is very stable. It takes an enzyme to unlock the energy that ATP stores.[10]

A resting cell has a high ATP concentration. An active cell has some ATP in it, as well as much ADP plus Pi. When a cell is active, it is constantly breaking down ATP in one part of the cell while rebuilding it in another part. An exhausted cell—a muscle cell, for example—will have a very high concentration of ADP and a very low concentration of ATP. When that happens, cell activity grinds to a halt. Only by resynthesizing needed ATP can the cell ready itself to go again. At rest a person's cells recycle ADP plus Pi to ATP and then reverse the cycle, reusing small amounts over and over. The amount of ATP used would be the equivalent of about 40 kilograms (88 pounds) per 24 hours. During physical activity, ATP use can reach the equivalent of 0.5 kilograms (1.1 pounds) per minute.[10]

Think about that the next time you race after a bus. When you finally sit down, you are exhausted. You breathe hard, and your heart races. Your muscle cells have used up most of their ATP and other high energy compounds. While you rest, muscle cells begin to resynthesize ATP by fusing the ADP and Pi created during the breakdown of ATP. If you sit long enough, you can then race to your class using the newly formed ATP. (To learn more about metabolism in exercise, as well as about diets for athletes, see Nutrition Perspective 7-1.)

Throughout this chapter we simplify many metabolic pathways by including only the most important steps. We mainly want you to understand the overall picture of metabolism. Future courses will cover the pathways step-by-step, enzyme-by-enzyme. If you want to look at any particular pathway in detail, see Appendix K.

CARBOHYDRATE METABOLISM

Let's now look at how ATP is generated in a human cell. All life forms have only two means for synthesizing ATP: using fuel molecules to supply the energy or trapping light energy by means of photosynthesis. You, of course, can do only the former. The easiest place to begin studying ATP generation in human cells is with

glycolysis
The breakdown of glucose into pyruvate (lactate) molecules.

carbohydrate metabolism. Next we'll look at fat metabolism and protein metabolism, and finish with alcohol metabolism in Nutrition Perspective 7-2. Again, all these compounds can be used to synthesize ATP.

Glycolysis

Glycolysis literally means "breaking down glucose." The glycolysis pathway has a dual role: it degrades monosaccharides to generate energy, and it provides building blocks for synthesizing needed cell compounds, such as glycerol for triglyceride synthesis. Before glycolysis can begin, a cell must obtain glucose molecules. Only liver and muscle cells store glucose to any extent. Recall that glucose is stored as glycogen. The liver and muscle cells break down the glycogen into a form of glucose; other body cells take glucose from the bloodstream. A few types of cells, such as liver cells, can even produce their own glucose from amino acids (see a later section in this chapter on gluconeogenesis). In these ways every body cell has glucose available to it.

The net result of glycolysis is the splitting of the 6-carbon compound glucose into two units of a 3-carbon compound called pyruvic acid (pyruvate). Some cells then convert pyruvate into lactic acid (lactate). But, for the most part, pyruvate is the end point of glycolysis. To begin glycolysis, glucose has a phosphate group added to it, which makes glucose more reactive. It also traps the glucose in the cell. Only liver cells and some kidney cells can reform free glucose once a phosphate group is attached. Now that the phosphate group is added, glucose is ready to participate in subsequent reactions.

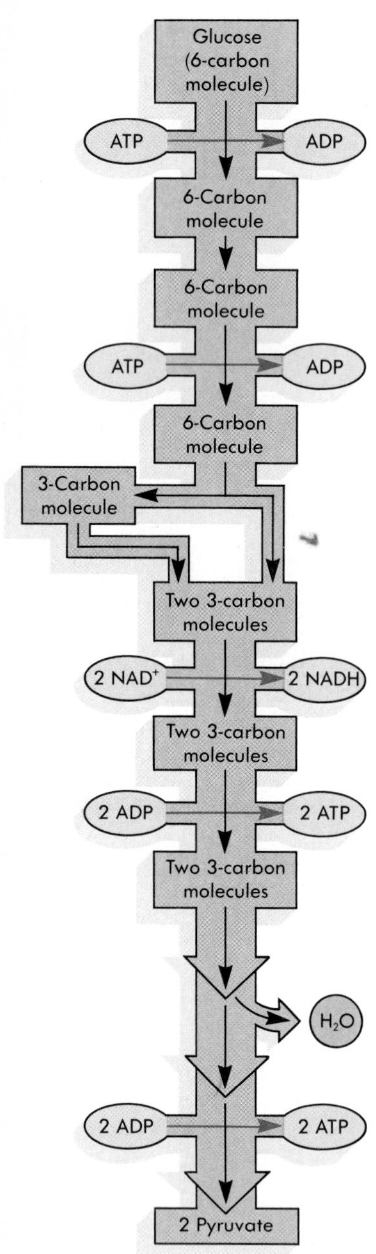

The synthesis of glucose into glucose-6-phosphate requires about 4 kcalories per mole of molecules. ATP yields about 7.3 kcalories per mole of molecules. Thus about 55% of the energy in ATP is used by the reaction (4 ÷ by 7.3) × 100; the rest is lost as heat.

The newly formed glucose-6 phosphate is changed to fructose 6-phosphate. Fructose 6-phosphate has another phosphate group added to it, and so becomes fructose 1,6-diphosphate. This compound splits into two 3-carbon compounds. These are then converted through a variety of steps into two molecules of the 3-carbon compound pyruvate. *Thus in glycolysis a cell starts with a 6-carbon glucose molecule and ends up with two molecules of the 3-carbon compound pyruvate.*

So where is the ATP?

In glycolysis, (Figure 7-7) one ATP molecule is used to add the first phosphate group to glucose; another ATP molecule is used to convert fructose-6-phosphate into fructose-1, 6-diphosphate. *So to begin glycolysis, a cell uses ATP energy.* As the two 3-carbon molecules are converted into pyruvate, each one generates two ATP molecules, for a total of four. The net energy produced thus far from glycolysis renders four ATP molecules minus two ATP molecules used, or two net ATP molecules. There are more to come.

As glucose breaks into two pyruvate molecules, four hydrogen atoms (containing a total of four electrons) are released. The hydrogen atoms are picked up by a carrier called **nicotinamide adenine dinucleotide (NAD).** The vitamin niacin forms part of the NAD molecule. Each NAD accepts two electrons but only one hydrogen ion. Thus an end result of glycolysis is also the synthesis of two NADH molecules and the release of two free hydrogen ions. The ions float freely in the cell fluid.

Chemical energy stored in the electrons of NADH can eventually be turned into ATP energy. So NADH is a form of potential energy for the cell: as chemical energy is released from the carbon-hydrogen bonds originally present in glucose, NADH traps some of it. A cell must then convert the energy in NADH into ATP energy. Later we will show how that happens.

Concerning other monosaccharides, much of the fructose from food is metabolized by the liver into successively different compounds that eventually yield a 3-carbon compound, the same product that glucose metabolism yields. As with glucose two ATP molecules are used. Any galactose from foods is converted into glucose-6-phosphate in a four-step process that uses one ATP molecule. Again, this is the same amount of energy used by glucose to form glucose-6-phosphate. Glycolysis can then proceed in both cases.

NAD is actually NAD^+, indicating it has one unpaired electron. By picking up two electrons and one hydrogen ion, NADH ends up with no charge. The extra electron provides electron balance in the molecule. We will ignore the charge on NAD to simplify the discussion.

Lactate production

Some body cells lack a pathway for converting NADH energy into ATP energy. The red blood cell is an example. As a red blood cell converts glucose into pyruvate, NADH molecules build up in the cell. Eventually the NAD concentration falls too low for glycolysis to continue because most of the NAD molecules present are in the form of NADH.

To compensate, a red blood cell reacts pyruvate with an NADH molecule and a free hydrogen ion to form lactate (Figure 7-3). In the process, NADH turns into NAD. This process allows the red blood cell to resupply itself with NAD. Exercising muscles produce lactate for the same reason (see below).

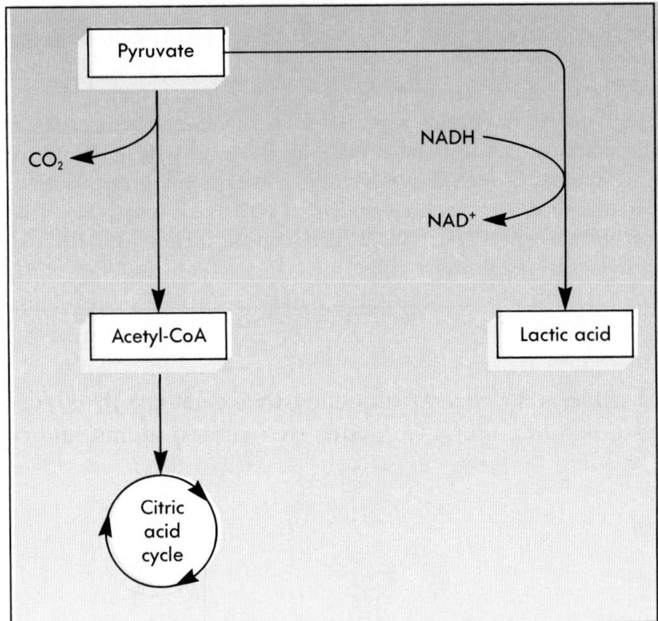

Figure 7-3

The metabolic fate of pyruvate. When the cell has oxygen available, pyruvate is usually broken down to acetyl-CoA. This enters the citric acid cycle. In the absence of oxygen, pyruvate, instead, takes the hydrogen ions and electrons yielded by glycolysis and carried by NADH. The product is lactic acid.

The production of lactate allows the glycolytic pathway to continue indefinitely: NAD is now always available. ATP is needed to begin glycolysis, but future ATP synthesis replaces that used in the beginning reactions and supplies extra for cell use. Since the entire pathway does not use oxygen, it is referred to as an **anaerobic** process. This pathway yields only two ATP molecules per glucose molecule. But for some cells—red blood cells, for example—it is the only method for making ATP. The lactate is released into the bloodstream and picked up primarily by the liver for resynthesis into glucose. Glucose then can reenter the bloodstream.

Regenerating NAD by using lactate represents a fermentation reaction. Some yeasts produce alcohol (ethanol) instead of lactate to regenerate NAD in anaerobic conditions. This is likewise a fermentation reaction.

Net energy production from glycolysis

Each glucose molecule has the potential to form 36 to 38 ATP molecules. So far, using glycolysis, we have made only two. However, it could be argued that we have really made six to eight. As you will see, each NADH molecule from glycolysis can yield two or three ATP molecules. Since we have two NADH molecules, we have really produced two actual and four to six potential ATP molecules using glycolysis.

Nevertheless, even 8 is nowhere near 36 to 38. Those two pyruvate (or lactate) molecules formed at the end of glycolysis still contain a lot of stored energy.

Acids commonly lose a hydrogen ion at the pH level found in human cells (pH 7.4). When that ion is lost, the name of the acid is changed by dropping the reference to acid and adding an "ate" ending. Thus lactic acid becomes lactate and pyruvic acid becomes pyruvate.

A cell must use another pathway to get the remaining energy from those molecules to form more ATP: it must use the citric acid cycle. Before the citric acid cycle can begin, however, pyruvate must lose a carbon dioxide group to form acetyl-CoA. As pyruvate turns into acetyl-CoA, another NADH molecule is produced, and in turn another three potential ATP molecules are produced. The conversion of pyruvate requires the vitamin thiamin. Carbohydrates in the diet increase thiamin needs. Now you know why.

Acetyl-CoA is basically the 2-carbon compound acetic acid, which gives the bite to vinegar. Attached to it is a large coenzyme A (CoA) molecule. CoA contains the vitamin pantothenic acid. The CoA molecule activates acetic acid similarly to the way a phosphate group activates glucose. Without a CoA molecule attached, acetic acid will not participate in the first reaction of the citric acid cycle.

Concept Check

Carbohydrate metabolism begins when a cell either forms glucose from glycogen or takes glucose from the bloodstream. Glucose is then degraded through a sequence of steps into two pyruvate molecules. The pathway, called glycolysis, yields NADH, a potential form of energy, and ATP, an actual energy source for a cell. Both fructose and galactose can also be metabolized via glycolysis to pyruvate molecules. Pyruvate then is broken down further or is converted into lactate. The conversion to lactate allows the cell to reform NADH back into NAD. This supports the needs for NAD by glycolysis. NADH can also be turned into NAD via oxygen-requiring pathways found in most cells.

The citric acid cycle

The citric acid cycle is an elegant sequence that cells use to convert carbon atoms into carbon dioxide. Acetyl-CoA adds two carbon atoms, and then two car-

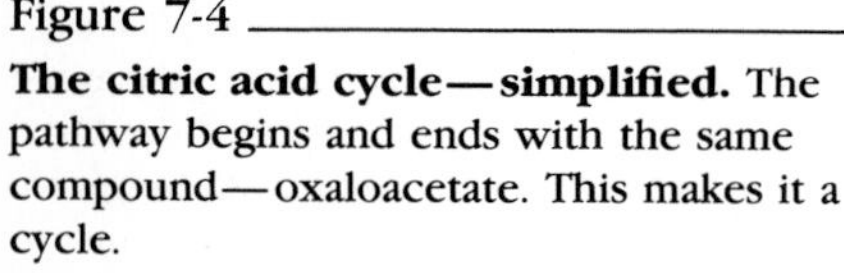

Figure 7-4

The citric acid cycle—simplified. The pathway begins and ends with the same compound—oxaloacetate. This makes it a cycle.

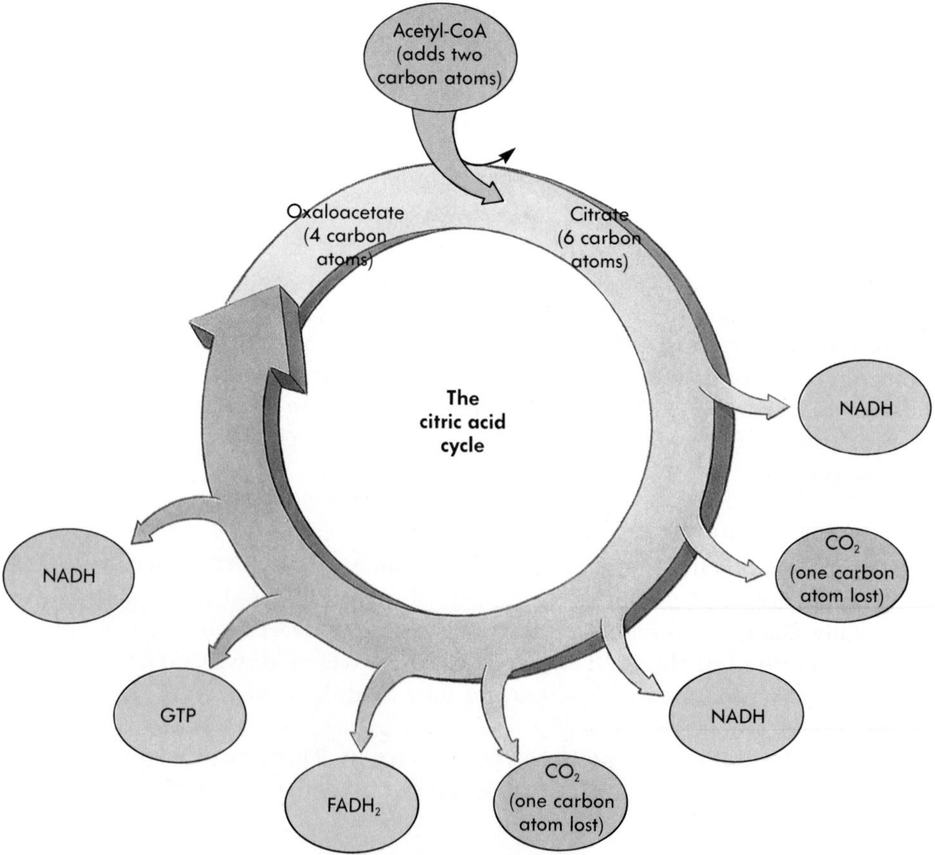

bon atoms are lost as carbon dioxide. In the process, the cell makes more NADH and other related molecules, which can eventually yield 12 more ATP molecules per acetyl-CoA molecule.

Other names of the citric acid cycle are the tricarboxyalic acid cycle (TCA cycle) and the Krebs cycle, named after Hans Krebs, the scientist who described it.

To begin the citric acid cycle, acetyl-CoA combines with a 4-carbon compound (oxaloacetic acid, or oxaloacetate) to form a 6-carbon compound (citric acid, or citrate) (Figure 7-4). The CoA molecule is released. Recall that the portion of acetyl-CoA that interests us, the acetic acid, had two carbon atoms. *The basic function now of the citric acid cycle is to take this 6-carbon citrate molecule and turn it back into a 4-carbon oxaloacetate molecule.* In the process, two carbon dioxide molecules are lost. More important, however, the process also produces potential ATP in the form of NADH and other compounds.

Overall, the citric acid cycle begins and ends with the same compound, oxaloacetate. The pathway adds two carbon atoms as acetic acid to oxaloacetate. As the citric acid cycle reactions occur, two carbon atoms from carbon dioxide are lost, and the process ends up where it started. As citrate is turned back into oxaloacetate, three more NADH molecules are formed. Another hydrogen carrier, **flavin adenine dinucleotide** (FAD), forms $FADH_2$. FAD contains the vitamin riboflavin. Finally, guanosine triphosphate (GTP, which is analogous to ATP) is made from GDP and Pi. In all, one acetyl-CoA molecule yields three NADH molecules, one $FADH_2$ molecule, and one ATP-like molecule.

GTP can be used to synthesize ATP.

Converting citrate back into oxaloacetate requires a variety of reactions in this citric acid cycle. *However, the important thing to remember is that two carbon atoms enter the citric acid cycle as acetyl-CoA, and two carbon atoms are then lost as carbon dioxide.* These steps ensure that the beginning and ending compounds are the same: oxaloacetate.

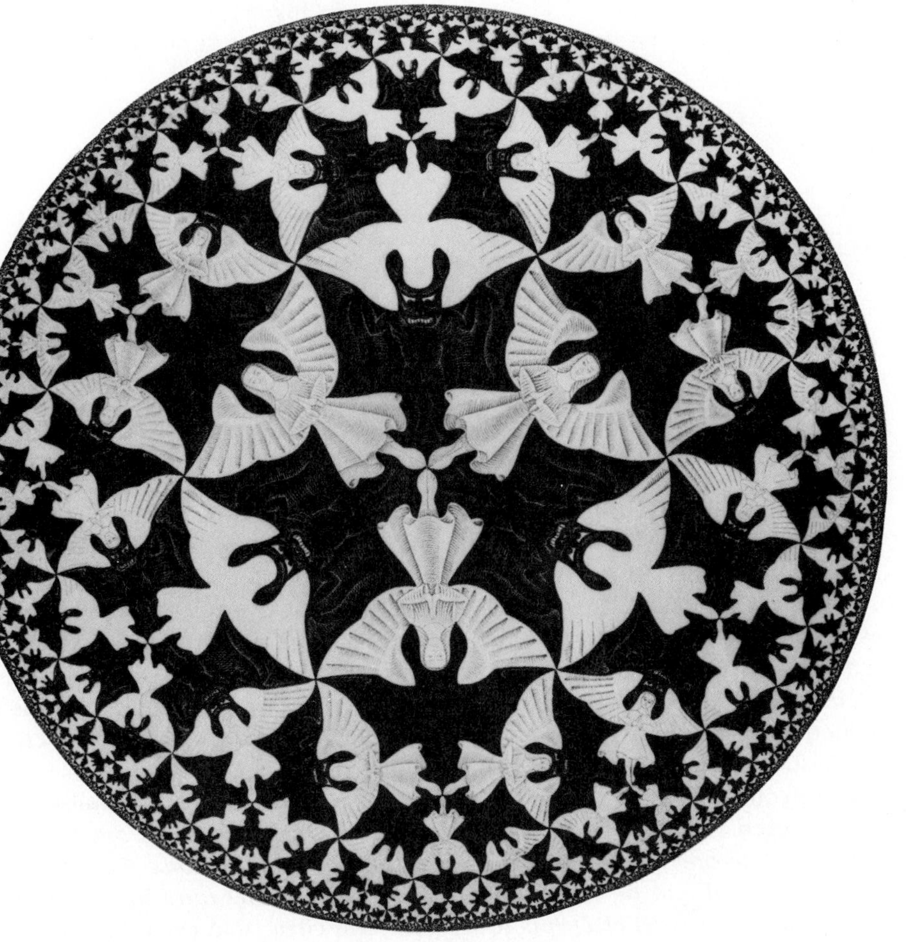

Figure 7-5

M.C. Escher. Circle Limit IV. 1960 (woodcut in two colors)

Exploring Issues and Actions

At first glance the citric acid cycle can be a stumbling block. To see it clearly requires time, effort, and some concentrated thinking and studying. The pathway is like the drawings of MC Escher: at first you see only the angels, not the devils. You look and look at the work until suddenly it is clear to you. The devils are now staring you in the face, and you wonder why you could not see them before. You may find that your perception of the citric acid cycle, and metabolism in general, works the same way.

To review: we started with glucose, stopped a while at pyruvate, detoured through acetyl-CoA, and ended up with carbon dioxide. We have taken all the carbon atoms in glucose and turned them into carbon dioxide. The carbon dioxide eventually leaves through the lungs. In the process, we have made three ATP molecules directly using both glycolysis and the citric acid cycle, as well as NADH molecules and $FADH_2$ molecules. These latter molecules can be "cashed in" for ATP—two or three each for NADH and two for each $FADH_2$—in the electron transport chain, which we discuss below.

We accomplished what we started out to do: we took the energy in the chemical bonds of glucose and turned it into ATP. In doing that, we converted the energy in foodstuffs into a form cells can use rather than just into heat, as would have happened if we had burned the food with a match. *In engineering terms, we captured about 40% of the chemical energy in glucose and stored it in a useful form for later use.* This same ratio applies for energy metabolism of fatty acids and amino acids. That's fairly efficient when you consider that an automobile engine captures only about 10% of the chemical energy in gasoline.

ELECTRON TRANSPORT CHAIN

electron transport chain
A series of reactions using oxygen that converts NADH and $FADH_2$ molecules into free NAD and FAD molecules, yielding water and ATP.

By putting protein, carbohydrate, fat, and alcohol through the citric acid cycle and/or glycolysis, cells generate NADH and $FADH_2$. Most cells can "cash in" these compounds for ATP. The pathway that performs this exchange is called the **electron transport chain.** The process is called oxidative phosphorylation (Figure 7-6). Both iron and copper are needed for this process.

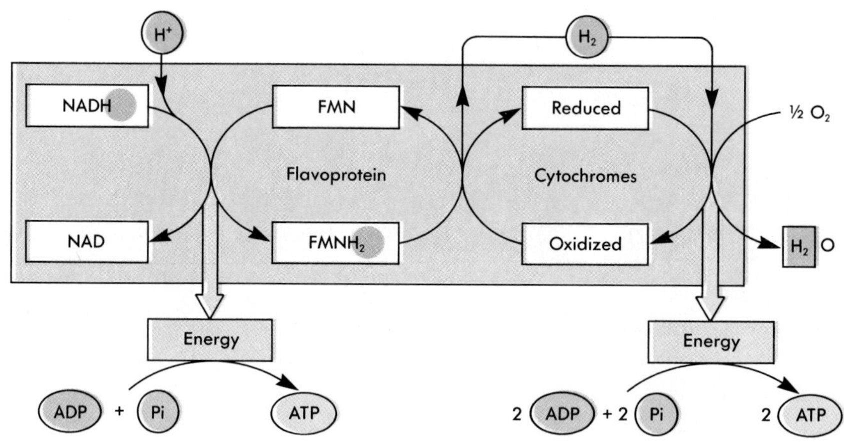

Figure 7-6
Electron-transport chain. NADH and $FADH_2$ transfer their electrons to electron carriers located on a mitochondrial membrane. The energy in the electrons is used to generate ATPs. The electrons and hydrogen ions combine with oxygen to form water.

Basically, in the electron transport chain NADH donates its chemical energy to an FAD derivative, called flavin mononucleotide (FMN). As the high-energy NADH becomes the low-energy NAD form, the reaction liberates some energy to form one ATP molecule and to yield $FMNH_2$ as well. The $FMNH_2$, through a series of steps that uses other electron carriers called **cytochromes,** donates its chemical energy to oxygen. Water, two more ATP molecules, and a free FMN molecule are formed. Thus the net result of the electron transport chain is the production of ATP and water. Although we can describe this process, there are still questions about how it works.

cytochromes
Electron-accepting compounds that participate in the electron transport chain.

aerobic
Requiring oxygen.

The electron transport chain represents the **aerobic** side of metabolism, since it uses oxygen. *Although oxygen does not participate directly in the citric acid cycle, the cycle operates only under aerobic conditions because the NADH and $FADH_2$ produced can be regenerated into NAD and FAD only by the eventual transfer of their stored electrons to oxygen.* The citric acid cycle has no way to

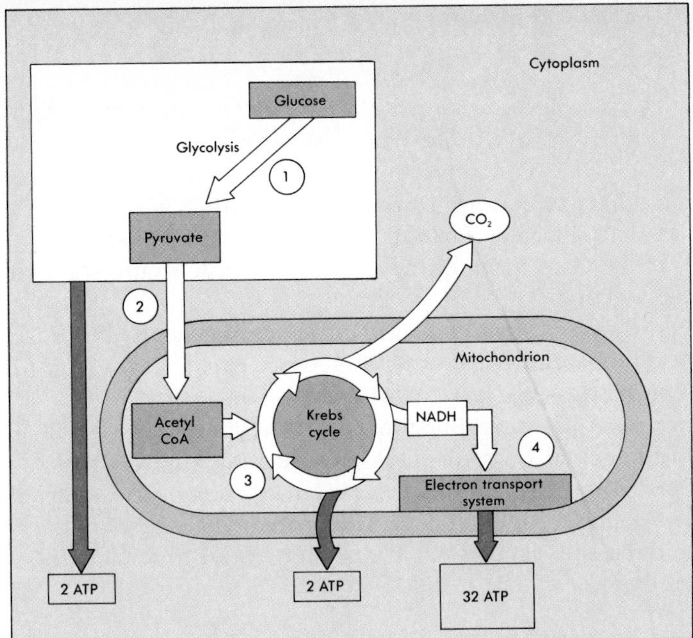

Figure 7-7

An overview of glucose metabolism. The citric acid cycle and the electron transport chain are located within the mitochondria, and glycolysis occurs in the cytoplasm. In glycolysis, each glucose molecule is broken down into two molecules of pyruvate. These enter a mitochondrion and, in turn, the citric acid cycle. All three carbon atoms of pyruvate eventually yield three carbon dioxide molecules. Chemical energy produced by the citric acid cycle is then transferred to the electron transport chain, which is located in a membranes of the mitochondrion. Most of the ATP that results from glucose metabolism is formed at this stage.

recycle NADH and $FADH_2$ analogously to the way that anaerobic glycolysis uses lactate: oxygen is a necessity.

You already knew that two by-products of cell metabolism are carbon dioxide and water. You now know where the carbon dioxide and water come from. The carbon dioxide comes from the citric acid cycle, and the water comes from the electron transport chain (Figure 7-7). In this metabolism, energy is produced in the forms of heat and ATP. That is the essence of metabolism. Cells need to release and then trap as much energy bound in foods as possible, and in a useful form. The body cannot afford to lose all energy as heat. *Some heat is necessary for warming the body, but the body also needs mobilizing energy.* Glycolysis, the citric acid cycle, and the electron transport chain accomplish many things. The greatest feat of these processes, however, is that they enable cells to capture the chemical energy in food as ATP energy. ATP energy then acts as the cellular energy currency. In effect, it allows cells to get up and do what needs to be done.

Glycogen metabolism

Glycogen synthesis uses a form of glucose to eventually add more glucose molecules to an existing glycogen molecule. This allows liver and muscle cells to store glucose for future needs. Later, when glucose is needed, glycogen breakdown yields glucose as glucose-1-phosphate. This then turns into glucose-6-phosphate to begin glycolysis. An enzyme in glycogen breakdown uses a form of vitamin B-6.

Concept Check

In the citric acid cycle the 2-carbon acetate molecule (in the form of acetyl-CoA) reacts with a 4-carbon compound (oxaloacetate) to form a 6-carbon compound (citrate). The cycle then, through numerous reactions, causes citrate to lose two carbon dioxide molecules, eventually yielding oxaloacetate, the starting material. This oxaloacetate molecule can then combine with another acetyl-CoA molecule to begin the process again. The NADH and $FADH_2$ molecules produced in the citric acid cycle donate their electrons and hydrogen atoms to the electron transport chain, yielding free NAD and FAD molecules, water, and numerous ATP molecules.

FAT METABOLISM

Lipolysis: fat breakdown

Lipolysis is the splitting—breakdown—of fat (lipid). It includes the breakdown of triglycerides into free fatty acids and glycerol and the further breakdown of the fatty acids for energy production. Almost all fatty acids in nature are composed of an even number of carbon atoms, usually 16 or 18 carbon atoms. *The*

lipolysis
The breakdown of lipids.

beta-oxidation
The breakdown of a fatty acid into numerous acetyl-CoA molecules.

first step in converting the energy in a fatty acid into ATP energy is to clip off all carbon atoms, two at a time, from the fatty acid. These 2-carbon clips form acetyl-CoA. The process of converting a free fatty acid into many acetyl-CoA molecules is called **beta-oxidation.** During beta-oxidation, NADH and $FADH_2$ are produced. So, as with glucose, a fatty acid is eventually degraded into the 2-carbon compound, acetyl-CoA. Some of the chemical energy is also trapped, in this case as NADH and $FADH_2$.

The acetyl-CoA will now enter the citric acid cycle and be broken down into carbon dioxide molecules, just as with glucose. *Thus glucose and fatty acids use a common pathway—the citric acid cycle.*

No matter how many carbon atoms a fatty acid contains, it will always be broken down into acetyl-CoA molecules. Occasionally a fatty acid has an odd number of carbon atoms. Then the cell forms many acetyl-CoA molecules, plus one 3-carbon compound, propionyl-CoA. The propionyl-CoA enters the citric acid cycle directly, bypassing acetyl-CoA. It can then go on to form carbon dioxide and other products.

Why fats burn in a "fire of carbohydrate"

In addition to its role in energy production, the citric acid cycle provides compounds that leave the pathway and enter biosynthetic pathways, such as those used to make the red blood cell protein hemoglobin. This means that even though oxaloacetate is reused in the cycle, a minimum level of it must be constantly replaced because the compounds removed from the citric acid cycle for biosynthetic reactions prevent the complete cycle back to oxaloacetate. The source of this additional oxaloacetate is pyruvate, a carbohydrate. *So as fatty acids create acetyl-CoA, they actually burn in a fire of carbohydrates: the carbohydrate is necessary to keep the concentration of oxaloacetate high in the citric acid cycle so that acetyl-CoA can enter the cycle.*[10]

Ketogenesis: producing ketones

ketone bodies
Products of acetyl-CoA metabolism containing three to four carbon atoms: acetoacetic acid, beta-hydroxybutyric acid, and acetone.

Ketone bodies—also called ketones—are normally produced in small quantities and then quickly metabolized for energy. *The production of large numbers of ketone bodies begins when excessive fatty acids flood the bloodstream, allowing acetyl-CoA molecules to overwhelm the liver's ability to metabolize them into carbon dioxide.*[8] The flood of fatty acids occurs when there is inadequate insulin production by the pancreas or an insufficient amount of dietary carbohydrate (see below and Chapter 4). The liver picks up the fatty acids and degrades them into acetyl-CoA. Then it joins two acetyl-CoA molecules together to form the 4-carbon compound acetoacetyl-CoA. This compound is further metabolized and eventually secreted into the bloodstream as the ketone acetoacetic acid. Before leaving the liver, acetoacetic acid may react with NADH to form the ketone beta-hydroxybutyric acid. In addition, acetoacetic acid may lose a carbon dioxide molecule and form the ketone acetone.

Cells pick up the first two types of ketones, acetoacetic acid and beta-hydroxybutyric acid, and turn them back into acetyl-CoA. These molecules are then pushed through the citric acid cycle to form ATP. Much of the acetone leaves via the lungs, giving the person in ketosis a characteristic "fruity" breath.

Ketosis in fasting. When a person fasts, liver cells must use much oxaloacetate to produce a glucose supply for the brain, red blood cells, and part of the kidney (see Chapter 4). Oxaloacetate is then generally unavailable in the liver cells for reacting with acetyl-CoA in the citric acid cycle. This scarcity of oxaloacetate—found in people in states of semi-starvation and with low carbohydrate diets—diverts acetyl-CoA from the citric acid cycle to form ketone bodies. Heart muscle and some parts of the kidney must then turn to ketone bodies for fuel. Given a few days, the brain also begins to metabolize ketones for energy.

Ketosis in diabetes can be harmful. The main problem in insulin-dependent forms of diabetes mellitus is that not enough insulin is produced to allow for normal fat metabolism in adipose cells. Without sufficient insulin, fatty acids flood out of the adipose cells, leading to an excess of free fatty acids in the bloodstream. Consequently metabolizing the fatty acids burdens the liver. The resulting buildup of acetyl-CoA molecules then stimulates ketone production. If the level of ketone bodies rises too high in the bloodstream, the excess pours into the urine, pulling sodium and potassium ions with it. Eventually it causes ion imbalances to mount in the body. The problem usually occurs only in ketosis due to diabetes mellitus; in fasting blood ketone levels usually do not rise high enough.

Lipogenesis: building fatty acids

Lipogenesis is the formation of fat (lipid). Ingested glucose or protein that the body does not use immediately is mostly stored as triglyceride. Some carbohydrate is stored as glycogen, but that amounts to only about 350 grams in the body. Some protein is stored in amino acid pools in the body, but that also does not amount to much (Figure 6-2). When a lot of glucose and amino acid molecules are left over from a large meal, most of their carbon atoms are used to synthesize triglyceride. This process requires ATP and the vitamins biotin, niacin, and pantothenic acid.

lipogenesis
The building of fatty acids using derivatives of acetyl-CoA molecules.

The major lipogenic (fat-making) organ in the body is the liver. In it, carbon atoms from glucose and carbon skeletons of amino acids become acetyl-CoA. Cells in the liver in effect bond the acetate parts of acetyl-CoA molecules together in a series of steps to eventually form a 16-carbon saturated fatty acid, palmitic acid. This 16-carbon fatty acid can later be lengthened to an 18- or 20-carbon atom chain. The fatty acids are then joined (esterified) to a form of glycerol (produced during glycolysis) to yield a triglyceride. That is later released as a very low density lipoprotein, or VLDL (see Chapter 5). Cells then use the synthesized fat for energy production, or it is stored in adipose cells along with fats from excess dietary fat intake.

Exploring Issues and Actions

You notice that one of your friends is trying to lose weight by cutting out all carbohydrates. You also know that if she doesn't eat enough carbohydrates, she may go into ketosis. Can you explain to her how this will change metabolism in her body?

Concept Check

Fatty acids are degraded into numerous acetyl-CoA molecules. These molecules participate in the citric acid cycle and electron transport chain to eventually yield carbon dioxide, water, and much ATP. To synthesize fat, a cell binds numerous acetate molecules (donated by a derivative of acetyl-CoA) together to form a fatty acid. Three fatty acids can then react with a form of glycerol to yield a triglyceride. If liver cells are overwhelmed with acetyl-CoA molecules, such as in cases of uncontrolled diabetes mellitus, acetyl-CoA forms into ketone bodies. These ketone bodies enter the bloodstream and are eventually metabolized to carbon dioxide and water (after being converted back into acetyl-CoA) by various body cells.

PROTEIN METABOLISM

Protein metabolism begins after proteins are degraded into amino acids. Then, to burn an amino acid for fuel, cells first split off the amine group ($-NH_2$) in a process called deamination. This often requires a form of vitamin B-6. Deamination leaves a carbon skeleton, which can usually directly enter the citric acid cycle. However, some carbon skeletons must enter the pathway at acetyl-CoA (Figure 7-8). In addition, often a cell must first metabolize the carbon skeleton into another compound or compounds before the parts can enter the citric acid cycle. So different parts of an amino acid carbon skeleton may enter at various points in the pathway. Any part of the carbon skeleton that can bypass acetyl-CoA and enter the citric acid cycle directly can eventually become part of glucose. You'll see how shortly.

Carbon skeletons of amino acids that enter directly into the citric acid cycle or become pyruvate are called glucogenic amino acids. This indicates that these carbon atoms can become the carbon atoms of glucose. Any parts of carbon skeletons that become acetyl-CoA are called ketogenic because these atoms cannot become parts of glucose molecules.

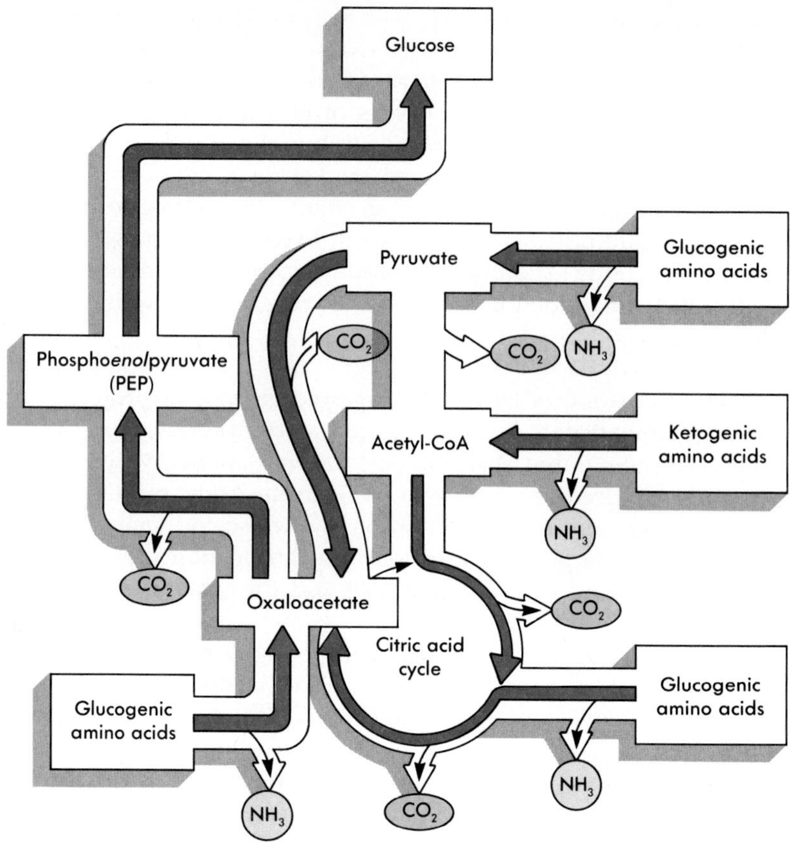

Figure 7-8

Gluconeogenesis. Glucogenic amino acids can yield net glucose while ketogenic amino acids cannot. The deciding factor is whether the amino acid yields a *new* oxaloacetate molecule during metabolism.

Gluconeogensis
The formation of new glucose molecules, primarily using carbon atoms from amino acids.

Gluconeogenesis: producing new glucose molecules

The starting material for gluconeogenesis is oxaloacetate, which is derived primarily from the carbon skeletons of some amino acids. The entire gluconeogenesis pathway is present only in liver cells and some kidney cells. ***The 4-carbon oxaloacetate loses a carbon dioxide molecule and converts to the 3-carbon compound. This then basically reverses the path back through glycolysis to form glucose*** (Figure 7-8). Some steps in gluconeogenesis are simply a reversal of glycolysis reactions, but others are variations of glycolysis. This entire process requires ATP, as well as forms of the vitamins biotin, riboflavin, niacin, and B-6.

Let's trace the path of gluconeogenesis by converting glutamic acid, an amino acid, into glucose. Glutamic acid is first deaminated to form its carbon skeleton. This enters the citric acid cycle directly and is converted by stages into oxaloacetate. Oxaloacetate loses a carbon dioxide molecule and then reverses through glycolysis to form glucose. Since a 3-carbon compound is used, a cell actually needs two of them to form a 6-carbon glucose molecule. So a cell needs two glutamic acid molecules to eventually form one glucose molecule.[6]

Recall from Chapter 4 that if there is an insufficient amount of carbohydrate in your body, the liver and kidneys are forced to make it from body protein to support the energy needs of your brain and red blood cells. We have just described one way that can happen. Liver and kidney cells start with carbon skeletons of some amino acids that can directly enter the citric acid cycle. These are converted to oxaloacetate, then to a 3-carbon compound, and finally to glucose. Over many weeks, the need for constant gluconeogenesis wastes away body protein. This in turn severely compromises health and eventually contributes to death if carried on long enough, usually about 50 to 60 days of total fasting (see Chapter 9 for further details).

Can we have gluconeogenesis from fatty acids?

Let's try to turn a fatty acid into glucose. A fatty acid breaks down into many acetyl-CoA molecules. *The step between pyruvate and acetyl-CoA is irreversible. Acetyl-CoA can never reform into pyruvate once the carbon dioxide molecule is lost.* The only option for acetyl-CoA, besides forming fatty acids or ketones, is to combine with oxaloacetate in the citric acid cycle. However, two carbon atoms of acetyl-CoA are added at the beginning of the citric acid cycle, and two carbon atoms are subsequently lost when citrate converts back to the starting material, oxaloacetate. So when we arrive at oxaloacetate, no carbon atoms are left to turn into glucose.

A cell could take the oxaloacetate out of the citric acid cycle and turn it into glucose, but then the citric acid cycle would not function. There would be no oxaloacetate left to react with new acetyl-CoA molecules. What the cell would have to do then is to take a pyruvate molecule and add a carbon dioxide molecule to it to form a new oxaloacetate molecule. Cells can do that, but overall it is futile. There is no reason to take an oxaloacetate molecule out of the pathway to make glucose, and then use a glucose derivative, pyruvate, to make a new oxaloacetate molecule.

Trying to convert fatty acids into glucose is pointless: it cannot be done. The only part of a triglyceride that can become glucose is the glycerol portion and any propionyl-CoA that is formed from odd-chain fatty acids. Glycerol enters into the glycolosis pathway, and propionyl-CoA directly enters the citric acid cycle. Both then can flow backward through the citric acid cycle and through the process of gluconeogenesis to convert to glucose. Neither of these compounds yields much glucose, since we form little propionyl-CoA, and only about 10% of a triglyceride is glycerol.

Some plants have a metabolic pathway that allows them to convert fatty acids into glucose, known as the glyoxalate pathway.

Disposing of excess amine groups

The breakdown of amino acids yields amine groups ($-NH_2$) that then form ammonia (NH_3). The ammonia must be excreted because its buildup is toxic for cells. The liver prepares the amines for excretion in the urea cycle. During the urea cycle, two ammonia groups react through a series of steps with carbon dioxide molecules to form urea ($H_2N\text{-}\underset{\underset{O}{\|}}{C}\text{-}NH_2$) and water. Urea is then excreted in the urine.

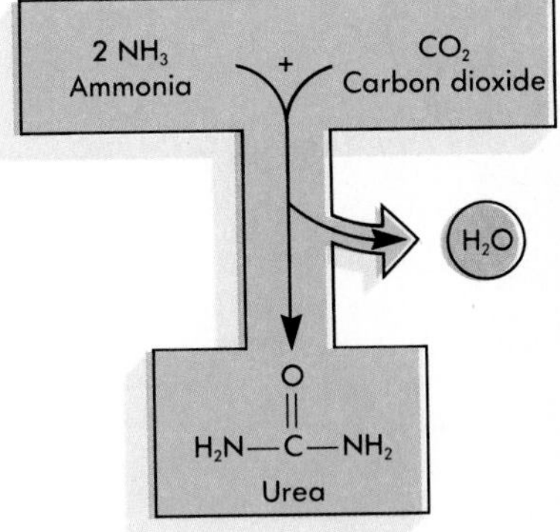

Concept Check

In the process of losing an amine group, individual amino acids form carbon skeletons. Many carbon skeletons can be further metabolized so that they enter either the citric acid cycle or glycolysis. If so, the carbon atoms can be pushed through gluconeogenesis to ultimately form new glucose molecules. If the carbon skeleton enters metabolism at acetyl-CoA, glucose production is not possible.

WHAT HAPPENS WHERE

Glycolysis takes place in the cytosol (Figure 7-1). Pyruvate then enters the mitochondria, where the citric acid cycle and electron transport chain occur. The NADH made in the cytosol from glycolysis must be shuttled into the mitochondria so that the electron transport chain can be used to convert NADH back into

For a final accounting, the ultimate production of ATP from glucose is 6 to 8 ATP molecules from glycolysis and 30 ATP molecules from the citric acid cycle. For a 16-carbon fatty acid, 35 ATP molecules are generated from beta-oxidation (to acetyl-CoA) and 96 ATP molecules are generated after all the acetyl-CoA molecules enter the citric acid cycle (with use of the electron transport chain).

NAD and produce ATP. Shuttle systems in some cells use no energy, but one shuttle system in some cells—the alpha glycerol phosphate shuttle—uses one ATP molecule per NADH molecule. In those cases, NADH yields only two net ATP molecules instead of three, since one is used by the shuttle system. Thus glucose may yield either 36 or 38 ATP molecules, depending on how each of two NADH molecules produced by glycolysis in the cytosol enter the mitochondria.

Beta-oxidation for the breakdown of fatty acids also occurs inside the mitochondria. Fatty acids have to be shuttled from the cytosol into the mitochondria, using a compound called **carnitine.** Athletes sometimes take carnitine pills hoping it will help them burn fat faster in exercise. But since our cells can make carnitine, the bother seems hardly worth it. Dr. David Lamb discusses this in his Expert Opinion section. The product of beta-oxidation, acetyl-CoA, is then metabolized by the citric acid cycle in the mitochondria. Fatty acids are synthesized in the cytosol.

carnitine
A compound used to shuttle fatty acids from the cytosol of the cell into mitochondria (see Chapter 12).

Gluconeogenesis begins in the mitochondria with the production of oxaloacetate. It eventually finishes in the cytosol with the production of glucose. The same is true for the urea cycle: some stages occur in the cytosol and some in the mitochondria.

Since the citric acid cycle produces most of the ATP for the cell, the mitochondria are the major energy-producing organelles in the cell. Cells that need to make a lot of ATP, such as muscle cells, have thousands of mitochondria. Cells that need very little ATP, such as adipose cells, have fewer mitochondria.

MUSCLE METABOLISM

The relationship between the citric acid cycle and glycolysis is quite special in the muscle cell. Muscle cells at rest burn primarily fat. Fat breaks down into acetyl-CoA, which enters the citric acid cycle to form carbon dioxide and eventually yield ATP. While the muscle cell is busy making ATP from fat, it cannot readily make ATP from glucose. That is because the high ATP and citrate concentrations in the cell inhibit the major enzyme in glycolysis, phosphofructokinase (PFK). Thus muscles at rest primarily burn fat.

See Chapter 4 for discussion of carbohydrate-loading to enhance glycogen storage for endurance exercise.

When someone exercises hard, fat metabolism may not keep up with the ATP demand of the cell. In that case, the ATP concentration in the cell drops, and the ADP concentration in the cell increases. The lower ATP concentration then allows the enzyme PFK to speed up, increasing the rate of glycolysis. Glycogen in the muscle eventually breaks down into glucose-6-phosphate, and in turn enters glycolysis to form pyruvate.

Much of the pyruvate, however, cannot become acetyl-CoA because the citric acid cycle is already busy metabolizing the acetyl-CoA from fat. In addition, partly because of insufficient oxygen in the muscle cells, some NADH formed in glycolysis cannot be handled by the oxygen-requiring electron transport chain. Besides that, the breakdown of pyruvate is inhibited by acetyl-CoA, NADH, and GTP—all products of fat breakdown. All these conditions force the pyruvate molecules to pick up NADH molecules and hydrogen ions to make lactate molecules. This then regenerates NAD for further glycolysis. The lactate molecules spill into the bloodstream (Figure 7-3). Cells in the heart and liver then pick these up and use them for fuel or convert them to other substances.

When you perform intense muscular exercise, such as running a 100-meter dash, the lactate level in both the bloodstream and muscles increases. Lactate in a muscle is a major cause of fatigue but it also has some value. Lactate must be produced to reduce the high NADH concentration caused by glycolysis so an ample NAD concentration can support further glycolysis.

If you start exercising regularly four or five times a week, you will experience a "training effect." At the start maybe you can exercise for 20 minutes before you tire. A month later you may be able to exercise an hour before you feel tired. During that month your muscle cells have produced more mitochondria.[5] They can now burn more fat and recycle NADH more rapidly. That means you will produce less lactate during exercise. Since lactate contributes to fatigue, you have now delayed the onset of fatigue and so extended your exercise capacity. Part of the training effect is also due to increased efficiency of the lungs and heart in supplying oxygen to muscles. Muscle fibers also enlarge and get stronger. However, *when you consider only metabolism, a very important result of training is the increase in the number of mitochondria in the muscle cells.*

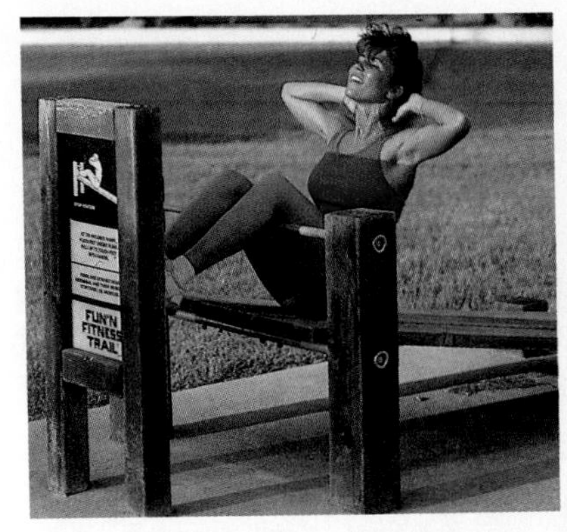

Regular exercise will allow your muscles to metabolize fat much more effeciently.

Putting it all together

By stringing together the glycolysis pathway and the citric acid cycle, cells can convert carbohydrates into fatty acids, convert carbohydrates into carbon skeletons for nonessential amino acids, and process carbohydrates to yield ATP energy (Figure 7-9). These pathways can also turn carbon skeletons from one amino acid into carbon skeletons for other amino acids. Furthermore, they can either convert carbon skeletons from amino acids to glucose or have them yield ATP energy. Finally, fatty acids can yield ATP energy or ketones, and the glycerol part of the triglyceride can either be converted into glucose or yield ATP energy. *"Feasting" encourages glycogen synthesis and fat synthesis. "Fasting" encourages fat breakdown, protein breakdown, gluconeogenesis, and ketone production.*

In all, acetyl-CoA plays a central role in energy metabolism. No matter what type of diet you eat—high-carbohydrate, high-protein, or high-fat—all energy metabolism passes through the acetyl-CoA stage. It is the common denominator that links all human diets (Figure 7-10).[10]

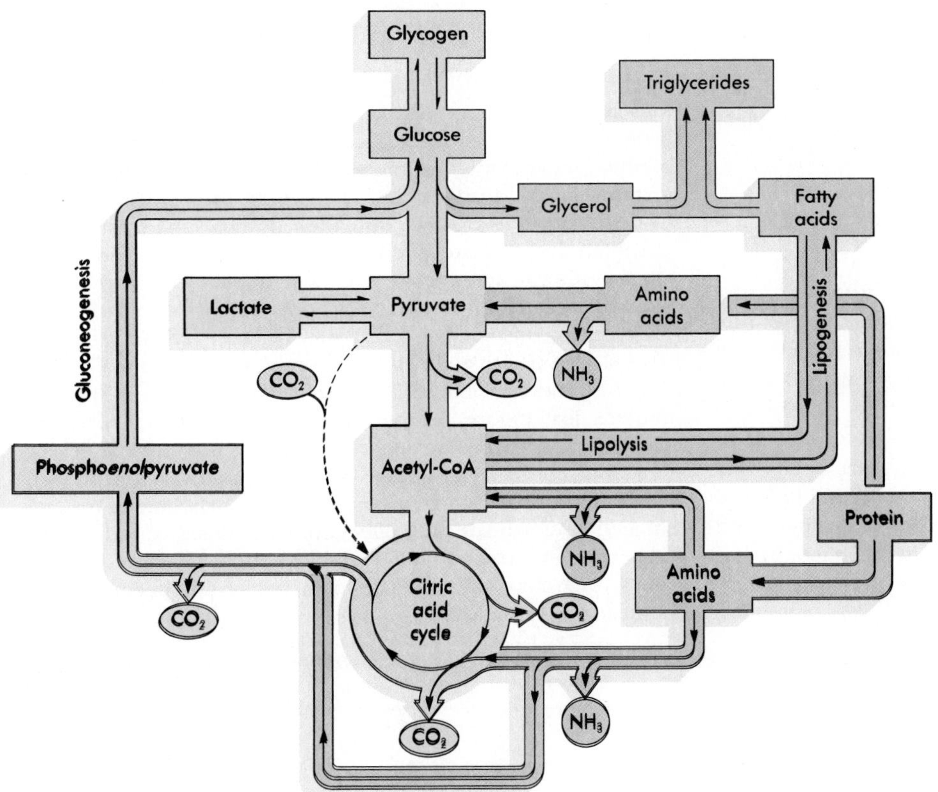

Figure 7-9

Cell metabolism—a bird's eye view. Note how acetyl-CoA forms a crossroads for many pathways. The citric acid cycle can also be used to help build compounds, such as amino acids.

Expert Opinion

Can Dietary Substances Enhance Athletic Performance?

DAVID R. LAMB, Ph.D.

Manipulation of the diet in hopes of enhancing athletic performance has a long and checkered history. As late as 30 years ago, American football players were encouraged on hot practice days to get "toughened up" for competition by liberally consuming salt tablets before and during practice and by not drinking water; it is now widely recognized that this practice can be fatal. Contemporary athletes are at least as likely as their ancestors to experiment with bee pollen, seaweed, freeze-dried liver flakes, artichoke hearts, and other untested ingestible "ergogenic" (work-producing) aids. However, these modern-day athletes can take advantage of rather recently documented scientific evidence that some dietary substances do have ergogenic properties, at least in some athletes in certain situations.

WATER AND PERFORMANCE

Athletes can lose more than 2 liters of sweat per hour during prolonged exercise in hot environments. If this fluid loss is not replaced, the resulting dehydration reduces blood volume, increases heart rate, raises body temperature, and impairs athletic performance. Muscle cramps, circulatory collapse, delirium, and life-threatening heat stroke are potential outcomes of serious dehydration. Numerous investigations have demonstrated that the consumption of water or other fluids before and during prolonged exercise can minimize these physiological problems and dramatically enhance performance. Because the sensation of thirst in human beings is quickly depressed by drinking even small amounts of water athletes must be repeatedly encouraged to drink to replace body weight losses (sweat) during practice and competition.

CARBOHYDRATES AND PERFORMANCE

Carbohydrate is an indispensable fuel for essentially all types of athletic performance because the energy demand in athletics exceeds the maximal rate of energy supply from fat or protein stores. There is ample evidence from muscle biopsy studies that carbohydrate (glycogen) depletion in muscle is a cause of fatigue in exercise that lasts longer than 60 to 90 minutes. It is probable, although not conclusively proven, that glycogen depletion in a small fraction of highly recruited muscle fibers also contributes to diminished performance in brief, high-intensity competition. Furthermore, a reduction in blood glucose during prolonged exercise has been associated with early fatigue. It is not surprising that dietary carbohydrate has been manipulated before and during exercise in hopes of improving athletic performance.

Carbohydrates during competition.
The emptying of ingested beverages from the stomach into the intestine is progressively slower for increasing concentrations of sugars in the beverages. A 2.5% glucose solution, for example, empties from the stomach about as fast as water, but most of a 40% glucose solution remains in the stomach for 1 hour or more before being emptied into the intestine, where the fluid is absorbed into the bloodstream. Consequently it is often claimed that carbohydrate solutions in concentrations greater than 2.5% are poor rehydrating agents that should not be consumed during prolonged exercise. The truth is that beverages containing approximately 5% to 8% carbohydrates (sucrose, glucose, and glucose polymers are equally effective) maintain cardiovascular function and body temperature regulation as well as water. Moreover, endurance performance is usually improved by the consumption of 150 to 250 milliliters of 5% to 8% carbohydrate solutions every 20 minutes during exercise, whereas flavored water placebos don't improve performance. In endurance athletes, this beneficial effect of carbohydrate ingestion may amount to a 30% improvement in endurance; less well trained athletes can expect a more modest improvement of 5% to 7% in an event lasting more than 45 minutes. Fortuitously, most commercial "sports rehydration drinks" include carbohydrates in the appropriate concentration range. Beverages containing more than 3% to 4% fructose or more than 10% glucose or sucrose tend to cause GI distress and are not well tolerated by most athletes.

BICARBONATE LOADING

Muscles that contract vigorously during athletic performance produce lactic acid. Lactic acid accumulation (reduced pH) inhibits the activity of numerous enzymes involved in energy metabolism and leads to early fatigue. In the 1930s, attempts to neutralize this acid accumulation by ingesting small doses of sodium bicarbonate failed to improve athletic performance. On the other hand, more recent experiments with large doses (300 milligrams per kilogram of body weight) of bicarbonate in capsules consumed 1 or 2 hours before exercise generally have shown positive effects on strenuous performance lasting 2 to 10 minutes. Submaximal exercise (warmup) for 20 to 30 minutes just before the performance trial seems necessary. The bicarbonate-loading apparently speeds the removal of lactate from contracting muscle cells; that is, there is a greater concentration of lactate in the blood of bicarbonate-treated subjects. Unfortunate side effects of large doses of sodium bicarbonate are nausea and diarrhea, often at unpredictable times. Therefore, bicarbonate-loading has not become very popular with athletes.

Carbohydrate-loading.

Carbohydrate-loading is the practice of gradually reducing the duration of athletic training sessions during the week before an important competition while progressively increasing the consumption of dietary carbohydrates. The athlete consumes 20% to 45% of dietary calories as carbohydrate for the first 3 days of the carbohydrate-loading protocol and then 70% to 85% for the 3 or 4 days immediately preceding competition. This procedure is designed to maximize the storage of muscle glycogen before competition, thereby extending the duration of high-level performance before the onset of fatigue. For the average athlete, carbohydrate-loading has been shown in both laboratory and field situations to significantly increase endurance time. Although some persons experience GI discomfort or a feeling of sluggishness with high-carbohydrate diets, most athletes and exercise physiologists vouch for the efficacy and reliability of carbohydrate-loading.

Carbohydrates just before competition.

In the 1970s and most of the 1980s, the conventional scientific wisdom was that the consumption of carbohydrates in the last 3 hours before competition would cause an overproduction of insulin (hyperinsulinemia) that would lower the blood sugar and adversely affect athletic performance. More recent and comprehensive research has shown that for most athletes, a rise in insulin and a transient depression of blood glucose (hypoglycemia) after pre-exercise carbohydrate ingestion does not harm performance—and that such feedings often improve athletic endurance. This is not the case for certain individuals who are particularly sensitive to hyperinsulinemia and hypoglycemia. Thus as with all "ergogenic" aids, practice trials are required to determine whether pre-exercise carbohydrate consumption is suitable for a given athlete.

CAFFEINE AND PERFORMANCE

The consumption of 3 to 4 cups of coffee (or the insertion of caffeine suppositories in the rectum) about 1 hour before a prolonged endurance competition enhances performance in some, but not all, athletes. The mechanisms underlying any improvement in performance—increased mobilization of fatty acids and sparing of muscle glycogen, psychoactive effects, enhancement of glycolysis in muscle—are controversial. Furthermore, some subjects experience cardiac arrythmias, nausea, or lightheadedness that can actually impair performance.

VITAMINS AND MINERALS

Many studies of possible ergogenic effects of vitamin and mineral supplements have been conducted throughout the last 100 years. In general, improved athletic performance as a result of ingesting such supplements occurs only when the subjects are deficient in vitamins and minerals before supplementation begins. In particular, supplements of thiamin and ascorbic acid may benefit performance in vitamin-deficient athletes, and iron supplementation improves performance in those suffering from iron-deficiency anemia (but not in those simply exhibiting low stores of iron in the blood).

SUMMING UP

Although most claims of ergogenic effects for dietary manipulations in athletes are unfounded, the exceptions we've described are based on systematic scientific investigations. This is not to say that there are no other potentially ergogenic substances in the diet, but only that such aids are not scientifically verified.

Dr. Lamb is Professor and Director of the Exercise Physiology Laboratory, School of Health, Physical Education, and Recreation, at Ohio State University.

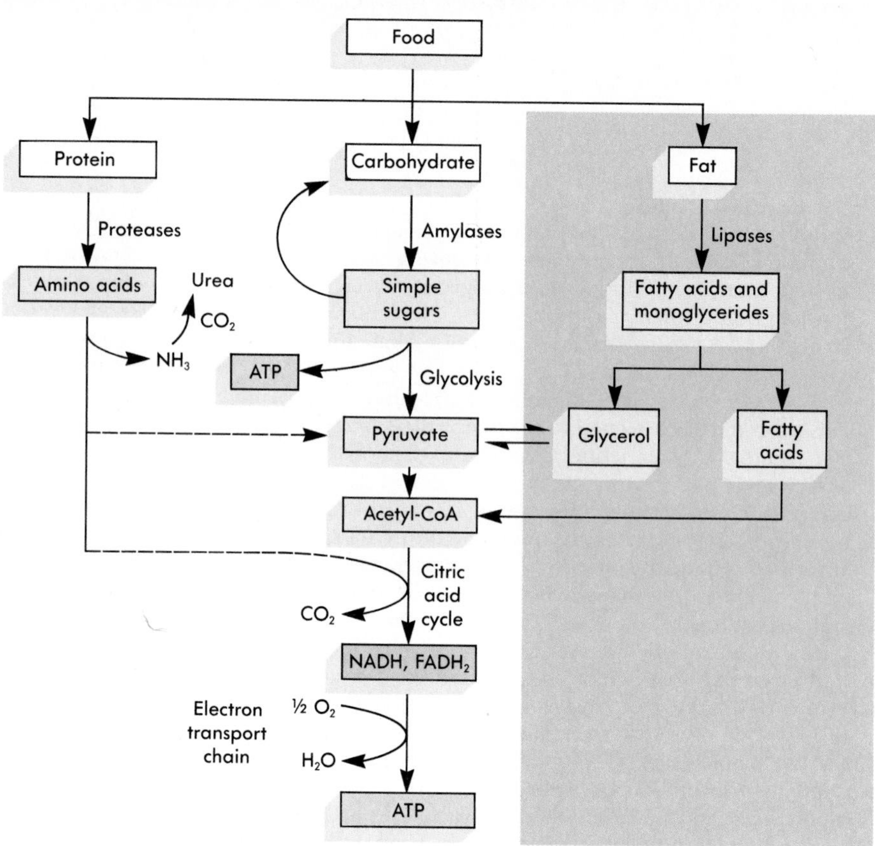

Figure 7-10

The fate of food. In terms of energy production, most food consists of carbohydrate, protein, and/or fat. During digestion, protein is broken down into amino acids, carbohydrate is broken down into single sugars, and fats are primarily broken down to fatty acids and monoglycerides. Various forms of these compounds then eventually enter a common metabolic pathway—the citric acid cycle.

Regulating metabolism

Metabolism is regulated by various means. Enzymes are the key to metabolic pathways: both their presence and rate of activity are critical to reactions and processes along the pathways. Synthesis of enzymes themselves and their activity levels are somewhat controlled by cells and by the products of the reactions in which the enzymes participate. The ATP concentration in the cell likewise serves to regulate metabolism. Generally, high ATP concentrations decrease energy-yielding reactions and promote synthetic reactions, which then use ATP. Another factor in regulating metabolism is the liver: both because it contains such a variety of enzymes, and most nutrients pass through the liver, providing an opportunity for metabolism there (Figure 7-11).

Epilogue

Figure 7-9 summarizes the major pathways we have considered. Don't be surprised if it takes you a little time to grasp it thoroughly. It illustrates a complicated system within which a lot is taking place. Study it part by part. Read this chapter again tomorrow, and maybe again in 2 or 3 days. We are sure that you can understand it if you take enough time.

You now know more about what happens in a cell than most people ever know. Knowledge is power. You can use this power right away to understand how vitamins and minerals function. You have already seen how thiamin, niacin, riboflavin, biotin, pantothenic acid, and vitamin B-6, as well as the minerals magnesium, iron, and copper, play important roles in the metabolic cycles. This introduction sets the stage for chapters 11 through 14. You can also use this knowledge to debunk fad diet claims, such as the touted long-term safety of low-carbo-

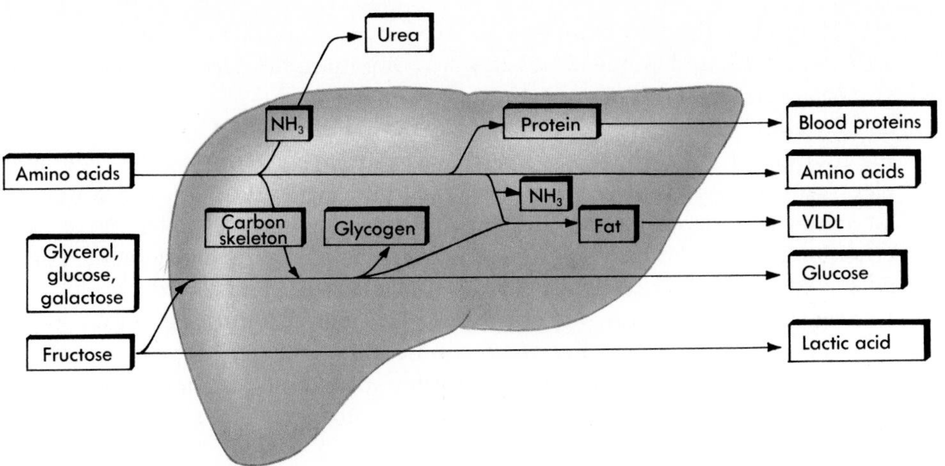

Figure 7-11

The liver is the crossroads for many nutrient interconversions. What leaves the liver is often not what entered it.

hydrate diets. Future classes in nutrition, nursing, biology, physiology, biochemistry, pharmacy, and medicine should also be a little easier, because all of them build on this subject of metabolic pathways.

Concept Check

Glycolysis takes place in the cytosol of the cell; the citric acid cycle and electron transport chain occur in the mitochondria. Fatty acids break down in the mitochondria, and they are synthesized in the cytosol. The urea cycle and gluconeogenesis take place in both parts of the cell. Since many metabolic pathways converge at acetyl-CoA, it represents a central compound in energy metabolism. Regardless of the diet, whether high-protein, high-fat, or high-carbohydrate, the processes used to release the energy from those diets usually include acetyl-CoA.

Summary

1. A cell is the basic unit of structure in the body. Within the cell membrane is a nucleus to direct protein synthesis and cell division, mitochondria to produce usable forms of energy, golgi bodies to package cell products, an endoplasmic reticulum whose various areas are involved in protein and fat synthesis, and storage granules of glycogen and droplets of fat.
2. ATP is the major form of energy for cellular metabolism. As ATP is breaking down into ADP plus Pi, energy is released. This energy is used to pump ions, promote enzyme activity, and contract muscles. All energy available to humans ultimately comes from solar energy. Plants capture solar energy using photosynthesis. Human metabolic pathways are able to extract that energy from foodstuffs and convert it into ATP energy.
3. In glycolysis, glucose is degraded into two pyruvate molecules, yielding NADH (a storage form of energy) and ATP. Pyruvate can then proceed to other metabolic pathways to form carbon dioxide and water or to react with NADH to form lactate. In both pathways, NADH is eventually reformed into NAD, supplying in turn the NAD needed to continue glycolysis.
4. In the citric acid cycle, the acetyl-CoA is formed when a carbon dioxide molecule is lost from pyruvate. Acetyl-CoA is then pushed through many metabolic steps, eventually yielding two more carbon dioxide molecules. In this way the citric acid cycle accepts two carbon atoms from acetyl-CoA and yields two carbon atoms as carbon dioxide. In the process, NADH, $FADH_2$, and a form of energy that can yield ATP directly (GTP) are formed. The

NADH and $FADH_2$ then enter the electron transport chain to yield numerous ATP molecules and water molecules by combining the electrons and hydrogen ions released with oxygen.

5. In fatty acid breakdown, 2-carbon fragments are clipped off a fatty acid, yielding multiple acetyl-CoA molecules. These then use the citric acid cycle and electron transport chain to yield ATP energy, carbon dioxide, and water. In fat synthesis, acetate molecules (in the form of a acetyl-CoA derivative) are combined to yield a fatty acid, primarily the 16-carbon palmitic acid. These fatty acids can then react with a form of glycerol to yield a triglyceride.
6. During starvation and uncontrolled diabetes mellitus, more acetyl-CoA molecules are produced in the liver than can be metabolized in the citric acid cycle. These acetyl-CoA molecules are turned into ketone bodies. Ketone bodies flood into the bloodstream and are metabolized by other tissues after being turned back into acetyl-CoA.
7. Amino acids can lose their amine group to form a carbon skeleton. These skeletons then can be metabolized into compounds that enter the citric acid cycle, eventually yielding energy. Some carbon skeletons can also be formed into oxaloacetate, a compound found in the citric acid cycle, which in turn can be converted to glucose. The process of converting carbon skeletons of amino acids into glucose is part of gluconeogenesis. Acetyl-CoA molecules, and thus fatty acids, cannot participate in gluconeogenesis.
8. Glycolysis occurs in the cytosol of a cell, and the citric acid cycle and electron transport chain occur in the mitochondria. Fatty acid breakdown occurs in the mitochondria, and fatty acids are synthesized in the cytosol. The synthesis of urea and the pathway for gluconeogenesis both take place partly in the cytosol and partly in the mitochondria.
9. Acetyl-CoA is a pivotal player in cell metabolism inasmuch as carbohydrates, proteins, amino acids, and fatty acids all can yield acetyl-CoA. The coordination of various metabolic pathways allows the carbon atoms of glucose to become the carbon atoms of fatty acids and the carbon atoms of amino acids to become the carbon atoms of glucose.
10. Vitamins such as thiamin, niacin, riboflavin, biotin, pantothenic acid, and B-6 and minerals such as magnesium, iron, and copper play important roles in the metabolic cycles.

Take Action

1. Your best friend has entered a marathon race covering 26 miles of rough roads. The race takes place in 2 weeks. She has asked you for nutritional help. Read Nutrition Perspective 7-1 and then design a 1-day menu to follow that will help her maximize her performance.

Breakfast: ______________________________

Snack: ______________________________

Lunch: ______________________________

Snack: ______________________________

Dinner: ______________________________

Snack: ______________________________

REFERENCES

1. ADA Reports: Position of the American Dietetic Association: nutrition for physical fitness and athletic performance for adults, Journal of the American Dietetic Association 87:933, 1987.
2. Aronson VA: Vitamins and minerals as ergogenic aids, The Physician and Sports Medicine 14:209, 1988.
3. Bower B: Alcoholism's elusive genes, Science News 134:74, 1988.
4. Drinkwater BL and others: Bone mineral content of amenorrheic and eumenorrheic athletes, New England Journal of Medicine 311:277, 1984.
5. Holloszy JO and Coyle EF: Adaptations of skeletal muscle to endurance exercise and their metabolic consequences, Journal of Applied Physiology 56:831, 1984.
6. Lieber CS: Alcohol and the liver, Liver Annual 5:116, 1986.
7. Lieber CS: Biochemical and molecular basis of alcohol-induced injury to liver and other tissues, New England Journal of Medicine 319:1639, 1988.
8. Linder MC: Nutritional biochemistry in metabolism, New York, 1985, Elsevier Science Publishing Co Inc.
9. Mitchell MC and Herlong HF: Alcohol and nutrition, Annual Reviews of Nutrition 6:457, 1986.
10. Murray RK and others: Harper's biochemistry, Norwalk, Conn, 1988, Appleton & Lange.
11. O'Neil FT and others: Research and applications of current topics in sports nutrition, Journal of the American Dietetic Association 86:1007, 1986.
12. Stryer L: Biochemistry, ed 3, New York, 1988, WH Freeman.
13. Williams MH: Nutritional ergogenic acids and athletic performance, Nutrition Today January/February: 7, 1989.

SUGGESTED READINGS

Two excellent biochemistry references, particularly useful for more detailed discussions of metabolism, are those by Murray and others and by Stryer. The articles by Aronson and Williams each summarize current research on vitamin and mineral use to enhance athletic performance. To round out your knowledge in this area, see the position paper by The American Dietetic Association. The accompanying text describes diets for athletes and is easy to understand.

CHAPTER 7

Answers to nutrition awareness scale

1. *True.* Carbohydrates provide both energy for the body and carbon atoms that can be synthesized into fat.
2. *True.* Fat can be stored in adipose tissue for future needs or used for energy by cells, such as muscle cells.
3. *False.* The carbon atoms in protein can become the carbon atoms of fat; high-protein diets can be fattening.
4. *True.* The brain uses glucose primarily for energy. Ketone bodies can be used under special circumstances, such as in cases of semi-starvation.
5. *True.* Ketone body levels in the bloodstream rise during fasting, partly because the liver is engaged in gluconeogenesis and is prevented from metabolizing fat efficiently. Ketone bodies are then synthesized from breakdown products of fatty acids.
6. *True.* High and low doses of ethanol are metabolized by alternate systems in the liver. The enzyme system that metabolizes high doses yields less energy than the enzyme system used for low doses.
7. *True.* An alcohol intake of seven beers a day over a long period of time can lead to gradual fat buildup in the liver. This fat reduces blood circulation in the liver, causing cell death that then leads to cirrhosis.
8. *False.* The carbon atoms in alcohol can become the carbon atoms of fat.
9. *True.* Caffeine can enhance fat use by muscles, which may improve athletic performance in some endurance events.
10. *False.* Carnitine is used to shuttle fatty acids into a cell's mitochondria for energy metabolism.
11. *False.* Ketones are primarily formed from acetyl-CoA, a breakdown product of fatty acids. Glycerol can form acetyl-CoA, but there is not enough glycerol in our diets to be of nutritional importance.
12. *True.* Mitochondria are the major sites of ATP production in the cell.
13. *True.* Carbon atoms of carbohydrate, fat, protein, and alcohol molecules can all become the carbon atoms of acetyl-CoA. This compound then has a pivotal role in energy metabolism. In essence, all roads lead to acetyl-CoA.
14. *True.* Using photosynthesis, plants trap solar energy and store it in the chemical bonds of glucose and other organic compounds.
15. *True.* Thirst is not a good indication for fluid replacement needs after hard exercise. A much better guide is weight loss: a general rule is to consume a pint of fluid for every pound of weight lost (or 1 liter per kilogram).

Nutrition Perspective 7-1

Diets for Athletes

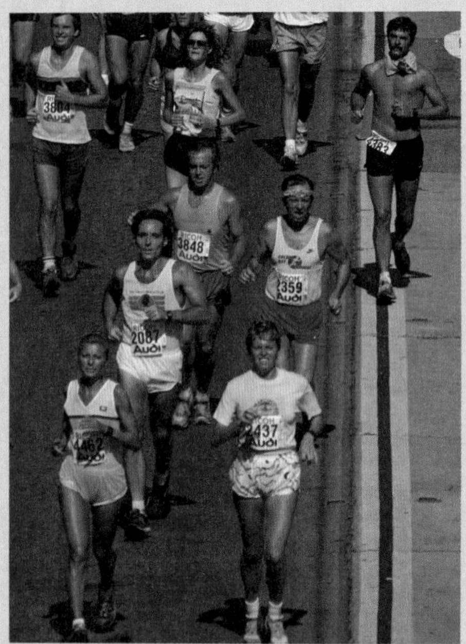

Triathletes and marathon runners should try to eat at least 600 grams of carbohydrates per day during training or when preparing for an event.

A diet can be used to boost athletic performance. We talked about carbohydrate-loading in Chapter 3. That technique may be used for endurance events. Now let's discuss general dietary recommendations for all athletes. Keep in mind, however, that athletic training and sheer genetic potential are two other very important determinants of athletic performance. A good diet won't be a substitute for either.

Athletes in hard training should consume about 400 grams of carbohydrates a day,[1] eating a variety of foods from the Daily Food Guide. This amount will help maintain adequate muscle glycogen stores and especially replace glycogen losses from the previous day. Triathletes and marathoners should consider eating closer to 600 grams of carbohydrates a day, even more if necessary. A large portion should be consumed within 2 hours of ending training, as that is when glycogen synthesis is the greatest.

During muscle-building phases athletes should consume 1 gram and maybe up to 1.5 to 2 grams of protein per kilogram of body weight. *Anyone eating a variety of foods and approximately 3000 kcalories a day will easily meet this recommendation. Thus protein supplements are not needed for athletes because they usually exceed this kcalorie level.*[11] Athletes who must limit their energy intake, such as ballet dancers or those who are vegetarians, should determine how much protein they eat and make sure it equals at least 1 gram per kilogram of desirable body weight. A close look at vitamin and mineral intake is also in order. In addition, the athlete eating few kcalories should focus on nutrient-dense foods: low-fat milk, broccoli, tomatoes, oranges, strawberries, lean beef, kidney beans, turkey, fish, and chicken, to name a few.

Athletes should consume enough water or other fluid replacements to keep their weight constant during exercise. By experimenting they can determine how much fluid is required. Thirst is not a reliable indicator of fluid need. A rule of thumb is to consume ½ liter (2 cups) of fluid about 15 minutes before a sports event. This is called "hyperhydration." Then consume approximately ¼ liter (1 cup) of fluid each 15 minutes for events that last longer than 30 minutes. The fluid can be water, fruit juice, or a "sports-type" drink. A homemade "sports-type" drink can be made of 30 grams (2 tablespoons) of sugar, ½ gram ($\frac{1}{10}$ teaspoon of salt), and ¼ gram ($\frac{1}{16}$ teaspoon) of potassium chloride (salt substitute) in 1 liter (1 quart) of water.[9] Cold liquids are absorbed faster.

Some athletes find that consuming caffeine (4 to 5 milligrams per kilogram of body weight) about an hour before an endurance event improves stamina and performance (Table 7-1). However, Olympic officials consider caffeine a drug and do not condone its use. A body level exceeding the equivalent of 5 to 6 cups of coffee is illegal.[11] Caffeine's action is due to its stimulation of lipolysis, or the burning of fat for energy. This process spares glycogen use, and so reduces lactate production. Besides the rules against use of large quantities of caffeine, another drawback to caffeine use is that caffeine can cause increased urination and anxiety. In addition, the advantage of improving stamina and performance is often not great in events lasting less than 2 hours, especially if the athlete has ample glycogen stores.[11]

VITAMINS AND MINERALS

Because athletes usually consume many kcalories, ample vitamins and minerals will naturally be part of the diet.[1] If a low-energy intake (less than 1200 kcalories) is needed, vitamin and mineral supplements can be used.[11] We will discuss this further in Chapter 11. *Extra vitamin and mineral intake well above the RDA is not needed. They supply no known ergogenic (work-producing) benefit.*[2,11] Special attention should be focused on iron intake, especially by female athletes, since sweat losses and increased blood volume,

Table 7-1

Caffeine content of beverages

Item and serving	Caffeine per serving (mg)
3-ounce cup	
Coffee—drip method	110-150
percolated	64-124
instant	40-108
decaffeinated	2-3
Tea—1-minute brew	9-33
3-minute brew	20-46
instant	12-28
Cocoa—mix	6
12-ounce container	
Tea—iced	22-36
Coca Cola; TAB	46
Shasta, all colas	44
Dr. Pepper, regular or diet	40
Pepsi, diet or light; RC cola	36

Note: Data abstracted from "Caffeine", a Scientific Status Summary by the Institute of Food Technologists, April 1983. Milk chocolate candy contains 6 mg caffeine/oz and baking chocolate contains 33 mg/oz.

coupled with menses, all lead to increased need for iron. See Chapter 14 to determine whether you are consuming enough iron.

Disturbing reports concerning calcium show that female athletes who do not menstruate regularly have far less dense spine bones than both nonathletes and female athletes who menstruate regularly. Researchers have just begun to understand the importance of regular menstruation for the promotion of bone maintenance (see Chapter 13). Female athletes who become irregular in their menses should decrease their level of training, and/or increase body weight in an attempt to restore regular menses. Either or both changes will bring back menses in most women. If irregular menses persist, severe bone loss and eventual osteoporosis will likely result. *Extra calcium in the diet does not compensate for this loss of menses.*[4]

PRE-EVENT MEAL

A pre-event meal should be eaten 3 to 4 hours before the event. It should consist primarily of starchy carbohydrate sources, such as spaghetti, rye bread, breakfast cereals, beans, and oatmeal, and contain approximately 500 kcalories. This will supply glycogen stores.

In all, a diet following the Daily Food Guide suggestions is a positive step all athletes should consider. Supplements should be reserved for correcting medically diagnosed nutrient deficiencies.

Nutrition Perspective 7-2

Alcohol Metabolism

Alcohol is not a nutrient, but it does supply energy for the body: 7 kcalories per gram. The liver metabolizes most of the alcohol consumed. A social drinker who weighs 150 pounds and has normal liver function metabolizes about 7 to 14 grams of alcohol per hour (100 to 200 milligrams per kilogram of body weight per hour). If a person drinks slightly less alcohol each hour than the amount that can be metabolized by the liver—about 8 to 12 ounces of beer or half an ordinary sized drink—the blood alcohol content remains low (Table 7-2). In that case, a person can drink large amounts of alcohol over long periods without becoming noticeably intoxicated. When the rate of alcohol consumption exceeds the liver's metabolic capacity, the blood alcohol content rises and symptoms of intoxication appear (Table 7-3).

Alcohol metabolism rates vary among people for genetic reasons.[3] The rate of alcohol metabolism in the liver also depends on body weight, the frequency of alcohol consumption, and other factors. Anyone who consumes alcohol should find their own tolerance level so that they can drink without significantly affecting their coordination or judgment. Food consumed along with alcohol slows its absorption and therefore moderates the rise in blood alcohol concentration. In addition, certain medications, such as many sedatives, affect alcohol metabolism: if metabolism is slowed, alcohol rises more quickly to high blood concentrations.

At a blood alcohol concentration of 0.1%, drinkers in most states are considered le-

Table 7-2

Caloric, carbohydrate, and alcohol content of alcoholic beverages

Beverage	Amount (ounce)	Alcohol (grams)	Carbohydrate (grams)	Energy (kcalories)
Beer				
Regular	12	13	14	150
Light	12	10	6	90
Extra light	12	8	3	70
Near	12	2	12	60
Distilled				
Gin, rum, vodka, whiskey	1.5	15	—	105
Brandy, cognac	1.0	11	—	75
Wine				
Red	4	12	1	85
Dry white	4	11	0.5	80
Sweet	4	12	5	103
Sherry	2	9	1.5	75
Port, muscatel	2	7	7	95
Vermouth, sweet	3	12	14	141
Vermouth, dry	3	13	4	105
Manhattan	3	21	2	165
Martini	3	19	1	140
Old-fashioned	3	21	1	180

From: Guthrie HA: Introductory nutrition, ed 7, St. Louis, 1989, The C.V. Mosby Company.

Table 7-3

Physiological effects of alcohol

Blood alcohol concentrations (percent)	Common behavioral effects	Hours required for alcohol to be metabolized
0.00-0.05	Slight change in feelings—usually relaxation and euphoria. Decreased alertness.	2-3
0.05-0.10	Emotional lability with exaggerated feelings and behavior. Reduced social inhibitions. Impairment of reaction time and fine motor coordination. Increasingly impaired during driving. Legally drunk at 0.08 in Utah and 0.10 in many other states.	4-6
0.10-0.15	Unsteadiness in standing and walking. Loss of peripheral vision. Driving is extremely dangerous. Legally drunk at 0.15 in all states.	6-10
0.15-0.30	Staggering gait. Slurred speech. Pain and other sensory perceptions greatly impaired.	10-24
More than 0.30	Stupor or unconsciousness. Anesthesia. Death possible at 0.35 and above.	More than 24

Source: Modified from U.S. Department of Health and Human Services, 1986.

gally drunk. A concentration greater than 0.3% makes death possible: the higher the level, the greater the risk.

Alcohol depresses the central nervous system. As the blood alcohol level rises, the person suffers from poor muscle coordination, confused speech, poor walking, and often mental confusion and lack of judgment. When consumed by a pregnant woman, alcohol can cause severe birth defects in the growing fetus (see Chapter 15). Alcohol may also lower inhibitions and therefore appear to act like a stimulant to the body. *But the depressant nature of alcohol is actually more powerful.* As William Shakespeare wrote: "It stirs up desire, but it takes away the performance."

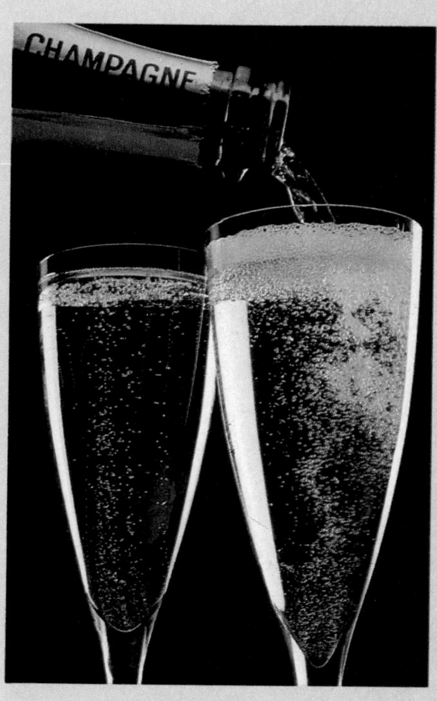

Alcohol may seem stimulating, but it is actually a depressant.

PATHWAYS FOR ALCOHOL METABOLISM

Alcohol at low doses first reacts with NAD to form the compound acetaldehyde. The enzyme used is **alcohol dehydrogenase** (Figure 7-12). This enzyme requires zinc for activity. Acetaldehyde is then converted into acetyl-CoA. Both reactions yield an NADH molecule. The acetyl-CoA enters the citric acid cycle, and the NADH, $FADH_2$, and GTP molecules produced in the citric acid cycle can then be used to generate ATP.

In structure, the end of ethanol with the hydroxyl group (−OH) resembles a carbohydrate. But since it breaks down directly into acetyl-CoA, alcohol carbons cannot become net carbons of glucose. So alcohol is metabolized more like a fat than like a carbohydrate, and thus is considered a fat in metabolic terms.

When a person drinks a lot of alcohol, the enzyme alcohol dehydrogenase cannot keep up with the demand to metabolize all of it into acetaldehyde. For this and other reasons, another enzyme system in the liver begins metabolizing alcohol. This system is called the **microsomal ethanol oxidizing system (MEOS).** The MEOS is usually used by the liver to metabolize drugs and other "foreign" compounds. The liver registers excessive molecules of alcohol as foreign compounds, and thus the MEOS kicks in.[5] Once the MEOS is active, alcohol tolerance increases because the rate of alcohol metabolism increases.

Continued.

Nutrition Perspective 7-2, cont'd

Alcohol Metabolism

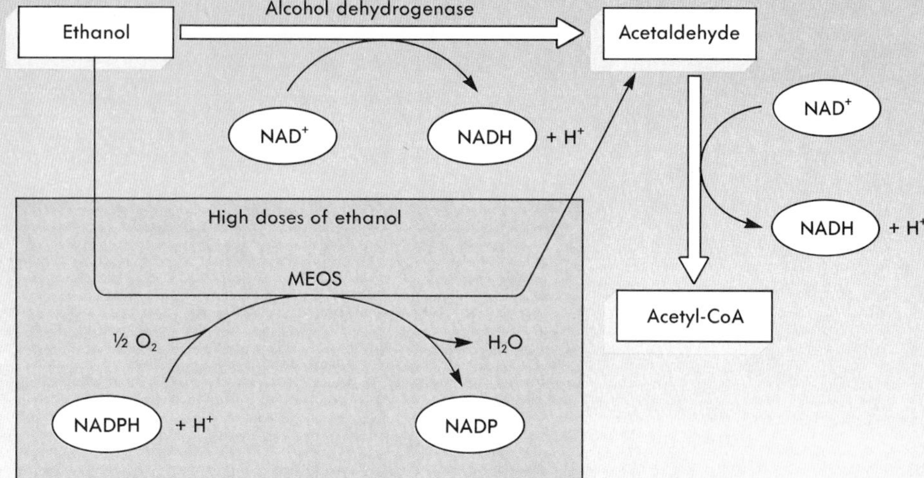

Figure 7-12

Ethanol metabolism. At low amounts of alcohol intake, the alcohol dehydrogenase pathway is used. At high amounts of alcohol intake, the microsonal ethanol oxidizing system (MEOS) is used. The MEOS uses rather than yields energy; use of the pathway also decreases the ability to detoxify drugs, increasing the risk of a drug overdose if large amounts of alcohol are consumed at the same time.

There are two interesting aspects about this use of the MEOS. First, instead of forming NADH as does alcohol dehydrogenase, the MEOS uses NADPH, a compound analogous to NADH. Now, instead of yielding three "potential" ATP molecules from the first step in alcohol metabolism, the MEOS uses three "potential" ATP molecules. This explains why people with alcoholism do not gain as much weight as expected from the amount of kcalories they consume via alcohol. High doses of alcohol are inefficiently used by the liver because they require energy for the first metabolic stop. The person with alcoholism basically wastes some alcohol kcalories by inducing this alternate metabolic pathway.

The use of the MEOS also increases the potential for an overdose of alcohol. *While the MEOS system is metabolizing alcohol, it has a reduced capacity to metabolize drugs such as many sedatives.* If high amounts of alcohol and these sedatives are mixed, the user may lapse into coma and die. The liver is not able to break down the sedatives in the body fast enough. *Alcohol itself is toxic in high quantities. Mix it with sedatives and an extremely toxic combination results.*

CIRRHOSIS OF THE LIVER

A long-term side effect of a high alcohol intake is fat infiltration of the liver and possible vitamin malnutrition (we will focus on the latter in Chapter 12).[7] Why fat builds up in the liver is still unknown, but the condition often accompanies alcoholism.[4] One theory is that the liver is so busy metabolizing alcohol that fatty acids are not burned, and so they build up and are synthesized into triglycerides. Or possibly not enough protein is available to transport fat from the liver as a lipoprotein. In addition, the large numbers of acetyl-CoA and NADH molecules generated from alcohol metabolism may force fatty acid synthesis. Other factors could be involved as well.

This buildup of fat in the liver eventually chokes off the blood supply—and therefore oxygen and nutrients—to the liver cells. Liver cells then die and are replaced by connective (scar) tissue. This scarring process is called cirrhosis. *Cirrhosis of the liver is a leading cause of death in alcoholism. Work with monkeys shows that no diet can protect against alcohol-induced cirrhosis.*

There is no specific dose relationship between alcohol consumption and cirrhosis. Some people are very susceptible to cirrhosis, while others are not. One rule of thumb is that cirrhosis results from a 15-year consumption of approximately 80 grams of ethanol per day. This is equivalent to 7 beers per day (Table 7-2). Some evidence suggests that the dose may even be as low as 35 grams a day for men and 20 grams a day for women. As the Dietary Guidelines suggest, if you drink alcoholic beverages, do so in moderation.

Exploring Issues and Actions

If you think you have an alcohol problem, the first person to see is your physician. College counselors can also offer advice. In addition, there may be some specific programs on your campus to help people overcome alcohol problems. If you do have an alcohol problem, you are not alone. Approximately 15 million adults do, as well as 3 million to 4 million teenagers.

Nutrition Perspective 7-3

Developing a Sports Nutrition Practice

BY NANCY CLARK, M.S., R.D.

Twenty years ago jogging was just becoming the "in" thing. Today exercise for fitness is an integral part of many persons' life-style. Ten years ago, 75 triathletes attempted Hawaii's Ironman Triathlon. Last year (1988), more than 1500 people entered this grueling test of human endurance (2.4 mile swim, 112 mile bike race, and then 26.2 mile run). Ten years ago when I started my sports nutrition practice, people were just waking up to sports nutrition and the fact that food affects performance. Today most athletes are more than eager to learn about what's best to eat.

Americans have not only become more conscious of health and fitness, they've also increased their interest in learning how to eat a healthful sports diet. Runners want to know what to eat before a marathon. Ballet dancers wonder how they can lose weight and still maintain energy for training. Wrestlers search for information about how to make weight and keep off the pounds without dehydrating themselves. Recreational athletes want information about the best pre-exercise sports snacks.

As the athletes demanding sports nutrition information have become more outspoken, nutritionists are being called upon to fill the void and feed the athletes the information they desire. Yet many nutritionists hesitate to step into this specialty area because they lack special training. For those interested in getting more involved in developing a practice as a sports nutritionist, I offer the following tips based on my entrepreneurial experiences at SportsMedicine Brookline, one of the largest sports medicine clinics in the Boston area and the United States.

PRACTICE WHAT YOU PREACH

To be an effective sports nutritionist, you should be sports-active yourself. You will be better able to relate to the athletes you counsel, and they'll have more respect for your knowledge, since it will be first-hand, rather than book-learned. One of the first questions my clients ask me is "What do *you* do for exercise?"

Since I've always been sports-active, I have a wide repertoire from which to draw: I've ridden my bicycle across America as well as through the Canadian Rockies: I've trekked in the Himalaya mountains, winter-camped and cross-country skied in the White Mountains, and competed in 10K road races, marathons, and even mountain marathons. As a bike commuter, cycling is an integral part of my daily routine. I'm a member of both the Charles River Wheelman Bike Club and the Greater Boston Track Club. Biking is for relaxation; running is for a competitive experience. Maintaining a fit body is important to me both personally and professionally, lending great credibility, as well as an understanding of my clients' needs.

GET SPECIALIZED EDUCATION

Every week, students and registered dietitians who want to specialize in sports nutrition write to me, inquiring about the wisest career path. They're undoubtedly active in sports and want to combine their personal sports interests with their professional nutrition career.

I recommend they complement their nutrition curriculum with additional classes in exercise physiology. Many state universities have exercise physiology departments that offer appropriate courses. Although it is not necessary for the nutritionist who wants to do counseling to have a degree in exercise physiology, it is important that he or she understands the basics and can answer in-depth physiological questions that a client might ask.

After getting my undergraduate degree in nutrition from Simmons College in Boston, completing an internship at Massachusetts General Hospital and working for 4 years, I

Continued.

Nutrition Perspective 7-3—cont'd

Developing a Sports Nutrition Practice

went to graduate school at Boston University for my master's degree in nutrition with a special emphasis on exercise physiology. Before I had this fundamental exercise physiology background, sports-active friends and athletes would ask me questions that I felt hesitant to answer. For example, I could tell them that they did not need a high protein diet to build up muscles, but I couldn't explain what *does* build muscles. I could say that water was fine for replacing sweat losses, but I didn't know how sports drinks fit into the picture. I had the surface answers to their questions, but not the in-depth theory and scientific background. Graduate school became an obvious need.

Conveniently for me, Boston University's Sargent College of Allied Health Professions offered graduate programs in both nutrition and exercise physiology—a perfect combination! Fortunately for me, the nutrition department's chairperson was Dr. Beverly Bullen, a pioneer in the area of sports nutrition. She understood my interests and helped me design a program that would fulfill my requirements.

Today several colleges offer the opportunity to combine nutrition with exercise; Columbia, Berkeley, Tufts (graduate), and several state universities are the names of a few. If you're interested in furthering your education in this area, it's important to talk with the professors to learn their areas of interest, what research opportunities are available, and the possibilities of coordinating between the nutrition and exercise physiology departments.

I thoroughly enjoyed the exercise physiology classes that I took. Since I'd previously studied only medical physiology, the exercise physiology classes clearly demonstrated that the active, healthy body is different than that previously emphasized. I learned about the biochemical, hormonal and muscular changes associated with training and strenuous exercise. I learned the scientific theory behind the nutrition recommendations, so that I could explain the "whys."

My thesis project, which looked at the effect of a high-fat diet on endurance performance, gave me an invaluable experience working with athletes. Only by counseling them, administering maximal performance tests, measuring oxygen uptake, observing muscle biopsies, and participating in the research process did I internalize a working knowledge of these textbook concepts. I've since learned that most athletes are also "exercise physiologists" . . . somewhat self-taught, but neverthless very knowledgeable. They understand their bodies remarkably. Since I can understand their lingo of fast twitch fibers, anaerobic threshold, max tests, and other such terms, I'm able to relate to them on their level.

The hours and hours of graduate study have paid off, but the need to keep learning is never-ending. Sports nutrition is a rapidly changing field. Each year, new facts replace old theories. To keep up to date is a full-time job in itself!

BECOME AFFILIATED WITH A LARGE FITNESS FACILITY OR SPORTS MEDICINE CLINIC

Being a member of the medical team at SportsMedicine Brookline has been a key to the survival of my sports nutrition practice. The clinic deals primarily with athletic injuries; my job is to address the nutritional concerns of the clients. The medical team includes orthopedists, podiatrists, physical therapists, athletic trainers—all with a sports background and the skills to focus upon the needs of both casual exercisers and competitive athletes. To my good fortune, Dr. William Southmayd, medical director, is very supportive of having me as a nutritionist on the team.

Although positions such as mine are few, they are growing in availability—and sometimes are just waiting to be created if the right nutritionist happens to come along. I highly recommend that registered dietitians knock on doors of their local sports medicine clinics to inquire about the possibilities of becoming associated on a professional basis.

Health clubs, universities, Y's, and other fitness facilities are also logical places to start

Nutrition Perspective 7-3—cont'd

Developing a Sports Nutrition Practice

a practice. Try to find one that has a large volume of flow-through traffic. This will enhance your visibility and potential client-base.

ENJOY WRITING AND PUBLIC SPEAKING

To generate business, you'll have to market yourself and let athletes know that: (1) you exist and (2) you're available for consultations. One of the best ways to become known is through writing for your local newspaper, track club newsletter, or other local sports publications. The second way is to set up talks with sports groups. With time, the athletes will become familiar with you/your name and know who to call when they are seeking professional advise.

Writing is a way not only to market sports nutrition services, but also to educate large numbers of people about the importance of eating healthfully. The written word also adds credibility to your name. For me, writing is also a way to express myself creatively; I enjoy it. The audience is there, ready and waiting, since most sports-active Americans are more than eager to read how to protect their health, to say nothing about how to run faster or become stronger through the powers of good nutrition.

PLAN ON THREE TO FIVE YEARS OF HARD WORK

Most people who are starting a business are warned that they'll need 3 to 5 years to develop it. Most of these same people, myself included, think "No, not me. I have more energy than the other entrepreneurs . . . I'll reach success far sooner." Well, I repeat that warning and encourage you to consider the possibility that you, too, will need those 3 to 5 years of energy! Only with time, hard work, public visibility, and written articles will the sports world get to know your name and respect your expertise.

In the 10 years that I've worked at SportsMedicine Brookine, I have learned that creating a sports nutrition practice demands an incredible amount of time, energy, and creativity. As any consultant knows, the work is never done—or so it seems. Yet, all the hard work and long hours are paying off. Although sports nutrition is a rewarding (and fun) speciality area, the disappointing news is that the average athlete prefers free nutrition information. They love to ask questions in group classes but hesitate to pay for individual consultations. You might get tired of living on beans and peanut butter before you tire of helping them win with good nutrition.

GO FOR IT!

I only hope that I have opened doors for other up-and-coming sports nutritionists. You have my support to knock on doors, create possibilities, and give it your all. By working together, we'll have greater success. As any entrepreneur understands, you have to do it yourself, but you can't do it alone.

Chapter 8

Energy Balance

Overview

Maintaining energy balance—regulating kcalorie intake so that it equals output—contributes to our health and well-being. Many adults in North America maintain desirable body weight by balancing their energy intake and output. Achieving that balance and maintaining it is an important goal for everyone who is interested in good health. Adulthood can be a time of creeping weight gain that turns into obesity and increases the likelihood of health problems. In this chapter we will discuss these health problems, review the major concepts underlying the theories of energy balance, and define obesity and learn how to assess it. Since obesity is a major health problem in North America, it is important for us all to understand more about the factors that lead to it.

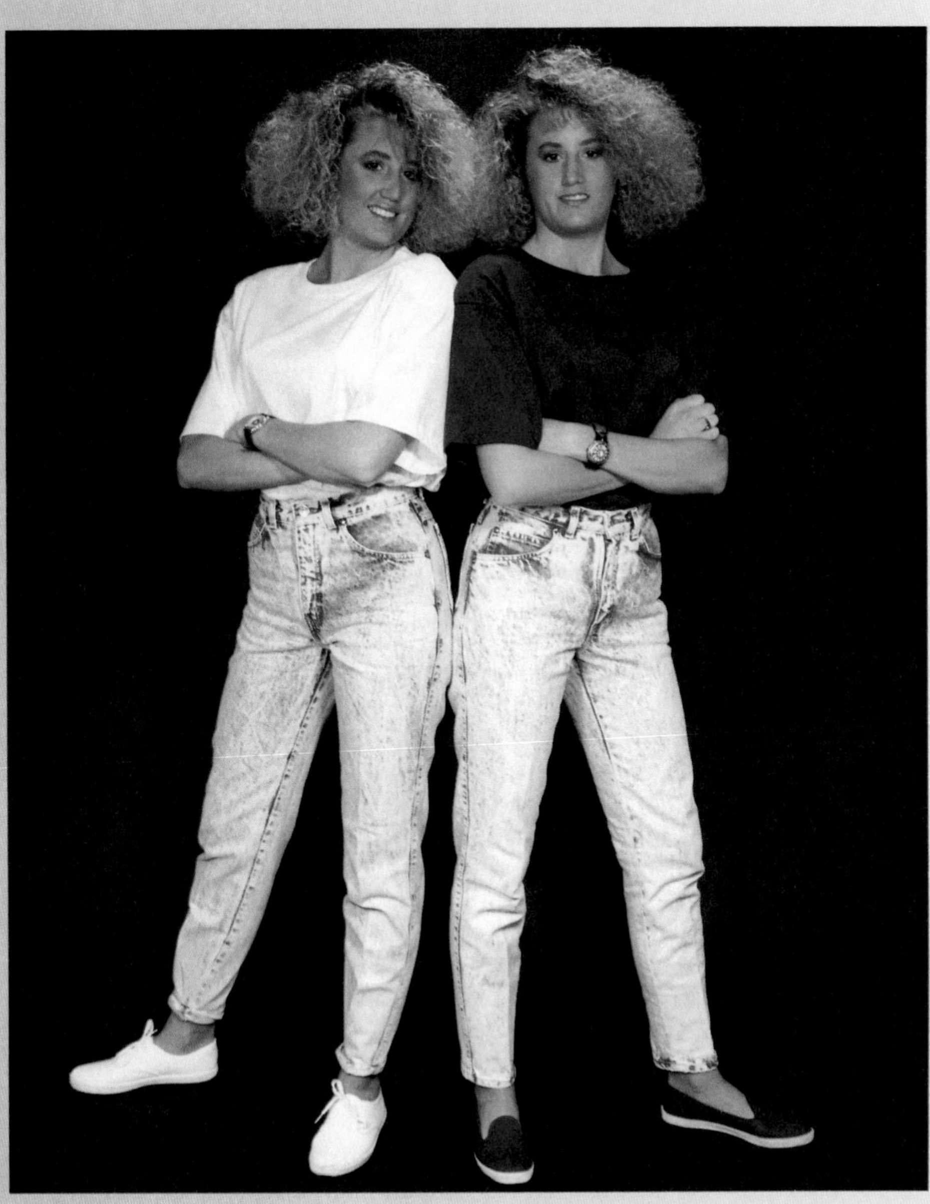

Nature or nurture—what causes these twins to have similar body weights?

Nutrition awareness inventory

Here are 15 statements about energy balance. Answer them to test your current knowledge. If you think the answer is true or mostly true, circle T. If you think the answer is false or mostly false, circle F. Use the scoring key at the end of this chapter to compute your total score. Take this test again after you have read this chapter. Compare the results.

1. **T F** Hunger is partially regulated by the liver.
2. **T F** "Set point" theory and blood pressure regulation work in a similar manner.
3. **T F** Total energy needs can be accurately estimated using the RDA.
4. **T F** The energy required to keep the resting body alive represents basal metabolism.
5. **T F** Brown adipose tissue is more active in adults than in infants.
6. **T F** That some obese people live past 80 years of age suggests that obesity probably doesn't affect longevity.
7. **T F** Body fat is a more important measure of risk for poor health than is body weight.
8. **T F** Men and women tend to add most fat to their bodies in the abdomen.
9. **T F** Health problems related to obesity occur when a person weighs about 20% over desirable weight.
10. **T F** The more muscle tissue one has, the higher the basal metabolism.
11. **T F** During physical activity, obese people burn more kcalories than lean people.
12. **T F** Adult obesity in men is usually tied to childhood obesity.
13. **T F** The major cause of obesity in North America is low thyroid hormone levels.
14. **T F** Most obesity is due to constant overeating.
15. **T F** Appetite often changes during a meal.

ENERGY INTAKE: THE FIRST HALF OF ENERGY BALANCE

hunger
The physiological drive to find and eat food.

appetite
The psychological drive to find and eat food, often in the absence of hunger.

satiety
A state in which there is no longer a desire to eat.

Energy balance depends on kcalorie input and kcalorie output. This balance then goes on to influence energy stores, primarily in adipose tissue (Figure 8-1). Let's look at the factors affecting these relationships.

Many factors influence our desire to eat. **Hunger** is a sign of the physiological drive to find and eat food. **Appetite** represents the psychological drive to find and eat food. Fulfilling both these drives should lead to a state of **satiety,** in which the desire to eat is extinguished for a short time. Together, these states—hunger, appetite, and satiety—and the factors that regulate them greatly influence body weight.[20]

The hypothalamus: a hunger regulator

The satiety center is often referred to as the ventromedial satiety center, and the feeding centers are often referred to as the lateral feeding centers.

The **hypothalamus,** which is part of the brain stem, plays a key role in regulating hunger. When specific groups of cells (nuclei) in the hypothalamus are stimulated by chemicals or electrical activity, hunger increases or decreases. We can refer to one group of cells as the **satiety center** and other groups of cells as the **feeding centers.** When the satiety center is stimulated, we no longer feel hungry. When the feeding centers are stimulated, we become hungry. Most likely these centers monitor the blood glucose level for a signal: a low blood glucose level

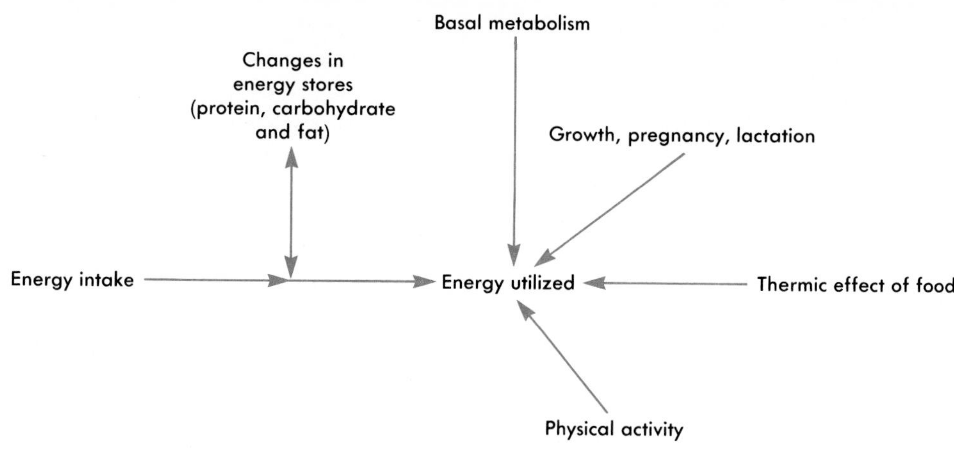

Figure 8-1

A model for energy balance. This model incorporates the variables that influence energy balance.

encourages feeding (this is indicated most clearly by work with laboratory animals). Amino acid levels in the bloodstream may also provide cues, as we will discuss further in the next section.[1]

The feeding and satiety centers can be destroyed by specific chemicals, surgery, and certain forms of cancer. When the satiety cells are destroyed, laboratory animals (and humans) continue to eat until they become quite obese. Once obesity is achieved, weight regulates around this new obese state.[1]

Researchers now think that the mechanism responsible for regulating weight—once a satiety-center lesion has developed—depends on the ability of adipose cells to respond to insulin; weight gain becomes more difficult as increasing obesity hampers the ability of the adipose cells to respond to insulin.[1] Normally, the hormone insulin increases fat uptake and storage in the adipose tissue cells. When adipose cell size increases so much that they ignore the signals from insulin, the metabolic changes associated with a satiety-center lesion are no longer powerful enough to cause further lipid storage (see Chapter 4). Another line of research suggests that adipose cells make a protein called **adipsin**, which reduces sensations of hunger. When full of fat, adipose cells appear to make a lot of adipsin, shutting off hunger controlled by the brain, and so further weight gain. More research is needed on this adipsin-hunger link.[16] See the Expert Opinion by Dr. Jules Hirsch in this chapter.

adipsin
A protein that appears to be made by adipose cells and acts as a communication link between adipose cells and the brain.

If the feeding-center cells are destroyed, animals lose the desire to eat and eventually lose weight. Their body weight then regulates around this new lower level.[1] A feeding-center lesion depletes fat stores (and body weight) only to a certain extent. If an animal's body fat is already reduced because of previous manipulations, such as semi-starvation, further depletion in the adipose cells is not possible.

Hunger regulation occurs at many body sites

The centers in the brain—satiety and feeding—interact with other groups of cells in the brain and liver that also form other important decision points for determining hunger and satiety. Hunger is actually regulated by a complicated network of numerous sites and systems. *For our purposes, it is important to remem-*

ber that there are specific sites in the brain and other organs that, when stimulated, greatly affect (increase and decrease) the desire to seek and eat food.

Accumulating evidence from studies on the regulation of hunger—especially from those using laboratory animals—suggests that an underlying hunger for food is never totally absent.[29] After a meal, glucose, fatty acids, amino acids, and other energy-yielding compounds increase in the bloodstream. At this point, and especially as monosaccharides and amino acids are metabolized by the liver, hunger is temporarily shut off. The satiety center in the brain registers that the satiation point is reached. Several hours after eating, when the concentrations of these compounds in the bloodstream begin to fall and liver metabolism slows, hunger returns because it is no longer inhibited by the metabolism of those energy-yielding compounds. Then the feeding centers begin to dominate again. This simplified model cannot totally account for the dynamics involved in hunger and satiation, but it is a start.

Hormonal regulation of feeding

Many hormones and hormone-like compounds affect feeding behavior and satiety (Table 8-1). After a meal, blood concentrations of cholecystokinin (CCK), secretin, gastrin, and other hormones increase.[20] These and various other hormone-related compounds increase satiety. In laboratory animal experiments CCK and stomach distention appear to work together to shut off hunger.

See Chapter 3 to review the role of CCK in digestion, especially in the release of enzymes, bile, and other substances from the pancreas and gallbladder.

Table 8-1

The following hormones, hormone-like compounds, and medications have been shown to affect feeding behavior[8]

Increase feeding	Cause satiety
Insulin*	Insulin*
Endorphins	Cholecystokinin (CCK)
Norepinephrine	Bombesin
Cortisol (required for norepinephrine action)	Serotonin
Neuropeptide Y	Calcitonin
Galadin	Glucagon
Tranquilizers	Somatostatin
Antidepressants	Vasoactive inhibitory peptide (VIP)
	Corticotropin-releasing factor
	Thyrotropin-releasing factor
	Neurotensin
	Amphetamines
	Antihistamines
	Fenfluramine
	Tumor necrosis factor (cachectin; a factor produced by immune cells)
	Nicotine

*Insulin leads to satiety as energy-yielding compounds are being put into use and storage. Once the energy-yielding nutrients fall in concentration in the bloodstream and their rate of liver metabolism slows, hunger returns. Since insulin action leads to both energy nutrient use and eventual depletion from the bloodstream, it needs to appear in both columns.

On the other hand, **endorphins,** the body's natural pain killers, and the hormones cortisol and insulin all lead to increased feeding.[4] The presence of cortisol is especially significant if animals are genetically prone to developing obesity. Insulin probably affects both hunger and satiety. As insulin increases liver metabolism of energy-yielding compounds, it promotes satiety. However, after insulin has done its job throughout the body, concentrations of energy-yielding compounds in the bloodstream are low. That probably causes hunger to return.[29] In general, then, the body's hormonal balance influences the tendency to feel hungry or satiated.

endorphins
Natural body tranquilizers that may be involved in the feeding response, as well as functioning in pain reduction.

Meal-to-meal regulation of feeding

Recent carbohydrate intake greatly influences later food intake in laboratory animals. When carbohydrate intake is reduced in animals for 1 day, they try to consume more carbohydrates the next day. On the other hand, if the animals consume a high-carbohydrate diet for 1 day, they tend to consume a diet higher in protein the next. Alterations in the protein or fat content of the diet have less effect.[1]

Studies suggest how diet might influence later food intake. Eating carbohydrates increases insulin levels in the bloodstream. Recall that insulin increases glucose uptake by cells. At the same time, it increases amino acid uptake by cells, especially uptake of the branched-chain amino acids—leucine, isoleucine, and valine—by muscle cells.

Before an examination you may wish to eat a high-protein diet rather than a high-carbohydrate diet. High-protein diets tend to make a person more attentive, whereas high-carbohydrate diets tend to make a person sleepier.

Clearing these branched-chain amino acids from the bloodstream acts to increase the relative concentration of another amino acid, tryptophan. As the tryptophan concentration in the bloodstream increases, more of it can pass into the brain, especially because its competitors—the branched-chain amino acids—are in low supply. The brain then synthesizes some of this tryptophan into the neurotransmitter **serotonin.** Serotonin, in turn, decreases carbohydrate craving, and it can induce sleep.[12]

serotonin
A neurotransmitter synthesized from the amino acid tryptophan that appears to both decrease the desire to eat carbohydrates and induce sleep.

For this mechanism to work in humans, a meal must be essentially protein-free. Tryptophan levels are generally low, even in high-protein foods, and would not be able to compete with the other amino acids in the diet for eventual uptake from the bloodstream into the brain. Even so, there is still debate about how powerful a high-carbohydrate meal really is in changing human feeding behavior. Studies have confused their findings about carbohydrates by using high-carbohydrate snacks that also are often high in fat. Putting this information into practice will require more research.[12]

Exploring Issues and Actions

How hungry are you most of the time? Is it really appetite? Which part of the day or night are you hungriest? Are you hungry after exercise, while studying, or before going to sleep? Are there any personal hunger patterns you can identify?

Long-term weight regulation—a set point?

Some scientists suggest that the hypothalamus monitors the amount of body fat in laboratory animals and humans and tries to keep that level constant over time. This level is often referred to as a **"set point."**[20] The protein produced by adipose cells, adipsin, may form the communication link between adipose cells and the brain that allows for this regulation.[16]

Analogies to the tight regulation of blood pressure and body temperature are used to support this concept of a set point for weight. *One researcher has described the set point as a coiled spring: the further you stray from your usual weight, the harder the force acts to pull you back to that weight.*[9]

There is sound evidence that body weight tends to be regulated. This is apparent after illness, for example, as the person regains lost weight.[5] If one reduces energy intake, the blood level of a thyroid hormone (T_3) falls, causing the metabolic rate to fall.[28] Due to these changes, the body resists further weight loss. In addition, the lower body weight decreases the energy cost of each future weight-bearing activity, and the total energy used by lean tissues falls because some of these tissues are also lost. Furthermore, the enzyme used by adipose cells and

set point
This refers to the close regulation of body weight. It is not known what cells control this set point or how it actually functions in weight regulation. There is no doubt, however, that there are mechanisms that help regulate weight.

muscle cells to pull in fat from the bloodstream (lipoprotein lipase) may increase its activity (see Chapter 9).

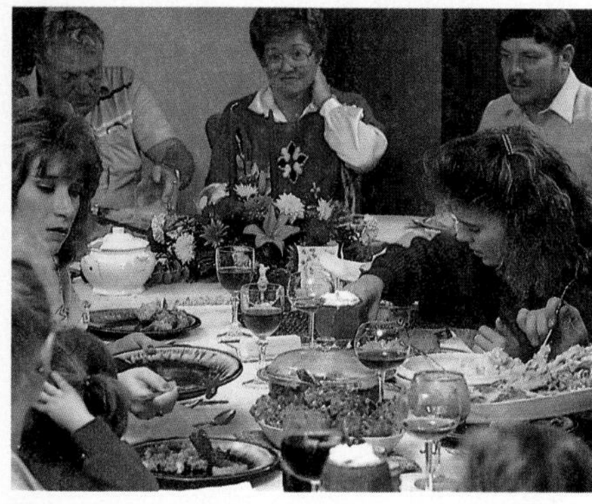

Because of the body's resistance to weight gain, a big holiday meal does not have as much effect on body weight as it should.

If a person overeats, in the short run the metabolic rate tends to increase because the T_3 hormone level increases.[28] This causes resistance to further weight gain. People often recognize the body's resistance to weight loss when dieting but do not think much about the resistance to weight gain after eating a big holiday meal.

Let's explore set point regulation of weight in concrete terms. The amount we eat varies from day to day. Daily energy intake varies from about 20% below to 20% above a person's 28-day average energy intake (about 400 kcalories).[28] In comparison, even as little as a 2% (40-kcalorie) overconsumption of energy per day, if continued for 20 years, could result in an 82-pound weight gain.[20] This significant effect from such a small error points out how easy it is to follow the road to obesity. But, the average weight gain between the ages of 18 and 54 years is only 15 to 20 pounds. It appears that some powerful factors encourage a balance of overeating with undereating. Thus, in the long run, daily energy imbalances cancel each other, with high-kcalorie intake days balancing the low-kcalorie intake days. When also considering that over a 35-year period an adult eats about 35 tons of food (yielding 30 million kcalories), the ability to regulate weight, though imperfect, is again still quite impressive.[16]

The concept of a set point has been widely touted in popular magazines and books. Proponents suggest that exercise or eating a low-fat diet lowers one's set point. However, whether a set point exists is immaterial. As we will discuss in Chapter 9, the reality is that exercise is important for weight maintenance,[15] a high-fat diet is often very high in kcalories, and dieting is very difficult. If these phenomena are easier to understand using the concept of set point, use it. However, very little valid evidence shows how set point operates. We must bear most of the responsibility for weight maintenance ourselves. *The odds are against the likelihood that—even with a set point helping us—we can avoid creeping weight gain in adulthood.*

Is appetite regulated?

The availability of food, the time of day, the taste, texture, and color of the food, emotional state, social custom, and mere suggestion all influence food intake (see Chapter 1 and Figure 8-2). Everyone has acted out this situation: "I saw it, so I ate it." Appetite may not be a biological process, but it is nevertheless an important factor in regulating food intake.

After a meal, appetite is reinforced by the pleasant tastes and feelings associated with satiety. The taste of food and the physical feelings associated with a meal are two important determinants of food choice. *If we find ourselves eating because of stress or depression, it is probably because eating often makes us feel good.*

The ample food supply in North America, coupled with relative prosperity, creates a situation in which many people eat primarily from appetite, rather than from hunger. Many of us do not often experience real hunger. You may want to try fasting for 1 day to see what real hunger feels like. Chances are now that you eat at noon, or 6 PM, or while watching television because of habit and custom, not from hunger.

Does appetite change?

Appetite changes even while we eat. At the beginning of a meal, we typically consume a variety of foods. By the end of a meal, food choices usually narrow. Consider the last time you went to a buffet. The first time past the food table you may have chosen some meat, pasta, salad, and something to drink. When you went through the line again, you probably steered toward the cake, pie, and ice cream.

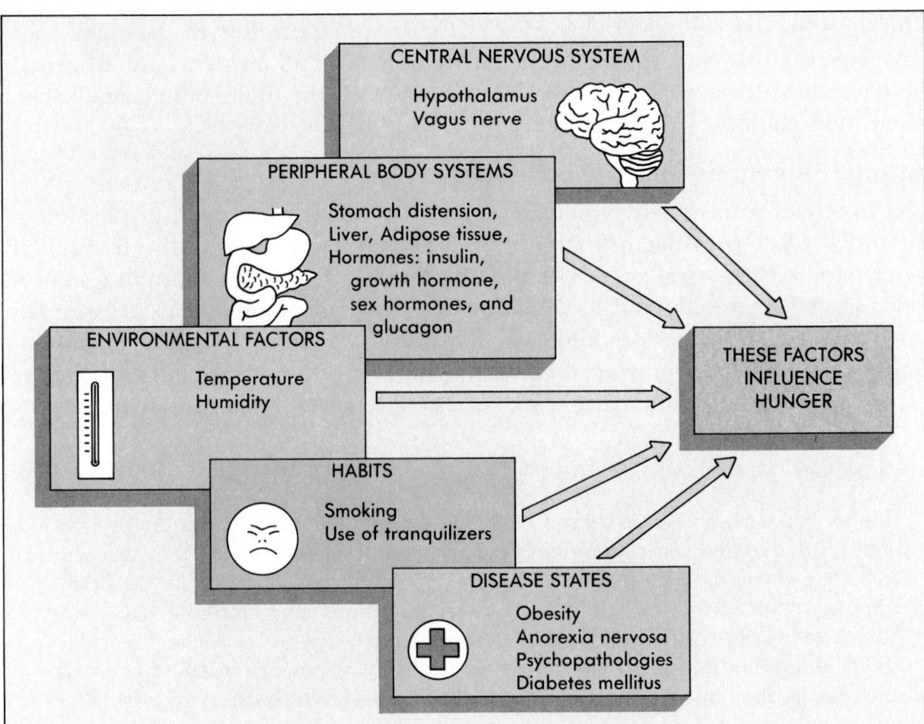

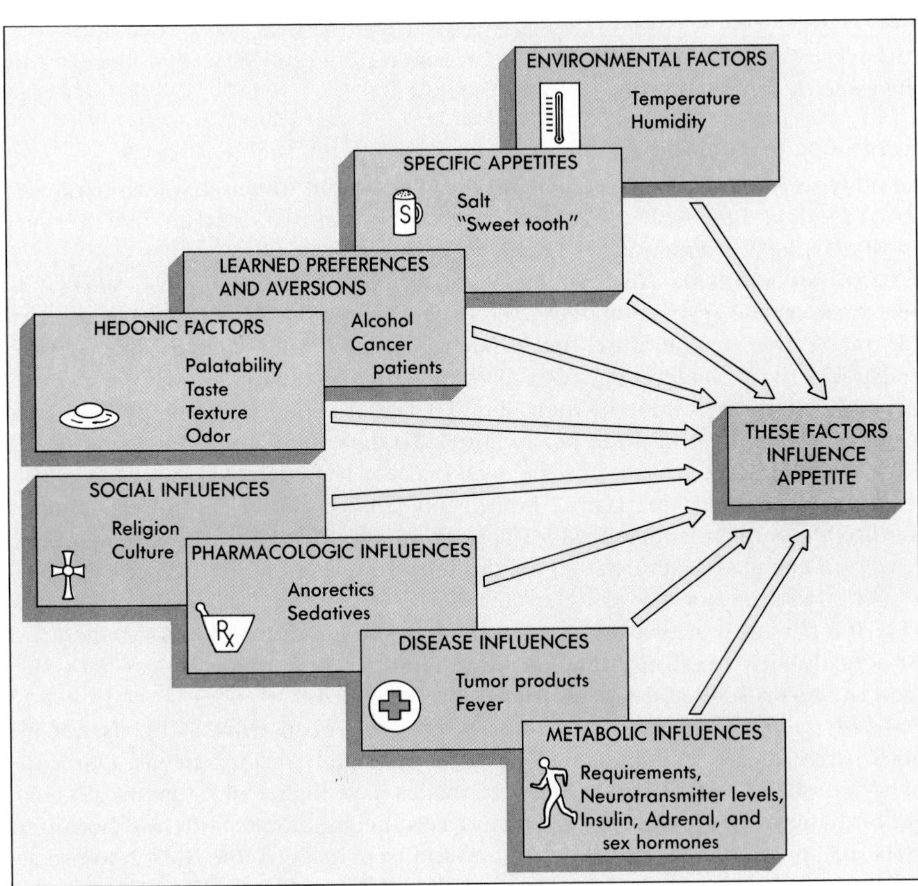

Figure 8-2

A model incorporating many factors that influence hunger and appetite.

Exploring Issues and Actions

Try eating salad after the entree, if you don't eat this way now. What do you think about this practice? Do you like mashed potatoes? How about for breakfast? If not, why not? Is your reaction physiological or psychological?

Although this may be partly due to social custom, research with laboratory animals suggests that this action is also partly biological. As nutrients are absorbed, the liver and surrounding organs communicate with the brain and change subsequent food choices.[1]

Putting hunger and appetite into perspective

Next time you wonder why you are hungry, you will know numerous physiological and psychological factors are involved (Figure 8-2). Cells in the brain, oral cavity, stomach, intestine, liver, and other organs, hormones (insulin), neurotransmitters (serotonin), and social customs all influence food intake.[20,29] Though appetite factors probably predominate in humans who have foods available, hunger mechanisms predominate in laboratory animals. Keep track of what drives you to eat food during the next few days. Is it primarily hunger or appetite?

Concept Check

Hunger is the physiological drive to find and eat food, and appetite is the psychological drive to find and eat food. Appeasing them both should leave you in a satiated state—you have no further desire to eat. Hunger is influenced by the brain, adipose tissue, liver, other organs, various hormones, and hormone-like compounds. Appetite is affected by social custom, time of day, food availability, palatability, and other factors. North Americans probably respond primarily to appetite cues, rather than hunger cues, in choosing what and when to eat.

ENERGY USE: THE OTHER SIDE OF ENERGY BALANCE

We have examined some stimuli for consuming energy. Now let's look at the other side of the relationship—energy output.

Other names for the thermic effect of food include specific dynamic action and diet-induced thermogenesis.

Energy use by the body

The body uses energy for three general purposes: **basal metabolism, thermic effect of food,** and physical activity. A fourth use—adaptive or facultative thermogenesis—is heat production when shivering due to cold.[24,28]

basal metabolism
The minimum energy the body requires to support itself when resting and awake. To have basal metabolic rate (BMR) measured, a person must fast for the previous 12 hours and must be maintained in a warm, quiet environment during the measurement. It amounts to roughly 1 kcalorie per minute, or about 1400 kcalories per day.

Basal metabolism. *Basal metabolism represents the minimum energy it takes to keep the resting awake body alive.* This includes maintaining a heart beat, respiration, temperature, and other functions. It does not include energy needs for activity or digesting foods. Basal metabolism amounts to about 1 kcalorie per kilogram per hour in men and 0.9 kcalorie per kilogram per hour in women (or roughly 1 kcalorie per minute). To determine a person's basal metabolic rate (BMR), he or she must lie awake in a warm room, as relaxed as possible, after not eating in the last 12 hours. Oxygen consumption (and usually carbon dioxide output) is measured for approximately 15 minutes. This then would be used to calculate kcalorie use (see the following section on indirect calorimetry). The best time of day to determine BMR is just after waking from a night's sleep. If a person is at rest but cannot meet all the conditions for BMR, then the test actually yields **resting metabolic rate** (RMR). These differ by less than 3%. Often the terms BMR and RMR are used interchangeably.[24]

While at rest about 40% of body energy is used by the brain and liver together, about 20% by muscle, and about 2% to 5% by adipose tissue.

Basal metabolism depends primarily on ***lean body mass.*** The tissues involved show high metabolic activity, and so have high kcalorie needs. Other influences on basal metabolism are gender (males have higher rates due to a higher lean body mass), temperature (fever increases metabolic rate), thyroid hormone levels, age, nutritional state, pregnancy, and muscle mass (Table 8-2). A low-kcalorie intake decreases BMR about 10% to 20% (about 150 to 300 kcalories per day). This reduction makes dieting even harder (see Chapter 9). In addition, it is hard to maintain a desirable body weight as we age because BMR declines approximately 2% every 10 years after age 30. This is mostly caused by a slow and

Table 8-2

Factors that increase and decrease basal metabolism

Increase	Decrease
Muscle mass (fat-free mass)	Age (primarily if lean body mass decreases)
Fever	Reduction in energy intake
Recent food intake	
Ovulation	
Surface area	
Recent exercise	
Thyroid hormone level	
Trauma	
Epinephrine	
Male gender (greater lean body mass)	
Pregnancy	

steady decrease in actively metabolizing cells, which is due to aging (see Chapter 17). *However, people who remain active into their elderly years do not show such a great decline in basal metabolism because lean body mass is better maintained.*

Thermic effect of food. Thermic effect of food represents the amount of extra energy used by the body during digestion, absorption, and associated metabolism of energy-yielding nutrients. The thermic effect of food is analogous to a sales tax, in this case, a charge of about 5% to 10% of total kcalories consumed. To supply the body 100 kcalories, a person must eat between 105 and 110 kcalories. The process of digestion, absorption, and metabolism uses the extra 5 to 10 kcalories to modify the nutrients so that they are more available for use. Given a daily kcalorie intake of 3000, the thermic effect of food would use 180 to 300 kcalories. The value for the thermic effect of food for either a pure-carbohydrate or pure-protein diet is higher than for a pure-fat diet. When you eat excess carbohydrate or protein, the liver turns it mostly into fat. Other organs are also involved in the metabolism. The energy needed contributes to the thermic effect.[28]

thermic effect of food The increase in metabolism occurring during the digestion, absorption, and metabolism of energy-yielding nutrients. This represents 5 percent to 10 percent of kcalories consumed.

In many animals—including humans to an undetermined extent—the thermic effect of food is also linked to the presence of **brown adipose tissue.** Recall that most fat is stored in white adipose tissue (see Chapter 5). Brown adipose tissue is a specialized form of fat storage found primarily in the shoulder area. For hibernating animals it is a main source of heat during their long winter sleep. The brown tint derives from the ample content of arteries and veins that supply the tissue with blood, plus the numerous mitochondria that are present to allow for enhanced energy metabolism.

brown adipose tissue A specialized form of adipose tissue that produces large amounts of heat by metabolizing energy-yielding nutrients without synthesizing much ATP. The energy released simply forms heat.

Brown adipose tissue yields heat by **uncoupling** the metabolism of energy-yielding nutrients with the formation of ATP. In Chapter 7 we noted that metabolism in the mitochondria helps turn the chemical energy inherent in glucose, fat, protein, and alcohol into ATP energy. In brown adipose tissue the mitochondria release this energy from foods, but little is used to make ATP. Most energy in the food is lost as heat. Thus these cells have the ability to make a lot of heat and, in turn, "waste" a lot of energy.

uncoupling The dissociation between liberation of energy from energy-yielding substances and the formation of ATP.

cafeteria-fed animal
A laboratory animal that is fed a high-fat and sugary diet to encourage it to overeat and become obese.

This manner of wasting energy is induced in **"cafeteria-fed" animals.** In response to consuming high-sugar, high-fat snacks, the animals show an enhanced thermic effect of food. This allows them to eat extra kcalories, presumably so that they can eventually obtain needed protein from these low-protein food sources without gaining as much fat as they would otherwise.

Whether brown adipose tissue works in adults—or is even present—is questionable. If you touch an infant's back, you can feel the heat produced by the brown adipose tissue. Sensitive instruments can demonstrate hotter spots around the shoulder area of adults, as well. However, it is difficult to determine how much heat production this represents in adults. Modern humans may be so coddled that the brown adipose tissue found in infancy mostly disappears by adulthood. Researchers in Finland suggest that brown adipose tissue is present in the shoulder area of lumberjacks and other people who spend the long winter months outdoors.

Tables listing the energy costs of various activities include values for the energy needs for basal metabolism and for the thermic effect of food (see Appendix J). Typical values are jogging at 5 to 10 kcalories per minute, tennis and cycling at 5 to 7 kcalories per minute, and swimming at 5 to 11 kcalories per minute. Reading this book takes about 1.5 kcalories per minute.

At this time the presence of brown adipose tissue in adults and its link to the thermic effect of food is open to question. Although it is unlikely that brown adipose tissue serves a pivotal role in weight regulation in adults, information is too sketchy to permit any definite conclusions.

Physical activity. Body energy also fuels physical activity. Physical activity level is the biggest variable in energy use among people. Basal metabolism is roughly the same in most people (usually ± 25% to 30%, though greater differences occur), as are the energy expenditures for the thermic effect of food.[24] Together, basal metabolism and the thermic effect of food represent about 60% to 75% of total energy use.[28] The big difference in energy use among people is due to different activity levels. Some people are very active physically and others are very sedentary.

Energy used for physical activity includes expenditures for sports such as handball and bicycling and for everyday activities. Using stairs rather than the elevator, walking rather than driving to the store, and standing in a bus rather than sitting—all increase physical activity and hence energy use. Recent studies show that people who fidget and can't sit still use more energy (an extra 100 to 800 kcalories per day in one study) than those who are generally quite relaxed.[25] As we will discuss in Chapter 9, the rates of obesity in North America are alarming. *We do not eat so many more kcalories than people did at the turn of this century, but as a group we are considerably less active. This inactivity contributes to our increased rates of obesity over those people of the early 1900s.*

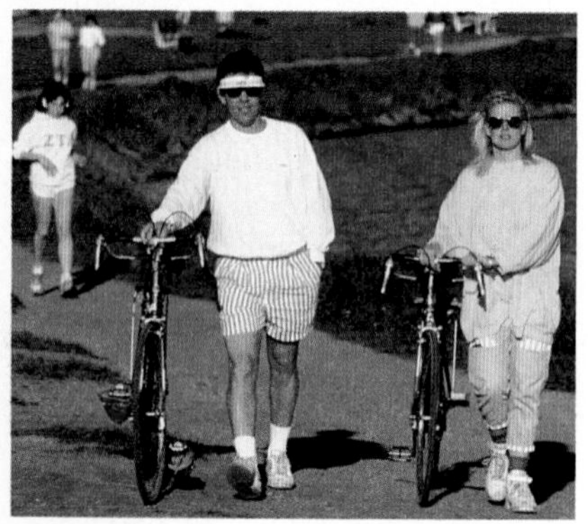

Bicycling is an excellent way to increase your energy output.

Concept Check

The body uses energy for three main purposes. Basal metabolism represents the minimum amount of energy needed to maintain a body in a resting state. The rate of a person's basal metabolism depends greatly upon the proportion of lean body mass, the amount of surface area, and thyroid hormone levels. The thermic effect of food represents the additional energy needed to digest, absorb, and process absorbed nutrients. This corresponds to about 5% to 10% of total kcalorie intake. Physical activity represents energy use above what is needed for basal metabolism and the thermic effect of food. In a sedentary person, 60% to 75% of energy is used for basal metabolism and the thermic effect of food; the remainder is used for physical activity.

direct calorimetry
A method to determine energy use by the body by measuring heat that emanates from the body, usually using an insulated chamber.

MEASURING ENERGY USE BY THE BODY

Direct and indirect calorimetry

There are two primary ways to measure the amount of energy the body uses: **direct calorimetry** and **indirect calorimetry.** When using direct calorimetry, a person is put into an insulated chamber, and the heat he or she releases is calculated by measuring the increase in the temperature of a layer of water surrounding the chamber. Recall that a kcalorie is defined as the amount of heat it takes to raise 1 liter of water 1° Celsius. By measuring the water temperature in the direct calorimeter before and after the study, the number of kcalories used can be determined. This method resembles that of using the bomb calorimeter to measure the kcalorie content of a food (see Chapter 1). Direct calorimetry works because all the energy used by the body eventually leaves as heat.[18]

Older direct calorimeters were quite large, about the size of a small room. Newer calorimeters are the size of a phone booth or smaller, about the size of a space suit. Nevertheless, few studies use direct calorimetry, mostly because of its expense and complexity.

indirect calorimetry
A method to measure the energy output by the body by measuring oxygen uptake and/or carbon dioxide output, and then using formulas to convert that gas exchange into kcalorie use.

In using indirect calorimetry, instead of measuring heat, a technician measures either the amount of oxygen a person takes up or the amount of oxygen taken up plus the quantity of carbon dioxide given off (Figure 8-3). There is a predictable relationship between the body's use of energy and its use of oxygen or carbon dioxide output. For example, when burning a mixed diet of carbohydrate, fat, and protein, the body uses 1 liter of of oxygen to burn about 4.85 kcalories. Generally, this mixture of nutrients is just the fuel the body uses.

The amount of energy that each liter of oxygen represents actually depends on a person's ratio of carbon dioxide output to oxygen uptake. This ratio is called the respiratory quotient, or RQ. However, it is possible to ignore the effect of the RQ because it is small.

Instruments used to measure oxygen consumption (and often carbon dioxide output, too) for indirect calorimetry are widely available. They can be mounted on carts and rolled up to a hospital bed or carried in backpacks while a person plays tennis or jogs. Tables showing the amount of energy used to perform various exercises rely on indirect calorimetry to calculate their figures (see Appendix J).

The newest approach to indirect calorimetry has a person to consume isotopically labeled water ($^2H_2{}^{18}O$). A technician measures the ^2H_2O and the $H_2{}^{18}O$ produced. Using formulas and some assumptions, total carbon dioxide (CO_2) output per day can then be estimated by measuring these forms of water in body fluids, such as urine. This CO_2 value then can be converted into energy use, just as is done with oxygen use in indirect calorimetry.[27] Both ^2H and ^{18}O represent stable isotopes of hydrogen and oxygen; special equipment can measure them.

This isotope method is quite accurate but also very expensive. With wider use, we expect it to soon extend our knowledge of variation in energy use by people over entire day periods. This information may further reveal why some people can more easily regulate their body weight than others.

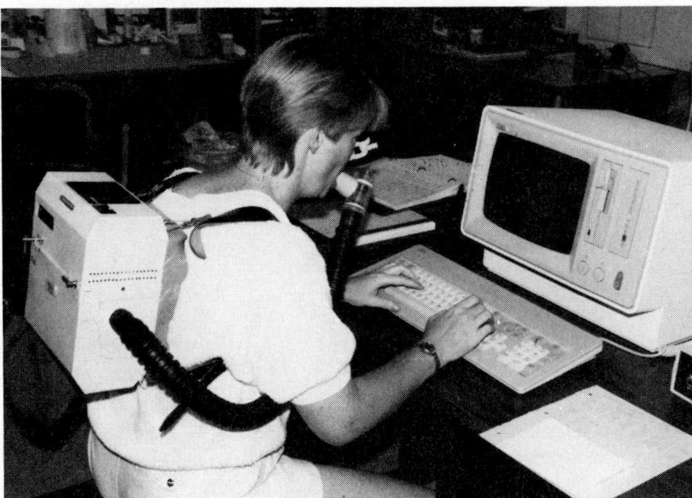

Figure 8-3

Indirect calorimetry. This method can be used to measure energy output during daily activities.

Harris-Benedict equation
An equation that predicts resting metabolic rate based on a person's weight, height, and age.

Estimating energy needs

A variety of formulas can estimate the body's resting energy needs (see Appendix M). The **Harris-Benedict equation,** widely used by registered dietitians for hospitalized patients, considers weight, height, and age. The value for resting energy needs is then increased by a predetermined factor to reflect a patient's degree of illness.[10] That value then gives total energy needs. Owen and others[23] have published standards for resting energy needs based on weight alone. The equations apply to both normal-weight and overweight people. Use of either formula yields reasonable estimates.

Total energy needs can be roughly estimated using the RDA. This provides average values for people who perform light activity (see inside this book's cover). Another rough estimate uses a person's weight and activity level. Sedentary energy needs are set at 9 to 10 kcalories per pound. The value is then decreased by 100 kcalories for every 10 years of age over age 30. Light activity starts with 12 to 13 kcalories per pound; heavy activity starts at 20 kcalories per pound, and values are then adjusted for age.

Concept Check

Energy use by the body can be measured by direct calorimetry as heat given off, and by indirect calorimetry as oxygen uptake (with or without carbon dioxide output). Energy needs, both resting and total, can be estimated using formulas based on a person's weight, height, and age, or simply on weight.

ENERGY IMBALANCE

Problems associated with the major type of energy imbalance in North America—obesity—go far beyond any social stigma (Table 8-3). Many health problems are caused by obesity.[7,19,21] These include an increased risk in surgery, non-

Table 8-3

Percent of overweight persons ages 20 to 74

	No. examined	Percent
Both sexes		
All races	11,765	25.7
Black	1,326	35.7
White	10,214	24.8
Male		
All races	5,604	24.2
Black	607	25.7
White	4,883	24.4
Female		
All races	6,161	27.1
Black	719	43.8
White	5,331	25.1

Note: Overweight in this study is defined as a sex-specific body mass index equal to or higher than the 85th percentile for examinees age 20-29 (Corresponds to a body mass index greater than 27–see text for details).
From: The NCHS report "Anthropometric Reference Data and Prevalence of Overweight, United States, 1976–1980, data from the second National Health and Nutrition Examination Survey (NHANES II), conducted 1976–1980. Data on body weight were obtained through height and weight examinations and anthropometric measurements.

Table 8-4

Health problems associated with excess body fat

Health problem	Partially attributed to:
Surgical risk	Increased anesthesia needs
Pulmonary disease	Excess weight over lungs
Adult-onset diabetes mellitus (NIDDM)	Enlarged adipose cells, which then poorly bind insulin and also poorly respond to the message insulin sends to the cell
Hypertension	Increased miles of blood vessels found in the fat tissue; however, no validated cause is yet known
Coronary heart disease	Increases in serum cholesterol and triglyceride levels, as well as a decrease in physical activity
Bone and joint disorders	Excess pressure put on knee, ankle, and hip joints
Gallbladder stones	An increase in cholesterol content of bile
Skin disorders	The trapping of moisture and microbes in fat folds
Various cancers	Estrogen production by adipose cells; animal studies suggest excess energy intake encourages tumor development
Shorter stature	An earlier onset of puberty

The greater the degree of obesity, the more serious these health problems can become. They are much more likely to appear in people who are greater than twice their desirable body weight.

insulin-dependent (adult-onset) diabetes mellitus, hypertension, heart disease, arthritis, gallstones, and various forms of cancer—such as colon, rectal, and prostate cancer in men and breast, uterine, and ovarian cancer in women. Possible explanations of why obesity causes these disorders are listed in Table 8-4. Let's now attempt to define obesity.

Defining obesity

Obesity can be defined using several different approaches. Here we will consider definitions based on body weight, body fat, fat distribution, and age of onset.

Using body weight. Overweight can be defined as weighing 10% more than desirable body weight. ***Obesity** is then defined as weighing 20% more than desirable body weight. Body weight is actually a crude measure because we are concerned about overfat, not simply overweight (obese) individuals.* However, overfat and overweight (obese) conditions almost always appear together: the husky athlete is the exception. We focus on body weight mainly because it is easier to measure than total body fat. More on this will be discussed.

obesity
A condition characterized by excess body fat, usually defined as weighing 20% above desirable weight.

To further define obesity, weighing 20% to 40% more than desirable body weight represents mild obesity, weighing 41% to 99% more than desirable body weight represents moderate obesity, weighing more than twice desirable body weight represents severe (morbid) obesity (Figure 8-4). In North America about 90% of cases of obesity are of the mild form. This condition carries little health

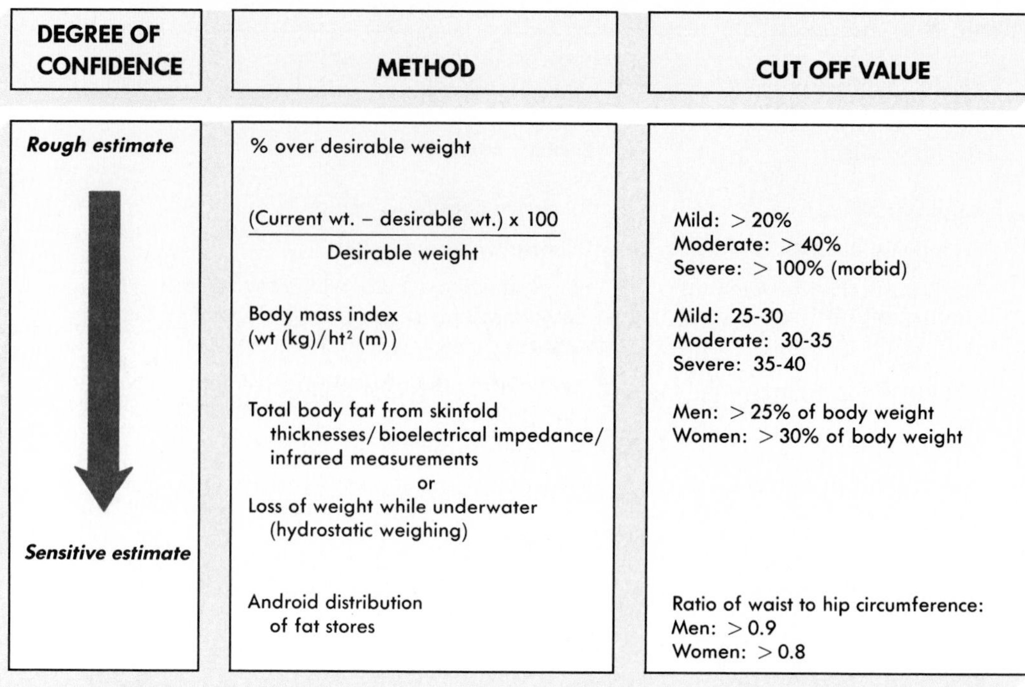

Figure 8-4
Diagnosing the extent of obesity to predict health risk. If one is obese by any of these measures and has an android distribution of fat stores, the risk of complications is more likely than if the fat distribution is gynecoid.

risk. *About 0.2% of cases are severe: this condition carries a twelvefold increase in health risk.*

Desirable body weight is usually based on the current Metropolitan Life Insurance Table (Table 8-5). This table lists for any height the weight that is associated with a maximum life span. *The table does not tell what weight will make one the healthiest while alive. It simply lists the weight most associated with longevity.*[31]

As a clinical tool, the Metropolitan Life Insurance Table is valuable. In 1985 a conference of physicians and research scientists supported its use.[21] However, nagging problems remain. The table's data are derived only from purchasers of life insurance. This results in under-representation for poor people and many minorities. People who smoke are included in the Table, and they often have both lower body weights and earlier ages of death because of their increased risk for lung cancer and heart disease. This distorted representation may mean that the table overestimates the best weight for maximum longevity. In addition, body weight was only determined at the time the insurance policy was purchased. No follow-up weights were recorded. A positive point is that the table does not include insured persons with significant diseases, such as heart disease, cancer, and diabetes.[31]

We mention this controversy because it helps put the desirable weight figure listed by the Metropolitan Life Insurance Table into perspective. If you weigh slightly more—or less—than the range listed but show no ill health, it is not

The term *desirable body weight* was first used in 1959 by the Metropolitan Life Insurance Company. At that time it replaced the term *ideal body weight.* The 1983 tables used neither the terms *desirable* nor *ideal.* Both are commonly seen in medical literature. The tendency today is to use the term *desirable* rather than *ideal.*

Table 8-5

1983 Metropolitan Life Insurance Co height and weight table

Height	Small frame	Medium frame	Large frame
		Weight in pounds	
Men*			
5′ 2″	128-134	131-141	138-150
5′ 3″	130-136	133-143	140-153
5′ 4″	132-138	135-145	142-156
5′ 5″	134-140	137-148	144-160
5′ 6″	136-142	139-151	146-164
5′ 7″	138-145	142-154	149-168
5′ 8″	140-148	145-157	152-172
5′ 9″	142-151	148-160	155-176
5′10″	144-154	151-163	158-180
5′11″	146-157	154-166	161-184
6′ 0″	149-160	157-170	164-188
6′ 1″	152-164	160-174	168-192
6′ 2″	155-168	164-178	172-197
6′ 3″	158-172	167-182	176-202
6′ 4″	162-176	171-187	181-207
Women†			
4′10″	102-111	109-121	118-131
4′11″	103-113	111-123	120-134
5′ 0″	104-115	113-126	122-137
5′ 1″	106-118	115-129	125-140
5′ 2″	108-121	118-132	128-143
5′ 3″	111-124	121-135	131-147
5′ 4″	114-127	124-138	134-151
5′ 5″	117-130	127-141	137-155
5′ 6″	120-133	130-144	140-159
5′ 7″	123-136	133-147	143-163
5′ 8″	126-139	136-150	146-167
5′ 9″	129-142	139-153	149-170
5′10″	132-145	142-156	152-173
5′11″	135-148	145-159	155-176
6′ 0″	138-151	148-162	158-179

*Weights at ages 25 to 59, based on lowest mortality. Weight in pounds according to frame (in indoor clothing weighing 5 lb, shoes with 1″ heels).
†Weights at ages 25 to 59, based on lowest mortality. Weight in pounds according to frame (in indoor clothing weighing 3 lb, shoes with 1″ heels).
Source: Courtesy of Metropolitan Life Insurance Company.

Other tables, such as those generated by the U.S. Nutrition Survey NHANES I, can be used to estimate desirable weight (see Appendix L). Appendix L also includes the Andres Table. This can be used for elderly people who show no diseases associated with obesity. It allows for a gradual increase in body fat as one ages through adulthood, noting this is of little concern if no health problems are associated with the weight gain.

necessarily cause for alarm. In addition, the weight ranges listed in Table 8-5 do not guarantee health when alive. They simply attempt to maximize the chances of living as long as possible.

The weight and height values in the Metropolitan Life Insurance Table assume one is wearing clothes and shoes. Note also that the table refers only to people under 60 years of age. It is not clear if overweight or obesity in elderly people follows the same pattern of association with disease as it does in younger people (see Chapter 17). An obese elderly person may have already avoided the typical causes of death, such as stroke, heart disease, and cancer, to which obesity contributes. The fact that they have survived into their 70s and 80s could suggest that they are more resistant to the effects of obesity than people who have already succumbed.

The Metropolitan Life Insurance Table adjusts for small, medium, and large frame sizes. Methods for estimating frame size use measurements of wrist width or elbow breadth (Table 8-6). The methods yield similar values.[22] *However, although these methods exist, frame size was never measured in the men and women used to develop the Metropolitan Life Insurance Table.* Researchers at the Metropolitan Life Insurance Company simply estimated that 25% of people are small frame, 50% of people are medium frame, and 25% of people are large frame based on other studies. They then arbitrarily put the weight data into small, medium, and large frame categories based on those percentages.

Therefore frame size may not be that important to these estimates. You can consider obviously small and thin people as having a small frame, and obviously big and bulky people who have large bones as having a large frame. Consider everyone else as having a medium frame.

One method for estimating desirable body weight for women is to allow 100 pounds for the first 5 feet and then add 5 pounds for every inch thereafter. A desirable body weight in men corresponds to starting with 106 pounds for the first 5 feet and then adding 6 pounds for every inch thereafter. Other, similar formulas exist.

Table 8-6

Determination of frame size

Method 1

Height is recorded without shoes.

Wrist circumference is measured just distal to the styloid process at the wrist crease on the right arm using a tape measure.

The following formula is used:

$$r = \frac{\text{height (cm)}}{\text{wrist circumference (cm)}}$$

Frame size can be determined as follows:

Males	Females
r > 10.4 small	r > 11.0 small
r = 9.6-10.4 medium	r = 10.1-11.0 medium
r < 9.6 large	r < 10.1 large

Source: Grant JP: Handbook of Total Parenteral Nutrition, Philadelphia, 1980, WB Saunders Co.

Method 2

The patient's right arm is extended forward perpendicular to the body, with the arm bent so the angle at the elbow forms 90° with the fingers pointing up and the palm turned away from the body. The greatest breadth across the elbow joint is measured with a sliding caliper along the axis of the upper arm, on the two prominent bones on either side of the elbow. This is recorded as the elbow breadth. The following tables give the elbow breadth measurements for medium-framed men and women of various heights. Measurements lower than those listed indicate a small frame size; higher measurements indicate a large frame size.

Men		Women	
Height in 1″ Heels	Elbow Breadth	Height in 1″ Heels	Elbow Breadth
5′2″-5′3″	2½″-2⅞″	4″10″-4′11″	2¼″-2½″
5′4″-5′7″	2⅝″-2⅞″	5″0″-5′3″	2¼″-2½″
5′8″-5′11″	2¾″-3″	5″4″-5′7″	2⅜″-2⅝″
6′0″-6′3″	2¾″-3⅛″	5″8″-5′11″	2⅜″-2⅝″
6′4″	2⅞″-3¼″	6″0″	2½″-2¾″

From: Metropolitan Life Insurance Co, 1983.

Using body mass index. Another way to define obesity is to calculate the **body mass index.**[8] This is a person's weight in kilograms divided by height in meters squared (Figure 8-5). For instance, a 70-kilogram man who is 1.78 meters tall has a body mass index of: $70 \div (1.78^2) = 22$. This particular value is the midpoint of the Metropolitan Life Insurance Table values and represents the lowest risk for mortality. Figure 8-5 shows that health risks from obesity for men and women begin when the body mass index exceeds about 25. At a value of about 27, the risk for diabetes or hypertension is 2.9 times greater than normal, and the risk for a high serum cholesterol level (greater than 250 milligrams per deciliter) is 2.1 times normal. *A body mass index above 30 poses an even greater risk for health problems and is often used as the cutoff for obesity* (Figure 8-4).[7] About 10% to 14% of North Americans exceed this value. A body mass index above 40 represents quite a high risk for health problems.[7,8]

body mass index
Weight in kilograms divided by height squared (in meters); a value of 30 or more indicates obesity.

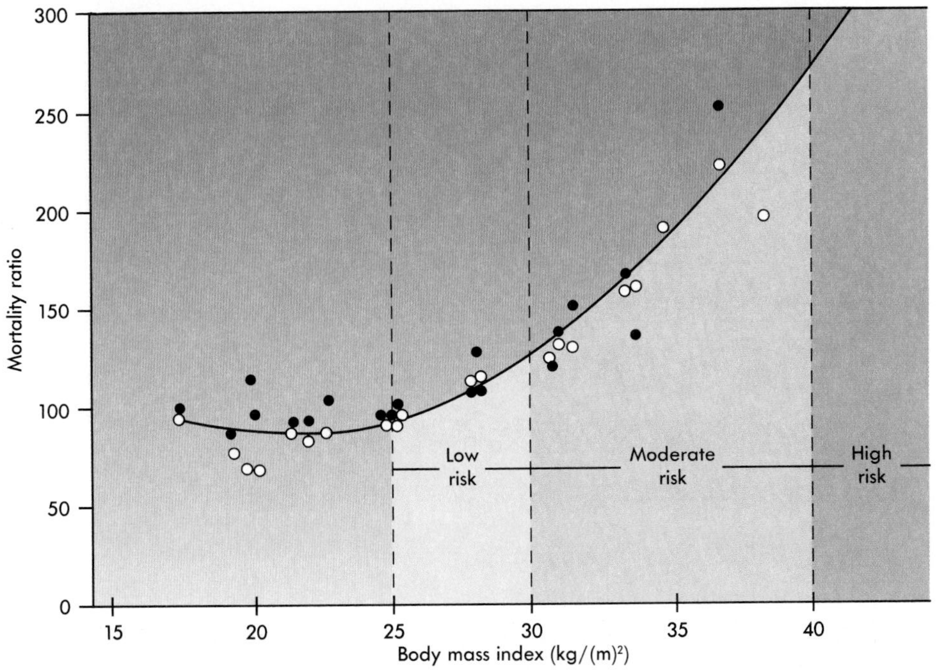

Figure 8-5
The relationship between body mass index and death rates (100 equals normal death rate). Solid circles show persons aged 20 to 29 years, and open circles show persons aged 30 to 39 years.

Do not be alarmed when you look at Figure 8-5 and see an increased risk of disease at very low values of body mass index. This increased risk of disease at a low body mass index probably reflects the poor health of people who smoke.

Notice that the graph in Figure 8-5 is curvilinear rather than linear. As one reaches a higher body mass index, health risk increases even more. Thus health risk increases at an even greater rate than does body mass index. The concept of body mass index is convenient to use because the cutoff values apply to both men and women, and no complicated table is needed.

Using body fat. References to the risks of being overweight usually refer only to people who are overfat. Specifically, *men having over 25% body fat and women having over 30% body fat are obese* (Figure 8-4). More desirable figures are 15% to 18% body fat for men and 20% to 25% fat for women.[8,17] Women need more body fat because some "sex-specific" fat is associated with their reproductive functions. This extra fat is normal and so factored into calculations of body composition.

A variety of methods can be used to determine how much fat a person contains. The most widely used method measures skinfold thicknesses. Over half of body fat lies directly under the skin. Clinicians use a special caliper to measure this fat layer. The amount of fat under the skin (subcutaneous) in turn reflects the fat composition of the body. Better methods use three or four skinfold measurements taken throughout the body to estimate total body fat (Figure 8-6).[17] With

Using skinfold thickness to predict body composition is one of the tools of anthropometry, which was discussed in Chapter 2. Anthropometry represents the measurement of lengths, weights, circumferences, and thicknesses on the outside of the body.

practice, these measurements take less than 10 minutes and the body fat values calculated are quite accurate.

bioelectrical impedance
A method to estimate total body fat that measures the impedance (resistance) of a low-energy electrical current by the body; the more fat storage a person has, the more impedance to electrical flow will be exhibited.

Clinicians have recently begun to measure body fat storage using **bioelectrical impedance** (Figure 8-7). This technique uses a low-energy electrical current. Fat resists the flow of electricity. Thus the more fat storage a person has per inch of height, the more resistance. Bioelectrical impedance analyzers convert body electrical resistance into an estimate of the percent of body that is fat. The test takes only about 5 minutes.

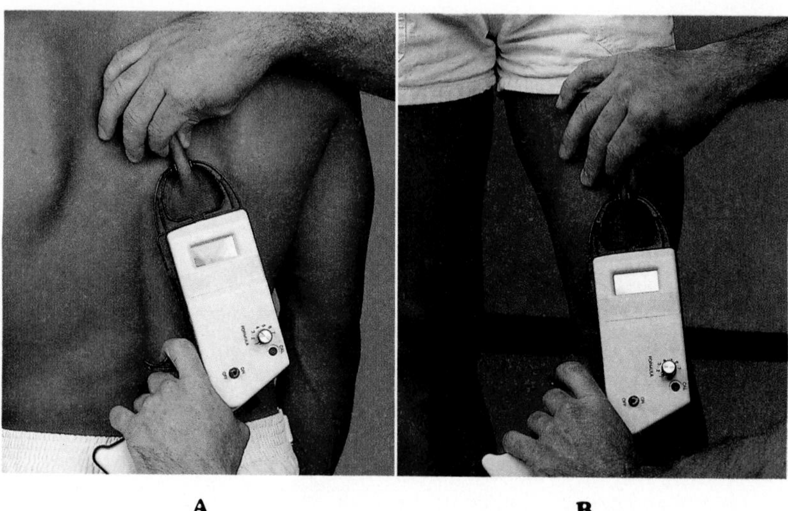

A B

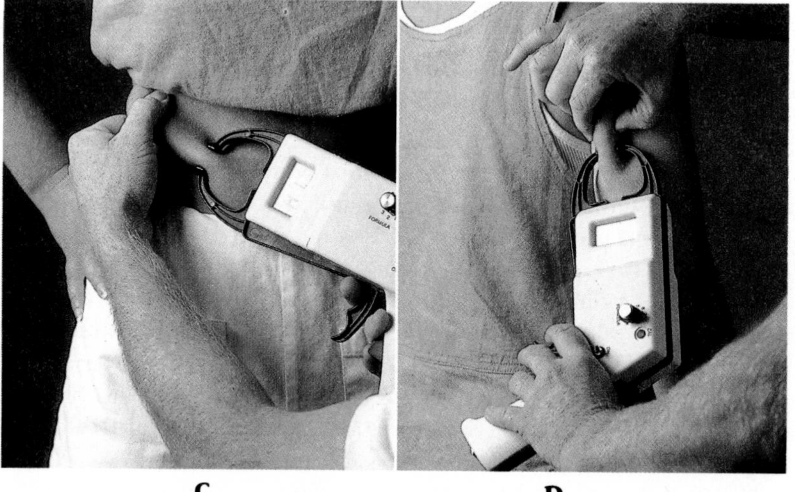

C D

Figure 8-6

Skinfold measurements. Using a proper technique, calibrated equipment, and standards, skinfold measurements can be used to accurately predict body fat content in about 20 minutes. Commonly measured skinfolds are: (A) subscapular. (B) Thigh. (C) Suprailiac. (D) Triceps.

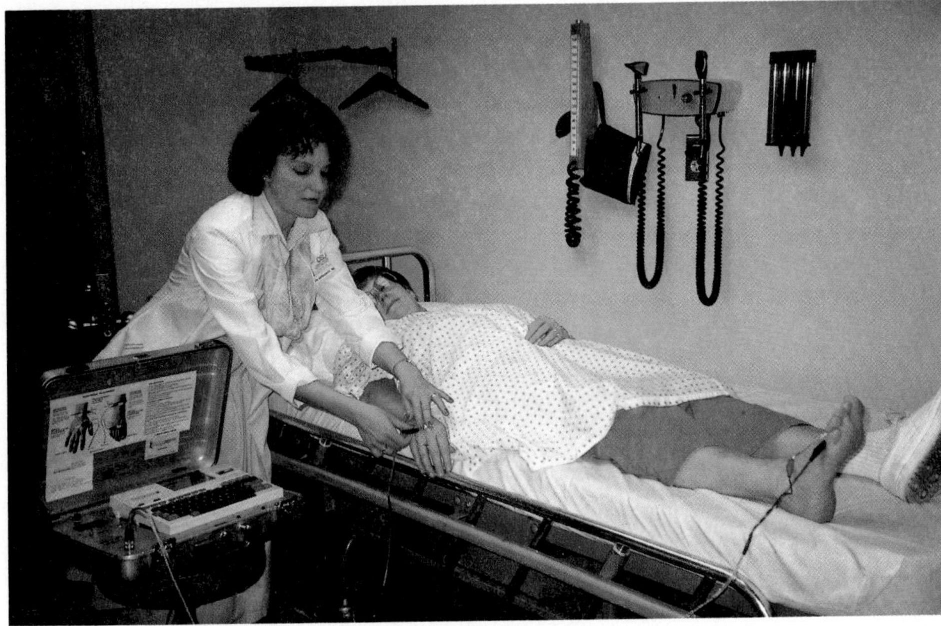

Figure 8-7

Bioelectrical impedence. This method can accurately be used to estimate total body fat in less than 5 minutes.

Both skinfold thickness and bioelectrical impedance methods were developed using body fat values determined by underwater weighing for comparison. Comparing a person's weight on land to his weight underwater can yield a very accurate estimate of body fat. This works because adipose tissue is less dense than lean tissue, and so the more adipose tissue in a body, the less a person weighs when submerged (the more he tends to float).

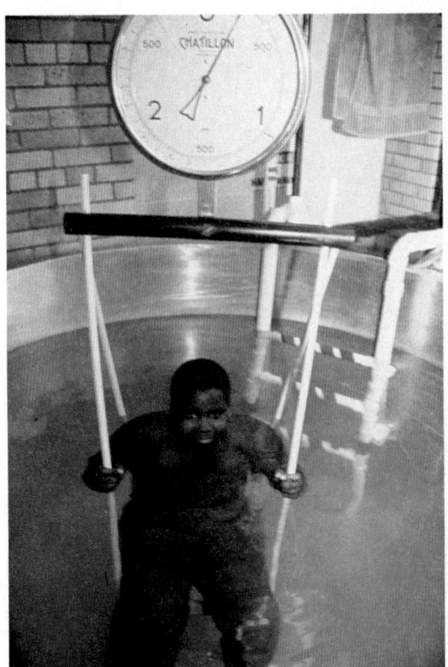

In addition, bioelectrical impedance values are affected by recent food intake, recent exercise, recent alcohol intake, and the use of certain medications, such as diuretics. To get an accurate value, the person must not have consumed alcohol within the last 24 hours, not have eaten within the last 4 hours, not have exercised hard within the last 12 hours, and not have recently taken medication that affects water balance in the body.

Another new method for estimating body fat uses infrared light interactions with the fat and protein in arm muscle. A device the size of a flashlight is held on the biceps muscle. Total body fat is then estimated after 2 seconds of infrared exposure.

Using body fat distribution. Calculating distribution of fat stores, in addition to the amount of fat, is also instrumental in assessing obesity—especially for predicting health risks (Figure 8-4). Obese people can be categorized as **android** or **gynecoid** (sometimes called gynoid). Android obesity is the characteristic male obesity with a large abdomen (pot belly) and a small buttocks and thighs (apple appearance).[8,14] High testosterone levels in men are thought to encourage upper body fat deposition. Fat storage in this area appears to be easier to lose than in the thigh area.

android obesity
The type of obesity in which fat is stored primarily in the abdominal area; defined as a waist-to-hip circumference ratio greater than 0.9 in men and 0.8 in women; closely associated with a high risk of heart disease, hypertension, and diabetes.

gynecoid obesity
Obesity in which fat storage is primarily located in the buttocks and thigh area.

Gynecoid obesity is the typical female obesity pattern showing a small abdomen and a much larger buttocks and thigh area (pear appearance). Women tend to have this type of obesity because the cells in this area contain more lipoprotein lipase, the enzyme that pushes fat from the bloodstream into fat cells. Furthermore, progesterone, a female hormone, increases the action of lipoprotein lipase in the lower torso region. Thus there are biological reasons why men tend to have android obesity and women tend to have gynecoid obesity.

A ratio of waist circumference (at the level of the umbilicus) to hip circumference greater than 0.9 in men and 0.8 in women indicates android obesity.[8,9] *The android form of obesity is associated with more heart disease, hyperten-*

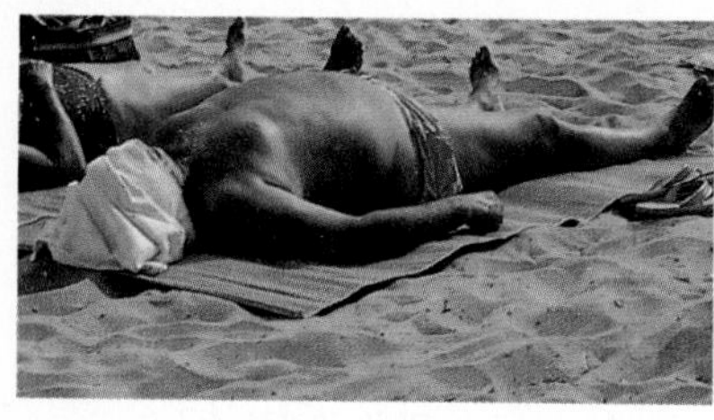

The android form of obesity is more common in men, and is associated with an increased risk for developing heart disease, hypertension, and diabetes mellitus.

sion, and diabetes than is gynecoid obesity. This may be because adipose tissue in the abdominal area more greatly resists the action of insulin, in turn increasing the risk of developing diabetes mellitus. Developing diabetes mellitus then leads to an increased risk of developing heart disease and hypertension. Data from the Honolulu Heart Study show that an android shape can increase health risk in men even if they are not obese.[11] Only a small percentage of women have android obesity.

Using age of onset. Obesity can be classified as **juvenile-onset, adult-onset,** or **endocrine-onset** (Table 8-7).[8] The latter includes obesity caused by relatively rare hormonal abnormalities and rare genetic disorders.

Table 8-7

Types of obesity	
Juvenile-Onset:	Hyperplastic—increased fat cell number Hypertrophic—larger fat cells
Adult-Onset:	Mainly hypertrophic About 80% to 90% of obesity is adult-onset
Endocrine:	Hypothyroidism, hypercorticoidism, brain tumors, Prader-Willi syndrome, Turner's syndrome, and others.

hyperplasia
An increase in cell number.

hypertrophy
An increase in cell size.

When obesity develops in infancy or childhood, the person develops more adipose cells, and each adipose cell grows greatly. When obesity develops in adulthood, the person usually ends up with a normal number of adipose cells, but each cell contains a large amount of fat. Adipose tissue consisting of a large number of cells shows **hyperplasia,** and adipose tissue consisting of large cells shows **hypertrophy.** Juvenile-onset obesity tends to be both hyperplastic and hypertrophic. Adult-onset obesity tends to be mainly hypertrophic, but in cases of extreme obesity can be both hyperplasic and hypertrophic.[18]

There has been concern for the last 20 years that in cases of juvenile-onset obesity it is more difficult for a person to lose weight than with the adult-onset type of obesity. This is because the increased number of fat cells accompanying juvenile-onset obesity may increase the body's resistance to greatly reducing fat stores. It is hard to rid oneself of these cells because they have a very long life span. It is possible, then, that each adipose cell needs to contain a certain amount of fat. In that case, more adipose cells automatically require more fat storage, and that condition would make it very hard to reduce total body fat to a desirable level. We are not sure whether such is the case. *It is clear that the longer one is obese, the more difficult it is to correct the problem.*

The individual path to obesity

Many paths lead to obesity, and each person with obesity has unique characteristics and problems. The clinician must tailor treatment to deal with these different problems. Dr. Kelly Brownell has published a list of possible characteristics of obese people that clinicians can use to begin to understand more about their clients.[9] Besides using body weight, body fat content, body fat distribution, and age of onset, other important factors to consider include family history of obesity, current energy expenditure, fasting blood glucose levels, and the extent of erroneous nutrition beliefs. *The variety of this list illustrates the many possible complications of an individual case of obesity.* Its multiple causes often make obesity a very heterogeneous disorder. As we discuss in Chapter 9, it requires consideration for individual treatment plans.

Dr. Brownell's research also indicates that a history of **yo-yo dieting**—losing and then regaining weight—can adversely affect obesity (see Dr. Brownell's Expert Opinion in Chapter 9). The chance for subsequent failure at weight loss may increase in these cases. Some experiments show that in a second bout of weight loss and regain, laboratory animals regain the lost weight in only half the time it took to regain it the first time they lost. Basal metabolism appears to dive even lower during a second dieting phase, setting up an energy-thrifty system that drives the animal to even more easily regain weight.

There are no data to suggest how long this yo-yo effect lasts in humans—that is, how long a cycle of dieting and weight regain affects future attempts at dieting. This is an active research area.

yo-yo dieting
The practice of losing weight and then regaining it, only to lose it and regain it again. This practice in animals (and probably humans) makes it more difficult to succeed in further attempts to lose weight because thyroid hormone levels drop very low in subsequent dieting, significantly slowing basal metabolism.

Concept Check

Obesity refers to a state of excessive body-fat storage. This usually corresponds to 20% over desirable body weight as predicted by the 1983 Metropolitan Life Insurance Table. A body mass index over 30 (calculated as weight in kilograms divided by height in meters squared) also indicates obesity. In addition, obesity corresponds to a percent of body fat greater than 25% in men and 30% in women. The actual amount of a person's body fat storage can be estimated using skinfold thicknesses or bioelectric impedance. Fat storage distribution further defines an obese state as android or gynecoid. Obesity in general leads to an increased risk for heart disease, some types of cancer, hypertension, adult-onset diabetes, bone and joint disorders, and some digestive disorders. The risks for some of these diseases are especially high if the fat storage is in an android distribution.

ENERGY USE IN OBESITY

Do obese and normal weight people differ in terms of energy use? Is there something inherent in an obese person that causes more or less efficient energy use

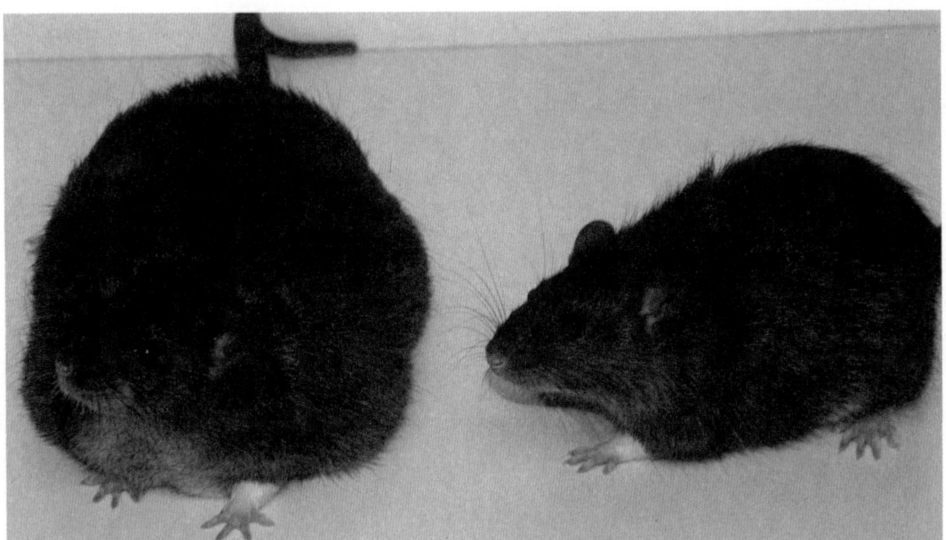

Figure 8-8

A rat with genetic obesity. No matter what type of diet the animal on the left eats, it will make more fat than the normal rat on the right. Genetics can have a powerful effect on the body composition of animals.

Expert Opinion

The Puzzle of Fat Cells

JULES HIRSCH, M.D.

Overweight and obesity are surely the most discussed—and probably the most prevalent—nutritional disorders in the United States today. More than 35 million Americans are sufficiently overweight or obese to be at serious risk for the development of diabetes mellitus, hypertension, heart disease, osteoarthritis, and very likely some types of cancer.

OVERWEIGHT VERSUS OBESITY

What's the difference between overweight and obesity? Someone with dense musculature may be overweight—that is, exceed the "desirable" weight on a weight chart—and yet not be fat (an athlete, for example). If weight exceeds 10% of the desirable weight, and the excess is due to fat storage, that person is only slightly obese, a condition that is sometimes called "overweight." If someone exceeds their desirable weight by 20% or more because of extra fat storage, that's significant and serious obesity. All the fat that causes either overweight or obesity is stored in a special tissue called adipose tissue. The fat, more correctly termed *triglyceride,* consists of long-chain fatty acids, each containing 16 to 18 carbon atoms—with or without double bonds—and all hooked to a small sugar called glycerol.

There is a good deal of triglyceride, and hence adipose tissue, even in people of perfectly normal weight. For example, a healthy, nonobese 68-kilogram (150-pound) man might carry as much as 9 kilograms (20 pounds) of fat. If he were to enter the ranks of the obese by gaining 13 kilograms (30 pounds), most of the weight gain would be an increase in the amount of stored fat, to roughly 18 kilograms (40 pounds). Some of the weight gain would be in nonfatty tissue, but the majority would be fat.

ADIPOSE TISSUES AND ITS CELLS

Like all tissues, adipose tissue is composed of many cells. Some are capillaries or ***fibroblasts*** that nourish and hold the characteristic cells (adipocytes) in place. About half the adipose tissue in an average person lies in subcutaneous depots just beneath the skin; the remainder is in deeper depots found in the abdomen. Smaller amounts are found around the kidneys, surrounding muscle fibers, and in such special areas as cushions behind the eyeballs and in joints.

The distribution of fat varies considerably from person to person, and there are notable differences between men and women. The male pattern, in which fat tends to be more centrally distributed in the abdomen, forms a pot belly when there's too much fat. This paunch is potentially dangerous because obese men, with excess fat storage primarily in and around the abdomen, are at greater risk for developing high blood pressure and diabetes mellitus than those in whom the fat is distributed in the more female pattern on the thighs and buttocks. But women can also develop a "male" pattern, which is just as hazardous to health for women as men.

Small samples of fat can be safely and easily obtained for scientific study by slipping a small needle just beneath the skin, much as one might do to obtain a blood sample. When the fat is examined under the microscope, it's clear that there are numerous round fat cells. These small cells are practically invisible to the naked eye; it would take several hundred lined up in a row to make one inch.

By volume, roughly 90% of the cell is a single droplet of fat. The fatty acids that are present closely reflect fat that has been eaten over long periods. Thus people who tend to eat more vegetable oils than animal fat will have an oily adipose tissue containing fatty acids with many double bonds. Fat that is made by eating excess carbohydrate tends to be much more saturated, with fewer double bonds.

The central oil droplet in each adipocyte is surrounded by a thin rim of cytoplasm (the protoplasm of a cell outside the nucleus) with the usual active cellular machinery. Although a nucleus is present in each cell, it is rare to find adipocytes dividing. So this tissue "turns over" very slowly, if at all, in adults—in sharp contrast to the rapidly dividing cells found in the liver, bone marrow, and the gastrointestinal tract.

The triglyceride in the oil droplet is released under the action of a particular enzyme known as hormone-sensitive lipase. The enzyme reacts to norepinephrine, epinephrine, and other hormones found in the bloodstream. When activated, this enzyme leads to the breakdown of fat and release of the fatty acids and glycerol. The tissue can also take up fatty acids, relink them with glycerol, and deposit this fat within the cell. The hormone insulin and the level of blood glucose help control the rate of fatty acid uptake and release from adipose tissue. This cycle of fat breakdown and reconstruction happens quite rapidly, thereby assuring that fatty acids and glycerol are always present in the bloodstream, even during fasts. During either a brief overnight fast or longer periods of starvation, most of the kcalories consumed by muscle and other tissues come from stored kcalories in fat.

LARGER CELLS—AND MORE OF THEM

An average fat cell contains about a half microgram (half a millionth of a gram) of triglyceride. To store the many pounds of fat present, it takes roughly 30 billion adipocytes in a normal, nonobese person. In all persons who become obese, these billions of cells tend to get larger. And the grossly obese are apt to have an even greater number of them. That is, morbidly obese people, who are more than double their desirable weight, are likely to have more and larger fat cells.

It is notable that with weight reduction the main change in adipocytes is a decrease in size. Fat cells, once filled with fat, do not disappear easily or at all in the adult state. Thus the formerly obese person persists in having a higher than normal cell number. Whether or not this increased number would ever disappear if the weight were kept down for many years remains arguable. Most evidence indicates that it wouldn't.

There has been a lively debate as to whether the increased number of small fat cells found in formerly obese individuals is implicated in the frequent weight regain. Is there such a thing as a starved fat cell? If so, how does this starved cell inform headquarters—the central nervous system with its feeding centers—that more food should be consumed and this obesity restored? These matters are under study, but there is as yet no proof that such signals from fat cells can influence food intake and the presence or absence of obesity.

Many studies have shown that neither animals nor humans are born with their full complement of fat cells. During various stages of growth and development, fat cells increase in number, and to some degree in size, much as do the cells of other tissues and organs. In general, fat cells tend to be made early in life, and the change in number dwindles over time. Yet, it has been shown that fat cells in experimentally overfed animals not only enlarge but also can increase in number. Some fat depots are more sensitive to this buildup than others. For example, fat cells surrounding the kidneys of overfed experimental rats have a particular proclivity to increase in number and in size. These cells, once formed, do not readily disappear.

FRONTIERS IN OBESITY RESEARCH

Several promising research developments may help unravel the relationship of adipocyte chemistry and structure to human obesity. Prominent among these studies are those that focus on adipocytes in the laboratory and the protein products that are isolated and examined from the cells.

An exciting chapter from obesity research has been the demonstration that the thin rim of cytoplasm around the droplet of oil in the adipocyte does more than release and take up fatty acids. It also is responsible for the synthesis of proteins. One of these, known as lipoprotein lipase, is an enzyme that leaves the fat cells and is transported to a nearby capillary, where it functions to break down triglycerides and make them available for deposit in adipose tissue. The amount of this special enzyme increases during abundant feeding and obesity and tends to decrease during starvation. What role this seesawing plays in shuttling fat in and out of adipocytes and in the control of fat-cell size is yet to be delineated. Another enzyme, adipsin, has recently been found to be made in fat cells and secreted into the bloodstream. Adipsin amounts are unusually low in certain obesities that occur genetically in rodents. What role this enzyme has, if any, in the production and perpetuation of obesity is yet to be defined.

Fat cells remain somewhat of a puzzle. We know that they are the cells for fat storage in the body and that in the obese they are always enlarged and sometimes more numerous than in leaner persons. But their biochemical activity and the steps in their development remain central features for study in human nutrition. Are they passive agents in the storage of fat in human obesity? Or do they play an active role in the control of food intake and energy balance? These questions can be answered only by further investigations.

Dr. Hirsch is professor of medicine and senior physician at Rockefeller University.

than in a lean person? For some obese people that is probably the case. It is clear that some laboratory and farm animals more efficiently turn food energy into fat storage (Figure 8-8). Farmers once selected cows and hogs based on their ability to acquire fat. Today we know that eating too much animal fat can increase the risk for heart disease, so farmers now select animals that acquire more lean and less fat tissue (see Chapter 5).

We humans are not so fortunate. Our parents did not choose each other based on genetic counseling. Some of us inherited a tendency for leanness and others probably inherited a tendency for obesity. There is no way to determine which kind of person you are without extensive testing of your resting energy needs. However, a person who is constantly struggling to maintain body weight probably has some genetic component to his weight problem. Unfortunately, nothing can be done to change genetic background. Nevertheless, we should all keep in mind that genetic differences do exist, and these can create a greater body-weight struggle for some people than for others.

Differences in basal metabolism

Basal metabolism tends to be higher in obese people because their extra fat stores require the addition of extra lean tissue, such as connective tissue, for support. The more lean tissue one has, the higher total basal metabolism is. Basal metabolism of an obese person would appear to be less if expressed as kcalories per pound, because adipose tissue has a low metabolic rate. However, when comparing two people, the obese person will have a higher total basal metabolism.[24] *Still, it doesn't take many more kcalories to maintain an obese state, just as it doesn't take many extra kcalories per day to become obese.*

Thermic effect of food in obesity

Thermic effect of food is lower in some obese people than in those at desirable weights. This could be partially caused by insulin resistance of adipose cells, a characteristic often present with obesity. Thus the thermic effect of eating carbohydrate will be decreased in the obese person because not enough insulin action is available to promote normal carbohydrate metabolism.[28]

Energy used in physical activity

Obese people burn more kcalories in activity than do lean people because their extra body weight requires more energy to perform muscular activity. Nevertheless, many obese people use fewer total kcalories in an activity because they are less active.[6] Studies of obese teenagers showed that when they played tennis they avoided rigorous activity. Studies using obese adults show that they also perform weight-bearing exercises, such as walking, less vigorously. A key component to either treating or preventing obesity is increasing the person's physical activity level.

Exploring Issues and Actions

How lean or overweight are your family members? How easy or difficult is it for you to maintain your weight?

WHY SOME PEOPLE ARE OBESE—NATURE VERSUS NURTURE

Both genetic traits and psychological influences can increase the risk for obesity. These two very different types of influences give rise to a "nature-nurture" question concerning causes of obesity.

How influential is nature in contributing to obesity?

Identical twins raised apart tend to have similar weight gain patterns.[30] Having been raised apart reduces the effect of nurture—what a person learns about eating habits and nutrition. If one twin is obese, the other is usually obese. Furthermore, people appear to have specific body types. These have been described by Dr. William Sheldon as **endomorphs, mesomorphs,** and **ectomorphs** (Figure 8-9). Endomorphs have short, stubby bones, short trunks, round heads, wide chest

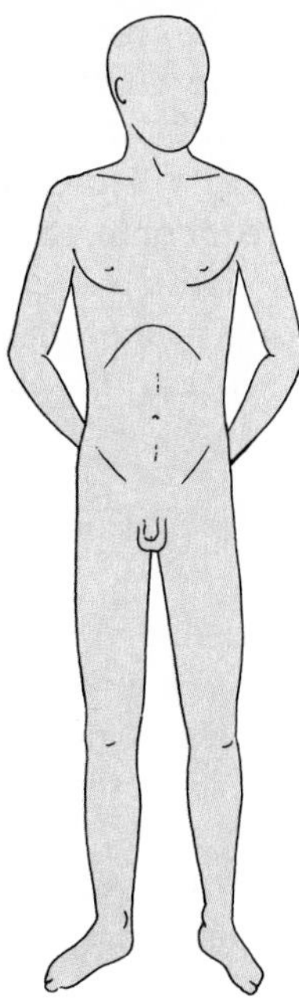

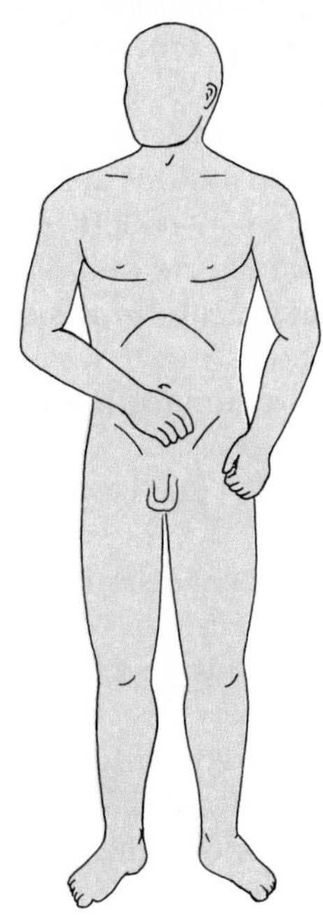

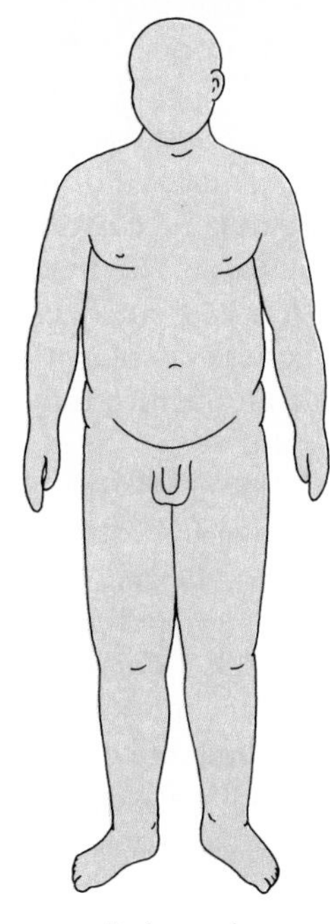

Figure 8-9

The three body types as proposed by the work of Dr. William Sheldon.

and hips, and very short fingers. They are essentially husky people. Mesomorphs are of average size. Ectomorphs are tall, slender individuals with very long, thin bones, and a narrow chest, hips, head, and fingers.

Ectomorphs appear to naturally have an easier time maintaining their body weight. Basal metabolism is affected by surface area. Tall people have more surface area (based on body weight comparisons) than short, stubby people.

As stated before, we think it is reasonable to assume that some people inherit a **thrifty metabolism.** Genetically obese mice and rats are good examples of animal species destined to become obese (Figure 8-8). Both species are much more efficient than the normal animal at turning energy intake into fat storage. Genetically obese rats and mice even make fat at the expense of synthesizing muscle tissue. That indicates how genetically prone they are to fat deposition and eventual obesity.

"thrifty" metabolism
A metabolism that characteristically conserves more kcalories than normal, such that the risk of weight gain and obesity is enhanced.

A very thrifty human metabolism would require less energy for body maintenance and activity. In earlier times, when food supplies were scarce, a thrifty metabolism would be a great advantage. Today, with food so readily available, a thrifty metabolism requires high physical activity and wise food choices to balance energy intake with output.

One important variable in this efficiency equation could be the degree to which food energy can be turned into ATP energy.[2] We cannot measure small differences in energy efficiency between people. In the long run, however, even a 1% or 2% difference in ability to turn food energy into ATP energy could mean massive weight gain or relative weight maintenance. People with thriftier metabolisms may more readily convert food energy into ATP energy, leaving extra kcalories to be synthesized more into more fat stores each day throughout their lives.

Work with Pima Indians in Arizona suggests that some families tend more toward low resting metabolic rates than do others. The families with lower resting metabolic rates show higher rates for obesity. Even after adjusting for the amount of fat a person has, research shows that resting metabolic rate can vary as much as 30% between leaner and more obese Indian families.[25]

So if you feel you have a thrifty metabolism, chances are that you inherited some of that characteristic. A child with no obese parent has only a 10% chance of becoming obese. With one obese parent, the child has about a 40% chance of becoming obese. A child who has two obese parents has about an 80% chance of becoming obese.

It can be argued that these probabilities are due to the way a child is raised. **Fraternal twins** show less variation in weight than two unrelated people. This supports the theory promoting the effects of environment, and the close association of body weights between identical twins supports the theory promoting a genetic explanation. This just shows how complicated it is to separate nature from nurture influences when searching for the cause of obesity.

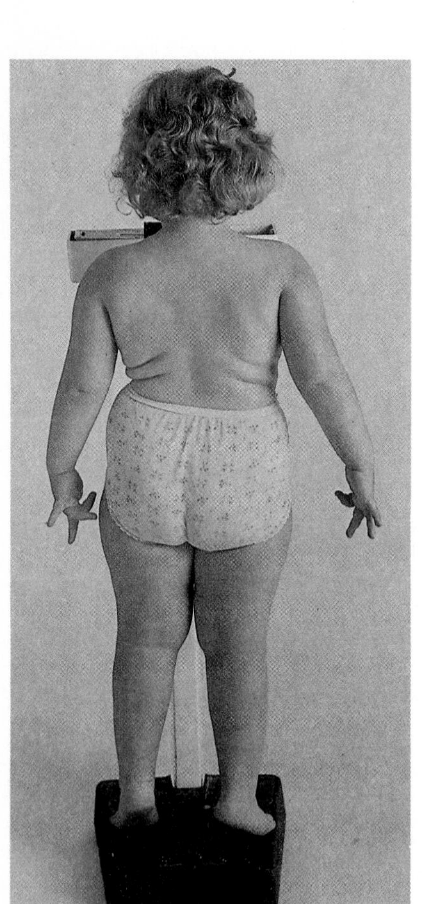

A child who is still obese after five years of age often faces a battle against obesity for the rest of his or her adult life.

Does nurture have a role?

As we just discussed, nurture—how a person is raised—can also strongly influence obesity. Family members often have similar eating habits, make similar food choices, and have similar degrees of fatness. They may find solace in being part of a "clan." This is true even for husbands and wives, two people who have no genetic commonality. So the environment in which a person is raised or now lives can influence food habits and ultimately fatness.[13]

Obesity is related to socioeconomic status in North America. Men and women in lower socioeconomic groups are more likely to be obese than people in upper socioeconomic groups. This is especially true for women.[8]

Gender also influences obesity risk. Adult obesity in women can often be tied to childhood obesity, but the same does not hold true for men. Men tend to become obese after age 30, probably as they become more financially successful and therefore more sedentary. This is probably the best evidence for a critical role of nurture in obesity. If nature is an important reason for obesity in men, obesity should be present much earlier in life.

Early research suggested that infant feeding practices may influence a child's chance to become obese in later life. Specifically, it was thought that both bottle feeding, as well as an early introduction of solid foods (before the age of 6 months), encouraged the infant to gain too much weight. This then increased the chance of becoming obese. However, many recent studies reexamining this issue show that very little relationship exists between feeding practices, or even obesity, in infancy and obesity in childhood. The exception could be the infant who gains weight very rapidly in the first 6 weeks of life.[8] Most overweight or obese infants become normal weight schoolchildren.

If a child remains obese at 5 years of age or has become obese by 5 years of age, immediate attention is necessary. Obesity in childhood is highly related to obesity in adulthood, especially in females. We discuss this further in Chapter 16.

Nature and nurture together

In summary, both nature and nurture influence the tendency for obesity (Figure 8-10). *We can view the development of obesity as nurture allowing nature to be expressed.* Some people may begin with a lower rate for energy metabolism. When these people are put into an inactive environment that is full of both high-kcalorie foods and social reinforcement, they are nurtured into expressing their natural tendency for obesity. This is speculation on our part, but it is a reasonable assertion.

We feel it is important for everyone to try to determine their own risk for obesity and to discover what specific factors in their life-style contribute to this risk. Only then can a person make an individual plan to reduce the risk for obesity. We will talk more about that plan in Chapters 9 and 18.

Keep in mind that although you may be fatter than you would like to be, a small amount of extra fat may pose no significant health risk. That fact may help a person put weight loss into perspective. *Knowing that weight loss is difficult and that current body weight poses no serious health threat, some people may*

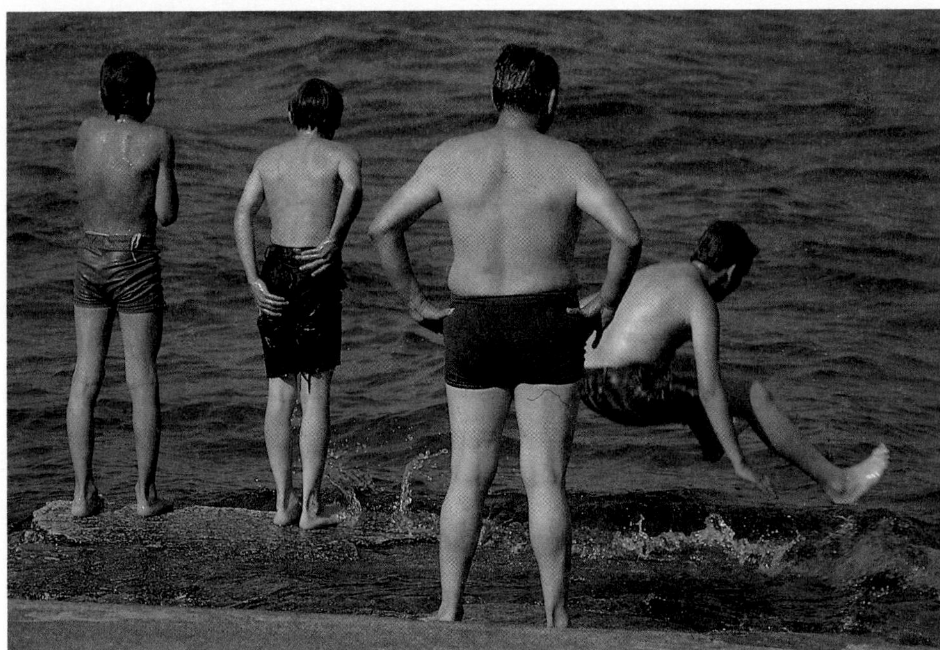

Figure 8-10

Is the difference in body fat due to nature or nurture, or both?

decide to just stay at their current weight and simply work to not gain any more. That alone would be a positive step for some people.

Concept Check

Genetic background plays a role in the cause of obesity. Your body shape and rate of basal metabolism is partially genetically determined. Nurture is also important. Family members often have similar eating habits, similar activity levels, and similar degrees of fatness. In addition, men tend to develop obesity after age 30 and women tend to develop it throughout their childhood and adult years. Putting both factors together we can speculate that a proper nurturing state may allow a genetic tendency for obesity to either be expressed or overcome.

Summary

1. Cells in the hypothalamus, called satiety and feeding centers, affect hunger, the physiological drive to find and eat food. When the satiety center in animals or humans is destroyed, overeating and eventual obesity results. If the feeding centers are destroyed, semistarvation results. These centers may monitor blood glucose and other nutrients and read low levels as a signal to promote feeding.
2. A set point for weight may be inferred when considering how closely weight is regulated. However, the set point cannot necessarily be relied upon to maintain a desirable weight because adults tend to gain about 15 to 20 pounds between the ages of 18 and 54. Factors contributing to the regulation of body weight, besides the feeding and satiety centers in the brain, include hormones and hormone-like compounds made by various cells.
3. Appetite, the psychological desire to find and eat food, is affected by time of day, food availability, social custom, palatability, and even what has recently been eaten. Appetite is an important determinant of food intake for North

Americans; because food is so readily available to most of us, for many, hunger is not a common experience.

4. Energy use by the body can be accounted for by basal metabolism, the thermic effect of food, and physical activity. Basal metabolism represents the minimum energy needed to keep the resting body alive. It is primarily affected by lean body mass, surface area, and thyroid hormone levels. The thermic effect of food represents the increase in metabolism to facilitate the digesting, absorbing, and processing of nutrients recently consumed. Physical activity represents energy use that is not due to the other two categories. About 60% to 75% of energy use goes for basal metabolism and the thermic effect of food.
5. Energy use by the body can be measured directly from heat output or indirectly by measuring oxygen uptake and/or carbon dioxide output. Energy use by the body can be estimated using formulas based on various combinations of body weight, height, and age.
6. Obesity is usually defined as 20% over desirable body weight as predicted by the 1983 Metropolitan Life Insurance Table. A body mass index (weight/height^2) over about 30 also represents obesity. In addition, a total body fat percent over 25% in men and 30% in women indicates obesity.
7. Fat distribution partially determines in the prediction of health risks due to obesity. An android fat storage distribution, in which the waist-to-hip circumference ratio is greater than 0.9 in men or greater than 0.8 in women, suggests higher risks of hypertension, heart disease, and diabetes associated with obesity.
8. Genetic factors influence the tendency to obesity. Basal metabolism and body shape both have genetic links. How one is raised (or nurtured) also influences the tendency for obesity, since family members often develop similar eating habits and activity patterns. Essentially, obesity can be viewed as nurture allowing nature to be expressed.

Take Action

Do you know your numbers? Complete the following table.

Height ________ centimeters ________ meters ________ inches
Weight ________ kilograms ________ pounds
Frame size (Table 8-6) (circle one): small medium large
Desirable body weight (Table 8-5): ________ pounds
(shortcut method, page 236): ________ pounds

Percentage of desirable weight:

$$\frac{(\text{current weight} - \text{desirable weight})}{\text{desirable weight}} \times 100 = \_\_\_\_\_\_\_\_$$

$$\text{Body mass index:} \frac{\text{weight (kilograms)}}{\text{height}^2\text{ (meters)}} = \_\_\_\_\_\_\_\_$$

Waist circumference: ________ centimeters ________ inches
Hip circumference: ________ centimeters ________ inches
Waist to hip ratio: ________
Shape (circle if appropriate): android gynecoid
Resting energy needs (Harris-Benedict equation, Appendix M)
(Owen formula, Appendix M)
H-B ________ kcalories; Owen ________ kcalories
Total energy needs: RDA ________ kcalories
based on weight (see page 232) ________ kcalories
Percentage of total energy needs due to resting metabolic rate:

$$\frac{\text{resting energy needs}}{\text{total energy needs}} \times 100 = \_\_\_\_\_\_\_\_ \%$$

Thermic effect of food in 24 hours:

total energy needs × either .06 or .10 = ________—________ kcalories

REFERENCES

1. Anderson GH: Metabolic regulation of food intake. In Shils ME and Young VR, eds: Modern nutrition in health and disease, Philadelphia, 1988, Lea & Febiger.
2. Anonymous: Genetic differences in mitochondrial ATPase, Nutrition Reviews 45:248, 1987.
3. Anonymous: Role of fat and fatty acids in the modulation of energy exchange, Nutrition Reviews 46:382, 1988.
4. Atkinson RL: Opioid regulation of food intake and body weight in humans, Federation Proceedings 46:178, 1987.
5. Beutler B: Cachexia: a fundamental mechanism, Nutrition Reviews 46:369, 1988.
6. Blair D and Buskirk ER: Habitual daily energy expenditure and activity levels of lean and adult-onset and child-onset obese women, The American Journal of Clinical Nutrition 45:540, 1987.
7. Bray GA: Complications of obesity, Annals of Internal Medicine 103:1052, 1985.
8. Bray GA: Nutrient balance and obesity: classification and evaluation of the obesities, Medical clinics of North America 73:29, 1989.
9. Brownell KD: The psychology and physiology of obesity: implications for screening and treatment, The Journal of the American Dietetic Association 84:406, 1984.
10. Daily JM and others: Human energy requirements: overestimation by widely used prediction equation, The American Journal of Clinical Nutrition 42:1170, 1985.
11. Donahue RP and others: Central obesity and coronary heart disease in men, Lancet, p 11, April 11, 1987.
12. Fernstrom JD: Tryptophan, serotonin, and carbohydrate appetite: will the real carbohydrate craver please stand up, Journal of Nutrition 118:1417, 1988.
13. Garn SM: Family-line and socioeconomic factors in fatness and obesity, Nutrition Reviews 44:381, 1986.
14. Haffner SM and others: Do upper-body and centralized adiposity measure different as-

pects of regional-fat body distribution? Diabetes 36:43, 1987.
15. Henson LC and others: Effects of exercise training on resting energy expenditure during calorie restriction, The American Journal of Clinical Nutrition 46:893, 1987.
16. Hirsch J and Leibel RL: New light on obesity, The New England Journal of Medicine 318:509, 1988.
17. Jackson AS and Pollock ML: Practical assessment of body composition, The Physician and Sports Medicine 13:76, 1985.
18. Leibel RL and Hirsch J: Metabolic characterization of obesity, Annals of Internal Medicine 103:1000, 1985.
19. Manson JE and others: Body weight and longevity, Journal of the American Medical Association 257:353, 1987.
20. Martin RJ and Mullen BJ: Control of food intake: mechanisms and consequences, Nutrition Today, p 4, September/October 1987.
21. National Institutes of Health Consensus Development Conference Statement: Health implications of obesity, Annals of Internal Medicine 103:1073, 1985.
22. Nowak RK and Schulz LO: A comparison of two methods for the determination of body frame size, The Journal of the American Dietetic Association 87:339, 1987.
23. Owen OE and others: A reappraisal of the caloric requirements of men, The American Journal of Clinical Nutrition 46:875, 1987.
24. Owen OE: Regulation of energy and metabolism. In Kinney JM and others, eds: Nutrition and metabolism in patient care, Philadelphia, 1988, WB Saunders Co.
25. Ravussin E and others: Determinants of 24-hour energy expenditure in man: methods and results using a respiratory chamber, Journal of Clinical Investigation 78:1568, 1986.
26. Ravussin E and others: Reduced rate of energy expenditure as a risk factor for body-weight gain, The New England Journal of Medicine 318:467, 1988.
27. Schoeller DA: Measurement of energy expenditure in free-living humans using doubly labeled water, Journal of Nutrition 118:1278, 1988.
28. Simms EAH: Storage and expenditure of energy in obesity and their implications for management, Medical Clinics of North America 73:97, 1989.
29. Striker EM: Biological bases of hunger and satiety: therapeutic implications, Nutrition Reviews 42:333, 1984.
30. Stunkard AJ and others: A twin study of human obesity, Journal of the American Medical Association 256:51, 1986.
31. Weigley ES: Average? Ideal? Desirable? A brief review of height-weight tables in the United States, Journal of the American Dietetic Association 84:417, 1984.

SUGGESTED READINGS

The article by Striker is a fascinating look at the processes that control hunger and satiety. It describes the feeding and satiety centers and shows how cells throughout the body affect feeding and behavior. Weigley's article details the evolution of height/weight tables. It provides the timeline for the versions of the Metropolitan Life Insurance Table and includes other tables developed from government surveys and by groups of researchers. To understand more about the physiology and psychology of obesity, see the article by Brownell. This paper reviews the concept of set point and provides an experienced clinician's view of the heterogeneity apparent in obese people. Finally, the articles by Bray detail the complications of obesity and of the use of body mass index in predicting health risks.

CHAPTER 8

Answers to nutrition awareness inventory

1. *True.* When the brain receives signals that the liver is metabolizing absorbed nutrients, it then signals less hunger.
2. *True.* Regulation of body weight has been compared with the regulation of blood pressure. Both appear to be "set" to some extent, with blood pressure even more so.
3. *False.* The RDA represents an average energy need for a person performing light activity. The range given may or may not accurately estimate a person's energy needs.
4. *True.* To keep a resting body alive, there is need to maintain heart rate, respiration, body temperature, and other functions. The energy used represents basal metabolism.
5. *False.* Brown adipose tissue mostly disappears between infancy and adulthood. Its role in the average adult is unclear.
6. *False.* In general, obesity increases risk for health problems and reduces life expectancy. The greater the obesity, the greater the effect it has on life expectancy. Occasionally a person may escape the health problems associated with obesity, but most people do not.
7. *True.* Your body weight may be greater than a desirable figure, as predicted from the Metropolitan Life Insurance Table, but excess weight yields a health risk only if it is due to excess body fat. Extra muscle mass poses no risk.
8. *False.* Women tend to store fat in the hip and thigh areas, whereas men tend to store fat in the abdominal area.
9. *True.* Health problems usually begin when a person exceeds desirable weight by more than 20%; the greater the difference, the greater the health risk.
10. *True.* Muscle tissue metabolizes at a high rate and thus has a great influence on the basal metabolism.
11. *True.* The extra weight carried by an obese person raises the kcalorie cost of physical activity.
12. *False.* There is little evidence that adult obesity in men is related to childhood obesity; however, there is a strong relationship between childhood and adult obesity in women.
13. *False.* Probably less than 10% of all cases of obesity in North America is due to diagnosed problems in thyroid or other hormone levels in the bloodstream.
14. *False.* Consuming no more than a few hundred extra kcalories daily for a few years can create an obese state. Once an obese state is achieved, it takes very few extra kcalories to maintain it.
15. *True.* At the beginning of a meal, people usually choose a variety of foods. At the end of a meal, appetite narrows and sweet food choices often predominate.

Nutrition Perspective 8-1

The True Energy Value of Fat

Scientists have recently questioned whether fats in foods actually yield 9 or 11 kcalories per gram when ingested.[24] In the bomb calorimeter, fats produce about 9 kcalories per gram. However, when metabolized in the body, fats are used very efficiently. Very little thermic effect is induced by dietary fats because fat bypasses the liver and liver metabolism on its way to the bloodstream via chylomicrons. Very little energy in fat is lost when it transfers from foods to fat storage.

This difference in the thermic effect of food between fats and either carbohydrates or proteins poses a dilemma for scientists. They can either reduce the amount of kcalories in carbohydrates and proteins to reflect the amount lost due to metabolism in the liver or increase the kcalorie value of fats to reflect their more efficient metabolism. If carbohydrates and proteins are to remain at their adjusted measured values of 4 kcalories per gram, then we really should increase the energy value of fats from the current value of 9 kcalories per gram to 11 kcalories per gram.

The issue is not purely academic. Scientists have noted for many years that growing rats fed high-fat diets gained more weight than rats fed low-fat diets, even though both diets contained the same amount of kcalories. If we assume that lipids actually yield 11 kcalories per gram, this explains the difference in weight gain. In animal experiments, to keep the total energy available to the animals on a low-fat diet equal to that available to those on a high-fat diet (these types of diets are often used in cancer research), it is important to consider the higher efficiency at which fats are used during animal growth.

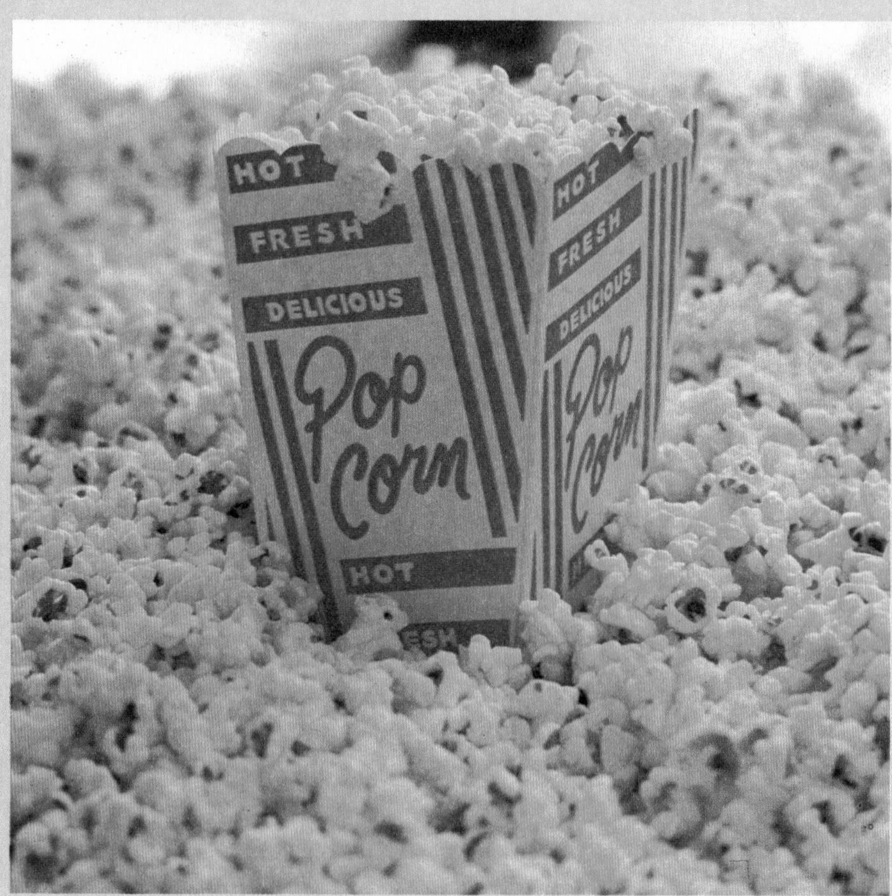

Chapter 9

Weight Control

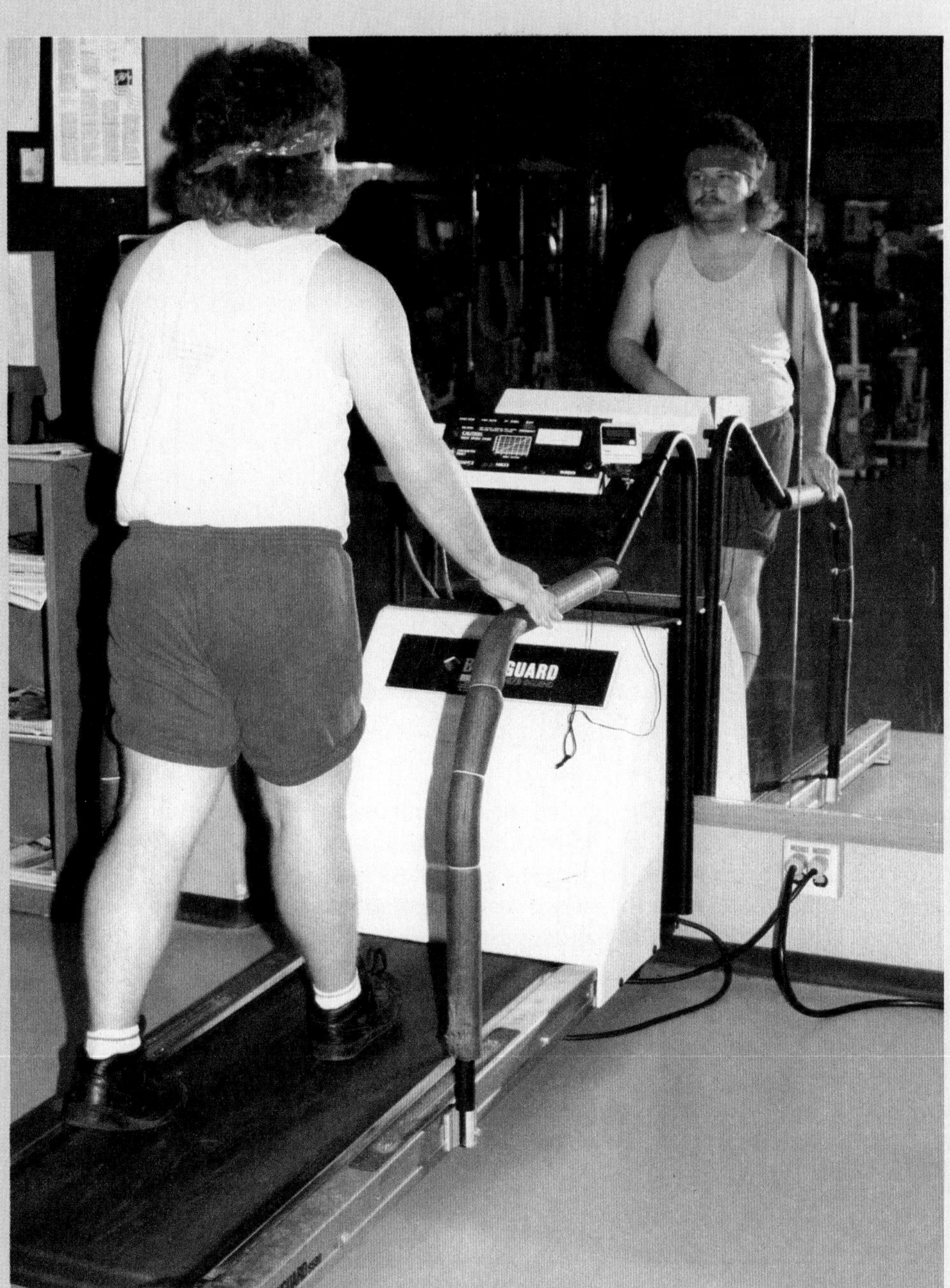

Exercise is important for weight loss and future weight control.

Overview

Diets come and go. At any given time about 27% of men and 46% of women are trying to lose weight—not to mention up to 75% of teenage girls. Still, the number of obese people in North America remains disturbing. Each new diet is promoted as the "diet of the century," or the "diet to end all diets." However, most diets fizzle; they are usually ineffective and monotonous and, worse, can be dangerous if followed for a long period or by the wrong people—especially by pregnant women, young children, and teenagers.

Fad diet books use come-ons like these: the routine is easy to follow, fast, and effective—perhaps even a scientific breakthrough previously available only in Europe. The descriptions sound terrific, almost too good to be true. And for the most part they are too good to be true. *The word fad is actually a shortened version of fiddle-faddle, which means "to play with and then cast aside."*[26]

This chapter will lead you through the issues of weight control. After reading it, you will be able to decide when diet books are telling the truth and when they are trying to deceive you.

Nutrition awareness inventory

Here are 15 statements about weight control. Answer them to test your current knowledge. If you think the answer is true or mostly true, circle T. If you think the answer is false or mostly false, circle F. Use the scoring key at the end of this chapter to compute your total score. Take this test again after you have read this chapter. Compare the results.

1. T F Physical activity is more important than diet in losing weight.
2. T F Scientists understand little about the physiology of weight regain after weight loss.
3. T F Weight-loss diets should contain at least 1000 kcalories per day.
4. T F Success rates of weight-loss programs are reasonably good.
5. T F Rapid weight loss is likely to mean the loss of muscle tissue.
6. T F A weight-loss program should include behavior modification.
7. T F A weight-loss program should encourage not eating meat after milk products.
8. T F The best foods to emphasize for weight loss are high-carbohydrate foods.
9. T F Feelings of hunger return quickly after a low-fat meal.
10. T F Changing habits is the single most important factor in keeping weight off.
11. T F Stimulus control refers to controlling factors that encourage eating.
12. T F You can lose 1 pound of fat storage each week by burning 200 extra kcalories per day beyond your normal activity.
13. T F Most obese children become obese adults.
14. T F A 20-minute brisk walk burns up about 100 kcalories.
15. T F Morbid obesity is defined as 100 pounds over desirable weight.

TREATMENT OF OBESITY

One of the 1990 Health Objectives for the United States is the reduction of obesity. Specifically, the goal of the National Institutes of Health (NIH) is to reduce the number of people who are obese (body mass index greater than 27.8 for men and 27.3 for women) to 18% of the male population and 21% of the female population. To do that, the NIH has suggested three specific actions:

1. Teach 90% of all adults that increasing physical activity while decreasing energy intake is the best way to lose weight.
2. Get 90% of the adults already at acceptable or desirable body weights to remain that way.
3. Motivate 90% of overweight Americans to adopt a plan to reduce energy intake and increase physical activity, ultimately attaining and then maintaining a desirable weight.

Improving the health of people in North America—and of others in most of the Western World—hinges on the possibility of reducing obesity rates. Reducing present rates of obesity would be one powerful tool providing a more healthful and fuller life for many people.

Some basic premises

Let's focus on three important principles concerning weight loss for adults (see Chapter 16 for weight-loss suggestions for children). First, *the body resists weight loss.*[3,11,17] We discussed this in Chapter 8. Thyroid hormone levels, and consequently basal metabolism, drop during weight loss.[11] This drop makes it difficult to lose weight. Recent studies also show that activity of the enzyme lipoprotein lipase increases in adipose cells after weight loss.[7] This enzyme is responsible for removing fat from lipoproteins and absorbing it into adipose cells (see Chapter 5). So after dieting, the body can more efficiently facilitate the uptake of fat from the bloodstream for storage.

Second, *preventing obesity should be emphasized, since curing the disease is very difficult.* The Canadian Dietetic Association strongly endorses this point.[4] *Only about 5% of those who diet actually lose weight and remain at that weight.* A weight-loss program should be considered successful only when its subjects remain at their lower weight for 3 to 5 years. Some programs have slightly higher success rates than 5%, but overall the statistics are grim. Dieting today often results in weight gain next month, creating yo-yo weight swings. The health consequences of these swings are discussed in the Expert Opinion by Dr. Kelly Brownell.

When you read brochures or research reports about specific diet plans, ask not only whether the people lost weight but also whether they maintained that weight loss for a period of a year or more. If the weight loss was not maintained, then the entire dieting program was in vain.

Third, *the weight should be lost from fat storage, not from muscle and other lean tissues.* Rapid weight loss at the start of a diet program often represents fluid lost due to a decreased salt intake, and loss of glycogen from the liver and muscles. Much muscle tissue may be lost as well. People are fooled when they weigh themselves after starting a fad diet. They have lost weight, but very little of it represents fat loss.

Wishful shrinking—why it can't be mostly fat

We know that rapid weight loss cannot be mostly fat loss because of the high-kcalorie deficit needed to lose fat tissue. Fat storage—adipose tissue plus support tissues—represents approximately 2700 to 3500 kcalories per pound.[22] To lose 1 pound of fat storage per week, energy intake must be cut by approximately 400 to 500 kcalories a day. *Diets that promise 10 to 15 pounds weight loss per week cannot ensure that the weight loss will be from fat storage alone.* Producing a kcalorie deficit sufficient to lose that amount of fat storage is simply not practical.

Although some books use 3500 kcalories per pound of fat gained or lost, newer evidence suggests that 2700 kcalories per pound of fat storage is a closer estimate. This is because when fat tissue is gained or lost, lean support tissue is lost as well. Lean support tissue includes muscle, connective tissue, blood supply, and other body components. This lean tissue is mostly water and therefore contains few kcalories. When a lot of fat tissue and some lean tissue is lost, the net result is approximately **2700 kcalories exchanged per pound of fat storage.**[22]

A sound weight-loss diet—what to look for?

A sound weight-loss diet should include management of three types of activities: control of kcalorie intake, changing problem food habits, and increased physical activity.[5,9,10,24] Focusing on just eating fewer kcalories is not enough, as we will show. Specifically, look for the following characteristics:[13,30]

1. The diet should meet nutritional needs, except for kcalories. To do that, it should follow the Daily Food Guide, emphasizing lower fat choices.
2. Slow and steady weight loss, as opposed to rapid weight loss, should be stressed. A loss of 1 to 2 pounds per week of fat storage is desirable.
3. The diet should allow adaptations to individual habits and tastes. No rigid rituals—such as only eating fruits in the morning or not eating meat after milk products—should be required.
4. The diet should minimize hunger and fatigue. To do this, it should contain at least 1000 kcalories per day. Even so, when kcalories are kept between 1200 to 1500 per day, consuming sufficient iron is difficult, especially for young women (see Chapter 2). If the diet calls for fewer kcalories than this per day, it should recommend either fortified foods (breakfast cereals, for example) or a balanced vitamin and mineral supplement to supply enough iron (see Chapter 11 for advice on using supplements).
5. The diet should contain readily obtainable foods. There is no magical food that

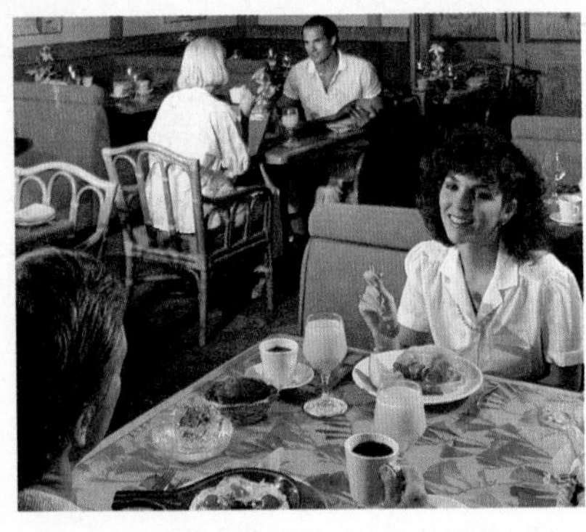

A sound weight loss diet should allow you to participate in social activities, such as eating at a restaurant.

Exploring Issues and Actions

Your best friend is overweight and searching for a rapid weight–loss program. Your friend becomes very interested in a popular high-protein program that promises more than it can probably deliver. What do you say to your friend?

can speed weight loss. If a diet suggests that there is—whether ginseng, tofu, or garlic—look elsewhere for advice.

6. The diet should be socially acceptable. It should allow the person dieting to attend parties, eat at restaurants, and participate in normal daily activities.
7. The diet should help change problem eating habits. It should promote reshaping food habits and life-style to make weight loss, and then weight maintenance, possible and so thwart further weight gain.
8. The diet should improve overall health. It should emphasize regular physical activity, proper rest, stress reduction, and other healthy changes in life-style.
9. The diet should insist that the dieter see a physician before starting the weight-loss program if the person has existing health problems, plans to lose weight as quickly as possible, or is over 35 years of age and plans to perform substantially greater than usual physical activity.

CONTROLLING ENERGY INTAKE

A goal of losing 1 to 2 pounds of fat storage per week usually requires an energy intake of 1000 to 1200 kcalories per day for women and 1200 to 1800 kcalories for men. Another approach is to allow 10 kcalories per pound of desirable weight for sedentary people and 13 kcalories per pound for active people, and then subtract 400 to 500 kcalories for each pound per week of fat loss desired. For example, a 140 pound woman who should weigh 120 pounds and wants to lose one pound per week could start with 1570 kcalories (13 × 120) and then subtract 400 kcalories. This yields about 1200 kcalories for her diet. Both methods are useful. *In any case, a dieter should not try to eat fewer than 1000 kcalories daily: that causes so much hunger that the person will probably not be able to stick to the plan.* A better idea would be to first increase activity level, which could then allow at least 1000 kcalories to be eaten.

Energy intake can be further adjusted to accommodate a high activity level. Look up the kcalorie needs of various activities in Appendix J and add those amounts to the kcalorie allowance after subtracting 1.5 kcalories per minute for resting energy needs.

Using the exchange system is an easy way for a dieter to monitor energy intake. See the menu patterns listed in Table 2-10 for some possible approaches. Another method is to write down food intake throughout the day and then calculate energy intake from food tables in the evening, adjusting future food choices as needed.

The best foods to eat when trying to lose weight are those high in carbohydrates. Carbohydrates provide less than half as many kcalories as fat. A weight-loss diet should include at least 150 grams of carbohydrate daily to both prevent ketosis and reduce the risk of bingeing on large amounts of food, particularly sweets, because of intense hunger.

It is best not to reduce fat content of a diet below 20% of kcalorie intake. *A diet too low in fat produces very little satiety, so hunger returns very quickly after eating.* One study showed that when diets were lowered from a fat level of 40% to 30% and then to 20% of kcalories, subjects compensated slightly. This means that they ate more food on the lower-fat diet. However, the end result was that the lower-fat diet provided far fewer kcalories, allowing the people on the lower-fat diet to lose more weight.[20]

A diet that contains 30% kcalories as fat permits a person to incorporate most commonly eaten foods into the diet. Even subtle changes in food habits can promote desired weight loss. The best diet is always one the dieter can continue practicing throughout life. Changing habits appropriately is the key to both losing weight and maintaining a desirable weight.

Table 9-1 addresses the question of what foods are appropriate for a diet. Table 9-2 shows how to start saving kcalories. Many plans suggest eating most foods

Table 9-1

What can I eat?

Minimum servings*	Food group	Some suggestions
4	Breads, cereals, and other grain products	Emphasize whole grains. Breads, yes; avoid those high in fat and sugar. Cereals with little or no sugar. Rice and pasta—but watch out for the sauces and second helpings.
4	Fruits	All except avocados and olives; don't add sugar or whipped cream.
	Vegetables	All kinds, but go easy on butter, margarine, and other sauces or toppings high in fat. Avoid fried vegetables.
2	Meat, poultry, fish, and alternates	Lean parts of meat; poultry without skin; fish. Broil, roast, simmer. Avoid items that are breaded and fried. Eggs, dry beans and peas, and tofu are good alternates.
2	Milk, cheese, and yogurt	Skim or low-fat milk and low-fat cheeses. Low-fat and nonfat plain yogurt.
Limit, but include at least one teaspoon of vegetable oil per day.	Fats, sweets, and alcoholic beverages	Watch out for these. They provide kcalories and little else—not what dieters want. Use spices and herbs instead of sauces, butter, and other fats. For dessert, try fresh fruit or choose baked products made with less fat and sugar—angel food cake, for example. Drink coffee or tea without cream or sugar; use low-fat milk.

*Based on the Daily Food Guide. The National Academy of Sciences recently recommended 6 or more servings of breads and cereals per day and 5 or more servings of fruits and vegetables per day. This is an excellent suggestion if the dieter can still lose weight with these extra kcalories in the diet (see Chapter 17).

Adapted from: USDA Home and Garden Bulletin No. 232-2, 1986.

Table 9-2

Saving kcalories: ideas to help get started

Check out the following kcalorie-saving ideas. Then think of other changes to help cut kcalories.

Instead of:	Try:	Kcalories saved:
3 ounces well-marbled meat (prime rib)	3 ounces lean meat (eye of round)	140
½ chicken breast, batter-fried	½ chicken breast broiled with lemon	175
½ cup beef stroganoff	3 ounces lean roast beef	210
½ cup home-fried potatoes	1 medium baked potato	65
½ cup green bean-mushroom casserole	½ cup cooked green beans	50
½ cup potato salad	1 cup raw vegetable salad	140
½ cup pineapple chunks in heavy syrup	½ cup pineapple chunks canned in juice	25
2 tablespoons bottled French dressing	2 tablespoons low-calorie French dressing	150
1/7 9-inch apple pie	1 baked apple	185
3 oatmeal-raisin cookies	1 oatmeal-raisin cookie	125
½ cup ice cream	½ cup ice milk	45
A Danish pastry	Half an English muffin	150
1 cup sugar-coated corn flakes	1 cup plain corn flakes	60
1 cup whole milk	1 cup 1% low-fat milk	45
7-fluid-ounce Tom Collins	6-fluid-ounce wine cooler made with sparkling water	150
1-ounce bag potato chips	1 cup plain popcorn	120
1/12 8-inch white layer cake with chocolate frosting	1/12 angel food cake, 10-inch tube	185

Adapted from: USDA Home and Garden Bulletin No. 232-2, 1986.

during the hours of greatest physical activity, between 7 AM and 5 PM. Then absorbed fat heads right to the active muscles, bypassing the adipose cells. Conversely, a large dinner eaten after physical activity has ceased or considerably slowed may leave excess fat in the bloodstream with no place to go but into fat storage. Even so the most important habit is to eat less and be more active.

Most people need to lose fewer than 50 pounds. By consuming a lower-kcal-

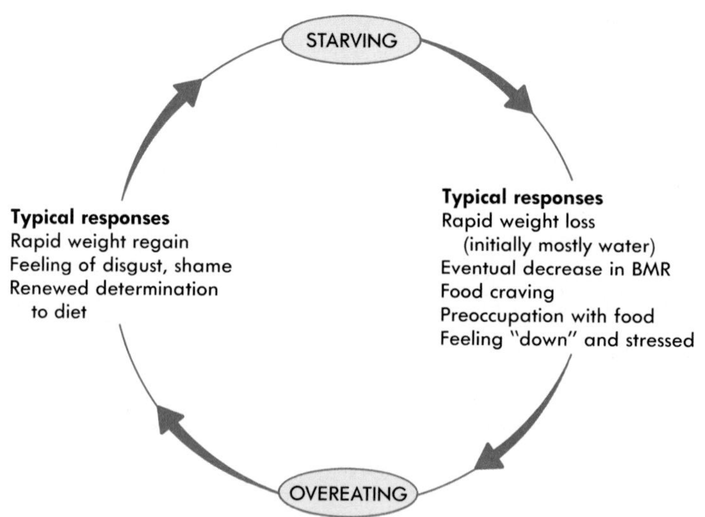

Figure 9-1

A poor start often leads to a poor finish. When considering dieting to lose weight, changing habits is often the key.

orie diet these people should be able to achieve a desirable body weight within 1 year. *It took time to gain weight. It takes time to lose it.* Figure 9-1 shows how starting out on the wrong foot, with limited food selections and rapid weight loss, can sabotage a person's effort to lose weight by encouraging the bingeing and feelings of failure that often accompany those types of dieting approaches.

Concept Check

Key points to consider when dieting to lose weight include these: (1) The body resists weight loss; (2) Emphasis should be placed on preventing obesity, since curing the disease is very difficult; (3) Weight should be lost from fat stores, not from lean tissues. Appropriate weight loss diets have the following characteristics in common: (1) They meet nutritional needs—this can be evaluated by referring to the Daily Food Guide; (2) They can adjust to accommodate the dieter's habits and tastes; (3) They emphasize readily obtainable foods; (4) They promote changing habits that lead to overeating; (5) They encourage an increase in physical activity.

BEHAVIOR MODIFICATION—WHAT MAKES US TICK?

Controlling energy intake is an important step in a weight-loss program. Another vital part is behavior modification.[14,21] Basically, each dieter must decide which behaviors contribute to his obesity and then find ways to modify those behaviors. In essence, *a person's life-style and environment should be reshaped so that weight maintenance—rather than weight gain—is the overwhelming thrust, and self-control is not constantly being tested.*

To do this, a person should consider the events that cause him to start eating, factors that influence food choices, and factors associated with stopping eating (Table 9-3). Psychologists often use terms like **chain-breaking, stimulus control, cognitive restructuring, contingency management,** and **self-monitoring** when discussing behavior modification. This terminology helps place the problem in perspective and organize the intervention strategy into manageable steps.

Chain-breaking deals with separating behaviors that tend to occur together, for example, snacking on chips and peanuts while watching television. While these activities do not have to occur together, they often do and need to be systematically separated.

Stimulus control involves controlling factors that encourage eating. That may mean hiding irresistible food in the back of the refrigerator, taking the light bulb out of the refrigerator, moving foods from the counter into cabinets, or avoiding the path by a certain vending machine on the way to class.

Cognitive restructuring aims to change a person's frame of mind appropriately. A hard day becomes—instead of a reason to binge—a reason to relax, perhaps walk and talk with a friend. *Contingency management* focuses on planning ahead for responses to possible pitfalls and high-risk situations. One strategy, for example, is to rehearse what to say when people press food on you and what to do when irresistible foods are within arm's reach at a party.

Self-monitoring, a key practice in behavior modification, usually begins with keeping a diary of foods eaten and the circumstances that lead to eating. The record can reveal general patterns that provide a better understanding of eating habits (Table 9-4). Self-monitoring is an efficient way to spot problems in eating habits, especially times of unconscious overeating. Self-monitoring can be a persuasive means of encouraging people to adopt new habits to counteract unwanted behaviors. These new habits might include limiting eating to only one place in the house. That could reduce snacking in front of the television and in the kitchen while preparing meals. People who eat very rapidly can put down their utensils while chewing. This slows the rate of eating and helps the hormone

chain-breaking
Breaking the link between two or more behaviors that encourage overeating, such as snacking while watching television (see Chapter 18).

stimulus control
Altering the environment to minimize the stimuli for eating, for example, removing foods from sight and storing them in kitchen cabinets.

cognitive restructuring
Changing one's frame of mind regarding eating, for example, instead of using a difficult day as an excuse to overeat, substitute other pleasures for rewards, such as a relaxing walk with a friend.

contingency management
Forming a plan of action to respond to an environment where overeating is likely, such as when snacks are within arm's reach at a party.

self-monitoring
A process of tracking foods eaten and conditions affecting eating; actions are usually recorded in a diary, along with location, time, and state of mind. This is a tool to help a person understand more about his or her eating habits.

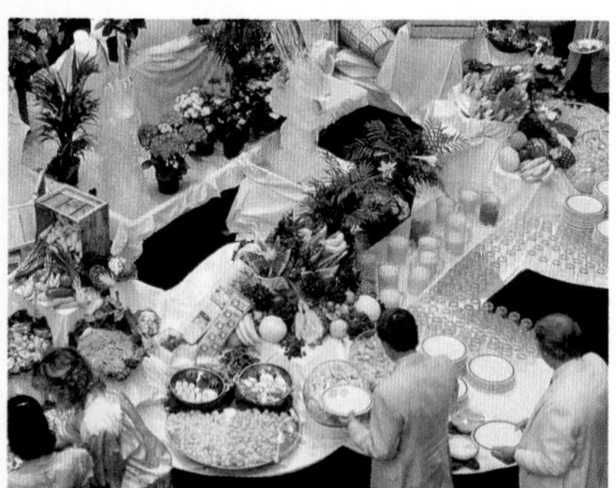

A contingency management plan might consist of learning to eat only healthful foods at a party, or eating a small snack beforehand.

Table 9-3

Behavioral principles of weight loss

Stimulus control

Shopping

1. Shop for food after eating—buy nutritious foods
2. Shop from a list; do not buy irresistible "problem" foods
3. Avoid ready-to-eat foods; let others who want them buy them and store them
4. Don't carry more cash than needed for shopping list

Plans

1. Plan to limit food intake
2. Substitute exercise for snacking
3. Eat meals and snacks at scheduled times; don't skip meals
4. Don't accept inappropriate foods offered by others

Activities

1. Store food out of sight, preferably in the freezer so that compulsive eating is discouraged
2. Eat all food in the same place
3. Remove food from inappropriate storage areas in the house
4. Keep serving dishes off the table, especially sauces and gravies
5. Use smaller dishes and utensils
6. Avoid being the food server
7. Leave the table immediately after eating
8. Don't save leftovers; empty leftovers directly into the garbage

Holidays and parties

1. Drink fewer alcoholic beverages
2. Plan eating habits before parties
3. Eat a low-calorie snack before parties
4. Practice polite ways to decline food
5. Don't get discouraged by an occasional setback

Eating behavior

1. Put fork down between mouthfuls
2. Chew thoroughly before swallowing
3. Prepare foods one portion at a time
4. Leave some food on the plate
5. Pause in the middle of the meal
6. Do nothing else while eating (read, watch television)

Reward

1. Solicit help from family and friends
2. Help family and friends provide this help in the form of praise and material rewards
3. Utilize self-monitoring records as basis for rewards
4. Plan specific rewards for specific behaviors (behavioral contracts)

Self-monitoring

Diet diary

1. Note time and place of eating
2. List type and amount of food eaten
3. Record who is present and how you feel

Nutrition education

1. Use diet diary to identify problem areas
2. Make small changes that you can continue
3. Learn nutritional values of foods
4. Decrease fat intake; increase complex-carbohydrate intake

Table 9-3, cont'd

Behavioral principles of weight loss

Physical activity

Routine activity

1. Increase routine activity
2. Increase use of stairs
3. Keep a record of distance walked each day

Exercise

1. Begin a very mild exercise program
2. Keep a record of daily exercise
3. Increase the exercise very gradually

Cognitive restructuring

1. Avoid setting unreasonable goals
2. Think about progress, not shortcomings
3. Avoid imperatives like "always" and "never"
4. Counter negative thoughts with rational restatements
5. Set weight goals

Table 9-4

A method for monitoring food habits

Time	Minutes spent eating	M or S*	H**	Activity while eating	Place of eating	Food and quantity	Others present	Feeling before eating
7:10 a.m.	15	M	2	standing, fixing lunch	kitchen	1 c orange juice 1 c corn flakes ½ c 2% milk 2 t sugar black coffee	—	anxious
10:00 a.m.	4	S	1	sitting, taking notes	classroom	12 oz. diet cola	class	rushed
12:15 p.m.	40	M	2	sitting, talking	union	1 chicken sandwich 1 pear	friends	good
2:30 p.m.	10	S	1	sitting, studying	library	12 oz. regular cola	friend	bored
6:30 p.m.	35	M	3	sitting, talking	kitchen	1 pork chop 1 baked potato 2 T margarine lettuce 1 oz ranch dressing 1 c whole milk 1 piece cherry pie	boyfriend	good, hungry
9:10 p.m.	10	S	2	sitting, studying	living room	1 glass mineral water	—	sleepy, thirsty

*M or S: Meal or snack

**H: Degree of hunger (0 = none; 3 = maximum)

Table 9-5

Setting a goal as part of behavior modification

I. Goal assessment

A ***Describe the goal in positive, behavioral terms:*** ______________________________

____

B ***To whom is the goal most important?***

_____ dieter

_____ friend

_____ family

_____ someone else: if so, whom? ______________________________

C ***Is the goal based on:***

_____ realistic expectations

_____ wishful thinking

_____ other factors, if so, describe: ______________________________

____

D ***How will attaining this goal affect the dieter's life?*** ______________________________

____

E ***Do you think the dieter can achieve this goal?***

_____ ***yes*** _____ ***no***

F ***What are the realistic problems the dieter will face in trying to achieve this goal?***

____

____

G ***Goal Roadblock Analysis. What is your understanding of the barriers the dieter must overcome to achieve this goal?***

_____ Knowledge roadblock. Describe: ______________________________

____

What does the dieter need to know? ______________________________

____

_____ Skill roadblock. Describe: ______________________________

____

What skills does the dieter need? ______________________________

____

_____ Risk-taking roadblock. Describe: ______________________________

____

What risks does the dieter have to take? ______________________________

____

_____ Social support roadblock. Describe: ______________________________

____

What social supports does the dieter need? ______________________________

____

_____ Some combination of knowledge, skills, risk-taking, and social support. Describe: ______________________________

____

cholecystokinin (CCK) to signal a natural satiety response, while giving the stretch receptors in the stomach time to signal fullness. People who tend to eat *anything available* can stop purchasing foods they cannot resist.

Dieters must analyze their own particular shortcomings; they should sensitize themselves to facets of their life-style that make dieting difficult. Is snacking, compulsive eating, or overeating at each meal a constant problem? Then specific problems must be addressed. Table 9-3 provides many options for changing shopping and eating behaviors. Table 9-5 shows step-by-step how to set goals and how to develop specific activities to meet these goals. It is usually best to develop a written plan and show it to a friend or spouse. Social support is important. A

Table 9-5, cont'd

Setting a goal as part of behavior modification

II. Goal attainment

A. *Identify the steps using the Goal Ladder. Are the steps small and manageable? If not, divide the most complex step. More than 10 steps are possible.*

GOAL LADDER

Goal: ______________________________

Step	Time Frame (in no. of weeks or by date)
10	
9	
8	
7	
6	
5	
4	
3	
2	
1	

B *With which steps if any, is the dieter likely to have trouble?* ______________________________

What kind of help will assist the dieter to overcome this trouble? ______________________________

Who can offer this assistance? ______________________________

From: Laquatra I and Danish SJ: A primer for nutritional counselling, In Frankle RT and Yang M, eds: Obesity and Weight Control, Rockville, MD, 1988, Aspen Publishers Inc.

system of rewards for following the plan can add incentive if it focuses on both short- and long-term successes. See Chapter 18 for a more detailed discussion of how to develop a plan to change behavior.

A dieter can tolerate an occasional lapse. Planning a response to lapses should be part of a diet plan, including encouragement to stay calm when errors are made, to take charge immediately, and to ask for help. When a dieter lapses from the diet plan, the newly-learned food habits should bring him or her back toward the plan, and enable the dieter to avoid the lapse to relapse to collapse trap. *Without a strong behavior plan, however, a lapse frequently turns into a relapse.* Once many poor food choices have been made, the dieter feels like a failure and tends to stray further and further from the plan. As the relapse lengthens, the diet plan eventually collapses, and the person stops short of achieving the weight-loss goal. Even with a good behavioral plan, a person may fail at a diet. Dieting is very difficult, and anyone who wishes to diet should be well aware of that. However, without a good behavioral plan, losing weight is even more difficult.

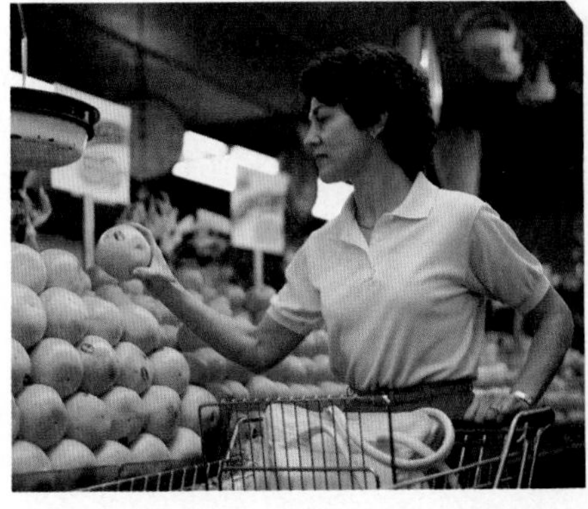

One way to avoid "problem" foods is to choose food wisely at the grocery store.

Concept Check

Several facets of behavior can be modified to improve conditions for losing weight. One behavior area that requires change involves breaking habit chains that encourage overeating, such as snacking while watching television. Another tactic is to modify the environment to reduce temptations, for example, by putting foods out of sight into cupboards. Planning how to handle and refuse food temptations is another strategy. In addition, rethinking attitudes about eating—for example, substituting pleasures other than food as a reward for coping with a stressful day—can be important for altering undesirable eating behavior. Finally, careful observation and recording of eating habits in a diary can reveal subtle behaviors that lead to overeating.

PHYSICAL ACTIVITY—ANOTHER KEY TO WEIGHT LOSS

Engaging in regular physical activity is very important for people who are trying to lose weight.[15] We use many more kcalories in activity than at rest (Figure 9-2). Burning only 200 to 300 extra kcalories per day—above and beyond the normal activity level—can eliminate about a half pound of fat storage per week: that's about 25 pounds of fat loss in a year.

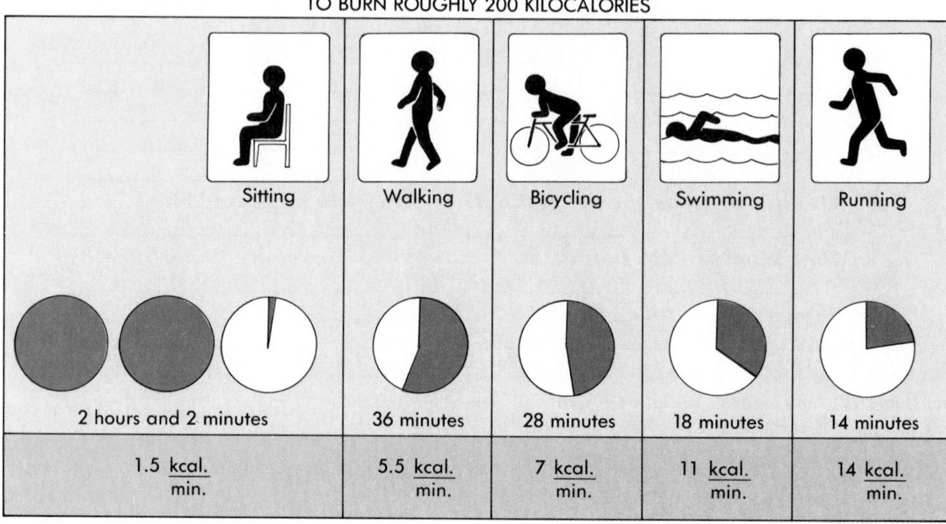

Figure 9-2

Exercise improves any diet. Weight loss will occur because we burn so many more kcalories than at rest.

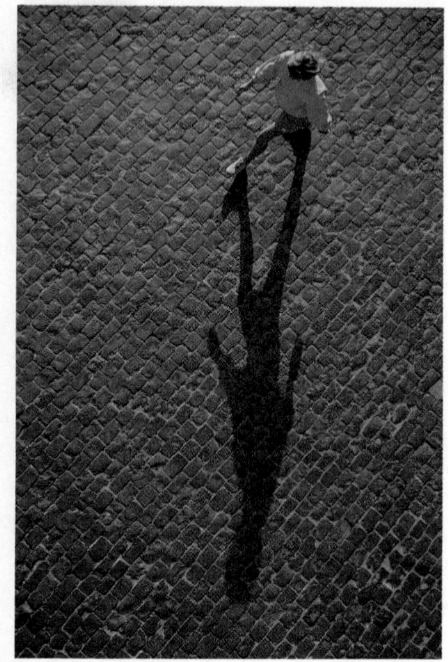

Make walking part of your daily routine.

The easiest way to increase physical activity is to make it part of a daily routine. Experts recommend an hour of brisk walking every day. Using a heel-to-toe motion eases the stress on the body by distributing the impact of shifting weight over the ball of the foot. Comparatively, jogging can be quite stressful for joints.

Besides using energy, exercise has the added advantage of reducing the stress and boredom of a diet. It takes the dieter out of the house and away from snacks. Eventually, an exercise program leads to increased muscle mass as well. More lean tissue raises basal metabolism so that, even while sitting quietly, one burns a few more kcalories than when the same body contains a higher proportion of fat tissue.

Recent studies suggest that activity does not cause the body to raise kcalorie use for hours after an activity, as was earlier thought. Nevertheless, the extra energy used while exercising, coupled with an increase in muscle mass, can pay dividends. Exercise can also help compensate for the loss of muscle mass when on a diet. Whatever means of increasing physical activity is chosen, the activities should be ones the dieter enjoys so that the person will practice them regularly. They should also be convenient, within the dieter's budget, and should provide options for bad weather.

Once a regular exercise program is established, the rate of weight loss begins to diminish. One cause of this slower weight loss is the lowered body weight, which reduces the energy cost of activity. At this point activity level should be increased. The dieter could consider walking 15 minutes more each day to receive the same exercise benefit.

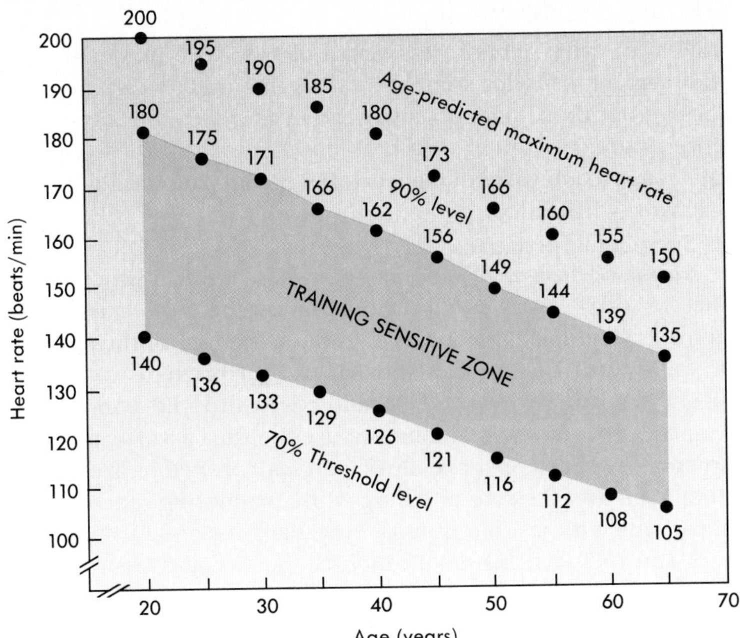

Figure 9-3

Target heart rates for cardiovascular fitness. These rates balance the need for cardiovascular stimulation with those of safety.

Exercise—an added benefit is heart health

One goal in exercising might be to increase **cardiovascular** fitness. To achieve that it is best to increase heart rate to 70% of the maximum rate for about 30 minutes per day at least 3 days per week. Figure 9-3 shows this training-sensitive zone for cardiovascular fitness for various ages. When following this exercise prescription, it is important to use at least 5 minutes to both warm-up and cool-down.

cardiovascular
Referring to the heart and blood vessels.

While heart health is a laudable goal, obese people may find it easier to concentrate on losing weight first. *When the goal is weight loss, the key word is duration—not intensity.* An activity should last long enough to burn 200 to 300 extra kcalories. To get an idea of how long that takes for different exercises, see Figure 9-2 and Appendix J.

Before embarking on a program of regular physical activity, it might be useful to have your body fat measured by bioelectrical impedance or by a skinfold thickness test. These measurements would enable you to track not only weight changes in dieting but also fat mass versus lean mass changes. Many people find their weight does not change as rapidly as their fat mass changes because some fat mass is replaced by lean tissue due to the exercise.

PROFESSIONAL HELP FOR WEIGHT LOSS

The first professional to see for advice about a weight-loss program is the family physician. Doctors are best equipped to assess overall health and the appropriateness of a weight-loss plan. The physician will probably refer the person to a registered dietitian for a specific plan and for answers to diet-related questions. *Registered dietitians are uniquely qualified to help design a weight-loss plan because they understand both food composition and what food means to people* (see Chapter 20).

Many communities have a variety of weight loss organizations. These may include self-help groups, such as Take Off Pounds Sensibly and Weight Watchers. Other programs, such as Nutri System, Diet Center, and Physicians Weight Loss Center among others, are often less desirable for the average dieter. These programs are generally expensive mainly because of their requirements for intense counseling and/or mandatory diet foods and supplements.

Exploring Issues and Actions

Your father is overweight and asks you to recommend an exercise program. He is out of shape and you suspect that he is likely to give up at the first sign of difficulty. What advice can you give? What activities can you recommend? What role can family support play?

Treating morbid obesity

Morbid obesity refers to the status of a body at least 100 pounds over desirable body weight, or twice someone's desirable body weight. Few people have morbid obesity, but those who do suffer the most severe obesity-related health problems. More drastic treatment measures may be used in these cases if the more conservative approach—reducing kcalorie intake, increasing exercise, and modifying behavior—has failed.

Local fat deposits can be reduced in size using suction lipectomy. Lipectomy simply means surgical removal of fat. A pencil-thin tube is inserted into an incision in the skin and the fat tissue, such as that in the buttocks and thigh area, is suctioned off. This procedure, developed in the early 1980s, carries risks such as infection, large depressions in the skin, and blood clots that can lead to kidney failure. Also, it is often quite painful. It is not designed to help a person lose 30 to 40 pounds, but it can be used as part of cosmetic surgery by an experienced physician to help a person reduce localized fat deposits that are very diet-resistant.

Surgical approaches

Stomach surgery. The most common surgical procedure for treating morbid obesity today involves modifying the stomach by **gastroplasty,** also known as stomach stapling.[6] The goal is to reduce the size of the stomach to approximately 50 milliliters, the size of a shot glass. That prevents overeating, except with liquids. Overeating solid foods would result in rapid vomiting. One of two specific surgical procedures is commonly used, either a vertical-banded gastroplasty or a Roux-en-Y gastric bypass. Both surgical procedures are effective. The smaller stomach slows the rate of eating while promoting more rapid satiety. About 75% of patients with morbid obesity eventually lose 50% of body weight after this surgery and they can maintain much of that weight loss over time.[12] This dramatic loss occurs because they can eat only small amounts of food throughout the day. So they are forced to do what was difficult to do before—eat less.

gastroplasty
Surgery on the stomach to limit its volume to approximately 50 milliliters, which is the size of a shot glass.

Stomach surgery for weight loss is costly and often not covered by medical insurance. *There is also nothing magical about the surgery. The person does not awaken from anesthesia thin.* Instead, torturous months must be endured while weight loss occurs. Thus the surgery should not be seen as an easy answer to obesity. The procedure is analogous to jaw-wiring to prevent overeating, but is more effective.

Intestinal bypass. In the 1970s, **intestinal bypass** surgery for weight loss was common. This procedure connected the first foot of the jejunum to the last 4 inches of the ileum, bypassing approximately 12 feet of intestinal absorptive area. This surgery profoundly reduces the body's capability to absorb nutrients, and so contributes to rapid weight loss. However, the physiological consequences of this surgery are staggering. They include electrolyte imbalances, gallstones, kidney stones, fat buildup in the liver, and anemia. Thus this surgical procedure is no longer advised.

intestinal bypass
A surgical procedure that causes intentional malabsorption of food by shortening the length of the intestine by about 12 of its normal 15 feet. This procedure is no longer used to treat obesity because of the major medical problems that resulted.

Gastric balloons. A new "answer to obesity" whose popularity has already waned is the **gastric balloon.**[18,19] It was inserted into the upper portion of the stomach. The balloon is only the size of a soda can, but by sitting in the upper part of the stomach, it was supposed to stimulate satiety receptors, and thus reduce food intake.

The Food and Drug Administration (FDA) originally allowed the balloons to stay in place for 4 months. But because of the high incidence of spontaneous deflations, the time limit was reduced to between 3 and 4 months. Each insertion and removal of the balloon costs approximately $600. Thus a person could spend a lot of money in a short time using this method to decrease eating. Also, if spontaneous deflation occurred, the balloon would pass through the intestinal tract, causing extreme pain. As of May 1988 this product is no longer available.

Dietary approaches

Very low calorie diets. If more traditional diet changes have failed, treating morbid obesity with a **very low calorie diet (VLCD)** is possible. Some researchers believe people with body weights greater than 40% above desirable weight are also appropriate candidates.[28] The diet allows a person to eat 400 to 700 kcalories per day, often in liquid form.[8] (These diets were known earlier as protein-sparing modified fasts.) Of this amount, about 30 grams are carbohydrates. The rest is high biological value protein, making up about 2 grams per kilogram of desirable body weight. This low-carbohydrate intake causes ketosis, which may

very low calorie diet (VLCD)
Also known as a protein-sparing modified fast (PSMF), this diet allows the consumption of 400 to 700 kcalories per day in liquid form. Of this, about 30 grams are made up of carbohydrate; the rest is high-biological value protein.

decrease appetite. However, the main reasons for weight loss are the few kcalories allowed and the absence of food choice. About 3 to 5 pounds can be lost per week: men tend to lose at a higher rate than do women.

Losing weight too rapidly on a VLCD can cause a significant loss of heart tissue, which may lead to sudden death from heart attack.[2] Therefore *anyone following this type of diet must be under a doctor's care and should use this type of diet only when more conservative approaches have failed.*[28] The dieter needs to consume at least 2 grams of potassium per day[2] and should participate in a behavior modification program designed to prevent weight regain once the diet is stopped. The Optifast program meets these stipulations but can cost over $100 per week. In addition, a recent study shows few people can maintain the weight loss: men had the best results, especially if they met their goal weights.[16] Newer behavior modification programs may improve long-term success.

Very-low–calorie diets should not be used with infants, children, teenagers, pregnant women, or elderly people. In addition, people with diseases such as gout, heart disease, hypertension, and diabetes mellitus are advised to seek alternate methods for weight reduction.

Researchers recommend limiting a VLCD to 12 weeks maximum.[1] The dieter should then take a 1-month vacation from the diet to minimize the loss of lean tissue. During the vacation a low-kcalorie but completely balanced diet is appropriate. The dieter can then return for another 12 weeks of the VLCD.

Instead, if one follows a VLCD for months at a time, the risk of sudden heart attack becomes very high. When this type of diet was marketed in the 1970s as a "liquid-protein diet" and promoted by a book called *The Last Chance Diet,* it became "the last chance" for the more than 60 people who died, primarily from heart failure.

Concept Check

When a person is faced with morbid obesity and previous failures with conservative weight loss strategies, other options can be considered. Either surgery to reduce the volume of the stomach to approximately 50 milliliters, or a very low calorie diet consisting of 400 to 700 kcalories per day may be used. In both cases, behavior modification must be part of the program to help the person to maintain the weight loss.

FAD DIETS—WHY ALL THE COMMOTION?

Many overweight people try to treat themselves using the latest fad diet book. But, as you will see, most of these diets do not help, and some can actually harm those who follow them (Table 9-6).

You may wonder why fad diet books exist at all. Why doesn't the government put a stop to them? Many contain blatant misinformation. However, the FDA concerns itself only when products are suspected of doing serious harm, as in the case of the liquid protein diets. The FDA is too busy to pursue every new fad diet plan. So, concerning fad diet books, ancient advice is still valid: "let the buyer beware." Responsibility rests with the authors and publishers, who want to sell a lot of books and earn a lot of money and know there is little risk involved. Making outrageous claims sells more books than writing "eat less and exercise more." Nutritional Perspective 9-1 discusses some common misconceptions associated with all types of quackery, including fad diets. Figure 9-5 shows dieting quackery has existed for years.

It is illegal in the United States to falsely represent worthless or dangerous cures and medical devices. Thus U.S. citizens can use their rights under federal law to have the FDA pursue a seller of a dangerous fad diet in an attempt to have it removed from the bookshelves.

How to recognize a fad diet

Fad diets typically share some common characteristics. We list a few here:[31]

1. They promote quick weight loss. As mentioned before, this loss is primarily due to glycogen, sodium, and lean muscle mass depletion. All lead to a loss of body water.

Figure 9-4

Rating the popular diets by Dr. Jack Yetiv.

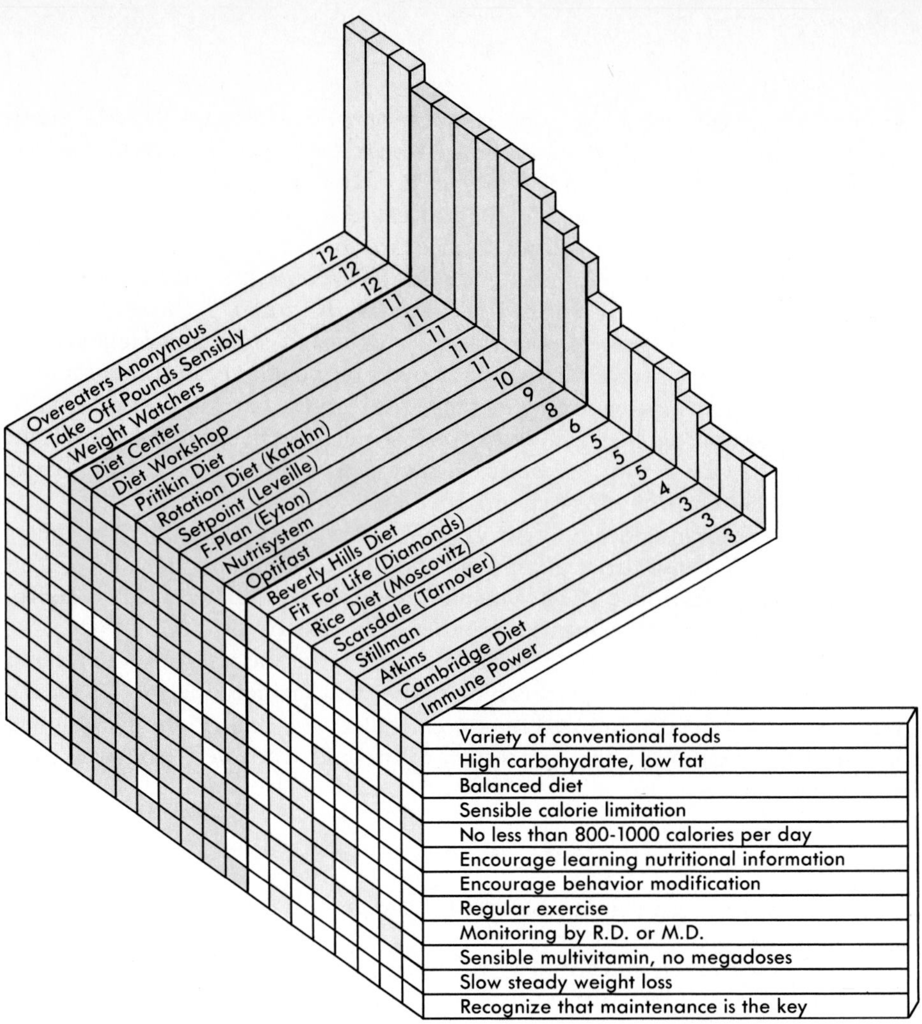

2. They limit food selections and dictate specific rituals, such as only eating fruit for breakfast.
3. They use testimonials from famous people and tie the diet to well-known cities, such as Beverly Hills and New York.
4. They bill themselves as "cure-alls." Whatever the type of obesity or whatever a reader's specific strengths and weaknesses, these diets claim to work for everyone.
5. They often recommend expensive supplements. Some of these supplements can be harmful, such as high doses of vitamin A, vitamin D, vitamin C, or vitamin B-6 (pyridoxine).
6. No attempts are made to permanently change eating habits. The dieter follows the diet until the desired weight is reached and then reverts to old eating habits. Eat rice for a month, lose weight, and then return to old habits.
7. They are generally critical of and skeptical about the scientific community. They suggest that physicians and registered dietitians do not really want people to lose weight. They encourage people to look outside the medical establishment for correct advice.

Probably the cruelest characteristic of fad diets is that they guarantee failure for the dieter.[13,25] *These diets are not designed for permanent weight loss.* Habits are not changed, and the food selection is so limited that the person cannot follow the diet for more than 1 or 2 weeks. Although dieters assume they have lost fat, they have actually lost mostly muscle and other lean tissue mass. As soon as they begin eating normally again, the lost tissue is replaced. In a matter of weeks, most of the lost weight is back. The dieter appears to have failed when

35 Pounds of Fat.

DR. EDISON'S OBESITY PILLS AND REDUCING TABLETS CURED MRS. MANNING.

No Other Remedies But Dr. Edison's Reduce Obesity—Take No Others.

SAMPLES FREE—USE COUPON.

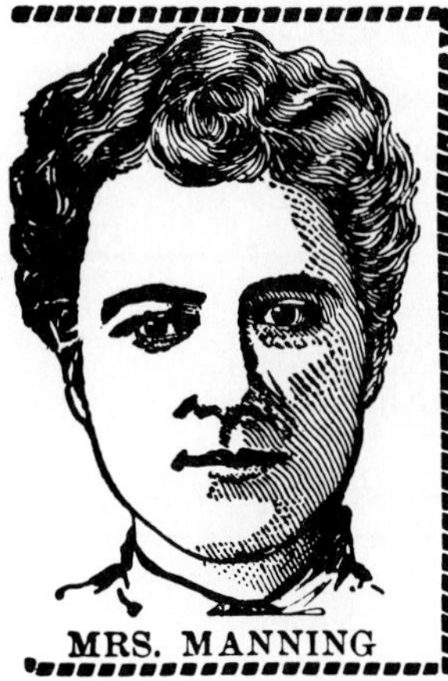

Mary Hyde Manning, one of the best known of Troy's, New York, society women, grew too fleshy, and used Dr. Edison's Obesity Remedies. Read the letter telling of her reduction and restoration to health:—"In six weeks I was reduced 35 pounds, from 171 to 136, by Dr. Edison's Obesity Pills and Reducing Tablets. I recommend these remedies to all fat and sick men and women."

The following well-known men and women have been reduced by DR. EDISON'S OBESITY REMEDIES:

Mrs. H. Mershon, 156 South Jackson St., Lima, O., 148 lbs.
Mrs. Josephine McPherson, 7916 Wright St., Chicago, 42 lbs.
Rev. Edward R. Pierce, 410 Alma St., Chicago, 42 lbs.
C. C. Nichols, 145 Clark St., Aurora, Ill., 36 lbs.
Mrs. W. Davlin, Whitemore, O., 149 lbs.
W. H. Webster, 618 2d Ave., Troy, N. Y., 26 lbs.
J. M. McKinney, 4504 State St., Chicago, 30 lbs.
Mrs. J. M. McKinney, 4504 State St., Chicago, 33 lbs.
Mrs. A. Walker, 1104 Milton Place, Chicago, 20 lbs.

Figure 9-5

Quackery has been with us for ages. Even at the turn of this century, people wanted to believe that fat could be lost without changing habits.

actually the diet has failed. This whole scenario can add more blame and guilt to the psyche of the dieter—and that is very unfortunate.[23] If someone needs help losing weight, professional help is the answer. That is something fad diets rarely offer.

Types of fad diets

Low-carbohydrate (ketogenic) approaches. This is the most common form of fad diet. The low-carbohydrate intake forces the liver to perform gluconeogenesis (see Chapters 4 and 7). The source of carbon atoms for gluconeogenesis is protein tissue. Thus a low-carbohydrate diet results in protein tissue loss, as well as urinary loss of essential electrolytes, such as potassium. Since protein tissue is mostly water, the person loses weight very rapidly. When a normal diet is resumed, the protein tissue is rebuilt and that weight comes right back.

There is nothing special about a low-carbohydrate diet in terms of weight loss. If the diet is also low in kcalories, then it is likely to result in weight loss. But a low-carbohydrate diet by itself does not result in more weight loss than any other type of diet.

Diet plans that use a low-carbohydrate approach are the *Dr Atkinson Diet Revolution, Dr Stillman's Calories Don't Count Diet,* the *Scarsdale Diet,* the *Drinking Man's Diet, Four Day Wonder Diet,* and the *Air Force Diet.* When you see a new fad diet advertisement, look first to see how much carbohydrate it contains. If breads, cereals, fruits, and vegetables are extremely limited, you are probably looking at a ketogenic diet.

Low-fat approaches. The very low fat diet turns out to be a very high carbohydrate diet. These diets contain approximately only 5% to 10% of kcalories as fat. The most notable is the *Pritikin Diet.* This approach is not harmful but it is extremely difficult to follow. People get bored with this type of diet very quickly because many of their favorite foods cannot be eaten. The dieter primarily eats grains, fruits, and vegetables, and most people cannot do this very long. Eventually, the person will want some foods higher in fat or protein. Thus the person is

Table 9-6

Summary of popular dietary approaches to weight control

Approach and Examples	Characteristics and possible negative health consequences
Moderate caloric restriction	
The Setpoint Diet Slim Chance in a Fat World Weight Watcher's Diet The American Heart Assoc. Diet Mary Ellen's Help Yourself Diet Plan The Beyond Diet	Usually 1000-1800 kcal per day Reasonable balance of macronutrients Encourage exercise May employ behavioral approach No consequences if vitamin and mineral supplement used and permission of family physician is granted
Macronutrient restriction	
Low carbohydrate:	Less than 100 grams carbohydrate per day
Atkin's Diet Revolution Calories Don't Count Drinking Man's Diet Woman Doctor's Diet for Women The Doctor's Quick Weight Loss Diet (Stillman's) The Complete Scarsdale Medical Diet Four Day Wonder Diet	Weakness due to ketosis; poor exercise capacity due to poor glycogen stores in the muscles; excessive animal fat intake
Low-fat:	Less than 20% of calories from fat Limited (or elimination of) animal protein sources, all fats, nuts, seeds
The Rice Diet Report The Macrobiotic Diet (some versions) The Pritikin Diet The Tokyo Diet The Palm Beach Lifelong Diet The James Coco Diet The 35+ Diet The Pasta Diet	Little satiety; flatulence, possibly poor mineral absorption from excess fiber; limited food choices → deprivation
Novelty diets	
Dr. Abravanel's Body Type and Lifetime Nutrition Plan Dr. Berger's Immune Power Diet Fit for Life The Rotation Diet The Beverly Hills Diet Dr. Debetz Champaign Diet Sun Sign Diet	Promote certain nutrients, foods, or combination of foods as having unique, magical, or previously undiscovered qualities Malnutrition; no change in habits → relapse; unrealistic food choices → leading to possible bingeing

Table 9-6, cont'd

Summary of popular dietary approaches to weight control

Approach and Examples*	Characteristics and possible negative health consequences
Very low calorie diets	
Optifast Cambridge Diet The Last Chance Diet Genesis	Less than 800 kcalories per day Also known as protein-sparing modified fasts Weakness; organ tissue loss—especially from the heart; low serum potassium level → heart failure; expense → must be under close physician scrutiny; kidney stones; gout
Formula diets	
U.S.A. (United Sciences of America), Inc. Optifast Genesis Cambridge Diet Herbalife The Last Chance Diet Slimfast	Based on formulated or packaged products Many are very low—calorie diet regimens (see above) No change in habits → increased chance of relapse; expensive; constipation
Premeasured diets	
Nutri System	Most food supplied in premeasured servings Expensive; may not allow for easy sound eating later

*Diets may be listed in more than one category if multiple characteristics apply.

bound to suffer a lapse, then a relapse, and probably a collapse. These diets are just too atypical of our usual diet to follow consistently.

Novelty diets. A whole variety of diets are built on gimmicks. *The Rotation Diet,* for example, rotates the amount of kcalories ingested in an attempt to prevent the usual drop in basal metabolism associated with dieting. A woman is supposed to eat 600 kcalories per day for 3 days, then 900 kcalories per day for 4 days, and then 1200 kcalories per day for 7 days, repeating this cycle over and over again. For men, the levels are 1200, 1500, and 1800 kcalories. No scientific data show that this diet works or even how it could work. Diets calling for fewer than 1000 kcalories are suspect because of their low-nutrient content. Thus it must be considered a fad diet.

Other novelty diets emphasize one food or food group to the exclusion of almost all others. A rice diet was designed in the 1940s to lower blood pressure; now it has resurfaced as a weight-loss diet. The first phase consists of eating only rice and fruit until you cannot stand them any longer. Another novelty diet is the egg diet. You eat all the eggs you want. On the *Beverly Hills Diet* you eat almost nothing but fruit.

The rationale behind these diets is that you can eat only eggs, or fruit, or rice for so long. You will soon become bored and, in theory, will reduce your energy intake. However, chances are that you will abandon the diet entirely before you lose much weight.

Numerous other gimmicks for weight loss have come and gone and are likely to resurface. These include blockers of starch digestion (discussed in Chapter 3), as well as various hormones and hormone stimulators. If in the future an important aid for weight loss is discovered, you can feel confident that major journals will report the finding, such as the *Journal of The American Dietetic Association,* the *Journal of the American Medical Association,* or the *New England Journal of Medicine.* You don't need to rely on paperback books or newspaper advertisements.

In the 1960s grapefruits were touted for their supposed unique ability to cause weight loss. To add appeal to the grapefruit diet, several "diet aids" were added: lecithin to help release fat from the tissues, vitamin B-6 to act as a diuretic, vinegar to provide potassium, and kelp to stimulate the thyroid glands. In the 1980s we had an entirely new product, *Herbalife.* This contains herbs high in caffeine; caffeine stimulates the metabolic rate. None of these aids is very effective. None of them substitutes for moderating food intake, modifying behavior, and increasing activity.

The most bizarre of the novelty diets propose that "food gets stuck in your body." *Fit for Life* and the *Beverly Hills Diet* are examples. The supposition is that food gets stuck in the intestine, putrefies, and creates toxins that invade the bloodstream and cause disease. This is utter nonsense.[31] Nevertheless, the same idea has been promoted in health food books since the 1800s. Today, *Fit for Life* suggests meat eaten with potatoes will not be digested, and to only consume fresh fruit before noon. These recommendations are absurd. They are gimmicks that appear controversial but are really designed to sell books. If weight loss does occur, it is because the books use such complicated combining rules and rituals that, by the time you have figured out what you can eat, it is the wrong time to eat it!

Finally, we should mention some commercial schemes used to sell diet books. Books describing the allergy approach to dieting, for instance, suggest that current diseases, including obesity, are due to food allergies. Supposedly, once your food allergies are found and treated, you will no longer have the disease. However, we know of no research that supports the claim that 30% of people have food allergies, as suggested in *Dr Berger's Immune Power Diet Book.* In addition, see the *Sun Sign Diet* if you believe in astrology, the *Champagne Diet* if you need a drink, or the *Body Type and Lifetime Nutrition Diet* if you have a "dominant" gland.

Exploring Issues and Actions

Why are diet books so popular? How many have you bought? What would prompt you to buy one, if you haven't so far?

Concept Check

Fad diets characteristically promote quick weight loss and limited food selections, use testimonials from famous people, bill the plan as a cure-all, include expensive supplements, and show little concern for permanently changing food habits. Typical approaches include low-carbohydrate regimens, low-fat regimens, and novel approaches, which consist of complex food-combining rules or a focus on one type of food, such as rice or fruit.

OVER-THE-COUNTER MEDICATIONS TO AID WEIGHT LOSS

Over-the-counter medications that claim to facilitate weight loss sell briskly. Some can be effective,[29] but so far none can substitute for the basic approach we have outlined in this chapter to promote weight loss. Diet aids include caffeine, fiber pills, **phenylpropanolamine,** and benzocaine. Caffeine tends to blunt appetite. Phenylpropanolamine is an epinephrine-like drug that can cause a slight decrease in food intake. Benzocaine numbs the tongue, so a person tends to eat less.

phenylpropanolamine
An over-the-counter stimulant that has a mild appetite-reducing effect.

Fiber pills can increase bulk in the stomach and ideally lead to satiety. A recent study showed that only soluble-type fiber, the type found in beans and oats, was effective in decreasing food intake after 2 weeks. Bran fiber, such as that found in fiber pills, was not effective. However, when the people in the study took enough soluble fiber (23 grams) incorporated into crackers to decrease food intake, they also had significant intestinal gas.[27]

Regarding prescription medications, physicians sometimes prescribe *amphetamines* for weight loss.[29] Amphetamines cause a person to eat less, but they are also possibly addictive. In addition, amphetamines can increase heart rate and nervousness and lead to insomnia. Thyroid hormone preparations were once popular, but these caused significant loss of lean tissue.

Fenfluramine and fluoxetine have been prescribed by physicians to promote weight loss. These drugs increase the action of serotonin in the brain, which may lead to less food craving, especially for high-carbohydrate foods (see Chapter 8). Rapid weight gain after discontinuing the drug is a problem.

Another class of experimental medications that reduce food intake are the *opiate-antagonists,* such as naloxone and naltrexone. These drugs cause a significant decrease in food intake in animals, but the results from human studies are very discouraging. Development of related drugs is continuing.

Overall, in skilled hands, prescription medications can aid weight loss,[29] however, they do not supplant the need for following more conservative approaches of reducing kcalorie intake, modifying problem behaviors, and increasing physical activity.

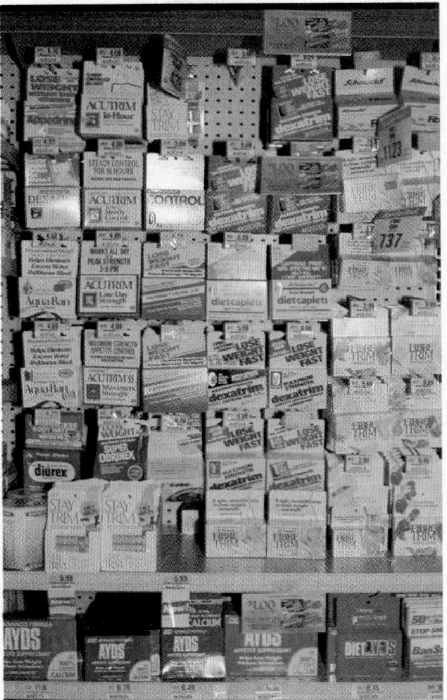

Although diet aids are popular, they are no substitute for a sound weight loss program.

PUTTING WEIGHT LOSS INTO PERSPECTIVE

A disturbing fact about dieting for weight loss is that often the weight is regained. People may end up heavier after their diet-and-regain cycle than when they began. Based on this information, *it appears that dieting itself can promote obesity. Thus dieting should not be undertaken lightly.* If a person is not highly moti-

Figure 9-6

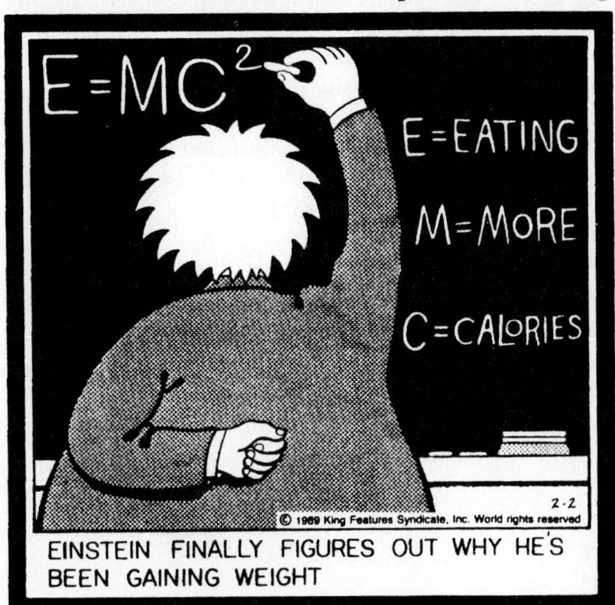

Expert Opinion

Dieters' Weight Regained: Are There Risks?

KELLY BROWNELL, Ph.D.

Just about everyone has been on a diet. And millions of us have learned that the weight we have lost is all too easily regained. Statistics tell the story: a recent Gallup poll revealed that 30% of American women between 19 and 39 diet *at least once a month.* If dieting really works, why repeat the process again and again?

We have become a nation of "yo-yo" dieters—our weight perennially cycling down, up, down, and up again. Still, despite their frustration, few dieters question the wisdom of dieting. After all, they reason, the worst that can happen is to regain the weight they've lost—in which case, they can just go on a diet again.

But new research shows there is a risk: yo-yo dieting can seriously distort the body's weight-regulation system. It seems that the more diets you go on, the harder it becomes to lose weight. Even worse, there is new evidence that repeated yo-yo dieting may increase your risk of heart disease.

For years we've suspected that yo-yo dieting—or "weight cycling"—can make it harder and harder to lose weight. Some people who come to our clinic at the University of Pennsylvania have already lost and regained hundreds of pounds. Now, even on near-starvation diets, many of these yo-yo dieters can lose little weight.

From our current research we're starting to see several disturbing possibilities why chronic dieting may cause problems:

- Yo-yo dieting may increase the proportion of fat to lean tissue on the body.
- The loss-gain cycle may increase the desire for fatty foods, which are themselves unhealthy.
- Yo-yo dieters may *redistribute* body fat—shifting it from the thighs and hips to the abdomen—in a way that is dangerous to health.
- Repeated cycles of losing and gaining may raise the risk of developing heart problems.

The last prospect is especially unsettling. Northwestern University researchers reported that men who showed the greatest up-and-down weight swings also had the highest risk of sudden death from coronary heart disease. The report was based on a major study of 1701 men who were tracked over a period of 25 years.

The Framingham Heart Study, which has monitored more than 5000 people in Framingham, Massachusetts for nearly 40 years, also provides troubling statistics: people who lost 10% of their body weight had a 20% reduction in risk of coronary heart disease—but people who then regained 10% *raised* the risk by *30%*. Going from 150 to 135 pounds, and back to 150 again could leave you with a higher heart-disease risk than you started with.

None of this means that dieting is necessarily futile or foolish. There are good reasons to reduce: successful weight loss can lower blood pressure and cholesterol and can help control blood sugar in adult-onset diabetes, as well as helping people feel better about themselves. But the new research does mean dieting is an activity to be taken seriously.

It also means that dieting alone is not the best route to weight control. When a weight-loss program includes exercise, you lose more fat and less muscle, and you're less likely to gain the weight back. Exercise may help counteract the physiological changes that tend to make yo-yo dieting so futile—starting with the metabolic changes that make it notoriously easy to regain the weight you lose.

WHAT OUR PATIENTS TAUGHT US

My interest in the yo-yo problem began in 1982, when my colleagues Thomas Wadden and Albert Stunkard and I were experimenting with very low-calorie diets (800 calories or fewer per day). We hoped that patients in our clinic could lose large amounts of weight rapidly on these diets, then sustain the weight loss with a good behavior modification program.

Suzanne Steen, a sports nutritionist with our group, and Robert Oppliger at the University of Iowa have studied elite high school wrestlers at Iowa's summer wrestling camp. We predicted that wrestlers whose weight fluctuated significantly—yo-yo dieters—would have lower metabolic rates than those who wrestled close to their natural weight. After accounting for differences in wrestlers' weights and body compositions, our suspicion was confirmed.

We have now started to look at other athletes who keep their weight chronically low—distance runners, gymnasts, figure skaters, divers, and ballet dancers. Remarkably enough, some elite women runners maintain their weight on a little over 1,200 calories a day—even when they're burning about 600 calories a day in exercise.

UP-AND-DOWN HEALTH HAZARD?

Though we understand yo-yo dieting much better than we did just a few years ago, we are especially concerned with the

Expert Opinion—cont'd

bottom-line question: How do weight cycles affect a person's health? For example, one woman, Marie, began a weight-loss program at 230 pounds, reduced to 192 pounds, and then "hit a wall," even though she stayed on her diet and walked two miles a day. Marie, like many others in our program, had been a yo-yo dieter. It was my impression that the yo-yo dieters tended to have the most difficulty losing weight.

To see if dieting could really change the body this way, we began to study weight fluctuations in animals. Our first study—conducted with Drs. Eliot Stellar and E. Eileen Shrager at Penn, and M.R.C. Greenwood at Vassar—involved a group of rats that we turned into yo-yo dieters. We first fattened them up by feeding them a high-fat diet. Then, after they became obese, we altered their diets repeatedly to make them lose weight, regain, lose again and regain again.

The results were striking. The first time the yo-yo-ing rats lost weight, it took 21 days for them to go from obese to normal weight. On their second diet, it took 46 days for the same loss, even though the rats ate exactly as many calories as they had the first time!

And with each yo-yo, it became easier for the rats to regain. After the first diet, they took 45 days to become obese again; after the second diet, they took only 14 days. In other words, on the second yo-yo cycle, *it took twice as long to lose weight, and only one-third as long to regain it.*

Our dramatic results fit with those of other researchers. Sweden's Dr. Per Bjorntorp and Mei-Uih Yang found that losing and regaining weight greatly increases food efficiency—the ease with which animals (or people) can maintain their weight on a given number of calories. After one yo-yo cycle of fasting and refeeding, Bjorntorp's rats became *five times* more food-efficient than animals who had not lost and regained weight.

Following our experiments with rats, we decided to look systematically at human yo-yo dieters as well. So Rutgers psychologist G Terence Wilson and I contacted Harvard surgeon George Blackburn, a pioneer in the use of very low calorie diets. Blackburn and his colleagues selected 140 dieters who had been through their clinic, had lost weight and then regained it—and had returned to the clinic for a second try. The records showed that they'd lost an average of 2.3 pounds a week the first time, but lost only 1.3 pounds a week the second time.

More recent studies, done as part of the Weight Cycling Project, have taught us to look at new aspects of yo-yo dieting. We're asking, for example, whether it can change the proportion of fat to muscle tissue.

People who lose weight by dieting—especially on a crash diet, or on a diet low in protein—can lose a substantial amount of muscle. But then, if they gain weight back, they may regain less muscle and more fat. While the reason isn't clear, it may be easier for the body to put fat on than to rebuild lost muscle.

Yo-yo dieting also appears to increase the desire for fatty foods. In animal experiments at Yale, psychologist Judith Rodin and student Danielle Reed gave rats a choice of different food sources—carbohydrate, protein, or fat—before and after weight cycling. For some time after dieting, the rats chose more fat.

In addition, yo-yo dieters may lose fat from one part of the body and gain it back somewhere else—a change that can pose a health hazard. Research shows that fat above the waist raises the risk of heart disease and diabetes more than fat below the waist. Weight cycling could shift fat to the abdomen, according to preliminary studies in both animals and people. When George Blackburn asked his yo-yo dieters where they regained the weight they had lost on the first diet, they said most of it had gone to their waists.

Thus the way in which you lose weight can make a big difference. The best approach is to eat a low-fat, high-complex-carbohydrate diet and get regular aerobic exercise. The combination gives you the best odds of *permanent weight loss,* and may lower the risk of heart disease, help normalize blood sugar and possibly prevent cancer.

One final point: If you've been a yo-yo dieter in the past, don't be too discouraged. You can still take control of your weight. It may just take a little more effort and a little more patience the next time around.

Dr. Brownell is professor of psychiatry at the University of Pennsylvania School of Medicine. A leading obesity researcher, he is president-elect of the Association for the Advancement of Behavior Therapy and the Society of Behavioral Medicine.

vated and does not have the needed social support, dieting for weight loss should be delayed until a more appropriate time.

Would-be dieters should choose and follow diet plans that are appropriate for them. There is a smorgasbord of options: kcalorie reduction, behavior modification, increased activity, and group and/or individual counseling. Many tools are effective, but some will be more useful than others, depending on the dieter's life-style, personality, and motivation. To discover which techniques promote the best chance of losing weight and maintaining the loss, the person must explore his or her own strengths and weaknesses.

Overall, in terms of both health and self-esteem, the life of the dieter should improve as weight is lost. All diets should be measured by that standard.

Concept Check

Neither over-the-counter drugs nor prescription medications dramatically improve the prospects for weight loss. The focus still remains a reduction in kcalorie intake, modification of problem eating behaviors, and increased physical activity. A dieter should realize that weight loss is difficult, and thus should only be attempted when there is a strong commitment to the goal of weight loss.

TREATING UNDERWEIGHT

Underweight, too, can be a problem that requires medical intervention. Underweight can increase the risk of a woman delivering a low birth weight baby (see Chapter 15), lead to complications in surgery, and slow recovery after illness. A physician should be consulted to rule out hormonal imbalances, depression, or other hidden disease in underweight people.

Treatments for underweight adults use several different approaches. The person could gradually increase consumption of kcalorie-dense foods, especially those higher in fat, with particular emphasis on vegetable fats. These are best eaten at the end of a meal so that they don't cause early satiety. Lowfat cheeses, dried fruit, bananas, nuts, and granola are good kcalorie sources, as these have a potential for a low content of saturated fat (read the label). The person should avoid diet soft drinks and other substitutes for good energy sources. It might be helpful to keep a daily food record and review it weekly to see whether higher kcalorie food choices could be made (see the left side of Table 9-2).

An underweight person who is very physically active could also consider reducing activity. If the person remains very lean, a body-building program might be considered, incorporating weight lifting to increase muscle development.

If these efforts fail to achieve the desired weight, they at least should prevent health problems associated with being underweight. After achieving that, the person may have to accept his or her very lean frame, and perhaps find some consolation in the exemption from a struggle against a disease possibly more difficult to overcome—obesity.

Summary

1. When considering a treatment for obesity, three points should be remembered: (1) The body resists weight loss; (2) The emphasis should be on preventing obesity, since curing the disease is very difficult; (3) Weight loss on a diet should represent a loss of fat storage, and not the loss of muscle and other lean tissues.
2. A sound weight-loss diet should meet the dieter's nutritional needs by following the Daily Food Guide; it should adapt to the person's habits, consist of readily obtainable foods, strive to change poor eating habits, recommend reg-

ular physical activity, and insist the person see a physician if weight is to be lost rapidly or if the person is over 35 years of age and plans to perform substantially greater physical activity than usual.

3. A pound of adipose tissue represents approximately 2700 to 3500 kcalories. Thus if energy output exceeds energy intake by 400 to 500 kcalories per day, a pound of fat storage can be lost per week. Decreasing the intake of high-fat foods is probably the best way to obtain this kcalorie deficit, along with increasing physical activity.
4. Behavior modification is a vital part of a weight-loss program because the dieter may have many habits that encourage overeating, and so discourage weight maintenance. Specific behavior modification techniques, such as stimulus control and self-monitoring, can be used to help change those problem behaviors.
5. Increasing physical activity is a vital part of a weight-loss program; the focus should be on duration rather than intensity. Ideally, approximately 200 to 300 extra kcalories should be expended in activity each day.
6. Treatment of morbid obesity includes stomach surgery to reduce stomach volume to approximately 50 milliliters, or very low calorie diets, containing 400 to 700 kcalories per day. Both these procedures should be reserved for people who have failed at more conservative approaches to weight loss. They require medical supervision.
7. Fad diets are easy to recognize. They often promote rapid weight loss, limited food selections, offer testimonials from famous people, are billed as "cure-alls," include expensive supplements, and make little or no attempt to permanently alter food habits. General criticism of and skepticism about the scientific community is also common.
8. Fad diets can be classed as low-carbohydrate approaches, low-fat approaches, and novel approaches. The latter category includes diets with complex food-combining rituals and those that focus on one type of food to the exclusion of most others, such as rice or fruit.
9. Medications to aid weight loss that are available over-the-counter in drug stores include caffeine and other mild stimulants and fiber pills. None of these, however, can substitute for a good diet, behavior, and exercise plan.

Take Action

Use a separate sheet of paper to develop a plan aimed at your problem food behaviors. Identify those behaviors that will be difficult to change and those that will be easy to change.

	Problem Food Behaviors	Corrective Action
Easy to Change		
a.______		
b.______		
c.______		
d.______		
Difficult to Change		
a.______		
b.______		
c.______		
d.______		

REFERENCES

1. Atkinson RL and others: A comprehensive approach to outpatient obesity management, Journal of the American Dietetic Association 84:439, 1984.
2. Atkinson RL: Very low calorie diets: getting sick or remaining healthy on a handful of calories, Journal of Nutrition 116:918, 1986.
3. Brownell KD: Obesity and weight control: the good and bad of dieting, Nutrition Today May/June:4, 1987.
4. Canadian Dietetic Association: Obesity: a case for prevention, Journal of the Canadian Dietetic Association 49:11, 1988.
5. Council on Scientific Affairs, American Medical Association: Treatment of obesity, Journal of the American Medical Association 257:1323, 1988.
6. Cronin BS and McDonough A: Nutrition management of morbid obesity in conjunction with surgical intervention, Topics in Clinical Nutrition 2:59, 1987.
7. Eckel RH and Yost TJ: Weight reduction increases adipose tissue lipoprotein lipase responsiveness in obese women, Journal of Clinical Investigation 80:992, 1987.
8. Fisler JS and Drenick EJ: Starvation and semistarvation diets in the management of obesity, Annual Reviews of Nutrition 7:465, 1987.
9. Frankel RT and Yang M: Obesity and Weight Control. Rockville, Md, 1988, Aspen Publishers Inc.
10. Fuller E: Helping your patient lose weight, Patient Care June 15:125, 1986.
11. Geissler CA and others: The daily metabolic rate of the post-obese and the lean, The American Journal of Clinical Nutrition 45:914, 1987.
12. Graney AS and others: Gastric partitioning for morbid obesity: postoperative weight loss, technical complications, and protein status, Journal of the American Dietetic Association 86:630, 1986.
13. Haggerty PA and Blackburn GL: A critical evaluation of popular low calorie diets in America, part 2, Topics in Clinical Nutrition 2:37, 1987.
14. Holli BB: Using behavior modification in nutrition counseling, Journal of the American Dietetic Association 88:1530, 1988.
15. Horton ES: Metabolic aspects of exercise and weight reduction, Medicine and Science in Sports and Exercise 18:10, 1986.
16. Kirschner MA and others: An eight-year experience with a very-low-calorie formula diet for control of major obesity, International Journal of Obesity 12:69, 1988.
17. Leibel RL and Hirsh J: Metabolic characteristics of obesity, Annals of Internal Medicine 103:1000, 1985.
18. Levine GM: Intragastric balloons: an unfulfilled promise, Annals of Internal Medicine 94:354, 1988.
19. Lindor KD and others: Intragastric balloons in comparison with standard therapy for obesity: a randomized, double-blind trial, Mayo Clinic Proceedings 62:999, 1987.
20. Lissner L and others: Dietary fat and the regulation of energy intake in human subjects, American Journal of Clinical Nutrition 46:886, 1987.
21. Loper JF and Barrows KK: Nutrition and weight-control program in industry, Journal of the American Dietetic Association 85:148, 1985.
22. Owen OE: In Kinney JM and others, eds: Obesity in nutrition and metabolism in patient care, Philadelphia, 1988, WB Saunders Co.
23. Pasulka PS: Is there a risk from recurrent dieting? Topics in Clinical Nutrition 2:1, 1987.
24. Rock CL and Coluston AM: Weight-control approaches: a review by the California Dietetic Association, Journal of the American Dietetic Association 88:44, 1988.
25. Schapell DS and others: A critical evaluation of popular low calorie diets in America: part 1, Topics in Clinical Nutrition 2:29, 1987.
26. Spillman D: Fiddle-faddle, mythos, and quacksalver, Topics in Clinical Nutrition 3:36, 1988.
27. Stevens J and others: Effect of psyllium gum and wheat bran on spontaneous energy intake, American Journal of Clinical Nutrition 46:812, 1987.
28. Wadden TA and Stunkard AJ: Letter to the editor on Weight-control approaches: a review by the California Dietetic Association, Journal of the American Dietetic Association 88:905, 1988.
29. Weintraub M and Bray GA: Drug treatment for obesity, Medical Clinics of North America 73:237, 1989.
30. Yetiv J: Popular diets: the good, the bad, and the ugly, Healthline 7:1, 1988.
31. Yetiv JZ: Popular nutritional practices: a scientific appraisal, Popular Medicine Press, Toledo, Ohio, 1986, Popular Medicine Press.

SUGGESTED READINGS

Excellent reviews on treating obesity by reducing kcalorie intake and modifying behavior can be found in the articles by the Council on Scientific Affairs of the American Medical Association, Fuller, Rock with Coulston, and Brownell. Together these articles provide a detailed account of all conservative options available for losing weight. The article by Holli contains numerous suggestions for behavior modification practices. The articles by Atkinson are excellent reviews on the use of very low calorie diets. In addition, see the letter to the editor in the Journal of the American Dietetic Association written by Wadden and Stunkard on this subject. Finally, for an in-depth and spirited look at fad diets, see both the article and book by Yetiv—the book is especially detailed and a valuable resource for a nutrition library.

CHAPTER 9

Answers to nutrition awareness inventory

1. *False.* Although physical activity is helpful, a low-kcalorie diet is equally important.
2. *True.* Diet relapse is a critical issue that is just now receiving focused attention.
3. *True.* A diet with fewer than 1000 kcalories is likely to cause hunger and fatigue.
4. *False.* Most people regain the weight they lost within 1 year.
5. *True.* It is impractical to lose fat tissue rapidly because of the high-kcalorie deficit required.
6. *True.* Behavior modification is likely to affect the tendency to relapse into bad habits.
7. *False.* There is no evidence that eating one affects the other.
8. *True.* High-carbohydrate foods generally contain fewer kcalories than high-fat foods.
9. *True.* Satiety is related to the fat content of foods.
10. *True.* People who can change their habits are able to exercise more control over their food choices and behavior.
11. *True.* An example might be to avoid a candy machine that is on the way to class.
12. *False.* You must burn about 3000 extra kcalories to lose 1 pound.
13. *True.* More than 70% of obese children become obese adults.
14. *True.* Brisk walking burns about 5 kcalories per minute.
15. *True.* Weighing twice one's desirable body weight is another measure of morbid obesity.

Nutrition Perspective 9-1

Ten Common Misconceptions About Quackery

BY STEPHEN BARRETT, M.D.

Although most Americans are harmed by quackery, few perceive it as a serious problem and even fewer are interested in trying to do anything about it. As a psychiatrist, I have been trained to look to hidden reasons why people act the way they do—especially when they fail to avoid trouble. Applying this technique to quackery, I have identified 10 misconceptions that I believe contribute to this situation:

MISCONCEPTION 1: QUACKERY IS EASY TO SPOT

Quackery is far more difficult to spot than most people realize. Modern promoters use scientific jargon, which can fool people unfamiliar with the concepts being discussed. Even health professionals can have difficulty in separating fact from fiction in fields unrelated to their expertise.

MISCONCEPTION 2: PERSONAL EXPERIENCE IS THE BEST WAY TO TELL WHETHER SOMETHING WORKS

When you feel better after having used a product or procedure, it is natural to give credit to whatever you have done. This effect can be misleading, however, because most ailments resolve by themselves, and those that don't can have variable symptoms. Even serious conditions can have sufficient day-to-day variation to enable quack methods to gain large followings. In addition, taking action often produces temporary relief of symptoms (a placebo effect). For these reasons, scientific experimentation is usually necessary to establish whether health methods are actually effective.

MISCONCEPTION 3: MOST VICTIMS OF QUACKERY ARE GULLIBLE

Gullibility implies a wish for magic. Individuals who buy one diet book or "magic" diet pill after another are indeed gullible. And so are many people who follow whatever health fads are in vogue. But the majority of quackery's victims are merely unsuspecting. People tend to believe what they hear the most. And quack ideas—particularly those regarding nutrition—are everywhere. Another large group of quackery's victims is composed of individuals who have serious or chronic diseases that make them feel desperate enough to try anything that offers hope.

Alienated people—many of whom are paranoid—form another victim group. These people tend to believe that our food supply is unsafe, that drugs do more harm than good, and that doctors, drug companies, large food companies, and government agencies are not interested in protecting the public. Such beliefs make them vulnerable to those who offer foods and healing approaches alleged to be "natural."

MISCONCEPTION 4: QUACKERY'S VICTIMS DESERVE WHAT THEY GET

This misconception is based on the feeling that people who are gullible should "know better" and therefore deserve whatever they get. This feeling is a major reason why journalists, enforcement officials, judges, and legislators seldom give priority to combat quackery. As noted earlier, however, most victims are not gullible. Nor do people deserve to suffer or die because of ignorance or desperation.

MISCONCEPTION 5: QUACKS ARE FRAUDS AND CROOKS

Quackery is often discussed as though all its promoters were engaged in deliberate deception. This is untrue. Most promoters of quackery sincerely believe in what they do. Most people think of quackery as being promoted by quacks, charlatans, or others who are deliberately taking advantage of others. Actually, most of it is promoted by victims of quackery who share their misinformation and personal experiences with others. Quackery is also involved in misleading advertising of nonprescription drugs. Again, no "quack" is involved—just hype from an advertising agency.

Dictionaries define quackery as "the practices or pretensions of a quack" and define quack as "a pretender to medical skill." I think it is better to define quackery as "anything associated with false claims in the field of health." This definition covers the broadest possible spectrum of quackery and avoids implying that its promoters intend to deceive.

MISCONCEPTION 6: MOST QUACKERY IS DANGEROUS

Quackery can seriously harm or kill people by inducing them to abandon or delay effective treatment for serious conditions. Although the number of people harmed in this manner cannot be determined, it is not large enough or obvious enough to arouse a general public outcry. Most victims of quackery are harmed economically rather than physically. Moreover, many people believe that an unscientific method has helped them. In most cases, they have confused cause-and-effect and coincidence. But sometimes an unproven approach actually relieves symptoms by lowering the person's tension level.

MISCONCEPTION 7: THE MEDIA ARE RELIABLE

Most people believe that statements about health issues "wouldn't be allowed" if they weren't true. Some media outlets—most notably *Consumer Reports* magazine—do achieve great accuracy. But most are willing to publish sensational viewpoints that they believe are newsworthy and will increase their audience. Radio and television talk shows abound with promoters of quackery. Even exposés on questionable methods are often "balanced" by including testimonials from satisfied customers.

MISCONCEPTION 8: ADVERTISING OUTLETS ARE ETHICAL

There is a widespread public belief that if something isn't legitimate, publications and broadcast outlets would not allow it to be advertised. Although most outlets have some limitations, few screen out misleading ads for health products.

MISCONCEPTION 9: EDUCATION IS THE ANSWER

Education can help unsuspecting people learn to recognize quackery. However, those who are desperate, gullible, or alienated may be difficult if not impossible to educate. Law enforcement is necessary to protect them.

MISCONCEPTION 10: GOVERNMENT PROTECTS US

Although various government agencies are involved in fighting quackery, most don't give it sufficient priority to be effective. Moreover, the agencies involved do not have a coordinated plan to maximize their effectiveness.

Dr. Barrett, a practicing psychiatrist and consumer advocate, is co-author/editor of 22 books including Vitamins and "Health" Foods: The Great American Hustle. *In 1984 he received the FDA Commissioner's Special Citation Award for Public Service in fighting nutrition quackery.*

Chapter 10

Anorexia Nervosa and Bulimia

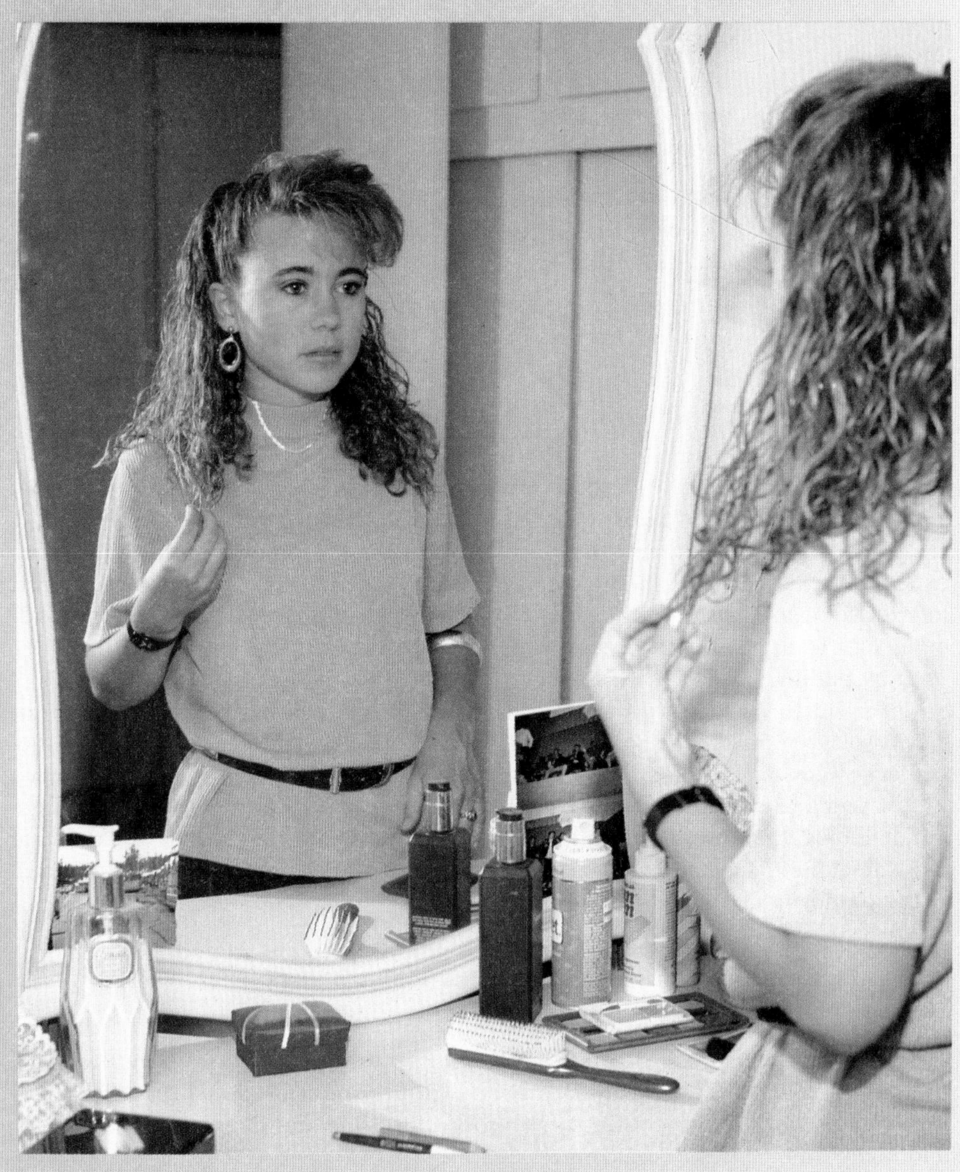

For those with eating disorders, the difference between the real and desired body image may be too difficult to accept.

Overview

Overeating that leads to obesity is a problem, but it falls within the guidelines of typical social behavior. The eating disorders we explore in this chapter, on the other hand, involve severe distortions of the eating process. What's most alarming about these disorders, *anorexia nervosa* and *bulimia*, is the rate at which they are increasing. Contemporary society provides a ready-made conflict: though food is abundant and our lifestyle is fairly sedentary, the "ideal" bodies flaunted before us are ultraslim and lean. Daily we are besieged by the images in television programs, billboard ads, magazine pictures, movies, and newspapers. We cannot escape them or the destructive comparison between the image of what is good and beautiful and our own—possibly thicker—bodies. Some people are more receptive and vulnerable to these messages than others. These are the people who may be more prone to eating disorders. Moreover, the messages are not aimed at all people equally; they are overwhelmingly beamed at women, and women account for almost all cases of anorexia nervosa and bulimia.

Nutrition awareness inventory

Here are 15 statements about eating disorders. Answer them to test your current knowledge. If you think the answer is true or mostly true, circle T. If you think the answer is false or mostly false, circle F. Use the scoring key at the end of this chapter to compute your total score. Take this test again after you have read this chapter. Compare the results.

1. T F Human societies deal irrationally with food.
2. T F Eating disorders are widespread in Western society.
3. T F People with anorexia nervosa have an intense fear of losing weight.
4. T F Bulimic people often engage in self-induced vomiting to control their weight.
5. T F People with anorexia nervosa are often overachievers.
6. T F People with anorexia nervosa have a distorted view of their own bodies.
7. T F People with bulimia are aware that their eating patterns are abnormal.
8. T F People with bulimia are easy to identify because of their openness about their problem.
9. T F North American society favors the lean and angular look.
10. T F The real problem underlying eating disorders is often how people feel about themselves.
11. T F People with eating disorders are often perfectionists.
12. T F Eating disorders are easier to treat at early stages.
13. T F Bingeing is characteristic of bulimia.
14. T F Treatment of bulimia emphasizes the immediate return to a strict diet.
15. T F Baryophobia is a new eating disorder found in children.

Every human society invests food with meaning and symbols that extend beyond its availability and nutritional value. Yams and sweet potatoes, for example, are highly nutritious and are part of the American Thanksgiving tradition. Other cultures, however, do not value them so highly; in England yams are considered inferior food and are rarely eaten by the middle or upper classes. Correspondingly, in Western cultures mineral water has prestige in some circles, but is rarely used by middle and lower classes.

From birth, we learn to link food with personal emotional experiences. An infant associates milk with security and warmth, and so the bottle or breast becomes a source of comfort, as well as of food. People are further exposed to the use of foods as rewards. On the surface, the practice appears harmless enough, but, eventually, both parents and children can build patterns of behavior that use foods to achieve unstated goals. Here are some typical statements one might hear at the dinner table:

"You can't play until you clean up your plate."
"I'll eat the broccoli if you let me watch TV."
"I'm only eating this because I love you."

While foods are sources of nutrients, society attaches far more significance to them than just their role as a link to good health. Food is used as a tool of expression—of power, bonding with some groups, prestige and class values, affection, and many other types of exchanges.

Exploring Issues and Actions

The next time you hear table conversation like the above, think about its real meaning. What is the person trying to achieve?

TWO COMMON TYPES OF EATING DISORDERS

Anorexia nervosa and ***bulimia*** (sometimes called bulimia nervosa) have been written about for centuries, as far back as the Middle Ages. Anorexia nervosa is characterized by extreme weight loss, poor body image, and an irrational—almost morbid—fear of obesity and weight gain. *The term* anorexia *implies loss of appetite; however, denial of appetite is a more accurate description.* By rough estimate, approximately 1 of every 250 teenage girls between the ages of 12 and 18 years suffers from anorexia nervosa.[2,13,16,18] Few men are affected, though no one yet knows why. The psychological profile of a woman who has this disorder reveals someone who sees herself as fat and having a protruding stomach, even though she is very, very thin.

anorexia nervosa
An eating disorder involving a psychological loss of appetite and self-starvation, partly due to a distorted body image and various social pressures associated with puberty.

Bulimia means "ox hunger," or being as hungry as an ox. It is characterized by episodes of bingeing followed by attempts to purge the food, usually by vomiting, fasting, and using laxatives or ***diuretics***. *Bulimic practices are difficult to identify because of the secretive aspect of this type of behavior and the lack of apparent symptoms.* Researchers think that approximately 1% to 4% of college-age women suffer from this disorder.[13,18,24]

bulimia
An eating disorder in which large quantities of food are eaten at one time (bingeing) and soon purged from the body by means of vomiting, use of laxatives, or other means.

The Diagnostic and Statistical Manual of Mental Disorders (3rd edition, revised) of the American Psychiatric Association lists specific criteria for diagnosing each of these disorders (Figure 10-1). A person may exhibit some characteristics of these disorders but not enough to qualify as a "true" case. Anorexia nervosa and bulimia overlap considerably (Figure 10-2), and a person may exhibit characteristics of both diseases. The overlaps can be categorized as anorexia nervosa–restrictive diet; anorexia nervosa with binge-purge cycles; bulimia; and bulimia with history of anorexia nervosa. These terms are not officially recognized.

diuretic
A substance which, when ingested, increases the flow of urine.

Figure 10-3 describes some characteristics of people with anorexia and bulimia.[9] Before you read on, look at them to determine whether you or someone you know may be at risk. If so, professional help is needed immediately, first to

CRITERIA FOR EATING DISORDER

Anorexia nervosa

A) Refusal to maintain body weight over a minimal normal weight for age and height, for example, weight loss leading to maintenance of body weight 15% below that expected; or failure to make expected weight gain during period of growth, leading to body weight 15% below that expected.
B) Intense fear of gaining weight or becoming fat, even though underweight.
C) Disturbance in the way in which one's body weight, size or shape is experienced. The person claims to "feel fat" even when emaciated, believes that one area of the body is "too fat" even when obviously underweight.
D) In females, absence of at least three consecutive menstrual cycles when otherwise expected to occur (primary or secondary amenorrhea). (A woman is considered to have amenorrhea if her periods occur only following hormone administration, such as estrogen.)

Bulimia nervosa

A) Recurrent episodes of binge eating (rapid consumption of a large amount of food in a discrete period of time).
B) A feeling of lack of control over eating behavior during the eating binges.
C) The person regularly engages in either self-induced vomiting, use of laxatives or diuretics, strict dieting or fasting, or vigorous exercise to prevent weight gain.
D) A minimum average of two binge eating episodes a week for at least 3 months.
E) Persistent overconcern with body shape and weight.

[1]Source: *Diagnostic and Statistical Manual for Mental Disorders, DSM IIIR* (14).

Figure 10-1
Diagnostic criteria for anorexia nervosa and bulimia nervosa.

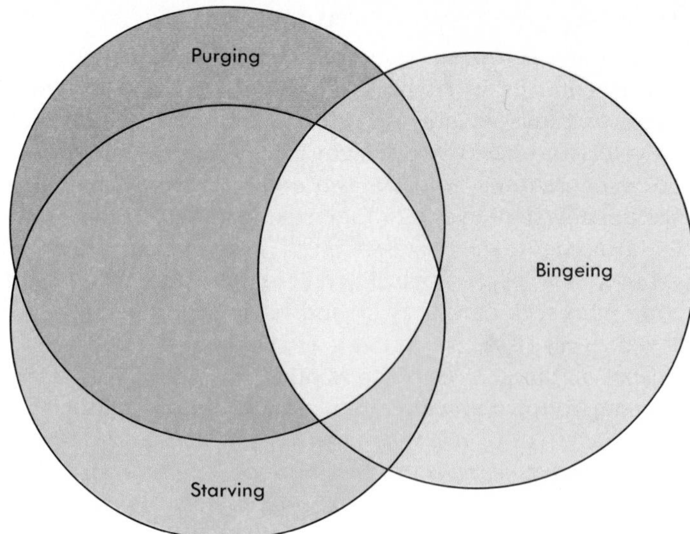

Figure 10-2

The overlap of eating disorders. A combination of bingeing, purging, and/or starving can be found in both anorexia nervosa and bulimia.

rule out other diseases, such as cancer, gastrointestinal disease, schizophrenia, and depression. If the psychological profile fits, consider immediate treatment for the diagnosed eating disorder. *The best a friend can do is to lead the person to treatment. Both problems require professional help, and that is often available at student health centers on college campuses.*

Eating disorders are complex and rooted in multiple causes—biological, psychological, and social.[12,13] *They have neither simple causes nor solutions.* In Nutrition Perspective 10-1 we review some sociological aspects of eating disorders. This information will help you understand why these disorders might develop, and how someone might fall into this trap.

ARE YOU AT RISK FOR AN EATING DISORDER?

Characteristics of anorexia nervosa

- Rigid dieting causing dramatic weight loss
- False body perception—thinking "I'm too fat," even when emaciated; relentless pursuit of thinness
- Rituals involving food, excessive exercise, and other aspects of life
- Maintenance of rigid control in life-style; security found in control and order
- Feeling of panic after a small weight gain; intense fear of gaining weight
- Feelings of purity, power, and superiority through maintenance of strict discipline and self-denial
- Preoccupation with food, its preparation, and observing another person eat
- Helplessness in the presence of food
- Lack of menses after what should be the age of puberty

Characteristics of bulimia

- Secretive binge eating; never overeating in front of others
- Eating when depressed
- Bingeing followed by fasting, laxative abuse, self-induced vomiting, or excessive exercise
- Shame, embarrassment, deceit, and depression; low self-esteem and guilt (especially after a binge)
- Fluctuating weight resulting from alternate bingeing and fasting
- Loss of control; fear of not being able to stop eating
- Perfectionism, "people pleaser"; food is the only comfort/escape in an otherwise carefully controlled and regulated life
- Erosion of teeth, swollen glands

Figure 10-3

Some characteristics of people with anorexia nervosa as an eating disorder.

ANOREXIA NERVOSA

Anorexia nervosa represents an extremely unhealthy mental and physical state, characterized by great weight loss, poor body image, and an intense fear of obesity and weight gain.[11,12] Of persons suffering from anorexia, 6% to 20% die prematurely—from suicide, heart ailments, or infections. About half the remaining persons recover; the rest simply exist with the disease. The longer one suffers from anorexia nervosa, the poorer the chances for complete recovery.[26] Some clinicians believe that no person with anorexia ever completely recovers. Some people are better able to cope with the disease, however, and minimize its future effects.

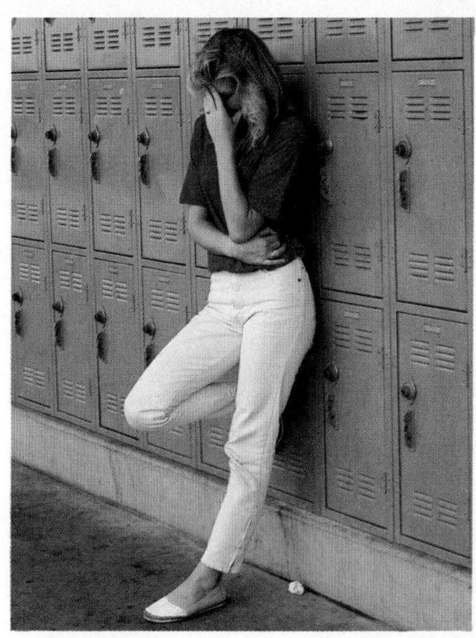

The stress of crossing from childhood into adulthood may trigger anorexia nervosa.

Anorexia nervosa may begin as a simple attempt at dieting to lose weight. The attempt may have been triggered by a comment from a friend, relative, or parent, suggesting that the person was gaining weight or was too fat. Physical changes around the age of puberty and the stress of crossing from childhood to adulthood may also spark the weight loss.[1] In addition, going away to boarding school or to college or starting a job may underscore the wish to make oneself more "socially acceptable."

Once the dieting begins, however, the person doesn't stop. The results are long periods of semistarvation practiced rigidly, almost with a vengeance. Anorexia nervosa may eventually lead to bingeing on large amounts of food in short periods, then purging oneself of the food. Purging is done primarily by vomiting, but laxatives, diuretics, fasting, and exercise are also used. Thus a person with anorexia may exist in states of semistarvation or may alternate periods of starvation with periods of bingeing and purging (Figure 10-3).

Once a person loses 15% of normal body weight, there is great risk for lifelong suffering from anorexia. After losing 25% of body weight, a cure becomes very difficult, hospitalization is almost always necessary, and premature death is more likely.

Warning signs

Anorexia nervosa exhibits important warning signs. First, dieting becomes the life focus. The person may feel, "The only thing I am good at is dieting. I can't do anything else." Or, "I never won at anything until I started losing weight." This innocent beginning often leads to very abnormal eating habits, such as cutting a pea in half before eating it (Figure 10-4). A woman with anorexia may cook a large meal and watch others eat it while refusing to eat any herself. As the disease progresses, she narrows her own food choices considerably. For someone developing anorexia these practices demonstrate, "I am in control." The anorectic person may be hungry but denies it. She may feel that good things will happen for her if she just becomes thin enough—that hope drives her on.

Some girls may use anorexia nervosa to try to delay puberty and remain childlike. Or they may use anorexia nervosa to gain attention in the family.

Soon the person becomes irritable and hostile and begins to withdraw from family and friends. School performance generally crumbles. The person refuses to eat out with family and friends, thinking, "I won't be able to have the foods I want to eat," or "I won't be able to throw up afterward." The person also tends to be excessively critical of self and others. Nothing is good enough. A sense of joylessness pervades life.

Eventually, as stress builds in an anorectic person's life, sleep disturbances and depression are common. In a female these problems, coupled with a lower and lower body weight, can result in a lack of menses, which may be the first sign of the disease a mother notices. Overall, the person usually falls into a "pit" where life appears meaningless and hopeless because it cannot be perfect.

Parents, teachers, friends, and coaches need to be aware of these early signs of anorexia nervosa.[1] This disease is much easier to treat when caught at an early stage. If not treated right away, it quickly becomes willful self-destruction.

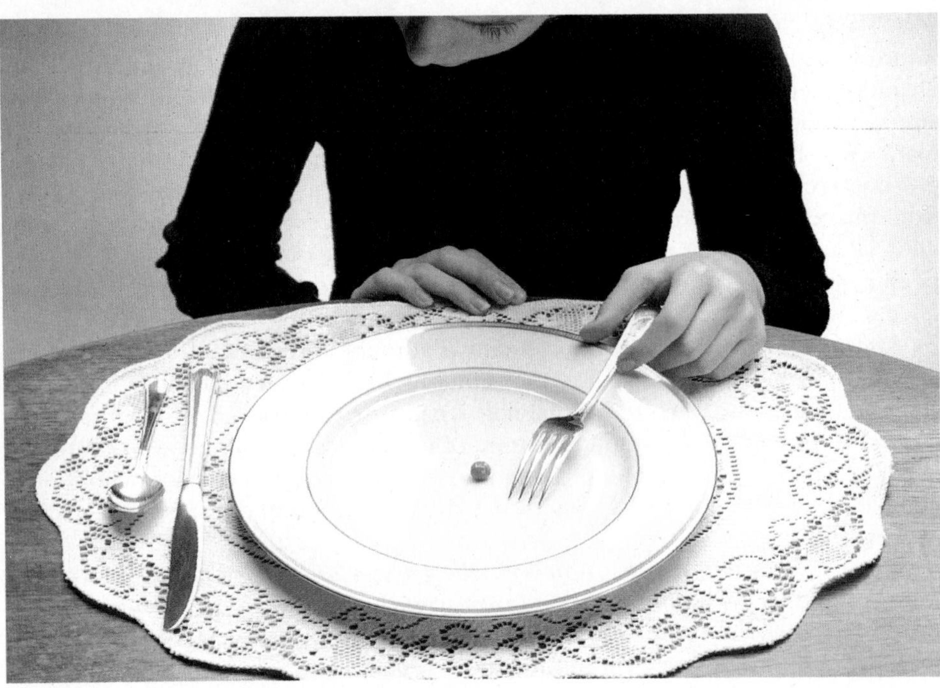

Figure 10-4
When life reaches this stage, one needs professional help.

Profile of a person with anorexia nervosa

The person with anorexia nervosa is usually a girl from the middle or upper socioeconomic class. She is often described by parents and teachers as "the best little girl in the world." She has high parental standards, is competitive, and is often obsessive. Physicians note that after a physical examination she may fold her examination gown very carefully and clean up the examination room before leaving. At home, she may not allow clutter in her bedroom. Still, it takes fine clinical judgment to separate a true case from other adolescent complaints, such as delayed puberty, fatigue, and depression.[1]

The major hallmark of anorexia nervosa is a refusal to eat. Other practices already mentioned may or may not appear, such as excessive energy output, vomiting, or the use of laxatives or diuretics. Ultimately, however, the person eats very little food; 300 to 600 kcalories per day is not unusual.[12] In place of food she may consume up to 20 cans of diet soft drinks per day.

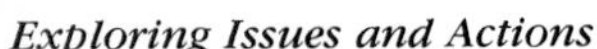

Exploring Issues and Actions

Do you know anyone who has anorexia nervosa? Can you imagine yourself with this problem? What should you do for this person?

Conflicting family structures are common among people with anorexia nervosa.[1] Frustration over unrealistic expectations causes family bickering. Rigidity, overprotection, and denial can also be seen in such families. Often the eating disorder allows the person to experience a feeling of control over an otherwise powerless existence.

Physical signs and symptoms

The major physical sign of anorexia is weight loss (Figure 10-5).[2,4] The anorectic person is 20% to 40% below desirable body weight and ends up essentially skin and bones. This state of semistarvation greatly disturbs many body systems as it forces the body to conserve as much energy as possible. Hormonal responses then cause an array of predictable physiological effects:

- Lowered body temperature resulting from loss of fat insulation and decrease in basal metabolism caused by decreased synthesis of active thyroid hormone.
- Decreased heart rate resulting from slowing of metabolism; this leads to easy fatigue, easy fainting, and an overwhelming need for sleep.
- Iron-deficiency anemia caused by poor nutrient intake, which leads to further weakness (see Chapter 14).

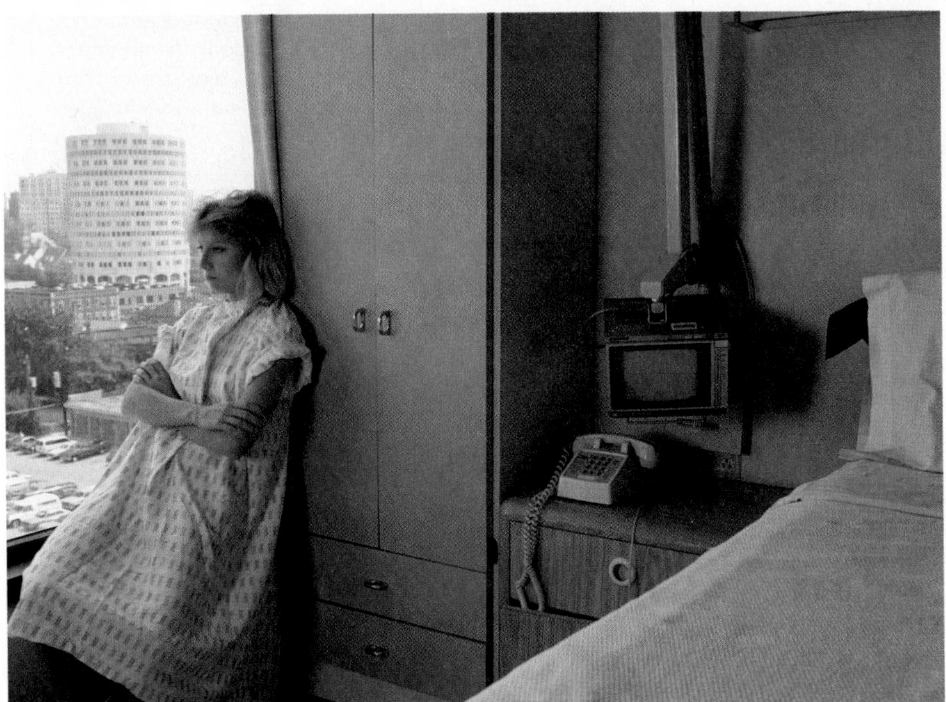

Figure 10-5

Anorexia nervosa. Treatment needs to start before this point is reached. This psychological condition can become life-threatening.

- Rough, dry, scaly, and cold skin resulting from poor nutrient intake and anemia.
- Low white blood cell count resulting from poor nutrient intake, especially protein. This condition increases the risk of infection, which is one cause of death in anorexia nervosa.
- Loss of hair caused by poor nutrient intake. To replace the insulating value of fat, the person grows downy hair, called ***lanugo,*** all over the body. As these small hairs stand erect they trap air, adding a layer of insulation to the body.
- Constipation, partly caused by semistarvation and partly a result of laxative abuse.
- Low blood potassium (hypokalemia) resulting from poor nutrient intake and use of some types of diuretics. This increases the risk of heart rhythm disturbances, another leading cause of death in anorexia.
- Loss of menstruation, partly caused by both low body weight and the stress of the disease. This causes a loss of bone mass, in turn increasing the risk of future osteoporosis (see Chapter 13).[7]
- Eventual loss of teeth caused by frequent vomiting. The loss of teeth and bone mass are lasting signs of the disease, even if the other physical and mental problems are resolved.

lanugo
Down-like hair that appears after a person has lost much body fat due to semistarvation. The hair stands erect and traps air, acting as insulation to the body to replace the insulation usually supplied by body fat.

A person with anorexia nervosa is psychologically and physically ill and needs help.

Concept Check

Anorexia nervosa is found primarily in girls at or around puberty. It is characterized by semistarvation leading to severe weight loss. The person ends up essentially "skin and bones," but often still thinks she is fat. This semistarvation state leads to hormonal and other changes that result in a lower body temperature, slower heart rate, decreased immune system status, loss of hair, and loss of menstruation. It is a very serious disease that, if not corrected, can lead to lifelong destructive effects, and even death.

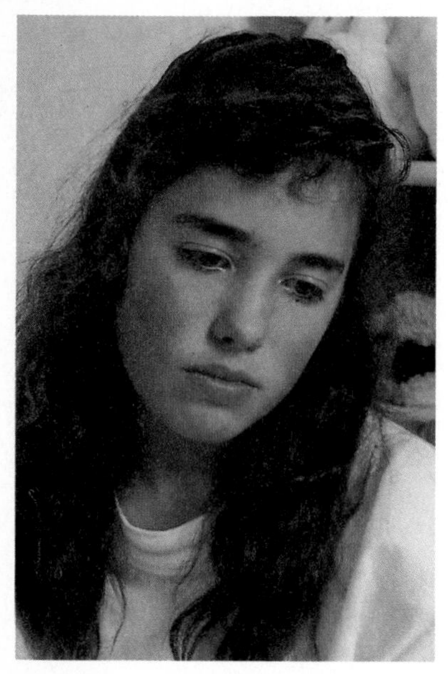

The therapy team often must break through isolation, fear, and loneliness before healing can begin.

Groups of people with long-standing histories of anorexia nervosa include models, ballet dancers, and gymnasts. These people often have a strong economic incentive to stay ultra-slim.[3,5]

Treatment of anorexia nervosa

Treatment requires a team of physicians, registered dietitians, psychologists, and other health professionals working together. [11,13,14] Before treatment can begin, the therapy team must first gain the cooperation of the anorectic person. Often the person has sunken deep into a shell of isolation, fear, and loneliness. It takes hard work from the person, family members, and the medical team to restore a sense of balance, purpose, and future to the person's life.

Nutrition therapy. The first goal of therapy is for the person to regain sufficient weight to both raise her metabolic rate to normal and reverse many physical signs of the disease.[28] An important treatment goal is to decrease the overwhelming mental fixation on food that semistarvation brings. Nutrient intake is designed to first stop further weight loss and then to restore regular food habits. After this is accomplished, the focus can switch to slow weight gain. Rewards, such as visits from friends, may be used to encourage desired eating behaviors.

The person does not need many kcalories to gain weight because her very low metabolic rate creates a high metabolic efficiency. A starting point can be set by the Harris-Benedict equation or the Boothby and Berkson Food Nomogram (see Appendix M). Once weight maintenance is established, a reasonable goal would be a weekly increase of 200 kcalories as treatment progresses. The person needs to be warned that weight gain will be rapid at first, due to a rebuilding of fluid and electrolyte stores, glycogen stores, and muscle and organ mass. In addition, weight swings of 2 to 3 pounds may be seen when menses resumes.

One critical goal at this stage of treatment is to allow the person a feeling of control over her life. Only by knowing what must be faced can the person keep a sense of control. It is important for the medical team to warn the person what to expect beforehand, especially any anticipated weight gain.

The medical team must also remember that semistarvation greatly narrows a person's focus of thinking. *A psychiatrist cannot counsel a starving person.* Extreme low body weight creates such a strong restorative desire for food that both dreams and morbid thoughts about food abound. This same mental state appeared in conscientious objectors in World War II who were purposely put into a state of semistarvation to study the effects of a "concentration camp" existence[13] (see Chapter 6).

Some clinicians use regular foods during the refeeding process. Others prefer liquid food supplements, which remove choices about eating, thereby freeing the anorectic person to think about issues she considers more important. A severely malnourished person may need to be fed by tube or vein to achieve necessary weight gain.[27] In that case, it is best to admit the person into a clinic that specializes in treatment of anorexia nervosa. However, people with less severe cases can be treated as ***outpatients,*** especially if binge-purge practices have not already begun.

outpatient
A person treated by medical personnel outside the hospital setting, for example, in a clinic or physician's office.

The medical team entrusted with the care of anorexia nervosa patients must be experienced in handling such people. An anorectic person may be on the edge of suicide and starvation. In addition, anorectic people are often very clever and resistant. They may try to hide weight loss by wearing many layers of clothes, putting coins in their pockets, and drinking numerous glasses of water.

Psychological therapy. Once a person's physical problems are being addressed, the therapists can focus on behavioral and psychological goals and attempt to understand the role that anorexia nervosa plays in the person's life. The therapist needs to determine how dieting became such a dominant force for this person, keeping in mind that the dieting is probably merely a sign of a deeper emotional illness.[20,21] To get well, the anorectic person must relinquish the pride she feels from the control she has achieved over her body and the resulting emaciation. To help her reach that point, the therapists need to know how she arrived there.

If the therapists can discover reasons for the anorexia nervosa, they can design and test alternate coping strategies and skills. These strategies aim to restore normal weight and eating habits by resolving psychological conflicts. Eventually, psychological therapy can be extended to include a nutrition and exercise plan to help the person function more appropriately in both clinical and social environments. Work with the person must proceed very slowly. It is easy to overstress these people, precipitating a new round of the practices everyone is trying to avoid.

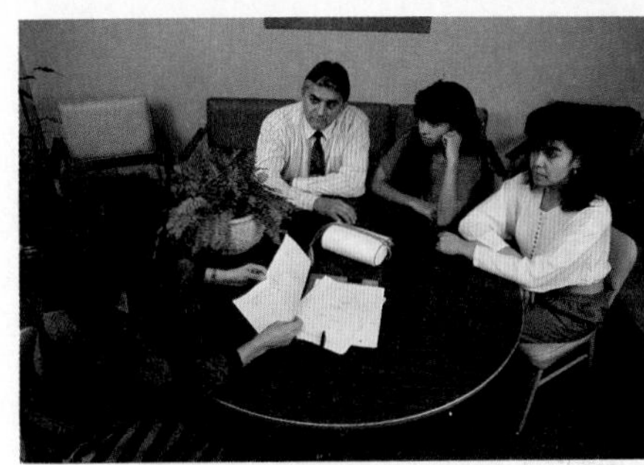

Patients must often work through family problems to discover the roots of their disorder.

A key aspect of psychological treatment is showing the person how to retain control of at least some facets of her life and how to cope with tough situations. Finding a better means to exhibit control than through dieting allows eating to become a normal life routine, in turn allowing renewed focus on previously neglected activities.

Therapists work to help people accept setbacks, and to regard these setbacks as opportunities to learn more about themselves rather than as sources of depression and frustration. Counselors can also provide background literature to clarify the issues of the disease and to encourage greater participation in the treatment. Furthermore, the counselor can lead the individual to focus on positive health goals, such as consuming more potassium, dietary fiber, and calcium.[1]

Family therapy can be an important part of the treatment of anorexia nervosa. Many times, a therapist finds that family struggles are at the heart of the problem. When anorexia disappears, the person has to relate to family members in new ways to achieve the attention she had before. Siblings often feel anger toward the anorectic sibling because of all the attention she received. The family needs to help the young person ease into adulthood and accept the responsibilities, as well as the advantages, of that stage. The family can help find new ways for the young person to gain attention and respect, other than by dieting, so that the young woman will not feel so trapped and dependent on old patterns of coping with problems.

With professional help, many people with anorexia nervosa can restore normalcy to their lives, creating instead lives that do not depend on unusual eating habits to cope with daily problems. *There are no set answers or approaches, however, because each case is individual.*

Exploring Issues and Actions

What or who do you feel is mostly responsible for anorexia nervosa: the anorectic person, the media, or society? What implications would this have for treatment?

Concept Check

Treatment of anorexia nervosa first requires a person to be brought back from a semistarvation state. Once a kcalorie intake sufficient to maintain basal metabolism is established, psychotherapy can begin to find the root causes of the disease and to help the person develop skills needed to return to a healthy life.

BULIMIA

Bulimia—with its episodes of bingeing followed by attempts to purge the food—is most commonly practiced by college-age students, usually women who have tried many weight-reduction diets throughout their teen years. These diets produce periods of intense hunger, which often lead in turn to periods of binge eating. A binge can be precipitated by a combination of stress, boredom, loneliness, and depression, or perhaps by a critical incident that imparts a sense of helplessness. The bulimic person may have both biological factors and life-style patterns that predispose to overweight.[10] In those who are susceptible, alternating feelings of accumulating hunger and of denial of their dietary disorder can push them into a desperation pattern of bulimia.

Pinpointing the number of people who practice bulimia is difficult when the strictest guidelines proposed by the revised third edition of the *Diagnostic and Statistical Manual of Mental Disorders* are followed (Figure 10-1). These guidelines indicate that a person must vomit at least twice a week for 3 months to be diagnosed as bulimic. Using this criterion, approximately 1% to 4% of college-age women suffer from the disease.[13] However, because of the secret nature of bulimic behaviors and the lack of obvious external symptoms, identifying bulimic practices depends on self-report, and that is often unreliable. The problem, especially of milder cases, may be much more widespread than has been thought.

Bingeing occurs first; later, purging begins in an attempt to control the increase in body weight. The person practicing bulimia is usually at, or slightly above, a normal weight, and is more likely to be sexually active than the person with anorexia nervosa. Some of your best friends may practice bulimia without your knowing it. Again, the disorder is often a very secret one.

Like people with anorexia nervosa, those with bulimia are usually female, successful, and perfectionists. They are also greatly preoccupied with food. The major difference is that the person with bulimia turns *to* food during a crisis or problem, not away from it. These people often have very low self-esteem. The world sees the person's competent side, while inside she feels out of control. The

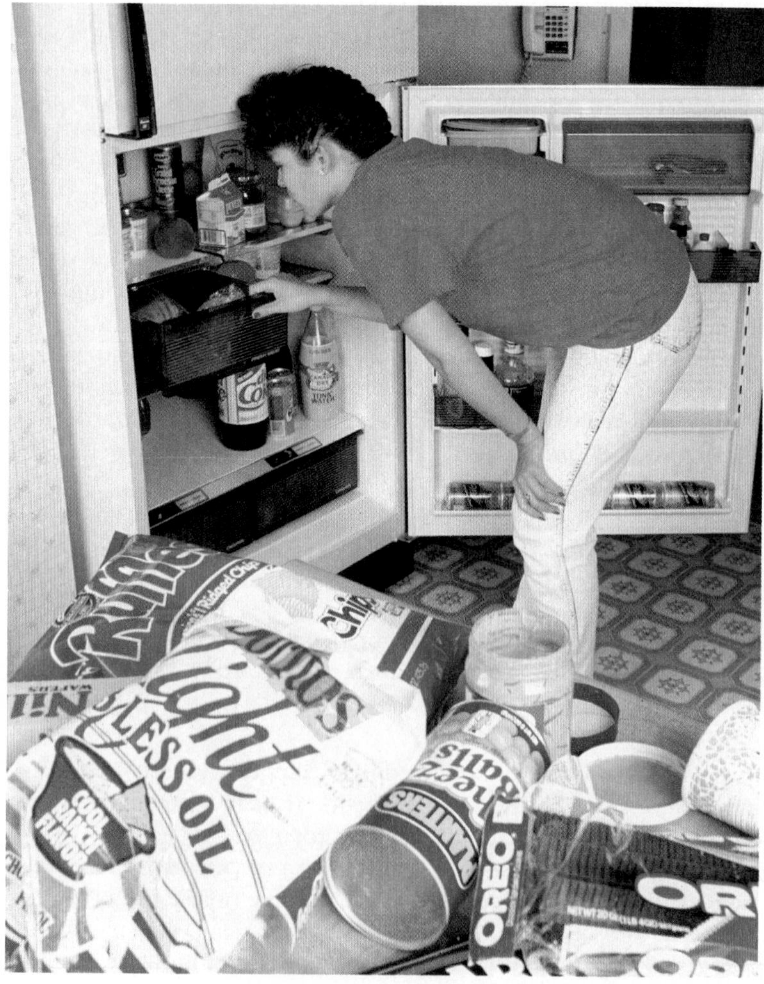

Figure 10-6

The binge-purge cycle. It can lead to a state of helplessness.

bulimic person may be very impulsive. Part of the problem may actually arise from an inability to control responses to impulse and desire.[12]

The binge-purge cycle may occur daily, weekly, or at other intervals. A special time is often set aside. Most bingeing occurs at night when other people are less likely to interrupt, and usually lasts from a half-hour to 2 hours. The foods chosen are usually high-kcalorie convenience foods—cakes, cookies, pies, ice cream, donuts, and pastries. As much as 20,000 kcalories might be eaten in a binge. *Approximately 20% to 33% of these kcalories are absorbed, even when vomiting follows very quickly. More kcalories are absorbed if laxatives are used for purging.* Thus practicing bulimia is actually a losing proposition. Bulimic people are mistaken in thinking that they are consuming tasty foods at no energy cost.

People suffering from bulimia are not proud of these actions (Figure 10-6). Over time they develop somber, intense, tragic, and often hopeless feelings about their situations. Compulsive lying and drug abuse can further intensify the feelings. Frequent mood swings are not unusual. If a person has just started a binge when somebody comes to visit, the response may be, "Get out of my house." The person eventually loses friendships and family relationships because of the preoccupation with bingeing and purging, which takes up a lot of time.[12]

Health problems stemming from bulimia

Most health problems in bulimia arise from vomiting.[12,17] Vomiting is the most effective way of purging. However, it is also the most physically destructive. To start, the acid in vomit demineralizes teeth. Dentists, in fact, are often the first health professionals to notice signs of bulimia. The person complains of very sensitive teeth that are painful when subjected to heat, cold, or acids. Eventually, the teeth may fall out or show severe decay.

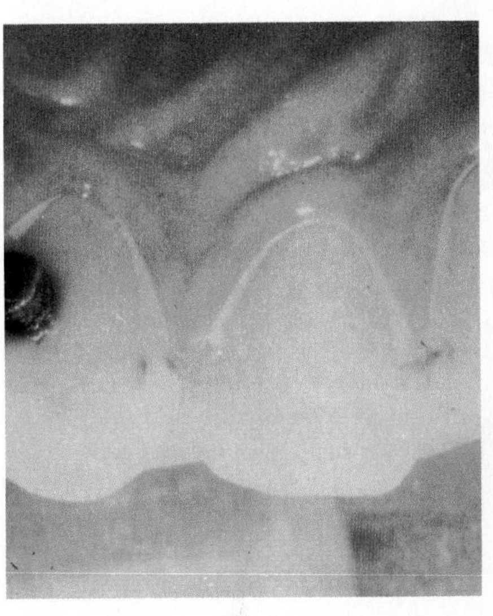

Tooth decay seen in a bulimic patient.

The blood potassium level often decreases in a bulimic person because a lot of potassium is lost in vomit. This can disturb the heart's rhythm and even lead to sudden death. The salivary glands can swell because of infection and irritation from the vomit. A link between the swelling and hormonal changes is also suspected. The person may even suffer from bleeding and tears in the esophagus, as well as stomach ulcers. Constipation may result from frequent laxative use.[1]

Since people with bulimia often use their fingers to induce vomiting, bite marks around the knuckles are a characteristic sign of this disorder. Therefore it is important for physicians to routinely examine this spot in young people. Once the disease is established, however, a person often can vomit by simply contracting the abdominal muscles, or the vomiting may occur automatically.

Ipecac syrup in excess is also used to induce vomiting. This substance is very toxic to the heart and has been the cause of accidental poisoning.[15]

Treatment of bulimia

Therapy for bulimia also requires a team approach.[1] Clinicians have yet to agree on the best method. Psychotherapy is used primarily to help a person develop a more realistic body and self-image. Because the bulimic person is often very embarrassed about the practice, the therapist needs to be accepting and nonjudgmental. A therapist can best help a person when both are totally honest with each other.

Therapy is usually managed on an outpatient basis so that the person can incorporate treatment into daily life. Involving the family often helps. The therapist needs to convince a bulimic person that it is normal to sometimes doubt oneself and feel depressed. *When needed, psychological help and counseling is available to all of us.* No one needs to seek solace in foods to avoid facing a hard problem. Therapists may also prescribe antidepressant medications to combat some of the depression associated with bulimia.

Expert Opinion

Psychological Treatment for Binge Eating

BRUCE ARNOW, PH.D.

Many of us overeat from time to time. In most cases we are apt to forgive ourselves, perhaps vowing not to overeat the next time. Often we attribute our overeating to the palatability of the food, reasoning that it tasted so good that it was simply difficult to stop. However, binge eating, or bulimia, is a problem distinct from overeating that frequently leads to serious physical and psychological difficulties. What distinguishes a binge from an episode of overeating are the following: (1) the food is consumed within a relatively brief period and (2) the person experiences a loss of control during the episode. Bulimic people frequently report negative emotional reactions following binges. Depression, guilt, and self-denigration are common. Binge eating usually occurs secretly and often involves the consumption of high-kcalorie food. The behavior has a driven, or compulsive, quality to it, and bulimic people often report that they do not really taste or enjoy the food once a binge is under way.

Binge eating is a feature of several different eating-related difficulties. It is encountered in 30% to 50% of people with anorexia nervosa—that is, those patients who demonstrate an intense drive for thinness, self-imposed starvation, a refusal to maintain body weight at a level adequate for healthy functioning, and a belief that they are overweight despite emaciation. Binge eating is also a significant problem among the overweight. A series of studies assessing binge eating among those applying for behavioral weight-loss treatment reported rates between 23% and 46%. A more recent study done at Stanford University shows that the incidence of binge eating increases substantially with increasing levels of obesity. Binge eaters are more likely to drop out of weight-loss programs prematurely and to regain weight more quickly than nonbingers.

Among sufferers of bulimia nervosa, binges often alternate with attempts to rigidly restrict food intake. Elaborate "food rules" are common. One frequently encountered rule is to avoid eating sweets. Thus if even one cookie or donut is consumed, the individual may feel that she has "broken a rule" and must "get rid of" the objectionable food. Usually this leads to further overeating, both because it is easier to regurgitate a large amount of food than a small amount and because "having blown it," a decision is made to "go all the way" and start over tomorrow. In some cases, binges are triggered by negative mood states such as depression or anger.

Most of the effort to develop effective psychological treatment for binge eating has been directed toward those bulimic people who both binge and purge—that is, those with bulimia nervosa. Cognitive-behavioral therapy has been the most extensively evaluated and appears at this point to be the most effective. This type of therapy focuses on helping patients alter those beliefs and assumptions that appear critical to maintaining bulimic behavior. The patient is asked to act as if she were a scientist testing assumptions and beliefs about food and weight as though they were hypotheses rather than absolute "truths." The patient and therapist engage in a collaborative effort to examine the evidence regarding the validity of such beliefs. Usually, the evidence gathering and hypothesis testing involves the patient in a series of tasks performed outside the therapy session. Among the procedures typical of cognitive-behavioral therapy for bulimia nervosa are the following:

Self-monitoring of food intake and purging episodes. Patients are asked to keep detailed records indicating when they eat, what and how much they have consumed, whether they consider what they ate to be a binge, whether they purged, and the thoughts and feelings they had surrounding each episode of eating and purging. This procedure allows the patient and therapist jointly to examine patterns of thinking, feeling, and behavior that become the focus of change efforts.

Normalization of the eating pattern. Patients are encouraged gradually to eat three adequate meals daily. This pattern breaks the binge/starve cycle that is so much a part of this problem. It also is a way of testing the validity of certain frequently reported beliefs among bulimic people, such as "I will gain weight if I don't starve myself."

The addition of "forbidden foods" in small quantities to the diet. Rigid food rules are important in maintaining bulimia. If a patient eats even a small amount of a forbidden food, it usually leads to a binge. Thus one way that patients are encouraged to experiment with a less rigid set of rules is by gradually adding to their diet in smaller quantities those foods that are forbidden.

Cognitive restructuring. This term refers to a set of procedures for identifying and attempting to correct "irrational" or maladaptive beliefs. All the preceding tasks are designed to challenge such assumptions. However, cognitive-behavioral therapy for bulimia nervosa also involves direct identification and challenge of distortions in thinking that are associated with the disturbance. For example, perfectionism and "all-or-nothing" thinking is common among this group. One is either eating perfectly or horribly; one's weight is "acceptable" at 125 pounds and "totally unacceptable" at 126 pounds. Helping patients become aware of such thinking patterns and attempting to alter them is an important part of treatment.

Identification of antecedents to binges and development of alternative coping strategies. One advantage of self-monitoring is that it enables a therapist and patient to identify events that seem to "trigger" binge episodes, and to explore alternative solutions for coping with those events. Sometimes, in addition to anxiety over a lapse in adherence to strict food rules, interpersonal situations may trigger bingeing; at other times, negative emotional states such as depression, anxiety, or anger precipitate binges. Once such patterns are identified, alternative coping strategies can be developed, and the patient can begin to experiment with them.

Several published studies have indicated reductions in the incidence of binge eating and self-induced vomiting ranging from 63% to 96% after cognitive-behavioral therapy. The percentage of participants who abstain from bingeing and vomiting following such treatment has generally ranged between 50% and 60%. In the most recent study completed at Stanford University, cognitive-behavioral therapy resulted in a 77% reduction in purging; 59% of the participants were abstaining from bingeing and purging 6 months after treatment. In addition, participants showed significant improvement in other areas, such as depression and food preoccupation.

While such results are most encouraging, not everyone benefits from such treatment. What can be said about those who do not derive benefit? One factor associated with poor outcome in cognitive-behavioral treatment for bulimia has been a history of anorexia. It is possible that those with a history of anorexia are prone to *more* extreme preoccupation and are unable to tolerate the anxiety associated with experimenting with eating forbidden foods and developing a less restrictive eating pattern.

In my experience, another major factor influencing success and failure is a patient's ability to enter into an open, collaborative relationship with the therapist. One characteristic of bulimic patients is preoccupation with the expectations of others. The therapy discussed here involves direct suggestions by the therapist. While many patients welcome such focus and direction, some respond as though they are being evaluated on their ability to carry out the therapeutic tasks. Such patients are likely to feel that they have let the therapist down if they experience difficulty, or may expect that the therapist will become angry or punitive if improvement is not rapid enough. Others respond to the suggestions as though they are being coerced and "rebel" against what they perceive as the therapist's attempts to control their behavior. Cognitive-behavioral therapy is action-oriented; the cognitive change, or insight, that leads to therapeutic success derives not only from discussions with the therapist, but also from actions carried out by the patient. To the extent that the patient is unable to collaborate with the therapist on the execution of those tasks, the therapy is undermined.

Dr. Arnow is director of the Behavioral Medicine Clinic at the Department of Psychiatry, Stanford University Medical Center.

Table 10-1

General protocol for outpatient dietary management of bulimia

Education	Weight issues	Food diary	Dietary plan
Aim: To inform/educate patient about bulimia and its consequences.	Aim: To reduce preoccupation and overconcern with body weight and develop an acceptance of normal body weight.	Aim: To gain a thorough understanding of patient's current eating habits.	Aim: To help patient gain control and establish a pattern of regular eating.
1. Patient education begins early in treatment and continues throughout. 2. Topics covered include: a. physical and health risks of bulimia and purging; b. physiological and psychological effects of starvation; c. ineffectiveness of various purging techniques in controlling weight; d. role of body fat in normal development; e. basic information on energy and nutrient processes; f. identifying misconceptions and dysfunctional attitudes about food, eating, and dieting.	1. Any desired weight loss must be delayed until after the bulimic/purging behaviors are under control and a normal eating pattern has been established. 2. For bulimics entering treatment in a starvation state, reversal of starvation must occur before psychotherapy begins. 3. Patients are instructed not to weigh themselves and are weighed once a week by a treatment team member. 4. Help patients accept a normative weight for themselves and give up an unrealistically thin body weight. 5. The concept of a "weight range" of 3 to 6 pounds is stressed.	1. Upon entering program, patients are given forms and instructed to keep a structured food diary of quantities of all foods eaten, eating environment, accompanying thoughts, feelings, and binge/purge episodes. 2. The diary is kept throughout treatment until eating habits are under control and is useful in monitoring progress and making dietary recommendations.	1. Dietary plan is three structured meals a day with one to two snacks eaten irrespective of patient's appetite and at the same time each day (when possible). 2. Patients are taught to use exchange lists for meal planning. Exchanges are based on calorie levels needed to maintain current weight (minimum of 1200 kcal per day). 3. Patients are taught behavior strategies to help regulate eating. 4. Patients are instructed to preplan meals. 5. Patients are initially told to avoid foods that are binge items. After treatment has progressed, those foods should be gradually reintroduced into their diets.

From: Story M: Nutrition management and dietary treatment of bulimia, Journal of the American Dietetic Association 86:517, 1986.

Nutritional counseling can help correct misconceptions about food and be used to plan a diet within the person's energy needs that still contains a reasonable amount of tasty foods (Table 10-1). In the early stages it may be best to avoid "binge" foods. *The primary goal is to develop a normal eating pattern so that food choices become more mechanical.*[17] Some nutrition specialists believe that using the exchange system is helpful as it enables a person with bulimia to more accurately assess the energy content of different foods. The person needs to understand that no food, when eaten in moderation, is necessarily fattening; the exchange system convincingly demonstrates that by listing kcalorie contents.

Nutritional counseling emphasizes setting up regular eating habits, rather than stopping the bingeing and purging. Once regular eating habits are established, the binge-purge cycle should stop by itself. Stressing the maintenance of healthful eating habits is a key to helping a person regain nutritional perspective.[25]

A recent survey of people with bulimia found that when seeking help, they preferred intensive treatment groups. The most important nutritional changes, the survey found, were eating a balanced diet of regular meals, increasing exercise, and avoiding binge foods, sugar, alcohol, and drugs. Involving family members in the treatment was also considered helpful.[8]

Bulimia is a serious health problem. If not treated, grave medical complications can result. Relapse is likely, so therapy should have a long-term focus. Years of treatment may be needed. A high risk of suicide is associated with bulimia. It is important for people who suffer from this disease to take advantage of the professional help available on their campus and/or in their community.

PREVENTING EATING DISORDERS

Professionals working with young adults, parents, and friends should consider the following advice for discouraging future cases of eating disorders:

1. Discourage restrictive dieting, meal skipping, and fasting.
2. Provide information about normal changes that occur during puberty.
3. Correct misconceptions about nutrition, desirable body weight, and healthy approaches to weight loss.
4. Carefully phrase any weight-related recommendations and comments.

Our society as a whole can benefit from a fresh focus on healthful food habits and a healthful outlook toward foods.

Concept Check

Bulimia is characterized by episodes of bingeing followed by purging, usually by vomiting. Vomiting is very destructive to the body, often causing severe dental decay, stomach ulcers, irritation of the esophagus, and blood potassium imbalances. Treatment using nutrition counseling and psychotherapy attempts to restore normal eating habits and to help the person find tools to tackle the stresses of life.

BARYOPHOBIA

Baryophobia, literally "the fear of becoming heavy," is a relatively new disorder. The term pertains to children who exhibit a reduced growth rate.[22] Decreased growth in a child usually reflects disease. If no hormonal or other abnormality can be found, the possibility of baryophobia should be investigated. It could be that the parents underfeed the child, fearing that obesity or heart disease might develop later in life. These parents put their children on the same low-fat, high-carbohydrate diet adults follow, but the adult diet does not provide enough kcalories for the child to maintain an adequate growth rate.

baryophobia
A disorder associated with a poor growth rate in a child because parents underfeed the child in an attempt to prevent development of obesity and/or heart disease.

In these cases, the parents need nutrition counseling concerning their child's nutritional needs. Including some sweets and higher-fat foods in a child's diet is appropriate (see Chapter 16). Selected foods can still be low in saturated fat, which should be the real focus of diets designed to reduce the risk of heart disease. Supplying adequate kcalories and protein and other nutrients is the key to promoting growth in childhood, and it can be done in a healthful manner.

Summary

1. The person with anorexia nervosa is usually a girl around the age of puberty who begins to diet but then finds it difficult to stop. The person is generally a perfectionist and a high achiever, often described as the "best little girl in the world."
2. Warning signs for anorexia nervosa include abnormal food habits, such as cutting a pea in half before eating it or cooking a large meal and watching others eat, while the anorectic person refuses to eat any herself. Later, school perfor-

mance crumbles, the person often refuses to eat out with family and friends, and she develops a very critical and joyless nature. Menstruation may also cease.

3. Physical effects of anorexia nervosa include a decrease in body temperature, a decrease in heart rate, iron-deficiency anemia, a low white blood cell count, loss of hair, constipation, a low blood potassium level, and a loss of menses. A person with anorexia nervosa is physically very ill.
4. Treatment of anorexia nervosa includes increasing food intake to at least a level sufficient to support basal metabolism (approximately 1200 kcalories/day). Psychological counseling attempts to help the person establish regular food habits and to find means of coping with the life stresses that led to the disorder. Hospitalization may be necessary, especially if a binge-purge cycle has been established.
5. Bulimia is characterized by bingeing on up to 20,000 kcalories at one sitting, and then purging by using vomiting, laxatives, exercise, or other means. Vomiting as a means of purging is especially destructive to the body; it can cause severe tooth decay, stomach ulcers, irritation of the esophagus, low blood potassium levels, and other problems. Bulimia poses a serious health problem and is associated with significant risk for suicide.
6. Baryophobia is a disorder in which a child fails to grow because the parents feed the child a low-fat diet in an attempt to reduce the risk that the child will develop obesity and/or heart disease. Counseling is needed for the parents regarding desirable nutrient intake and weight gain patterns for a child.

Take Action

Examine Figure 10-3. List your own behaviors that would put you at risk for an eating disorder. Rank them according to importance in your life. What insights have you achieved that will affect your future behavior? What new food habits might you begin? Do you need to discard any? Should you seek counseling to address any of your problems?

"At risk" habit	Importance of habit to life-style	Corrective action to consider

REFERENCES

1. Adams LB and Shafer MD: Early manifestations of eating disorders in adolescents: defining those at risk, Journal of Nutrition Education 20:307, 1988.
2. ADA Reports. Position of the American Dietetic Association: Nutrition intervention in the treatment of anorexia nervosa and bulimia nervosa, Journal of The American Dietetic Association 88:68, 1988.
3. Borgan J and Corbin C: Eating disorders among female athletes, Physicians and Sports Medicine 15:89, 1987.
4. Casper RC: The pathophysiology of anorexia nervosa and bulimia nervosa, Annual Reviews of Nutrition 6:299, 1986.
5. Evers CL: Dietary intake and symptoms of anorexia nervosa in female university dancers, Journal of the American Dietetic Association 87:66, 1987.
6. Feldman W and others: Culture versus biology: children's attitudes toward thinness and fatness, Pediatrics 81:190, 1988.
7. Frisch RE: Fatness and fertility, Scientific American 62:88, 1988.
8. Ganan MA and Mitchell JE: Subjective evaluation of treatment methods by patients treated for bulimia, Journal of the American Dietetic Association 86:520, 1986.
9. Garner DM and Garfinkel PE: The eating attitudes test: an index of the symptoms of anorexia nervosa, Psychological Medicine 9:273, 1979.
10. Geraciot TD and Liddle RA: Impaired cholecystokinin secretion in bulimia nervosa, The New England Journal of Medicine 319:683, 1988.
11. Health and Public Policy Committee, American College of Physicians: Eating disorder: anorexia nervosa and bulimia. Nutrition Today March/April 29, 1987.
12. Herzog D and Copeland P: Eating disorders, The New England Journal of Medicine 318:295, 1985.
13. Herzog D and Copeland P: Bulimia nervosa—psyche and satiety, The New England Journal of Medicine 319:716, 1988.
14. Huse DM and Lucas AR: Dietary treatment of anorexia nervosa, Journal of the American Dietetic Association 83:687, 1983.
15. Isner JM: Effects of Ipecac on the heart, The New England Journal of Medicine 314:1253, 1986.
16. Kapoor S: Treatment for significant others of bulimic patients may be beneficial, Journal of the American Dietetic Association 88:349, 1988.
17. Killen JD, and others: Self-induced vomiting and laxative and diuretic use among teenagers, Journal of the American Medical Association 255:1447, 1986.
18. Kirkley BG: Bulimia: clinical characteristics, development, and etiology, Journal of the American Dietetic Association 86: 468, 1986.
19. Mackenzie M: The pursuit of slenderness and addition to self-control: an anthropological interpretation of eating disorders: Nutrition Update Volume 2, p 173, Briggs, editor, New York, 1985, John Wyley & Sons Inc.
20. Nicholi AM, editor: The new Harvard guide to psychiatry, Cambridge, Mass, Harvard University Press, 1988.
21. Omizo SA: Anorexia nervosa: psychological considerations for nutritional counseling, Journal of the American Dietetic Association 88:49, 1988.
22. Pugliese MT, and others: Fear of obesity: a cause of short stature and delayed puberty, The New England Journal of Medicine 309:513, 1983.
23. Rigotti N: Osteoporosis in women with anorexia nervosa, The New England Journal of Medicine 311:1601, 1984.
24. Schotte DE and Stunkard AJ: Bulimia versus bulimic behaviors on the college campus, Journal of the American Medical Association 258:1213, 1987.
25. Story M: Nutrition management and dietary treatment of bulimia, Journal of The American Dietetic Association 86:517, 1986.
26. Toner B, and others: Long-term follow-up of anorexia nervosa, Psychosomatic Medicine 48:520, 1986.
27. Winston DH: Treatment of severe malnutrition in anorexia nervosa with enteral tube feedings, Nutrition Support Services 7:24, 1987.
28. Woo LMH: Diet counseling: treatment of anorexia nervosa and bulimia, Topics in Clinical Nutrition 1:73, 1986.

SUGGESTED READINGS

The articles by Herzog and Copeland and that by the American College of Physicians provide a detailed medical perspective of eating disorders. These articles contain numerous references for your further reading. The articles by Kirkley and Story demonstrate the registered dietitian's perspective on eating disorders and their own role in treatment. This role is further developed in the position paper by the American Dietetic Association. These references supply a detailed account of the causes, development, and treatments for these disorders.

CHAPTER 10

Answers to nutrition awareness inventory

1. *True.* Some cultures use certain foods as aphrodisiacs. In the United States waffles are a breakfast food, while in England they are dessert.
2. *True.* About 5% of young women suffer from an eating disorder.
3. *False.* They have an intense fear of gaining weight.
4. *True.* This is referred to as purging.
5. *True.* People with anorexia nervosa tend to be extremely competitive.
6. *True.* People with anorexia nervosa see themselves as fat, even when they are thin.
7. *True.* But they don't like to admit it.
8. *False.* Bulimia is extremely secretive.
9. *True.* This attitude is reflected in advertisements.
10. *True.* Most people with eating disorders see themselves as inadequate.
11. *True.* People with eating disorders are often obsessively neat and highly aware of imperfections.
12. *True.* The damaging effects of late stages of these conditions increase the risk of permanent injury.
13. *True.* Bingeing and purging characterize bulimia.
14. *False.* Treatment should emphasize choice as opposed to restriction.
15. *True.* This should be suspected in children who exhibit poor growth rates.

Nutrition Perspective 10-1

Eating Disorders: A Sociological Perspective

We evaluate ourselves in many ways. One way is based on body image. We identify our bodies with ourselves and judge it as we think others see us, knowing that our appearances affects their opinions of us.

Early in life, we learn to recognize what "acceptable" and "unacceptable" body types look like. Of all attributes that constitute attractiveness, body weight is probably perceived as the most important—partly because it is an aspect over which we have control somewhat.

Yet body weight is probably the aspect of image that dissatisfies us most. Fatness has been ranked as the most dreaded deviation from our cultural ideals of body image, the one most derided and shunned, even among schoolchildren. Children often describe other overweight children as lazy, stupid, filthy, sloppy, mean, and ugly. Girls often associate overweight with poor social acceptance; they tend to add adjectives such as "worried," "sad," and "lonely" to descriptions of pictures of obese girls.[6]

CHANGING TIMES

The "full-bodied" woman as a cultural ideal did not survive into the twentieth century (Figure 10-7).[19] Over the course of this century, a woman's "ideal" body form has become thinner and thinner. Our passion for thinness may have its roots in the Victorian era, which specialized in denial of "unpleasant" physical realities such as appetite and sexual desire. Flappers of the 1920s cemented a trend for thinness (Figure 10-8). Annette Kellerman, a movie star of this period, stated, "Fleshiness and obesity . . . are only soft-pedal euphemisms for clumsy, unhealthy, ugly, and awkward." These trends for women can be documented by studying the Miss America winners and fashion magazines. Barbie and Ken dolls are the ultimate in the long and lean look. Over the past 20 years, the ideal has gradually moved toward a thinner, more angular body shape, while the population as a whole has gained weight. The same holds for men in general: a lean, slightly muscular physique characterizes men in advertisements and movies.

Researchers have linked this acceptance of leanness as the desirable body type to the recent surge in eating disorders.[29] As the more full-figured woman (earth mother) was re-

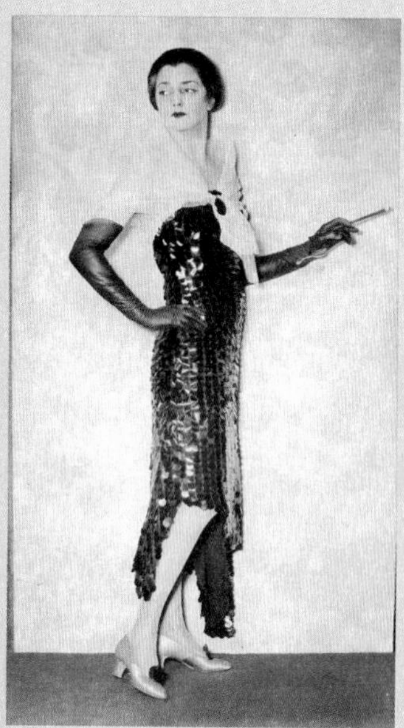

A

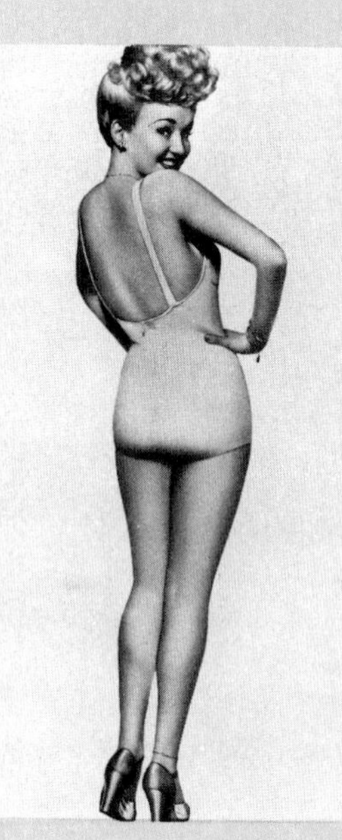

B

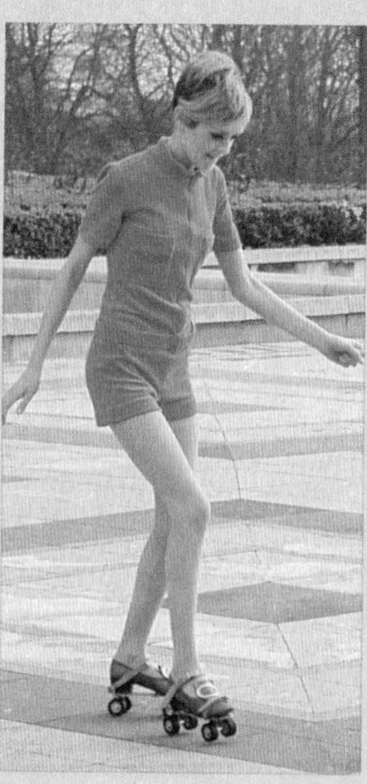

C

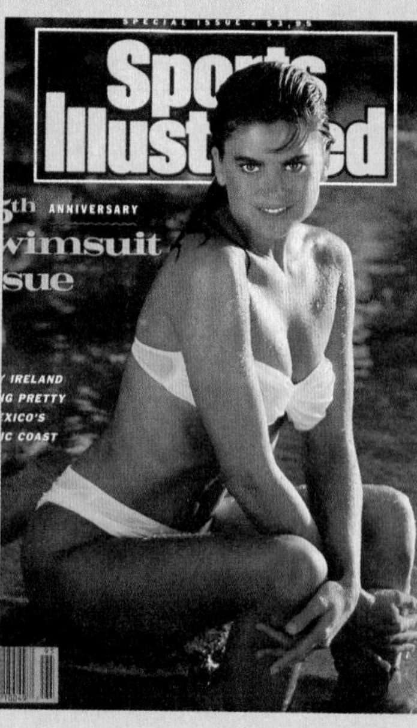

D

Figure 10-7

The changing views of desirable body weight. American society has imposed varying stereotypes for desirable body weight, especially for women. (A) The svelt flapper of the 1920's. (B) The "thin but curvaceous" look of the 1940's. (C) Ultra-thin was in during the 1960's. (D) Lean and well-toned physiques grace magazine covers of the 1980's and 1990's.

placed by the ultra-thin, gaunt woman, our preoccupation with obesity and the incidence of eating disorders has increased. It appears that these cultural pressures for thinness are stretching the physiological capabilities of many women and men. We discussed in Chapter 8 the variability among people in basal metabolism, rates for the thermic effect of food, and activity levels. Lower rates and activity levels, especially encouraged by sedentary jobs and living conditions, set up some of us to gain weight. Some other body types may more easily resist. People with biological and emotional predispositions to eating disorders may be forced "over the edge" by a change in social values to which they are not physically equipped to conform.

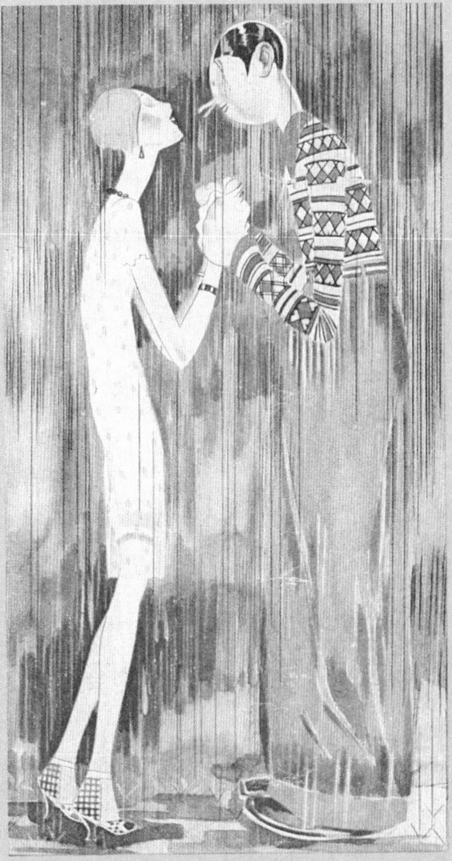

Figure 10-8
A fasting girl made the perfect flapper.

THE PURSUIT OF POWER

Today, obesity is viewed by society as a failure of control, willpower, competence, and productivity. At stake is social acceptance and even access to scarce resources, such as good jobs, an attractive spouse, and social recognition. Whether we like it or not, our appearance says a lot about us. We no longer know many people on a one-to-one basis, as we did when we lived in mostly small towns. Appearance is now more important. It is one's calling card, and the question implicit in our society's values is this: if a person cannot control himself enough to stay slim, can he supervise employees, organize the work day, and reliably bear heavy responsibilities?

MIXED MESSAGES

On top of the pressure for thinness, we receive mixed messages. Half the advertisements in women's magazines may be for diets, and the other half for tasty foods such as chocolate cake. Movie and television stars are almost always perfect physical specimens. Yet television advertisements encourage us to visit our local fast food restaurant, where a hamburger, french fries, and milk shake can quickly add up to 1200 kcalories—about the equivalent of what our daily basal metabolism uses. We may know that bingeing and purging are not healthy, yet film stars such as Jane Fonda now admit that these practices were part of their life-styles early in their careers.

NEW PRESSURES

Divorce now ends about one half of all marriages. This increases the stress on children and adolescents, who, like adults, can turn to food under stress.[1] Considering other prevalent stresses—alcoholism, school and work pressures, traffic, and crowded urban conditions—many of us face family and social environments that encourage us to find a pressure release valve. That valve may be food. Food in excess, however, creates a new problem—a socially unacceptable appearance. While attempting to defuse stress in one part of life, some of us add another whole network of problems.

THIN IS IN!

All in all, fat has lost favor in our society. Today's myth is that thin people are better than obese people—more beautiful, more competent, more healthy, and more strong-willed. A lean physique may provide a nice backdrop for designers to show off their creations, but the image is tough on their customers. Thin may be in, but this fashion does not always lead to good health.

Drive-up windows in fast-food restaurants allow a person to pick up and eat 1200 or more kcalories without ever leaving the car. This availability makes overeating just that much more possible.

Eating disorders are usually only a symptom of greater emotional trauma in a person's life. When psychiatrists are able to dig deeper, they find that eating disorders mask serious questions of self-worth, family struggles, and possibly fear of puberty and the future. The real illness is not the eating disorders—though they eventually contribute to poor health—but rather, the way people feel about themselves. Current social values contribute to these disturbing views. How can you help?

Nutritional Perspective 10-2

Thoughts of a Person with Bulimia

I am wide awake and immediately out of bed. I think back to the night before when I made a new list of what I wanted to get done and how I wanted to be. My husband is not far behind me on his way into the bathroom to get ready for work. Maybe I can sneak onto the scale to see what I weigh this morning before he notices me. I am already in my private world. I feel overjoyed when the scale says that I stayed the same weight as I was the night before, and I can feel that slightly hungry feeling. Maybe IT will stop today, maybe today everything will change. What were the projects I was going to get done?

We eat the same breakfast, except that I take no butter on my toast, no cream in my coffee and never take seconds (until Doug gets out the door). Today I am going to be really good and that means eating certain predetermined portions of food and not taking one more bite than I think I am allowed. I am very careful to see that I don't take more than Doug. I judge by his body. I can feel the tension building. I wish Doug would hurry up and leave so I can get going!

As soon as he shuts the door, I try to get involved with one of the myriad of responsibilities on my list. I hate them all! I just want to crawl into a hole. I don't want to do anything. I'd rather eat. I am alone, I am nervous, I am no good, I always do everything wrong anyway, I am not in control, I can't make it through the day, I know it. It has been the same for so long.

I remember the starchy cereal I ate for breakfast. I am into the bathroom and onto the scale. It measures the same, BUT I DON'T WANT TO STAY THE SAME! I want to be thinner! I look in the mirror, I think my thighs are ugly and deformed looking. I see a lumpy, clumsy, pear-shaped wimp. There is always something wrong with what I see. I feel frustrated, trapped in this body, and I don't know what to do about it.

I float to the refrigerator knowing exactly what is there. I begin with last night's brownies. I always begin with the sweets. At first I try to make it look like nothing is missing, but my appetite is huge and I resolve to make another batch of brownies. I know there is half of a bag of cookies in the bathroom, thrown out the night before, and I polish them off immediately. I take some milk so my vomiting will be smoother. I like the full feeling I get after downing a big glass. I get out six pieces of bread and toast one side in the broiler, turn them over and load them with patties of butter and put them under the broiler again till they are bubbling. I take all six pieces on a plate to the television and go back for a bowl of cereal and a banana to have along with them. Before the last toast is finished, I am already preparing the next batch of six more pieces. Maybe another brownie or five, and a couple of large bowlfuls of ice cream, yogurt, or cottage cheese. My stomach is stretched into a huge ball below my ribcage. I know I'll have to go into the bathroom soon, but I want to postpone it. I am in never-never land. I am waiting, feeling the pressure, pacing the floor in and out of the rooms. Time is passing. Time is passing. It is getting to be time.

I wander aimlessly through each of the rooms again, tidying, making the whole house neat and put back together. I finally make the turn into the bathroom. I brace my feet, pull my hair back and stick my finger down my throat, stroking twice, and get up a huge pile of food. Three times, four and another pile of food. I can see everything come back. I am glad to see those brownies because they are SO fattening. The rhythm of the emptying is broken and my head is beginning to hurt. I stand up feeling dizzy, empty, and weak. The whole episode has taken about an hour.

Part IV
The Vitamins and Minerals

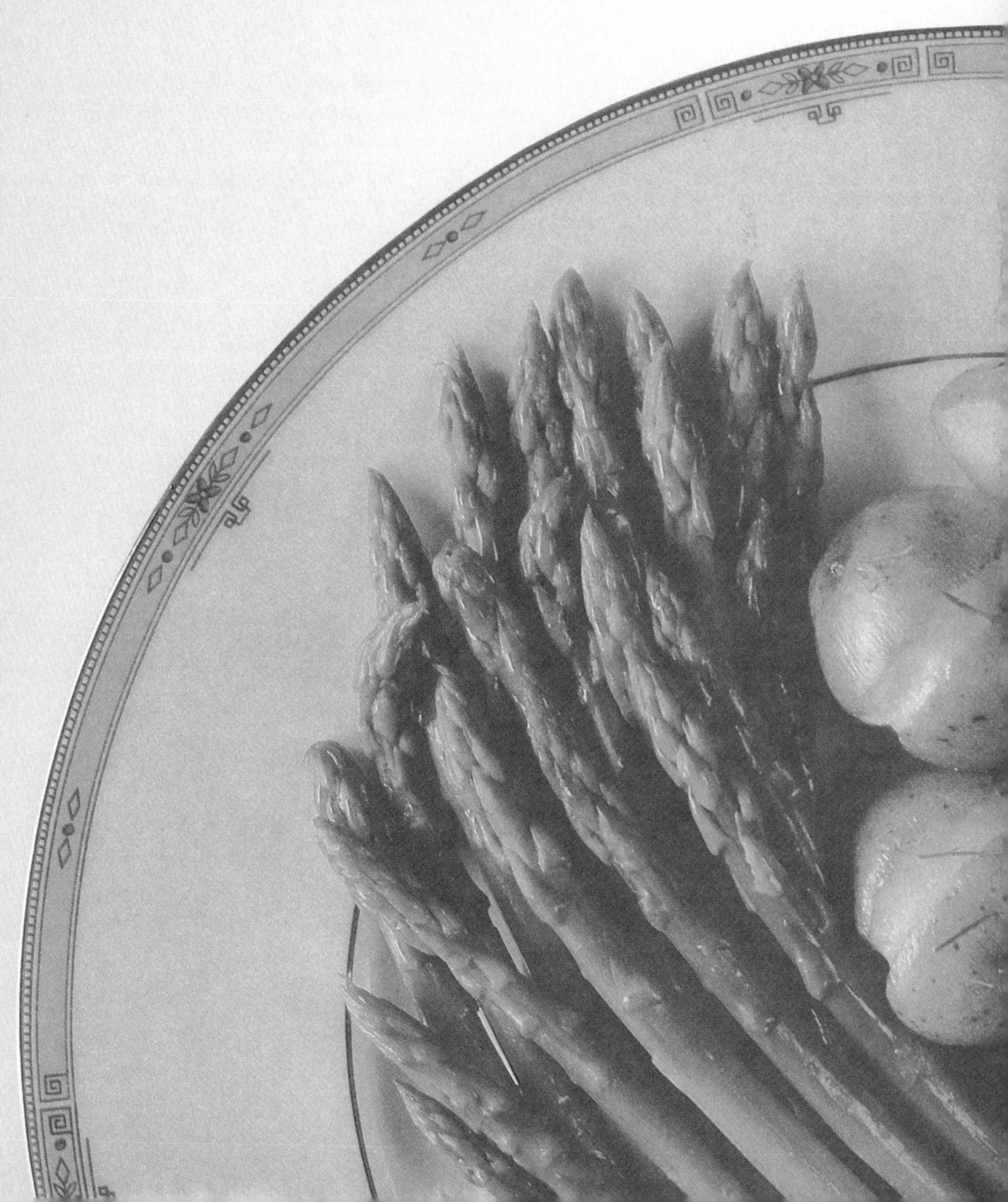

Chapter 11

Vitamins in General, and the Fat-Soluble A, D, E, and K

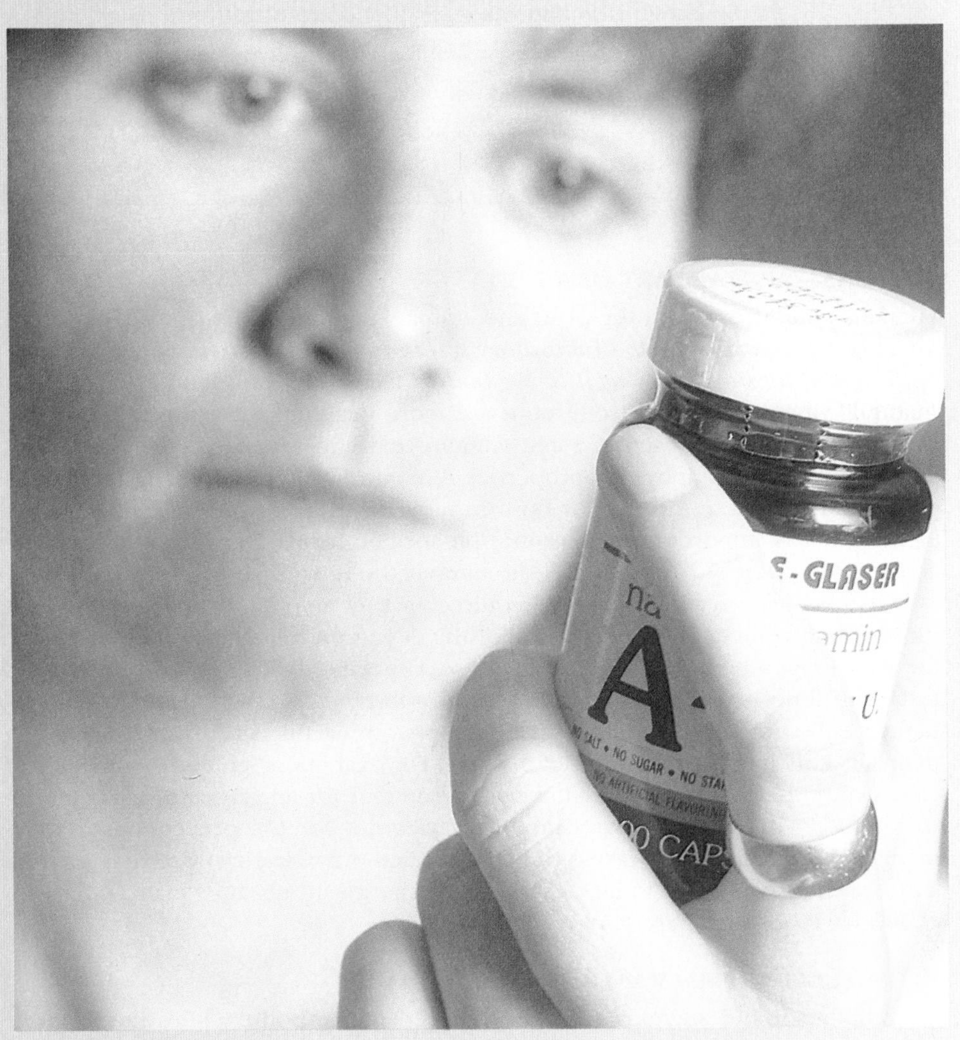

Most North Americans have diets that supply enough vitamins for good health.

Overview

Vitamins are organic (carbon-containing) compounds needed for important metabolic reactions in the body. Most plants can synthesize all the vitamins they need. But human bodies cannot make them, and so we rely on our diets. However, we need vitamins in only small quantities, about 28 grams (1 ounce) for every 70 kg (150 pounds) of food we eat.

Vitamins yield no energy for the body. Instead, they facilitate energy-yielding chemical reactions and promote body growth and development. Vitamins A, D, E, and K dissolve in fat, while the B vitamins and vitamin C dissolve in water. In addition, the B vitamins and vitamin K function as parts of coenzymes: these are molecules that directly help enzymes function.

Let's look at the vitamins—important contributors to health, and so to life.

Nutrition awareness inventory

Here are 15 statements about vitamins in general and fat-soluble vitamins in particular. Answer them to test your current knowledge. If you think the answer is true or mostly true, circle T. If you think the answer is false or mostly false, circle F. Use the scoring key at the end of this chapter to compute your total score. Take this test again after you have read the chapter. Compare the results.

1. **T F** There is a danger of deficiency if a vitamin is missing in your diet for 1 week.
2. **T F** Vitamin K is stored in the body more efficiently than other vitamins.
3. **T F** People who use mineral oil as a laxative at mealtimes are susceptible to fat-soluble vitamin deficiencies.
4. **T F** Fat-soluble vitamins are easily lost in cooking.
5. **T F** It is extremely unlikely that all vitamins have been discovered.
6. **T F** Vitamin D improves calcium absorption.
7. **T F** Vitamin A is important for night vision.
8. **T F** Toxic levels of vitamin A may appear at five times the RDA.
9. **T F** Vitamin D is a hormone.
10. **T F** Vitamin D is synthesized by sunlight.
11. **T F** Vitamin E is a free radical.
12. **T F** Vitamin K is important for blood clotting.
13. **T F** Antibiotic use can provoke a vitamin K deficiency.
14. **T F** Vegetables are good sources of vitamin K.
15. **T F** A safe dosage for a supplement is generally 50% to 150% of the U.S. RDA.

VITAMINS—A VITAL PART OF A DIET

Vitamins come from both the plant and animal kingdoms. *Whether isolated from foods or synthesized in the laboratory, vitamins are the same chemical compounds and work equally well in the body.* Claims by health food literature that "natural" vitamins isolated from foods are more healthful than those synthesized in a laboratory are nonsense. Some vitamins exist in several related forms that differ in chemical or physical properties. Vitamin E, for example, has alpha and gamma forms. These forms exist both in nature and in synthesized vitamin supplements. It is important to consume the specific forms that the body can use, and we will point out those forms throughout the next chapters.

Vitamins are organic nutrients required in tiny amounts to promote one or more specific biochemical reactions. For the definition to fit, lack of the substance for a prolonged period of time must cause a specific deficiency disease that—if caught in time—is quickly cured when the substance is resupplied. Doses of vitamins well above the RDA also have been proven useful as pharmacological medicinal agents in a small number of diseases. For example, high doses of niacin are an accepted part of cholesterol-lowering treatment for appropriately selected individuals.[8,11] Other various applications of vitamins for the prevention or treatment of nondeficiency diseases are being studied. Any claims concerning vitamin supplement treatment should be looked at cautiously because many unproven claims have been, and are continually, made.

FAT-SOLUBLE VERSUS WATER-SOLUBLE VITAMINS

Overall, fat-soluble vitamins are readily stored in the body, while water-soluble vitamins are not. This occurs partly because the water in cells dissolves water-soluble vitamins and flushes them out of the body via the kidneys. Notable exceptions are the fat-soluble vitamin K and the water-soluble vitamin B-12: vitamin B-12 is stored much more readily than vitamin K. *Vitamins in foods should be consumed daily, but an occasional lapse in the intake of one or more water-soluble vitamins should cause no harm.* It takes an average person 10 days to develop the first symptoms of a thiamin deficiency and 20 to 40 days for a vitamin C deficiency to develop when these vitamins are completely lacking in the diet. This shows that all vitamins are stored to some extent in the body.

Because fat-soluble vitamins are not readily excreted, some can build up in the body and cause toxic reactions. Vitamins A and D are especially likely to do so, from heavy and regular consumption of supplements or foods such as liver. Regular use of a "one-a-day" type of multivitamin and mineral supplement will not cause toxicity problems if this yields less than two times the RDA, except perhaps during pregnancy, and then only because of the vitamin A content (see p. 315 for a discussion). But consuming many vitamins, especially highly potent sources of vitamins A and D, can cause problems. In the 1930s fish oils such as cod liver oil became sources of vitamin toxicity because of their very high concentrations of vitamins A and D. Today major sources of vitamin toxicity are found in grocery, drug, and health food stores, where very concentrated forms of vitamin A and vitamin D are sold.

Isolated reports in the scientific literature show that vitamin E and the water-soluble vitamins B-6 and niacin also can be toxic, but only when consumed in very high amounts (50 to 100 times the RDA). So except for vitamin pill use these three vitamins are unlikely to cause toxic symptoms. In comparison, vitamins A and D can cause toxicity with long-term use at just five to ten times the RDA.

People with extra vitamin needs

People who experience fat malabsorption—for example, those with cystic fibrosis, celiac disease, or Crohn's disease—also experience fat-soluble vitamin malabsorption (see Chapter 3). Unabsorbed fat carries fat-soluble vitamins to the colon and into the feces. Such a person is especially susceptible to a vitamin K deficiency because it is not as readily stored as are the other fat-soluble vitamins. People who use mineral oil as a laxative at mealtime are also susceptible to fat-soluble vitamin deficiencies. The mineral oil collects fat-soluble vitamins and pulls them into the colon, from which they are expelled. Some B vitamins (such as folate) and minerals (such as calcium and magnesium) are also susceptible to malabsorption during intestinal disease. See Nutrition Perspective 11-1 to find out whether you should take a vitamin supplement.

Vitamin losses in cooking

Water-soluble vitamins can be lost in cooking due to heat, alkalinity, and leaching into the cooking water.[28] Steaming, stir-frying, microwaving, or simmering vegetables in minimal moisture allows them to retain most of the B vitamins and vitamin C. Although baking soda is sometimes added to vegetables during cooking to make them greener, or to beans to make them softer, it is not a good nutritional practice: the alkalinity destroys much of the thiamin and vitamin C found in the vegetables (Table 11-1). Cooking loss for other vitamins is generally less likely. Important examples will be discussed as we review specific vitamins.

Have we found all the vitamins?

You may wonder if there are still more vitamins lurking in foods, waiting to be discovered. After all, the structure and chemical formula of the first known vitamin (thiamin) was not determined until 1937, and the last known vitamin (vitamin B-12) was characterized in 1948. Though some optimistic researchers

Table 11-1

Suggestions for retaining the maximum amount of vitamins when harvesting, storing, and cooking foods

Consume or process vegetables immediately after harvest

- More vitamins, especially vitamin C and folate, are lost the longer vegetables are kept before they are eaten or processed.

Store vegetables and fruits properly

- The best method is to freeze fruits and vegetables when possible. Blanch them first (briefly simmer them in water) to retain more flavor. Consult a cookbook for directions. This method preserves the vitamin content best because it stops the enzyme activity that destroys the vitamins. However, watch out for texture changes.
- If you cannot eat fruits and vegetables immediately after harvesting them, but plan to do so within a few days, keep them in the refrigerator. Place them in covered containers or plastic bags to stop moisture loss.
- Canning fruits and vegetables is possible, but this method causes a greater nutrient loss because of the high temperatures required. In addition, it can require a lot of work.

Reduce preparation and cooking of vegetables

The more preparation and cooking of vegetables, the greater the nutrient loss. To reduce the losses:

- Avoid soaking vegetables in water.
- When possible, cook vegetables in their skins.
- Cook in as little water as possible.
- Bake, steam, or broil vegetables. A microwave oven retains vitamins.
- When boiling, use tight-fitting lids to diminish evaporation of water.
- Cook vegetables in as short a time as possible. Develop a taste for a more crunchy texture.
- Cook frozen vegetables in the frozen state: don't thaw beforehand.
- Reduce cutting up of vegetables and fruits before cooking. The more vegetables and fruits are cut up before cooking, the more exposure to air they receive and the greater the loss of vitamins, especially vitamin C and folate.
- Don't add baking soda to vegetables. It produces an alkaline pH that destroys much vitamin C, thiamin, and other vitamins.

hope to discover one more vitamin,[2] most scientists are confident that all vitamins needed by humans have been discovered: we can already maintain human life for years on total parenteral nutrition if it is properly designed and the person is closely monitored. No food needs to be eaten. A person can receive all nutrients by vein. By receiving protein, carbohydrate, fat, all the known vitamins, and the essential minerals in this manner, a person can continue not only to live but to build new tissue, have a baby, heal wounds, and fight existing diseases. *Experiences with total parenteral nutrition have also taught us that some lesser known vitamins, such as biotin, are still very important to health.*

THE FAT-SOLUBLE VITAMINS—A, D, E, AND K

Let's turn to the fat-soluble vitamins—A, D, E, and K. Table 11-2 summarizes much of what we know about each of them. Figure 11-1 shows their chemical structures.

Table 11-2

Summary of the fat-soluble vitamins, their functions, deficiency conditions, and food sources

Vitamin	Major functions	Deficiency symptoms	Dietary sources	RDA	Toxicity symptoms
Vitamin A (retinol) and pro-vitamin A (carotenoids)	1. Adapt to dim light (formation of rhodopsin); color vision 2. Promote growth 3. Prevent drying of skin and eye 4. Promote resistance to bacterial infection	1. Night blindness 2. Bitot's spots 3. Xerophthalmia 4. Poor growth 5. Dry skin (keratinization)	Vitamin A Liver Fortified milk Provitamin A Sweet potatoes Spinach Greens Carrots Cantaloupe Apricots	Females: 800 RE* (4000 IU†) Males: 1000 RE* (5000 IU†)	Fetal malformations, hair loss, skin changes, pain in bones
D (chole- and ergocalciferols	1. Facilitates absorption of calcium and phosphorus 2. Maintain optimum calcification of bone	1. Rickets 2. Osteomalacia	Vitamin D Fortified milk Fish oils	5-10 micrograms (200-400 IU)	Growth retardation, kidney damage, calcium deposits in soft tissue
E (tocopherols)	1. Antioxidant: prevents oxidation of vitamin A and unsaturated fatty acids	1. Hemolysis of red blood cells 2. Nerve destruction	Vitamin E Vegetable oils Some greens Some fruits	Females: 8 Alpha-tocopherol equivalents Males: 10 Alpha-tocopherol equivalents	Muscle weakness, headaches, fatigue, nausea, inhibition of vitamin K metabolism
K (phyllo- and menaquinones)	1. Form prothrombin and other factors for blood clotting	1. Hemorrhage	Vitamin K Green vegetables Liver	60-80 micrograms‡	Anemia and jaundice

*Retinol equivalents
†International units

Absorption of fat-soluble vitamins

The vitamins A, D, E, and K in the diet are absorbed along with dietary fat. These vitamins then travel in chylomicrons with other dietary fats through the lymphatic system and reach the bloodstream. They are then carried by the chylomicrons and other lipoproteins (VLDL and LDL—see Chapters 3 and 5) to body cells. Other carriers in the bloodstream also help distribute vitamins A and K.

When fat absorption is efficient—that is, the actions of bile salts and lipase promote adequate digestion and there is adequate absorptive capacity from a healthy intestinal wall—about 40% to 90% of the fat-soluble vitamins are absorbed. As the blood lipoproteins are metabolized by cells lining the bloodstream, the lipoprotein remnants (remains) are picked up by the liver. In this way the fat-soluble vitamins contained in the remnants also enter the liver, which is a major storage site, especially for vitamin A.

In disease states in which fat digestion is poor or lipoprotein synthesis is hampered, fat-soluble vitamin status may be deficient, especially for vitamins E and K.

Supplements may then be appropriate, with a physician's guidance (see Nutrition Perspective 11-1).

Concept Check

Fat-soluble vitamins—A, D, E, and K—are generally more readily stored and less likely to be lost in cooking than are the water-soluble vitamins—B vitamins and vitamin C. When a person ingests a vitamin-free diet, the first deficiency signs are due to a thiamin deficiency after about 10 days. This shows that even water-soluble vitamins are stored to some extent in the body, and so an occasional poor daily consumption should be of no health concern. It is prudent, however, to regularly consume foods rich in both water-soluble and fat-soluble vitamins. Fat malabsorption decreases fat-soluble vitamin absorption; this has the greatest effect on vitamin K status in the body. Fat-soluble vitamins pose the greatest risk for toxicity, especially vitamins A and D. Water-soluble vitamins known to show toxic effects are vitamin B-6 and niacin, but only at very high doses.

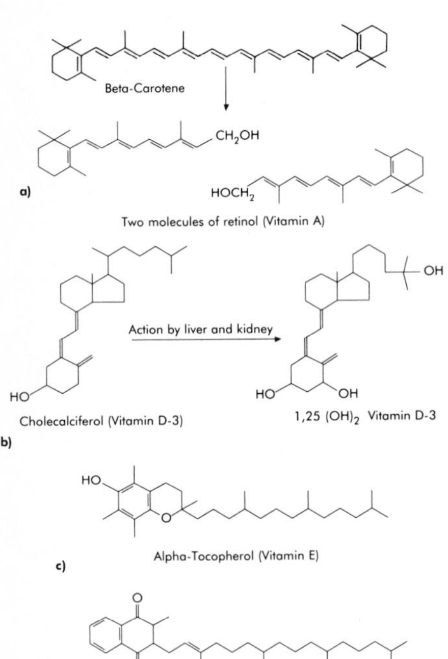

Figure 11-1
The fat-soluble vitamins.

retinoids
Chemical category for preformed vitamin A; one source is animal foods.

VITAMIN A

Vitamin A comes in a variety of forms: retinal (aldehyde form), retinol (alcohol form), retinoic acid (acid form), and others. These forms are found in the diet and to some extent can be converted into each other. As a family these compounds are called **retinoids.** Vitamin A activity in the diet is also present in the form of the common plant pigments, such as beta-carotene, also called provitamin A (Figure 11-1). Carotenoids are actually the original source of all vitamin A. Over 600 carotenoids are found in nature; 50 of them have vitamin A activity, and so serve as provitamin A. The most potent form is beta-carotene.

In the intestinal cells, most carotenes are split, yielding in turn some vitamin A. Some of the beta-carotene in the diet is not split to form vitamin A. About 30% is absorbed intact and deposited into adipose cells. The carotene stored in adipose tissue gives the characteristic yellow-orange tone to the skin of people who are especially fond of carrot juice. Combining the retinoids with the provitamin A carotenoids yields what is generically referred to as vitamin A.[22]

Most vitamin A is stored in the liver. To leave the liver, retinol must bind to a retinol-binding protein, which requires zinc for its synthesis. Thus a zinc deficiency will result in a **secondary** vitamin A deficiency.

Functions of vitamin A

Vitamin A performs many important functions in the body. Its importance to night and color vision is perhaps its best-known role. Vitamin A's link to vision has been known since ancient Egyptian times, when juice extracted from liver was used as a cure for night blindness.

The visual cycle. To participate in vision, one form of vitamin A—retinal—combines with a protein in the eye, called opsin, forming **rhodopsin** (Figure 11-2). When light strikes rhodopsin, retinal is changed from a cis isomer form to a trans isomer form. Now retinal can no longer attach to the protein portion of the rhodopsin molecule (opsin), so it comes off. This then alters the structure of rhodopsin, which in turn allows ions to enter cells in the eye. The change in ion balance in the cells of the eye stimulates nerve fibers. This signals the brain that light is striking the eye.

See Chapter 2 for a description of cis and trans isomer forms.

The cells in the eye recover from a flash of light by first turning the trans retinal back into the cis form, and then rhodopsin is reformed. This series of actions constitutes the visual cycle. Not all retinal can be recycled: a certain amount is lost and must be replaced by retinol from the bloodstream, which originally came from the diet. Retinol is converted to retinal in the eye.

If an adult's diet is deficient in vitamin A for many years, the retinol level in

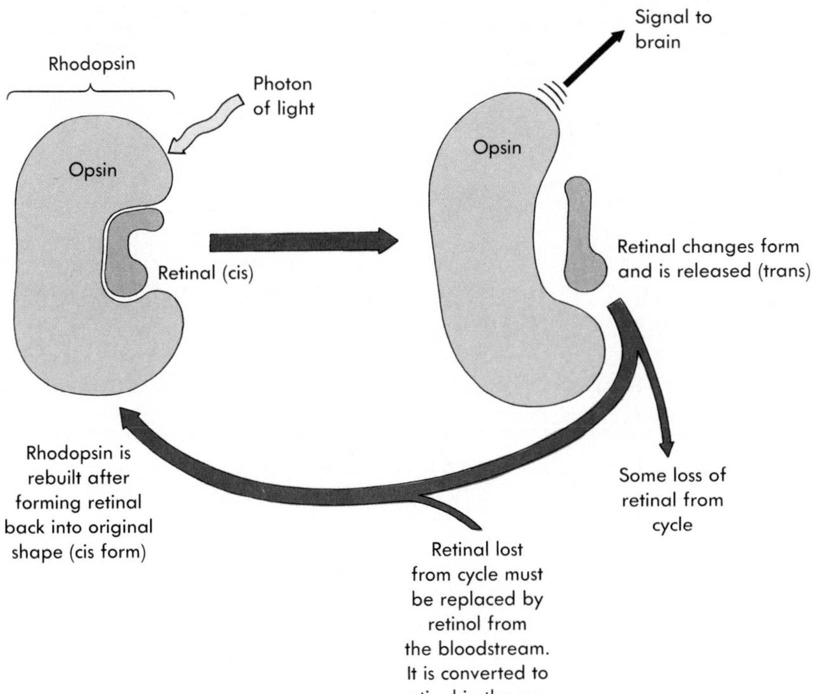

Figure 11-2

Vitamin A participates in the visual cycle. Light (photons) hits rhodopsin. This causes retinal to change form, and so it is released from opsin. Opsin then changes shape and allows the ion balance in the retina membrane to change. This ion change signals "light" to the brain.

the bloodstream decreases. In children this decrease happens sooner, since body stores are less. When retinol in the bloodstream is insufficient to replace that lost from the visual cycle, the cells in the eye recover from flashes of light more slowly, because there is less rhodopsin stored in the eye cells. Night blindness increases and the ability to adapt to darkness decreases. It takes longer to see light again once it has already struck the eye, such as after seeing headlights of an oncoming car. An injection of vitamin A into the bloodstream can cure night blindness in a matter of minutes!

Xerophthalmia. Vitamin A is very important for the maintenance of mucus-forming cells and synthesis of various **mucopolysaccharide** substances. Without vitamin A, mucus-forming cells deteriorate and no longer synthesize mucus, a lubricant needed throughout the body. The cells then make a hard protein, called keratin, which is typically found in hair and nails. The organ first affected by this loss of mucus-synthesizing capacity are the eyes, especially the cornea. Mucus in the eye is critical for lubricating its surface and washing away dirt and other particles that land on the eye. Mucus also contains a protein—lysozyme—that can degrade bacteria.

mucopolysaccharides Substances containing protein and carbohydrate parts, as found in bone and other organs.

In vitamin A deficiency, the surface of the eye dries out, partly because of a lack of mucus production. This symptom appears as night blindness develops. Eventually, when dirt particles scratch the dry surface of the eye, bacteria invade the scratch and cause an infection. White blood cells finally arrive and make matters worse by synthesizing degradative enzymes to attack the infection. These enzymes also attack the eye. Lesions on the eye that develop in a vitamin A deficiency are first referred to as Bitot spots. Soon the infection spreads from one spot to the entire surface of the eye, eventually leading to blindness (Figure 11-3). This disease process is called **xerophthalmia,** which means "dry eye."

xerophthalmia Literally "dry eye." A cause of blindness that results from a vitamin A deficiency. The specific cause is a lack of mucus production by the eye, which then leaves it more vulnerable to surface dirt and bacterial infections.

Vitamin A deficiency is the second-leading cause of blindness in the world after accidents. North American children are at little risk because of generally good diets. Children in less-developed nations, however, are especially susceptible to vitamin A deficiency because their poor intakes and stores of the vitamin fail to meet their high needs due to rapid childhood growth. Over 500,000 children in poorer nations of the world become blind each year because of vitamin A

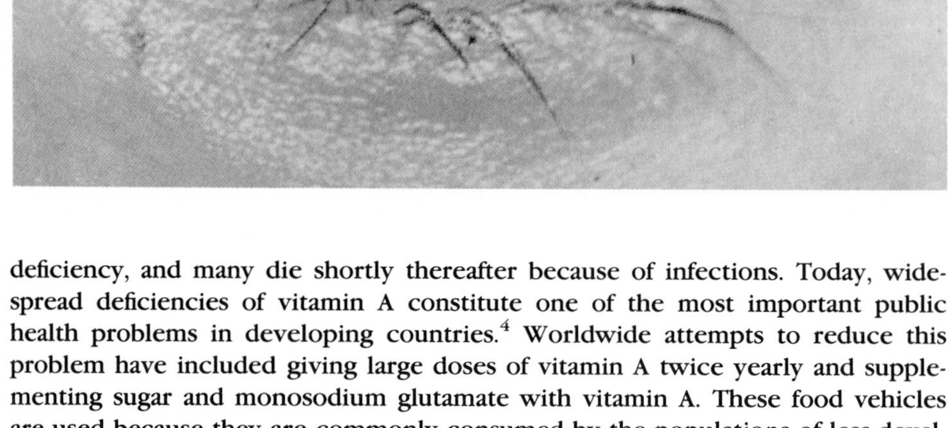

Figure 11-3

A vitamin A deficiency can eventually lead to blindness. Note the severe scar on this eye.

In North America, the leading cause of blindness in adults is diabetes, and in children it is accidents.

deficiency, and many die shortly thereafter because of infections. Today, widespread deficiencies of vitamin A constitute one of the most important public health problems in developing countries.[4] Worldwide attempts to reduce this problem have included giving large doses of vitamin A twice yearly and supplementing sugar and monosodium glutamate with vitamin A. These food vehicles are used because they are commonly consumed by the populations of less-developed nations.

epithelial cells
The surface cells that line the outside of the body and all external passages within it.

Immune function. During vitamin A deficiency, insufficient mucus production in the intestines and lung cells and poor health of **epithelial** cells in general increases the risk of infection. A vitamin A deficiency also reduces the activity of some immune cells, such as T-lymphocytes. Together, these effects leave the vitamin A–deficient person more vulnerable to infections.[20] That is why night blindness in children is accompanied by two to three times the normal risk for respiratory tract infections.[30]

Growth and development. Vitamin A is necessary for the growth and development of cells. This is most easily demonstrated with laboratory animals, but human growth is also enhanced.[34] The resorption of old bone, which precedes deposition of new bone, requires bone cells that may be stimulated by vitamin A. The synthesis of some components of bone also requires vitamin A (the section on vitamin D and Chapter 13 contain more information about bone metabolism).

This proposed action of vitamin A interacting with DNA in a cell works similarly to the way steroid (cholesterol-derived) hormones, such as active vitamin D, influence cell protein synthesis (see the section on vitamin D).

Vitamin A–deficient animals cannot reproduce. Vitamin A can travel into a cell and interact with the DNA in the cell nucleus. By doing so, vitamin A causes the DNA to increase the synthesis of some cell proteins that in turn stimulate proper growth and development. Alternately, vitamin A may help synthesize mucopolysaccharides that also influence cell metabolism.

Cancer prevention. *The ability of retinoids to influence epithelial cell development, coupled with its ability to increase immune system activity, could make it a valuable tool in the fight against cancer, especially skin, lung, bladder, and breast cancer.* Researchers have been encouraged by work using animals and also by the fact that most forms of cancer arise from epithelial cells. Active research with humans using forms of vitamin A is now under way in many centers in North America.[19] However, wait for those results before embarking on personal experimentation as toxicity is a possible result. The Daily Food Guide is still the best tool for identifying vitamins to reduce cancer risk.

Carotenoid precursors of vitamin A, especially beta-carotene, may also help prevent cancer because they are excellent antioxidants.[5] The many double bonds present in some carotenoid molecules make them effective traps for free oxygen atoms and peroxides.[21] These are two of many **oxidizing agents** that can probably initiate the cancer process. Some evidence shows that regular consumption of vegetables high in carotenes decreases risk of lung cancer in smokers.[35] However, much investigation is needed in this area before specific recommendations regarding carotenes and cancer prevention—other than eating fruits and vegetables regularly—can be made.

oxidizing agent
A compound capable of capturing an electron from another compound or supplying an oxygen atom to a compound.

Vitamin A in foods

Vitamin A in foods exists in the two forms already discussed: animal (preformed vitamin A) and plant (provitamin A). Preformed vitamin A is found in liver, fish oils, fortified milk, and eggs. Butter and margarine are also fortified with vitamin A, but we don't eat enough of either to make them significant sources. Provitamin A carotenoids are mainly found in dark green and orange vegetables and some fruits. Carrots, spinach, squash, broccoli, papayas, and apricots are examples of sources. About 50% of the vitamin A in the North American diet comes from animal sources; the rest comes as provitamin A.

Exploring Issues and Actions

What type of study would convince you that carotenoid consumption decreases the risk of lung cancer?

The major contributors of vitamin A—either preformed or provitamin A—to the U.S. diet are liver, carrots, eggs, tomatoes, vegetable soups, whole milk, and greens. Foods with the highest nutrient density (per kcalorie) for vitamin A are carrots, liver, spinach and other greens, sweet potatoes, yellow squash, and romaine lettuce (Table 11-3). Beta-carotene accounts for some of the major yellow-orange color of carrots. The yellow-orange color is often masked, however, by

Table 11-3

Good food sources of vitamin A activity, ranked by nutrient density

Food	Serving size to yield 1000 RE*	Kcalories needed to yield 1000 RE
Fried beef liver	⅓ ounce	10
Whole carrot	½ each	30
Baked sweet potato	½ each	48
Baked butternut squash	½ each	50
Cooked spinach	⅔ cup	60
Romaine lettuce	7.5 cups	70
Chopped green onions	1 cup	100
Cooked tomatoes	3 cups	120
Cantaloupe	⅔ each	130
Cooked turnip greens	1-⅓ cups	150
Mango	1-¼ each	175
Papaya	2 each	191
Apricots	11 each	200
Cooked broccoli	4 cups	210
Cooked mustard greens	1-½ cups	250
Cooked asparagus	6 cups	293
Skim milk	7 cups	620
2% milk	7 cups	820

*Adult male RDA
Note how few kcalories you need to consume to obtain the RDA if you choose the right vegetables and fruits.

Not all the carotenoids in fruits and vegetables yield vitamin A: an example is lycopene in tomatoes.

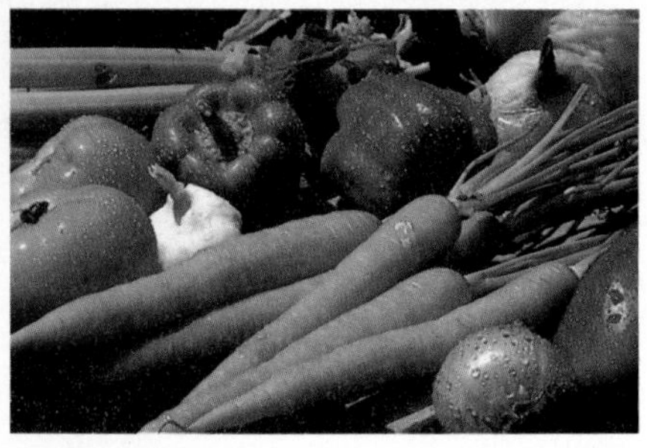

Carrots are rich in beta-carotene.

dark-green chlorophyll pigments in vegetables such as broccoli. *Consuming a varied diet rich in green vegetables and carrots ensures sufficient sources for meeting vitamin A needs.*

Retinol equivalents (RE)

Most nutrient levels in foods were formerly expressed in crude **international units (IU).** These were usually based on the different growth rates animals showed when fed different amounts of a specific nutrient. Today we can precisely measure nutrient quantities, and so milligrams and micrograms have replaced international units. Some food labels still show the older IU values for nutrients because the US RDA is based on the RDA from 1968, which used the IU system. The current RDA does not.

international unit (IU)
A crude measure of vitamin activity often based on the growth rate of animals. Today these units have been replaced by more precise milligram and microgram quantities.

For vitamin A the new unit of measurement is the retinol equivalent (RE). In this system, 6 milligrams of beta-carotene yields 1 milligram of vitamin A activity. In addition, 12 milligrams of any other provitamin A carotenes (alpha, delta, or others) are needed to yield 1 milligram of vitamin A activity. Retinol equivalents (RE) are calculated by adding actual weight of dietary retinol (preformed vitamin A) to the adjusted weight values for the provitamin A carotenoids in the food (Appendix N).

Relative to preformed vitamin A, the beta-carotene measurement is divided by 6 to compensate for both its poorer absorption and its incomplete conversion into vitamin A. The other carotene measurements are divided by 12 because these forms are not so active as the beta form. Actually, these values—6 and 12—are our best educated guesses, based on incomplete knowledge.

RDA for vitamin A

The current RDA for vitamin A for adults is 1000 RE for men and 800 RE for women. (Throughout the next four chapters, refer to the inside cover for vitamin recommendations for other ages and to Appendix G for Canadian recommendations). The recommendation approximates the average intake for adult men and women in the United States. A more regular intake of green vegetables among women could raise intakes to RDA levels.

In the older system, the RDA value is 5000 IU for men and 4000 IU for women. A good translation formula equates 1 RE of vitamin A to 5 IU of vitamin A if based on a mixture of preformed and provitamin A. Otherwise, 3.3 IU of preformed vitamin A alone equals 1 RE.

Measuring serum vitamin A levels is one way to assess a person's status. However, this is an insensitive measure, since serum levels often won't fall until vitamin A stores in the liver are very low.

North Americans at risk for a vitamin A deficiency. In North America, poor vitamin A status may be seen in preschool children who do not eat enough protein or vegetables, especially in Hispanic communities.[26] The urban poor, the elderly, and adults who are alcoholics or who have liver disease (which limits vitamin A storage) also show poor vitamin A statuses, especially with respect to stores. Finally, children with severe fat malabsorption, as in cases of cystic fibrosis, may also show a vitamin A deficiency.

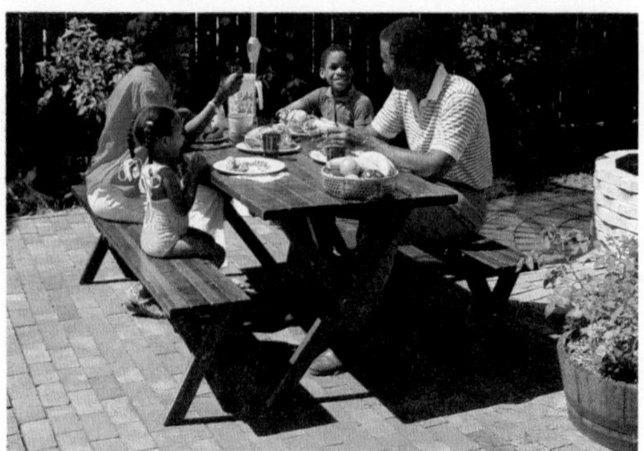

Parents can be good role models by eating what they want their children to eat.

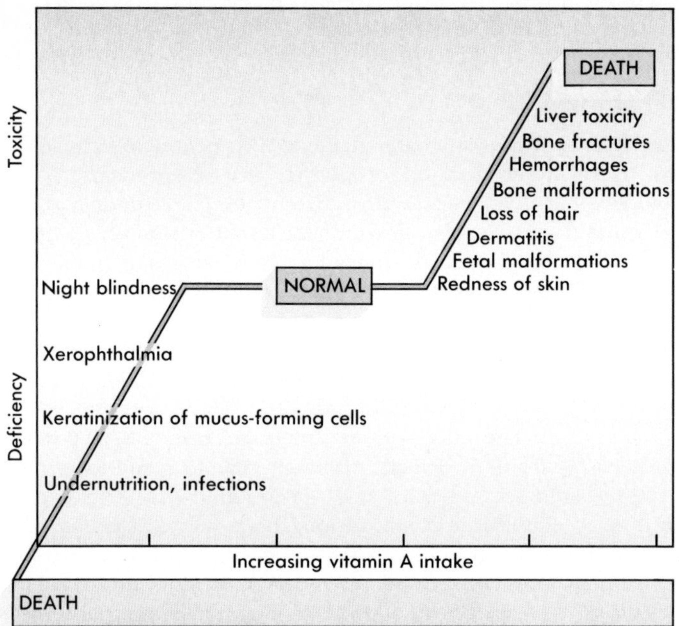

Figure 11-4

Consuming the right amount of vitamin A is critical to overall health. A very low (deficient) and a very high (toxic) vitamin A intake can produce damaging symptoms and even lead to death. The severity of effects and the intake range vary for individuals.

Parents often encourage their children to eat vegetables. Besides contributing to good food habits, this practice helps them take in enough vitamin A. Parents provide important role models for children, and they can positively influence their children's eating interests by eating as they want their children to eat (see Chapter 16).

Toxicity from excessive vitamin A. *Toxicity symptoms from excessive vitamin A can appear with long-term supplement use at just 10 times the RDA* (Figure 11-4). High vitamin A intakes are especially dangerous during pregnancy because they can cause fetal malformation.[16] See the Expert Opinion by Dr. James Olson for a detailed discussion.

In children, *one* single dose of 60,000 RE has been used for the possible prevention of vitamin A deficiency. This treatment, which causes mild, short-lived side effects in some children, is common as part of medical practice in countries where foods high in vitamin A are not often consumed. It should last the child for 3 to 6 months. However, if such large doses are taken regularly by either children or adults for months at a time, many toxicity symptoms may appear. Even regular consumption of large quantities of chicken livers by infants can lead to toxic side effects. The symptoms range in infants and adults from bone pain, loss of appetite, headache, dry skin, and hair loss to high blood triglyceride levels, increased liver size, and vomiting. Treatment is simply to withdraw the supplement. Symptoms then decrease over the next few weeks to a month as blood levels fall to normal range.

Vitamin A for acne: is it safe?. A derivative of vitamin A—13-cis retinoic acid (Accutane)—is an oral drug used in high doses to treat serious acne. Taking high doses of vitamin A itself would not be safe. Even with this derivative physicians walk a fine line between treating the acne and inducing toxicity symptoms. The person must also limit sun exposure because skin is quite sensitive to sunburn when this drug is used. Furthermore, women must not be pregnant or become pregnant while using this medication because it carries a very high risk for fetal malformations, especially for those of the central nervous system.

Recently, derivatives of vitamin A have been put into creams (Retin-A) that manufacturers claim will reduce some effects of aging on the skin. Note that if one is already deeply wrinkled, these creams won't be the answer. Taking care of the skin by limiting sun exposure and using sun blocks is a much better preventive measure.

Hypercarotenemia. If someone consumes large amounts of carrots, in the form of carrot juice, for example, or if infants eat a great deal of squash, the high

Vitamin A: How Much Is Too Much?

JAMES ALLEN OLSON, PH.D.

Vitamin A is a required nutrient that is present in two forms in foods: preformed vitamin A, originating primarily from liver and other animal products, and provitamin A carotenoids, mainly coming from dark green leafy vegetables and fruits with a yellow-to-orange color. In the less industrialized world (mainly in parts of Asia and Africa) vitamin A deficiency causes blindness in 250,000 to 500,000 preschool-aged children each year. Because very little vitamin A is required to maintain sight in children—0.2 to 0.4 milligrams daily or 70 to 150 milligrams per year—many efforts are currently being made to reduce the ravages of this terrible condition.

The other side of the coin is vitamin A toxicity (hypervitaminosis A). Perhaps more so than for any other required nutrient, the old fallacious adage, "If a little is good, more is better," leads to very serious consequences in the case of vitamin A overconsumption.

Before the specific consequences of vitamin A toxicity are cosidered, however, the difference between carotenoids and preformed vitamin A must be stressed. The ingestion of large amounts of carotenoids does *not* cause vitamin A toxicity. Nonetheless, individuals who drink large amounts of carrot or tomato juice or who ingest pills containing beta-carotene (more than 30 milligrams) daily often assume a yellowish coloration, particularly the palms of the hands and soles of the feet. Although resembling jaundice in many ways, the condition is harmless and disappears after excessive intakes of carotenoids are stopped. The reasons that provitamin A carotenoids are useful nutritionally in small amounts but do not cause hypervitaminosis A are that: (1) their rate of conversion into vitamin A is relatively slow and regulated, and (2) the efficiency of carotenoids absorption from the small intestine decreases markedly as the oral intake increases. Thus Nature protects us from any serious toxic effects from dietary carotenoids.

Let's now turn to the toxicity of preformed vitamin A. Three kinds of vitamin A toxicity exist: acute, chronic, and teratogenic (causing fetal deformities). Acute toxicity is caused by the ingestion of one very large dose of vitamin A or of several large doses taken over several days. The signs of acute toxicity, as indicated in the table, are largely manifestations of central nervous system abnormalities. Once the dosing is stopped, these signs disappear. Extraordinarily large doses, however, can cause death. For example, a single intramuscular dose that caused death in 50% of treated young monkeys was 68 milligrams of retinol (560,000 IU_a) per kilogram of body weight. (See first note to the following table for explanation of IU_a values.) In humans, the only known case is a 2.25 kilogram infant who died from the ingestion of 1,000,000 IU during an 11-day period, or a total dose of 147 milligrams of retinol (440,000 IU_a) per kilogram of body weight.

Chronic toxicity, which is much more common than acute toxicity, results from ingesting excessive doses of vitamin A on a regular basis during a period of weeks to years. As shown in the table, the skin, hair, internal organs, and the central nervous system are affected. Most of the adverse signs disappear after cesation of dosing. Permanent damage to the liver, bones, eyes, and recurrent joint and muscle pain, however, can occur. A few individuals suffer signs of chronic vitamin A toxicity on relatively low daily intakes of vitamin A, for example, less than 6000 micrograms of retinol, or less than 20,000 IU_a. Such persons probably suffer from vitamin A intolerance, which seems to have a genetic basis and often is exacerbated by other clinical problems. These cases, although rare, are nonetheless worthy of note.

The most serious and tragic effects of hypervitaminosis A are birth defects. Although vitamin A and its acidic forms, all-*trans* retinoic acid (tretinoin) and 13-*cis* retinoic acid (isotretinoin), have long been known to cause abortion and birth defects in experimental animals, the risk in humans was only highlighted in 1985 by Professor Edward Lammer and his colleagues in a study of a group of pregnant women taking large doses of isotretinoin for acne. Although only a few cases of a clear relationship between birth defects and excessive intakes of vitamin A, as distinguished from isotretinoin, have been reported in the literature, birth defects have been *associated* with daily vitamin A intakes of greater than or equal to 18,000 IU taken early in pregnancy.

Let's be careful, however, of the way we interpret this association. It does *not* mean that the ingested vitamin A has definitely *caused* the abortion or birth defect, but only that higher intakes of vitamin A occur more often in women that produce defective babies. Many other completely different factors may be involved. Nonetheless, the association must be considered seriously, particularly in view of the known causal relationship between birth defects and high doses of vitamin A in humans and the relationship between abortion and birth defects and intake of acidic retinoids in experimental animals.

Most birth defects relate to the head, probably because neural crest cells, which are important in the development of the head and brain, are known to be very sensitive to excess amounts of vitamin A. Retinoid-related birth defects are listed in the following table.

Obviously, too much vitamin A can cause a lot of trouble. But how much is too much? Two questions might be raised here that have subtly different, but important, distinctions. First, how much vitamin A is needed to maintain physiological function and provide for an adequate reserve in most healthy adults? And second, how much vitamin A can be safely ingested?

The answer to the first question, provided in the following table, is an average of 600 to 1000 micrograms of retinol daily, depending on whether you accept the World Health Organization's Recommended Daily Intake (RDI) or the U.S. Recommended Daily Allowance (U.S. RDA). Because most adults in the United States have liver reserves that are three to five times greater than they need to provide for good health, the use of supplements of vitamin A by most people is completely unnecessary, as indicated in a joint statement in 1987 of the American Institute of Nutrition, the American Society for Clin-

Intakes and Signs of Vitamin A Needs and Toxicity in Adults

Retinol (in micrograms)	Retinol in IU_a*	Daily Intake* Category	Major signs
50	167	Deficiency	Night blindness, skin abnormalities, and xerophthalmis (dryness and thickening of the membranes of the eyelid and eye).
150	500	Marginal status	Cures night blindness and other visual abnormalities.
300	1000	Marginal status	Corrects most, if not all, effects of vitamin A deficiency in individuals.
600	2000	Satisfactory status	Provides adequate total body reserves in most persons in a population. Currently, the RDI of the World Health Organization.‡
1000	3333	Satisfactory status	Provides generous reserves for most persons in a population. Currently, the RDA for the adult male in the United States.‡
5400 to 150,000	18,000 to 500,000	Teratogenicity	Abortion; prominent facial and cranial abnormalities, including the brain, ears, eyes, jaw, mouth, and lips; and defects of the heart, kidney, and gastrointestinal tract.
7500 to 210,000	25,000 to 700,000	Chronic toxicity	Headache, loss of hair, cracking of lips, dry and itchy skin, enlarged liver, bone abnormalities, muscle and joint pain, and visual defects.
300,000 or more	1,000,000 or more	Acute toxicity	Nausea, vomiting, headache, dizziness, blurred vision, and muscular incoordination.

*Amounts of vitamin A are expressed both in micrograms of retinol, or micrograms retinol equivalents, and in international units (IU). To distinguish between IU of vitamin A and of beta-carotene, which have different values nutritionally, subscripts are used: IU_a for vitamin A and IU_c for carotenoids. Thus 0.3 micrograms of retinol = 1 IU_a, whereas 0.6 micrograms of beta-carotene = 1 IU_c.

‡The RDI (RDA) for women is usually about 80% of that for men, based primarily on differences in body weight.

ical Nutrition, and the American Dietetic Association. Nonetheless, premature infants and young growing children—who start life with poor vitamin A reserves and people with liver or kidney disorders or lipid malabsorption syndromes do need special attention.

The second question does not deal with need but with safety—that is, an absence of toxic effects. In this regard, the Teratology Society of the United States recommended in 1987 that women of childbearing age limit their total daily intake of preformed vitamin A to 2400 micrograms (8000 IU_a), and that any supplements be in the form of provitamin carotenoids. The National Academy of Sciences recommends in its 1989 report on *Diet and Health* that daily supplements of any nutrient not exceed one U.S. RDA value: 1000 micrograms (3333 IU_a) of vitamin A. The International Vitamin A Consultative Group, which deals primarily with third world deficiency problems, recommended in 1986 that pregnant women—only in areas where vitamin A deficiency is common—be given supplements of preformed vitamin A of 10,000 IU_a or less. Finally, the Council for Responsible Nutrition, a trade association of the nutritional supplement industry, advises pregnant women to limit their daily supplements of preformed vitamin A to 10,000 IU_a.

The net result of all of these recommendations is clear: If you are healthy and eat a balanced diet, you don't need vitamin A supplements, nor indeed, of any other nutrient. But if, for whatever reason, you wish to take supplements of preformed vitamin A, limit your daily intake to 10,000 IU_a or less. Whatever you do, keep clearly in mind that preformed vitamin A, when ingested in excess, can cause a lot of trouble. Why seek trouble? Doesn't life pose enough challenges?

Dr. Olson is a Distinguished Professor of Sciences and Humanities in the Department of Biochemistry and Biophysics, Iowa State University.

hypercarotenemia
High level of carotene in the bloodstream, usually caused by a diet high in carrots or squash, or by taking beta-carotene supplements.

carotene levels in the bloodstream that result can turn skin yellow-orange. The result is **hypercarotenemia** (or just carotenemia). The person appears to have **jaundice,** but unlike a case of jaundice, the sclerae (whites of the eyes) are white (instead of yellow), and the liver does not enlarge. Hypercarotenemia is thought to cause no harm.[29]

Concept Check

Vitamin A in the diet comes in two forms: preformed vitamin A and provitamin A carotenoids. Vitamin A is important for maintaining vision and mucus-forming cell activity in the body, ensuring the health of the immune system, and directing aspects of growth and development; and carotenoid intake is associated with a reduced risk of developing some forms of cancer. Major food sources of vitamin A include liver, carrots, eggs, tomatoes, milk, and many vegetables. North Americans most at risk for poor vitamin A status are preschool children, because of insufficient intakes or fat malabsorption, and adults with alcoholism. Vitamin A can be quite toxic, even at dosages only 10 times the RDA, especially during pregnancy.

VITAMIN D

Vitamin D is not just a vitamin—it is also considered hormone because skin cells can make it in the presence of sunlight. It is then metabolically activated by other cells. The amount of sun-time needed to produce vitamin D depends on the darkness of the skin: young light-skinned people need approximately 15 minutes a day in the sun, while dark-skinned people need more sun exposure. The process is also more efficient in younger people than in the elderly. *Anyone who does not receive enough sunshine to make vitamin D must consume vitamin D instead. For these people, vitamin D is a vitamin.* To discover why the vitamin nature of vitamin D is emphasized more than its hormonal nature, see Nutrition Perspective 11-2, which discusses the history of vitamin D.

Synthesis of vitamin D

The starting product for vitamin D synthesis in the body is 7-dehydrocholesterol, a derivative of cholesterol (Figure 11-5). In a two-step process, sunshine (specifically, ultraviolet light at 282 nanometers) first strikes the skin and opens up a ring on the 7-dehydrocholesterol molecule. The compound produced will then slowly convert itself in the second step into vitamin D (cholecalciferol) over a span of 36 hours.[3]

Staying too long in the sun causes the skin to make, in addition to vitamin D, other related compounds, such as lumisterol.[33] These other products probably protect us from making too much vitamin D, which otherwise could then result in vitamin D toxicity. Over time, these other compounds can be converted back into vitamin D (Figure 11-5).

Forming the active hormone

calcitriol
The active hormone form of vitamin D (1,25-dihydroxyvitamin D)—not to be confused with calcitonin, the hormone that also affects calcium utilization.

To form the active hormone, vitamin D has to have two hydroxyl groups (-OH) added to it. The liver adds the first hydroxyl group to form 25-hydroxyvitamin D. The second hydroxyl group is then added primarily by the kidney to form 1,25-dihydroxyvitamin D. The final compound depends on which form of vitamin D begins the process. The animal form (the one humans make), cholecalciferol, makes 1,25-dihydroxycholecalciferol, known as **calcitriol.** The plant form of vitamin D, ergosterol, yields 1,25 dihydroxyergocalciferol. Both compounds work effectively in humans.

Functions of vitamin D

The main function of the vitamin D hormone calcitriol is to help regulate calcium and bone metabolism. To do this, it performs a variety of functions: Vita-

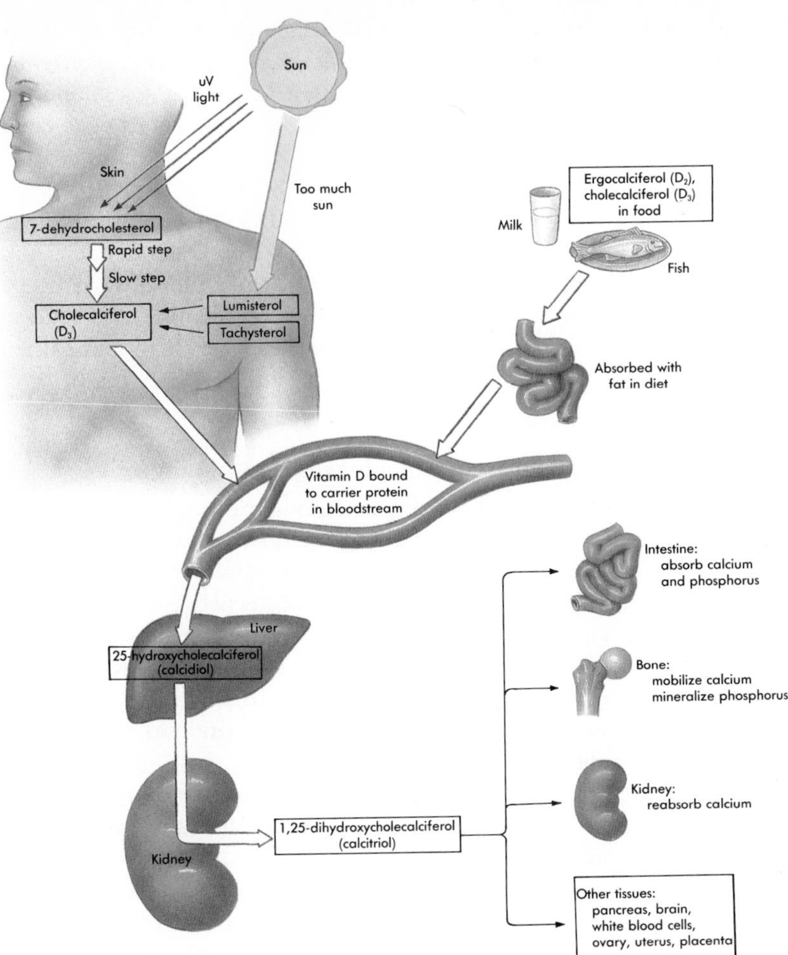

Figure 11-5
The many facets of vitamin D metabolism.

min D helps regulate absorption of calcium and phosphorus from the intestine, it reduces kidney excretion of calcium, and it helps regulate the deposition of calcium in the bones.[27]

The vitamin D hormone calcitriol probably increases calcium and phosphorus absorption in the small intestine by means of two separate mechanisms. In one process, calcitriol traveling into the nucleus of the intestinal cell to direct the DNA to synthesize a variety of calcium-transport proteins, including one that binds calcium. These proteins then increase calcium and phosphorus absorption from the intestine.[3,9] In the other process, calcitriol alters the characteristics of intestinal cell membranes, allowing more passive calcium absorption into the intestinal cells. Researchers think this second mechanism is at least partially responsible for enhanced calcium absorption because absorption increases even before the calcium-binding proteins appear in the cell.[27]

Many cells besides intestinal cells and bone cells contain cell surface **receptors** for calcitrol and therefore respond to calcitriol.[13] These cells are found in the pancreas, pituitary, brain, white blood cells, ovary, uterus, and placenta. In all these cases, calcitriol probably affects calcium metabolism.[27]

receptor
A site on or in a cell where compounds (such as hormones) bind. Cells that contain receptors for a specific compound are influenced by that compound.

Rickets and osteomalacia

The net result of calcitriol action is to increase calcium and phosphorus deposition in bones. Without adequate calcium and phosphorus deposition, bones weaken and bow under pressure. When these symptoms occur in a child, the disease is called **rickets** (Figure 11-6). Symptoms of rickets include enlarged head, joints, and rib cage, a deformed pelvis, and bowed legs.

rickets
A disease characterized by softening of the bones due to poor calcium deposition. This deficiency disease arises from lack of vitamin D activity in the body.

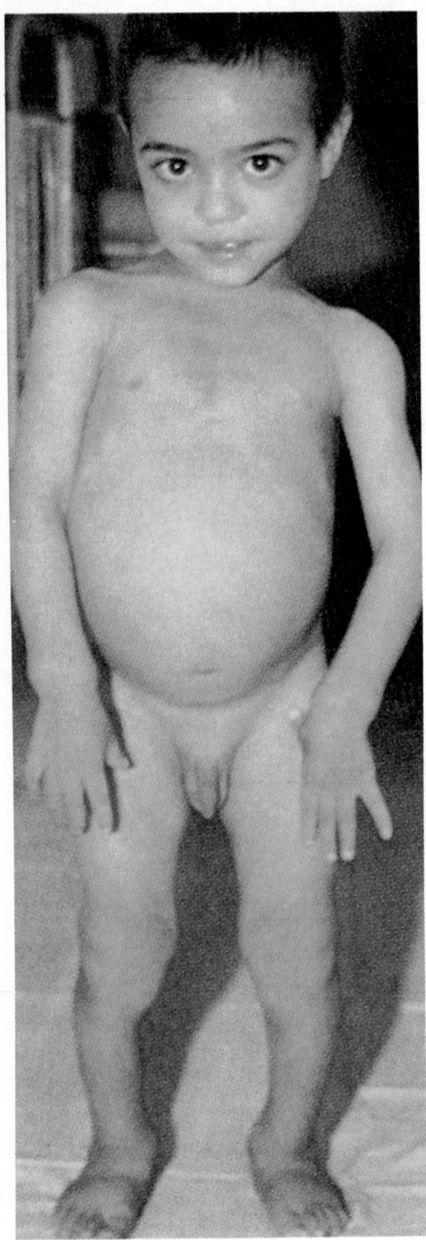

Figure 11-6
The bowed legs of rickets.

The diets of infants, particularly, and of others as well, should contain a food or supplement source of vitamin D if sufficient exposure to sunlight is not possible (Figure 11-7). This is especially important for breast-fed infants in their first 6 months of life. Today, rickets is most commonly associated with fat malabsorption, as is seen in children with cystic fibrosis.

Rickets in adults is called **osteomalacia,** which means "soft bones." It can cause fractures in the hip, spine, and other bones. (Do not confuse this with the disease osteoporosis, which we discuss in Chapter 13). Osteomalacia in adults most likely occurs in people with kidney, stomach, gallbladder, or intestinal disease (especially when most of the intestine has been removed), and with cirrhosis of the liver. These diseases affect both vitamin D metabolism and calcium absorption. Combinations of sun exposure and/or treatment with calcitriol can be used in these cases.

Calcitriol, parathyroid hormone, and calcitonin: a balance

The vitamin D hormone calcitriol works in conjunction with parathyroid hormone and the hormone calcitonin to maintain proper bone mineralization and proper serum calcium levels (see Chapter 13 for a detailed description of bone mineralization). Calcitriol needs parathyroid hormone present to increase bone resorption and reduce calcium loss in the kidneys. The net effect of both these actions is to increase serum calcium. Parathyroid hormone also increases the synthesis of calcitriol. When these hormonal actions eventually raise serum calcium, further production of parathyroid hormone decreases, and this in turn reduces further calcitriol synthesis.

On the other hand, the hormone calcitonin inhibits bone demineralization by halting the action of the bone-resorbing cells. It also reduces the synthesis of calcitriol. Together, these actions lower serum calcium.

As you might suspect, parathyroid hormone responds to a decrease in serum calcium, while calcitonin responds to an increase in serum calcium. Both hormones cause their metabolic effect in part by altering synthesis of calcitriol, the active vitamin D hormone.

Vitamin D in foods

When exposure to sunshine does not create vitamin D sufficient to meet a person's needs, fatty fish (fish oils) and fortified milk serve as the most nutrient-dense

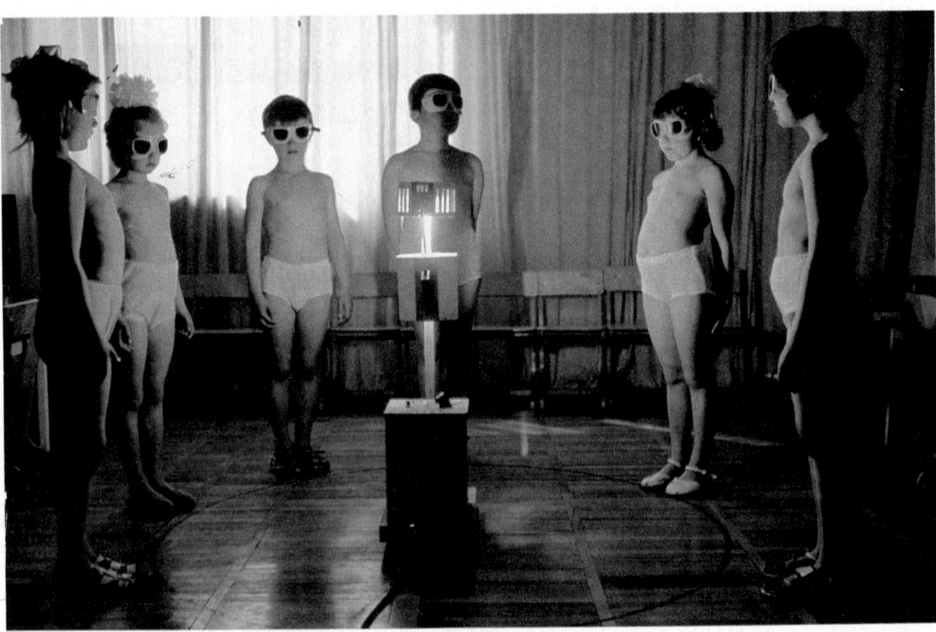

Figure 11-7
Who's got the tanning oil? Southern Russia endures a long winter. These Stayropol kids are exposed to a quartz lamp to provide the vitamin D synthesis they would normally experience from playing outdoors.

Table 11-4

Food sources of vitamin D, ranked by nutrient density

Food	Serving size to yield* 10 micrograms	Kcalories needed to yield 10 micrograms
Eel, smoked	¼ ounce	15
Cod liver oil	1 teaspoon	45
Baked salmon	3-½ ounce	190
Tuna fish	3-½ ounce	190
Milk (fortified, skim)	4 cups	360

*Adult RDA (higher limit)
Aside from fish and fortified milk, no other foods are good kcalorie bargains for vitamin D.

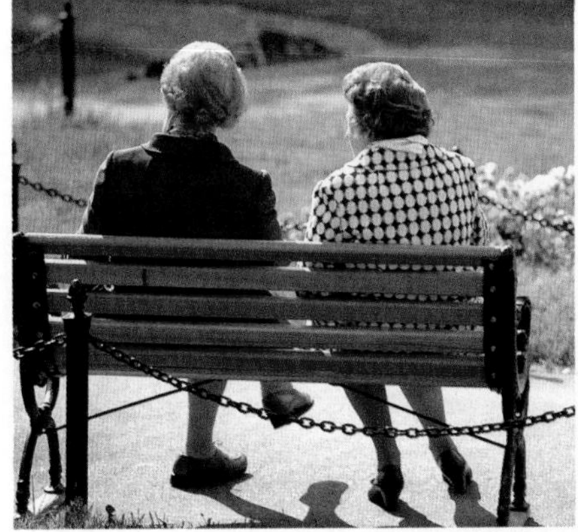

Older adults should get some exposure to the sun or dietary source to ensure they get enough vitamin D.

sources (Table 11-4). In the United States, milk is fortified with 10 micrograms (400 IU) per quart, and in Canada 9 micrograms (360 IU) per quart are added. Eggs, butter, and liver contain vitamin D, but require too great a serving size to be considered significant sources. So few other foods contain vitamin D that food tables do not list sources.

RDA for vitamin D

The RDA for adults for vitamin D varies from 5 to 10 micrograms per day (200 to 400 IU per day). Recall that young light-skinned people can make this amount of vitamin D in about 15 minutes of sun exposure on just the face and hands.

North Americans at risk of vitamin D deficiency

Studies suggest that particular groups—totally breast-fed infants, prisoners, and elderly people,—anyone who both stays inside most of the day and ingests little or no vitamin D—are at risk for developing a vitamin D deficiency.[15,31] These people need either a more predictable amount of sun exposure or a regular food source of vitamin D. People who suffer from severe fat malabsorption, such as children with cystic fibrosis, should concentrate on getting their vitamin D from the sun.

Exploring Issues and Actions

You are visiting your grandmother in a nursing home. She never leaves the building and does not drink milk or consume other vitamin-D fortified foods. You suspect she might be vitamin D deficient. What should she do?

Vitamin D resistance

Some human bodies resist the action of vitamins, including vitamin D. Resistance to vitamin D can be caused either by a lack of calcitriol synthesis in the kidney or by an inability of calcitriol to bind to receptors throughout the body. In both cases, the treatment is a large daily dose of calcitriol. This treatment works fine in the first case but is not so successful in the other.

Toxicity of vitamin D

Vitamin D is a very toxic substance. An intake of just 5 times the RDA can be toxic in children if consumed regularly. Anyone who needs to supplement the diet should consider a dosage not higher than the RDA, 5 to 10 micrograms per day. Consuming more than 25 micrograms (1000 IU) of vitamin D per day requires close scrutiny by a physician. The main symptom of toxicity is overabsorption of calcium, and eventual calcium deposits in the kidneys and other organs. The person will also suffer the typical symptoms of **hypercalcemia**—weakness, loss of appetite, diarrhea, vomiting, mental confusion, and increased urine output. Calcium deposits in organs cause local cell death, and then other symptoms result from this cell death.

hypercalcemia
A high level of calcium in the bloodstream that can lead to loss of appetite, calcium deposits in organs, and other health problems.

Measuring the serum 25-hydroxycholecalciferol is the best way to assess vitamin D status in the body.

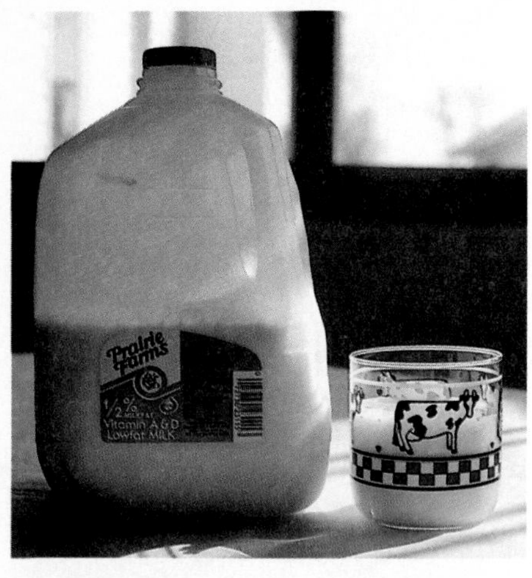

Milk is often fortified with vitamin D.

Concept Check

Vitamin D is a vitamin only for people who fail to produce enough from sunlight. Using a form of cholesterol, most people can synthesize adequate vitamin D by the interaction of sunlight on their skin. The vitamin D is later activated by the liver and kidneys to form the active hormone calcitriol. This compound increases calcium absorption in the intestine and works with other hormones to maintain proper calcium metabolism in bones and other organs in the body. Significant food sources of vitamin D are fish oils and fortified milk. Vitamin D is quite toxic: intakes greater than 5 times the RDA should be consumed only with a physician's guidance. Sun exposure appears to pose no risk of vitamin D toxicity.

VITAMIN E

What we call vitamin E is actually a family of compounds—the **tocopherols** and the tocotrienols. Various forms exist for both these major types of compounds. Some forms are more active than others, as you will soon see.

Functions of vitamin E

Vitamin E is one of the body's fat-soluble antioxidants: vitamin C is one water-soluble counterpart. As noted in Chapter 5, an antioxidant has the ability to step between a compound seeking electrons and the compound's target molecule, such as a fatty acid in a cell membrane (Figure 11-8). *The antioxidant donates electrons and/or hydrogens to the electron-seeking compound, thus neutralizing it.* This then protects other molecules or parts of the cell from an attack by the electron-seeking compound.

If vitamin E does not step in, the electron-seeking compound can pull electrons from cell membranes, DNA, and other electron-dense cell parts. That either alters the cell DNA, which may increase the risk for cancer, or destroys the cell membrane, causing cell death and possibly speeding the aging process.

tocopherols
The chemical name for some forms of vitamin E.

One group of electron-seeking compounds likely to be found in cells are **free radicals.** These short-lived forms of compounds exist in a state in which an oxygen or carbon atom in the molecule contains an unpaired electron in its outer shell. Consequently, it seeks an electron to fill that outer shell. The special chem-

free radical
Short-lived form of compounds that exists with unpaired electrons in the outer shell. This imbalance causes it to have an electron-seeking nature, which can be very destructive to electron-dense areas of a cell, such as the DNA and cell membranes.

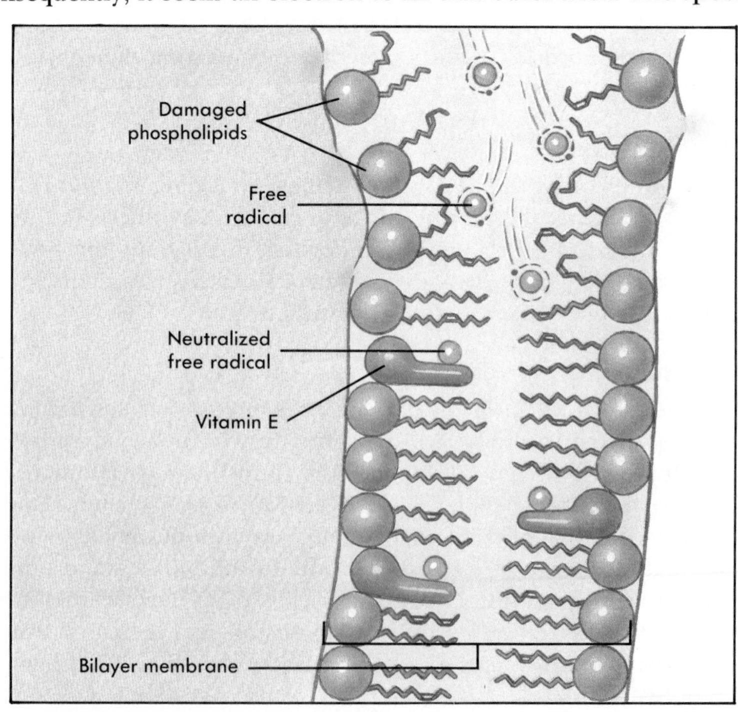

Figure 11-8
Vitamin E helps stop free radical chain-reactions. This should happen before much cell damage takes place.

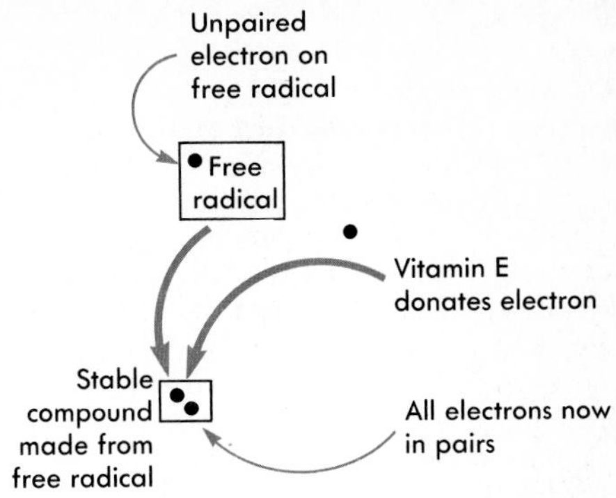

ical natures of oxygen and carbon atoms allow them to readily form a free radical structure. Often a free radical is generated by breaking a covalent bond, from which each breakdown product takes an electron (see Chapter 2). That yields two compounds, each having one unpaired electron in the outer shell of an end atom.

Free radicals are a necessary part of cell metabolism. But because free radicals cause chain reactions, it is very important for vitamin E to buffer their assault on cell membranes to prevent significant cell destruction. Within minutes, one free radical can generate thousands of others: a small amount of cell destruction can lead to great destruction. Other enzyme systems in the cell, such as superoxide dismutase, aid vitamin E in neutralizing free radicals. After vitamin E donates two electrons, it is broken down itself and can no longer function.

High levels of vitamin E are found in the lungs, which is good because oxygen is concentrated there. The lung needs protection from the oxygen. People who smoke need even more vitamin E because of the oxidant stress that smoking puts on the lung. A recent study, however, showed that even when consuming 240 times the adult RDA, smokers still had lower vitamin E concentrations in their lung fluids.[24] Thus the safest way to protect the lungs is to not smoke.

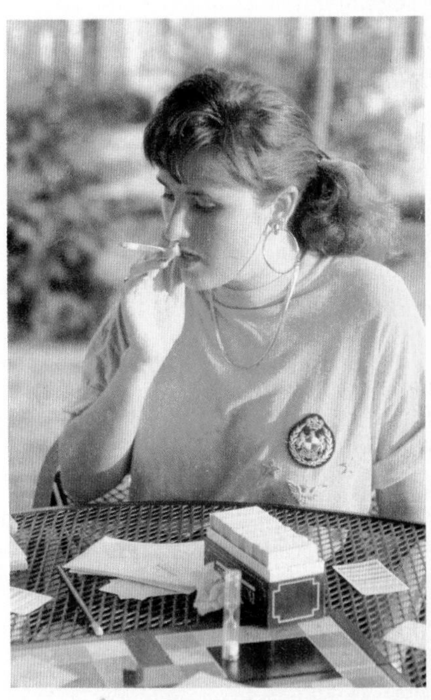

Among other health problems, smokers often have very low levels of vitamin E in their lungs.

Protecting red blood cell membranes

A deficiency of vitamin E causes breakdown **(hemolysis)** of red blood cells, especially in infancy. The polyunsaturated fatty acids in the red blood cell membrane are very sensitive to attack by free radicals. Since vitamin E can neutralize these agents, it can protect the red blood cell membrane from damage.

Red blood cell hemolysis is common in **premature** infants because they did not receive sufficient vitamin E from their mothers. The rapid growth of the premature infant, coupled with the high oxygen concentration found in infant incubators, greatly increases the stress on red blood cells, raising the risk of free-radical damage. Special formulas and supplements for premature infants compensate for their lack of vitamin E. These products can reduce hemolysis of red blood cells and other deficiency symptoms, such as some eye disorders. But vitamin E treatment does not totally prevent the vitamin E–related disorders of prematurity.[25] Hemolysis of red cells also occurs in adults who are deficient in vitamin E.

Other roles for vitamin E

Vitamin E can help improve vitamin A absorption if the dietary intake of vitamin A is low. In this case vitamin E acts to protect the double bonds in vitamin A from damage. Vitamin E can also help protect the double bonds in dietary unsaturated fatty acids. Vitamin E also is needed for iron metabolism in the cell and the maintenance of nervous tissues[32] and immune function.[1]

Popular health food literature attests to many other benefits of vitamin E. None has been shown to be true for humans. A vitamin E deficiency in laboratory animals can result in muscular dystrophy, fetal resorption, and impotence. The link between vitamin E deficiency and fetal resorption in rats, noted in 1922, gave vitamin E its chemical name tocopherol, which means "to bring forth birth." However, vitamin E supplementation in humans is unable to cure any of these conditions. Vitamin E has also been promoted as an anti-aging vitamin. This is because as cells age, they accumulate lipid breakdown products called **lipofuscin (ceroid pigments)**, which appear as brown spots on the skin. The ceroid pigments may then eventually reduce cell metabolism and lead to cell death. Unquestionably, consuming the RDA for vitamin E is important for minimizing lipid destruction by free radicals and peroxides and, in turn, maintaining cell health. However, there is no evidence that supplementation beyond this amount stops aging.[12]

One way to assess the vitamin E status of a person is to incubate a sample of red blood cells with peroxide. After 3 hours measure how much red blood cell destruction occurred. A newer method uses the same procedure but instead measures the amount of a breakdown product of polyunsaturated fatty acids. These tests can be used in addition to measuring the serum vitamin E level.

Any mystery surrounding vitamin E stems from our incomplete understanding of this family of compounds. Many functions of vitamin E depend on its antioxi-

We suggest that if you really want to prevent the effects of aging, you begin by following the Daily Food Guide, see your physician regularly (for early diagnosis of health problems), don't smoke, limit your alcohol intake, maintain a desirable body weight, and stay physically active. These factors have a much greater influence on the rate of aging of North Americans than does a lack of vitamin E (see Chapter 17).

dant ability. But others, such as the maintenance of male sexual function in rats, are unrelated to its antioxidant system. *When questions persist concerning a vitamin's function, promoters of fad diets and health food zealots are quick to suggest that the mystery powers of such vitamins can cure many diseases or provide other physical benefits.* Such is the case with vitamin E.

The mineral selenium can spare some of the need for vitamin E

An enzyme in cells—**glutathione peroxidase**—converts peroxides into harmless forms of alcohols and water, in turn reducing the peroxide load in a cell. Peroxides tend to form free radicals. So with a decreased peroxide load, the tendency to form free radicals likewise decreases. Consequently the need for vitamin E decreases because fewer free radicals will be made. The cellular enzyme catalase also helps destroy peroxides, specifically hydrogen peroxide.

glutathione peroxidase
A selenium-containing enzyme that can destroy peroxides.

The enzyme glutathione peroxidase contains the mineral selenium. Adequate levels of selenium in the diet allow this enzyme to function at full speed, destroying peroxides, thereby sparing some of the need for vitamin E. Thus an adequate dietary intake of selenium reduces the need for vitamin E, whereas low selenium intake in the diet increases it.

Vitamin E in foods

The most nutrient-dense food sources of vitamin E are plant oils, some fruits and vegetables, such as peaches and asparagus, and margarine (Table 11-5). Animal fats have practically no vitamin E. Careful processing of plant oils to remove pesticide residues does not reduce much of the vitamin E present.[14] One reason to eat a variety of foods is to obtain the vitamin E spread throughout selections from the Daily Food Guide. *The presence of a tablespoon of plant oil in foods eaten each day is especially helpful.*

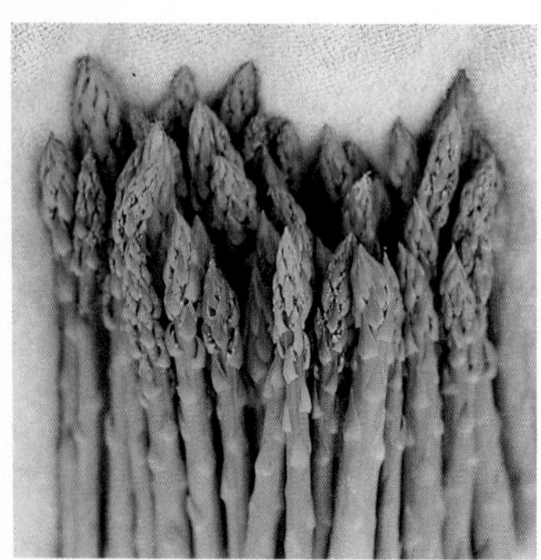

Asparagus is a nutrient-dense source of vitamin E.

Table 11-5

Good food sources of vitamin E, ranked by nutrient density

Food	Serving size to yield 10 milligrams*	Kcalories needed to yield 10 milligrams
Corn oil†	1 tablespoon	120
Sunflower oil	1-¼ tablespoons	150
Soybean oil	1-¼ tablespoons	150
Cooked asparagus	3-½ cups	176
Canned peaches	2-½ cups	354
Margarine	7 tablespoons	700

*Adult male RDA.
†Vitamin E is in other plant oils as well; these are just some examples.
This shows how important a tablespoon of oil a day is to our diets. For other sources of vitamin E, either the serving size and/or the kcalorie cost is too great.

The actual vitamin E content of a food depends on how it was harvested, processed, stored, and cooked because vitamin E is very susceptible to destruction by oxygen, metals, light, and especially repeated use of oils in deep-fat frying. For healthy people, a varied diet that includes vegetable oils should supply the vitamin E they need. Thus the likelihood of finding a poor vitamin E status in North America among nonsmokers is very low. Selenium, which spares the need for vitamin E, is found in cereals, meats, and seafood.

RDA for vitamin E

The RDA for adults for vitamin E is 10 milligrams per day for men and 8 milligrams per day for women. This is about how much we usually eat each day. To convert from the older IU system, 10 milligrams equals about 15 IU. A variety of forms of vitamin E exist. The RDA is based on alpha-tocopherol equivalents. Beta-, delta-, and gamma-tocopherol are not as active. Appendix N shows how to determine the amount of vitamin E activity in a food by using the potencies of different forms. Once a food's content is calculated in alpha-tocopherol equivalents, this amount can be called vitamin E.

In 1980, the RDA for vitamin E was decreased from previous recommendations. However, the U.S. RDA still uses the older 1968 value (20 milligrams). So food labels, because they are based on a percentage of the older, larger value, understate (2 times) the vitamin E contribution of foods in terms of % U.S. RDA.

Diets high in polyunsaturated fatty acids need to contain more vitamin E (about double) to protect all the double bonds present. When consuming more vegetable oils, a person needs to also consume more vitamin E. It turns out, however, that plant oils high in polyunsaturated fatty acids are also often high in vitamin E; so in this case, things usually balance out. One exception is highly unsaturated fish oil, which has been currently used in greater amounts lately; this often contains very little vitamin E.

Toxicity of vitamin E

Vitamin E is relatively nontoxic. Some studies show that amounts in excess of approximately 500 milligrams (800 IU) per day of vitamin E can cause nausea, weakness, headache, diarrhea, and fatigue, as well as antagonize vitamin K metabolism, especially if medications that decrease blood clotting are being used. However, other studies show that intakes up to 2100 milligrams (3200 IU) may be safe for months. People with diseases such as phlebitis, in which blood clots form easily, sometimes benefit from large supplements of vitamin E but should follow such a regimen under the careful eye of a physician. Otherwise, hemorrhages may result. Part of the mechanism here may be the antagonism of vitamin K's role in blood clotting (see the next sections on vitamin K).

Concept Check

Vitamin E functions primarily as an antioxidant. It can donate electrons to electron-seeking compounds, such as free radicals. By neutralizing free radicals, vitamin E helps prevent cell destruction, especially the destruction of red blood cell membranes. The breakdown of red blood cell membranes occurs with a vitamin E deficiency. The best sources of vitamin E are plant oils. The more plant oils consumed, the more vitamin E needed to protect the double bonds found in plant oils. However, the vitamin E content in plant oils is usually high. One reason to eat a variety of foods is to obtain the vitamin E spread throughout selections from the Daily Food Guide. For adults, people who smoke run the biggest risk of a vitamin E deficiency. In that case, the best therapy is to stop smoking. Supplements are not that helpful.

VITAMIN K

The family of compounds known as vitamin K include **phylloquinone** from plants and the **menaquinones** found in fish oils and meats. The menaquinones are also synthesized by bacteria in the human small intestine.[23]

Functions of vitamin K

Vitamin K is vital for blood clotting. The K stands for *koagulation,* as it is spelled in Denmark, because a Danish researcher, Dam, first noted the relationship between vitamin K and blood clotting. Vitamin K contributes specifically to the syn-

phylloquinone
A form of vitamin K that comes from plants.

Figure 11-9
Forming a blood clot. This requires the participation of vitamin K in both the intrinsic and extrinsic blood clotting pathways.

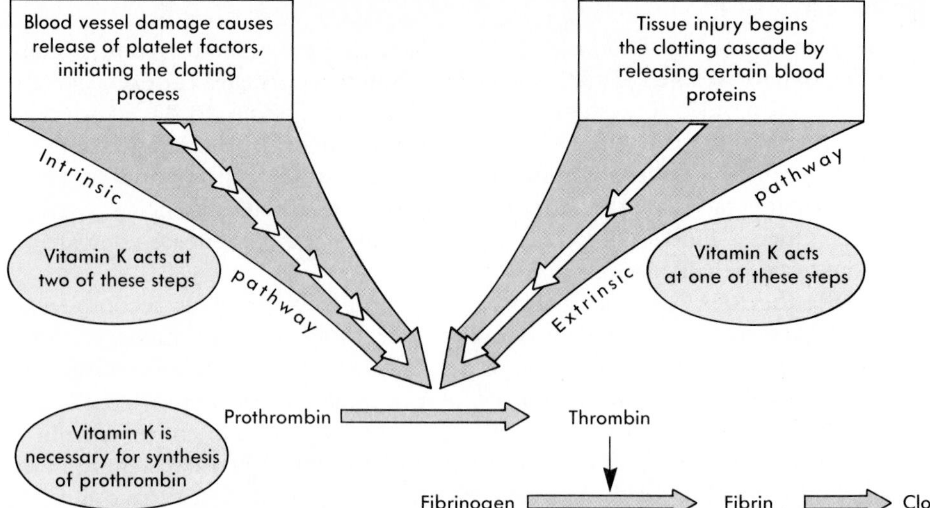

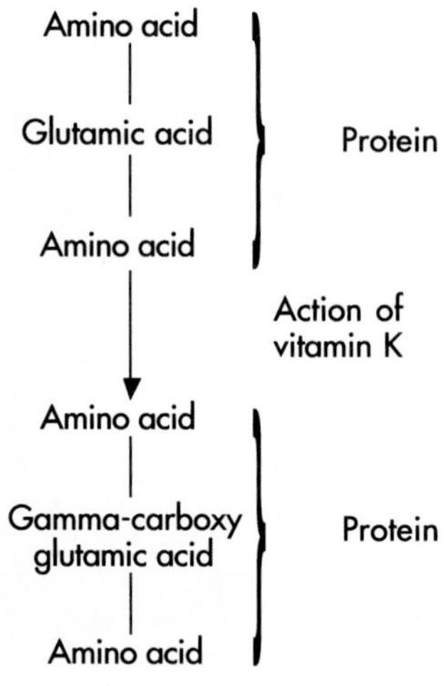

H H O
—N—C—C—
CH_2
O
C—CH
O⁻
C=O
Ca^{++} 2 ---O⁻

(Acid group)

Positive calcium ion attracted to two negative charges on gamma-carboxyglutamate.

thesis of several blood-clotting factors, including **prothrombin**[23] (Figure 11-9). *Vitamin K is needed for adding carbon dioxide molecules to these compounds,* specifically on the amino acid glutamic acid (glutamate). This forms gamma-carboxyglutamate. In turn, these gamma-carboxyglutamate molecules give a protein its calcium-binding potential, an important ability if prothrombin is to participate in the blood-clotting cascade. Vitamin K also adds carbon dioxide molecules to glutamate residues on proteins found in the bones, muscles, and kidneys, in turn imparting calcium-binding potential to those organs.

A deficiency of vitamin K most likely occurs when a person takes antibiotics or has severe fat malabsorption. It is critical to establish this is not the case before a person undergoes surgery otherwise excess bleeding is likely in this instance. Antibiotic use destroys many bacteria in the intestines that normally account for half the vitamin K absorbed.

Physicians use vitamin K's link to blood clotting to a practical advantage. Because the structure of vitamin K resembles those of the drugs dicumarol and warfarin, the drugs can antagonize the action of vitamin K and so act as potent anticoagulants. People who tend toward increased blood clotting greatly benefit from these drugs. However, *people taking these drugs must be warned against consuming supplements of vitamin K and foods especially rich in vitamin K, since that would reduce the action of the drugs.*

Food sources of vitamin K

The most nutrient-dense food sources of vitamin K are green, leafy vegetables, other vegetables such as peas and green beans, and liver (Table 11-6). Vitamin K

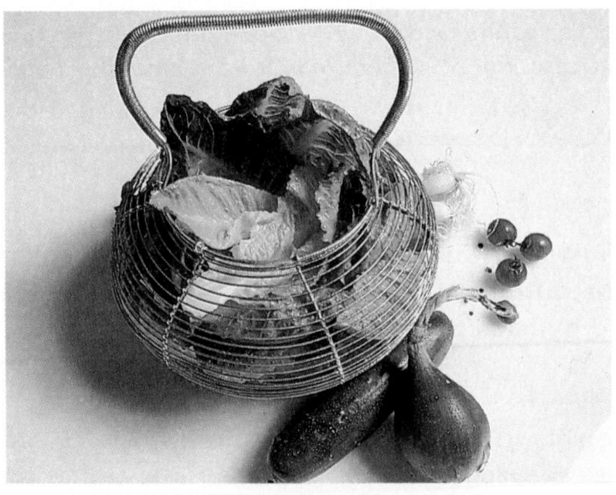

Green, leafy vegetables are the most nutrient-dense food sources of vitamin K.

Table 11-6

Good food sources of vitamin K, ranked by nutrient density

Food	Serving size to yield 80 micrograms*	Kcalories needed to yield 80 micrograms
Cooked turnip greens	1/7 cup	10
Cooked kale	1/7 cup	10
Cooked spinach	1/7 cup	10
Cooked green peas	1/7 cup	10
Raw cabbage	7/8 cup	15
Cooked green beans	1/4 cup	15
Cooked broccoli	3/8 cup	25
Fried beef liver	3 ounces	200

*Adult male RDA

Make a serving of green vegetables a regular part of your diet to get a concentrated and low kcalorie source of vitamin K.

is yet another reason to consume a diet rich in fruits and vegetables. Vitamin K is quite resistant to cooking losses.

Most vitamin K consumed in a day is gone by the next. However, vitamin K is so abundant in the diet that there is low risk of suffering a deficiency.

Not much vitamin K is found in human milk. In addition, an unborn child is not well adapted to store or has bacteria to synthesize vitamin K. So at birth, infants run the risk of poor blood clotting and eventual hemorrhage. To prevent this possible vitamin K deficiency condition, physicians routinely treat infants at birth with a form of vitamin K. This protection is intended to last until the infant's intestinal bacteria begin to synthesize vitamin K.

The best clinical sign of a vitamin K deficiency is an increase in blood clotting or prothrombin formation time. The latter is a measure of how quickly prothrombin in the blood can form a clot. In addition, today the actual vitamin K and prothrombin levels in the bloodstream can be measured.

RDA for vitamin K

The RDA vitamin K for adults is 60 to 80 micrograms per day. The U.S. diet contains 300 to 500 micrograms per adult per day of vitamin K, so a deficiency is very unlikely.

Toxicity from vitamin K is likewise highly unlikely because, although it is fat-soluble, it is poorly stored in the body. One form of vitamin K, menadione, can be toxic if taken in high amounts. Symptoms include jaundice and a type of anemia.

Concept Check

Vitamin K is important for blood clotting because it imparts a calcium-binding ability to certain blood proteins, such as prothrombin. To do this, vitamin K helps add a carbon dioxide molecule to the protein-bound amino acid glutamate. About half the vitamin K we absorb every day comes from bacterial synthesis in the intestines and about half from the diet. The amount in the diet alone is generally about five times higher than our needs. Thus, except for newborns, a deficiency of vitamin K is unlikely, even though it is poorly stored in the body.

Take Action

1. On a piece of paper create a menu that is low in vitamins A, E, and K. Then suggest four to six good food sources that could be eaten to help improve the menu for these nutrients.

MEALS	DIET: Poor content of vitamins A, E, and K	DIET: Rich in vitamins A, E, and K
Breakfast:		
Lunch:		
Dinner:		

Summary

1. Vitamins are organic (carbon-containing) compounds needed for important metabolic reactions in the body. They yield no energy themselves, but instead contribute to energy-yielding chemical reactions in the body, whereas promoting growth and development. Vitamins A, D, E, and K are fat-soluble, while the B vitamins and vitamin C are water-soluble. Fat-soluble vitamins are generally stored more readily in the body and are less susceptible to cooking loss than are water-soluble vitamins.
2. Some fat-soluble vitamins pose a potential for toxicity. Vitamins A and D are especially likely to build up to toxic levels. The water-soluble vitamins B-6 and niacin can also induce toxic symptoms, but only at very high doses.
3. Fat-soluble vitamins are absorbed along with dietary fat. They travel through the lymphatic system into the bloodstream and are then bound by lipoproteins. In disease states in which fat digestion is poor or lipoprotein synthesis is hampered, fat-soluble vitamin status may be compromised, especially with vitamins E and K.
4. Vitamin A consists of a family of compounds: retinal, retinol, and retinoic acid. A plant derivative known as beta-carotene, along with some other carotenoids, yields vitamin A after metabolism by the intestine. Vitamin A contributes to the maintenance of vision, the proper development of cells (especially mucus-forming cells), and proper immune function. Vitamin A is found in liver, fish oils, and fortified milk; carotenoids are especially plentiful in dark green and orange vegetables and in some fruits.
5. North Americans at risk for poor vitamin A status are children with poor fat absorption and adults with alcoholism. Vitamin A can be quite toxic when taken at just 5 to 10 times the RDA. High vitamin A intakes are especially dangerous during pregnancy because they can lead to fetal malformations.
6. Vitamin D is usually a hormone rather than a vitamin. It can be synthesized by the skin using sunshine and a form of cholesterol. This vitamin D is then metabolized by the liver and kidney to yield the active hormone, calcitriol. Calcitriol is important for calcium absorption from the intestine, and with other hormones it helps regulate bone metabolism. Vitamin D in foods is found in fish oils and fortified milk. Vitamin D is a very toxic substance. An intake just two and a half to five times the RDA can be toxic in children if taken regularly. Anyone who feels a need to use a supplement should consult a physician first.
7. Vitamin E primarily functions as an antioxidant. By donating electrons to electron-seeking compounds, it neutralizes them. One group of electron-seeking compounds, known as free radicals, can cause widespread cell destruction, both to cell membranes and to DNA, if not stabilized. Vitamin E is plentiful in

plant oils. The more plant oils one consumes, the more vitamin E one needs, but this need is usually met by those same plant oils. Fish oils, in contrast, often contain little vitamin E.

8. Vitamin K contributes to blood clotting: it imparts calcium-binding capability to certain blood proteins by adding carbon dioxide molecules to the protein-bound amino acid glutamate. About half the vitamin K absorbed each day comes from bacterial synthesis in the intestine, whereas the other half comes from foods, primarily green leafy vegetables. Vitamin K is poorly stored in the body, but our intake from diet alone is about 5 times our need.

REFERENCES

1. Anonymous: The effect of vitamin E on immune responses, Nutrition Reviews 45:27, 1987.
2. Anonymous: Is pyrroloquinoline quinone a cofactor derived from an undiscovered vitamin? Nutrition Reviews 46:139, 1988.
3. Audran M and Kumar R: The physiology and pathophysiology of vitamin D, Mayo Clinic Proceedings 60:851, 1985.
4. Bauernfeind JC: Vitamin A deficiency: a staggering problem of health and sight, Nutrition Today March/April:34, 1988.
5. Burton GW: Antioxidant action of caretenoids, Journal of Nutrition, 119:109, 1989.
6. Callaway CW and others: Statement on vitamin and mineral supplements, Journal of Nutrition 117:1649, 1987.
7. Council on Scientific Affairs: Vitamin preparations as dietary supplements and as therapeutic agents, Journal of the American Medical Association 257:1929, 1987.
8. Draper HH: Nutrients as nutrients, and nutrients as prophylactic drugs, Journal of Nutrition 118:1420, 1988.
9. Francis R and Peacock M: Local action of oral 1,25-dihydroxycholecalciferol on calcium absorption in osteoporosis, American Journal of Clinical Nutrition 46:315, 1987.
10. Goodwin GW: Metabolism, nutrition, and function of carotenoids, Annual Reviews of Nutrition 6:273, 1986.
11. Greger JL: Food, supplements, and fortified foods: scientific evaluations in regard to toxicology and nutrient bioavailability, Journal of the American Dietetic Association 87:1369, 1987.
12. Hale WE and others: Vitamin E effect on symptoms and laboratory values in the elderly, Journal of the American Dietetic Association 86:62 5, 1986.
13. Haussler MR: Vitamin D receptors—nature and function, Annual Review of Nutrition 6:527, 1986.
14. Hunter JE: Nutritional consequences of processing soybean oil, Journal of the American Oil Chemist Society 58:283, 1981.
15. Lamberg-Allardt C: Vitamin D intake, sunlight exposure and 25-hydroxyvitamin D levels in the elderly during one year, Annals of Nutrition and Metabolism 28:144, 1984.
16. Lammer EJ and others: Retinoic acid embryopathy, The New England Journal of Medicine 313:837, 1985.
17. Lips P and others: Determinants of vitamin D status in patients with hip fracture and in elderly control subjects, American Journal of Clinical Nutrition 46:1005, 1987.
18. Mederios OM and others: Vitamin and mineral supplementation practices of adults in seven western states, Journal of the American Dietetic Association, 89: 389, 1989.
19. Menkes MS and others: Serum beta-carotene, vitamins A and E, selenium, and the risk of lung cancer, The New England Journal of Medicine 315:1250, 1986.
20. Milton RC and others: Mild vitamin A deficiency and childhood morbidity—an Indian experience, American Journal of Clinical Nutrition 46:827, 1987.
21. Moon RC: Comparative aspects of carotenoids and retinoids as chemopreventive agents for cancer, Journal of Nutrition 119:127, 1989.
22. Olson JA: Recommended dietary intakes (RDI) of vitamin A in humans, American Journal of Clinical Nutrition 45:704, 1987.
23. Olson RE: Vitamin K. In Shils ME and Young VR, eds, Modern nutrition in health and disease, Philadelphia, 1988, Lea & Febiger.
24. Pacht ER and others: Deficiency of vitamin E in the alveolar fluid of cigarette smokers, Journal of Clinical Investigation 77:789, 1986.
25. Phelps DL and others: Tocopherol efficacy and safety for preventing retinopathy of prematurity: a randomized controlled double-masked trial, Pediatrics 79:489, 1987.
26. Pilch SM: Analysis of vitamin A data from the Health and Nutrition Examination Survey, Journal of Nutrition 117:636, 1987.
27. Reichel H and others: The role of the vitamin D endocrine system in health and disease, The New England Journal of Medicine 320:980, 1989.
28. Sauberlich HE: Vitamins—how much is for keeps? Nutrition Today January/February:20, 1987.
29. Schwenk TL and others: Carotenemia, Amer-

ican Family Physician 36:135, 1987.
30. Sommer A: New imperatives for an old vitamin (A), Journal of Nutrition, 119:96, 1989.
31. Sowers MR and others: Parameters related to 25-OH-D levels in a population-based study of women, American Journal of Clinical Nutrition 43:621, 1986.
32. Traber MG and others: Lack of tocopherol in peripheral nerves of vitamin E-deficient patients with peripheral neuropathy, The New England Journal of Medicine 317:262, 1987.
33. Webb AR and Holick MF: The role of sunlight in the cutaneous production of vitamin D_3, Annual Reviews of Nutrition 8:375, 1988.
34. West KP and others: Vitamin A supplementation and growth: a randomized community trial, American Journal of Clinical Nutrition 481257, 1988.
35. Ziegler RG and others: Carotenoid intake, vegetables, and the risk of lung cancer among white men in New Jersey, American Journal of Epidemiology 123:1080, 1986.

SUGGESTED READINGS

The articles by both the Council on Scientific Affairs of the American Medical Association and Callaway and others review current recommendations for vitamin and mineral supplement use. The article by the Council on Scientific Affairs is particularly detailed. The article by Bauernfeind and that by Lammer and others outline the result of vitamin A deficiency and toxicity, respectively. Worldwide, vitamin A deficiency is a much more serious problem. Audran and Kumar review the physiology of vitamin D. Articles such as this in the Mayo Clinic Proceedings are often interesting and easy to understand. Finally, RE Olson reviews vitamin K nutrition in *Modern Nutrition in Health and Disease.* As suggested earlier, the chapters in this book are detailed and contain numerous references for further research.

CHAPTER 11

Answers to nutrition awareness inventory

1. *False.* No vitamin missing from a diet for a week leads to deficiency symptoms. Earliest signs of deficiency appear with a thiamin-free diet after about 10 days. The first symptoms of a vitamin C deficiency are seen after about 20 to 40 days.
2. *False.* Although fat-solubility should enhance storage capability, fat-soluble vitamin K is very poorly stored in the body.
3. *True.* Mineral oil is not absorbed by the intestine. During its passage, mineral oil can dissolve fat-soluble vitamins and pull them into the colon for eventual elimination.
4. *False.* Because fat-soluble vitamins do not dissolve rapidly in boiling water, they are not leached out of foods during cooking to the same extent as most water-soluble vitamins.
5. *True.* There is a slight chance that one more vitamin remains to be discovered, but for the most part nutrition scientists feel they have isolated all the vitamins necessary for human health.
6. *True.* When in the active form, vitamin D, through a variety of mechanisms, can improve calcium absorption from the small intestine.
7. *True.* Vitamin A enhances night vision by participating in the formation of the compound rhodopsin.
8. *True.* Vitamin A has a high potential for causing toxicity, especially in pregnant women and children.
9. *True.* Aided by the action of sunlight, the skin produces vitamin D, which can then be metabolized by the liver and kidneys to form the active vitamin D hormone. By definition this compound is a hormone, since it is made in one part of the body and acts in another.
10. *True.* As mentioned above, sunlight striking the skin converts a modified form of cholesterol into vitamin D. This is then slowly transferred from the skin into the bloodstream.
11. *False.* Vitamin E is able to stabilize free radical compounds by donating an electron, thus decreasing the tendency for the free radicals to steal electrons from fatty acids and other electron-dense compounds.
12. *True.* Vitamin K is able to add hydroxyl groups (−OH) to one type of amino acid, in turn imparting calcium-binding properties to the proteins that contain those acids.
13. *True.* Antibiotics can reduce the growth of bacteria in the small intestine and colon. These bacteria synthesize a form of vitamin K that we absorb and use.
14. *True.* Vegetables are a good source of vitamin K. This is another reason why we should "eat our vegetables."
15. *True.* The American Medical Association recently recommended that a proper nutrient supplement dosage is generally 50% to 150% of the U.S. RDA for most vitamins.

Nutrition Perspective 11-1

Vitamin Supplements—Who Needs Them?

Our opinions about vitamins have changed since the turn of the century when Casimir Funk first coined the term from the words "vital amine" (an amine has a carbon atom bonded to a nitrogen atom). In the early 1900s, vitamins were first a curiosity and then the subject of intense scientific scrutiny and research. Today, they are promoted as cure-alls by many health food enthusiasts and consumed as supplements by as many as 45% of adults in the United States.[18] Supplements are such big business, in fact, that their sales more than doubled between 1976 and 1986 from $1.2 billion to almost $3 billion.

Exploring Issues and Actions

Do you take vitamin supplements? If so, why? If not, why not?

Should you take a vitamin and mineral supplement? To answer that question, you first need to look closely at your diet. Does it follow the Daily Food Guide outlined in Chapter 2, especially emphasizing low-fat products, lean meats, whole grains, leafy and dark green vegetables, fruits containing vitamin C, and vegetable oils? If so, men are probably meeting their needs; some women (those with heavy menstrual flows) may still need more iron. Secondly, do you regularly consume a fortified breakfast cereal? Most breakfast cereals have extra vitamins and mineral added, some even matching the adult U.S. RDA.

Nutrition scientists generally agree that most people can obtain the vitamins and minerals they need if they eat a healthy diet. We think you should start there first. Improve your diet where needed, as suggested in Chapter 2. After that, consider whether you need a supplement. We advise talking to your doctor as well, who may refer you to a registered dietition.

Recently a panel of scientists from the American Institute of Nutrition and the American Society for Clinical Nutrition suggested a few cases in which vitamin and mineral supplementation should be considered:

- Women with excessive bleeding during menses may need extra iron
- Women who are pregnant or breastfeeding may need extra iron, folate, and calcium
- People with very low kcalorie intake need the range of vitamins and minerals
- Some vegetarians may need extra calcium, iron, zinc, and vitamin B-12
- Newborns, under the direction of a physician, need a single dose of vitamin K
- People with specific other illnesses or diseases, such as vitamin-resistance diseases, and those who use certain medications may require supplementation of specific vitamins and minerals, at the direction of a physician. Examples of medications requiring supplemental vitamins or minerals would be a thiazide diuretics, that often require extra potassium, and the treatment of osteoporosis, which may require extra vitamin D.

Supplementation during illness and drug therapy needs to be directed by a physician because use of some vitamins and minerals counteracts the actions of certain medications. Vitamin B-6 can counteract the action of L-dopa (used in treating Parkinson's disease) and isoniazid (used in treating tuberculosis), whereas high intakes of vitamin E can inhibit vitamin K metabolism, and therefore increase the action of anticoagulants, such as warfarin.

WHICH SUPPLEMENT SHOULD YOU CHOOSE?

If you decide to take a vitamin and mineral supplement, which one do you choose? We suggest following the guidelines set forth by the Council on Scientific Affairs of the American Medical Association.[7] They recommend that a supplement contain between 50% and 150% of the adult U.S. RDA for vitamins A, D, E, and C, folate, thiamin, riboflavin, niacin, vitamin B-6, and vitamin B-12. They do not recommend that this supplement contain biotin or pantothenic acid, two other nutrients that have a U.S. RDA, because a deficiency is so unlikely, and vitamin K can disturb anticoagulant therapy. For minerals, we suggest using the same guideline, 50% to 150% of the U.S. RDA (Table 2-6), or up to 100% of the estimated safe and adequate daily dietary intake (see the inside cover). This amounts to a one-a-day type, but read the label to be sure.

A balanced formulation in a multivitamin and mineral supplement is important because it minimizes chances of vitamin and mineral competition, and therefore of an eventual vitamin and mineral imbalance and other toxicity problems. For example:

- High amounts of vitamin C can cause overabsorption of iron and lead to iron toxicity in susceptible people. Consuming high amounts of vitamin C can also decrease the ability of certain diagnostic tests to assess the development of diabetes or colon cancer and inhibit copper absorption.
- Large amounts of vitamin E inhibit vitamin K metabolism and carotenoid absorption.
- Large amount of fish oil can lead to poor blood clotting.
- Large amount of copper can inhibit zinc absorption and vice versa.
- Excess fluoride exposure in childhood can cause staining and even weaken the teeth (see Chapter 14).
- Large amounts of folate can mask symptoms of a vitamin B-12 deficiency, preventing early diagnosis while it becomes potentially life-threatening. Large doses of folate, approximately 100 times the RDA, can also inhibit the action of anticonvulsants. Patients with epilepsy who require anticonvulsant therapy jeopardize their health if they also consume many folate supplements. This is another reason to discuss vitamin and mineral supplementation beyond the RDA or ESADDI with a physician and registered dietitian. Only then can you appropriately evaluate whether supplementation is in your best interest.

Definitions of supplements

supplement— to enhance nutrient intake	= 50% to 150% of the RDA
therapeutic agent— used under medical supervision to correct a nutrient deficiency	= 2 to 10 times the RDA
pharmacological megadose dose	= usually greater than 10 times the RDA

We will discuss these and other potentially toxic effects of vitamin and mineral overuse throughout Chapters 11 to 14. Keep in mind that the intake level set by the Food and Nutrition Board for vitamins or minerals, as outlined in the RDA and ESADDI, is important for good health. But that does not suggest that taking higher doses (greater than twice the RDA) will be any more beneficial. Furthermore, the chances are great that as doses increase, toxic symptoms will probably result.

Surveys of people who use vitamin and mineral supplements find that they generally consume multivitamin and mineral preparations. About 50% of the supplement market consists of these. For single supplemental doses, vitamins E and C, and calcium are the most common. Some supplementation may be appropriate, if it is designed to counteract a limited food intake when dieting (below about 1200 kcalories/day), or possibly to retard some bone loss with calcium supplements (see Chapter 13). But most of this practice is inappropriate, such as when using vitamin E to cure arthritis or supplementing nutrients already adequate in the diet.

The Food and Drug Administration (FDA) does not regulate all vitamin and mineral supplements closely, and is prevented from doing so by the Proxmire Amendment to the 1938 Food, Drug, and Cosmetic Act, unless it has evidence that the supplements are inherently dangerous or marketed with illegal claims. (see the section in Chapter 12 on folate for one example). So Americans cannot rely on the federal government to protect them from vitamin and mineral supplement overuse. People have to know what they are doing and preferably rely on the advice of physicians and registered dietitians for guidance.

A popular practice in Japan today is to consume tonics that are promoted as producing high energy and greater health. These tonics are often laced with ethanol, caffeine, nicotine-derivatives, and vitamins, along with bizarre substances such as extract of cobra and essence of seal. This practice has not invaded North America, but keep an eye out for it. *Remember that Americans cannot blindly trust any supplements, since the FDA has limited jurisdiction over them. Nor do most people need supplements.* The situation actually is, "Let the buyer beware."

Nutrition Perspective 11-2

Solving the Rickets Mystery

Rickets was first described in England about 1650. The "English disease" spread throughout Europe in the years following, mostly due to the pall of coal smoke that flooded Europe during the Industrial Revolution. In the early 1800s, a German town, Wezlar, was described as follows: "The children must sit indoors . . . which ends in death, or if they continue to live, they develop thick joints, cease to be able to walk, and have deformed legs. The head becomes large and even the vertebral column bends. It comes to pass that such children sit often for many years without being able to move: at times they cease to grow and are merely a burden to those about them." William Hogarth further sketched the eighteenth-century European view of the long-term effects of rickets (Figure 11-10).

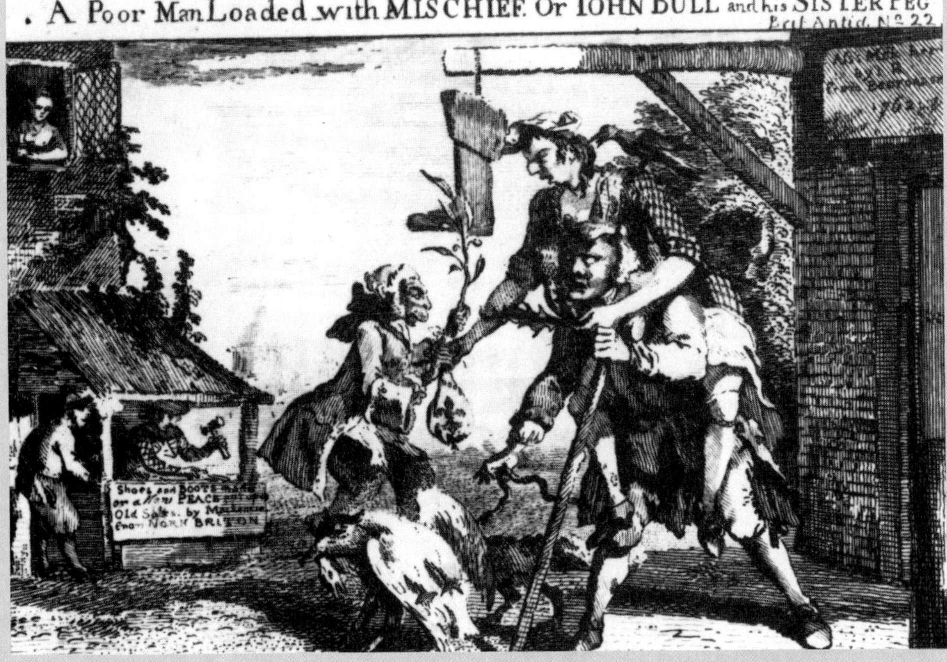

Figure 11-10
William Hogarth depicts how rickets left many an Englishman in a contorted state.

As early as 1888, researchers noted that animals in the London Zoo contracted rickets, while those in the wild never did so. This gave rise to the hypothesis that rickets was due to confinement. The long, cold winter months in Europe kept people indoors, and this was thought to bring on rickets. Physicians in Germany noted that children born in the fall who died in the spring had rickets, while those who were born in the spring and died in the fall were free of the disease.

When missionary Theobald Palm traveled to Japan in 1890, he was struck by the absence of rickets among the Japanese compared with the children of England and Scotland. He, too, deduced that rickets was caused by confinement, especially by isolating the children from the benefits of sunlight.

By early 1900s, it became increasingly clear to many physicians that sunlight had the power to prevent and cure rickets. However, there was no way to provide this sunlight during the long European winters. Then in 1919, a Berlin physician tried the light from a mercury-vapor quartz lamp—which includes the ultraviolet wavelengths—on four cases of advanced rickets in children. He found that this exposure completely cured rickets within 2 months.

In 1924, other researchers found that ingesting linseed, cottonseed, or yeast radiated with ultraviolet wave lengths cured rickets. It became increasingly clear that there was a relationship between sunlight and rickets. To further make that point, scientists showed that rickets in England was closely tied to the major smoke-filled industrial areas of England, and was not found as frequently in rural areas.

VITAMIN D BECOMES A VITAMIN

In 1919, Sir Edward Mellanby showed that a particular diet could cause rickets in dogs. He then found that cod liver oil could cure the rickets. He hypothesized that a substance or "vitamine" in cod liver oil cured rickets.

The idea that rickets was due to a vitamin deficiency reflected the tenor of the times. Funk and others had recently established the "vitamine" theory—that substances vital to health were contained in foods. The British Medical Research Committee was excited about this work on rickets and in turn endorsed the notion that rickets was a nutritional deficiency.

IS VITAMIN D A VITAMIN?

It is clear that sunlight alone, irrespective of diet, can cure rickets. But because of the influence of important researchers, such as Mellanby, and powerful organizations, such as the British Medical Research Committee, people now think of vitamin D as primarily a vitamin. As mentioned at the outset of this chapter, vitamin D is not a vitamin for many people. It is a vitamin for the homebound and shut-in and maybe for people who live in very northern climates, especially the elderly, and who receive little sunlight. But many of us in the temperate world can make enough vitamin D every sunny day we step outside.

Chapter 12

The Water-Soluble Vitamins: B Vitamins and Vitamin C

Overview

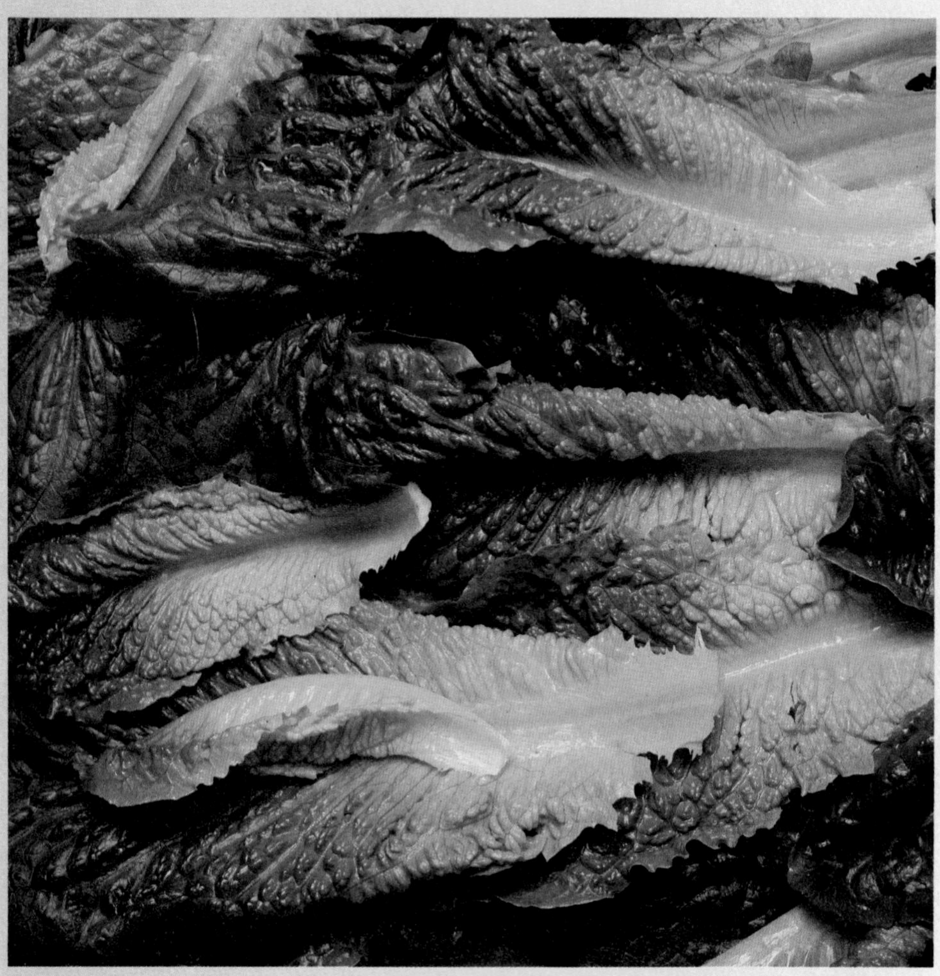

Romaine lettuce is an excellent choice for salad greens because it is rich in vitamins such as riboflavin and folate.

The B vitamins and vitamin C play critical roles in cell metabolism. Many metabolic pathways in a cell could not function without an ample supply of the B vitamins in the diet (Figure 12-1). Every student of nutrition should understand how these vitamins function, what foods supply them, and how either a deficiency or toxicity affects the body. The B vitamins form coenzymes, which are compounds that enable specific enzymes to function. You do not need to consume the vitamins in the coenzyme form because coenzymes break down to the actual vitamins in the small intestine before absorption.

At the end of this chapter we discuss vitamin-like compounds. People may need these substances under certain unusual circumstances, but they cannot be called vitamins because the average healthy person does not need them. *The term vitamin is often misused by health food enthusiasts who want to promote a substance that is not truly an essential part of a diet.*

Nutrition awareness inventory

Here are 15 statements about water-soluble vitamins. Answer them to test your current knowledge. If you think the answer is true or mostly true, circle T. If you think the answer is false or mostly false, circle F. Use the scoring key at the end of this chapter to compute your total score. Take the test again after you have read the chapter. Compare the results.

1. **T F** Thiamin needs are related to the amount of fat intake.
2. **T F** Thiamin is found in pork.
3. **T F** Enriched white rice is a good source of thiamin.
4. **T F** Milk is a good source of riboflavin.
5. **T F** A deficiency in riboflavin suggests a deficiency in thiamin, niacin, and vitamin B-6.
6. **T F** Physicians should investigate the possibility of poor absorption of vitamin B-12 in their elderly patients.
7. **T F** Using an amino acid, the body can make niacin.
8. **T F** A niacin deficiency causes severe skin inflammation.
9. **T F** Nicotinic acid can lower serum cholesterol levels.
10. **T F** Alcohol decreases the absorption of vitamin B-6.
11. **T F** The term *folate* comes from the word foliage.
12. **T F** Vitamin B-12 is present only in animal foods.
13. **T F** A deficiency in vitamin C causes pinpoint hemorrhages in the skin.
14. **T F** Vitamin C enhances iron absorption.
15. **T F** Vitamin C can prevent the common cold.

The B vitamins were assigned serial numbers as each was isolated from liver tissue. The only numbers we still use for the B vitamins are B-6 and B-12. Nutritionists no longer refer to thiamin as vitamin B-1, riboflavin as vitamin B-2, or niacin as vitamin B-3.

THE B VITAMINS

After being ingested, B vitamins are first broken down from their coenzyme forms into free vitamins in the stomach and small intestine. The vitamins are then absorbed, primarily in the small intestine. About 50% to 90% of B vitamins in the diet are typically absorbed. Once inside cells, the coenzyme forms are resynthesized[23] (Figure 12-1).

THIAMIN

Thiamin is a compound made up of two rings connected by two bonds between a carbon atom. This bond between the two rings is easily broken by prolonged cooking of food, and especially by heating foods in alkaline solutions, such as when baking soda is added to water. The name *thiamin* comes from the sulfur (thio-) and amine ($-NH_2$) groups in the molecule. Note that in modern spelling the "e" has been dropped from *thiamin,* although the FDA and some others retain it.

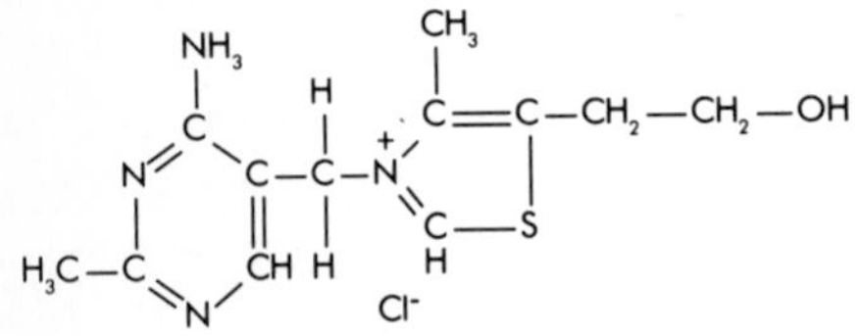

Thiamin

Thiamin has two phosphate molecules added to form the coenzyme (thiamin pyrophosphate).

Functions of thiamin

The coenzyme thiamin pyrophosphate (TPP) participates in reactions in which a carbon dioxide molecule is lost from a larger molecule. An example of this reaction is the conversion of pyruvate to acetyl-CoA to prepare a pyruvate molecule to enter the citric acid cycle. During metabolism of most carbohydrates, pyruvate is formed (see Chapter 7). The TPP found inside nerves may also help in the synthesis of neurotransmitters, such as acetylcholine.[23]

An alternate metabolic pathway for carbohydrate found in some cells, the hexosemonophosphate shunt, uses TPP. This pathway allows cells to make the monosaccharide ribose for RNA. TPP also participates in the citric acid cycle and reactions in which carbon dioxide molecules are removed from branched-chain

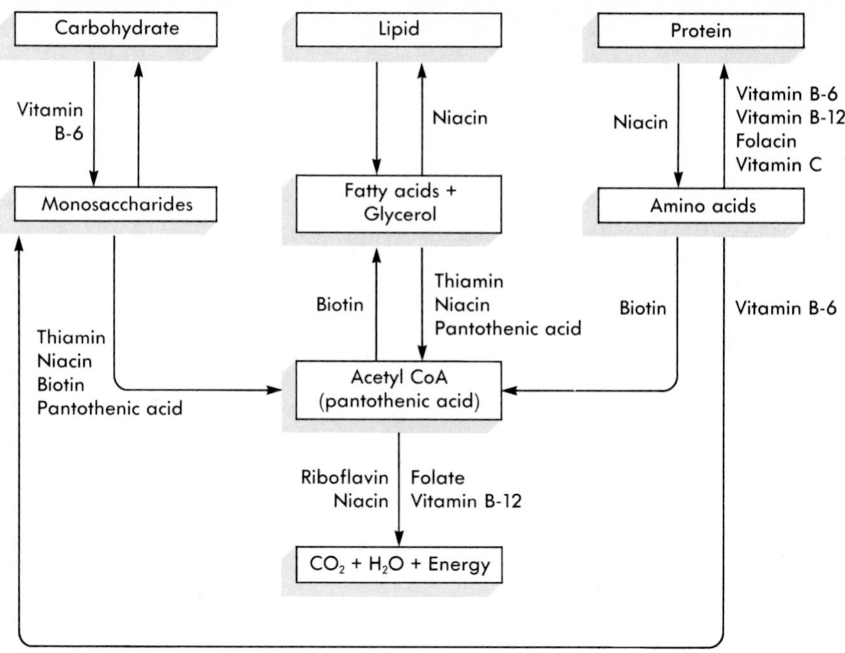

Figure 12-1

Examples of metabolic reactions for which vitamins are essential. The metabolism of energy-yielding nutrients requires vitamin input.

Enzyme activities in red blood cells that require vitamins to function can be used to test vitamin status. The tests are categorized as functional biochemical tests. Enzyme tests are available for thiamin (transketolase), riboflavin (glutathione reductase) and vitamin B-6 (aminotransferase) status.

amino acids. *Although thiamin is used by a variety of cellular metabolic pathways, the most important pathway is its link with carbohydrate metabolism.*

Beriberi

The thiamin deficiency disease is called **beriberi,** which means "I can't, I can't" in Sinhalese. The signs and symptoms include weakness, loss of appetite, irritability, nervous tingling throughout the body, poor arm and leg coordination, and deep muscle pain in the calves. A person with beriberi often develops an enlarged heart and sometimes severe edema ("wet" beriberi).

beriberi
The thiamin deficiency disorder characterized by muscle weakness, loss of appetite, nerve degeneration, and sometimes edema.

Brain and nerve cells convert pyruvate into acetyl-CoA and then push the acetyl-CoA through the citric acid cycle to obtain ATP energy. The thiamin coenzyme, TPP, participates in these metabolic pathways. So body functions associated with brain and nerve action quickly show signs of a thiamin deficiency.

Symptoms of depression and weakness can be seen after only 10 days on a thiamin-free diet. This shows how poorly our bodies store thiamin. It is best to consume ample thiamin daily from foods. Also, note that all these symptoms of beriberi are partially due to a thiamin deficiency, but can also result from concurrent B-vitamin deficiencies. *Since the B vitamins are often found in the same foods, a lack of one B vitamin may mean other B vitamins are deficient as well.*

Beriberi is traditionally associated with people who eat polished (white) rice. Brown rice, which has its bran and germ layer intact, is a good source of thiamin. White rice, which has had its bran and germ layer removed, is a poor source of thiamin. However, thiamin is often replaced (during the enrichment process; see Chapter 2) in rice available in North America.

Thiamin in foods

Foods containing a very high nutrient density of thiamin are pork products and sunflower seeds. Whole grains (wheat germ), enriched grains, green beans, organ meats, peanuts, dried beans, and other seeds are also good sources. *However, aside from pork products, there is really no one excellent source of thiamin in the North American diet. The foods we eat tend to contribute small amounts of thiamin* (Table 12-1). Following the Daily Food Guide is the best way to obtain enough thiamin.

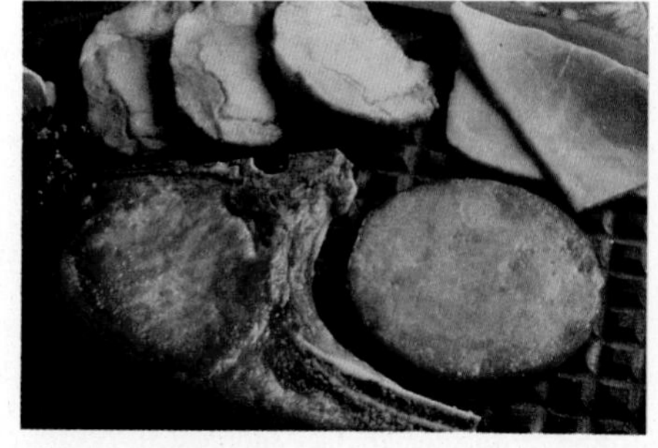

Pork is a good source of thiamin.

Table 12-1

Good food sources of thiamin, ranked by nutrient density

Food	Serving size to yield 1.5 milligrams*	kcalories needed to yield 1.5 milligrams
Brewers yeast	1-¼ tablespoons	30
Ham, canned roasted	5-½ ounces	252
Wheat germ, raw	1 cup	268
Cooked Canadian bacon	8 pieces	340
Sunflower seeds, dry	½ cup	369
Green peas, cooked	3-¼ cups	466
Pork chop, broiled	5-½ ounces	468
Watermelon	4 slices	585
Oatmeal, cooked	5 cups	745

*RDA for adult male, ages 19 to 24 years.
Sunflower seeds, pork, and ham yield much thiamin for both a limited serving size and kcalorie cost. Other foods contain small amounts, but they add up as servings from the Daily Food Guide are consumed.

Major contributors of thiamin to the U.S. diet are white bread and rolls, crackers, pork, hot dogs, luncheon meat, cold cereals, orange juice, and dairy products. White bread, bakery products, and cereals are usually enriched with thiamin and serve as important sources of it because many people eat them so often. Laboratory animal studies show that the thiamin in these products is as available as that found in whole grains. Some fish and shellfish contain an enzyme called thiaminase, which destroys thiamin. Cooking inactivates thiaminase.

RDA for thiamin

The RDA for thiamin for adults is approximately 1.5 milligrams per day for men and 1.1 milligrams per day for women. (Throughout the rest of this chapter refer to the inside cover for vitamin recommendations for other age groups and to Appendix G for Canadian recommendations.) The U.S. food supply yields approximately one-and-a-half times the RDA for thiamin per person per day, but that does not consider the thiamin lost in food preparation and in cooking.

The more carbohydrate consumed and the greater one's energy output, the more thiamin is required for metabolism. The RDA can even be expressed in terms of energy intake: 0.5 milligrams of thiamin per 1000 kcalories, but no less than 1 milligram per day if a person is on a low-kcalorie diet. No cases of toxicity have been associated with consumption of vitamin supplements of thiamin.

North Americans at risk for a thiamin deficiency

Some groups of people, such as the poor and the elderly, probably barely meet their needs for thiamin. *A diet dominated by highly processed and unenriched foods, sugar, fat, and alcohol also creates a potential for a thiamin deficiency.* Women should be especially careful to consume good sources of thiamin. Their average intakes barely meet the RDA.

When physicians see a person suffering from unexplained delirium in the emergency room, they must consider whether it may be caused by a thiamin deficiency due to alcoholism. The treatment is an injection of thiamin. Dietary supplementation will not suffice because thiamin is only slowly absorbed, especially in a person with alcoholism.

People with alcoholism are at great risk for thiamin deficiency because absorption and utilization of thiamin is profoundly diminished. Furthermore they often eat poorly. Recall that thiamin is very poorly stored in the body. If an alcohol binge lasts 1 to 2 weeks, the person may quickly deplete already poor stores of thiamin. Thiamin deficiency in alcoholism can lead to a combination of symptoms, including mental confusion, memory loss, and poor nervous system control of arms and legs.

RIBOFLAVIN

Riboflavin is a three-ringed structure with a monosaccharide-like compound (ribitol) attached. The name *riboflavin* comes from its yellow color—*flavus* means "yellow" in Latin. Riboflavin forms the coenzymes flavin mononucleotide (FMN) and flavin adenine dinucleotide (FAD). Riboflavin is present as FMN and FAD in food, except in enriched grain products, where riboflavin is present as the vitamin itself. Either form is well utilized.

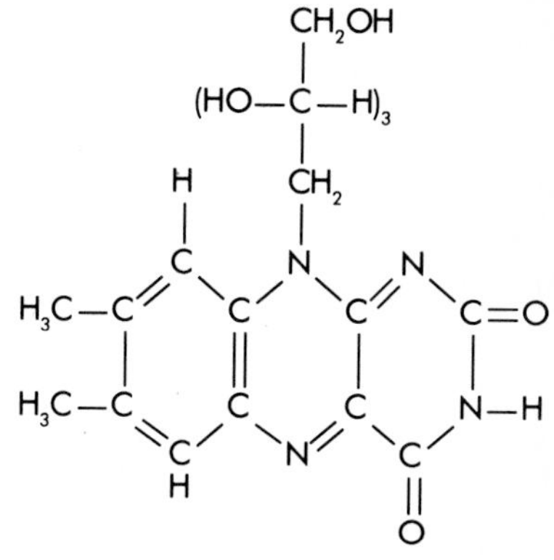

Riboflavin

Functions of riboflavin

The coenzymes of riboflavin participate in many cellular metabolic pathways. Both the citric acid cycle and the pathway for breaking down fatty acids (beta-oxidation) use FAD to form $FADH_2$. The electron transport chain in the mitochondria uses these coenzymes and FMN and $FMNH_2$, as well. In all these examples, the coenzymes act as both electron and hydrogen ion donors and acceptors. When cells form ATP using aerobic pathways or fatty acids are broken down and burned for energy, the coenzymes of riboflavin are used. Some vitamin metabolism also requires riboflavin.[23]

Ariboflavinosis

The symptoms associated with **ariboflavinosis,** a riboflavin deficiency, include inflammation of the mouth and tongue, dermatitis, cracking of tissue around the corners of the mouth (cheilosis), various eye disorders, and confusion (Figure 12-2). The first symptoms of a deficiency are inflammation of the mouth and tongue. The complete picture of deficiency symptoms develops after approximately 2 months of consuming a riboflavin-poor diet (consuming one fourth of the RDA).

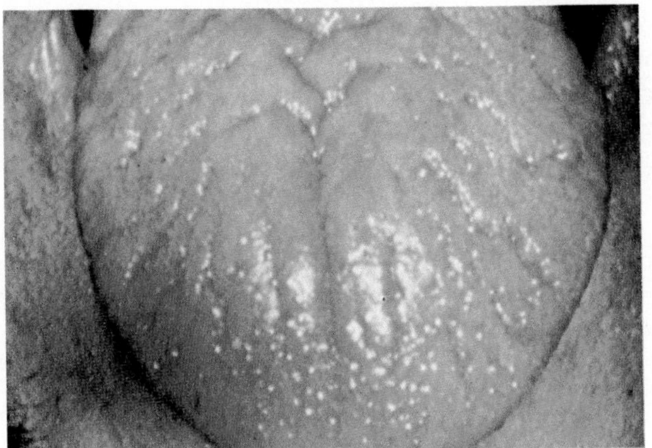

Figure 12-2
An inflamed tongue (glossitis) can signal a vitamin deficiency. A painful and inflamed tongue can be seen in a niacin, vitamin B-6, riboflavin, folate, or vitamin B-12 deficiency. Often more than one deficiency may be the cause. Since other medical conditions can also cause glossitis, the person needs a further evaluation before a nutrient deficiency can be established.

Clinicians have great difficulty identifying true riboflavin deficiencies because clinical signs and symptoms are not specific for riboflavin. Other B vitamins, such as thiamin, vitamin B-6, and folate, also cause similar effects. In addition, isolated riboflavin deficiencies probably do not exist. *A riboflavin deficiency often occurs with deficiencies of niacin, thiamin, and vitamin B-6. Again, these nutrients are often found in the same foods.*

Table 12-2

Good food sources of riboflavin, ranked by nutrient density

Food	Serving size to yield 1.7 milligrams*	kcalories needed to yield 1.7 milligrams
Beef liver, fried	1-½ ounces	92
Brewers yeast	5-½ tablespoon	138
Mushroom pieces, cooked	3-¾ cups	158
Spinach, cooked	4 cups	164
Broccoli, cooked	5-⅓ cups	243
Nonfat milk + solids	4 cups	360
Braunschweiger sausage	4 pieces	360
1% low-fat milk	4 cups	410
Buttermilk	4.5 cups	440
Oysters, Eastern	4 cups	640
Whole milk	4-¼ cups	648
Cottage cheese, low-fat	4 cups	820
Steak, beef	16 ounces	945
Pork, roasted	16 ounces	1120

*RDA for adult male, ages 19 to 24 years.
By eating vegetables and drinking milk, the RDA is easy to obtain using very few kcalories.

The enrichment of refined flours includes riboflavin. However, grains do not naturally provide amounts of riboflavin as high as that in enriched flours. Thus riboflavin-enriched grains have a greater riboflavin content than whole grains.

Riboflavin in foods

The most nutrient-dense sources of riboflavin are liver, mushrooms, spinach and other green leafy vegetables, and low-fat and nonfat milks (Table 12-2). Lean meats, poultry, and eggs are also good sources.

Most riboflavin in the U.S. diet comes from milk and milk products. Riboflavin is a major contribution of the Daily Food Guide's milk and cheese group. Including dairy products in your diet is the best guarantee for a good riboflavin intake. The rest of the U.S. riboflavin intake comes from enriched white bread, rolls, and crackers; meat; and eggs. For some people, high meat consumption partially offsets the low intake of dairy products.

Riboflavin is very stable at temperatures used to pasteurize milk and reheat foods in a microwave. However, its sensitivity to light causes riboflavin to break down rapidly when exposed. To protect milk products from light, paper and plastic cartons—not glass—work well.

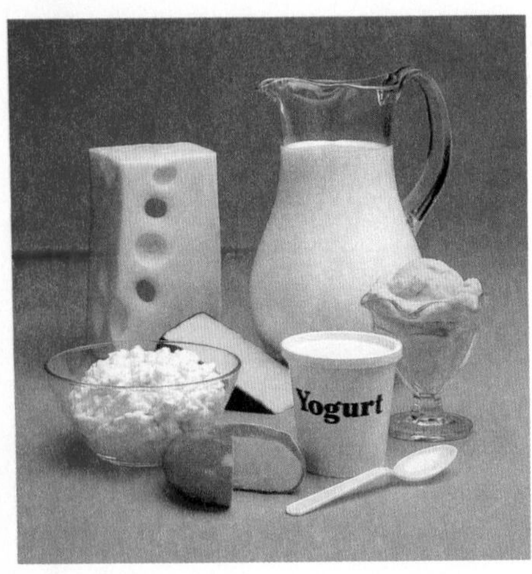

Milk products are major sources of riboflavin.

RDA for riboflavin

The RDA for riboflavin for adults is 1.4 to 1.7 milligrams per day for men and 1.2 to 1.3 milligrams per day for women. Another way of expressing the RDA is 0.6 milligrams per 1000 kcalories, but no less than 1.2 milligrams per day. People in the United States consume on average the RDA for riboflavin. Athletes may need extra riboflavin because of their increased use of fat for fuel (the metabolic pathways use FAD), and their greater use of all the energy-yielding pathways in the cell.[5] However, the RDA will still suffice, according to the Food and Nutrition Board. There are no specific signs or symptoms that indicate riboflavin toxicity is a concern.

North Americans at risk for a deficiency of riboflavin

Riboflavin deficiencies are rare, but some people hardly consume an adequate amount, especially those who do not regularly consume milk and milk products. People with alcoholism also risk riboflavin deficiency because they often eat very nutrient-poor diets. We suggest that if you do not use milk and milk products, you should search for another adequate dietary source of riboflavin. Enriched breakfast cereals are good sources.

NIACIN

Niacin is actually composed of a pair of compounds—nicotinic acid and nicotinamide. Both compounds can function as niacin in the body, but only nicotinic acid lowers serum cholesterol levels when taken in very high doses. The two coenzyme forms of niacin are nicotinamide adenine dinucleotide (NAD) and nicotinamide adenine dinucleotide phosphate (NADP).

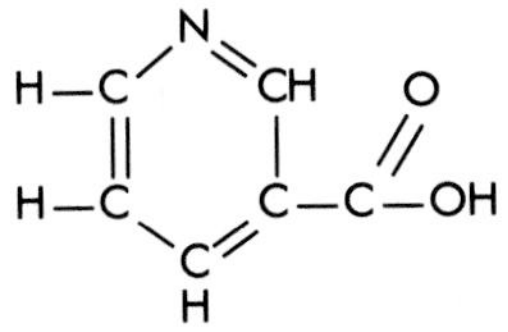

Nicotinic acid

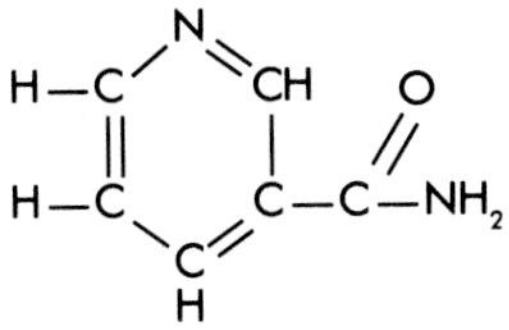

Nicotinamide

Functions of niacin

The coenzyme forms of niacin, NAD and NADP, function in many cellular metabolic pathways. In general, when ATP is being formed, NAD is used first as an electron and hydrogen ion receptor and then as an electron and hydrogen ion donor. This is true for glycolysis, the citric acid cycle, and the electron transport chain.[23]

Synthetic pathways in the cell—those that make new compounds—often use NADPH. This is especially true of the pathway for fatty acid synthesis. Cells that synthesize a lot of fatty acids, such as those in the liver and female mammary gland, have higher concentrations of enzymes needed to synthesize NADPH than do cells that do not synthesize fat, such as muscle cells.

Pellagra

Since almost every cellular metabolic pathway uses either NAD or NADP, a niacin deficiency causes widespread changes in the body. The entire group of symptoms is known as *pellagra,* which means "rough" or "painful skin." The symptoms of the disease are known as the four "Ds"—dementia, diarrhea, dermatitis, and death (Figure 12-3). Early symptoms include poor appetite, weight loss, and weakness. Pellagra decimated corn-eating populations beginning in the 1700s in southern Europe. It spread to the southeastern United States in the late 1800s and persisted until the late 1930s. Nutrition Perspective 12-1 discusses the history of this disease. The pellegra epidemic in the United States in the early 1900s gave impetus to the federally sponsored program in 1941 to enrich grains.

Niacin in foods

The most nutrient-dense sources of niacin are mushrooms, wheat bran, tuna and other fish, chicken, asparagus, and peanuts (Table 12-3). Most niacin in the American diet comes from enriched white bread, rolls, crackers, and breakfast cereals (niacin is added as part of the enrichment process); beef, chicken, and turkey. Niacin is very heat stable: little is lost in cooking.

Besides the preformed niacin found in protein foods, each 60 milligrams of extra dietary tryptophan—leftover after protein synthesis—yields approximately 1 milligram of niacin. This conversion requires participation from thiamin, riboflavin, and vitamin B-6 coenzymes. We can assume that 1% of dietary protein is tryptophan. To estimate the number of milligrams of niacin supplied by dietary protein, just divide extra grams of dietary protein intake by 6. About half the niacin we use is produced by this process. Animal proteins (except gelatin) are especially rich in tryptophan.

Food tables list only the actual niacin content. Therefore they often underes-

Figure 12-3

The dermatitis of pellagra. Dermatitis on both sides of the body (bilateral) is a typical result of pellagra. Sun exposure worsens the condition.

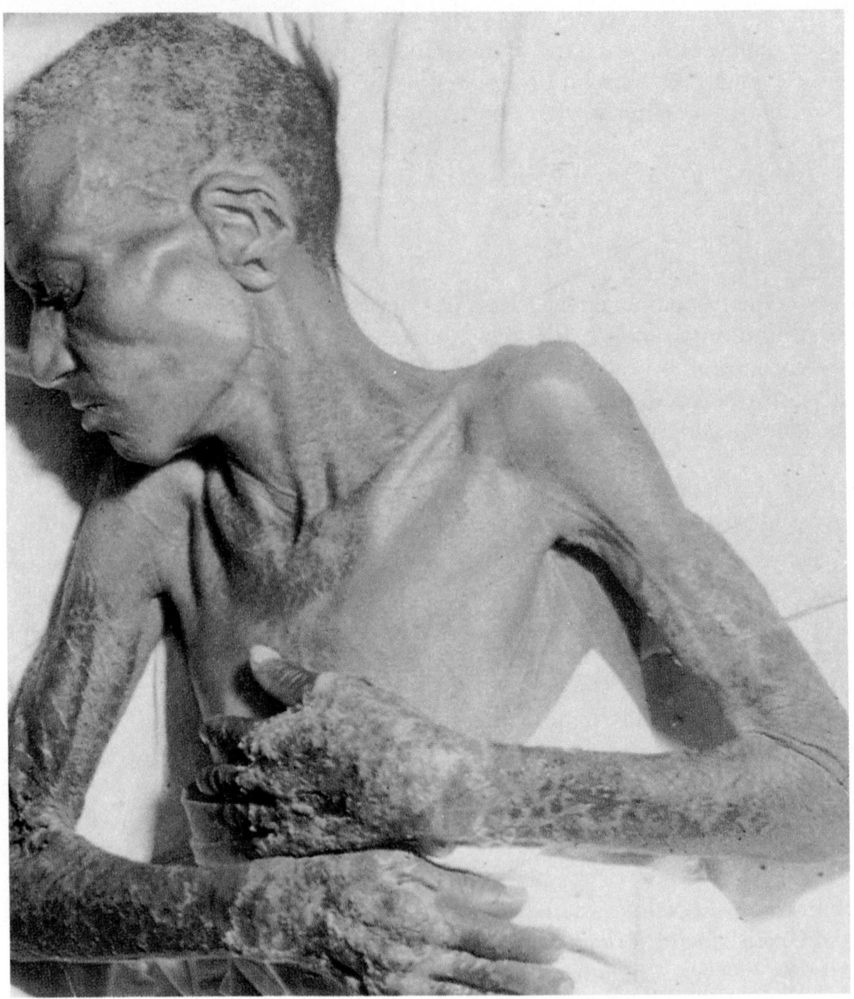

timate the total niacin contribution in protein foods, since protein foods yield the vitamin niacin and also contribute niacin from the conversion of tryptophan.

Niacin in corn is bound by a protein, so it is poorly absorbed. Soaking corn in an alkaline solution such as lime water (water and calcium hydroxide) releases bound niacin and renders it more usable. Hispanic populations soak corn in lime water before making tortillas. The soaking treatment is one reason Hispanic populations never suffered much pellagra, in contrast to Europeans and Caucasian Americans. Unaware of the importance of soaking the corn in lime water, Spanish explorers failed to inform Europeans how to prepare corn properly when they brought it back from the New World.

RDA for niacin

The RDA for niacin for adults is 15 to 19 milligrams per day for men and 13 to 15 milligrams per day for women. The difference in muscle mass between genders accounts for the different recommendations. The RDA is expressed as niacin equivalents to account for niacin received intact from the diet, as well as that synthesized from tryptophan.

Niacin status is determined by measuring the amount of its breakdown product, N-methyl nicotinamide, in the urine. Low amounts suggest poor status.

The U.S. food supply contains 1.4 times the RDA (26.8 milligrams of niacin) per person per day, without considering the contribution from tryptophan.[29] *As long as you follow the Daily Food Guide, developing a niacin deficiency is*

Table 12-3

Good food sources of niacin, ranked by nutrient density

Food	Serving size to yield 19 milligrams*	kcalories needed to yield 19 milligrams
Mushroom pieces, cooked	2-½ cups	109
Wheat bran	1-¾ cups	140
Brewers yeast	6 tablespoons	142
Tuna, canned	4 ounces	183
Chicken breast, roasted	¾ each	214
Beef liver, fried	4-½ ounces	270
Pink salmon, canned, raw	8 ounces	317
Halibut, broiled w/ butter and lemon juice	7 ounces	326
Salmon, broiled/baked	10 ounces	462
Sardines, canned	12 ounces	482
Turkey, roasted	11-½ ounces	562
Peanuts, dried unsalted	4 ounces	720
Lamb chops	10 ounces	800
Peanut butter	10 ounces	840
Steak, beef	16 ounces	950
Hamburger, lean	12 ounces	950

*RDA for adult male, ages 19 to 24 years.

Mushrooms, chicken, beef, pork, and salmon supply ample niacin within both a reasonable serving size and kcalorie cost.

highly unlikely. People with alcoholism are generally the only group to show niacin deficiency.

Toxicity of niacin

Intakes of 100 milligrams or more of nicotinic acid can lead to an increase in blood flow to the skin, causing a general blood vessel dilation or "flushing" of the body. Headache and itching also may result. This excessive intake is sometimes used, under a physician's guidance, to lower elevated blood cholesterol levels.

Concept Check

The B vitamins thiamin, niacin, and riboflavin are all important in the metabolism of carbohydrates, proteins, and fats. Enriched grains are adequate sources of all three vitamins. Otherwise, pork is an excellent source of thiamin, milk is an excellent source of riboflavin, and protein foods in general, such as chicken, are excellent sources of niacin. Deficiencies of all three vitamins can occur with alcoholism, and a thiamin deficiency is the most likely. Only niacin shows toxicity symptoms when consumed in high doses.

PANTOTHENIC ACID

Pantothenic acid forms part of coenzyme A. To do so the vitamin must combine both with a part of ATP and with the amino acid cysteine. This last addition provides the sulfur atom, which is the "business end" of the coenzyme.

Pantothenic acid

Functions of pantothenic acid

By forming coenzyme A (CoA), pantothenic acid allows many important metabolic actions of the citric acid cycle to take place. This happens because the CoA molecule can make other molecules much more reactive. For example, CoA activates fatty acids before they break down and enter the citric acid cycle as acetyl-CoA. Coenzyme A is also used in the beginning steps of fatty acid synthesis. In addition, pantothenic acid forms a part of a compound called the acyl carrier protein. This attaches to fatty acids and shuttles them through the pathway designed to increase their chain length.

Pantothenic acid is too widespread in foods to ever allow a nutritional deficiency. To study the possible consequences of a pantothenic acid deficiency, researchers must induce it in subjects by having them consume an antagonist to the vitamin. When antagonists are given, people suffer from tingling hands, fatigue, headache, sleep disturbances, nausea, and abdominal distress.[23]

Pantothenic acid in foods

Pantothenic acid is present in all foods. "Pantothen" actually means "from every side" in Greek. Nutrient-dense sources of pantothenic acid are mushrooms, yeast, liver, peanuts, and eggs (Table 12-4). Other good sources are meat, milk, and many vegetables. Because pantothenic acid is not added to enriched grains, they are not especially good sources of the vitamin.

ESADDI for pantothenic acid

The estimated safe and adequate daily dietary intake for pantothenic acid is 4 to 7 milligrams per day for adults. The current U.S. intake is about 6 milligrams of pantothenic acid per person per day. In a recent study, women were found to consume about 2.75 milligrams per 1000 kcalories.[35]

Table 12-4

Good food sources of pantothenic acid, ranked by nutrient density

Food	Serving size to yield 7 milligrams*	kcalories needed to yield 7 milligrams
Raw mushrooms	4-½ cups	82
Brewers yeast	10 tablespoons	228
Fried beef liver	4-½ ounces	272
Broccoli, cooked	7 cups	343
Cooked lobster	14 ounces	632
Cooked eggs	8 each	640
1% milk	9 cups	809
Cooked chicken, roasted	4.5 cups	993
Wheat bran	8 cups	1004
Blue cheese	14 ounces	1428
Baked salmon	22 ounces	1260
Peanuts, oil-roasted	2-⅓ cups	1878
Dates	5 cups	2444
Pecans	3-½ cups	3031

*Top range of ESADDI

Some vegetables supply the greatest nutrient density, but nuts and meats offer the most reasonable serving size relative to their nutrient density.

A deficiency of pantothenic acid might occur in cases of alcoholism in which a very nutrient-deficient diet is consumed. However, the symptoms would probably be hidden among deficiencies of thiamin, riboflavin, vitamin B-6, and folate, so the pantothenic acid deficiency might be unrecognizable. There is no known toxicity level for pantothenic acid.

BIOTIN

Biotin exists in two forms—the vitamin itself and biocytin, an inactive form that is simply biotin with the amino acid lysine attached.

Biotin

Absorption of biotin

Both forms of biotin are absorbed. Once in the intestinal cells or bloodstream, a biotinidase enzyme cleaves the lysine from biocytin, yielding free biotin. Occasionally, infants are born with a genetic defect that leaves them very low levels of the biotinidase enzyme (about 1 in 8000 to 12,000 births). They develop biotin deficiency symptoms. Clinicians debate whether infants should be screened at birth for a biotinidase deficiency, as they are for phenylketonuria (see Chapter 6).[36] If a deficiency is found, the infant is treated with 50 to 200 times the ESADDI.

Functions of biotin

Biotin acts as a coenzyme in fat and carbohydrate metabolism. Specifically, biotin assists the addition of carbon dioxide molecules to other compounds. By doing so, it provides the high oxaloacetate concentration needed in the citric acid cycle for gluconeogenesis, contributes to the synthesis of fatty acids, helps in the breakdown of some amino acids, and participates in the synthesis of one of the two types of bases (purines) needed for constructing DNA and RNA. Biotin is also important for the metabolism of the 3-carbon fatty acids so that they can enter the citric acid cycle.[23] Altered serum fatty acid profiles occur in a biotin deficiency.

One problem in assessing biotin status is that there is no accurate measure for it. Symptoms of an overt biotin deficiency include a scaly inflammation of the skin, changes in the tongue and lips, decreased appetite, nausea, vomiting, anemia, depression, muscle pain, muscle weakness, and poor growth.

Biotin in foods

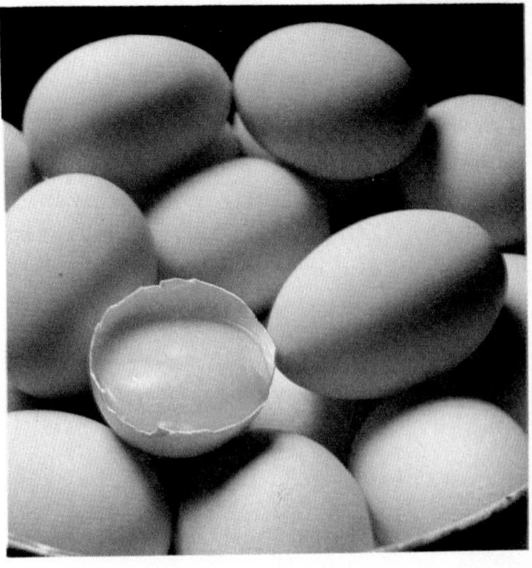

Egg yolks are a nutrient-dense source of biotin.

Cauliflower, egg yolks, yeast, liver, peanuts, and cheese are the most nutrient-dense sources of biotin (Table 12-5). Fruits are generally poorer sources. *Intestinal synthesis of biotin by bacteria probably supplies part of our needs, especially considering that a biotin deficiency is so unlikely.* There is even more biotin in our feces than we eat. However, questions remain about the amount of biotin we actually absorb of that synthesized by bacteria in our intestines.[21] Some researchers think it might be bound inside the bacteria and therefore be unavailable. Still, if a person lacks a large part of the small intestine or needs to take antibiotics for many months, special attention should be paid to eating good food sources of biotin.

A protein called **avidin** in raw egg whites can bind biotin and inhibit its absorption. Feeding many raw egg whites to animals leads to the classic "egg white injury" deficiency symptoms as described above. An occasional raw egg in eggnog is of no concern because it would take a regular daily consumption of 12 to 24 raw eggs to produce a biotin deficiency. In cases of alcoholism, however, biotin deficiency symptoms resulting from raw eggs have been reported in people with a regular consumption of just three raw eggs a day. These people probably had very poor diets. Nevertheless, consuming raw eggs is still a concern when you consider the increased risk for *Salmonella* bacteria food poisoning (see Chapter 19).

avidin
A protein found in raw egg whites that can bind biotin and inhibit absorption; cooking destroys avidin.

Table 12-5

Good food sources of biotin, ranked by nutrient density

Food	Serving size to yield 100 micrograms*	kcalories needed to yield 100 micrograms
Brewers yeast	5-½ tablespoons	141
Cooked cauliflower	6-½ cups	158
Egg yolk	4 each	252
Cooked beef liver	4-½ ounces	278
Cheese, American	5 ounces	470
Wheat bran	4 cups	618
Canned sardines	16 ounces	771
Broiled chicken, roasted	22 ounces	1237
Peanut butter	1 cup	1500
Baking chocolate	11 ounces	1555
Peanuts	10 ounces	1725

*Top range of ESADDI; bacterial synthesis probably also yields some contribution. Egg yolks, liver, and cheese provide the most reasonable balance of kcalorie cost and serving size. Cauliflower, peanut butter, and chicken are probably the best choices if a low cholesterol, low saturated fat intake is desired.

ESADDI for biotin

The estimated safe and adequate dietary intake for biotin is 30 to 100 micrograms per day for adults. The U.S. food supply is thought to contain 100 to 300 micrograms per person per day. It is important to avoid a biotin supplement that exceeds the ESADDI, unless a physician recommends it. We know very little about this vitamin, especially its potential for toxicity.

Exploring Issues and Actions

Much of your grandmother's small intestine was removed during recent surgery. What should she do to ensure an adequate intake of biotin?

North Americans at risk for a biotin deficiency

A diet designed to decrease the risk of heart disease may call for reducing egg and organ meat consumption. This diet may then be low in biotin. Again, current thinking is that bacterial synthesis of biotin in the intestine probably compensates for the difference between our biotin needs and what our diets supply, but we can't be absolutely sure. Seeking alternate food sources is a wise measure.

VITAMIN B-6

Vitamin B-6 is actually a family of compounds: pyridoxal, pyridoxine, and pyridoxamine. All three forms can be changed to the active vitamin B-6 coenzyme, pyridoxal phosphate (PLP). The general vitamin name is pyridoxine.

Functions of vitamin B-6

Vitamin B-6 is needed for the activity of more than 50 enzymes involved in carbohydrate, protein, and fat metabolism.

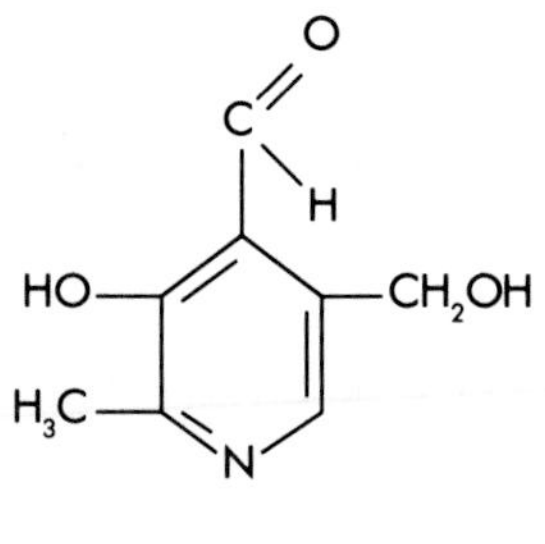

Protein metabolism. *The most important function of vitamin B-6 concerns protein, because the metabolism of every amino acid requires the active coenzyme PLP.*[23] This includes transamination reactions (see Chapter 6). Essentially, the PLP coenzyme plus some enzymes it works with ease the splitting of the amine group from an amino acid.

If vitamin B-6 were missing from the body, every amino acid would become an "essential" amino acid—that is, every amino acid would have to be supplied by the diet. In normal circumstances, however, we can make 11 of the 20

O
C
H
HO
CH_2OH
H_3C
N

Pyridoxal

types of amino acids our diets supply. None of that synthesis would be possible without PLP. Poor cell synthesis, as evidenced by skin changes and a sore tongue, occurs with vitamin B-6 deficiency.

Blood cell synthesis. The coenzyme PLP is important for the synthesis of hemoglobin, the oxygen-carrying part of the red blood cell. Vitamin B-6 is also necessary for the synthesis of white blood cells, which perform a major role in the immune system. An anemia resembling iron-deficiency anemia occurs in a vitamin B-6 deficiency (see Chapter 14).

Neurotransmitter metabolism. The syntheses of many neurotransmitters, such as serotonin, gamma amino butyric acid (GABA), and norepinephrine, require PLP. These compounds allow nerve cells to communicate with each other. A deficiency of vitamin B-6 results in depression, headaches, confusion, and seizures.[26] These results are predictable, given the importance of PLP in metabolism of key nervous system regulators. In the 1950s, infants fed oversterilized commercial formulas developed deficiency symptoms, particularly convulsions. Heat destroyed vitamin B-6 in the formulas, possibly contributing to the infants' decreased ability to synthesize the neurotransmitter GABA. Today, manufacturers are more careful to maintain adequate vitamin B-6 levels in formulas (see Chapter 16).

The link between vitamin B-6 and neurotransmitters suggested to some researchers that vitamin B-6 might be helpful in the treatment of **premenstrual syndrome.** This disorder appears in some women a few days before a menstrual period begins and is characterized by depression, headache, bloating, and mood swings. Researchers thought that increasing vitamin B-6 intake might increase the synthesis of serotonin, and in turn decrease the depression and confusion associated with premenstrual syndrome.

premenstrual syndrome
A disorder found in some women a few days before a menstrual period begins, which is characterized by depression, headache, bloating, and mood swings.

However, researchers now know that vitamin B-6 is not effective and also has a great potential for toxicity.[38] *Some women have suffered toxic side effects of vitamin B-6 (see the section on toxicity) in attempting to treat themselves for premenstrual syndrome.* A better approach to treatment is to eat a nutrient-rich diet; decrease alcohol, caffeine, nicotine, and salt use to decrease nervousness, depression, and bloating; and increase exercise to stimulate relaxation. If that therapy is not helpful, women with premenstrual syndrome should seek a physician's advice.[9]

Vitamin B-6 in foods

The most nutrient-dense sources of vitamin B-6 are some fruits and vegetables, such as bananas, cantaloupe, broccoli, and spinach (Table 12-6). Protein foods, especially meat, fish, and poultry (vitamin B-6 is stored in muscles), are also good sources, and the vitamin B-6 present in animal foods is often more absorbable than that in plant foods. *This makes meats, fish, and poultry our best sources of vitamin B-6.* Note that vitamin B-6 is not part of the enrichment process. If it were, we would probably see breads, cakes, and cookies listed as major sources. Food tables listing vitamin B-6 are often incomplete because measuring this vitamin in foods is difficult.

RDA for vitamin B-6

The RDA for vitamin B-6 for adults is 2 milligrams per day for men and 1.6 milligrams per day for women. The RDA is set high in response to high protein intakes found in the United States. The more protein eaten, the more vitamin B-6 needed. The recommendations can also be expressed as 0.016 milligrams of vitamin B-6 per gram of protein. This corresponds to 2 milligrams per 126 grams of protein—twice the RDA for protein for adult men.

Athletes may need more vitamin B-6 because of their increased use of glycogen for fuel (glycogen metabolism requires vitamin B-6), their increased use of

Table 12-6

Good sources of vitamin B-6, ranked by nutrient density

Food	Serving size to yield 2.0 milligrams*	kcalories needed to yield 2.0 milligrams
Brewers yeast	5 tablespoons	125
Spinach, cooked	4½ cups	186
Broccoli, cooked	6⅓ cups	292
Banana, peeled, slices	2 cups	318
Salmon, broiled/baked	8½ ounces	440
Watermelon	2¾ slices	440
Salmon, broiled	9 ounces	455
Chicken breast, roasted	2 whole	600
Cantaloupe	3 each	605
Tuna, water packed	13½ ounces	614
Turkey	14½ ounces	700
Sunflower seeds, oil-roasted	1 cup	945

*RDA for adult male, ages 19 to 24.
Some vegetables provide more vitamin B-6 per kcalorie than meat and fish, but the serving size for many vegetables presents quite a challenge, and the vitamin B-6 present is often less absorbable. Thus meats, fish, and poultry are ultimately our best sources of vitamin B-6.

amino acids for fuel, and their high protein intakes. Dietary protein should easily supply any extra vitamin B-6 needed.

Average consumption of vitamin B-6 in the United States is 2.06 milligrams per person per day, or about the RDA.[29] A national average intake that equals the RDA is of concern because that means that about half the intakes are below the value. In such cases, some people are probably not meeting their needs.

North Americans at risk for vitamin B-6 deficiency

Vitamin B-6 status can be assessed by measuring the amount of coenzyme PLP in the bloodstream.

Numerous studies show that about 35% to 40% of adolescent, adult, and elderly women have poor vitamin B-6 intakes.[12] However, since the vitamin B-6 values of many foods are not known, they are consequently not counted. True intakes, then, may be better. Poor vitamin B-6 status is often found in women who use oral contraceptives. While this relationship has been known for the last 15 years, there is still no consensus about whether the problem requires vitamin B-6 supplements.[27] Today, it is not possible to reliably separate adequate vitamin B-6 status from an abnormal or deficient state. Still, there is much concern that the vitamin B-6 status for many women is poor. Further research is needed.

People with alcoholism are susceptible to a vitamin B-6 deficiency because acetaldehyde, a metabolite formed in ethanol metabolism, can displace the coenzyme PLP from its enzyme. This increases the tendency for PLP to be broken down. In addition, alcoholism decreases the absorption of vitamin B-6 and decreases its synthesis into PLP. Cirrhosis and hepatitis disable liver tissue from actively metabolizing vitamin B-6, thus the synthesis of PLP is inefficient. Both cirrhosis and hepatitis accompany alcoholism.

Toxicity of vitamin B-6

Intakes of 2 to 6 grams of vitamin B-6 per day for 2 to 40 months can lead to irreversible nerve damage. These high doses have mostly been used by women with PMS. Symptoms include walking difficulties and hand and foot numbness. Some nerve damage in individual sensory neurons is probably reversible, but damage to the ganglions (where many nerve fibers converge) is probably permanent.[3]

That vitamin B-6 can cause nerve damage may account for its erroneous reputation in health food literatures as a cure for **carpal tunnel syndrome.** This is a disease in which nerves traveling to the wrist are pinched, causing numbness in the hands. High doses of vitamin B-6 cause nerve damage. Possibly the hand no longer feels numb because the nerve is dead. People with carpal tunnel syndrome should seek the advice of a neurologist. Self-medication with vitamin B-6 is dangerous.

Before deciding to take a supplement of vitamin B-6, or any supplement to treat a disorder, make sure that double-blind studies published in medical journals, such as the ones we cite in the references, support your decision. Then discuss your plans with your physician. To review the characteristics of a double-blind study, see Chapter 1.

There is concern about toxicity from doses of vitamin B-6 as low as 25 milligrams per day. This concern deserves note, since 1000 milligram tablets of vitamin B-6 are available in health food stores. It is quite easy to take a toxic dose.

Concept Check

Pantothenic acid and biotin both participate in metabolism of carbohydrate and fat. A deficiency of neither vitamin is likely: pantothenic acid is found widely in foods, and our need for biotin is probably partially met by intestinal synthesis from bacteria. Vitamin B-6 is important for protein metabolism, neurotransmitter synthesis, and other key metabolic functions. Headache, anemia, nausea, and vomiting can result from a vitamin B-6 deficiency. Women, in general, should consume a diet richer in vitamin B-6, using foods such as animal protein foods, broccoli, spinach, and bananas. Doses in excess of 25 times the RDA can cause nerve destruction.

Exploring Issues and Actions

Should vitamins be treated like drugs? Who should control their availability?

FOLATE

In the past, folate was known as folic acid and folacin. Today, the term *folate* is preferred because it encompasses the variety of food forms of the vitamin. Only a few food forms are in the true folic acid configuration, but vitamin supplements often contain this form.

Folate is built of three parts—a pteridine group, paraaminobenzoic acid, and glutamic acid (an amino acid). If one glutamate molecule is present, it is in the folic acid form. However, in foods, over three quarters of the folate molecules have more than one glutamate added. These are called **polyglutamate forms.** Folate is turned into active coenzyme derivatives of tetrahydrofolic acid (THFA).

polyglutamate form
Folate with more than 1 glutamate molecule attached.

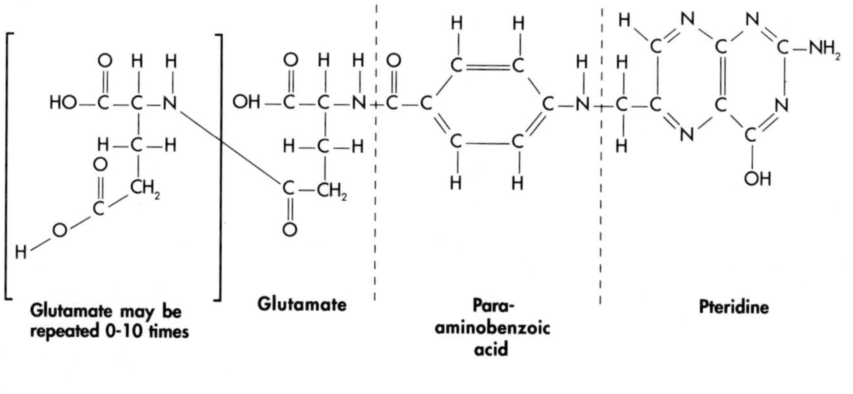

Glutamate may be repeated 0-10 times
Glutamate
Para-aminobenzoic acid
Pteridine

Folate is built of three parts.

Absorption of folate

Absorption of folate occurs with both the monoglutamate (folic acid) and the polyglutamate forms. Approximately 85% of true folic acid is absorbed, and 20% to 70% of the polyglutamate forms are absorbed. All but the last glutamate molecule must eventually be released during absorption. The cells that line the small intestine accomplish that, aided by the enzyme system called **conjugase.** When absorbed, most folate is stored in the liver. This makes liver a good food source. Once inside the body's cells, folate quickly forms coenzyme forms of THFA.

conjugase
An intestinal enzyme system that enhances folate absorption by removing glutamate molecules from polyglutamate forms.

Functions of folate

When it participates in metabolic reactions, the active coenzyme forms of THFA are always accepting or donating single-carbon molecules. Transfers of single-carbon molecules are needed for the synthesis of DNA and RNA, as well as for the metabolism of various amino acids and their derivatives.

Probably the most important role of folate is to contribute to the formation of purine and pyrimidine bases in RNA and DNA. One major change caused by a folate deficiency is that in the early phases of red blood synthesis, the precursor cells cannot divide because they cannot form new DNA. The cells grow larger and larger because they can still synthesize enough protein and other cell parts to make new cells. But when it is time for the cells to divide, there is insufficient DNA to form two nuclei. The cells then remain in a large immature form, known as a **megaloblast.** Megaloblasts can convert to abnormally large red blood cells, called **macrocytes** (Figure 12-4).

Single carbon molecules include methyl groups ($-CH_3$), formyl groups ($-\overset{\overset{\displaystyle O}{\|}}{C}-H$), methylene groups ($-CH_2-$), and methynyl groups ($-CH=$).

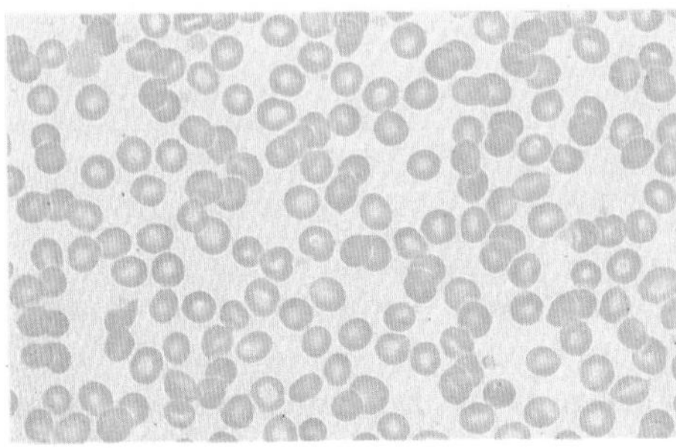

A

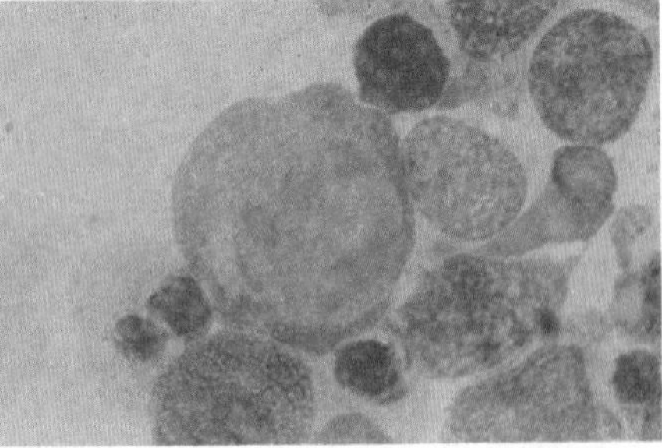

B

Figure 12-4
Macrocytic anemia. (A) Normal blood cells. Both size and color are normal. (B) Macrocytic anemia. The large red blood cells have been arrested at an immature stage of development, leaving them quite large.

Since the bone marrow of a folate-deficient person produces mostly immature megaloblast cells, few mature red blood cells (erythrocytes) arrive in the bloodstream. Since fewer mature red blood cells are present, oxygen-carrying capacity decreases, causing anemia. In short, a folate deficiency causes megaloblastic anemia.

The changes in red blood cell formation occur after 7 to 16 weeks on a folate-free diet, depending on the folate stores of the person. White blood cell formation is also affected, but not as much as red blood cell formation. In addition, cell division throughout the entire body is disrupted. We focus primarily on red blood cells because they are easy to examine.

megaloblast
A large, immature red blood cell that results from a cell's inability to divide when it normally should.

macrocyte
A greatly enlarged mature red blood cell; they have short life spans.

Clinical signs and symptoms of folate deficiency are inflammation of the tongue, diarrhea, poor growth, mental confusion, and problems in nerve function. Some forms of cancer therapy provide a vivid example of the effects of a folate deficiency on DNA metabolism. A cancer drug, methotrexate, closely resembles folate. Because of this resemblence, when methotrexate is taken in high doses, it hampers folate metabolism. DNA synthesis then decreases throughout the body. Since cancer cells are among the most rapidly dividing cells in the body, they are among those affected first. However, other rapidly dividing cells, such as intestinal cells and skin cells, are also affected. Typical side effects of methotrexate therapy are diarrhea, vomiting, and hair loss. You could predict these signs—they are all signs of a folate deficiency.

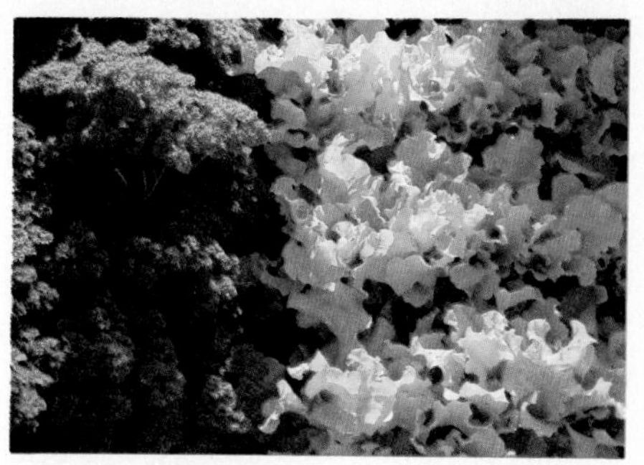

Green leafy vegetables are an excellent source of folate.

Folate in foods

Green leafy vegetables (the term *folate* is derived from the Latin word *folium,* which means foliage), organ meats, sprouts, other vegetables, and orange juice are the most nutrient-dense sources of folate (Table 12-7). In fact, 1 cup of orange juice contains about 100 micrograms of folate, which is approximately one half of the RDA. While orange juice is promoted for its vitamin C content, an added benefit of orange juice is its substantial folate contribution. The vitamin C in the juice also reduces folate destruction.

Food processing and preparation destroy 50% to 90% of the folate in food. Folate is very susceptible to destruction by heat. *This underscores the importance of regularly eating fresh fruits and lightly cooked vegetables—or raw when appropriate—as part of the Daily Food Guide regimen.* Vegetables are best cooked quickly in minimal water—steaming, stir-frying, or microwaving.

RDA for folate

The RDA for folate for adults is 180 to 200 micrograms per day. Because of new data showing that polyglutamate forms of folate are better absorbed than once thought, our current RDA is about half the value given in the ninth edition.[31] These newer figures are much more in line with the current folate content of the North American food supply, which is approximately 225 micrograms per day per person (not accounting for losses in preparation and cooking). *We need to emphasize fresh fruits and minimally cooked vegetables in our diets to meet our folate needs.*

Table 12-7

Good food sources of folate, ranked by nutrient density

Food	Serving size to yield 200 micrograms*	kcalories needed to yield 200 micrograms
Brewers yeast	½ tablespoon	16
Spinach, fresh chopped	1¾ cups	22
Romaine lettuce, chopped	2½ cups	23
Spinach, cooked	¾ cup	31
Turnip greens, cooked	1 cup	34
Asparagus, cooked	1 cup	48
Broccoli, cooked	1¾ cups	86
Beets, cooked	2 cups	104
Orange juice	1¾ cups	205
Wheat germ, raw	¾ cup	219
Cantaloupe melon	1¼ each	235
Beef liver, fried	4 ounces	246
Liver, beef	4½ ounces	377
Beans, pinto	1½ cups	398
Sunflower seeds, oil-roasted	½ cup	525

*RDA for male adults.

Spinach, asparagus, broccoli, and orange juice are some good nutrient-dense folate sources. Other fruits and vegetables also contribute to total dietary folate.

Expert Opinion

The Race to Discover Folic Acid

ROBERT STOKSTAD, Ph.D.

The history of folic acid research constitutes a fascinating account of many independent lines of research converging on the ultimate discovery. Folate functions as a coenzyme in single carbon metabolism and is essential for nucleic acid formation (part of DNA and RNA) and cell division. What we know now as folic acid deficiency was described in humans by Wills in 1931, in monkeys (called vitamin M deficiency) by Day and coworkers in 1938, and in chicks (called vitamin B_c conjugase deficiency) by Hogan and O'Dell in 1939.

My own involvement began in 1939 as a chemist at the Western Condensing Company (a dried milk factory) with a description of an unidentified growth factor for chicks. My 1939 assay method, which was based on the growth of chicks, was very slow. In 1940, however, Snell and Peterson at the University of Wisconsin described a new, unidentified growth factor for the bacterium *Lactobacillus casei.* Subsequently, Mitchell, Snell, and Williams at the University of Texas described a growth factor for the bacterium *Streptococcus lactis,* which they termed folic acid because of its abundance in leafy material. Since it seemed possible that this bacterial growth factor could also be the nutritionally important one we were studying in animals, we discontinued our chick assays and began isolation of the growth factor using *L. casei* assay.

When I joined Lederle Laboratories as a chemist in 1941, the isolation of the *L. casei* factor continued using liver as a source, since large amounts of liver by-products were available from Lederle's commercial production of injectable liver extracts. However, only small amounts of folic acid could be isolated from liver. At this time, Lederle also began the commercial production of antibiotics and riboflavin by fermentation, and scientists believed that other vitamins might also be made this way. Dr. Brian Hutchings, who had worked on the *L. casei* factor at the University of Wisconsin and recently joined Lederle, began looking for an organism that would make folic acid. Many bacteria cultures were examined, and a few were found that had variable activity. It was then determined that a rod-shaped *Corynebacterium,* which was present as a cotaminant in our cultures, was the organism responsible for the folic acid biosynthesis. By culturing this organism in fermentation tanks, it was possible to produce the large amounts of material necessary for chemical studies.

The folic acid produced by this organism was termed the fermentation *L. casei* factor. However, this factor was biologically different from the factor obtained from liver. Although both factors were approximately equally active for *L. casei,* the fermentation factor for *Cornebacterium* was less active than the liver factor for *Streptococcus faecalis.*

During the final stages of purification of this factor from liver, scientists tested for various chemical groups on the molecule. In discussing this with members of the analytical control laboratory, researchers mentioned the Bratton and Marshall test for certain types of amines. This test was used for the analysis of sulfonamide tablets (sulfa drugs), which were then an important antibiotic promoted by Lederle. Since the reagents were readily available, this test was applied to highly active *L. casei* factor preparations. A faint pink color, similar to that given by sulfanilamide, was obtained. We know now that the color was due to *p*-aminobenzoylglutamic acid that formed during the slow breakdown of folic acid. The color seemed to correlate roughly with biological activity and so was used occasionally to follow isolation procedures and the course of various degradation reactions.

Other experiments with this *L. casei* factor continued. For example, when hydrolysis (molecular breakdown using the addition of water) was carried out under anaerobic conditions, an interesting effect occurred. Liver folic acid is active for both *L. casei* and *S. faecalis.* Fermentation folate, however, is about 70% as active as liver folic acid for *L. casei,* but only 6% as active for *S. faecalis.* It was observed that when fermentation folic acid was heated anaerobically with concentrated sodium hydroxide at 120° C for 10 hours, the *S. faecalis* activity markedly increased to the point where it now had

Expert Opinion—cont'd

the same relative activity for these two organisms as did liver folic acid. This suggested that fermentation folic acid had been converted into the liver folic acid form. Accompanying this increase in activity for *S. faecalis,* 25% of the nitrogen in the fermentation of folic acid appeared as an amino acid, which Dr. Hutchings identified as glutamic acid. Thus we found that the elimination of glutamic acid from fermentation folate converted it into liver folic acid form.

We also found a breakdown product—again, using a hydrolysis reaction—formed from liver folic acid that had an absorption spectrum similar to *p*-aminobenzoic acid, but which was found to be more polar when measured by comparisons between water and organic solvents. Subsequently, it was identified as *N-(p*-aminobenzoyl)glutamic acid. The identification of the amine component was made with little difficulty because Lederle had the good fortune of being near a control laboratory that did sulfonamide assays by the Bratton and Marshall test.

A fluorescent pigment of folate from aerobic alkaline oxidation was identified as 2-amino-4-hydroxy-6-carboxypteridine by Dr. John Mowat. The parallel appearance of the fluorescent pterin and the aromatic amino group suggested that the pterin fragment was linked to the amino group of *p*-aminobenzoic acid. The susceptibility of the linkage to aerobic, but not to anaerobic cleavage, and the behavior of model compounds, suggested a methylene bridge ($-CH_2-$) between the two components.

Liver folic acid was, therefore, postulated to consist of a pteridine linked by a methylene bridge to *N-(p*-aminobenzoyl) glutamic acid. On the basis of this proposed structure, Dr. Coy Waller achieved the synthesis of folic acid using dibrompropionaldehyde, 2,4,5-triamino-6-hydroxypyrimidine and *N-(p*-aminobenzoyl)glutamic acid in a single reaction mixture. The structure and synthesis of folic acid were reported in 1945, and folic acid was given the chemical name of pteroylglutamic acid. This work was made possibly by the collaboration of two groups working on different aspects of the problem. These included Drs. Angier, Boothe, Hutchings, Mowat, Semb, Stokstad, SubbaRow, and Waller from Lederle Laboratories and Cosulich, Fahrenbach, Hultquist, Kuh, Northey, Seeger, Sickles, and Smith from the Calco Chemical Divisions of the American Cyanamid Co.

While this work was proceeding at Lederle, Dr. Hogan collaborated with Dr. Pfiffner and Dr. O'Dell at Parke Davis and Co. They were the first to report the isolation of vitamin B_c conjugase (folic acid) from liver. They also identified yeast folic acid as pteroylheptaglutamate, thus calling attention to the existence of the longer polyglutamates of folate. When synthetic folate acid became available, its role in human and animal nutrition was quickly established. Biochemical studies showed that the reduced form due to the addition of hydrogen atoms (tetrahydrofolate) functioned as a coenzyme in the transfer of single carbon units, such as in the formation of nucleic acids and the amino acid methionine.

Once folic acid has been synthesized, structural analogues were quickly made. This opened new avenues of research as some of the potent antifolates were found to be effective as antitumor agents. The best known is methotrexate, which was synthesized by Cosulich, Hultquist, and Seeger in 1948. This contains an extra amino and methyl group in the structure. It is a potent inhibitor of the conversion of dihydrofolate to tetrahydrofolate. In the synthesis of thymidylate (used in DNA), the methylene group of methylene-tetrahydrofolate is converted to a methyl group with a corresponding oxidation of tetrahydrofolate to dihydrofolate. Methotrexate blocks the conversion of dihydrofolate back to tetrahydrofolate, thus inhibiting the synthesis of more thymidylate, and, in turn, the formation of DNA. This inhibition of thymidylate synthesis by methotrexate is the basis of its anti-tumor activity. The elucidation of the function of folic acid in nucleic acid formation then opened up a new field of tumor chemotherapy based on other folate antimetabolites.

Dr. Stokstad is Professor Emeritus of Nutritional Sciences at the University of California, Berkeley. He has worked in the folic acid field since 1938.

North Americans at risk for folate deficiency

Folate deficiencies sometimes appear in pregnancy. Pregnant women need extra folate to meet the greater cell division rate, and therefore greater DNA synthesis, for themselves and the fetus. Prenatal care routinely includes vitamin and mineral supplements enriched with folate to compensate for extra pregnancy needs. This is one important reason why women need to see their physicians early in pregnancy. They need to increase the folate sources in their diet and/or start their folate supplements as soon as possible.

Folate status can be assessed using blood levels of the nutrient.

Even young women often register low serum folate values, especially those on oral contraceptives.[11] It is important for women to seek good sources of folate that they enjoy eating and then eat those foods regularly.

Folate deficiencies also often occur in alcoholism. In fact, a folate-related (megaloblastic) anemia often tips off a physician to the possibility of alcoholism. Alcohol disrupts folate absorption, probably by inhibiting the conjugase enzyme system in the small intestine that is needed for efficient absorption.[6,33]

Toxicity of folate

There are no documented symptoms of folate toxicity, probably because it is difficult to consume large doses of folate. In the United States, the FDA limits the amount of folate in nonprescription vitamin supplements to 400 micrograms when no statement of age is listed on the label. When age-related doses are listed, there can be no more than 100 micrograms for infants, 300 micrograms for children, or 400 micrograms for adults. Therefore consuming a large amount of folate would require eating many, many vitamin pills.

The FDA limits the amount of folate in a vitamin supplement to prevent its masking a vitamin B-12 deficiency. The metabolism of folate and vitamin B-12 are linked, as we will soon discuss. For now, note that the major early detectable symptom of a vitamin B-12 deficiency is the alteration in blood cell formation, mainly resulting in megaloblastic anemia.[14] However, if a large amount of folate is consumed regularly, this symptom does not occur—despite a vitamin B-12 deficiency.

A vitamin B-12 deficiency, for other reasons, can also eventually result in paralysis and death. So if a vitamin B-12 deficiency is developing in a person, it is important for a physician to diagnose and treat it early. *The FDA wants to ensure that the early warning sign of a vitamin B-12 deficiency (altered red blood cell formation) is not "masked" by an overzealous folate supplementation practice.* Therefore the FDA limits the amount of folate manufacturers can put into vitamin supplements. Since only about 100 micrograms of folate are usually needed to treat a true folate deficiency, the limits set by this FDA mandate are appropriate.[14]

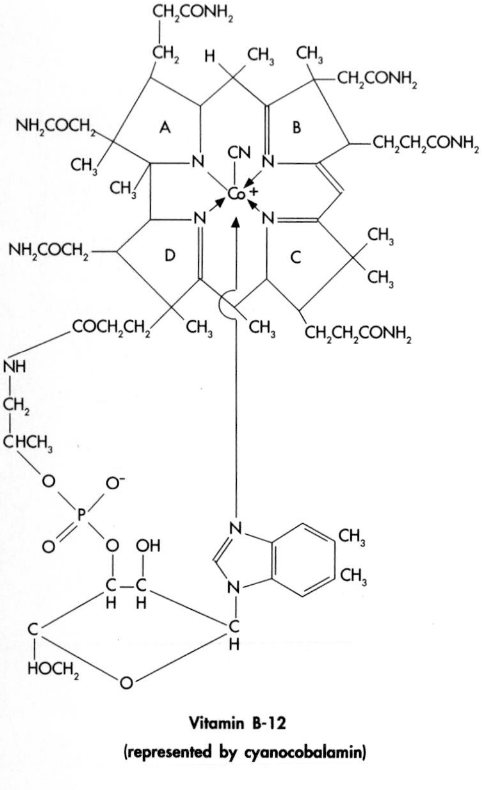

VITAMIN B-12

Vitamin B-12 actually represents a family of compounds that contain cobalt. They form the active coenzymes such as methylcobalamin. All vitamin B-12 compounds are synthesized by bacteria, fungi, and other lower organisms.

Vitamin B-12
(represented by cyanocobalamin)

Absorption of vitamin B-12

Vitamin B-12 in food enters the stomach and is liberated from other materials by digestion, especially by the action of stomach acid. The free vitamin B-12 then binds with a protein called **R-protein,** produced by salivary glands in the mouth (Figure 12-5). Researchers think the R-protein prevents bacteria in the small intestine from absorbing and using the vitamin B-12. The R-protein/vitamin B-12 complex travels to the small intestine, where the pancreatic enzyme trypsin removes the R-protein.

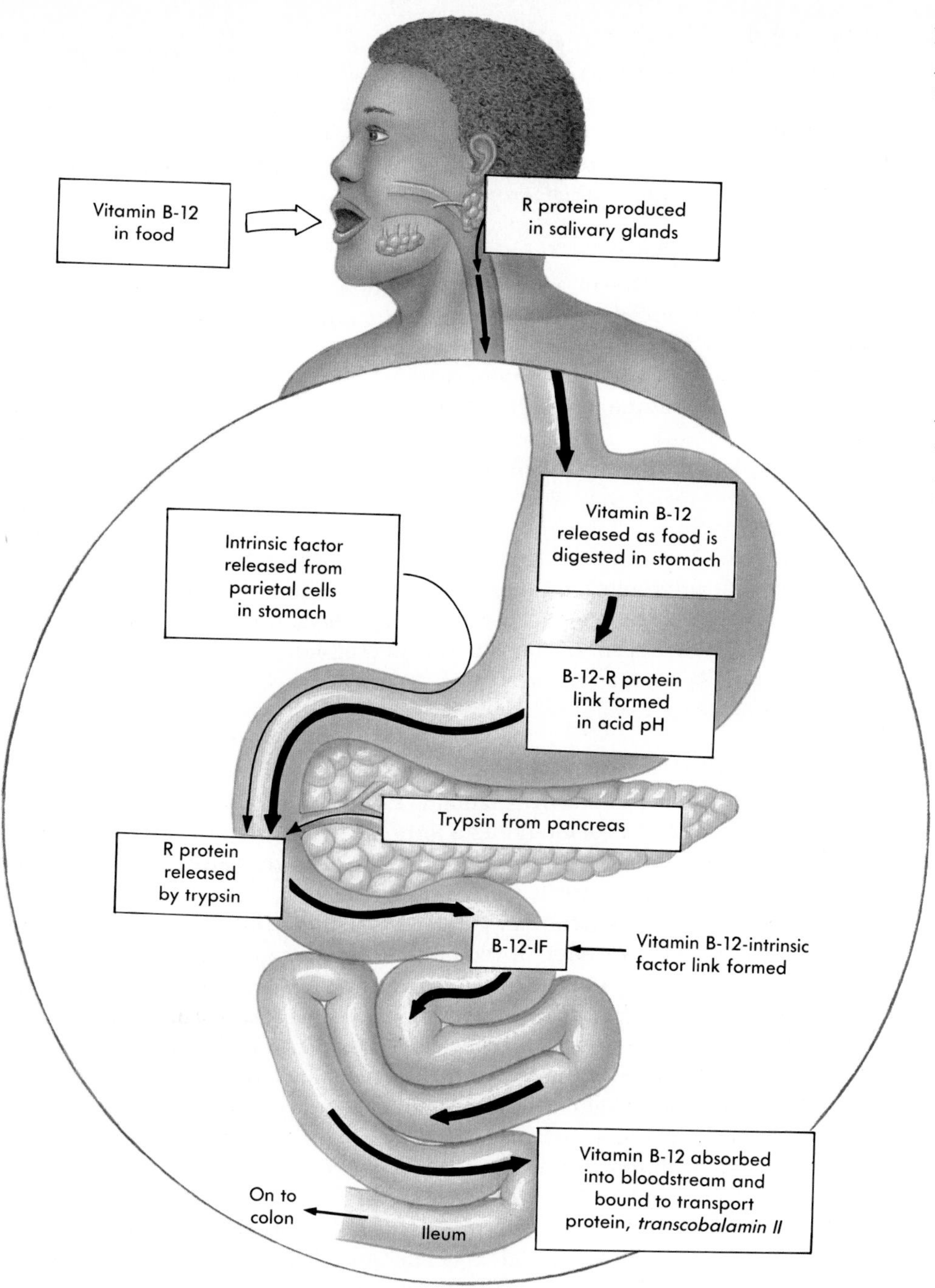

Figure 12-5
Absorption of vitamin B-12. Many factors and sites in the GI tract participate.

R-protein
A protein produced by the salivary glands that enhances vitamin B-12 absorption possibly by protecting it during its passage through the stomach.

Once vitamin B-12 is free again, it binds to **intrinsic factor,** a type of protein made by the stomach's acid-producing parietal cells. The resulting intrinsic factor/vitamin B-12 complex travels to the last portion of the small intestine, the ileum. Ileum cells absorb vitamin B-12 and transfer it to a special blood transport protein. Using this system, approximately 30% to 70% of dietary vitamin B-12 is absorbed, depending on the body's need for it. Any failure in this system results in only 1% to 2% absorption of dietary vitamin B-12.

intrinsic factor
A protein-like compound produced by the stomach that enhances vitamin B-12 absorption.

Vitamin B-12 absorption can be disrupted by inefficient synthesis of intrinsic factor, a genetic deficiency in R-protein synthesis, a lack of trypsin synthesis by the pancreas, poor binding of the intrinsic factor/vitamin B-12 complex in the ileum, or the absence of an ileum or stomach. In addition, a host of other variants prevents vitamin B-12 absorption, including surgical removal of key parts of the stomach, bacterial overgrowth of the small intestine, and tape worm infestations.

In the 1920s, researchers noted that they could cure a vitamin B-12 deficiency with massive amounts of liver or with concentrated water extracts of liver. In this case, the researchers cured a vitamin B-12 absorption defect by providing enough vitamin to allow simple diffusion to suffice. No R-protein/intrinsic factor system was needed.

Once a defect in absorption is established, the person must then take monthly injections of vitamin B-12 to bypass the need for absorption, use a vitamin B-12 nasal gel (nasal absorption does not require the intrinsic factor), or take very potent vitamin B-12 supplements weekly (300 times the RDA). *95 percent of all cases of vitamin B-12 deficiencies in healthy people result from a defect in vitamin B-12 absorption, rather than from inadequate intakes.*

FUNCTIONS OF VITAMIN B-12

Vitamin B-12 participates in a variety of reactions. Probably its most important function is in folate metabolism. Once the folate coenzyme is bonded to a methyl group ($-CH_3$), a form of vitamin B-12 is needed to remove the methyl group. Without vitamin B-12, the folate coenzymes are quickly bound by methyl groups. The cell then has insufficient free folate coenzymes for metabolic needs. This shortage prevents other important metabolic reactions, such as DNA synthesis, from taking place in the cell. Thus *a vitamin B-12 deficiency contributes to a secondary folate deficiency.* The metabolism of vitamin B-12 and of folate are closely intertwined.

Another vital function of vitamin B-12 is maintaining the myelin sheaths that insulate nerve fibers from each other. People with vitamin B-12 deficiencies show patchy destruction of the myelin sheaths.[4] While the actual cause is unknown, alterations in the metabolism of the amino acid methionine and other compounds may contribute. Whatever the cause, this destruction eventually causes paralysis, and perhaps death.

Pernicious anemia

pernicious anemia
The anemia that results from a lack of vitamin B-12 absorption; it is pernicious because of associated nerve degeneration that can result in eventual paralysis.

In the past, the inability to absorb vitamin B-12 eventually led to death. Researchers in mid-19th century England noted a form of anemia that caused death within 2 to 5 years of initial illness. They called this **pernicious anemia** (pernicious literally means "leading to death"). Clinically, the anemia looks much like a folate deficiency anemia. You can probably guess why—the folate/vitamin B-12 connections. Many macrocytes are seen in the bloodstream (Figure 12-4). Thus the vitamin B-12 anemia is called a macrocytic anemia. Strictly speaking, a lack of vitamin B-12 in the diet alone cannot cause pernicious anemia. Only a decreased ability to absorb vitamin B-12 can cause it, because it takes too long to develop significant nerve destruction due to a true dietary deficiency. Once pernicious anemia is noted, an injection of vitamin B-12 reverses changes in red blood cell synthesis and other clinical signs in 1 to 2 days.

Pernicious anemia and its resulting nerve destruction often occur in elderly people. The average age in whites is 68 years. In blacks and Hispanics it appears about a decade sooner.[7] As stomach parietal cells age, they lose their ability to synthesize the intrinsic factor, which is needed for vitamin B-12 absorption. Current research suggests that this failure is due to an autoimmune reaction—people make white blood cells and other factors that attack their own parietal cells. Because parietal cells make acid, pernicious anemia is often accompanied by a decrease in stomach acid production, called **achlorhydria.**

achlorhydria
Decrease in stomach acid primarily due to age-associated loss of acid-producing stomach cells.

Besides anemia, clinical signs and symptoms of pernicious anemia include weakness, sore tongue, back pain, apathy, and tingling in the extremities. It takes about 3 years for symptoms of nerve destruction to develop.

Other functions of vitamin B-12

Vitamin B-12 has other important functions. One is to rearrange carbon atoms in derivatives of odd chain fatty acids so that they can eventually enter the citric acid cycle. The synthesis of the amino acid methionine from homocysteine also requires vitamin B-12.

Vitamin B-12 in foods

The most nutrient-dense sources of vitamin B-12 are liver, clams, oysters, and hot dogs. Beef, pork, eggs, and milk are also good sources (Table 12-8). *Vitamin B-12 is present only in animal foods.* While plants do not contain vitamin B-12, bacteria and soil contamination of vegetables and the process of fermentation may contribute some to the vegan's diet. However, these are not reliable sources (see reference no. 9 in Chapter 6). Animals, such as cows and sheep, obtain vitamin B-12 from either bacterial synthesis in their multiple stomachs (rumens) or from soil they ingest while eating and grazing.

Table 12-8

Good food sources of vitamin B-12, ranked by nutrient density

Food	Serving size to yield 2 micrograms*	kcalories needed to yield 2 micrograms
Beef liver, fried	1/16 ounce	3
Oysters	1½ each	10
Clams, canned	⅛ cup, 0.12 ounce	150
Roast beef	1½ ounces	65
Egg	1¾ each	140
1% milk, low-fat	1¾ cups	180
Frankfurter, beef	3 each	240
Ham, baked	7½ ounces	350

*RDA for adults.
Manytypes of animal protein provide ample vitamin B-12 within a reasonable energy intake.

RDA for vitamin B-12

The RDA for vitamin B-12 for adults is 2 micrograms per day. The U.S. food supply yields approximately 8 micrograms of vitamin B-12 per person per day. This high intake provides the average meat-eating person with 2 to 3 years' storage of vitamin B-12 in the liver. *Thus if you eat animal foods regularly and can absorb vitamin B-12, a vitamin B-12 deficiency is highly unlikely.*

It takes approximately 20 years of consuming a diet essentially free of vitamin B-12 for a person to exhibit nerve destruction caused by a deficiency. However, as mentioned before, it takes only approximately 2 to 3 years to see the same nerve destruction if a person develops an inability to absorb vitamin B-12. That shows the degree to which the body can reclaim the vitamin B-12 it secretes into the small intestine if absorption is possible. Supplements of vitamin B-12 are virtually nontoxic.

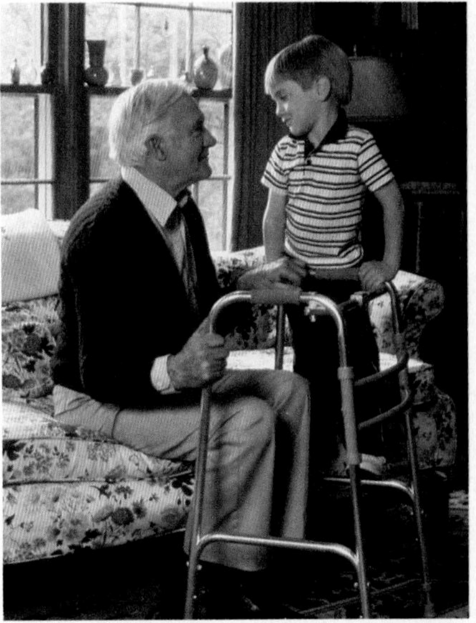

Due to poor vitamin B-12 absorption, older adults have a greater risk for pernicious anemia than younger adults.

North Americans at risk of a vitamin B-12 deficiency

Vegans who eat no animal products should find a source of vitamin B-12. Options include a vitamin supplement, fortified soy milk, and special yeast grown in media rich in vitamin B-12. Otherwise, a vitamin B-12 deficiency is possible. The elderly are at risk for developing pernicious anemia. Regular physical exams should especially look for enlarged red blood cells, low blood levels of vitamin B-12, and nervous tingling in the extremities.[16]

VITAMIN C

Vitamin C (ascorbic acid) is a puzzling vitamin. It is found in all living tissues, and most animals synthesize their own from glucose. Note the similarity in structure

Concept Check

Folate is needed for cell division because it is tied to RNA and DNA synthesis. A folate deficiency results in anemia, as well as inflammation of the tongue, diarrhea, and poor growth—all signs of poor cell division. Folate is found in fresh vegetables and organ meats. It is important to emphasize "fresh" and "lightly cooked" with vegetables, because much folate is lost during cooking. Folate needs during pregnancy are especially high. Otherwise, a deficiency appears most often in alcoholism. Vitamin B-12 is necessary for folate metabolism. Without dietary vitamin B-12, folate deficiency symptoms, such as anemia, develop. In addition, vitamin B-12 is necessary for maintaining the nervous system: paralysis can develop from a vitamin B-12 deficiency. Vitamin B-12 is found only in animal foods; meat eaters generally have a 3 to 5 year supply stored in the liver. Vitamin B-12 absorption may decline in the elderly years, requiring monthly injections.

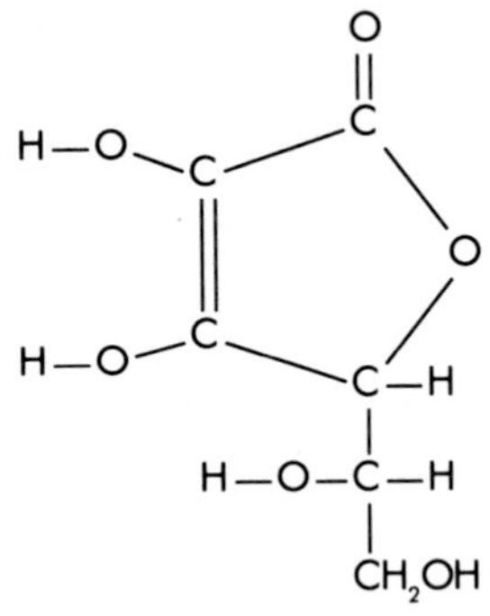

Ascorbic acid

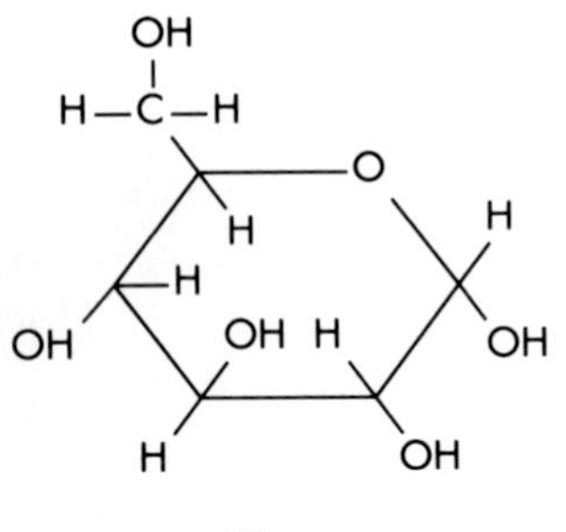

Glucose

between vitamin C and glucose. Only guinea pigs, monkeys, some birds, a few fish, and humans need vitamin C in their diets. What is strange is that animals who synthesize vitamin C often make quite a lot of it. For instance, a pig produces 8 grams per day (though we do not benefit from it when we eat pork, since it is lost in processing). This amount is over 130 times our human RDA of 60 milligrams, and even 60 milligrams appears to be quite a generous intake for humans. As little as 10 milligrams daily can prevent scurvy, the vitamin C deficiency disease. Why some animals make so much vitamin C, while a few other animals, including humans, appear to need so little, has fueled much controversy surrounding this vitamin.

Absorption and metabolism of vitamin C

Absorption of vitamin C occurs in the small intestine by means of an active transport system. About 80% to 90% of vitamin C is absorbed when a person eats between 30 and 180 milligrams of it per day. If someone ingests 6 grams per day, absorption efficiency drops to about 20%. *A common side effect of high vitamin C intakes is diarrhea.* The unabsorbed vitamin C stays in the small intestine and attracts water until it finally causes diarrhea. Some health food enthusiasts even claim that the ideal dosage of vitamin C is one that produces diarrhea.

Vitamin C can be reversibly changed by losing 2 hydrogen ions to form dehydroascorbic acid. Dehydroascorbic acid can then regain 2 hydrogen ions to re-form ascorbic acid. When vitamin C is broken down in the body, dehydroascorbic acid is irreversibly converted into diketogulonic acid. This acid is then converted into oxalic acid and other products. When high levels of vitamin C are consumed, most of it is excreted in the urine as vitamin C itself or a slight derivative. Oxalic acid is a major breakdown product at low doses (100 milligrams).

Functions of vitamin C

Collagen synthesis. Vitamin C performs a variety of very important cellular functions. It does this primarily by providing electrons to activate metal and oxygen ions—especially iron in the Fe^{+2} state—so that enzymes can use these "activated" ions to perform additions of hydroxyl groups (−OH) to other molecules.[20] *Probably its most notable reaction is the addition of a hydroxyl group to the amino acid proline within a protein to form the hydroxyproline residue.* There is also an analogous reaction where the amino acid hydroxylysine is synthesized from the amino acid lysine within some proteins. The synthesis of these two amino acid residues is important for the formation and cross-bonding of the protein collagen, which plays a crucial role in body protein support systems.

Collagen is found in high concentrations in connective tissues, bone, and

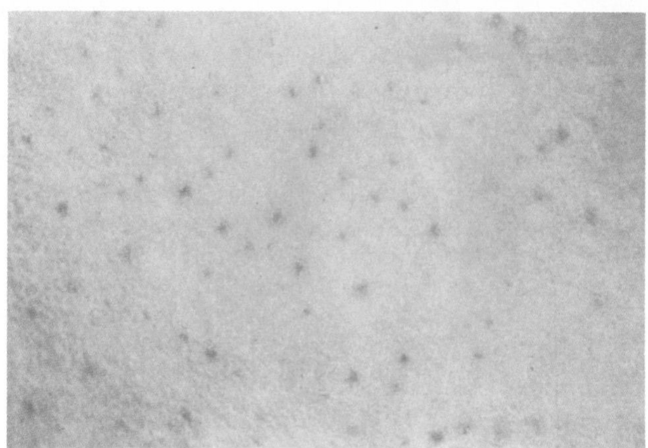

Figure 12-6

Pinpoint hemorrhages on the skin—an early stage of scurvy. The spots are caused by slight bleeding into hair follicles. The person will also often show poor wound healing—all signs of poor collagen synthesis.

blood vessels, and is very important for wound healing. The cross-bonding of collagen, which is increased by vitamin C, stabilizes collagen and so greatly strengthens the tissues it helps form. Widespread changes in tissue metabolism and structure occur when a person is deficient in vitamin C. One symptom of scurvy is a reduction in the rate of wound healing.

Other symptoms of scurvy include weakness, opening of previously healed wounds, bone pain, fractures, bleeding gums, diarrhea, and pinpoint hemorrhages (petechiae) around hair follicles on the back of the arms and legs (Figure 12-6).[24] Most of these symptoms are linked to a decrease in collagen synthesis.

The first symptoms of scurvy appear after about 20 to 40 days of no vitamin C intake and include weakness and tiny hemorrhages in the skin. In addition, gums bleed and joints become painful.[2]

Scurvy was the bane of sailors throughout the 19th century. On long sea voyages a captain often lost half or more of his crew to scurvy. From 1556 to 1857, more than 114 scurvy epidemics were reported in Europe. Soldiers in the U.S. Civil War died of scurvy. In 1740, Dr. James Lind, working aboard the HMS Salisbury, showed that citrus fruits—two oranges and one lemon a day—could cure scurvy. Fifty years after Lind's discovery, rations for British sailors included limes to prevent scurvy. That is why the British today are often called "limeys."

Antioxidant. Vitamin C is one of the cell's water-soluble antioxidants. Recall that vitamin E is a fat-soluble antioxidant in the cell membrane. Using its antioxidant capabilities, vitamin C can reduce the formation of carcinogenic nitrosamines in the stomach and also keep the folate coenzymes intact and so prevent their destruction. If vitamin C is found effective in preventing cancer, its effectiveness will probably be due to its antioxidant capabilities.

Enhancing iron absorption. Vitamin C is important for iron absorption because it keeps iron in the Fe^{+2} form. This conversion renders the iron much more soluble in the small intestine's alkaline environment, and thus increases iron absorption. To produce this effect, about 50 milligrams of vitamin C (about 4 ounces of orange juice) must be consumed at the same meal with the iron.

Increasing vitamin C intake is very beneficial if one has poor iron stores. However, some people suffer from a disease characterized by an overstorage of iron (hemochromatosis; see Chapter 14). These people are actually harmed if, by increasing their vitamin C intake, they likewise increase their iron absorption. This is just one of many examples in which recommending a vitamin intake above the RDA may have conflicting results. Some people may benefit, whereas others may be injured.

Synthesis of vital cell compounds. Vitamin C is necessary for the synthesis of thyroxine—the thyroid hormone—as well as epinephrine, carnitine, norepinephrine, serotonin, bile acids, steroid hormones, and purine bases used in DNA synthesis. The synthesis of many of these compounds requires the addition of hydroxyl groups.

Vitamin C is vital for the function of the immune system, especially for the activity of certain cells in the immune system. In addition, vitamin C is used by chemical-detoxifying mechanisms in cells. *Thus both disease states and drug use can increase the need for vitamin C, but we don't know how much vitamin C intake above the RDA to prescribe.*

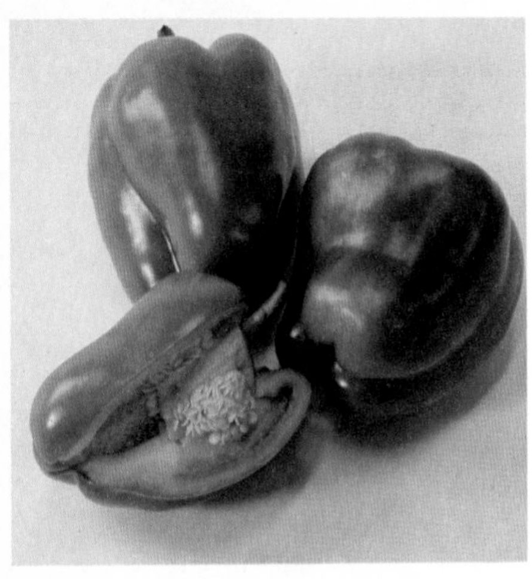

Many people may be surprised to learn that green peppers are a good source of vitamin C.

Vitamin C in foods

The most nutrient-dense sources of vitamin C are green peppers, cauliflower, broccoli, cabbage, strawberries, papayas, and romaine lettuce (Table 12-9). Citrus fruits, potatoes, and other green vegetables are also good sources of vitamin C. *The four servings of fruits and vegetables from the Daily Food Guide should easily provide enough vitamin C.* The major contributors of vitamin C to the U.S. diet are orange juice, grapefruit and grapefruit juice, tomatoes and tomato juice, fortified fruit drinks, oranges, tangerines, and potatoes. Note that the isoascorbate (erythrobate) that is used as a food preservative in fruits and vegetables has no vitamin C value.

Vitamin C is easily lost in processing and cooking. Juices are good foods to fortify with vitamin C because their acidity reduces vitamin C destruction. Vitamin C is very unstable when in contact with heat, iron, copper, or oxygen.

Table 12-9

Good sources of vitamin C, ranked by nutrient density

Food	Serving size to yield 60 milligrams*	kcalories needed to yield 60 milligrams
Green peppers, whole, raw	⅔ each	12
Cauliflower, cooked	1 cup	26
Bok choy cabbage, cooked	1-⅓ cups	27
Broccoli, cooked	⅔ cup	28
Strawberries, fresh	¾ cup	32
Mustard greens, cooked	2 cups	37
Brussel sprouts, cooked	⅔ cup	37
Papaya, whole fresh	⅓ each	38
Romaine lettuce, chopped	4-½ cups	41
Grapefruit pink/red	1-⅓ each	48
Cantaloupe	¼ each	50
Orange, fresh, medium	1 each	52
Asparagus, cooked	1-¼ cups	53
Orange juice, fresh	½ cup	53
Tomato juice, canned	1-⅓ each	56
Grapefruit white	1-½ each	60
Grapefruit juice, fresh	⅔ cup	61
Spinach, cooked	1-½ cups	62
Tomato, whole raw	2-¾ each	65
Sauerkraut, canned	2 cups	75

*RDA for adults.
All these foods provide ample vitamin C within both a limited serving size and kcalorie cost. Emphasize these fruits and vegetables for a nutritious diet.

RDA for vitamin C

The RDA for vitamin C for adults is 60 milligrams per day. The current RDA suggests cigarette smokers consume 100 milligrams per day because they greatly stress their lungs. The U.S. food supply yields about twice the adult RDA (120 milligrams) of vitamin C per day, of which approximately 82 milligrams is derived naturally from foods. The rest comes from food supplements. So probably almost all of us are meeting our daily need for vitamin C.

North Americans at risk for vitamin C deficiency

Today vitamin C deficiency appears mostly in alcoholic persons who eat very nutrient-poor diets and in elderly men who live alone and also eat poorly. Men are more susceptible than women because they smoke more and are less apt to consume vitamin supplements. Smokers also generally have lower vitamin C stores.[17] Studies show that 14% to 20% of adult and elderly men have low serum vitamin C levels. Worldwide, scurvy is associated with poverty. It is especially common in infants who are fed boiled milk (all forms of milk are poor sources of vitamin C) and not provided with a good food source of vitamin C or a supplement.

Vitamin C status is assessed by its concentration in white blood cells. A diet history of limited fruit and vegetable consumption also suggests a deficiency.

Toxicity of vitamin C

Vitamin C is probably not toxic when consumed in amounts less than 1 to 2 grams. Regularly consuming more than that can cause stomach inflammation, diarrhea, overabsorption of iron, oxalate kidney stones, and possibly a syndrome called "rebound" or "withdrawal" scurvy. What may happen in "rebound" scurvy is that the body, when receiving a high vitamin C intake, develops enzyme systems to rapidly excrete it. If one abruptly reduces the intake to normal, the enzyme systems take a while to readjust.[22] One may even find "rebound" scurvy in an infant born to a mother who consumed large amounts of vitamin C during pregnancy. When born, the child's daily dose of vitamin C drastically decreases. If a person has a history of a high vitamin C intake, slowly tapering it is recommended, rather than abruptly cutting down.

Many attributes of large doses of vitamin C—consisting of 2 grams or more per day—have been suggested. *The mistaken notion is that if 60 milligrams of vitamin C are enough for good health, and higher doses may produce even better health. This assertion is not established by reputable research.*[37]

Most vitamin C consumed in large doses just ends up in the stool or the urine. The body is totally saturated at intakes of 150 milligrams per day. In any event, maladies such as common colds are rarely severe enough, nor last long enough, to merit megadose vitamin C therapy. Consuming vitamin C may decrease a cold's severity somewhat, so we see no reason to discourage people from drinking a few glasses of orange juice when they have a cold. If it doesn't help them physically, it may help them psychologically. *Psychological effects can often work wonders. However, there is no striking evidence from double-blind studies that large amounts of vitamin C greatly decrease the severity or duration of a cold.*

In addition, no credible evidence suggests that a dose even as high as 10 grams a day will cure colon cancer.[28] Early studies that suggested this were too poorly controlled to be credible. If people with cancer want to dabble with large doses of vitamin C, they should alert their physician, primarily because high doses of vitamin C can change reactions to medical tests for diabetes or blood in the stool. Physicians may misdiagnose conditions when large doses of vitamin C are consumed without their knowledge.

As suggested earlier, there is a possibility that vitamin C, acting as an antioxidant, may help prevent cancer. For that reason, we encourage you to regularly consume fruits and vegetables. However, there are no data to support a stronger suggestion.

Now that we have discussed the vitamins, review the Daily Food Guide in Chapter 2 and note how each group makes an important vitamin contribution. Also, see Table 12-10.

VITAMIN-LIKE COMPOUNDS

The various vitamin-like compounds—choline, carnitine, inositol, taurine, and lipoic acid—are necessary to maintain proper metabolism in the body. They can be synthesized by the body, but that often occurs at the expense of important essential nutrients, such as essential amino acids. The needs for these compounds also often increases in times of rapid tissue growth, as for the premature infant.[34]

There is no concern that these vitamin-like compounds are needed by the average healthy adult. But more research is needed for certain disease states,

Table 12-10

A summary of the water-soluble vitamins

Name and coenzyme	Major functions	Deficiency symptoms	People most at risk
Thiamin; TPP	TPP is involved with enzymes in glycolysis, the citric acid cycle, hexosemonophosphate shunt; nerve function	Beriberi; nervous tingling, poor coordination, edema, heart changes, weakness	Alcoholism, poverty
Riboflavin; FAD and FMN	Coenzymes involved in citric acid cycle, electron transport chain, fat breakdown; drug-detoxifying pathways	Ariboflavinosis; inflammation of mouth and tongue, cracks at corners of the mouth, eye disorders	Possibly people on certain medications if no dairy products consumed
Niacin; NAD and NADP	Coenzymes involved in glycolysis, citric acid cycle, electron transport chain, fat synthesis, fat breakdown	Pellagra; diarrhea, bilateral dermatitis dementia	Severe poverty where corn is the dominant food; alcoholism
Pantothenic acid; Coenzyme A, acylcarrier protein	Citric acid cycle, fat synthesis, fat breakdown	Using an antagonist causes tingling in hands, fatigue, headache, nausea	Alcoholism
Biotin, biocytin	Glucose production, fat synthesis, purine (part of DNA, RNA) synthesis	Dermatitis, tongue soreness, anemia, depression	Alcoholism
Vitamin B-6, pyridoxine and other forms; PLP	Protein metabolism, neurotransmitter synthesis, hemoglobin synthesis, many other functions	Headache, anemia, convulsions, nausea, vomiting, flaky skin, sore tongue	Adolescent and adult women; people on certain medications; alcholism
Folate (folic acid); THFA	DNA and RNA synthesis, amino acid synthesis, choline synthesis	Megaloblastic anemia, inflammation of tongue, diarrhea, poor growth, mental disorders	Alcoholism, pregnancy, use of certain medications
Vitamin B-12 (cobalamins)	Folate metabolism, nerve function	Macrocytic anemia, poor nerve function	Elderly due to poor absorption; vegans
Vitamin C (ascorbic acid)	Collagen synthesis, hormone synthesis, neurotransmitter synthesis	Scurvy; poor wound healing, pinpoint hemorrhages, bleeding gums, edema	Alcoholism, elderly men living alone

Concept Check

Vitamin C deserves a credible scientific evaluation because of the high interest in it. Only guinea pigs, monkeys, some birds and fish, and humans need dietary vitamin C. It is used mainly to help synthesize collagen, a major connective tissue protein. A vitamin C deficiency, known as scurvy, causes many changes in the skin and gums, such as small hemorrhages. This is due to poor collagen synthesis. Vitamin C also improves iron absorption and is involved in synthesizing certain hormones and neurotransmitters. Citrus fruits, green peppers, cauliflower, broccoli, and strawberries are good sources of vitamin C. As with folate, fresh or lightly cooked foods are important to emphasize, since loss of vitamin C in cooking can be high. At doses greater than about 15 times the RDA (1 gram), vitamin C can lead to diarrhea. These high doses do not prevent the common cold or cure cancer; however, consuming the RDA of vitamin C is part of the overall approach to good health.

RDA or ESADDI	Dietary sources	Toxicity
1.1-1.5 milligrams	Sunflower seeds, pork, whole and enriched grains, dried beans	None possible from food
1.2-1.7 milligrams	Milk, mushrooms, spinach, liver, enriched grains	None reported
15-19 milligrams	Mushrooms, bran, tuna, chicken, beef, peanuts, enriched grains	Flushing of skin at > 100 milligrams
4-7 milligrams	Mushrooms, liver, broccoli, eggs; most foods have some	None
30-100 micrograms	Cheese, egg yolks, cauliflower, peanut butter	Unknown
1.8-2 milligrams	Animal protein foods, spinach, broccoli, bananas	Nerve destruction at doses > 100 milligrams
180-200 micrograms	Green leafy vegetables, orange juice, organ meats, sprouts	None, nonprescription as vitamin dosage is controlled by FDA
2 micrograms	Animal foods, especially organ meats	None
60 milligrams	Citrus fruits, strawberries, broccoli	Doses > 1-2 grams causes diarrhea and can alter some diagnostic tests

specifically concerning their addition to infant formulas and total parenteral nutrition solutions. Presently, manufacturers often add these vitamin-like compounds to infant formulas.

Choline

Choline is widely distributed within the plant and animal kingdoms. So much choline naturally occurs in the diet that a deficiency is hardly possible. Choline has a very simple structure. It can be built in the liver using carbon atoms from the amino acid methionine, along with the help of folate and vitamin B-12. Under normal circumstances, if enough choline is not in the diet, the body can make the rest if enough methionine-containing protein is eaten.[25]

Choline forms part of the emulsifier lecithin (actually called phosphatidylcholine) and the neurotransmitter acetylcholine, as well as other compounds. Lecithin is widely distributed in blood lipoproteins, cell membranes, and bile. The name choline actually comes from "chole," which means bile.

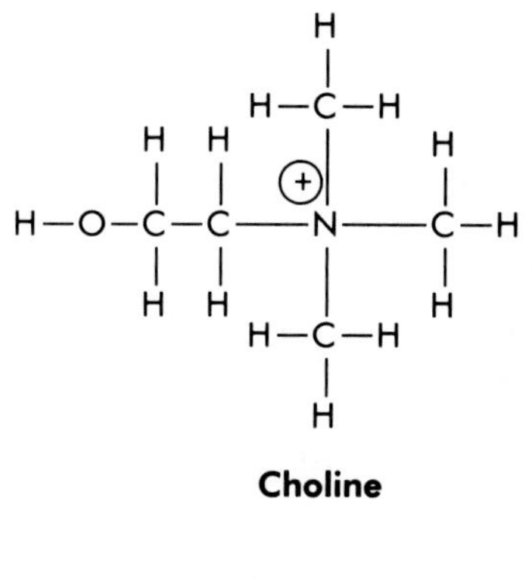

Choline

A choline-free diet in animals probably causes a choline deficiency, of which a major symptom is a fatty liver. Animals evidently cannot make enough to supply all their needs. This type of fatty liver is not the same type as that seen in alcoholism. Attempts to treat alcoholic fatty liver with high doses of choline or lecithin have failed. Scientists have attempted to treat some neurological disorders, such as Alzheimer's disease and other forms of senile memory loss, with lecithin. It is too early to say if these problems can benefit from that treatment. This is an active research area.[34]

We consume probably 400 to 900 milligrams of choline per day. Doses as high as 20 to 30 grams per day have been administered. The side effects include a "fishy" body odor, especially when choline itself, rather than lecithin, is used. Gastric distress, vomiting, and diarrhea may also result. There is some concern that these high doses of choline may also increase the risk of developing stomach cancer, since choline can be metabolized to compounds that then form nitrosamines. These are very powerful carcinogens.

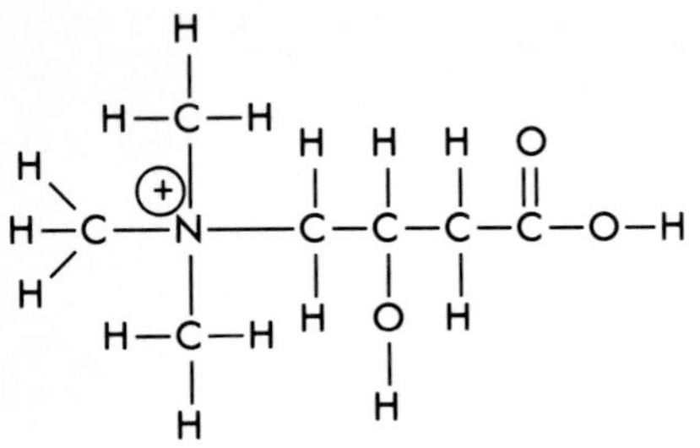

Carnitine

Carnitine in the cell primarily shuttles long chain fatty acids from the cytosol into the mitochondria so that fatty acids can be burned to provide energy. Carnitine also shuttles the breakdown products of some amino acids into the mitochondria. With the help of vitamin B-6 our liver cells make carnitine using the amino acids lysine and methionine. People with very low protein intakes, such as people with kwashiorkor (see Chapter 6), appear to have lower levels of carnitine in the bloodstream. Thus it is important to eat an adequate amount of protein to supply the building blocks needed for making this compound. There is concern that people with cirrhosis of the liver may need carnitine supplements because carnitine is made in the liver. See the Expert Opinion in Chapter 7 to see if this is also true for athletes.

Carnitine

Meat and dairy products are the main sources of carnitine. We consume about 100 to 300 milligrams per day. Vegetarian diets are very low in carnitine because it is not found in plant foods. However, vegetarians show normal blood levels of carnitine. Consequently, nutritionists doubt whether carnitine is necessary for maintaining health.[13] In times of recovery from disease or serious trauma, carnitine supplements may be important.[8]

Inositol

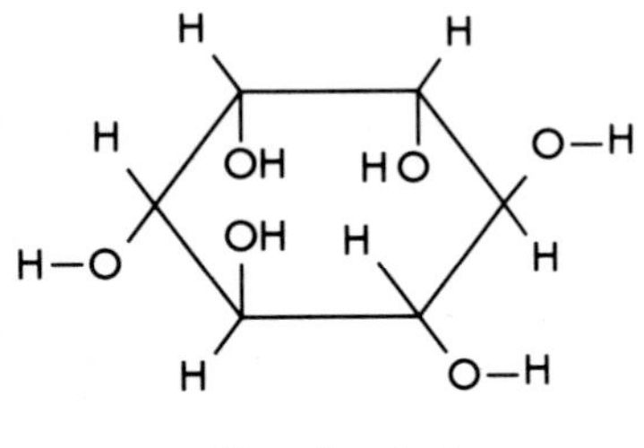

There are 9 forms of inositol. The one used by humans is called myo-inositol. Inositol has a structure similar to that of glucose. We make inositol from glucose. This compound functions as part of phosphotidylinositol, which is found in high concentrations in the brain and forms part of the structure there. Inositol also forms a basic part of phytic acid, a substance that binds minerals in plant foods, such as wheat bran. We eat about 1 gram of inositol per day. It is widely found in both plant and animal products.[15]

Myo-inositol

Taurine

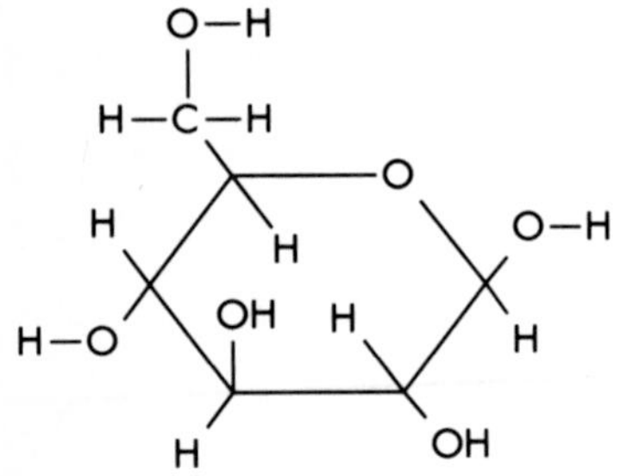

Taurine performs many vital functions. It forms part of some bile acids, is necessary for nerve function, and is important for vision. It is synthesized from the amino acids methionine and cysteine, and is found only in animal foods. Taurine looks like the amino acid glycine except for the substitution of a sulfur-containing group. It is the only free amino acid readily found in nature (others are combined into proteins).

No clear cases of taurine deficiencies have been diagnosed in vegans, and again it is not found in plants. Thus it appears that healthy people need not worry about consuming taurine. Synthesis by the body apparently meets our needs.

During rapid growth we seem to need more taurine.[10] Once growth rates level off in adulthood, the need for taurine decreases. Premature infants now have taurine added to their formulas, primarily because the taurine concentration in human milk is very high.

Glucose

```
   O H H
   ‖ | |
H—O—S—C—C—H
   ‖ | |
   O H N
      / \
     H   H
```

Taurine

```
     O H
     ‖ |
H—O—C—C—H
       |
       N
      / \
     H   H
```

Glycine

Lipoic acid

Lipoic acid is used in reactions in which a carbon dioxide molecule is lost, as when pyruvate is converted into acetyl-CoA. Health food stores sell this compound, but our bodies can make lipoic acid.

```
  H H H H H H H O
  | | | | | | | ‖
H—C—C—C—C—C—C—C—C—OH
  |  H |  | | | |
  S————S  H H H H
```

Lipoic acid

Bogus vitamins

A variety of bogus vitamins is promoted by health food enthusiasts.[14] None of these compounds is important in human nutrition. Some may increase growth in less complex forms of life, so vitamin hucksters try to pass them off as necessary for humans.

The list of these pseudo-vitamins changes frequently. The following list shows some of the more persistent pseudos:

- **Para-aminobenzoic acid**—Recall that this compound is part of folic acid. If people consume this drug in conjunction with sulfa antibiotics, they can defeat the effect of the antibiotic.
- **Laetrile**—This cyanide-containing compound—wrongly labeled "vitamin B-17"—is promoted as a cure for cancer, but the FDA does not recognize it as a legitimate therapy.
- **Bioflavonoids**—These compounds—wrongly labeled "vitamin P"—include rutin and hesperidin. They were originally thought to be more effective than vitamin C alone for treating fragile blood vessels in scurvy. Today, there is no recognized nutritional or medical need for bioflavinoids, although they may enhance vitamin C absorption.
- **Pangamic acid**—This bogus compound—wrongly labeled "vitamin B-15"—has no link to nutrition and deserves no attention.

Other compounds will come and go in the next few years. Again, since people have been maintained for years on parenteral feedings containing all the known essential nutrients without developing deficiency symptoms, it is unlikely that any vitamin remains to be discovered. You can be sure that if a "new" compound has the potential to be a vitamin, the Food and Nutrition Board of the National Academy of Sciences will closely examine it. *If it then appears with the rest of the nutrients that have an RDA or ESADDI, you can be confident the compound can be called a vitamin and is worth your attention.*

Concept Check

A variety of vitamin-like compounds are found in the body. They can be synthesized by cells using common building blocks, such as amino acids and glucose. In disease states synthesis may not meet needs, and therefore dietary intake can be crucial. The need for choline, carnitine, and taurine in certain conditions, such as for premature infants or in total parenteral nutrition, are current areas of research.

Summary

1. Thiamin has a key role in carbohydrate metabolism. A deficiency results in problems in nervous system functions, primarily because nervous tissues use mostly carbohydrate for energy. Deficiencies are most likely in alcoholism. Pork, dried beans, and enriched grains are excellent sources of thiamin.
2. Riboflavin participates in the metabolism of all energy-yielding nutrients because it plays key roles in the citric acid cycle, electron transport chain, and fat breakdown. A deficiency results in mouth and tongue inflammation, but is quite unlikely unless a person does not consume dairy products and takes medication that hampers riboflavin availability. Enriched grains are a good source of riboflavin.
3. Niacin is a key nutrient used in many pathways for metabolism of energy-yielding nutrients. A deficiency results in severe skin lesions, dementia, diarrhea, and death. Alcoholism and the poor diets consumed by the impoverished can lead to a deficiency. High niacin concentrations are found in protein foods commonly consumed by North Americans.
4. Pantothenic acid participates in many aspects of cell metabolism, including fat metabolism and the citric acid cycle. A deficiency is unlikely since it is widely found in foods.
5. Biotin participates in glucose production and fat synthesis and contributes to DNA synthesis as well. A deficiency results in anemia and inflammation of the skin and tongue. It may appear with alcoholism. Synthesis by intestinal bacteria probably suffices for much of our needs and adds to the biotin found in eggs and cheese.
6. Vitamin B-6 forms a vital role in protein metabolism, especially in the synthesis of nonessential amino acids. It also participates in the synthesis of neurotransmitters and performs other metabolic roles. Headaches, anemia, nausea, and vomiting result from a deficiency. Generally, women are most likely to have poor vitamin B-6 stores. Regular consumption of animal protein foods, cauliflower, and broccoli provides needed vitamin B-6. Destruction of nervous system tissues appears from high doses, specifically at 12 times the RDA.
7. Folate plays an important role in RNA and DNA synthesis. Signs of poor cell division, such as anemia, tongue inflammation, diarrhea, and poor growth, appear in a deficiency. Pregnancy puts high demands for folate on the body. Otherwise, a deficiency occurs most likely in alcoholism. Excellent food sources are leafy vegetables, organ meats, and orange juice. Since the amount of folate lost in cooking can be great, dietary emphasis is on lightly cooked vegetables.
8. Vitamin B-12 is needed for metabolizing folate and maintaining the insulation surrounding nerves. A deficiency results in anemia (because of its relationship to folate) and nerve degeneration. Poor absorption of vitamin B-12 often occurs in the elderly. In these cases, monthly injections of the vitamin can be used. For others, a deficiency is unlikely because it is present in high concentrations in animal foods, which constitute a major part of the North American diet. Vitamin B-12 does not occur in plant foods, except through minor soil contamination. Vegans need to find a supplemental source.
9. Vitamin C is needed mainly to synthesize collagen, a major protein used in building connective tissue. A vitamin C deficiency results in scurvy, which is evidenced by poor wound healing, pinpoint hemorrhages in the skin, and bleeding gums. Vitamin C also enhances iron absorption and is needed for the synthesis of some hormones and neurotransmitters. Fresh fruits and vegetables, especially citrus fruits, are generally good sources. Since the amount of vitamin C lost in cooking is high, the dietary emphasis—as with folate—is on fresh or lightly cooked vegetables. Deficiencies often occur in people with

alcoholism and in elderly men whose diets lack enough fruits and vegetables. High doses of vitamin C often cause diarrhea.

10. A variety of vitamin-like compounds are found in the body. Cells synthesize them using common building blocks, such as amino acids and glucose. In disease states, synthesis may not meet needs, and therefore dietary intake becomes more critical. The need for choline, carnitine, and taurine in some conditions, such as for premature infants or for total parenteral nutrition, are current areas of research.

Take Action

Visit a health food store and browse through their magazines. How many statements about vitamins can you find that you consider fraudulent? Record at least 4 below. Discuss these statements with your friends and explore their point of view.

1. ______________________________

2. ______________________________

3. ______________________________

4. ______________________________

REFERENCES

1. Anonymous: Biotin deficiency due to total parenteral nutrition alters serum fatty acid composition, Reviews 47:121, 1989.
2. Anonymous: Experimental scurvy in a young man, Nutrition Reviews 44:13, 1986.
3. Albin RL and others: Acute sensory neuropathy-neuronopathy from pyridoxine overdose, Neurology 37:17, 29, 1987.
4. Beck WS: Cobalamin and the nervous system, New England Journal of Medicine 318:752, 1988.
5. Belko AZ and others: Effects of exercise on riboflavin requirements of young women, American Journal of Clinical Nutrition 37:509, 1983.
6. Blocker DE and Thenen SW: Intestinal absorption, liver uptake, and excretion of ^{3}H-folic acid-deficient, alcohol-consuming nonhuman primates, American Journal of Clinical Nutrition 46:503, 1987.
7. Carmel R and others: Pernicious anemia in Latin Americans is not a disease of the elderly, Archives of Internal Medicine 147:1995, 1987.
8. Carroll JE: Carnitine deficiency revisited, Journal of Nutrition 117:1501, 1987.
9. Casey V and Dwyer JT: Premenstrual syndrome: theories and evidence, Nutrition Today, p 4, November/December 1987.
10. Chesney RW: Taurine: is it required for infant nutrition? Journal of Nutrition 118:6, 1988.
11. Clark AJ and others: Folacin status in adolescent females, American Journal of Clinical Nutrition 46:302, 1987.
12. Driscoll JA and others: Longitudinal assessment of vitamin B-6 status in southern adolescent girls, Journal of The American Dietetic Association 87:307, 1987.
13. Feller AJ and Redman D: Role of carnitine in human nutrition, Journal of Nutrition 118: 541, 1988.
14. Herbert VD: "Folic acid" and "vitamin B-12" and "Pseudovitamins." In Shils ME and Young VR, eds: Modern Nutrition in Health and Disease, ed 7, Philadelphia, 1988, Lea & Febiger.
15. Holub BJ: Metabolism and function of myoinositol and inositol phospholipids, Annual Reviews of Nutrition 6:563, 1986.
16. Karnaz DS and Carmel R: Low serum cobalamin levels in primary degenerative dementia, Archives of Internal Medicine 147:429, 1987.
17. Kallner AB and others: On the requirements of ascorbic acid in man: steady-state turnover and body pool in smokers, American Journal of Clinical Nutrition 34:1347, 1981.
18. Koplin JP and others: Nutrient intake and supplementation in the United States (NHANES II), American Journal of Public Health 76:287, 1986.
19. Leklein JE: Vitamin B-6: of reservoirs, receptors and requirements, Nutrition Today, p 4, September/October, 1988.
20. Levine M: New concepts in the biology and biochemistry of ascorbic acid, New England Journal of Medicine 314:892, 1986.
21. Marshall MW: The nutritional importance of biotin—an update, Nutrition Today, p 26, November/December, 1987.
22. Maye ST and others: Rebound effect with ascorbic and in adult males, American Journal of Clinical Nutrition. 48:379, 1988.
23. McCormick, DB: "Thiamin," "riboflavin," "niacin," "vitamin B-6," "pantothenic acid," and "biotin". In Shils ME and Young VR, eds: Modern Nutrition in Health and Disease, ed 7, Philadelphia, 1988, Lea & Febiger.
24. McLaren DS: Out of sight, out of mind, Nutrition Today, p 4, January/February, 1985.
25. McMahon KE: Choline, an essential nutrient? Nutrition Today, p 18, March/April, 1987.
26. Merrill AH and Henderson JM: Diseases associated with defects in vitamin B-6 metabolism or utilization, Annual Reviews of Nutrition 7:137, 1987.
27. Miller LT: Do oral contraceptive agents affect nutrient requirements—vitamin B-6? Journal of Nutrition 116:1344, 1986.
28. Moertel CG and others: High-dose of vitamin C versus placebo in a treatment of patients with advanced cancer who have had no prior chemotherapy, New England Journal of Medicine 312:137, 1985.
29. Nutrition Monitoring Division, Human Nutrition Information Service, Nationwide Food Consumption Survey: Nutrition Today, p 18, May/June 1986; p 23, May/June, 1986; p 31 November/December, 1986; p 36 September/October, 1987.

30. Ranhotre G and others: Bioavailability for rats of thiamin in whole wheat thiamin-restored white bread, Journal of Nutrition 115:601, 1985.
31. Reisenauer AM and Halsted CH: Human folate requirements, Journal of Nutrition 117:600, 1987.
32. Roe DA: A plague of corn, Ithaca, New York, 1962, Cornell University Press.
33. Said MH and Strum WB: Affect of ethanol and other aliphatic alcohols on the intestinal transport of folates, Digestion 35:129, 1986.
34. Sheard NF and Zeisel SH: Choline: an essential dietary nutrient, Nutrition 5:1, 1989.
35. Song WO and others: Pantothenic acid status of pregnant and lactating women, Journal of the American Dietetic Association 85:192, 1985.
36. Sweetman L and Nyhan WL: Inheritable biotin-treatable disorders and associated phenomena, Annual Reviews of Nutrition 6:317, 1986.
37. Truswell AS: Ascorbic acid, New England Journal of Medicine 315:709, 1986.
38. Van den Berg H and others: Vitamin B-6 status of women suffering from premenstrual syndrome, Human Nutrition:Clinical Nutrition 40C:441, 1986.

SUGGESTED READINGS

McCormick reviews our current understanding of many water-soluble vitamins in the textbook by Shils and Young. Casey and Dwyer discuss premenstrual syndrome and the possible role of nutrition—including vitamin B-6—in its treatment. Finally, Truswell and McLaren both provide an updated look at vitamin C in their articles. McLaren's insights are especially interesting in the description of his experiences with scurvy during early medical training. Truswell, more concerned with the medical uses of vitamin C, provides numerous references to refute the desirability of using it to treat the common cold and cancer.

CHAPTER 12

Answers to nutrition awareness inventory

1. *False.* Thiamin needs are more closely tied to carbohydrate intake because the conversion of pyruvate to acetyl-CoA requires thiamin. Carbohydrate foods generate pyruvate.
2. *True.* Pork is an excellent source of thiamin, along with sunflower seeds and dried beans.
3. *True.* Enriched grains in the United States contain extra thiamin, niacin, riboflavin, and iron.
4. *True.* Milk is the best source of riboflavin in the North American diet.
5. *True.* A deficiency in a major B vitamin, such as riboflavin, suggests other B vitamins will also be deficient, since most are found in similar foods.
6. *True.* In the elderly years, cells in the stomach commonly decrease the synthesis of a factor that is vital for vitamin B-12 absorption. The treatment is usually monthly injections of vitamin B-12.
7. *True.* The amino acid tryptophan is converted into niacin in the body. Niacin needs then are met by consuming both niacin-containing foods and protein in the diet.
8. *True.* A niacin deficiency causes severe dermatitis and skin redness, especially where the sun strikes, as well as diarrhea and dementia.
9. *True.* Nicotinic acid in pharmacological (high) doses can lower serum cholesterol levels. At the same time, it often causes redness of the skin and itching.
10. *True.* Alcohol decreases the absorption of vitamin B-6, thiamin, and folate. Alcoholism is a major cause of B vitamin deficiencies.
11. *True.* Good sources of folate include green leafy vegetables and sprouts, organ meats, and orange juice.
12. *True.* Vitamin B-12 is not found in plants unless its presence is due to fermentation or contamination of the product from bits of soil or insects.
13. *True.* Pinpoint hemorrhages in the skin near hair follicles is an early sign of scurvy. These occur after about 20 to 40 days of no vitamin C intake.
14. *True.* Vitamin C converts Fe^{+3} into Fe^{+2}; the Fe^{+2} form of iron is absorbed more readily.
15. *False.* High doses of vitamin C may moderately reduce the symptoms and duration of a cold; no medication can prevent colds.

Nutrition Perspective 12-1

Pellagra

MAL DE LA ROSA

The symptoms associated with the disease pellagra—inflammation of the skin where the sun has struck, diarrhea, dementia, and hallucinations—have been described since the 14th century. The first official record of pellagra was made by the Spanish physician Casal in 1735, when it was named mal de la rosa or "red sickness." Pellagra was commonly seen in people who worked on farms. Redness around the neck was called the "Casal's necklace."[32]

Columbus and the explorers of the New World took corn (maize) back to Europe. Until 1550, it was used for medicinal purposes. By the 17th century, corn cultivation spread throughout southern Europe, and by the 18th century it reached all of Europe. As soon as corn was cultivated in an area, pellagra appeared. The disease usually appeared in the aftermath of poverty and famine.

In Europe, pellagra typically progressed through four phases. After Christmas, people began to feel unwell. They suffered from anorexia, joint pain, headaches, and other nonspecific symptoms. In Spring, sun exposure brought on severe skin lesions that caused the skin to peel heavily. After 3 to 4 months, the skin redness would disappear, and the disease appeared to be cured. But by the following Christmas the disease would reappear, and by Spring it would be back in full force. As this recurred year after year, the afflicted people became increasingly weaker. Eventually, the victim would suffer constant headaches, dizziness, depression, and eventual delusion. Body wasting and weakness would ensue, and the person would be bedridden and then catch other diseases. Death, eventually, was caused by heart failure or tuberculosis. People thought that an infectious agent caused the disease.

PELLAGRA COMES TO AMERICA

The first cases of pellagra in the United States may have been described as early as 1864, but certainly by 1902 to 1906 the outbreak of pellagra in the southeastern United States had begun. This has been the only widespread vitamin deficiency disease to reach epidemic proportions in the United States. The first clear cases were found in patients in a mental institution in Alabama. Very quickly, by 1917 to 1918, over 200,000 people in the United States had pellagra, and many of these people ended up with such severe dementia that they were relegated to spend the rest of their lives in mental institutions. Over 10,000 Americans died of pellagra in 1915.

A physician from the U.S. Marine Hospital, Joseph Goldberger, was given the task around 1910 of unraveling the mystery of the cause of pellagra. Goldberger noticed that prisoners in the South suffered from pellagra, but that jailers, physicians, and nurses who worked in the prisons never did. He found that he could cure pellagra in mental asylums by feeding the patients more milk, meat, and oatmeal. Goldberger was also able to cause pellagra in prisoners in 1915 by feeding them a corn-based diet. One problem in Goldberger's early work was that he often treated patients in which the disease had developed to such an extent that no cure was possible. Thus not everyone was cured by a better diet.

THE DECISIVE EXPERIMENT

Even after Goldberger's early experiments with improved diets, many physicians still believed that pellagra was an infectious disease. They noticed again that its incidence increased in the spring when mosquitoes were more common, and many cases often occurred within families. Both events supported the idea that pellagra was a contagious disease. Goldberger found himself in a difficult position. He had to conclusively disprove that pellagra is not an infectious disease, but is instead a dietary deficiency disease. To do this, he enlisted himself and other volunteers. They consumed the blood, feces, urine, and infectious skin secretions from people with pellagra. After 6 months, none of the volunteers had contracted pellagra. This evidence was then powerful enough to convince physicians that pellagra resulted from a poor diet.

NIACIN IS "DISCOVERED"

Goldberger noticed that people with pellagra often had dogs with a disease called blacktongue. In 1937, CV Elvehjem and others showed that nicotinic acid cured blacktongue in dogs. This compound had been sitting on the chemists' shelves for almost 100 years! Once researchers were aware of the relationship between niacin and blacktongue, they immediately tested nicotinic acid on humans. They found that nicotinic acid also cured pellagra in humans. Unfortunately, Goldberger died of cancer in 1929,. and never saw the ultimate outcome of his research—establishing the factor in food that prevented pellagra.

Even as late as 1930, there were still 200,000 cases of pellagra in the United States. *Discovering the cure for pellagra still did not lead to a cure for poverty and poor diets.* The Depression eased the epidemic of pellagra somewhat, because when cotton prices dropped, sharecroppers switched to growing more food for their families, making them less dependent on corn. The prosperity of milltowns and farmers in southeastern United States following World War II and the enrichment of refined grains in 1941 dealt the final blow to the epidemic that Goldberger helped unravel.

THE LINK TO PROTEIN IS ESTABLISHED

An important link in the pellagra story was supplied in 1948 when researchers showed that tryptophan was converted into niacin in the body. This helped explain why diets high in protein but not high in niacin cured pellagra. It also explained why pellagra was much more commonly seen in the wintertime and early spring. In the winter, food low in protein would be consumed for months and months because the bountiful fall harvest was already consumed. People would exist on staples alone, such as corn. This diet provided both insufficient protein and niacin.

Pellagra is still found today throughout Southeast Asia and Africa, associated with diets very low in protein and niacin. Poverty, when combined with a high reliance on corn, still promotes pellagra.

Nutrition Perspective 12-2

Alcoholism and Vitamin Status in the Body

Imagine that you have walked into a hospital room where a man is suffering from anemia, inflammation of the tongue (glossitis), hair loss (alopecia), diarrhea, edema, and muscle wasting. Your first thoughts might take you back to Chapter 6. He might have kwashiorkor. The problem could result from too much intravenous glucose water (D_5W), and not enough protein during the hospital stay.

To investigate your original impression further, you consult his chart. He has been admitted many times in the last 10 years to this hospital. The reasons for admission involve one central cause—alcoholism.

Continued.

Nutrition Perspective 12-2—cont'd

Alcoholism and Vitamin Status in the Body

ALCOHOL AND NUTRITION—ANOTHER LOOK

The nutritional problems of a person with alcoholism result from deficiencies of a variety of nutrients. As we have seen, people with alcoholism exhibit the gamut of vitamin deficiencies, including:

- **Vitamin A deficiency.** This may be caused by a poor diet, an inability of the liver to produce retinol-binding protein, or poor zinc status, which reduces retinol-binding protein synthesis. In addition, the chemical-detoxifying systems in the liver induced by chronic alcohol consumption may have increased the rate of vitamin A degradation in the liver.
- **Thiamin deficiency.** This can be caused by decreased thiamin absorption or decreased synthesis by the liver of the active coenzyme TPP. People with alcoholism often exhibit neurological symptoms similar to those seen in a thiamin deficiency (Wernike-Korsokof syndrome).
- **Vitamin B-6 deficiency.** This is one of the most common deficiencies of alcoholism, probably stemming from a poor dietary intake and an increased degradation of PLP. PLP can be displaced from the enzymes it works with by large amounts of acetaldehyde, a by-product of alcohol metabolism.
- **Folate deficiency.** A deficiency can be caused by a poor diet and poor nutrient absorption.[6,33] This, along with vitamin B-6 deficiency, are the two most common vitamin deficiencies of alcoholism.
- **Vitamin D deficiency.** This deficiency is usually due to the liver's decreased capacity to convert vitamin D into 25-hydroxyvitamin D.
- **Vitamin C deficiency.** It is not clear if this deficiency is usually caused by a decrease in dietary intake, altered liver metabolism, or both.
- **Vitamin K.** This deficiency is probably due to a combination of decreased synthesis by intestinal bacteria, decreased dietary intake, and decreased absorption.

Often accompanying the practice of alcoholism is a combination of a poor dietary intake, poor absorption, and altered metabolism of vitamins, as well as the direct toxic effects of ethanol on various organ systems, such as the liver and small intestine. These effects eventually lead to a very poor nutritional status, which then probably increases the rate of liver destruction by alcohol because it decreases the liver's ability to regenerate new tissue. In addition, this reduced regeneration decreases the liver's ability to counteract other toxic substances, such as free radicals, because the supplies of antioxidants, such as vitamin E, vitamin C, and the other nutrient-dependent antioxidant enzyme systems, are depleted.

A nutritious diet can help prevent some complications associated with alcoholism, but usually alcoholism eventually results in serious destruction of the body, with or without an adequate diet. The research is very clear in monkeys—even when consuming a nutritious diet, alcoholism often leads to cirrhosis of the liver.

In the past, it was easier to stereotype people with alcoholism as "skid-row bums." This is no longer possible. *Alcoholism cuts across all levels of society.* Financially successful people and very poor people are both often affected by this disease. The registered dietitian must be vigilant in seeking all possible deficiencies present in people with alcoholism, in consultation with the attending physician, when recommending proper diets to meet those deficiencies.

Chapter 13

Water and the Major Minerals

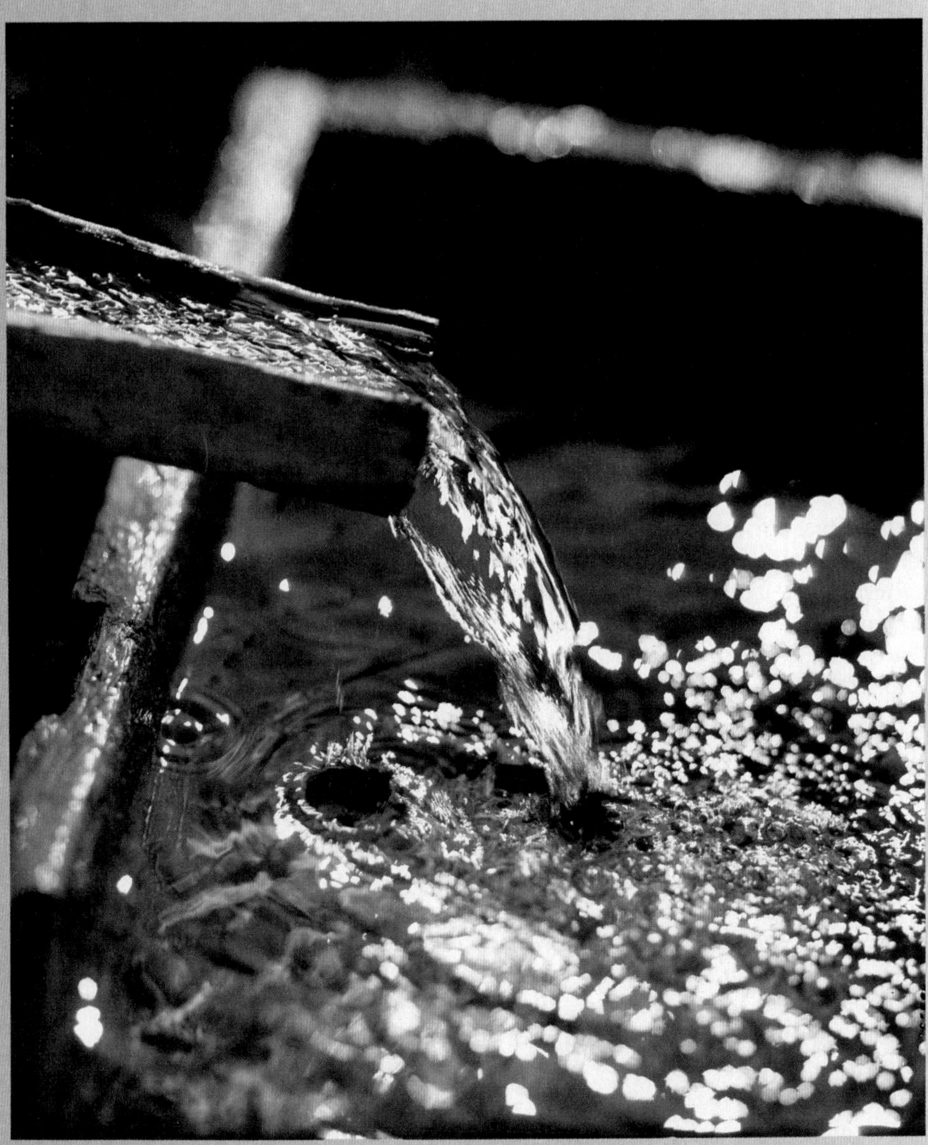

The water we drink is often a source of minerals, such as magnesium.

Overview

Minerals, like vitamins, are vital to health. As free atoms, they are considered inorganic because they are not bonded to carbon atoms. Figure 13-1 lists the amounts of some minerals found in the human body. We know that animals require many minerals for survival, but we are not sure that all the minerals found in our bodies—for example, vanadium and nickel—are necessary to sustain human life. Some minerals, such as lead and cadmium, may be found in humans only because of environmental pollution. The mere presence of a mineral in our bodies is not proof that we need it. Nevertheless, we know that some mineral deficiencies can cause severe health problems. For this reason the study of minerals is critical to understanding human nutrition.

Nutrition awareness inventory

Here are 15 statements about water and electrolytes. Answer them to test your current knowledge. If you think the answer is true or mostly true, circle T. If you think the answer is false or mostly false, circle F. Use the scoring key at the end of this chapter to compute your total score. Take the test again after you have read this chapter. Compare the results.

1. **T F** Water is an electrolyte.
2. **T F** "Major" minerals are more important to health than "trace" minerals.
3. **T F** Vitamins often need minerals to help perform metabolic reactions.
4. **T F** Plant foods are usually the best sources of minerals.
5. **T F** You can survive longer without food than without water.
6. **T F** When water evaporates from your skin, you feel cooler because evaporating water takes heat with it.
7. **T F** The estimation of dietary water needs is 1 milliliter per kcalorie.
8. **T F** You can never drink too much water.
9. **T F** Sodium is often added to processed foods.
10. **T F** Oranges are alkaline ash foods.
11. **T F** A preference for salty foods is partially learned.
12. **T F** Most foods in the same food group, such as milk and cheese, contain similar amounts of sodium.
13. **T F** Perspiration has a lower sodium concentration than blood.
14. **T F** Calcium supplements can prevent osteoporosis.
15. **T F** Salt is "bad" for most people.

MINERALS

major mineral
A mineral vital to health that is required in the diet in amounts greater than 100 mg per day.

trace mineral
A mineral vital to health that is required in the diet in amounts less than 100 mg per day.

Minerals are categorized as **major** and **trace** minerals based on the amount humans need per day. If we require 100 milligrams or more per day of a mineral, it is considered a major mineral; otherwise, it is considered a trace mineral. Using this basis, calcium and phosphorus are major minerals and iron and zinc are trace minerals. The total of all trace minerals in the body is less than 15 grams (½ ounce). *Nevertheless, trace minerals, such as iron and zinc, are very important. The small amount needed does not necessarily reflect a mineral's nutritional importance.*

The metabolic roles of minerals vary considerably. Some, such as magnesium and manganese, work as cofactors, enabling enzymes to function. Minerals also contribute to important body compounds. For example, iodine is a component of the hormone thyroxine, and iron is a component of hemoglobin in the red blood cell. Sodium, potassium, and calcium enable the transfer of nerve impulses throughout the body. Calcium is also a key participant in muscle contraction.

Body growth and development also depend on certain minerals, such as calcium and phosphorus. Water balance utilizes sodium, potassium, calcium, and phosphorus. At all levels—cellular, tissue, organ, and whole body—minerals clearly play important roles in maintaining body functions.

Mineral bioavailability

Although foods contain and supply many nutrients to a body, bodies vary in their capabilities to absorb and use available nutrients. While minerals may be present

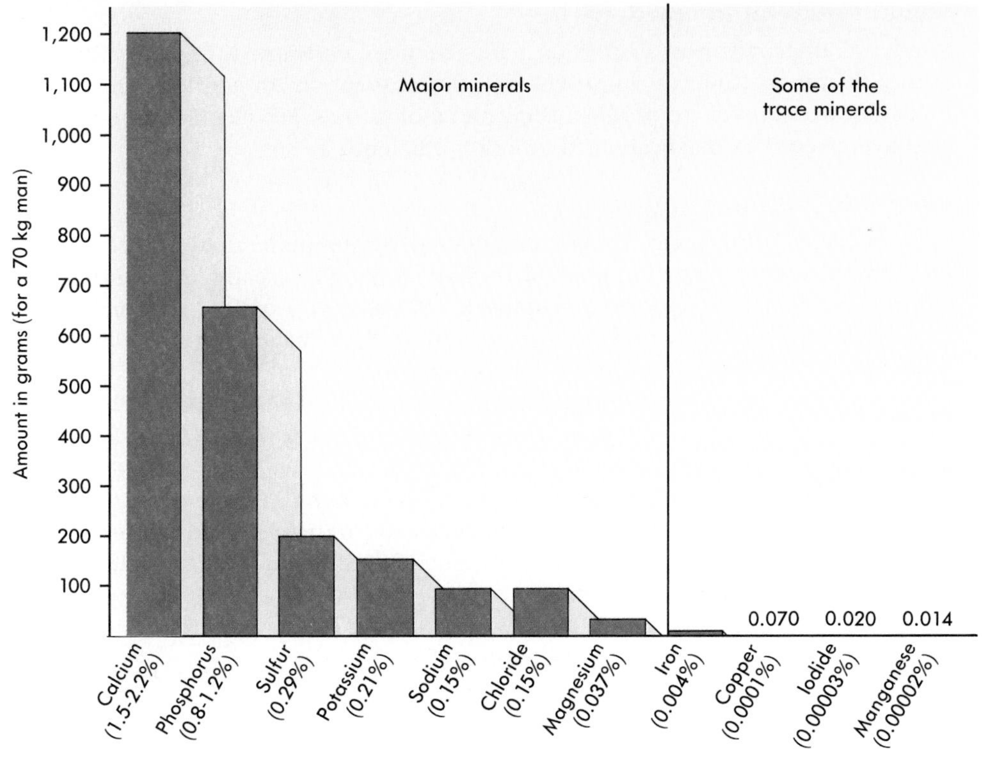

Figure 13-1

A list of minerals found in a 60 kilogram man. The percent figures represent percent of body weight.

in foods, they are not **bioavailable** unless a body can absorb them. The ability to absorb minerals from a diet depends on many factors.[8] A value listed in a food composition table is just a starting point for estimating the true contribution a food makes to our mineral needs. *One of the most important factors in determining a mineral's contribution to a body is the body's need for that mineral.* Other factors are discussed below.

bioavailability
The degree to which the amount of an ingested nutrient is absorbed and so is available to the body.

Mineral-mineral interactions

Many minerals have similar molecular weights and charges (valences). Magnesium, calcium, iron, and copper can exist in the +2 state. Having similar sizes and the same charge causes these minerals to compete with each other for absorption, and so they affect each other's bioavailability. Nutritionists caution people against taking individual mineral supplements, unless a medical condition specifically warrants it, because *an excess of one mineral influences the absorption and metabolism of other minerals.*

For example, the presence of a large amount of zinc in the body decreases copper absorption. Oral zinc can even be used to minimize copper absorption, if a medical diagnosis warrants that. However, mineral interactions are generally not desirable. We are only beginning to see the negative effects of the recent surge in calcium supplement use: it appears calcium supplements can interfere with magnesium and iron absorption.

Exploring Issues and Actions

Are you taking mineral supplements? What prompts you or others to do this?

Vitamin-mineral interactions

Vitamin C improves iron absorption when they are consumed together. The vitamin D hormone calcitriol improves calcium absorption. In addition, many vitamins require minerals to perform their metabolic roles. For example, the thiamin coenzyme requires magnesium to function efficiently.

Fiber-mineral interactions

Spinach contains plenty of calcium, but only about 5% of it can be absorbed because of the vegetable's high concentration of oxalic acid. Usually, about 25% to 35% of calcium is absorbed from foods.

Mineral bioavailability can be greatly affected by nonmineral substances in the diet. Phytic acid (phytate) in grain fibers binds minerals, greatly limiting their absorption, as does the oxalic acid in spinach and other vegetables.[9] High-fiber diets can decrease the absorption of iron, calcium, zinc, magnesium, and probably other minerals. Especially in diets that contain more than 35 grams of dietary fiber, decreased mineral absorption can be a problem. *We know very little about the long-term effects of high-fiber diets on mineral status in the body.* Scientists are actively researching this area.

If grains are leavened with yeast, as they are in bread, enzymes produced by the yeast can break some of the bonds between phytic acid and minerals. This increases mineral absorption. The zinc deficiencies found among some Middle Eastern populations can be attributed partly to low dietary zinc and partly to their unleavened breads. Phytic acid binds so much of the zinc from unleavened breads that little is absorbed (see Chapter 14).

Food sources of minerals

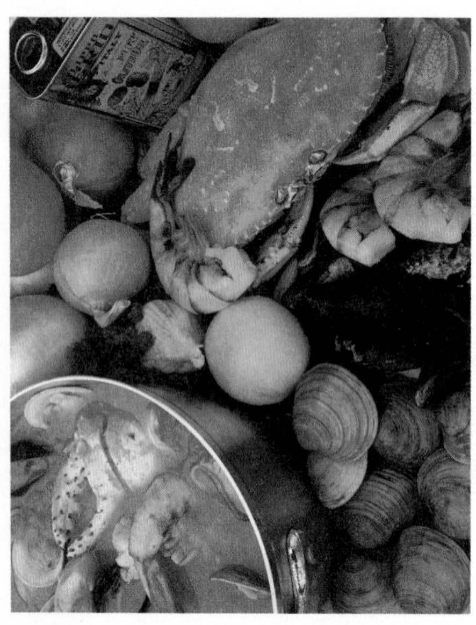

Minerals in animal products, such as seafood, are often more bioavailable than minerals in plants.

In general, *the best dietary mineral sources are animal products, especially seafood.* This is mainly because minerals in animal tissues are more concentrated than in plant tissues. As an animal eats plants year after year, minerals from the plants concentrate in the animal's body tissues. Likewise, sea animals, such as clams, oysters, and shrimp, concentrate the minerals found in seawater. Minerals in animal foods are also more bioavailable than in plant foods because there are less mineral-binding substances in animal foods than in plant foods.

A diet devoid of animal products is very likely to be low in minerals. The only exception is magnesium, which is far more plentiful in plant than in animal sources. Otherwise, some plants are good, but not excellent, sources of most minerals.

Mineral toxicity

Minerals can be quite toxic. Toxicity is yet another reason to carefully consider the use of mineral supplements. Miners have suffered the ill-effects of minerals, especially from manganese. Selenium also can cause many toxic side effects (see Chapter 14).

Concept Check

Many minerals are vital to health, though our needs for some remain uncertain. The bioavailability of minerals depends on many factors, including a body's need for the mineral and the mineral's interaction with fiber and other minerals. Taking an individual mineral supplement can greatly affect the absorption and metabolism of other nutrients. Animal products are generally the best sources of minerals because animals concentrate the minerals they consume from plants. Some minerals are potentially toxic. This is another reason to carefully consider any dietary mineral supplementation.

WATER

To appreciate how minerals operate, the nature of water and its characteristics must be understood. Water is the base of operations for minerals, and it forms the major part of the human body.[19] An adult can probably survive about 8 weeks without eating food (depending on fat stores), but only a few days without drinking water. This is not because water is more important than energy, protein, vitamins, or minerals, but rather because we can neither store nor conserve water as well as we can those other components of our diet.[29]

Water has some fascinating properties. It can dissolve most substances. It expands when cold so that a jar full of water cracks when frozen. Water has a high heat capacity; it takes much more energy to heat water than it does to heat fat. Foods with high water content heat up and cool down slowly. Compare the time it takes to heat water with the time it takes to heat butter in a microwave oven. Because water requires so much energy to change from a liquid to a gas, it forms an ideal medium for removing heat from the body. We will discuss that shortly.

Functions of water

Because of its unique chemical and physical characteristics, water plays several key roles in our life processes.

The fluid of life. Between 50% and 70% of body weight is made up of water. Lean muscle tissue is made up of about 73% water. The more body fat, the less body water a person has. As fat content increases, the percentage of lean tissue decreases in the body and total body water then drifts down toward 50%.

Two major roles of water involve chemical reactions. For example, water serves as a solvent for many chemical compounds and it provides a medium in which many chemical reactions occur. It also actively participates in chemical reactions, such as the hydrolysis reaction used to split one maltose molecule into two glucose molecules.

Intracellular and extracellular fluid. Water migrates in and out of body cells. When functioning inside cells, water is part of the **intracellular fluid.** When outside the cells, water is part of the **extracellular fluid.** Extracellular fluid is further divided into **interstitial fluid**—water between cells—and **intravascular fluid**—water in the bloodstream (Figure 13-2). Interstitial fluid forms an important transport link between tissue cells and the bloodstream.

The ratio of intracellular to interstitial to intravascular water is about 25:14:3. Water shifts freely from one compartment to another. For example, if blood volume falls, water can shift from the areas both inside and around cells to the bloodstream to increase blood volume. On the other hand, if blood volume increases, water can shift out of the bloodstream into cells and the areas between them.

The body controls the amount of water in each compartment mainly by controlling the ion concentrations in each compartment. Ions are charged par-

intracellular fluid
Fluid contained within a cell.

extracellular fluid
Fluid present outside the cells; it includes intravascular and interstitial fluids.

interstitial fluid
Fluid between cells.

intravascular fluid
Fluid within the bloodstream (that is, in the arteries, veins, and capillaries).

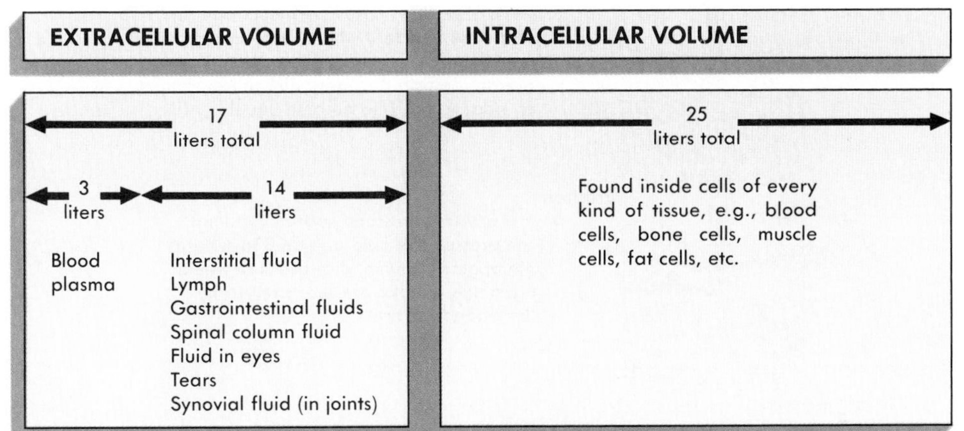

Figure 13-2
The fluid compartments in the body.

Both kidney function and proteins present in body fluids contribute to fluid balance (see Chapter 6).

ticles. Because of its polar nature, water attracts sodium, potassium, chloride, phosphate, magnesium, calcium, and other ions. In a water molecule, the oxygen atom tends to be more negative and the hydrogen atoms tend to be more positive. The slightly negative oxygen atom attracts positive sodium and potassium ions, and the slightly positive hydrogen atoms attract negative chloride and phosphate ions (PO_4^{-2}). By shifting ions in and out of the cellular compartments, the body can maintain a desirable amount of water in each compartment. Where ions go, so goes water.

Osmosis. Varying ion concentration to control the amount of water in cells and the bloodstream requires the action of osmosis. Osmosis occurs where a semipermeable membrane separates two bodies of fluid. In this case, *semipermeable* means water can pass through the membrane but particles cannot. In the body, these particles are usually ions, and the membranes are cell membranes. If the number of particles—or total ion concentration—in both compartments is the same, then osmosis works to equalize the amounts of water in each compartment.

Figure 13-3 illustrates osmosis. Adding particles to a compartment increases its particle concentration. Since particles cannot easily pass through the membrane, water shifts from the diluted compartment to that with a high ion concentration. The term **osmotic pressure** refers to the amount of force needed to prevent dilution of the compartment with a higher ion concentration. Examples of osmosis are sugar pulling fluid from strawberries, a salty salad dressing wilting lettuce, and red blood cell behavior when put into solutions of various salt concentrations.

osmotic pressure
The exerted pressure needed to keep particles in a solution from drawing liquid across a semipermeable membrane.

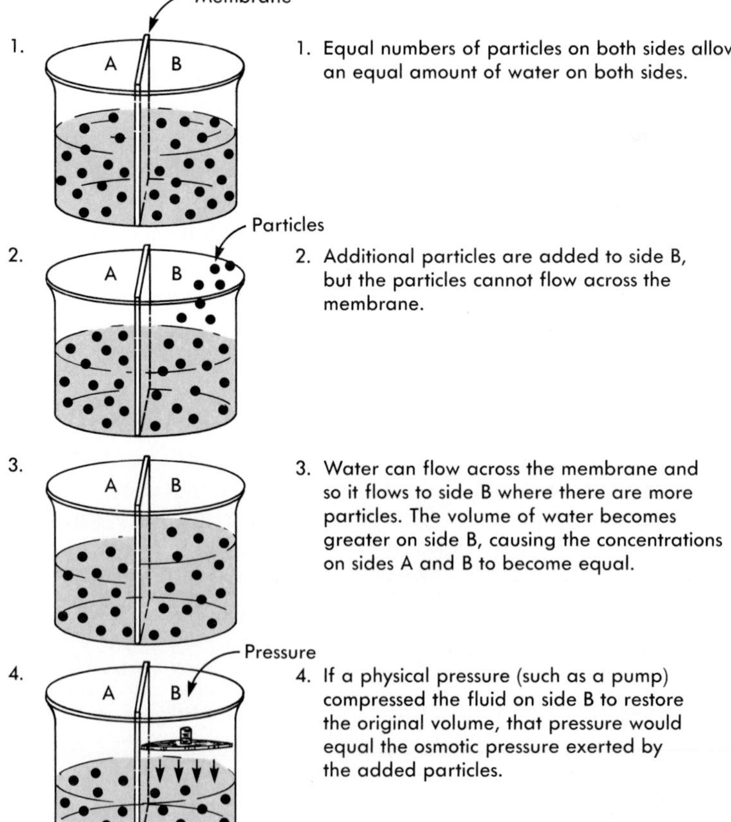

Figure 13-3

A graphic representation of osmosis and osmotic pressure. (1) Equal number of particles on both sides allows equal amounts of water. (2) Now additional particles are added to side B, but the particles cannot flow across the membrane. (3) Water can flow across the membrane and so it flows to side B where there are more particles. The volume of water becomes greater on side B, causing the concentrations on sides A and B to again become equal. (4) If physical pressure (such as a pump) compressed the fluid on side B to restore the original volume, that pressure would equal the osmotic pressure exerted by the added particles.

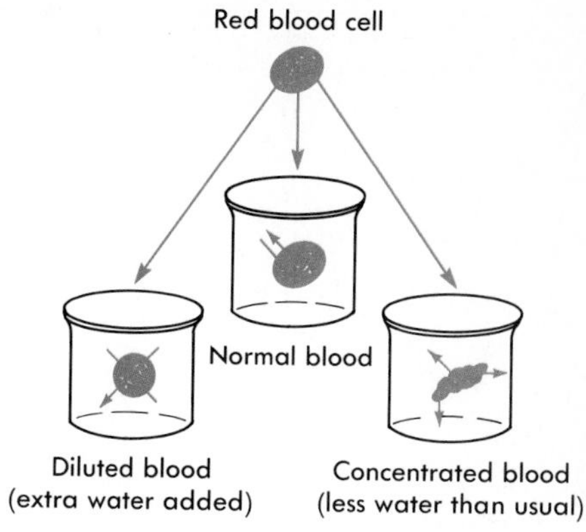

Water and ions in the body—a balancing act. Adding water—instead of particles—to a compartment dilutes its ion concentration, and so the compartment tends to donate water to more concentrated compartments nearby. Again, this equalizes the ion concentrations in the compartments. *Overall, then, due to the action of osmosis, water is forced to shift across membranes in response to changes in ion concentrations.*

Cell membranes differ slightly from this model: they are permeable to many ions. However, they also have pumping mechanisms that constantly draw potassium ions into the cell and pump sodium ions out. Other ion exchanges also take place. This pumping action, in effect, leaves cell membranes permeable to water but not to many ions. Ions, such as sodium, may cross into the cell, but the cell quickly pumps them back out.

Positive ions, such as sodium and potassium, pair with negative ions, such as phosphate and chloride. Intracellular water volume depends primarily on intracellular potassium and phosphate concentration. Extracellular water volume depends primarily on the extracellular sodium and chloride concentration.

Besides balancing the ion concentrations between the inside and outside of cells, the body must also balance ion charges. If a negative ion enters a cell, a positive ion also must enter the cell or another negative ion must leave it.

Temperature regulation. The body secretes fluids in the form of perspiration, which evaporates through skin pores. Evaporating water requires heat energy. So as perspiration evaporates, heat energy is taken from the skin, cooling it in the process. *Each liter of perspiration lost represents approximately 600 kcalories of energy lost from the skin and surrounding tissues.* In Chapter 8 we mentioned that fever increases basal metabolism, and now you know the reason. As extra heat dissipates from the body, energy is lost in the form of perspiration.

Humans tolerate hot, dry climates far better than they do hot, humid climates, because dry climates allow perspiration to work as it should. In hot, humid climates, not all perspiration can evaporate: some of it simply rolls off the skin or soaks into clothing. This perspiration does little to cool the body because water must evaporate to do its job. And so people just feel hot and sticky.

Recall from Chapter 7 that 60% of the chemical energy in food is turned directly into body heat. Only 40% becomes ATP energy, and even that energy eventually leaves the body in the form of heat. When we work hard or stay in a hot climate, we need a way to release extra heat. Otherwise, an increased body temperature would prevent enzyme systems from functioning efficiently. Perspiration is the primary way to rid oneself of that heat.

Removal of waste products. Water is an important vehicle for ridding the body of waste products. Most unwanted substances in the body are water-soluble, and can leave the body via the urine. In addition, when possible, liver metabolism can convert fat-soluble compounds into water-soluble compounds so that they too can be excreted in the urine.

A major body waste product is urea, made from the amine groups ($-NH_2$) of amino acids. The more protein eaten, the greater the necessity for excreting nitrogen (in the form of urea) in the urine. Likewise, the more sodium consumed, the more sodium excreted in the urine. *Total urine production is primarily determined by protein and sodium chloride (salt) intake.* By limiting excess protein and sodium intakes it is possible to limit urine output—a useful practice, for example, in space flights.

A healthy urine volume to aim for is 1 to 2 liters per day. More than that is fine, but less—especially less than 600 milliliters—forces the kidneys to form a very concentrated urine. The kidneys can accommodate to a point, but very concentrated urine increases the risk of kidney stones in susceptible people. Kidney stones are simply minerals that have precipitated out of the urine and eventually lodge in kidney tissues.

Lubrication and miscellaneous functions. Water helps form the lubricants found in knees and other joints of the body. It is the basis for saliva, bile, and **amniotic fluid.** Amniotic fluid acts as an important shock absorber surrounding the growing fetus before birth. Ion concentrations vary in each fluid compartment to accommodate specific needs.

amniotic fluid
Fluid contained in a sac within the uterus that surrounds and protects the fetus during its development.

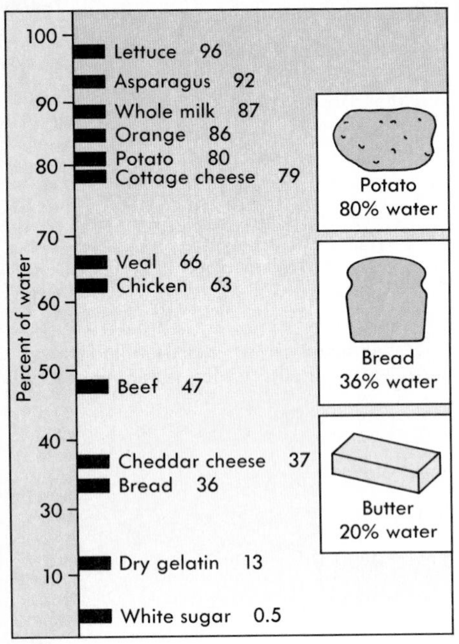

Water content of various foods (percent of total weight).

Water needs

Water needs for adults are roughly estimated as 1 milliliter per kcalorie in the diet. This works out to 2.4 liters (10 cups) for a 2400 kcalorie diet. Of this, about 1 liter is due to typical water losses from the lungs (400 milliliters), feces (150 milliliters), and skin (500 milliliters) (Figure 13-4). Since people are not normally aware of these water losses, they are called **"insensible"** water losses.

The loss of only 150 milliliters of water from feces per day is an incredible feat, considering that about 8000 milliliters enter the gastrointestinal (GI) tract daily via secretions from the stomach, intestine, pancreas, and other organs. An additional 2000 milliliters is added through diet. Absorption of all but 150 milliliters makes the GI tract a significant site of water conservation. The kidneys also conserve water by reabsorbing 97% of the water filtered from waste products.

We consume about 1 liter of water per day in various liquids (Figure 13-4). Foods supply another liter of fluid, and water as a byproduct of metabolism provides approximately 350 milliliters. This yields a total of about 2.4 liters. Note that this is very similar to estimates of water needs based on 1 milliliter per kcalorie if a person requires a diet of 2400 kcalories.

Thirst. If a person doesn't consume enough water, the body first signals so by registering thirst. The hypothalamus in the brainstem communicates to higher brain centers that the person needs to drink. The thirst mechanism is not always reliable, however, especially during illness, in elderly years, and when participating in vigorous athletic events. We have already mentioned in Chapter 7 that athletes should weigh themselves before and after training sessions to determine their rate of water loss and thus their water needs. Children who are ill, espe-

It is important to drink plenty of water, especially when you exercise vigorously.

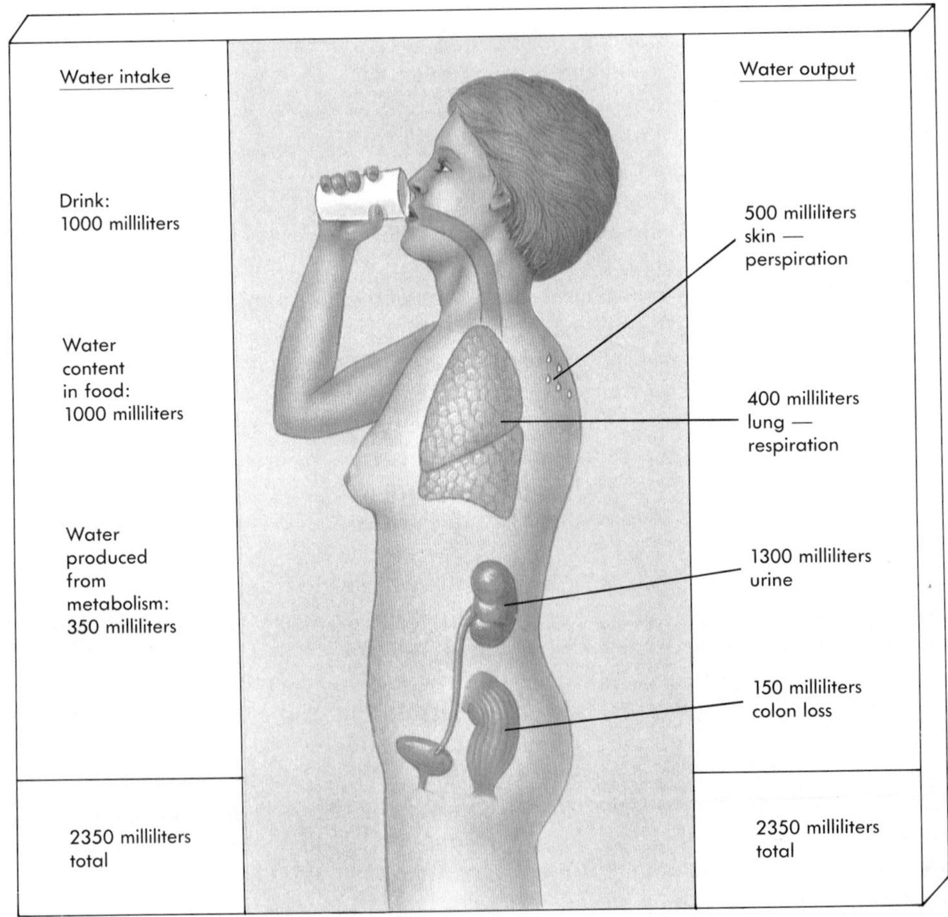

Figure 13-4

Water balance—intake versus output. We maintain body fluids at an optimum level by adjusting water intake and output. Most water comes from the liquids. Some comes from the moisture in more solid foods, and the remainder is manufactured in metabolism. Water output includes that via lungs, kidneys, skin, and bowels.

cially those with fever, diarrhea, and increased perspiration, need to be reminded to drink plenty of fluid. Elderly people in hospitals and nursing homes should have fluid intake and output monitored. One other situation that demands extra fluid for the body is long airplane flights: a traveler can lose approximately 1.5 liters (6 cups) of water during a 3-hour flight. The dehumidified air in the airplane is so dry that excessive "insensible" perspiration and evaporation occur.

What if the thirst message is ignored?. When the body registers a shortage of available water, fluid conservation increases. The pituitary gland releases **antidiuretic hormone (ADH)** to force the kidneys to conserve water. As its name implies, ADH stops diuresis. In addition, as fluid volume drops in the bloodstream, blood pressure falls. The fall signals the kidneys to release an enzyme called **renin,** which acts on a protein in the bloodstream to form the compound **angiotensin I.** Angiotensin I converts to **angiotensin II.** That triggers the adrenal gland to release more of the hormone **aldosterone,** which signals the kidneys to retain more sodium and therefore more water (Figure 13-5). Remember that water always follows ions. Thus low blood pressure, through this roundabout measure, causes increased water conservation in the body.

The effectiveness of ADH and aldosterone is limited. Fluid is constantly lost via the insensible routes—feces, skin, and lungs. Those losses must be replaced. In addition, urine can become only so concentrated. Eventually, if fluid is not consumed, the body becomes dehydrated and suffers ill effects.

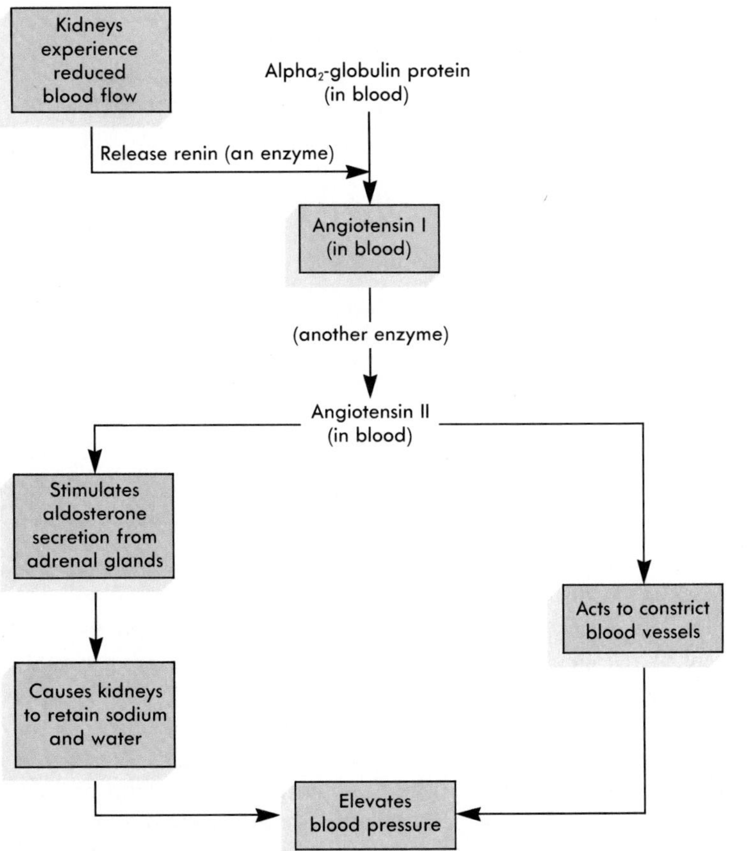

Figure 13-5

The renin-angiotensin system. This is one regulator of blood pressure.

Alcohol inhibits the action of ADH. One reason people feel so bad the day after heavy drinking is that they are very dehydrated. Even though they may have consumed a lot of liquid in their drinks, they have lost even more liquid because alcohol has inhibited ADH.

A disease known as diabetes insipidus results from an inability of the pituitary gland to produce the hormone ADH. Trauma to the head, such as from a car accident, and some cancer tumors can lead to diabetes insipidus. This condition leads to production of copious amounts of urine, causing dehydration unless the person drinks water quite regularly.

antidiuretic hormone (ADH)
A hormone secreted by the pituitary gland that acts on the kidneys to cause a decrease in water excretion.

renin
An enzyme formed in the kidneys in response to low blood pressure; it acts on a blood protein to produce angiotensin I.

angiotensin I
An intermediary compound, produced during the body's attempt to conserve water and sodium; it is converted to angiotensin II.

angiotensin II
A compound produced in response to low blood pressure that increases blood vessel constriction and triggers production of the hormone aldosterone.

aldosterone
A powerful hormone produced by the adrenal glands; it acts on the kidneys to cause sodium reabsorption and water conservation.

The effects of dehydration. By the time a person loses 2% of body weight in fluids, he or she will be thirsty. At a 4% loss of body weight, muscles undergo a significant drop in strength and endurance. *By the time body weight is reduced by 10% to 12%, heat tolerance is decreased and the person feels very weak.* At a 20% reduction, the person may lapse into a coma and soon die (Figure 13-6).

Water intoxication. Mental disorders such as schizophrenia sometimes encourage a person to drink copious amounts of water. Excessive drinking of water can quickly overwhelm the kidneys' capacity to excrete it. Water then accumulates in the body, causing headache, blurred vision, cramps, and eventually convulsions.

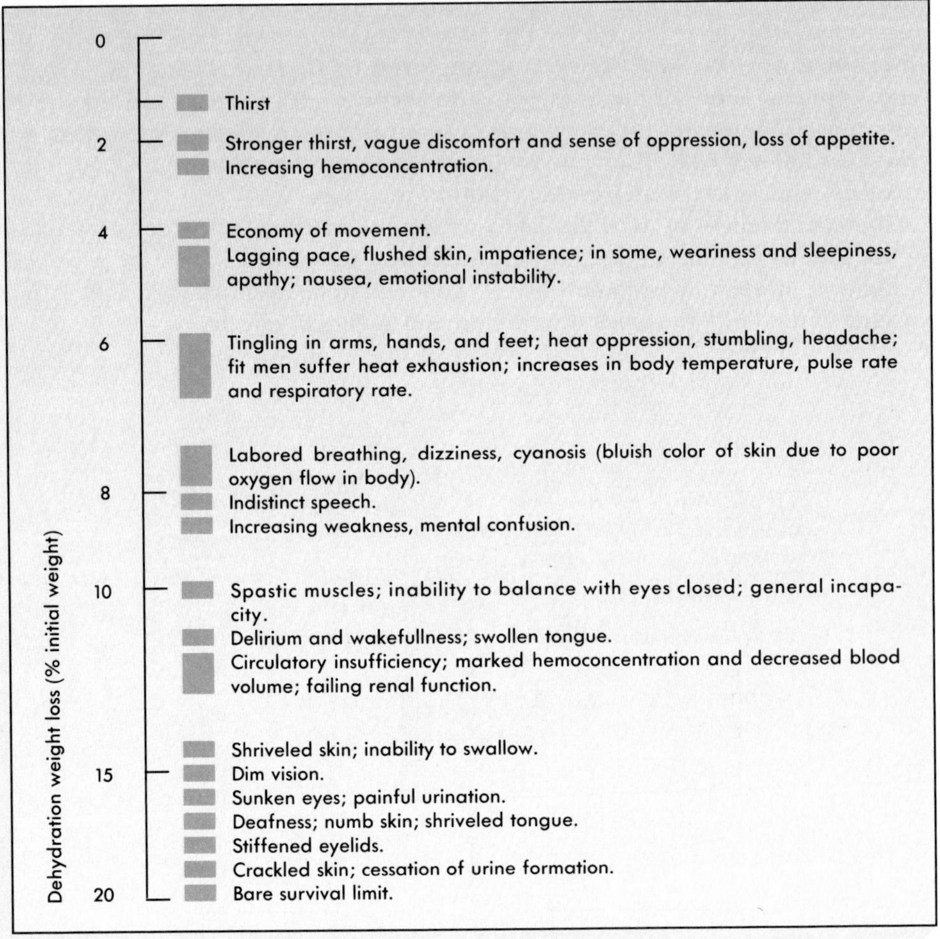

DEATH

Figure 13-6
The effects of dehydration. These range from thirst to death.

ACID-BASE BALANCE

In addition to balancing ion charges between body compartments, the body carefully regulates hydrogen ion balance using a variety of physiological responses. Recall from Chapter 2 that pH is the negative logarithm of the hydrogen ion concentration in a solution. The pH of the blood is kept between 7.35 and 7.45, just slightly on the alkaline (basic) side. To do this, the body uses the dilutional effects of total body water and the actions of lungs, kidneys, and blood proteins.

Diet mildly affects the acid-base balance in the body. Foods high in protein also frequently contain much sulfur and phosphorus. These ions remain after the rest of the protein is metabolized and eventually form acids in the body, namely sulfuric acid and phosphoric acid. These acids can cause a slight decrease in the blood's pH.

Most fruits and vegetables create a more alkaline effect. These foods contain sodium and potassium ions often attached to acids. When the food is metabolized, these ions remain and eventually form sodium hydroxide and potassium hydroxide, two bases.

Although fruits contain acids, their metabolism results in the formation of bases. Because sulfur, phosphorus, sodium, and potassium ions are the residue of a metabolic "burning" process, they are known as either **acid ash** or **alkaline ash** products. In either case, physiological mechanisms more than compensate for this effect on pH balance. It requires no attention in diet planning.

acid ash
Acid compounds that form from the residue of metabolized sulfur- and phosphorus-containing foods, such as protein foods.

alkaline ash
Alkaline compounds that form from residue of metabolized potassium- and sodium-containing foods, such as fruits and vegetables.

Concept Check

Since the body can neither readily store nor entirely conserve water, we can survive only a few days without it. Water functions as a solvent, a medium for chemical reactions, a thermoregulator, and a lubricant. Water constitutes 50% to 70% of body weight and is prevalent in lean tissue, intracellular and extracellular fluid, urine, and all other body fluids. For adults, water needs can be estimated as 1 milliliter per kcalorie consumed. Thirst is the body's first sign of dehydration. If a thirst mechanism is faulty, as it may be with illness or vigorous exercise, hormonal mechanisms also help conserve water. Too much water in a diet can be toxic.

MAJOR MINERALS

We have discussed some general characteristics of minerals and how some of them interact with water in the body. Now let us review the individual properties of the major minerals.

Sodium

North Americans both crave and fear sodium (chemical symbol is Na) and its primary dietary source, table salt. Some of this fear is warranted, and some is not.

Functions of sodium. Almost all dietary sodium is absorbed. It then becomes the major positive ion in extracellular fluid, and so a key electrolyte for retaining water in that compartment. Fluid balance throughout the body depends partly on varied sodium concentrations in body water compartments.

Sodium ions are important for nerve conduction. Impulses are transmitted down the nerve by sodium ions rushing into nerve cells. This reverses the charge of the cell membrane—**depolarizes** it—as positive sodium ions rush in, generating an electrical current. The electrical current travels from nerve cell to nerve cell. After the electrical wave passes through a nerve cell, sodium ions are pumped back out of the cell and potassium ions are pumped back in. This process requires ATP energy. When the ions regain their usual concentrations, the net charge along the membranes returns to its resting value and the nerve cell is ready to "fire" again.

depolarize
To create a neutral or uncharged condition.

Sodium regulation. A low-sodium diet, coupled with high perspiration losses or diarrhea, can deplete the body of sodium. This state can lead to muscle cramps, nausea, vomiting, and dizziness and later to shock and coma. The kidneys are the major organs to respond to this depletion. They begin a variety of reactions that eventually trigger the release of the hormone aldosterone, as we covered before (Figure 13-5). Aldosterone then increases sodium retention by the kidneys.

Even in cases of high rates of perspiration, sodium depletion in the body is very unlikely because our diets contain ample sodium. Only when weight loss from perspiration exceeds 6 pounds (2.7 kilograms) should sodium losses raise concern. Even then, merely salting foods—not a salt tablet—is needed. Perspiration has two thirds the sodium concentration of blood (about 2 grams of sodium per liter of perspiration versus 3 grams for blood). Although perspiration tastes salty on the skin, it is not because perspiration is highly concentrated in sodium: rather, in evaporating from the skin, water leaves concentrated sodium behind.

To assess sodium, potassium, chloride, calcium, magnesium, or phosphorus status in a person, serum levels can be measured. We will point out other methods, often more sensitive, when appropriate.

Sodium in foods. About one third to one half the sodium we consume is added during cooking or at the table (Table 13-1). Most of the rest is added dur-

Table 13-1

Sodium content of food varies with method of preparation

½ Cup of cooked peas	Sodium (milligrams)
Fresh	2
Frozen	70
Canned	185
Frozen with 2 tablespoons of cheese sauce	205
Frozen with 2 tablespoons of hollandaise sauce	310

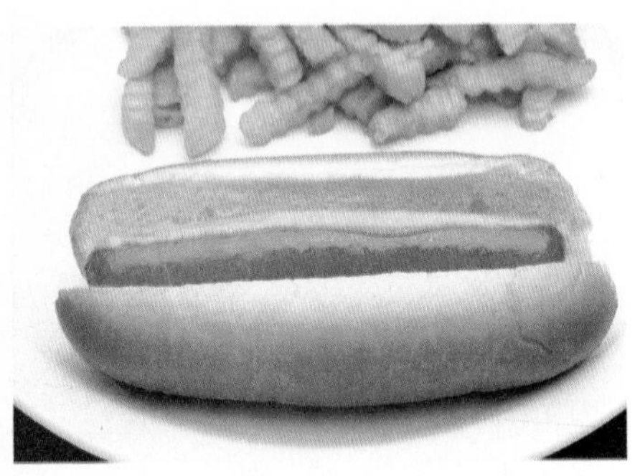

Hot dogs have a very high salt content.

Commercially prepared condiments, sauces, and seasoning are often high in sodium. Look first for the word sodium. In addition, those listed below are high in sodium:
Onion salt
Celery salt
Garlic salt
Seasoned salt
Baking powder
Sea salt
Salad dressings
Pickles
Soy sauce
Steak sauce
Barbecue sauce
Meat tenderizer
Baking soda
Salt pork
Brine
Chili sauce
Catsup
Mustard
Worcestershire sauce
Bouillon
Monosodium glutamate (msg)
Chili sauce
Relish

ing food manufacturing. Most foods naturally contain little sodium; milk is one exception. The more home-cooking available, the more sodium control a person has. Major contributors of sodium to the U.S. diet are white bread and rolls, hot dogs and lunch meats, cheese, soups, and spaghetti with tomato sauce, partly because these foods are eaten so often. Other foods especially high in sodium are tomato-based products in general, salted snack foods, French fries and potato chips, and sauces and gravies. Many condiments also contain large amounts of sodium.

If we ate only unprocessed foods and added no salt, sodium intake would be about 500 milligrams per day. By comparing that range with a typical North American intake—3000 to 7000 milligrams—it is clear that food processing and cooking contributes most of our dietary sodium.

A nutrition label lists a food's sodium content. In addition, a number of descriptive terms are used on labels, such as "sodium free" (less than 5 milligrams sodium), "very low sodium" (35 milligrams or less per serving), "low sodium" (145 milligrams or less per serving), and "reduced sodium" (a 75% reduction in sodium content). The terms "unsalted," "no salt added," or "without added salt" on labels describe food products processed without salt when it normally would be used. Many medicines contain sodium, and they must be limited if dietary sodium is restricted. Similarly, when sodium is severely restricted, contributions from tap water (especially softened water) must be considered.[11]

Minimum sodium requirements. The minimum sodium requirement is 500 milligrams per day for adults. (Throughout this chapter, see the inside cover for other age groups and Appendix G for Canadian recommendations.) This is a generous amount considering that we really need only about 100 milligrams.

Table salt is 40% sodium and 60% chloride. So the North American range of intake of 3 to 7 grams of sodium per day translates to 7.5 to 18 grams of salt. A teaspoon of salt contains about 2 grams of sodium (a teaspoon of most dry substance equals approximately 5 grams).

Most humans can adapt to various dietary salt levels. *For most of us, today's sodium intake is simply tomorrow's urine output. However, approximately 10% of North American adults are sodium sensitive.*[12] For these people, high-sodium intakes contribute to hypertension, and lower sodium diets (about 2 grams daily) often correct hypertension (see Nutrition Perspective 13-1 on Minerals and Hypertension). Scientific groups suggest that all adults limit daily sodium intake to 2.4 to 3 grams, mostly to limit the risk of hypertension.

If you have hypertension, you should try to reduce your sodium intake. If you don't have hypertension, you might still consider slowly reducing your intake to build good habits for the future. If your daily sodium intake range is already within 2 to 3 grams, you are doing enough. See Tables 13-2 and 13-3 to evaluate your sodium habits and intake.

Lowering your sodium intake. If you choose to lower your sodium intake, you can eventually adapt to a low-sodium diet.[1] At first foods will taste quite bland, but eventually you will perceive more flavor and your tongue will have a lower salt threshold. The tongue's salt receptors will be triggered by less salt.

By slowly reducing dietary sodium and substituting garlic, oregano, lemon juice, and other herbs and spices for it, you can eventually consume a diet that has only 2 to 3 grams of sodium daily, but which is still very flavorful. Many newer cookbooks can guide you to excellent recipes for flavorful foods. Except for yeast breads, omitting salt from food preparation can still yield an excellent product. For some people, this low-sodium approach to eating makes the difference between normal and high blood pressures.

Exploring Issues and Actions

Why do some people salt foods so heavily even before tasting them? Do you think you sometimes use too much salt? What was your blood pressure at your last checkup?

Table 13-2

Examining your sodium habits

Examine how the foods you eat and the way you prepare and serve them affect the amount of sodium in your diet.

How often do you:	Less than once per week	1 or 2 times per week	3 to 5 times per week	Almost daily
1. Eat cured or processed meats, such as ham, bacon, sausage, frankfurters, and other luncheon meats?	☐	☐	☐	☐
2. Choose canned or frozen vegetables with sauce?	☐	☐	☐	☐
3. Use commercially prepared meals, main dishes, or canned or dehydrated soups?	☐	☐	☐	☐
4. Eat cheese?	☐	☐	☐	☐
5. Eat salted nuts, popcorn, pretzels, corn chips, and potato chips?	☐	☐	☐	☐
6. Add salt to cooking water for vegetables, rice, or pasta?	☐	☐	☐	☐
7. Add salt, seasoning mixes, salad dressings, or condiments, such as soy sauce, steak sauce, catsup, and mustard to foods during preparation or at the table?	☐	☐	☐	☐
8. Salt your food before tasting it?	☐	☐	☐	☐

The more checks you have in the last two columns, the higher your dietary sodium intake. However, not all of the items listed contribute the same amount of sodium. For example, many natural cheeses are relatively low in sodium. Most process cheeses and cottage cheese are higher.

To cut back on sodium intake, you can start by having some items less often, particularly those you checked as "3 to 5 times a week" or more. This does not mean eliminating foods from your diet. You can moderate your sodium intake by choosing lower sodium foods from each food group more often and by balancing high-sodium foods with low-sodium ones. For example, if you serve ham for dinner, plan to serve it with fresh or plain frozen vegetables cooked without added salt.

From USDA Home and Garden Bulletin No. 232-6, April 1986.

Table 13-3

A short guide to sodium content of foods

Foods	Approximate sodium content (in milligrams)
Breads, cereals, and grain products:	
Cooked cereal, pasta, rice, unsalted	Less than 5 per ½ cup
Ready-to-eat cereal	100-360 per ounce
Bread, whole-grain or enriched	110-175 per slice
Biscuits and muffins	170-390 each
Vegetables:	
Fresh or frozen vegetables, cooked without added salt	Less than 70 per ½ cup
Vegetables, canned or frozen with sauce	140-460 per ½ cup
Fruit:	
Fruits (fresh, frozen, or canned)	Less than 10 per ½ cup
Milk, cheese, and yogurt:	
Milk and yogurt	120-160 per cup
Buttermilk, salt added	260 per cup
Natural cheeses	110-450 per 1-½ ounces
Cottage cheese, regular and low-fat	450 per ½ cup
Process cheese and cheese spreads	700-900 per 2 ounces
Meat, poultry, and fish:	
Fresh meat, poultry, fish with fins	Less than 90 per 3 ounces
Cured ham, sausages, luncheon meat, frankfurters, canned meats	750-1,350 per 3 ounces
Fats and dressings:	
Oil	None
Vinegar	Less than 6 per tablespoon
Prepared salad dressings	80-250 per tablespoon
Unsalted butter or margarine	1 per teaspoon
Salted butter or margarine	45 per teaspoon
Salt pork, cooked	360 per ounce
Condiments:	
Catsup, mustard, chili sauce, tartar sauce, steak sauce	125-275 per tablespoon
Soy sauce	1,000 per tablespoon
Salt	2,000 per teaspoon
Snack and convenience foods:	
Canned and dehydrated soups	630-1300 per cup
Canned and frozen main dishes	800-1400 per 8 ounces

From USDA Home and Garden Bulletin No. 232-6, April 1986.

Table 13-3, cont'd

A short guide to sodium content of foods

Foods	Approximate sodium content (in milligrams)
Nuts and popcorn, unsalted	Less than 5 per ounce
Salted nuts, potato chips, corn chips	150-300 per ounce
Deep-fried pork rind	750 per ounce
Hamburger with bun	450-750 each
French fries, salted	200 per 20
Fried chicken	50 per drumstick
Hot dog with bun	750 each

Concept Check

Sodium is the major positive ion of the extracellular fluid. It is important for maintaining fluid balance and conducting nerve impulses. Sodium depletion is unlikely, since the North American diet has abundant sources and most sodium consumed is absorbed. The more foods we prepare at home, the more control we have over our sodium intakes. The minimum sodium requirement per day for adults is 500 milligrams. The average North American consumes 3 to 7 grams daily. About 10% of the population is sensitive to sodium. In these people, hypertension can develop as a result of high-sodium diets. To reduce the effects of hypertension, they can limit sodium intake to 2 to 3 grams per day as suggested by scientific groups. This practice may reduce the risk for future hypertension.

Potassium

Potassium (chemical symbol is K) performs many of the same functions as sodium, but it operates inside rather than outside cells. It is also associated more with lowering—rather than raising—blood pressure.[27] We absorb about 90% of the potassium we eat. Once inside the cell, much of the potassium is bound by phosphate ions (PO_4^{-3}) and proteins. Some of these proteins are enzymes that function more efficiently with potassium ions. The intracellular fluid contains 95% of the potassium in the body. Potassium participates in fluid balance and nerve transmission. After the transmission of a nerve impulse, when sodium ions are pumped back out of the nerve cell, potassium ions are pumped back into the nerve cell.

Results of a potassium deficiency. A potassium deficiency is more likely than a sodium deficiency because we generally do not add potassium to foods. Such deficiencies occur in some disease states, such as when long bouts of vomiting and diarrhea deplete potassium stores. A continually poor food intake, as may be the case in alcoholism, can also result in a potassium deficiency.

A low blood potassium level is a life-threatening problem. Results often include a loss of appetite, muscle cramps, confusion and apathy, and constipation. Eventually, the heart will beat irregularly, decreasing its capacity to pump blood.

Potassium in foods. Leafy and other vegetables are all nutrient-dense sources of potassium (Table 13-4). Milk, whole grains, dried beans, and meats are also good sources of potassium. Major contributors of potassium to the U.S. diet include coffee, tea, milk, potatoes (French fries and other potato products), and orange juice.

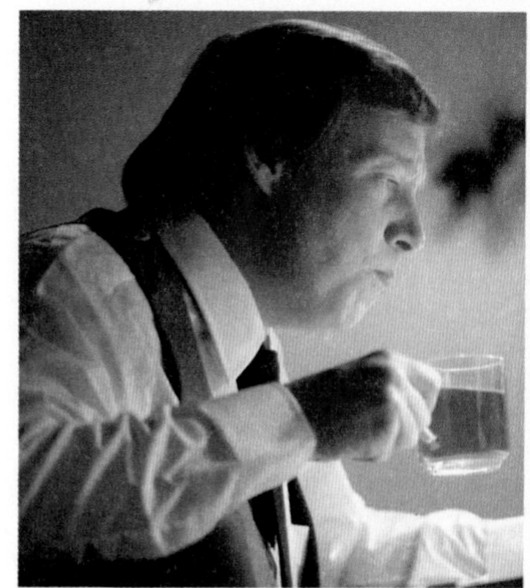

Coffee is a major contributer of potassium to the U.S. diet, primarily because so much coffee is consumed.

Minimum Potassium requirements. The minimum potassium requirement for adults is 2000 milligrams (2 grams) per day. *Diets of North Americans supply enough potassium if a variety of foods is eaten.* Intakes average 2 to 4 grams per day; women consume amounts near the lower intake level.[18]

Table 13-4

Good sources of potassium, ranked by nutrient density

Food	Serving size to yield 2000 milligrams*	kcalories needed to yield 2000 milligrams
Spinach, cooked	2½ cups	98
Lima beans	1½ cups	120
Zucchini squash, cooked	4 cups	127
Asparagus, cooked	3½ cups	158
Winter squash, baked	2 cups	187
Cantaloupe	1 each	225
Orange juice	3½ cups	410
Potato, baked	2 each	480
Pinto beans	2 cups	530
Bananas	2½ each	530
Kidney beans	4½ cups	660

*Minimum adult requirement.
A diet rich in vegetables and fruits provides ample potassium.

North Americans at risk for a potassium deficiency. People who take potassium-wasting diuretics, such as thiazides and furosemide, need to monitor their potassium intakes carefully. These diuretics deplete body potassium. Water follows the excreted potassium, eventually reducing blood volume and blood pressure. In such cases, high-potassium foods, such as fruits, fruit juices, and vegetables, are good additions to a diet, and perhaps potassium chloride supplements will also be recommended by a physician.

Several other groups are at risk for potassium deficiency and need blood potassium levels monitored. These groups include anorexia nervosa and bulimia patients. Poor diets and losses from vomiting cause the problem. People on very low calorie diets (protein-sparing modified fasts) are also at risk, as well as athletes who perspire heavily. These people can avoid the detrimental side effects of low potassium levels by consuming potassium-rich sources.

Toxicity of potassium. If kidneys function normally, typical intakes of dietary potassium are not toxic. When kidneys function poorly, potassium levels build up in the bloodstream (creating a condition called hyperkalemia) and inhibit heart function by causing irregular heart beats, (arrythmias). This eventually can cause the heart to stop beating. Consequently, in cases of poor kidney function, close monitoring of potassium intake is required.

Chloride

Chlorine (chemical symbol is Cl) is a very poisonous gas. Public water utilities often rely on this gas to kill bacteria in water supplies. Consequently many waterborne diseases are rare in North America.

Chloride, an ionic form of chlorine, forms an important negative ion for the extracellular fluid. These ions are a component of the hydrochloric acid produced by the parietal cells in the stomach and are also used during immune responses as white blood cells attack foreign cells. Most of the body's chloride is excreted by the kidneys; some is lost in perspiration.

A chloride deficiency is unlikely because our dietary sodium chloride intake is so high. Frequent and lengthy bouts of vomiting, if coupled with a nutrient-poor diet, can contribute to a deficiency because stomach secretions contain chloride. In 1978 to 1979, not enough chloride was added to a brand of infant formula. Infants who consumed it suffered severe convulsions and other health problems. This incident shows what can happen when the need for a nutrient normally abundant in our diets is not given adequate attention.

Chloride in foods. A few fruits and some vegetables are naturally good sources of chloride. However, most chloride comes from the addition of salt to food. If we know a food's salt content, we can predict closely its chloride content (sodium content × 1.5). Naturally occurring sodium or chloride doesn't significantly affect this calculation.

Minimum chloride requirement. The minimum chloride requirement for adults is 700 milligrams per day. Assuming that the average North American consumes at least 7.5 grams of salt daily, that yields 4.5 grams (4500 milligrams) of chloride, an abundant intake of this ion.

Toxicity of chloride. The chloride ion itself may be an important part of the blood pressure–raising action of sodium. Together, then, the sodium and chloride components of salt are implicated in the high rates of hypertension in North America. One researcher suggests that chloride supplies a negative ion that allows the body to retain the positive sodium ion. Since chloride ions tend to remain in the body, they trap the positive sodium ions to balance the equation. The result is the same either way: for hypertension, control salt intake. (See Nutrition Perspective 13-1.)

Concept Check

Potassium has functions similar to those of sodium, except it is the main positive ion of intracellular, not extracellular, fluid. Potassium is vital to fluid balance and nerve transmission. A potassium deficiency caused by poor intake, persistent vomiting, or use of certain diuretics can lead to loss of appetite, muscle cramps, confusion, and heart arrhythmias. Leafy vegetables, melons, tomatoes, and potatoes are rich sources of potassium. A risk of toxicity accompanies impaired kidney function. Chloride is the major negative ion of extracellular fluid. It functions in digestion as part of hydrochloric acid and in immune system responses. Deficiencies are unlikely because dietary sodium chloride intake is so high.

Calcium

All cells need calcium (chemical symbol is Ca), but over 99% of calcium in the body operates inside bones and teeth, strengthening them. This represents 40% of the mineral present in the body and equals about 1200 grams (Figure 13-1). As calcium circulates in the bloodstream, it supplies the calcium needs of other body cells. Growth and bone development in laboratory animals is closely tied to calcium intake. This link is seen in humans, too, but we can probably better adapt to a low calcium intake.

Absorption of calcium. Calcium is absorbed primarily in the upper part of the small intestine (duodenum) because calcium requires a pH below 6 to stay in solution. The duodenum tends to remain at this acidic pH because it takes time for the acidic stomach contents to be fully neutralized by bicarbonate ions released from the pancreas (see Chapter 3). Calcium absorption in the upper small intestine depends on the active vitamin D hormone calcitriol. Some additional calcium absorption occurs throughout the lower small intestine.

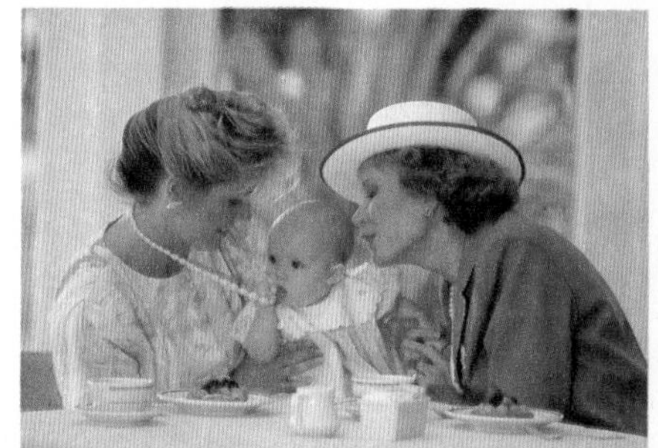

As a woman enters different stages of life, her calcium needs change.

Calcium absorption varies from about 25% to 40% of dietary intake, but can increase to as high as 50% during pregnancy and at other times of high-calcium needs. Young people tend to absorb calcium better than older people. The lowest rates of absorption occur in postmenopausal women who do not receive supplements of the hormone estrogen. Estrogen therapy increases the synthesis of calcitriol, which increases calcium absorption.

Table 13-5

Absorption of calcium from the intestinal tract

Factors favoring absorption	Factors hindering absorption
Acid nature of upper intestinal tract	Alkaline reaction in lower intestinal tract
Normal digestive activity and motility of intestinal tract	Large amounts of dietary fiber
Dietary calcium and phosphorus in about equal amounts	Laxatives or any circumstances that induce diarrhea or hypermotility of the intestine
Vitamin D	*Great* excess of phosphorus or magnesium in proportion to calcium
Need for higher amounts by the body, as during pregnancy	Phytate, oxalic acid, and unabsorbed fatty acids: they all bind calcium in the intestine
Low calcium intake	Vitamin D deficiency
Parathyroid hormone	Menopause
Lactose	Old age
Glucose	Tannins in tea

Many factors facilitate calcium absorption, such as the acidic environment of the small intestine; the presence of calcitriol, parathyroid hormone, dietary glucose, and lactose; and normal intestinal motility (flow) (Table 13-5). Factors limiting calcium absorption include large amounts of phytate, fiber, magnesium, or phosphorus in the diet, and tannins in tea; a vitamin D deficiency; menopause; diarrhea; and old age.[2]

One problem in setting the RDA for calcium is predicting the extent to which calcium will be absorbed.[10] The RDA is based on an estimated 30% to 40% absorption. Some people absorb calcium more efficiently than that, and others less efficiently. Less efficient absorption raises needs. However, deciding who is consuming sufficient calcium to accommodate body needs—even if they are not meeting the RDA—is not practical. That requires measuring calcium absorption, a complex task.

Bone loss caused by insufficient calcium in the diet proceeds slowly. Only after many years are clinical signs apparent. By not meeting the RDA for calcium, some people, especially women, may be setting the stage for future bone fractures. But, because we don't know how efficiently individuals absorb calcium, we often cannot predict who is at high risk. It is naive to assume that everyone can adapt to a calcium intake far lower than the RDA.

Regulating serum calcium. Each cell has a critical need for calcium, as we will discuss. This is probably the reason humans have such excellent hormonal systems to control blood calcium levels. A normal blood calcium level can be maintained despite a poor calcium intake. The bones, however, pay the price. *This makes serum calcium levels generally a poor measure of calcium status.* Measuring bone density over short periods isn't much more useful, however, because changes in bone density develop very slowly (see Nutrition Perspective 13-2 on calcium and osteoporosis).

As discussed in Chapter 11, when the serum calcium level falls, the parathyroid gland releases parathyroid hormone. This hormone increases calcium absorption by increasing synthesis of calcitriol, the active vitamin D hormone. It also increases the kidney's retrieval of calcium before possible urine excretion. In addition, parathyroid hormone causes increased calcium release from bones. In all, then, parathyroid hormone action increases the serum calcium level.

When serum calcium levels are too high, the thyroid gland secretes the hormone calcitonin. Calcitonin decreases calcium loss from bones and decreases the synthesis of the calcitriol. This causes the calcium level in the bloodstream to fall into the normal range.

Sometimes these hormonal controls do not work properly to hold serum calcium levels within the desired range. In the case of high parathyroid hormone levels, which occur with some kidney diseases, eventually severe bone loss takes place. Certain dietary manipulations, such as limiting dietary phosphorus, can be tried first. But many times a physician is forced to remove a person's parathyroid gland to prevent further calcium loss from the bones.

Functions of calcium. Bone formation and maintenance is a major role for calcium in the body. We will develop bone metabolism further in a later section. However, the importance of calcium in the body does not stop there. Calcium is essential for blood clotting. It participates in a reaction whereby prothrombin contributes to the synthesis of fibrin so that a blood clot can form. Without sufficient calcium in the bloodstream, blood will not clot.

Calcium is critical for muscle contraction. It allows the proteins in muscles, actin and myosin, to interact properly during muscle contraction. If the blood calcium level falls below a certain level, muscles cannot relax after contraction. The body then stiffens and shows signs of **tetany.**

tetany
A syndrome marked by sharp contraction of muscles and failure to relax afterward; usually caused by abnormal calcium metabolism.

Normal nerve transmission requires calcium. It permits the release of neurotransmitters, as well as the flow of ions in and out of nerve cells. Tetany can also occur when nerve transmission fails because insufficient calcium is available.

Finally, calcium helps regulate metabolism in the cell by participating in the **calmodulin** system. When calcium enters a cell (often because of hormone action) and binds to the protein calmodulin, the protein/calcium-complex formed then goes on to regulate activity levels of various enzymes, including those that synthesize glycogen (Figure 13-7).

calmodulin
A cell protein that, once bound to calcium, can influence the activity of some enzymes in the cell.

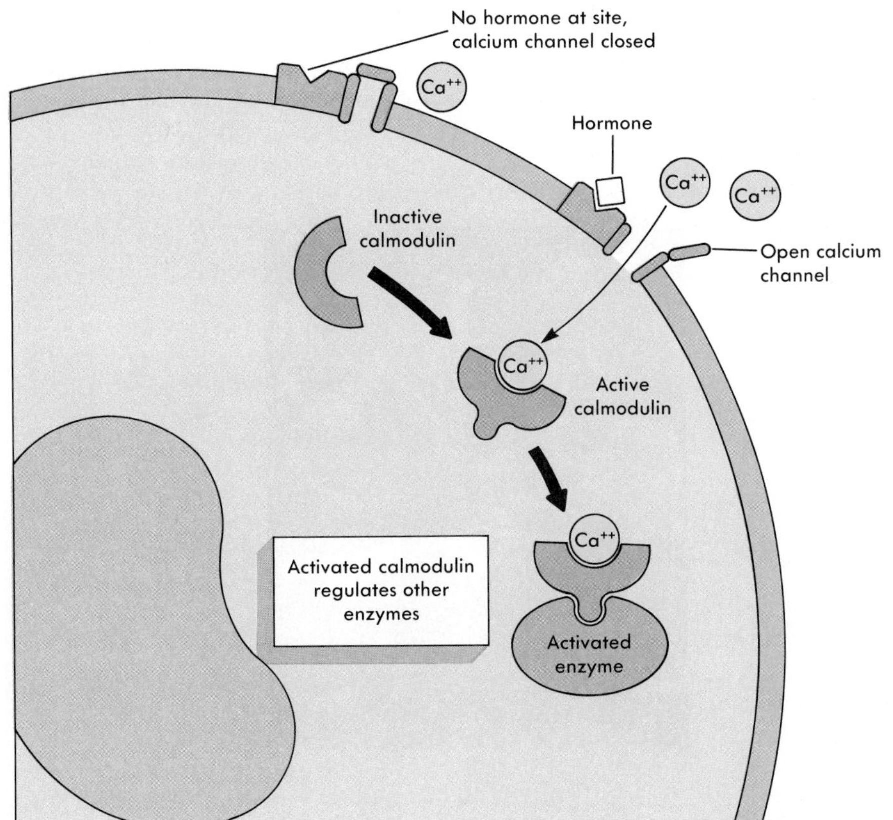

Figure 13-7
The calmodulin system. Certain hormones bind to receptors on the cell membranes of target cells. This allows calcium to enter the cell. Some calcium binds to calmodulin. This protein can then regulate enzymes, like those used in glycogen metabolism.

A Closer Look at Bone

A glance at a steak bone gives the impression that it is devoid of life. However, observing a bone while it is alive in the body would show that it is an actively metabolizing organ. Inside bone is a central cavity where marrow cells busily produce red and white blood cells and other blood components. Within the bone itself are osteo*c*last cells. These cells are continually breaking down the bone network. In essence, osteoclasts break down bone in areas where it is not needed. These osteoclasts are very active when a diet is deficient in calcium, because their action releases calcium from the bone so it can enter the bloodstream. *Remember, a supply of calcium is vital to all cells, not just to bone cells.*

Bone also contains osteo*b*last cells. These cells secrete a collagen protein matrix that forms the support structure of bone. They then secrete bone mineral, which strengthens the bone. This mineral matures and eventually approaches the composition of $Ca_{10}(PO_4)_6(OH)_2$, called **hydroxyapatite.**

Bone turnover refers to a cycle of bone breakdown by the osteoclasts, and then bone rebuilding by the osteoblasts. In this way, bone is remodeled when necessary. Once bone has been created in an area, osteoclast activity always precedes osteoblast activity. Before new bone can be built, the old bone in that area must be partially broken down.

During human growth, total osteoblast activity exceeds osteoclast activity, so we make more bone than we break down. In the first year of life, all bones in the body are rebuilt. In the young adult, 15% to 30% of the skeleton is rebuilt each year, with more bone being built in areas of high stress. A right-handed tennis player, for example, will lay down more bone in that arm in comparison with the left arm.

BONE STRUCTURE

The outer surface of an entire bone is composed of a very dense type of bone, called **cortical (compact) bone.** The shafts of bones, such as those of the arm, are almost entirely cortical bone.

Trabecular (spongy) bone is found in the ends of the bones, inside the spinal vertebrae, and inside the flat bones of the pelvis. Trabecular bone forms an internal scaffolding network for a bone (Figure 13-8). It supports the outer cortical shell of the bone, especially in heavily stressed areas, such as joints.

BONE STRENGTH

Bone strength is determined primarily by its density. The more densely packed the bone crystals are, the stronger the bone structure. The next important determinant is the rate at which the bone can heal itself. **Microfractures,** so small they cannot be seen on an x-ray or any type of bone scan, are constantly developing in bone. These microfractures must be knitted back together with collagen and bone crystal. Otherwise, they can accumulate and eventually allow a major fracture.

The third important element of strength is the trabecular bone network inside the bone. It is especially critical for the trabeculae to extend continuously—without breaks—throughout the bone. Any break weakens the support of the outer edge of the bone, and increases the risk for bone fracture.

Of those three factors—bone density, rate of self-healing, and integrity of the trabecular support—the only one that can

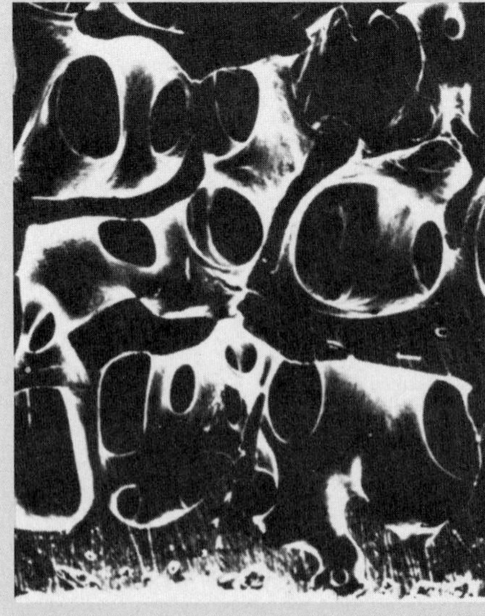

Figure 13-8
Cortical and trabecular bone. In the center you can see the lacy trabecular bone. Notice the dense cortical bone shell around the perimeter.

A Closer Look at Bone—cont'd

be measured when the bone is inside a person is bone density. *The bone density value can predict fracture risk, but it is not perfect because it cannot account for other factors that also determine bone strength.* Not all people with low-bone density suffer fractures, and some people with high-bone densities do suffer fractures, probably because these other factors come into play, as well.

BONE DENSITY AT DIFFERENT AGES

Rapid and continual bone growth and calcification occur throughout the adolescent years. Scientists are not sure when it stops. Additions to bone density may stop by age 18 years, or may continue through the ages of 20 to 30 years. This question of the age at which bone density peaks concerns women mainly: they make less bone than men, lose it at a faster rate, and live longer. Thus they start their adult years with less bone, and have a longer time to lose it. About one third of women eventually experience osteoporosis-related fractures (see Nutrition Perspective 13-2).

Bone loss, especially in trabecular areas, begins around age 30 years in women. The rate of bone loss between age 30 years and menopause (approximately age 50 years) appears to be slow and continuous. It often speeds up at menopause, and continues at a high rate for the next 5 to 10 years. By age 65 years, bone-loss rate has fallen to about the same rate as before menopause. *Estrogen replacement at menopause can stop this bone loss. Bones with a high trabecular content—those in the wrist and the spine—are the first to fracture in osteoporosis* (Figure 13-9).

In the very elderly, hip fractures due to osteoporosis commonly occur. The neck of the femur bone contains trabecular bone, but also quite a bit of cortical bone. It takes until about age 75 to 80 years to lose enough total bone in this area to increase the chances of a fracture.

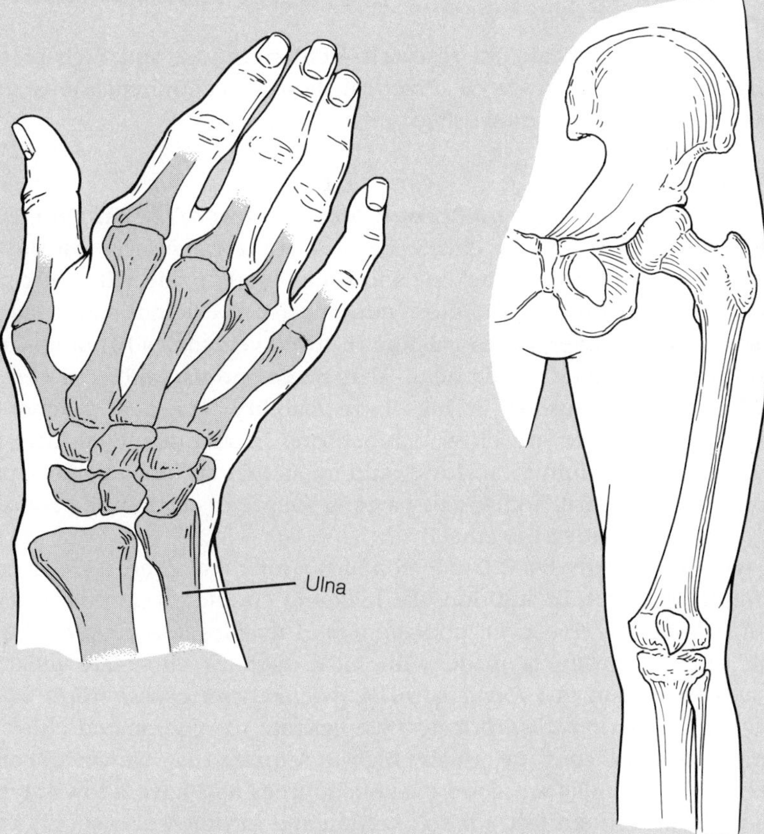

Figure 13-9
Major sites of osteoporosis-related fractures.

osteopenia
Decreased bone mass due to cancer, hyperthyroidism, or other reasons.

Osteoporosis. Failure to maintain enough bone mass in the body eventually results in **osteopenia,** which means "little bone." When a person has osteopenia, and no cause can be found—such as osteomalacia (see Chapter 11), the use of certain medications, or cancer tumors—then the diagnosis is osteoporosis. Osteoporosis can be further classified as Type I (postmenopausal), which appears in the years right after menopause, and Type II (senile), which is found in people of advanced ages.

Bone composition in osteoporosis is essentially normal. The bone may contain some extra sodium, but basically there is just less bone throughout the body. Because these bones have lesser substance, osteoporosis can lead to hip fractures in old age, as well as to loss of teeth. Recall from Chapter 11 that in osteomalacia the bone is abnormal, in that it is poorly calcified. Nutrition Perspective 13-2 discusses calcium and osteoporosis in detail.

Other possible benefits of calcium in the diet

Besides contributing to bone strength, dietary calcium may reduce the risk of colon cancer.[25] It appears that a high-calcium content in the stool can bind free fatty acids and bile acids found there. These compounds, when unbound, tend to irritate the colon. The irritation may increase cell turnover and in turn increase the risk of cancer (see Chapter 5). A daily dietary calcium supplement of 1250 milligrams reduces cell turnover in the colon. High calcium levels in the colon may also increase the tendency of cancer cells in the colon to clump together and decrease their tendency to metastasize to other areas.

Supplemental calcium intakes of 1 gram or more per day may also slightly decrease blood pressure.[13] It takes about 8 weeks to see the effect. (See Nutrition Perspective 13-1).

Both these areas of calcium research—colon cancer and high blood pressure—are new areas of research. Practical dietary recommendations stemming from this research are not established.

Calcium in foods

Dairy products, such as milk and cheese, provide most of the calcium in the U.S. diet. The exception is cottage cheese because most calcium is lost during production. White bread, rolls, crackers, and other foods made with milk products are secondary contributors. The most nutrient-dense calcium sources are green leafy vegetables. However, much calcium in these vegetables is not absorbed because of the presence of oxalic acid. That makes nonfat milk the best overall source of calcium because of its high bioavailability. The new calcium-fortified versions of orange juice are close competitors. In addition, new high-calcium milks increase the calcium to kcalorie ratio for nonfat and low-fat dairy products even more. Soybean curd (tofu) is also a good source of calcium if it is made with calcium carbonate (check the label).

To review options for dairy product use in lactose intolerance, see Chapter 3.

One reason the Daily Food Guide contains a milk and cheese group is to supply calcium to the diet. In addition, the milk and cheese group provides protein, vitamin A, vitamin D, riboflavin, potassium, and magnesium. People who do not like milk can use products made with milk, such as chocolate milk, yogurt, cheese, and ice cream. *All forms of milk, yogurt, and cheese allow about the same degree of calcium absorption.*[21] We hesitate to recommend either cheese or ice cream because they are usually high in saturated fat. However, some low-fat cheeses and ice milks are good calcium sources and have a low saturated-fat content. Bones in canned fish, such as salmon and sardines, also supply calcium.

Calcium supplements

Calcium supplements can be used by people who don't like milk or cannot incorporate into their diets either enough milk products or foods made with milk. Cal-

Table 13-6

Good sources of calcium ranked by nutrient density

Food	Serving size to yield 800 milligrams*	kcalories needed to yield 800 milligrams
Turnip greens, cooked	4 cups	120
Spinach, cooked	3-¼ cups	133
Beet greens, cooked	5 cups	200
Broccoli, cooked	4-½ cups	207
Parmesan cheese	¾ cups	266
Shrimp, boiled	9 ounces	272
1% low-fat milk	2-½ cups	275
Buttermilk	2-¾ cups	275
Romano cheese	2-½ ounces	275
Swiss cheese	3 ounces	321
Muenster cheese	4 ounces	416
Sardines, canned w/ bones	8 ounces	500

*RDA for adults 25 years of age.
Green leafy vegetables supply the fewest kcalories, but the calcium in nonfat milk is more bioavailable. So nonfat milk is actually the best nonfortified food source.

cium carbonate is the supplement form usually recommended because it contains 40% calcium. Thus the dosage can be of smaller or fewer pills. For elderly people who have lost much of their stomach acidity, calcium citrate—which is acidic itself—might be a better choice. The lower percent of calcium in that preparation, however, requires a greater number or size of pills. These supplements should be taken in divided doses with meals so that the acid produced by the stomach can aid digestion and absorption.

We hesitate to encourage calcium supplement use, even though supplements are as well absorbed as milk calcium. We know that many people have difficulty adhering to a supplement regimen. *Regular food habits can be integrated more easily into a routine compared with remembering to take several pills a day.* In addition, calcium carbonate acts as an antacid, and so interferes with the stomach's normally acidic environment.

Some calcium supplements are poorly digested because they do not readily dissolve. To test a supplement for this, put one in 6 ounces of cider vinegar. Stir every 5 minutes. It should dissolve within 30 minutes.

Taking 1000 milligrams of calcium in the form of calcium carbonate or calcium citrate is probably safe, but only long-term studies can confirm that. There appears to be no risk from high dietary calcium: foods supply a natural balance of other minerals, in addition to calcium, decreasing the likelihood of mineral imbalance.

RDA for calcium

The RDA for calcium for adults is 800 milligrams per day. The current RDA extends the 1200 milligram level used in teenage years to age 25, in hopes that these higher calcium intakes will help women build and maintain a higher bone mass. There is reason to believe that this may be a good idea. At 800 milligrams a day, young adult women have enough calcium to maintain bone, but some may not have enough to keep building more bone, if that is possible.

A recent National Institutes of Health (NIH) committee also recommended that postmenopausal women who do not take estrogen replacements consume 1500 milligrams of calcium daily. However, some research shows that even this amount will not be enough for these elderly women. Nutrition Perspective 13-2 provides some help in sorting out this controversy.

Expert Opinion

Nutrition and Bone Mass

VELIMIR MATKOVIC, M.D., Ph.D.

The human skeleton develops through infancy and childhood to a peak bone mass during late adolescence or early twenties. Thereafter, bone loss gradually occurs, resulting eventually in a bone mass value that increases fracture risk after minimal or moderate trauma. Research suggests the main determinants of osteoporotic-related fractures are the peak bone-mass level reached at skeletal maturity and the subsequent rate of bone loss. Besides these variables, abnormalities in microstructure and bone tissue repair also could lead to bone fragility and changes in bone quality, contributing to the overall incidence of fractures among the elderly.

PEAK BONE MASS

Since bone mass is a principal determinant of fracture risk, a high bone mass at skeletal maturity is considered important protection against age-related bone loss. Besides well-known factors influencing body stature, such as protein and zinc intake, very little is known about the mechanisms for increasing peak bone mass. Peak bone mass is clearly the result of age, gender, and probably other genetically determined factors. We do know that men have higher bone mass values than women, and that blacks have heavier skeletons than whites. As a direct consequence, men and blacks have a lower incidence of fractures than other populations. Peak bone mass could also be related to calcium nutrition.

The ages between 9 and 20 years seem critical for achievement of peak bone mass. From birth until about age 20 years, bones grow rapidly. After this period, the skeleton constantly remodels itself throughout life. The adolescent growth spurt is probably the most important period for bone growth. That is when bone mineral content is increasing at the rate of about 8.5% per year.

The average male begins his growth spurt at around 12 years of age, reaching his maximum velocity in height growth at about 14 years of age. At this time, he will be growing at nearly twice his childhood or preadolescent rate. His growth will be almost completed by age 18. Females begin puberty approximately 2 years earlier (at 8 to 10 years of age) and reach maximum velocity in height growth around 12 years of age. Cessation of linear growth in girls will be around age 16 years. There is about a 2% increase in body length thereafter in both boys and girls, extending to the early twenties of the young adult period. This increase is accounted for primarily by continued vertebral growth. Skeletal bone mass, based on skeletal weight measurements, is then achieved by the beginning of the third decade.

Total body calcium is also greatest at age 20 years. The external diameter of tubular (cortical) bones plateaus by the age of 20 years in males, and a few years earlier in females. Bone mineral content of the forearm also approaches its highest level by the beginning of the young adulthood, indicating once again that adolescence can be a critical period for cortical peak bone mass formation. There are few data regarding changes in trabecular bone mass in the adolescent period, but present literature suggests that peak bone mass for the vertebral column has been achieved by the age of 20 years. Postmortem data, using bone ash measurements and compressive strength measurements, indicate an increase in the vertebrae figures after the beginning of the third decade and a decline thereafter. Bone mineral density in the lower spine and pelvic area also declines after its maximum at about the age of 20 years in both males and females.

To accumulate total body calcium of about 1000 grams during the first 20 years of life (7300 days), females need an average daily accretion of calcium into the skeleton of about 140 milligrams per day. Males need 165 milligrams per day for total body calcium of 1200 grams in 20 years. During the adolescent growth spurt, the required calcium retention (milligrams/day) is 2 to 3 times higher than the average value.

CALCIUM AND BONE DENSITY

Among nutritional factors, low-calcium, low-vitamin D, high-protein, high-phosphate, and high-caffeine intakes are considered risk factors for developing osteoporosis. These factors can influence either peak bone mass formation and/or the subsequent rate of bone loss. Experiments with laboratory animals show that a calcium deficiency can cause osteoporosis.

Expert Opinion—cont'd

In the majority of the experiments, animals were fed a low-calcium diet during the growing period and skeletons were examined when the animal reached adulthood. The results indicated that calcium deficiency can cause osteoporosis by decreasing peak bone mass formation, rather than affecting later adult bone mass. Experimental calcium deficiency can cause growth retardation in animals, affecting bone volume and decreasing bone density (bone mass per bone volume). We have no clear-cut evidence that skeletons of growing humans will react to inadequate calcium intake in the same way as laboratory animals, although older growth studies of children suggest that they could. A group of British children who received milk supplementation at the turn of the century grew taller than a non-supplemented group. Unfortunately, bone mass measurements were not done in this study.

The Ten State Nutrition Survey done in the United States in the late 1960s found that children from more affluent families had a 5% higher rate of skeletal mass and bone formation than children from lower socioeconomic classes. However, it is not quite clear if those differences were due to inadequate protein and/or mineral nutrition. Malnutrition certainly can lead to growth retardation and, conversely, with correction of the nutritional deficit, growth rate rapidly can return to normal. At present, we don't know if there is adequate "catch-up mineralization" of the skeleton, particularly after the growth spurt period. It was also reported recently that some children who suffered an accidental fracture have decreased bone mineral density, as well as decreased calcium intake.

A study performed of the calcium intake, bone mass, and fracture rates in two populations in Croatia, Yugoslavia revealed that people who consume higher amounts of calcium throughout their lifetimes (1000 to 1200 milligrams/day) had denser skeletons and lower hip fracture rates than people with lower calcium intakes (400 to 500 milligrams per day). Since differences were present at the age of 30 years, this study suggests calcium is probably more important to peak bone mass formation, rather than to protect people from bone loss.

Adolescent females in the United States often have poor calcium intake compared with their calcium needs for skeletal growth. To satisfy their need for a high skeletal retention, supply enough to replace unavoidable calcium excretion into the urine, and account for variable absorption efficiency, calcium intake during adolescence should exceed 1000 milligrams per day. The RDA is 1200 milligrams per day. If the calcium intake is lower than 1200 milligrams per day with a subsequent decrease in calcium retention by 100 milligrams per day per 5 years, this should lower the peak whole body calcium by 182 grams. That same amount of bone calcium will allow negative calcium balance in postmenopausal women of 30 milligrams per day for 16 years and 15 milligrams per day for 32 years, (the typical figure for calcium loss in elderly women is about 30 milligrams per day). My hypothesis is that residents of the low-calcium district in Croatia did not have adequate calcium intake during adolescence and ended the bone growth period with decreased peak bone mass level. It was also recently reported that postmenopausal women who had decreased dairy product consumption during adolescence had decreased bone mass in the postmenopausal period.

CONCLUSION

Late childhood and adolescence represents the ideal time to build a dense skeleton, and both laboratory animal and human research points to an adequate calcium intake as an important goal. The RDA of 1200 milligrams per day for calcium in adolescence should represent a critical objective in diet planning. Moderation in protein, phosphorus and caffeine intakes and regular sun exposure (or Vitamin D intake) are also important. As a final caution, alcoholism is probably a risk factor of greater relative importance than has been commonly recognized. Prevalence of significant alcohol abuse in the adult U.S. population ranges between 8% and 16%. It was demonstrated several years ago that bone mass is seriously depleted in both male and female alcoholics. Defective osteoblastic function rather than increased bone resorption has been reported in patients with alcoholism.

Dr. Matkovic is Assistant Professor of Physical and Internal Medicine at The Ohio State University. His main research interest is in osteoporosis and calcium nutrition.

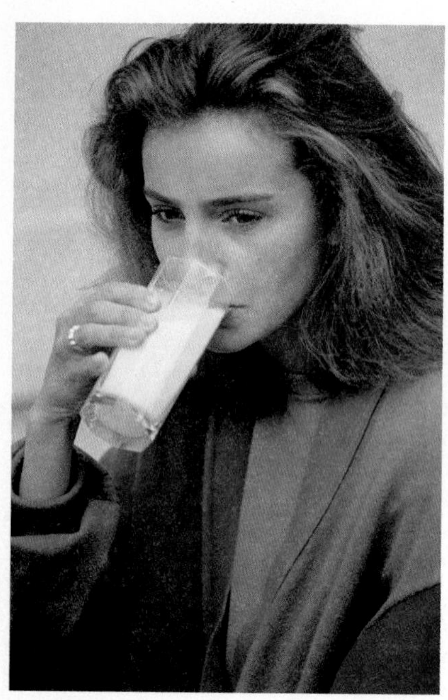

It is important for women, especially through age 24 years, to make sure they are regularly consuming enough calcium.

North Americans at risk of a calcium deficiency

The average calcium intake of women in North America ranges from approximately 500 to 650 milligrams per day, while it is 800 to 900 milligrams per day for men. *About 25% of women consume less than 300 milligrams per day.* So women's diets tend to be deficient in calcium, while men's do not. Men eat more food in general to support their higher kcalorie outputs, and that accounts for part of the difference. An easy way for women to increase calcium intake is to increase activity level and in turn their food consumption.

To estimate your calcium intake, use the rule of 300s. Give yourself 300 milligrams to start with. This accounts for small amounts of calcium provided by a moderate kcalorie intake from foods scattered throughout the Daily Food Guide. Add to that another 300 milligrams for every cup of milk or yogurt or 1.5 ounces (45 grams) of cheese.

If you eat a lot of tofu, almonds, or sardines, food composition tables will give you a more accurate account of your calcium intake. Our shortcut method underestimates it, especially in the case of vegans. It is important for vegetarians to focus on eating good plant sources of calcium, as well as on the total amount of calcium ingested.

Toxicity of calcium

The major risk from taking excess calcium supplements is kidney stones. A good rule of thumb is that calcium intake should not exceed 2500 milligrams per day. Any more and extra calcium in the urine can increase the risk, especially in people who tend to form kidney stones. The body absorbs calcium less efficiently as calcium intake increases, but overzealous use of calcium supplements can overwhelm the control of absorption.

If calcium/antacid supplements and milk intake together become exceedingly high, a milk-alkali syndrome can result.[28] With this condition, serum calcium climbs so high that calcium precipitates into tissues all over the body, causing local tissue death. Sticking to an intake of 1500 to 2500 milligrams, however, poses no risk for developing this problem.

Concept Check

About 99% of calcium in the body is found in the bones. Aside from its critical role in bone, calcium also functions in blood clotting, muscle contraction, nerve transmission, and cell metabolism. Calcium requires a slightly acid pH and the vitamin D hormone calcitriol for efficient absorption. Factors that reduce calcium absorption include large amounts of dietary fiber, decreased estrogen levels, and excess magnesium or phosphorus. Serum calcium level is regulated by parathyroid hormone and calcitonin and does not closely reflect daily intake or bone stores. Osteoporosis is bone loss with no specific cause. Women are particularly at risk for osteoporosis because they make less bone than men, lose it faster, and live longer. Dairy products are the best sources of calcium. Supplemental forms such as calcium carbonate are well-absorbed. However, supplements may interfere with the absorption of other minerals. Overzealous supplementation may also result in kidney stones.

Phosphorus

The body absorbs phosphorus (chemical symbol is P) quite efficiently and can increase absorption from 60% to 90% as body needs vary. This high absorption rate plus its wide availability in foods makes phosphorus a lesser concern in diet planning than calcium. The active vitamin D hormone calcitriol enhances phosphorus absorption, as it does for calcium. Excretion by the kidneys is primarily responsible for maintaining body levels. This is unlike calcium, where changes in the rates of absorption are also very important.

Functions of phosphorus. Phosphorus plays many important roles in the body. It is a component of enzymes, other key metabolic compounds, ATP, cell membranes, and the bone mineral hydroxyapatite. About 85% of phosphorus in the body is found in bone. The rest circulates freely in the bloodstream and operates inside cells. No deficiency disease is currently associated with a poor phosphorus intake, but a poor intake may contribute to bone loss in elderly women.

Phosphorus in foods. Milk, cheese, bakery products, and meat provide most of the phosphorus in the U.S. diet. Cereals, bran, eggs, nuts, and fish are also good sources (Table 13-7). About 20% to 30% of dietary phosphorus comes from food additives, especially those found in baked goods, cheeses, and processed meats, as well as in soft drinks (about 75 milligrams per 12 ounce serving). *Phosphorus is one of the most difficult nutrients to limit in the diet because it is found in so many foods.*

RDA for phosphorus. The RDA for phosphorus is the same as the RDA for calcium—800 milligrams per day for adults. The North American diet provides 1400 to 1500 milligrams of phosphorus per day. Thus *deficiencies of phosphorus are unlikely in adults, especially when considering its highly efficient absorption.*

Table 13-7

Good sources of phosphorus, ranked by nutrient density

Food	Serving size to yield 800 milligrams*	kcalories need to yield 800 milligrams
Cereal, bran	1 cup	163
Skim milk	3-½ cups	260
Cheese, American	4 ounces	403
Milk, 2%	3-½ cups	420
Salmon, broiled	9 ounces	450
Sardines, canned in oil w/ bones	5-¾ ounces	507
Trout, cooked	10 ounces	576
Eggs, yolks	9 each	581
Cheese, Swiss	5 ounces	620
Liver, calf, fried	7 ounces	650
Wheat flour, whole	2 cups	650
Herring, smoked, kippered	11 ounces	670
Chicken, light meat	12 ounces	682
Cheese, Colby	6 ounces	691
Wheat flour, whole	2 cups	776
Turkey, roasted	14 ounces	810
Almonds, dried	1 cup	850
Pork loin, broiled	12 ounces	850
Beef	12 ounces	949
Nuts, mixed, shelled	1-½ cup	1122

*RDA for adults 25 years of age.

Phosphorus is more widely distributed than calcium in the Daily Food Guide. Diet soft drinks are another nutrient-dense choice.

North Americans at risk for a phosphorus deficiency. Marginal phosphorus status can be found in premature infants, vegans, people with alcoholism, elderly people on nutrient-poor diets, cases of long-standing diarrhea, and people who daily use aluminum-containing antacids (usually to treat peptic ulcers). These types of antacids bind phosphorus in the small intestine. If you suspect a low dietary phosphorus intake, calculate the diet's phosphorus content.

Toxicity of phosphorus. If serum phosphorus levels are too high, the phosphate ions bind calcium, which leads to tetany and convulsions. Inefficient kidney function can cause detrimentally high levels. However, there is no known toxicity in healthy adults associated with phosphorus consumption. Formerly, scientists believed that a high-phosphorus intake coupled with a low-calcium intake led to bone loss. Recent research casts doubt on the importance of the calcium to phosphorus ratio in a diet, as long as the RDA for calcium is met.[26] If not met, then a high phosphorus intake may compound the bone loss from poor calcium intake.

Magnesium

Magnesium (chemical symbol is Mg) is best found in plant, rather than animal, products. Magnesium in the plant pigment chlorophyll and iron in hemoglobin in the red blood cell both serve similar roles in respiration. We absorb about 30% to 40% of the magnesium in our diets, but absorption efficiency can increase to 75% if intakes are low. The active vitamin D hormone calcitriol may enhance magnesium absorption.

Functions of magnesium. Bone contains 60% of the body's magnesium. The rest circulates in the blood and operates inside cells. Over 300 enzymes use magnesium as a cofactor. Without magnesium, many enzymes would function less efficiently. In addition, magnesium binds to ATP to form "active ATP." A magnesium ion bridges between the second and the last phosphate groups on an ATP molecule.

Proper nerve function and cardiac function require magnesium. Animals deficient in magnesium become very irritable. Eventually, if the deficiency becomes severe, the animals suffer convulsions and often die. In humans, a magnesium deficiency causes an irregular heart beat, which is sometimes accompanied by weakness, muscle pain, disorientation, and seizures.[24] However, a magnesium deficiency develops very slowly because we have large stores. A link between magnesium deficiency and sudden heart attacks has been observed, but its validity is not established.[20] *There is no test for magnesium deficiency both sufficiently accurate and available for routine clinical practice. Consequently, clinicians often fail to detect a poor magnesium status in a person when it exists.*

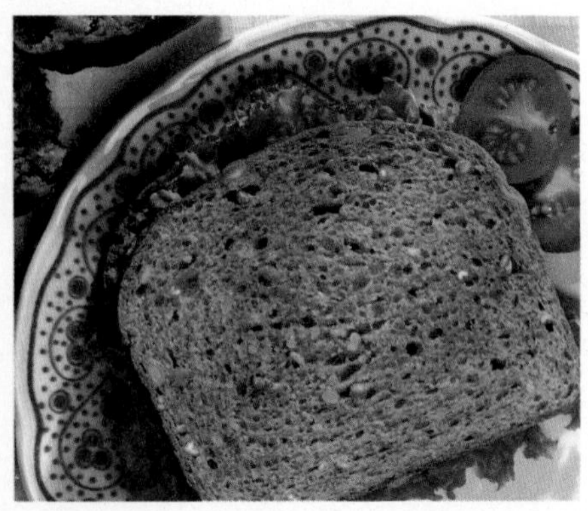

Not only are whole-grain breads high in dietary fiber, they are an excellent source of magnesium.

Magnesium in food. Good food sources for magnesium are whole grains (wheat bran), broccoli, squash, beans, nuts, and seeds (Table 13-8). *Magnesium is one reason why registered dietitians emphasize the importance of whole grains and vegetables in a diet: these are excellent magnesium sources.* Dairy products, chocolate, and meats also contribute magnesium to the diet. "Hard" tap water often contains a high concentration of magnesium, and so can be considered a source.

RDA for magnesium. The adult RDA for magnesium is 350 milligrams per day for men and 280 milligrams per day for women. The North American diet supplies about 350 milligrams of magnesium per person per day (about 120 milligrams per 1000 kcalories). Adult men consume an average of 330 milligrams daily, while women consume an average of 200 milligrams daily. The low intake for women causes concern, especially because many women have increased calcium consumption in response to the fear of osteoporosis. We have mentioned that as calcium in the diet increases, magnesium absorption decreases. We suggest women find some good sources of magnesium that they like, and eat them regularly.

Table 13-8

Good sources of magnesium, ranked by nutrient density

Food	Serving size to yield 350 milligrams*	kcalories needed to yield 350 milligrams
Spinach, cooked	2 cups	82
Beet greens, cooked	3-½ cups	140
Wheat bran	2 cups	152
Broccoli, cooked	3-½ cups	171
Tofu (soybean curd)	10 ounces	226
Shrimp, boiled	11 ounces	375
Wheat germ, raw	1-¼ cups	377
Popcorn, air popped	15 cups	450
Sunflower seeds, dry	⅔ cups	512
Blackeyed peas, cooked	3 cups	670
Cashews	5 ounces	800
Kidney beans	4 cups	920

*RDA for adult male.
Plant foods provide the most nutrient-dense sources of magnesium.

North Americans at risk for a magnesium deficiency. Besides a risk for women in general, a magnesium deficiency is also possible if one uses thiazide diuretics because they increase magnesium loss in the urine. In addition, heavy perspiration for weeks in hot climates and long-standing diarrhea or vomiting both cause significant magnesium loss. Alcoholism also increases the risk of a deficiency because dietary intake may be poor, and alcohol increases magnesium excretion in the urine. The disorientation and weakness from alcoholism is similar to that seen when magnesium is low in the blood. Presently, we have more questions than answers about the role of magnesium in human diseases. Again, magnesium status is tedious to determine.

To perform a sensitive measure of magnesium status in the body, first, a large dose is given. Then, total magnesium excretion in the urine must be measured over 24 hours. This is not a practical test and so is not often performed.

Toxicity of magnesium. Magnesium toxicity does not occur in healthy people who eat typical foods. Toxicity is associated with kidney failure because the kidneys primarily regulate serum magnesium levels. A high serum magnesium level leads to weakness, nausea, and eventual malaise.

SULFUR

Sulfur (chemical symbol is S) is a component of many important compounds in the body, such as the amino acids methionine and cysteine and the vitamins biotin and thiamin. Sulfur participates in acid-base balance in the body and is an important part of the drug-detoxifying pathways found in the liver. Finally, disulfide bridges, which occur when 2 sulfur atoms bind to each other, give important stability to many protein molecules (see Chapter 6).

We actually do not need to consume sulfur directly in our diets. Proteins supply the sulfur we need, so sulfur is naturally a part of a healthful diet. Sulfur compounds are also used to preserve foods (see Chapter 19).

OXYGEN

Oxygen (chemical symbol is O) is in a class by itself: it is not a nutrient in a dietary sense, but is still vital for sustaining life. We use oxygen for aerobic respiration in the electron transport chain. In addition, some cellular metabolic reactions incorporate oxygen directly into compounds. All oxygen in the atmosphere either is produced by plants and microbes that perform photosynthesis or is released by chemical breakdown in rocks.

Table 13-9

A summary of water and the major minerals

Name	Major functions	Deficiency symptoms	People most at risk	RDA or minimum requirement	Dietary sources	Results of toxicity
Water	Medium for chemical reactions, removal of waste products, perspiration to cool the body	Thirst, muscle weakness, poor endurance	Infants with a fever, elderly in nursing homes	1 milliliter per kcalorie* in diet	As such and in foods	Probably only in mental disorders, headache, blurred vision, convulsions
Sodium	A major ion of the extracellular fluid, nerve transmission	Muscle cramps	People severely restricting sodium to lower blood pressure (250-500 milligrams/day)	500 milligrams	Table salt, processed foods	High blood pressure in susceptible individuals
Potassium	A major ion of intracellular fluid, nerve transmission	Irregular heart beat, loss of appetite, muscle cramps	Use of potassium-wasting diuretics, poor diets seen in poverty and alcoholism	2000 milligrams	Vegetables, fruits, milk	Slowing of the heart beat, seen in kidney failure
Chloride	A major ion of the extracellular fluid, acid production in stomach	Convulsions in infants	No one, probably, if infant formula manufacturers control product quality adequately	700 milligrams	Table salt, some vegetables	High blood pressure in susceptible people when combined with sodium
Calcium	Bones, teeth, blood clotting, nerve transmission, muscle contractions, cell regulation	Poor intake probably increases the risk for osteoporosis	Women in general, especially those who constantly restrict their energy intake and consume few dairy products	800 milligrams	Dairy products, canned fish, leafy vegetables, tofu, fortified orange juice	Very high intakes may cause kidney stones in susceptible people
Phosphorus	Bones, teeth, metabolic compounds such as ATP, ion of intracellular fluid	Probably none; poor bone maintenance possible	Elderly consuming very nutrient-poor diets, total vegetarians? alcoholism?	800 milligrams	Dairy products, processed foods, soft drinks	Induces high levels of parathyroid hormone in kidney failure; poor bone mineralization if calcium intakes are low
Magnesium	Bones, enzyme function, nerve and heart function	Weakness, muscle pain, poor heart function	People on thiazide diuretics, women in general	Men: 350 milligrams Women: 280 milligrams	Wheat bran, green vegetables, nuts, chocolate	Causes weakness in kidney failure
Sulfur	Part of vitamins and amino acids, drug detoxification, acid base balance	None	No one who meets their protein needs	None	Protein foods	None likely

*Just an approximation; best to keep urine volume greater than 1 liter (4 cups).

Nutritionists are sometimes accused of forgetting that the lungs are a part of our physiological machinery. Breathing is much more automatic than eating, and so it is easy to forget that oxygen is essential for us. However, it is important to remember the critical role that oxygen plays. About 21% of air is oxygen, a vital resource on which we all depend.

Concept Check

Phosphorus absorption is quite efficient and is enhanced by the active vitamin D hormone calcitriol. Urinary excretion maintains body levels. Phosphorus aids enzyme function and is part of ATP molecules and cell membranes. No deficiency symptoms caused by poor intake have been reported. Good food sources include dairy products, baked goods, and meat. The RDA is met by most North Americans. Magnesium is found mostly in plant sources where it functions in chlorophyll. Magnesium is important to humans for nerve and cardiac function and is a cofactor for many enzymes. Women in general, people on thiazide diuretics, and people with alcoholism are at risk of developing a deficiency. Toxicity is mainly found in people with kidney failure. Sulfur is a component of certain vitamins and amino acids. It plays an important role in drug-detoxification and protein structure. Our diets naturally supply sulfur via the protein and vitamins normally consumed.

See Table 13-9 for a review of the major characteristics of water and the minerals we have covered so far.

Summary

1. Many minerals are vital for sustaining life. For humans, animal products are the best sources of most minerals. Supplements exceeding 150% of the U.S. RDA should be taken only under a physician's supervision, since toxicity and nutrient interactions are a real possibility.
2. Water constitutes 50% to 70% of the human body. Its unique chemical properties enable it to function as a solvent, a medium for chemical reactions, a thermoregulator, and a lubricant. It also helps regulate the acid-base balance in the body. For adults, daily water needs are estimated at 1 milliliter per kcalorie in the diet.
3. Sodium, the major positive ion of the extracellular fluid, is vital in fluid balance and nerve impulse transmission. The North American diet provides abundant sodium through processed foods and table salt. About 10% of the population is sodium-sensitive and is at risk for hypertension from consuming excessive sodium.
4. Potassium, the major positive ion of the intracellular fluid, functions similarly to sodium. Milk, fruits, and vegetables are good sources.
5. Chloride is the major negative ion in extracellular fluid. It functions in digestion as part of gastric hydrochloric acid and in immune function. Table salt supplies most of the chloride in our diets.
6. Calcium forms a vital part of bone structure and is also very important in blood clotting, muscle contraction, and nerve transmission. Calcium absorption is enhanced by stomach acid and calcitriol. Dairy products are important calcium sources.
7. Osteoporosis is defined as bone loss with no apparent cause. Women are particularly at risk and should maintain adequate calcium intake and regular exercise. Estrogen replacement at menopause is currently the most accepted way to stop significant adult bone loss.
8. Phosphorus aids enzyme function and forms part of ATP molecules, numerous metabolites, and cell membranes. It is efficiently absorbed, and deficiencies are

rare, although there is concern about the intake of elderly women. Good food sources are dairy products, bakery products, and meats.

9. Magnesium is the only mineral found mostly in plants, where it functions in chlorophyll. For humans, magnesium is important for nerve and heart function and as a cofactor to many coenzymes. Good food sources are whole grains (bran), vegetables, nuts, and seeds.
10. Sulfur is incorporated into certain vitamins and amino acids. Its ability to bond with other sulfur atoms enables it to stabilize protein structure.

Take Action

1. Develop a family history of bone fractures in your grandparents, aunts and uncles, and immediate relatives after age 60 years. This will give female students some idea of their relative risk for fractures when they get older. The more relatives who have had hip fractures, for example, the higher will be the risk, and the more women in that family should try to prevent osteoporosis.
2. Measure your height accurately. Plan to do this every few years. If you begin to lose more than 1 inch in height, you should suspect bone loss.
3. Using the rule of 300's, estimate your daily calcium intake for the next 3 days. Did your intake meet your RDA? What foods could you incorporate into your diet to meet your RDA?

1. Relatives (older than 60) with bone fractures:________

2. Current height:________

3. Day one:________

Day two:________

Day three:________

Foods to add to diet:

1. ________ serving size ________
2. ________ serving size ________
3. ________ serving size ________
4. ________ serving size ________

REFERENCES

1. Blais CA and others: Effect of dietary sodium restriction on taste responses to sodium chloride: a longitudinal study, American Journal of Clinical Nutrition 44:232, 1986.
2. Bronner F: Intestinal calcium absorption: mechanisms and applications, Journal of Nutrition 117:1347, 1987.
3. Dalesky GP and others: Weight-bearing exercise training and lumbar bone mineral content in post-menopausal women, Annals of Internal Medicine 108:824, 1988.
4. Drinkwater BL and others: Bone mineral density after resumption of menses in amenorrheic athletes, Journal of the American Medical Association 256:360, 1986.
5. Fishman JA: Control of hypertension through life style and nutrition, Topics in Clinical Nutrition 3:47, 1988.
6. Frost HM: The pathomechanics of osteoporosis, Clinical Orthopedics and Related Research 200:198, 1985.
7. Garraway WM and Whisnant JP: The changing pattern of hypertension and the declining incidents of stroke, Journal of the American Medical Association 258:214, 1987.
8. Greger JL: Mineral bioavailability/new concepts, Nutrition Today July/August:4, 1987.
9. Heaney RP and others: Calcium absorbability from spinach, American Journal of Clinical Nutrition 47:707, 1988.
10. Heaney RP and others: Variability of calcium absorption, American Journal of Clinical Nutrition 47:262, 1988.
11. Hoffman CJ: Does the sodium level in drinking water affect blood pressure levels? Journal of the American Dietetic Association 88:1432, 1988.
12. Houston MC: Sodium and hypertension, Archives of Internal Medicine 146:139, 1986.
13. Karanja N and McCarron DA: Calcium and hypertension, Annual Reviews of Nutrition 6:475, 1986.
14. Khaw K and Barrett-Connor E: The association between blood pressure, age, and dietary sodium and potassium: a population study, Circulation 77:53, 1988.
15. Klatsky AL and others: The relationships between alcoholic beverage use and other traits to blood pressure: a new Kaiser Permanente Study, Circulation 73:628, 1986.
16. National Nutrition Institute in Canada: dietary calcium and the prevention of post menopausal osteoporosis, Nutrition Today May/June:33, 1988.
17. Nelson L and others: Affect of changing levels of physical activity on blood-pressure and haemodynamics in essential hypertension, Lancet 2:474, 1986.
18. Pennington JAT and others: Nutritional elements in U.S. diets: results from the total diet study, 1982-1986, Journal of The American Dietetic Association 89:659, 1989.
19. Randal HT: Water, electrolytes, and acid-based balance. In Shils ME and Young VR editors: Modern nutrition in health and disease, Philadelphia, 1988, Lea & Febiger.
20. Rasmussen HS and others: Magnesium deficiency in patients with ischemic heart disease with and without acute myocardial infarction uncovered by an intravenous loading test, Archives of Internal Medicine 148:329, 1988.
21. Recker, RR and others: Calcium absorbability from milk products and imitation milk and calcium carbonate, American Journal of Clinical Nutrition 47:93, 1988.
22. Riggs BL and Melton LJ: Involutional osteoporosis, New England Journal of Medicine 314:1676, 1986.
23. Riis B and others: Does calcium supplementation prevent postmenopausal bone loss? New England Journal of Medicine 316:173, 1987.
24. Shils ME: Magnesium in Health and Disease, Annual Reviews of Nutrition 8:429, 1988.
25. Sorenson AW and others: Calcium and colon cancer: a review, Nutrition and Cancer 11:135, 1988.
26. Spencer H and others: Do protein and phosphorus cause calcium loss? Journal of Nutrition 118:657, 1988.
27. Tobian L Potassium and hypertension, Nutrition Reviews 46:273, 1988.
28. Tolstoi LG and Fosmire G: Milk-alkali syndrome revisited: a review of 63 years, Nutrition Today March/April:22, 1987.
29. Vokes T: Water homeostasis, Annual Reviews of Nutrition 7:383, 1987.
30. Wardlaw GM: The effect of diet and life-style on bone mass in women, Journal of The American Dietetic Association 88:17, 1988.

SUGGESTED READINGS

For an excellent review of osteoporosis, see the review article by Riggs and Melton. Wardlaw's article looks at diet and its relationship to bone health. The Houston article covers various issues surrounding sodium and hypertension. The article by Fishman shows how life-style changes can help control hypertension. Finally, Shils' article is a good look at magnesium, a mineral whose role in overall health nutritionists continue to question.

CHAPTER 13

Answers to nutrition awareness inventory

1. *False.* An electrolyte is a substance that dissociates into ions and so is able to conduct electricity. Although, in a water molecule, the hydrogen atoms are slightly positive and the oxygen atom negative, each water molecule does not break down into individual ions.
2. *False.* The terms *major* and *trace* are not designations of nutritional importance. They are classifications referring only to the amount needed for daily functioning.
3. *True.* For example, the coenzyme for the vitamin thiamin (TPP) requires magnesium to function efficiently.
4. *False.* Animal foods are often the best mineral sources, since animals concentrate the minerals they consume from plants. The exception is magnesium, which is plentiful in green plants.
5. *True.* The body can conserve water, but some must be lost every day. Thus after only a few days, severe dehydration and death can result from lack of water intake. Death from starvation can take as long as 50 or more days in an adult.
6. *True.* Water evaporation from the skin requires heat energy. So when perspiration evaporates, heat energy is taken from the skin, leaving you feeling cooler.
7. *True.* This simple method of estimation yields results similar to those derived by totaling all typical water losses via lungs, skin, feces, and urine.
8. *False.* In cases of some mental disorders, such as schizophrenia, people may drink tremendous amounts of water in a short time. This can overwhelm the kidneys' excretion capacity and lead to headaches, blurred vision, and cramps.
9. *True.* About one half of the sodium consumed by North Americans is supplied by processed foods. Sodium is prevalent in foods such as frozen dinners, canned soups, and convenience entrees.
10. *True.* Most fruits and vegetables are considered alkaline "ash" foods. After they are metabolized, the potassium and sodium left behind form alkaline compounds. The body's mechanisms that regulate acid-base balance, however, can compensate for the alkaline products formed.
11. *True.* Although part of our preference for salt is related to the sodium receptors on the tongue, habit also has a role. If you grow up consuming salty foods, you are more likely to prefer salty foods. Preferences can be relearned by gradually decreasing added salt.
12. *False.* Cheese has added salt unless it is a "low salt" cheese. Milk does not have added salt and so is lower in sodium per kcalorie.
13. *True.* Perspiration on the skin tastes salty, not because it has a higher sodium concentration than blood, but because once the water evaporates, concentrated sodium is left behind.
14. *False.* The effectiveness of dietary calcium in entirely preventing osteoporosis has been disproven, but adequate dietary amounts can slow some bone loss in old age.
15. *False.* It is estimated that only 10% of the population is at risk for developing hypertension from sodium intake. These people can benefit from restricting sodium. No data support the need for consuming a low-sodium diet if blood pressure is normal.

Nutrition Perspective 13-1

Minerals and Hypertension

Blood pressure is expressed by two different numbers. The higher number represents systolic blood pressure, which is the pressure in the arteries when the heart actively pumps blood. The second value is for diastolic pressure, which is the artery pressure when the heart is relaxed. Normal systolic blood pressure values vary from 100 to 140 millimeters of mercury (mm Hg). Normal diastolic blood pressure values varies from 60 to 90 mm Hg.

Hypertension is defined as sustained high blood pressure, usually with systolic pressure exceeding 140 mm Hg or diastolic blood pressure exceeding 90 mm Hg. Most hypertension (90% to 95%) has no apparent cause. It is called primary or **essential** hypertension. Kidney disease often causes the other 5% to 10% of cases and is known as secondary hypertension.

essential
Having no obvious, external cause.

About 30% of adults have "essential" hypertension. This is called a "silent" disease because, unless blood pressure is measured periodically, no one knows it is developing.

A physician usually does not treat hypertension with medication until the diastolic blood pressure measures at least 95 mm Hg on three or more occasions. But any value over 90 mm Hg is actually too high and deserves dietary and life-style interventions.

Hypertension		
Mild	Diastolic	90 to 104 mm Hg
	Systolic	140 to 159 mm Hg
Moderate	Diastolic	105 to 114 mm Hg
	Systolic	> 160 mm Hg
Severe	Diastolic	≥ 115 mm Hg

A systolic blood pressure value between 140 and 160 mm Hg should be treated with diet and exercise. Values above 160 mm Hg are often treated with medications. Usually anyone who has a high systolic blood pressure value will also have a high diastolic blood pressure value.

WHY CONTROL HYPERTENSION?

Hypertension needs to be controlled mainly to prevent heart disease, kidney disease, and strokes. All three diseases are much more likely to be found in people with hypertension than in people with normal blood pressure.

People with hypertension need to be diagnosed and treated as soon as possible. We now know the value of aggressively treating hypertension. In the last 20 years, blood pressures have fallen, as have the number of strokes.[7]

CAUSES OF HIGH BLOOD PRESSURE

A variety of factors affect blood pressure. Blood pressure usually increases as a person ages. Some increase is due to atherosclerosis (see Chapter 5). As plaque builds up in the arteries, the arteries become less flexible and cannot expand. When vessels remain rigid, blood pressure remains high. Eventually the plaque begins to choke off blood supply to the kidneys, decreasing their ability to control blood volume, and in turn, blood pressure.

Obesity often is associated with high blood pressure, especially in women. The same is true for inactivity. If an obese person can lose weight and become more physically active, exercising 3 to 4 times a week, blood pressure often returns to normal. A weight loss of as little as 10 pounds can help. *Often a minor change in life-style can greatly reduce, or even eliminate, the need for medications.*

High blood pressure is more likely in blacks than in whites. In addition, alcohol has a greater tendency to raise blood pressure in blacks than it does in whites. Finally the enzyme renin, and some hormone-like compounds, affect blood pressure (Figure 13-5). Medications are available to reduce the effect of the renin-angiotensin system.

SODIUM AND BLOOD PRESSURE

Sodium intake tends to increase blood pressure. The average North American intake of 3 to 7 grams can elevate blood pressure, particularly in those who are susceptible to the effect. However, nutritionists believe that only some of the 30% of North Americans with hypertension are very susceptible to sodium-linked hypertension. So sodium in the diet is not a problem for everyone, even among people with hypertension. Nevertheless, in populations that eat 1500 milligrams or less of sodium daily, hypertension is rare.[12] Although some physicians recommend that all people with hypertension reduce sodium intake, ideally, dietary advice should be decided on an individual basis, once the response to treatment is verified.

Continued.

Nutrition Perspective 13-1—cont'd

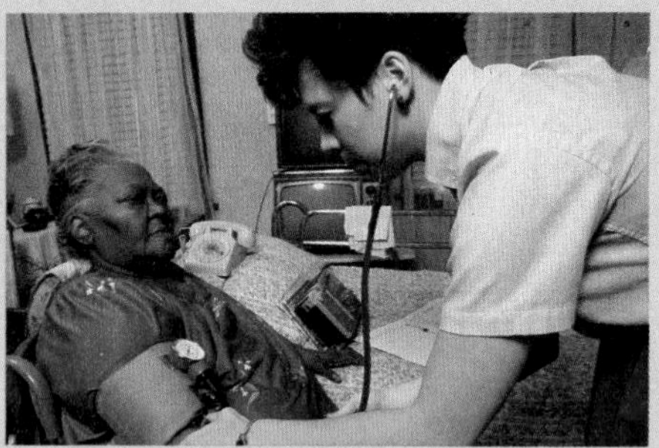

It is well worth the effort to attempt to reduce a diastolic blood pressure to below 95 mm Hg by practicing a few life-style changes: reducing body weight, moderating sodium and alcohol intake, increasing intakes of calcium, potassium, and magnesium, and increasing physical activity. Even if drugs are still needed, a proper diet and life-style approach can often reduce the dosage, and in turn the expense and side effects of medications. Nutritional therapy is a key to treating hypertension.

Minerals and Hypertension

If a person has hypertension, it is a good idea to reduce sodium. *Approximately 2 grams of sodium daily is the point at which sodium restriction usually improves hypertension.* While an intake less than that may lower blood pressure even more, people find it difficult to restrict sodium intake so severely for any length of time.

CALCIUM AND BLOOD PRESSURE

Since 1983 there has been debate concerning whether calcium intake can affect blood pressure. Careful studies show that about 50% of people register slightly lower blood pressures when they consume at least 1000 milligrams of supplemental calcium per day. Systolic blood pressure is affected more than diastolic blood pressure, so the actual importance of the change can be questioned. It is reasonable for a person with hypertension to experiment, in consultation with a physician, by increasing calcium intake to see if that produces a benefit worth the trouble and expense.

PREVENTING HYPERTENSION

To prevent hypertension we recommend maintaining an active life-style and a desirable body weight.[17] Epidemiological evidence suggests that a low-sodium diet may lead to less hypertension in later life. Hypertension does develop in many adults, especially in those with family histories of hypertension. So you may want to keep your sodium intake under 3 grams, as suggested by the American Heart Association. But, if your blood pressure is normal, there may be no reason to worry about sodium intake. As we saw with cholesterol in chapter 5, sodium appears to be a villain only for some of us. *In all, most of us need to be prudent—not paranoid—about dietary sodium.*

In addition, we suggest consuming a diet outlined by the Daily Food Guide, especially one rich in fruits and vegetables. This provides ample potassium, calcium, and magnesium—all of which may contribute to a lower blood pressure.[14]

Nutrition Perspective 13-2

Calcium and Osteoporosis

Widespread advertising has made it almost impossible for women to ignore osteoporosis. Its crippling effect on elderly women is now recognized as a medical emergency. The disease affects hundreds of thousands of people and is taxing our health care system (approximately $7 billion to $10 billion in 1986). The disease affects 20 million to 25 million people in the United States.

Osteoporosis leads to approximately 1.2 million bone fractures per year, usually in the hip, spine, and wrist. The slender, inactive woman who smokes is more susceptible to osteoporosis, but any woman who lives long enough can suffer from the disease. As women age into their 80s and 90s, osteoporosis becomes the rule—not the exception. Furthermore, osteoporosis is not only debilitating, it can be fatal. Between 12% and 20% of all elderly persons who suffer hip fractures eventually die from fracture-related complications.

CAN OSTEOPOROSIS BE PREVENTED?

Since 1985, estrogen replacement therapy has been recommended at menopause to prevent osteoporosis. It is also used to reduce symptoms of menopause. Studies to date show that estrogen replacement at menopause virtually stops further bone loss in women. Thus *it is reasonable to assume that estrogen replacement therapy will eliminate risk for significant osteoporosis in women who begin it right after menopause and take it for the rest of their lives.* However, we really need long-term studies to be sure. This therapy is thought to be very safe. Estrogen replacement therapy also reduces the risk of heart disease in women.

IS ESTROGEN THERAPY THE ONLY ANSWER?

Some women cannot take estrogen because they have estrogen-sensitive breast and uterine tumors. Other therapies, such as taking the active vitamin D hormone calcitriol or the hormone calcitonin, are available and quite effective. But for these women—and other women—will increasing calcium intake substitute for taking either estrogen or other medications?

Studies from the United States and Denmark have found that taking even 2000 milligrams of extra calcium (equal to 7.5 glasses of milk) does not prevent bone loss after menopause in the spine, hip, or wrist as successfully as estrogen replacement does. Extra dietary calcium more effectively reduces bone loss in the total skeleton than doing nothing at all.[23] *But a high-calcium intake may be no better for reducing bone loss in the spine than just meeting the RDA.* For those elderly women who do not consume even their RDA for calcium, we suggest they change their habits.

Spine fractures in women cause considerable pain and deformity and decrease physical ability. In addition, no cure exists for osteoporosis. So preventing these fractures is very important. Unfortunately, calcium therapy alone will probably not be enough. Increasing calcium intake to 1500 milligrams per day, however, can reduce the dose of estrogen needed to prevent bone loss. *Overall, for most women it is not estrogen versus calcium, but probably estrogen plus calcium that constitutes the most effective treatment.*

ARE ALL WOMEN AT RISK?

About one third of all women experience osteoporosis-related fractures in their lifetimes. Some women just do not live long enough to suffer from osteoporosis. They may experience bone loss, but their bones still remain strong enough throughout their life. This is especially true of women who die before the age of 75 years.

In addition, some women have much denser bone then others. They probably built more bone when they were young, and so they can endure greater bone loss without ex-

Continued.

Calcium and Osteoporosis

periencing more fractures. Also, some women may more easily adapt to lower-calcium diets.

Actually, the reason for such variation in bone density and fracture risk in women at any age still needs more research. However, numerous factors, such as physical activity, calcium intake throughout life, ability to adapt to low-calcium diets, and fluoride intake, are associated with higher bone density values in some studies (Table 13-10). On the other hand, a lack of regular menstruation, premature menopause, use of some medications, and prolonged bed rest are all associated with low bone density values in women. We can't focus only on calcium when discussing this disease—many factors are involved.[22]

Table 13-10

Factors associated with bone maintenance versus bone loss

Maintenance	Loss	
Normal menses	Lack of menses	Excessive aluminum consumption
Estrogen replacement	Amenorrhea	Alcoholism
Black race	Early menopause	Cigarette smoking
Thiazide diuretics	Glucocorticoid use	Slender figure
Fluoride (1-6 milligrams)	Hyperparathyroidism	Bed rest (months)
Physical activity*	Hyperthyroidism	Dietary fiber
Dietary Calcium†	Thyroid hormone replacement	
	Factors made by white blood cells	Anorexia nervosa

*The degree of effect remains to be established.
†Suspected, but not established.

AM I AT RISK?

Medical and nutritional recommendations concerning osteoporosis are best made when the individual status of a person is known. The bone density of a woman's spine, hip, and wrist can aid decisions. Special bone densitometers are available in medical centers for these measurements. Unfortunately, these density measurements don't reveal anything about bone architecture. Recall that bone relies upon its mineral density, trabeculae cross-bracing, and its ability to heal microfractures for its strength. So a bone-density measurement tells part of the story, not the whole story.

WILL A NUTRITIOUS DIET IN YOUTH PREVENT OSTEOPOROSIS LATER?

The importance of calcium intake in building and maintaining dense bones in the years before menopause (before about age 50 years) is still unknown. A study from Yugoslavia showed that women who normally consume about 950 milligrams of calcium a day had a lower rate for hip fractures than women who consumed about 450 milligrams of calcium daily.

In contrast, a variety of studies in the United States has shown a very weak relationship between usual calcium intake and bone density in middle aged and elderly women. It makes biological sense that a good calcium intake throughout a woman's life would help build and maintain a strong bone structure. However, at this time few data support this position.[30]

We still do not know enough about calcium's role in building a strong bone structure in childhood and early adulthood to make a statement about this age group. It is logical to assume that a good calcium intake would build a stronger bone structure than a poor one.

The RDA committee supports this. It is a very active research area, and we expect more studies soon. Until definite evidence is available, *we think it is prudent to assume that an intake of calcium at the RDA for young women (1200 milligrams) is a reasonable measure to recommend for possible prevention and/or minimization of osteoporosis.*

A PLAN FOR FRACTURE PREVENTION

As women mature from young children to their elder years, different strategies for preventing osteoporosis are needed.[30] Young women should see a physician at any sign of irregular menstruation and pursue an active life-style that includes sun exposure and weight-bearing exercise.[3] Note that exercise does not prevent the bone loss associated with irregular menstruation. *Regular menstruation is the overwhelming key to bone maintenance in young women, as evidenced by poor bone density in non-menstruating female athletes.*[4] Following the RDA for calcium is also important. If foods from the milk and cheese group are not usually consumed, it is wise to find another calcium source.

Avoidance of smoking and alcoholism are also important. Alcohol is toxic to bone cells. Alcoholism is probably a major undiagnosed and unrecognized cause of osteoporosis today.

At menopause, women need to discuss estrogen replacement therapy with a physician. They also need to accurately track their height (Figure 13-10). A decrease of more than 1 inch from premenopausal values is a sign that significant bone loss is taking place. If a plan to prevent osteoporosis is not in effect, a loss in height is the signal to see a physician and establish a plan.

Elderly women need to stay as physically active as possible. *They also need to minimize the risk for falls, especially by limiting their use of medications and alcohol which might disturb coordination.* Regular sun exposure and consuming food sources of vitamin D is also a good idea.

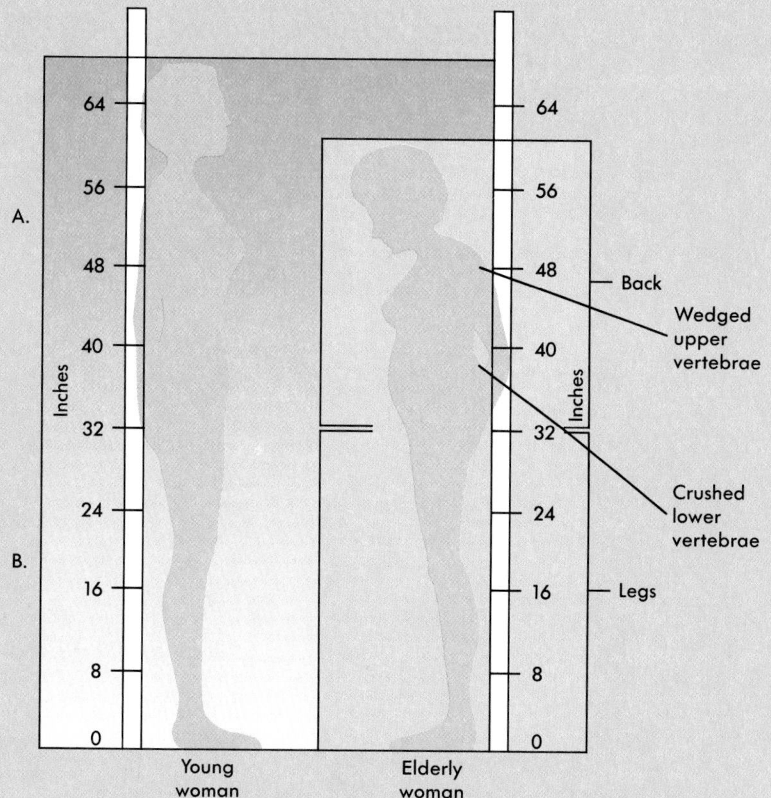

Figure 13-10

A loss of height and distorted body shape are common signs of osteoporosis. Monitor your adult height changes to detect early osteoporosis.

Chapter 14

The Trace Minerals

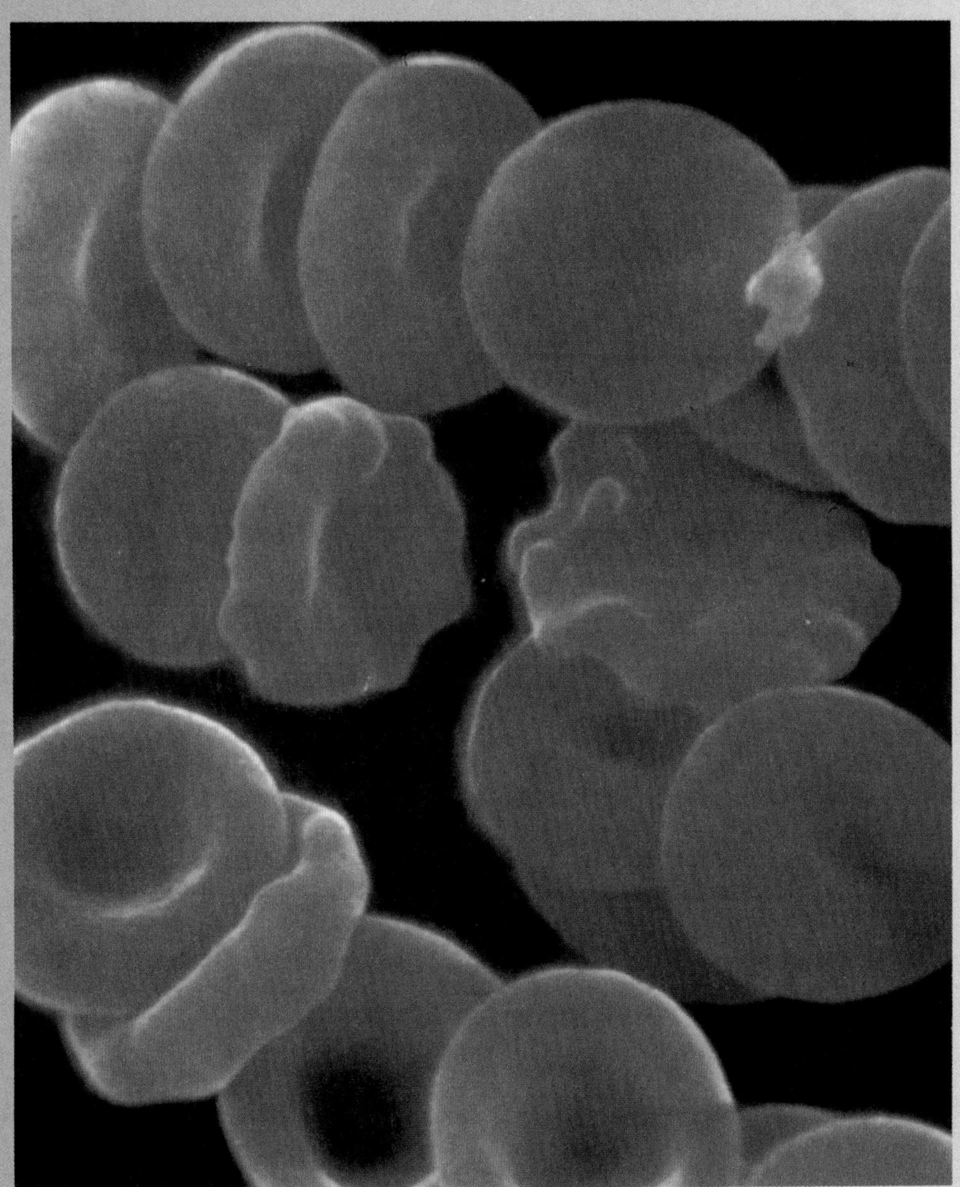

Most iron in the body is present in the hemoglobin molecules in the red blood cells.

Overview

Trace minerals constitute less than 1% of all minerals in your body. As noted in Chapter 13, a trace mineral is defined as one for which our daily nutritional need is less than 100 milligrams. Grouping them together this way, however, is too simplistic because trace mineral functions and means of absorption and metabolism all vary. For example, the body carefully regulates absorption of iron, copper, and zinc, but not selenium and iodide. So selenium and iodide levels in the body depend more than the others mentioned on the mineral content of a food eaten. The trace minerals are also very interactive: the abundance of one mineral in the diet and body can affect the absorption and metabolism of several others.[10]

Information about trace minerals is perhaps the most rapidly expanding area of knowledge in nutrition. With the exception of iron and iodide, the importance of trace minerals to humans has been recognized only within the last 30 years since most of your parents were in school. Let's examine some of these new findings.

Nutrition awareness inventory

Here are 15 statements about trace minerals. Answer them to test your current knowledge. If you think the answer is true or mostly true, circle T. If you think the answer is false or mostly false, circle F. Use the scoring key at the end of this chapter to compute your total score. Take this test again after you have read this chapter. Compare the results.

1. **T F** Trace mineral deficiencies are difficult to detect.
2. **T F** Some trace minerals interfere with the absorption of other minerals.
3. **T F** Trace mineral concentrations in plants usually depend on the trace mineral concentrations in the soil in which the plants are grown.
4. **T F** Enriched grains contain less of many trace minerals than whole grains.
5. **T F** Iron is the only nutrient with a higher RDA for adult women than for adult men.
6. **T F** Iron is easily excreted from the body when consumed in excess.
7. **T F** Zinc is important to the growth of children.
8. **T F** Zinc can be assessed using hair analysis.
9. **T F** High doses of zinc supplements can reduce immune function.
10. **T F** Copper plays an important role in iron metabolism.
11. **T F** A copper deficiency could result from consuming too much zinc.
12. **T F** The ultimate sources of most of our iodide intake are unprocessed foods.
13. **T F** Fluoride inhibits the growth of the bacterium that causes dental caries.
14. **T F** Consuming excess chromium supplements is not dangerous, since there is little chance of chromium toxicity.
15. **T F** The terms *iron deficiency* and *anemia* are synonymous and interchangeable.

TRACE MINERALS

Discovering the importance of each trace mineral to humans is a fairly recent and still unfolding drama that, in some cases, reads like a detective story. As recently as 1961 researchers linked dwarfism in villagers in the Middle East to a zinc deficiency[26] and recognized that an obscure form of heart disease in an isolated area of China was linked to a selenium deficiency.[25] In North America, some trace mineral deficiencies were first observed in the late 1960s to early 1970s when they were not added to synthetic formulas used in total parenteral nutrition.[26] *The lack of early human research means our understanding of trace mineral metabolism still relies mostly on knowledge of farm and laboratory animal nutrition.*

Researching our trace minerals needs is difficult because we need only minute amounts. Highly sophisticated technology is required to measure such small amounts in both food and body tissues. Rigorous protocols are required to produce a deficiency in animals (all animal research referred to in this text was conducted with farm and/or laboratory animals). They must be raised in ultraclean environments. Their diets must be carefully produced from individual essential nutrients to ensure that no mineral contamination occurs. Stainless steel and plastic cages must be used so that the animals do not obtain any trace minerals, such as zinc, from chewing on the cages. Minerals must often be filtered from the air, and the water must be as mineral-free as possible. In addition, glassware used for chemical analysis may need to be rinsed repeatedly in acid to eliminate trace mineral contamination; sometimes only plastic bottles are appropriate.

Because producing most trace mineral deficiencies in laboratory animals requires so much effort, human deficiencies are unlikely, considering all our mineral sources in food, air, and water. However, *for some trace minerals, such as iron, zinc, copper, and chromium, there is considerable concern that marginal dietary intakes do occur and mild deficiencies go undetected.*

We need far more research on trace minerals. Much has been and is being done. But because many questions remain, we caution you to be very careful when considering using trace mineral supplements. You can easily harm your body by using these types of supplements.

SETTING NUTRIENT NEEDS FOR TRACE MINERALS

The difficulty in measuring trace mineral nutrition in humans makes setting the RDA for them problematic. Most trace minerals have only an estimated safe and adequate daily dietary intake; only a few trace minerals have an RDA.

The major method used to set trace mineral nutrient needs is the balance study. The same basic technique used for nitrogen balance studies works for minerals. (See Chapters 2 and 6.) Researchers try to determine the lowest mineral intake that meets all mineral losses from urine, feces, hair, skin, perspiration, menses, and so on. These studies are very expensive to perform and often inconclusive because laboratory results frequently contradict each other. In addition, a balance study tells only the level of dietary intake needed to maintain a specific **pool** of the mineral in the body, but this pool does not necessarily represent the amount needed to maintain the best health.

pool
The amount of a mineral stored within the body that can be easily mobilized when needed.

There are further problems in setting nutrient needs for trace minerals. Symptoms often appear only with severe deficiencies. *We lack knowledge of subtle signs of most trace mineral deficiencies, so we cannot always detect when people are compromising their health.* They may consume just enough mineral to prevent obvious symptoms from being expressed. Besides lacking sensitive clinical signs, we also often lack sensitive laboratory assays to measure trace minerals. The main factor limiting chromium research today is the lack of a sensitive measure of it in body tissue and fluids.

A final complication is that trace minerals interact with each other.[10] An overabundance of zinc, copper, or iron in the body can interfere with absorption of the other minerals. Thus to set the RDA for zinc, nutrition scientists must estimate the amounts of copper and iron that will be consumed to predict how much zinc the body will actually absorb.

TRACE MINERALS IN FOODS

The trace mineral content of plants depends primarily on trace mineral concentration in the soil. *Because soil concentrations of trace minerals vary greatly, food composition tables can give misleading values for trace mineral contents of plant foods.* This is not as true for foods from animals because animals often eat a variety of plant products and are often shipped from one area to another during their growth, processing, and finishing in a feed lot. They then can consume foods from multiple soil conditions.

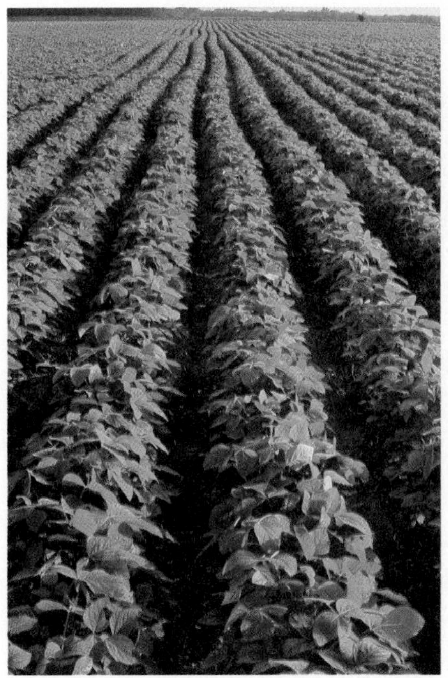

The trace mineral content in plant foods reflects the trace mineral concentration of the soil in which they were grown.

The bioavailability of trace minerals is another issue in planning diets. Finding a mineral-rich food does not ensure that you can absorb a particular mineral from it. Many factors in food inhibit mineral absorption. Mineral absorption from some plant foods often amounts to only 3% to 5% of the total present. In general, animal sources of minerals are superior because they contribute to more efficient absorption. Animal sources often contain factors that enhance mineral absorption, even for the trace minerals supplied by plant foods in a meal.

Throughout this book we repeatedly recommend *eating a variety of foods.* By doing that you eat plants and animals that have derived nutrients from a variety of soils, and you thus maximize your chances of consuming an adequate amount of trace minerals. In addition, *it is best to consume as many whole foods as possible.* Generally, the more refined a food—as in the case of white flour—the lower its content of trace minerals. The enrichment process adds only the trace mineral iron. The selenium, zinc, and copper lost when grains are refined are not replaced.

IRON

hemoglobin
The iron-containing part of the red blood cell that carries oxygen to the cells and carbon dioxide away from the cells. It is also responsible for the red color of blood.

myoglobin
Iron-containing compound that transports oxygen and CO_2 in muscle tissue.

The importance of dietary iron (chemical symbol is Fe) has been recognized for centuries. The Persian physician Melampus in 4000 BC gave iron supplements to sailors to compensate for the iron lost from bleeding during battles. Today, iron deficiency is one of the most common nutrient deficiencies worldwide. Iron is the only nutrient for which adult women have a greater RDA than adult men. It is found in every living cell; total body content is about 5 grams (1 teaspoon).

Absorption and distribution of iron

The body uses several mechanisms to regulate iron absorption.[22] Controlling absorption is important because the body cannot easily eliminate excess iron once it is absorbed. Iron absorption from foods varies from about 3% to 40%, depending upon a variety of factors (Table 14-1).

heme iron
Iron provided from animal tissues as hemoglobin and myoglobin. Approximately 50% of the iron in meat is heme iron; it is readily absorbed.

Table 14-1

Dietary factors that affect iron absorption

Increase	Decrease
Vitamin C	Phytate fiber
Acid in the stomach	Oxalate
Heme iron	Tannins (in tea)
High body demand for red blood cells (blood loss, high altitude, physical training, pregnancy)	Full body stores
Low body stores	Excess of other minerals (Cu, Zn, Mn, Ca)
Meat protein factor (MPF)	Lack of stomach acid
	Some antacids

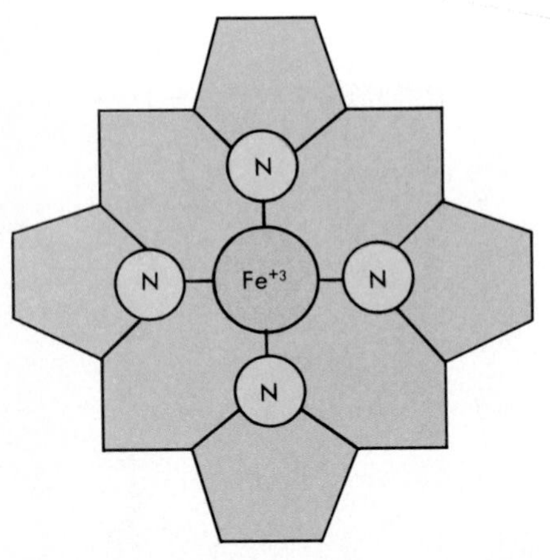

Heme iron

nonheme iron
Iron provided from plant sources and animal tissues other than hemoglobin and myoglobin. Nonheme iron needs to be ionized prior to absorption and is less efficiently absorbed than heme iron.

The form of iron in foods greatly influences its absorption. Iron that is still part of the **hemoglobin** and **myoglobin** molecules in animal flesh (40% of total iron present), called **heme iron,** is absorbed over twice as efficiently as the simple elemental iron, known as **nonheme iron.** Nonheme iron is also present in animal flesh, eggs, milk, vegetables, grains, and other plant foods.

About 10% to 15% of iron in the North American diet is heme iron, and usually 25% to 35% is absorbed. Nonheme iron makes up the rest, and usually 2% to 20% is absorbed. That makes animal flesh, especially red meat, the best source of iron in the North American diet, considering both its iron content and the increased efficiency of absorption for the iron present in the heme form.

Consuming heme iron and nonheme iron together increases nonheme iron absorption. One of several possible nonheme absorption facilitators may be a meat protein factor in meat. This factor appears to consist of amino acids that bind iron atoms and enhance their absorption. Overall, eating meat with vegetables and grain products enhances the absorption of their nonheme iron.

Organic acids, such as vitamin C, can increase nonheme iron absorption by changing Fe^{+3} (ferric form) to Fe^{+2} (ferrous form). The ferrous form of iron is better absorbed. Consuming more foods rich in vitamin C is particularly desirable if dietary iron is inadequate or serum iron levels are low. *When using an iron supplement, it's a good idea to take it with a glass of orange juice.*

Several dietary factors interfere with our ability to absorb iron. Phytic acid and other factors in grain fibers and oxalic acid in vegetables can all bind iron, reducing its absorption. A long-term consideration if you increase dietary fiber intake above 35 grams per day is the tendency for fiber components to bind iron (and other trace minerals), decreasing absorption. Tannins found in tea also reduce iron absorption. When trying to rebuild iron stores it is a good idea to reduce tea consumption, particularly at mealtimes. Finally, high-dose calcium supplements can also bind much iron—an important disadvantage to weigh when considering it an option instead of regularly consuming dairy products.

The most important factor influencing iron absorption is the body's need for it. In a deficiency state, nonheme iron absorption can increase about tenfold, and heme iron absorption can increase twofold. When iron stores are adequate, the main serum protein that carries iron, called transferrin, is full (saturated). This condition reduces iron transfer from the intestinal cells to the bloodstream. When intestinal cells are sloughed at the end of their 2 to 5 day life cycle, the iron returns to the intestinal tract for excretion.

When iron stores are low, transferrin in the bloodstream readily binds more iron, shifting it from intestinal cells into the bloodstream. By this means—under normal circumstances—iron is absorbed only if needed. This block against excess iron absorption is termed a "mucosal block" (Figure 14-1).

Heme iron is absorbed intact into the intestinal cell. The iron atoms released then combine with the nonheme iron atoms. Some of this iron will be bound by transferrin and ushered directly into the bloodstream, depending on body needs. The rest combines with a protein called **apoferritin** to form **ferritin** in the intestinal cells. This gives us a short-term form of iron storage for intestinal cells. First, however, the copper-containing protein called **ceruloplasmin** first converts Fe^{+2} to Fe^{+3} so that it can bind to apoferritin. *Thus copper metabolism and iron metabolism are closely linked.* Eventually, the iron is either absorbed or sloughed with the intestinal cell.

Most iron in the body is present in the hemoglobin molecules in the red blood cells. Some iron is stored in the bone marrow, and a small portion goes to other body cells or to the liver for storage as part of the protein ferritin. As liver

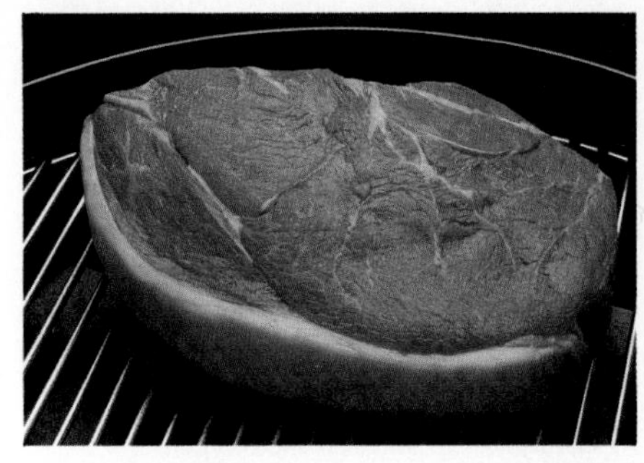

Red meat is our best source of iron.

apoferritin
A protein in intestinal cells that binds with the ferric form of iron (Fe^{+3}) to make ferritin.

ferritin
A protein compound that serves as the storage form of iron in the blood and tissues.

ceruloplasmin
A blue, copper-containing protein component of plasma that converts Fe^{+2} to Fe^{+3} (ferric form) so that it can bind with apoferritin.

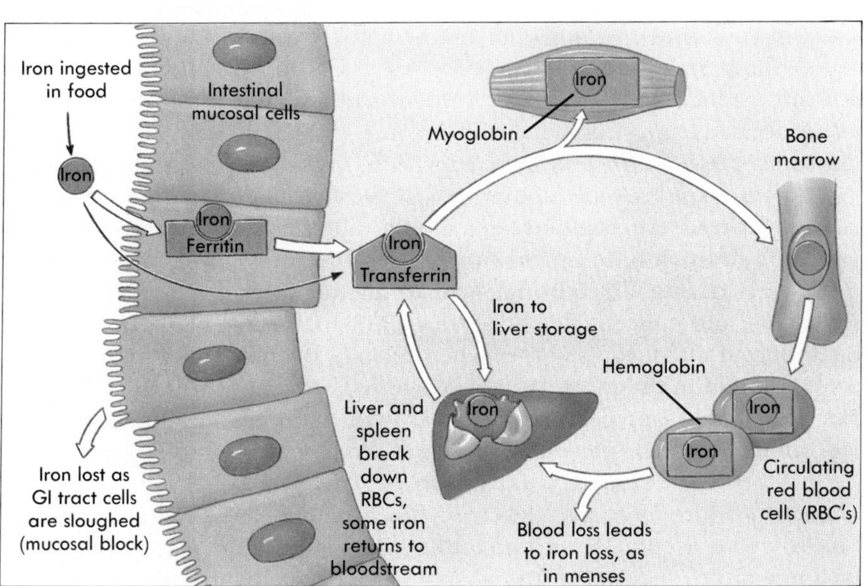

Figure 14-1
Iron absorption and distribution. Iron binds with a protein to form ferritin when stored in cells. If the intestinal absorption cells are shed before iron is absorbed from them, the iron is not absorbed into the bloodstream. This is one way the body can limit overabsorption of iron.

concentration of ferritin increases, it is partly digested by the liver cells, and the iron forms a more insoluble product called **hemosiderin.** As iron is needed, it can be mobilized (with the help of ceruloplasmin) from body stores. If dietary intake is inadequate, these iron stores become depleted. Only then do signs of an iron deficiency appear.

Function of iron

A key attribute of iron is its ability to both take up and release oxygen atoms and electrons. This allows it to participate in carrying oxygen in the bloodstream and in transferring electrons in the electron transport chain.

Iron forms part of hemoglobin in red blood cells and myoglobin in muscle cells. Iron is also necessary for the synthesis in the mitochondria of cytochromes used for the electron transport chain and for other systems found elsewhere. Iron is used to synthesize some enzymes and is needed for immune function (see Nutrition Perspective 14-1 entitled "Nutrients and Immunity"). Iron is involved in the synthesis of the protein collagen and contributes to drug detoxification pathways in the liver.

Hemoglobin molecules in red blood cells carry oxygen from the lungs to cells, and carry back carbon dioxide (CO_2) from cells to the lungs for excretion. Bone marrow cells in adults synthesize red blood cells when stimulated by the hormone **erythropoietin,** which comes from the kidneys. Erythropoietin is released in response to a decrease in oxygen concentration in the bloodstream, blood loss, or carbon monoxide binding to red blood cells.

erythropoietin
A protein secreted by the kidneys that enhances red blood cell synthesis and stimulates red blood cell release from bone marrow.

As a red blood cell matures in the bone marrow, it expels its nucleus, which contains DNA. That limits its life span to approximately 120 days because without DNA it can't direct new protein synthesis to replace cell parts such as enzymes. *A rapid cell turnover such as this puts great nutrient demands on the body, and iron is one of those greatly demanded nutrients.*

Iron-deficiency anemia

If neither the diet nor body stores can supply the iron needed for hemoglobin synthesis, red blood cell synthesis is reduced. Eventually, the red blood cell number falls so low that the amount of oxygen carried in the bloodstream is decreased. Such a person has anemia, which is defined as a decreased oxygen-carrying capacity of the blood. *While there are many types of anemia, the major type found worldwide is iron-deficiency anemia.* About 30% of the world's population is anemic, and about half of those cases are due to an iron deficiency.[12]

In iron-deficiency anemia, the percentage of red blood cells in the blood **(hematocrit)** falls below 34% to 37%. In addition, the hemoglobin concentration in the bloodstream falls below 10 to 11 grams per 100 milliliters of blood. A variety of diseases can reduce hemoglobin and hematocrit values, but usually, if both are reduced, the person has iron-deficiency anemia. If the volume of each red blood cell is also reduced, this is further evidence of anemia.[11] Probably about 8% of North Americans have iron-deficiency anemia.

hematocrit
The percentage of total blood volume occupied by red blood cells.

Iron-deficiency anemia in men is usually due to ulcers, colon cancer, or hemorrhoids.

More people have an iron deficiency than iron-deficiency anemia, especially in North America. Probably about 30% of women in North America have scant or no iron stores.[12] Their blood hemoglobin values are still normal, but they have no stores to draw from in times of pregnancy or illness.

Life stages during which iron-deficiency anemia often appears are infancy, preschool years, and puberty for both males and females. Women are also more vulnerable during childbearing years when menses occurs.[12] In addition, anemia is also often found in pregnant women, as we will discuss in Chapter 15. These life stages are singled out because either growth, with the resulting expansion of blood volume and muscle mass, increases iron needs, or total kcalorie intakes make it difficult to consume enough iron.

Much anemia in the Mediterranean area, Southeast Asia, and other parts of the world is due to a group of diseases called thalassemia. This genetic disease causes a person to synthesize incorrect forms of hemoglobin. The red blood cell then lacks the normal ability to carry oxygen.

Clinical symptoms of iron-deficiency anemia include pale skin and brittle finger nails, which eventually turn up into a spoon shape. The person suffers fatigue, poor temperature regulation, loss of appetite, and apathy. Insufficient iron for the synthesis of red blood cells and cytochromes may cause the fatigue.[13]

Researchers suspect that poor iron stores may also decrease learning ability, work performance, and immune status even before a person is actually anemic.[12] However, there is debate over this point: some researchers feel that unless a person has clinical anemia, concern about poor iron status is unwarranted. However, it makes sense to maintain good iron stores so that the body is able to respond to critical times for iron needs, such as during blood loss from disease, an increased need for blood synthesis when moving to a higher altitude, or the demands of pregnancy.

Exploring Issues and Actions

Your close friend complains that she is always run down. She also complains of heavy menstrual periods (menses) each month. You notice that she looks pale. Should you suggest she visit the student health center? What elements of her lifestyle should she examine and possibly change?

Causes of iron-deficiency anemia

A poor dietary intake of iron can lead to iron-deficiency anemia. Other causes include chronic blood loss from heavy menses, ulcers, hemorrhoids, and colon cancer, among others. The donation of one pint (0.5 liter) of blood represents a loss of 250 milligrams of iron. It generally takes several months to replace that iron. So it is wise, especially for women, to limit blood donations to two or three times a year. Remember that many people are iron deficient without showing symptoms of anemia. It takes a long time for iron-deficiency anemia to develop.

Blood loss due to intestinal and blood-borne parasite infections is a common additional cause of anemia in poverty, especially when people do not wear shoes. Parasites, such as hookworms, can easily penetrate the soles of the feet and enter the bloodstream.

Measuring iron status

The best way to assess iron status is to measure iron stores in the body. *The most sensitive measure of iron storage is the serum ferritin level.* If the serum ferritin level is low, iron stores in the liver are low. Because most extra iron is stored in the liver, low liver stores indicate that total body storage is also low.[11]

As iron deficiency proceeds, total iron-binding capacity of the blood increases. Many iron-binding sites on the blood proteins become free, leaving more room than usual for extra iron to bind. At the same time, the bone marrow, which synthesizes red blood cells, begins releasing immature red blood cell products called **free erythrocyte protoporphyrins.** Finally, as the iron deficiency worsens, hemoglobin and hematocrit values fall (Figure 14-2). The red blood cells will now be very small and pale. We refer to this as a **microcytic** (small cell) **hypochromic** (pale) anemia. Only very severe cases of iron deficiency reach this point.

free erythrocyte protoporphyrins (FEP)
Immature red blood cells released from the bone marrow. An increased serum level of FEP reflects a decreased ability to make red blood cells and suggests iron-deficiency anemia. Lead poisoning also raises blood FEP levels.

microcytic
Literally means "small cell." Red blood cells that are smaller than normal.

hypochromic
Pale red blood cells lacking sufficient hemoglobin due to an iron-deficiency. Hypochromic cells have a reduced oxygen-carrying ability

Treating iron-deficiency anemia

To speed the cure of iron-deficiency anemia, medicinal iron needs to be ingested. A physician should also find the cause so that the anemia does not recur. A good diet may prevent iron-deficiency anemia, but medicinal iron is a better cure.

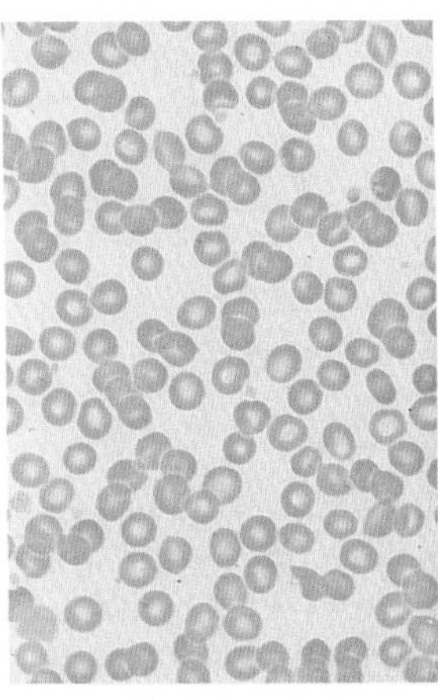

A

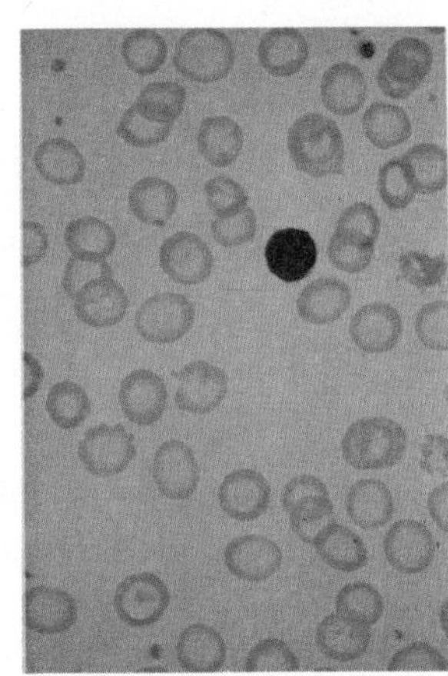

B

Stages of iron deficiency	Symptoms
poor iron stores	low serum ferritin level;
poor iron saturation in blood	low serum transferrin high total iron binding capacity in the blood
poor red blood cell synthesis	increased serum free erythrocyte protoporphyrins
anemia	low hemoglobin level and hematocrit level in the bloodstream; pale skin

Figure 14-2

Iron-deficiency anemia. (A) Normal cells: both cell size and color are normal. (B) Iron-deficient cells: both cell size and color are decreased. The loss of color stems from the lower amount of the pigment hemoglobin.

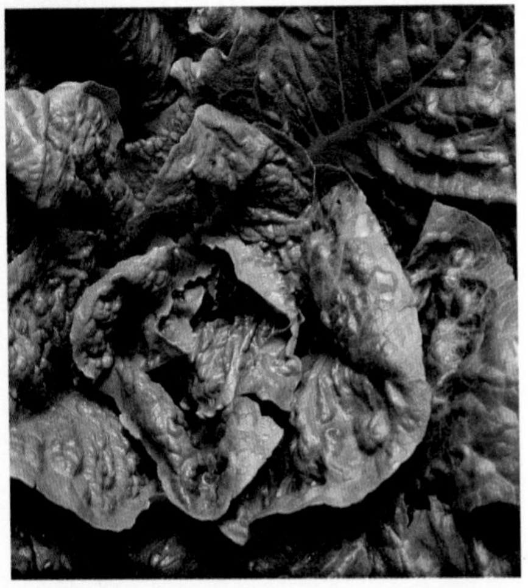

Spinach is rich in iron, but the bioavailability of iron from spinach is low.

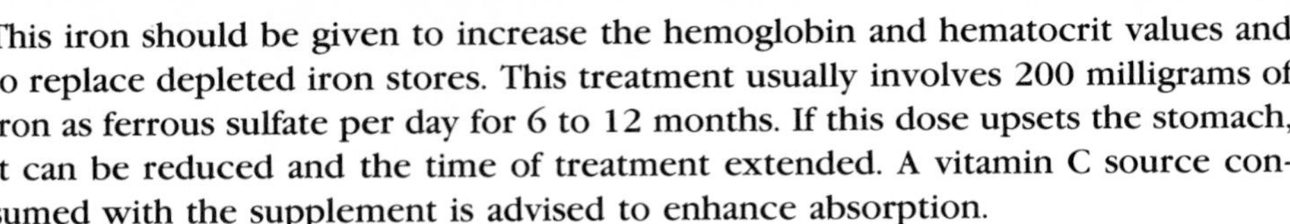

This iron should be given to increase the hemoglobin and hematocrit values and to replace depleted iron stores. This treatment usually involves 200 milligrams of iron as ferrous sulfate per day for 6 to 12 months. If this dose upsets the stomach, it can be reduced and the time of treatment extended. A vitamin C source consumed with the supplement is advised to enhance absorption.

Iron in foods

The most nutrient-dense iron sources are spinach, oysters, liver, clams, peas, and legumes (Table 14-2). However, total iron content of foods and nutrient density are not the only considerations when choosing dietary iron sources. Serving size and bioavailability are probably more important. For example, although spinach is iron rich, the body can absorb only very little of it. Animal sources contain some heme iron, the most bioavailable form. These are our best iron sources. The major iron sources in the U.S. diet are animal sources—beef steak, roasts, and hamburger. The next greatest sources are bakery products—white breads, rolls, and crackers. Most of this iron is added to refined flour to enrich it. Today, about 25% of the iron in the U.S. food supply comes from enriched bakery products. But there is debate about the value of iron enrichment: only about 3% of this iron is absorbed, both because of the form used and because other substances in flour bind iron.[10]

Table 14-2

Good sources of iron, ranked by nutrient density

Food	Serving size to yield 15 milligrams*	kcalories needed to yield 15 milligrams
Spinach, cooked	2½ cups	96
Oysters, raw	¾ cup	130
Sauerkraut, canned	4 cups	190
Green peas, cooked	5 cups	315
Beef liver, fried	8 ounces	525
Braunschweiger sausage	5½ pieces	575
Kidney beans, cooked	2½ cups	585
Lima beans, cooked	2½ cups	650
Navy beans, cooked	3 cups	660
Steak, beef	16 ounces	850
Prune juice	5 cups	935
Pot roast	13 ounces	1040

*The RDA for adult females, ages 11-50 years.
Bioavailability must be considered, as well as nutrient density. Due to the presence of heme iron and the meat protein factor, liver and meat are superior sources of iron compared with plants.

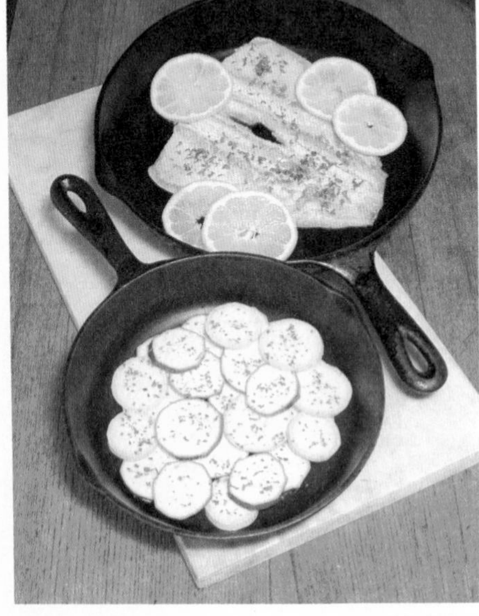

Foods cooked in iron pots and pans can pick up additional iron.

The use of iron-fortified formulas and cereals in the Women, Infant, and Children Program (WIC) in the United States is probably a major contributor to decreasing rates of iron-deficiency anemia in preschool children (see Chapters 15 and 16).[29] Another possible iron source is cooking utensils. When acidic foods, such as tomato sauce, are cooked in iron pots and frying pans, some iron from the cookware is taken up by the food.[6]

Milk is a very poor source of iron. A common cause of iron-deficiency anemia in children is an over-reliance on milk, coupled with an insufficient meat intake. Total vegetarians (vegans) are also susceptible to iron-deficiency anemia because of their lack of dietary heme iron.

RDA for iron

Iron needs are about 0.9 milligrams daily for men and 1.4 milligrams daily for women. The adult RDA for iron is 10 milligrams daily for men and 15 milligrams daily for women (throughout the rest of this chapter see the inside cover for other age groups and Appendix G for Canadian recommendations). The RDA value assumes that about 10% of dietary iron is absorbed. If iron absorption exceeds that, less dietary iron is needed.

The higher RDA for women is primarily due to menstrual blood loss. Women who menstruate more heavily and longer than the "average" menstruation may need even more dietary iron, and those who have lighter and shorter flows may need less iron. *The variation in menstrual blood loss makes it difficult to set an RDA for iron for women.*

By recording dietary intakes from a variety of women, we find that most women do not consume 15 milligrams of iron daily. The average value is closer to 11 milligrams per day. Of course, not all women need 15 milligrams of iron daily because the RDA is set high enough to meet the needs of most women. In addition, varied amounts of menstruation plus wide differences in iron absorption (recall it varies with need) further complicates evaluating a dietary intake. The RDA for a person absorbing 20% of dietary iron could be half that of the person absorbing 10% of it.

Thus a registered dietitian who finds that a person is not consuming the RDA for iron should be concerned, but not alarmed. This person should try to consume a diet that meets the RDA for iron. But whether a lower intake is actually harming this person's health is difficult to determine. Although we have very sensitive measures of iron stores in the body, we lack the knowledge to translate them into predictors of health status.[12]

North Americans at risk for an iron deficiency

As stated earlier, an iron deficiency is most common when iron needs greatly exceed normal intake—during infancy, preschool years, and puberty and during the child-bearing years for women. Pregnancy and disease also increase iron needs and therefore the risk for deficiency. Repeated pregnancies pose a special challenge to women to maintain adequate iron stores.

The North American diet contains about 5 to 7 milligrams of iron per 1000 kcalories. Thus men generally achieve a good iron status because a daily energy intake of 2000 to 3000 kcalories meets their RDA for iron. Most women, on the other hand, have difficulty eating 3000 kcalories daily while maintaining desirable weight. They then have difficulty consuming 15 milligrams of iron daily unless they seek out nutrient-dense forms of iron for their diets, such as is found in fortified breakfast cereals. If that does not suffice, a supplement should be used. *Iron-deficiency anemia, and especially poor iron stores, is not just a disease of the poor: it cuts across all social strata.*

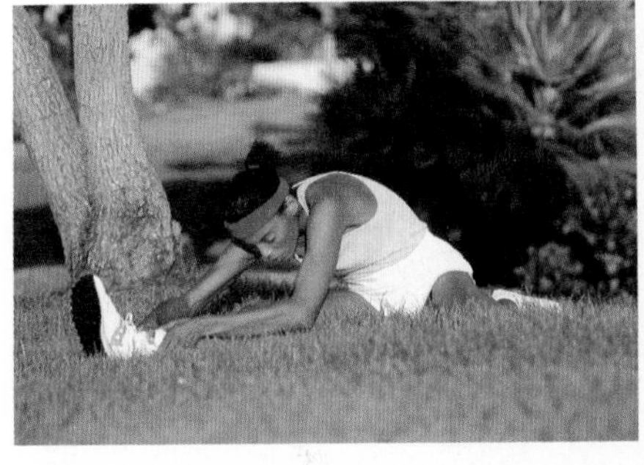

Runners following heavy training schedules should have their hemoglobin checked regularly to spot runner's anemia.

"Runner's Anemia"

Athletes incur a special type of anemia called **runner's anemia.** Three possible factors contribute to it: additional iron losses via increased perspiration, red blood cell destruction from trauma endured as red blood cells pass through the foot during exercise, and the increase in blood volume associated with athletic fitness. Runner's anemia can decrease sports performance, and so should be avoided. Athletes should have their hemoglobin levels and other iron status indicators monitored, and they should attempt to meet their iron needs by either dietary means or iron supplementation.

runner's anemia
A decrease in the blood's ability to carry oxygen found in athletes that may be caused by iron loss in perspiration, red blood cell destruction due to the impact of exercise, or increased blood volume and iron needs.

Toxicity of iron

Although iron deficiency is a common problem, an overabundance of iron can also be a serious problem because it is toxic. Even a large single dose of iron can be life-threatening. Iron pills and vitamin supplements containing iron commonly poison children. Smaller doses (but still greater than what is needed) over a long period can also cause problems. A form of iron toxicity has been observed in an African tribe that brews beer in iron pots.

hemochromatosis
A disorder of iron metabolism characterized by increased absorption, saturation of iron-binding proteins, and deposition of hemosiderin in the liver tissue.

Iron toxicity also accompanies the genetic disease called **hemochromatosis.** People with this disorder overabsorb iron, and throughout time the amount of iron in their bodies builds up to high levels especially in the bloodstream and liver. If not treated, excess iron is deposited in inappropriate tissues, contributing to severe liver and heart damage.[15] Researchers think that about 1 of 13 North Americans has one of the two genes needed to cause hemochromatosis. About 1 in 300 North Americans may have both hemochromatosis genes and therefore the disease.[16]

Probably the only factor keeping many people with hemochromatosis from experiencing serious effects of the disease is that they consume such a low amount of iron. For many years some nutrition interest groups have recommended increasing iron enrichment in grains to decrease the incidence of iron-deficiency anemia.[4] However, for people with hemochromatosis, that would probably increase the numbers who actually develop disease symptoms.

Treatment for hemochromatosis involves frequent bleeding and the use of medications to bind iron in the bloodstream to increase urinary excretion. If a case of hemochromatosis is found, the physician should also examine the affected person's brothers, sisters, and children. There is a good chance that other cases exist in the family.

Today, physicians do not routinely screen people for serum iron levels or transferrin saturation levels to look for hemochromatosis. Many physicians still believe it is a rare disease, but it is not.[15] In the future, you will probably notice a more aggressive approach in diagnosing hemochromatosis because with appropriate treatment, the disease process can be stopped, and the person can live a healthy and normal life. A first sign of hemochromatosis is arthritis-like symptoms.

Concept Check

Iron absorption depends on its form and the body's need for it. Absorption is controlled by a "mucosal block," but excess iron intake can override the control, leading to toxicity. Iron absorption increases in the presence of vitamin C and decreases in the presence of calcium and some components of grain fiber, such as phytic acid. Iron is most important in synthesizing hemoglobin and myoglobin and supporting immune function. An iron deficiency can cause decreased red blood cell synthesis, which can lead to anemia. It is particularly important for women of childbearing age to consume adequate iron, primarily to replace that lost in menstrual blood. Good sources include meat, enriched grains and cereals, and seafoods.

ZINC

Although zinc (chemical symbol is Zn) has been recognized as an essential nutrient in animals since the early 1900s, zinc deficiency was first recognized in humans in the early 1960s in Egypt and Iran. Zinc deficiencies were determined to be the cause of growth retardation and poor sexual development in many people. Curiously, the zinc content of the diet was fairly high. However, the customary diet contained almost exclusively unleavened bread and little animal protein. Unleavened bread is very high in phytates and other factors that decrease zinc bioavailability. Parasite infestation and the practice of eating dirt also probably contributed to the severe zinc deficiency.

In North America, zinc deficiencies were first observed in the early 1970s in hospitalized patients on total parenteral nutrition.[27] Zinc was not added to solutions prior to this time, but the protein source in the solutions was based on milk protein or blood fibrin, which are naturally rich in zinc. When the solutions were changed to include mostly synthetic amino acids as the protein source in the 1970s, deficiency symptoms quickly developed. This source of protein is very low in zinc content.

Absorption of zinc

Like iron, zinc absorption is influenced by foods ingested. About 25% to 40% of dietary zinc is absorbed; the higher figure is more likely when animal protein sources are used and the body's zinc needs are elevated. Zinc absorption, despite extensive study, is not clearly understood, but probably involves a compound that works in the intestine to help transport zinc into the intestinal cells.

When zinc is absorbed into intestinal cells, it induces the synthesis of the protein **metallothionein.** This binds zinc in much the same way that apoferritin binds iron. If zinc is not transferred to the bloodstream from the intestinal cells within 2 to 5 days, it is sloughed along with the cell and excreted. Thus a "mucosal block" works against overabsorption of zinc and iron (Figure 14-3). However, if large doses of zinc are taken, it overrides the mucosal block. Luckily for overconsumers, zinc is also excreted via the pancreas to the intestinal tract, unlike iron.

metallothionein
A protein that binds and regulates the release of zinc and copper (and other positive ions) in intestinal and liver cells.

Zinc intakes worldwide are generally poor. Supplementary iron competes with zinc for absorption,[10] and toasting cereals also reduces zinc absorption. Because most people worldwide rely on cereal grains for their source of protein, kcalories, and zinc, finding adequate zinc sources and maintaining adequate zinc intakes are a problem. More research on zinc status is needed worldwide.

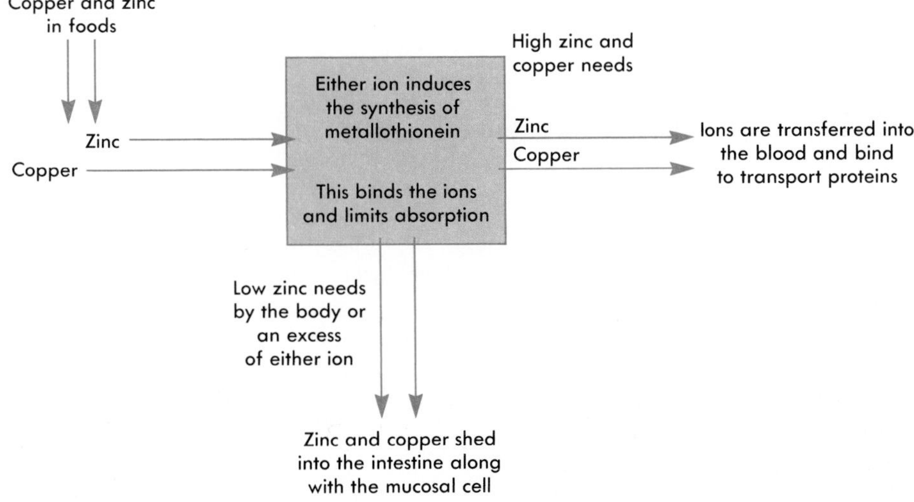

Figure 14-3

Zinc and copper absorption. Both influence the absorption of the other. The short life span of the intestinal absorptive cells also influences absorption.

Functions of zinc

Over 200 enzymes require zinc as a cofactor for optimum activity. Adequate zinc intake is necessary to support many bodily functions, such as:

- Nucleic acid and protein metabolism, wound healing, and growth
- Vitamin A mobilization from the liver
- Proper immune function (intakes in excess of the RDA do not provide any extra benefit to immune function[9])
- Proper development of sexual organs and bone
- Storage and release of insulin
- Prostaglandin synthesis (see Chapter 5)

Vitamin A deficiency symptoms in starvation can appear even though adequate vitamin A stores are found in the liver. This is because not enough zinc is available to help vitamin A bind to its transport protein. In the 1980s, when several men starved themselves to support a political cause, they developed blindness associated with a vitamin A deficiency. The primary deficiency, however, was of zinc, which induced a secondary vitamin A deficiency.

A recent study emphasizes the importance of zinc for growth. Children recovering from malnutrition gained weight much faster when they consumed zinc supplements containing approximately 3 times the RDA.[27]

Two important enzymes that require zinc are carbonic anhydrase and alcohol dehydrogenase. Carbonic anhydrase helps balance acid-base in the blood and aids stomach acid production in the parietal cells. Alcohol dehydrogenase breaks down alcohol.

Symptoms of zinc deficiency in adults include an acne-like rash, diarrhea, lack of appetite, reduced sense of taste and smell, hair loss, and poor growth and sexual development in children and adolescents[30] (Figure 14-4). Poor learning ability may result. A persistent rash, especially in the presence of a poor diet, should prompt a clinician to evaluate zinc status in a person.

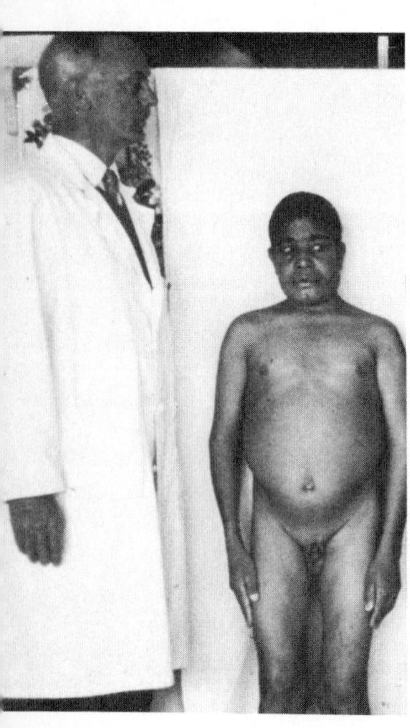

Figure 14-4

An example of zinc deficiency. An Egyptian farm boy, age 16 years and 49″ tall, with dwarfism and poor sexual development associated with a zinc deficiency.

Zinc in foods

In general, protein-rich diets are also rich in zinc. The most nutrient-dense sources of zinc are oysters, shrimp, crab, beef, turkey, greens, and mushrooms (Table 14-3). As with iron, nutrient density is not the only issue: bioavailability is probably more important. *Animal foods are our best zinc sources because zinc from animal sources is neither bound by phytates, nor so affected by local soil conditions.* Animal foods supply almost half our zinc intake, but their cost makes zinc a very expensive nutrient. We shouldn't discount good plant sources of zinc, such as whole grains, peanuts, and beans, however, because studies show they

Table 14-3

Good sources of zinc, ranked by nutrient density

Food	Serving size to yield 15 milligrams*	kcalories needed to yield 15 milligrams
Oysters, raw	¼ cup	32
Wheat germ, raw	1-⅓ cups	374
Crab meat, canned	2-¾ cups	380
Shrimp, boiled	14 ounces	445
Sirloin steak, lean	9 ounces	530
Beef liver, fried	10 ounces	640
Beef pot roast, lean	9 ounces	680
Lamb chop	12 ounces	744
Corned beef, canned	12 ounces	760
Turkey, all meat roasted	17 ounces	830
Blackeyed peas, cooked	5 cups	950

*Adult male RDA.

Seafoods are good, readily bioavailable sources of zinc.

can deliver substantial amounts of zinc to body cells. Zinc is not part of the enrichment process, so refined flours are not a good source.

RDA for zinc

The adult RDA for zinc is 15 milligrams daily for men and 12 milligrams daily for women. The average adult American intake of zinc is 8 to 12 milligrams daily. This raises concern that some people have marginal intakes.[24] Still, there are no indications of moderate or severe zinc deficiencies in an otherwise healthy adult population.[27]

North Americans at risk for a zinc deficiency

In North America, zinc deficiencies are most commonly found in hospital patients with severe malabsorption. Sickle-cell disease increases zinc needs by destroying massive amounts of red blood cells, which contain a great deal of zinc. In addition, people with alcoholism, elderly people, and total vegetarians can be deficient in zinc because of either a poor overall nutrient intake, or a diet low in animal foods. Greater zinc intake in these people can sometimes increase their appetite and sense of taste. In the United States, symptoms of zinc deficiency have been observed in groups of middle- and low-income children with poor growth. Supplementation with zinc improved growth and appetite (see the Expert Opinion on zinc by Drs. Janet King and Jean Weininger).

A rare disease, acrodermatitis enteropathica, results from an inherited inability to absorb zinc. Symptoms in infants include rash, hair loss, depressed immune response, poor sense of taste, lack of appetite, and poor growth. This disease can be treated with supplements of zinc in amounts of about twice the RDA.

The link between zinc and appetite, taste acuity, wound healing, and immune response underscores zinc's importance in the diets of elderly people. Immune status is often depressed in elderly people. Because of poorly fitting dentures or low-income status, elderly people may not eat enough animal products. This reduces zinc intake, and throughout months and years, can cause a zinc deficiency.

There are probably many cases of marginal zinc status in North America. However, we lack a sensitive marker for zinc status. The body must be very zinc-depleted for clinical tests to register a deficiency. Assessment of zinc status is difficult because serum zinc levels do not reflect body stores, and no test using a zinc-containing enzyme is accepted. *Measuring hair zinc may be a good measure of long-term zinc intake in albino laboratory rats, but hair analysis is not a reliable measure of zinc status in humans who color, perm, straighten, shampoo, and use an infinite array of other products that alter the zinc content of hair* (see Nutrition Perspective 14-2 on hair analysis). For your overall health, it is important to evaluate your zinc intake and to regularly consume foods that are good sources.

Toxicity of zinc

A high consumption of zinc works against iron and copper absorption. Recall that iron, copper, and zinc can all exist with a +2 charge. Oversupplementation with zinc can cause a copper deficiency. One study has shown that zinc supplements at approximately three to five times the RDA can reduce HDL cholesterol levels by about 15%.[5] In that case, excess zinc may interfere with copper metabolism. That is disturbing for two reasons. First, low HDL cholesterol levels are associated with an increased risk of developing heart disease (see Chapter 5). Second, it is common for people who take zinc supplements to consume this amount. So some North Americans, by unwittingly lowering their HDL cholesterol levels, may be increasing their risk for developing heart disease—even though they think that supplementing zinc in the diet contributes to overall health. Again, this shows why mineral supplements should not be consumed except under close scrutiny of a physician. Otherwise, more harm than good may result. Zinc intakes over 2 grams daily also result in diarrhea, cramps, nausea, vomiting, and sometimes depresses immune system function.[9]

Exploring Issues and Actions

You subscribe to a popular health magazine and notice an ad that strongly recommends zinc supplements to boost immune function. What is wrong with this ad? What are possible negative effects of following this advice, if any?

Expert Opinion

Zinc in Human Nutrition

JEAN WEININGER, Ph.D. AND JANET C. KING, Ph.D.

In the early 1960s, Investigators found that young men in Iran and Egypt who were severely retarded in growth and sexual maturation responded well to treatment with zinc. Since then, we've learned that zinc is essential in the human diet, not only for growth and development, but also for critical functions in every cell of the body.

Zinc promotes normal growth of the genital organs, healthy skin, wound healing, and the proper functioning of the immune system. Zinc and vitamin A work together to enable us to see, especially at night, and may affect our capacity to taste and smell. Zinc is necessary for numerous enzyme systems to function properly, and it is especially important in metabolizing DNA and synthesizing proteins.

Zinc is called a trace element because it's required in such small—though critical—quantities. There is only about 2 grams (2000 milligrams) of zinc in the whole body, about as much as is in a galvanized nail.

Severe zinc deficiency, which is rare in the United States, most commonly results from malabsorption caused by a genetic condition known as **acrodermatitis enteropathica.** However, some reports suggest mild zinc deficiency in otherwise healthy people in this country. Growing children and adolescents are at special risk, as are the elderly, and, possibly, pregnant women.

Certain conditions and diseases can also predispose a person to zinc deficiency. In cases of diabetes mellitus, alcoholic liver disease, and sickle-cell disease, for example, zinc is excreted in the urine. Signs of zinc deficiency are also found where intestinal absorption is decreased, such as in cases of inflammatory bowel disease and cystic fibrosis. Zinc deficiency has also occurred when it was inadvertently omitted from feeding solutions of hospitalized patients.

Various claims are made for the "powers" of zinc. In several studies near Denver, Colorado, researchers found that a small zinc supplement improved the growth rates of some children. Other proponents report that zinc supplements improve immune status in the elderly, but they have not been able to link that with zinc deficiency in the people studied. Some people claim that zinc deficiency may contribute to complications of pregnancy and delivery, birth defects, and low birth weight in infants, but again, no strong evidence relates these conditions to zinc deficiency. Researching these problems would be difficult because of the large number of women—over 1000—needed to obtain useful results.

Recent work shows that production of interleukin-2, a substance that plays a key role in the cellular immune system, is impaired in cases of mild and severe zinc deficiency. Another area of very active research is the role of zinc and its mobilization and redistribution throughout the body during trauma and tissue breakdown.

The best food sources of zinc are animal foods, such as red meat, poultry, and seafood. Oysters are one of the richest sources. Unrefined whole-grain cereals are also good sources of zinc, but refining processes destroy most zinc. Many breakfast cereals are excellent sources of zinc if zinc is added back after refining. Legumes and nuts are fairly good sources, and fruits and vegetables are generally poor sources. Zinc from animal sources is also more readily absorbed than zinc from plant sources because substances in plant foods—such as fiber and phytate—tend to bind zinc, interfering with its absorption.

Expert Opinion—cont'd

The Recommended Dietary Allowance for zinc—intended to cover the needs of most healthy adults—is 15 milligrams per day for men and 12 milligrams per day for women and is slightly more during pregnancy and lactation. While the average daily intake for many people in the United States is only about 8 to 12 milligrams, it appears that we have a tremendous ability to adapt to these lower intakes. When less zinc is consumed, relatively more zinc is absorbed and retained by the body. Since we don't have accurate methods to assess zinc requirements, it remains unclear whether mild zinc depletion is widespread in this country.

How much zinc do you eat? You can get an idea of your daily zinc intake by calculating a one day intake (see Take Action in Chapter 17). If you come within a few milligrams of the RDA, you probably do not need to be concerned. But if you are below 8 milligrams, you should probably pay more attention to your zinc sources.

If you take a vitamin/mineral supplement, avoid those containing more than 15 milligrams of zinc without first checking with your doctor. Although zinc is relatively nontoxic, high doses can interfere with the body's utilization of copper, and can cause adverse reactions, such as nausea and vomiting.

Zinc status in the body can be determined by measuring either the activity of zinc-requiring enzymes or the level of zinc in various blood components, urine, and hair. But the results of all these techniques can be confounded. For example, taking certain drugs, such as oral contraceptives, may decrease blood zinc levels, and certain conditions, such as diabetes mellitus, may elevate urine zinc levels, regardless of zinc status. While hair is easy to sample and its analysis is popular, the interpretation of hair zinc levels is difficult because the relationship of hair zinc to zinc status is unclear, analytical techniques are unreliable in some laboratories, and possible zinc contamination results from shampoos, dyes, and other sources. Currently, there are no good specific indicators of zinc status, and so it is difficult to evaluate zinc adequacy in individuals or populations.

There is a popular notion that zinc is a "sexy" nutrient, both because human zinc deficiency was first documented in sexually underdeveloped men, and because zinc is found in high levels in seminal fluid. But for adults whose diet is already adequate in zinc, there is no evidence that extra zinc increases the size of sexual organs or affects fertility or sex life in any way.

Another popular notion is that zinc can remedy the common cold, and people take zinc lozenges in hopes this is true. Although zinc does affect cold viruses in the laboratory, there is no convincing evidence that zinc is useful in treating colds. Some investigators have shown that taking large doses of zinc may even interfere with the body's natural immune response. There is currently no indication that zinc supplements have any value for people with AIDS and related syndromes.

Dr. King is Professor and Chair, Department of Nutritional Sciences, University of California, Berkeley. Dr. Weininger is a Research Associate in the same department.

COPPER

Copper (chemical symbol is Cu) contributes to the activity of many enzymes and aids in iron absorption and metabolism.[1] When a person with microcytic hypochromic anemia does not respond to iron supplements, the anemia can, although rarely, be due to a copper deficiency.

Functions of copper

Copper increases iron absorption by helping form a protein called ceruloplasmin (also known as ferroxidase). As we said earlier, this compound helps mobilize iron by converting Fe^{+2} into Fe^{+3}. To cross cell membranes (intestinal and other body cells) any Fe^{+2} must be converted to Fe^{+3}. Thus ceruloplasmin can enable iron to leave the intestinal cells and sites of iron storage in the liver and bind to the protein transferrin in the bloodstream. The iron is then transported to bone marrow and other cells.[1]

There is still some debate about the mechanism used in this iron copper relationship.

Copper is important for the function of enzymes that cross-bond collagen, a connective tissue protein. In a copper deficiency, blood vessels in laboratory animals rupture because collagen is not available to form the important connective tissue network needed to strengthen blood vessels.[14]

Copper facilitates the activity of enzymes that synthesize norepinephrine and dopamine, two neurotransmitters. In addition, copper is needed by enzymes that cause myelination (insulation) of the nervous system, cholesterol release from the liver, and the scavenging of electron-seeking (free radical) compounds. One of the body's major free radical scavengers, the enzyme superoxide dismutase, can contain copper and other minerals. Finally, copper is important for proper immune system function and blood clotting.[14]

Symptoms of copper deficiency include anemia, low white blood cell count (specifically, the neutrophils), bone loss, increased serum cholesterol levels, poor growth, and heart disease.[14]

Copper in foods

Copper is primarily found in seafood, liver, cocoa, legumes, nuts, and whole-grain breads and cereals (Table 14-4). It is not added to breakfast cereals since it speeds fat breakdown in the product. Milk is also a very poor source of copper. About 25% to 40% of dietary copper is absorbed.[28] High-fructose diets decrease copper absorption in rats, especially males, but we don't know if humans are affected the same way. *Food tables often list few values for copper, and even those values may not be reliable because soil conditions greatly affect the copper content of plant foods.*

ESADDI for copper

Copper has an estimated safe and adequate daily dietary intake of 1.5 to 3 milligrams daily for adults. Studies of young men show a minimum intake should be 1.3 milligrams daily. The average intake in North America is about 1 milligram daily. Women generally have marginal intakes.[24] Even so, the copper status of adults in North America appears to be good, though this may be because we lack sensitive measures for copper status. So some cases of marginal deficiencies may be missed. We suggest you find good sources of copper for your diet.

Several groups of people at the greatest risk for a copper deficiency include premature infants, infants recovering from malnutrition on a diet dominated by milk (which is a poor source of copper),[8] people recovering from intestinal surgery (during which time copper absorption decreases), and long-term total parenteral nutrition when insufficient copper is added. Use of large doses of antacids may also bind enough copper in the intestine to cause a deficiency.

An inherited condition known as Menkes' kinky hair syndrome is characterized by slow growth, brain degeneration, kinky white hair, and low serum copper levels. This condition results from a defect of copper absorption and ceruloplasmin metabolism. Supplemental copper is given in an attempt to reverse this condition.

A copper deficiency can result from overzealous supplementation of zinc,

Table 14-4

Good sources of copper ranked by nutrient density

Food	Serving size to yield 2 milligrams	kcalories needed to yield 2 milligrams
Oysters, raw meat	.75 ounce	14
Pecans	1.5 cups	80
Lobster	4.5 ounces	152
Brewer's yeast	7 tablespoons	175
Liver, beef or calf, fried	3 ounces	185
Cocoa powder, low-fat	2.5 ounces	185
Molasses, blackstrap	7 tablespoons	297
Wheat germ, toasted	1.25 cup	539
Sunflower kernels, dry hulled	3.5 ounces	578
Brazil nuts, shelled	.75 cup	689
Beans, red kidney, dry, cooked	4 cups	904
Walnuts, English	1.5 cup	963
Peanut butter	1.5 cup	2287

For comparison, the adult ESADDI is 1.5 to 3 milligrams.
Seafoods, nuts, seeds, and beans are good sources of copper.

since zinc and copper compete with each other for absorption (Figure 14-3). Both minerals increase the synthesis of the protein metallothionein, which binds them both—but particularly copper—in the intestinal cells, reducing future transfer into the bloodstream.

We have now seen that the absence of many nutrients from the diet can lead to anemia:

- Vitamin E deficiency can lead to hemolytic anemia (see Chapter 11).
- Vitamin K deficiency, especially coupled with use of antibiotics, can lead to blood loss and so to hemorrhagic anemia (see Chapter 11).
- Vitamin B-6 deficiency can lead to microcytic anemia (see Chapter 12).
- folate deficiency—megaloblastic anemia
- Vitamin B-12 malabsorption can lead to pernicious anemia (see Chapter 12).
- An iron deficiency can lead to microcytic hypochromic anemia.
- A copper deficiency can lead to a secondary iron-deficiency anemia, as copper aids in iron metabolism.

Toxicity of copper

Copper tends to cause vomiting at single doses greater than 10 to 15 milligrams. When copper is used to treat a deficiency, it must be given in divided doses to limit this effect. An inherited condition called Wilson's disease results in accumulation of copper in the liver, brain, kidneys, and cornea of the eye. If recognized early, treatment that binds copper in the bloodstream and increases its excretion in the urine can prevent damage to these tissues and reduce the mental degeneration commonly seen in active cases.

Concept Check

Similar to iron absorption, zinc absorption is regulated by a mucosal block. Both animal protein sources and increased body needs lead to increased zinc absorption. Copper and iron compete with zinc for absorption. Zinc functions as a cofactor for many enzymes and is important for growth, immune function, and sense of taste. Beef, seafood, and whole grains are good food sources. Copper functions mainly in iron metabolism, cross-bonding of collagen, myelination of nerve cells, and neurotransmitter synthesis. A deficiency can result in a microcytic hypochromic anemia. Good food sources of copper are meats, liver, legumes, and whole grains.

SELENIUM

Selenium (chemical symbol is Se) exists in many ionic forms. Most selenium in foods is bound within the amino acid derivatives of methionine and cysteine. These forms are readily absorbed from the diet.[25] There appears to be no physiological control of how much we absorb, so selenium shows a high toxic potential.

Functions of selenium

Selenium's most important role is as cofactor for the activity of a major form of the enzyme glutathione peroxidase. Each enzyme molecule can have 4 selenium atoms attached to it. This enzyme participates in a system that metabolizes peroxides into less toxic alcohols and water. In Chapter 11 we discussed how important this action of glutathione peroxidase is: peroxides tend to become free radicals that can then attack and break down cell membranes, causing cell death.

Recall that vitamin E also functions to prevent attacks on cell membranes by free radicals. *Thus vitamin E and selenium work together.* Selenium participates in an enzyme system that prevents free radical production by reducing peroxide concentration in the cell, and vitamin E stops the action of free radicals once they are produced. So an adequate selenium intake spares some of the body's need for vitamin E.

Selenium's role in reducing free radical production gives it a potential for reducing cancer. At one time, high dietary levels of selenium were considered carcinogenic, but after further studies, this is in doubt. In Chapter 5 we discussed how electron-seeking compounds can alter DNA. Alterations in DNA are known to cause cancer. By reducing the concentration of free radicals, it appears that an adequate selenium intake could be an important cancer prevention measure. Animal studies in this area are encouraging, and scientists hope results of human studies currently under way will clarify selenium's role in cancer prevention.[7] Until then, *recommending selenium supplementation to possibly prevent cancer in humans is premature.*[10] Selenium may have yet other metabolic functions, but none has been firmly established.[25]

Selenium deficiency symptoms in animals and humans include muscle pain, muscle wasting, and heart disease.[21] Farm animals in areas with low selenium soil concentrations, such as New Zealand, and humans in some areas of China develop characteristic muscle and heart disorders associated with poor selenium intake.[25] Other factors may also contribute. These same symptoms are noted when insufficient selenium is added to total parenteral nutrition solutions.

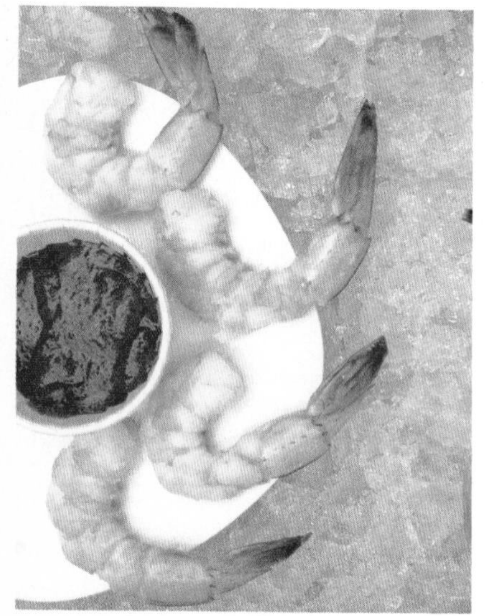

Selenium is found in shellfish.

Selenium in foods

Fish, meats—especially organ meats—eggs, and shellfish are good animal sources of selenium. Grains and seeds grown in soils containing selenium are good plant sources. A recent survey found the major selenium contributors in the U.S. diet are tuna, beef, white bread, chicken, eggs, noodles, and milk (Table 14-5). *Since we eat a varied diet supplied from many geographic areas of North America, it is unlikely that selenium deficiency in the soil in a few areas will cause a selenium deficiency in our diets.*

RDA for selenium

The RDA for selenium is 55 to 70 micrograms daily for adults. About 40 micrograms daily probably represents our minimum needs. North American diets probably include this much selenium, since the average intake is 80 to 130 micrograms daily. Nutritionists consider selenium intake adequate in most Western diets. However, we do not have sensitive measures of selenium status, and cannot accurately distinguish between a good and a marginal status.[25]

Toxicity of selenium

Excess selenium can be toxic.[25] Daily intakes as low as 2 to 3 milligrams (just 35 times the RDA) can cause toxicity symptoms if taken for many months. These

Table 14-5

Good sources of selenium, ranked by nutrient density

Food	Serving size needed to 70 micrograms*	kcalories needed to yield 70 micrograms
Tuna, canned in water	2¾ ounces	125
Whole wheat bread	2¾ slices	240
Ham, roasted, cooked	9 ounces	400
Egg noodles	2 cups	420
Eggs, poached	5½ each	440
Oatmeal, cooked	3½ cups	510
White bread	6½ slices	630
Hamburger with bun	10 ounces	695
Beef, sirloin steak, cooked	12 ounces	950
Chicken, meat, all, cooked	19½ ounces	1055
Meat loaf, beef and pork	15½ ounces	1064
Milk, 2% fat	100 ounces	1457
Luncheon meat, beef	22½ ounces	1945

*Adult male RDA.
Meats, bread and grain products, and eggs are good sources of selenium.

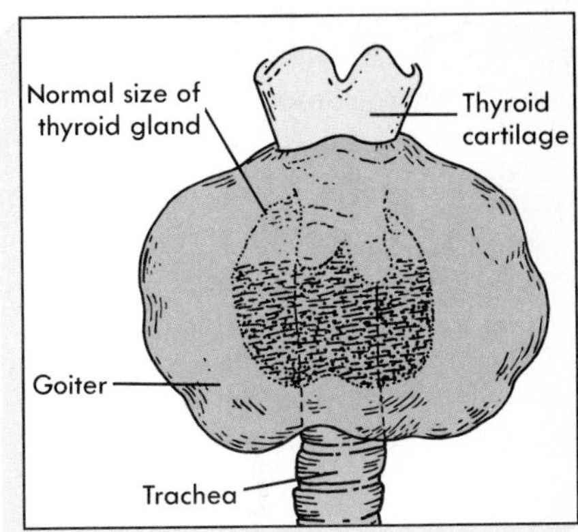

symptoms include a garlicky odor of the breath, hair loss, nausea and vomiting, and a general weakness. Rashes and cirrhosis of the liver may also develop. Selenium illustrates the saying: "It's the dose that makes the poison."

Animals show selenium toxicity symptoms if they eat plants containing high selenium levels. Some plants naturally concentrate selenium from the soil. Birds who live in water polluted with selenium leached from nearby fields also have exhibited toxicity symptoms.

Selenium is now the focus of much research. The FDA has limited supplemental doses in studies to 200 micrograms per day, based on our lack of knowledge of this mineral.

IODIDE

Iodine (chemical symbol is I), present in food as iodide and other non-elemental forms, was linked to the presence of an enlarged thyroid gland (goiter) during World War I. Men drafted from the Pacific Northwest and the Great Lakes Region of the United States had a much higher rate of goiter than men from other areas of the country. The soils in these areas are very low in iodide content. Researchers in Ohio then fed a large group of children low doses of iodide in the 1920s for 4 years. They found that could prevent goiter in children. That finding led to the addition of iodide to salt beginning in the 1920s.

Many times the term Iodine (I_2) is used instead of iodide (I^-). The ion iodide is what is essential in the diet. The element iodine itself is quite poisonous. To emphasize this point, we will use the term iodide exclusively.

Today, many nations, such as Canada, require iodide-fortification of salt. In the United States, salt can be purchased either fortified or plain. By law, the label on a salt container sold in the U.S. must clearly state if iodide is present or not. *Some areas of Europe, like Northern Italy, have very low iodide levels in the soil, but have yet to adopt the practice of fortifying salt with iodide. People in these areas, especially women, still suffer from goiter, as do people in areas of Central America, South America, and Africa.*

Function of iodide

The thyroid gland actively accumulates and traps iodide from the bloodstream to support its hormone synthesis. Thyroid hormones, such as thyroxine, are synthe-

Thyroxine **(T_4)**

sized from the amino acid tyrosine and iodide and help regulate metabolic rate, growth, and development, in addition to promoting bone and protein synthesis.

If a person's iodide intake is insufficient, the thyroid gland enlarges as it attempts to take up more iodide from the bloodstream. The hormone that stimulates thyroid hormone production, **thyroid-stimulating hormone,** also stimulates the growth of the thyroid gland. Usually, enough thyroid hormone is made to limit production of thyroid-stimulating hormone. However, in an iodide deficiency, insufficient thyroid hormone is produced to shut off the synthesis of this hormone. The constant release of thyroid-stimulating hormone by the pituitary gland causes continual growth of the thyroid gland, eventually producing a greatly enlarged thyroid gland, or **goiter** (Figure 14-5). Goiters have occurred in people since 3000 BC, usually in women.

thyroid-stimulating hormone
Regulates the uptake of iodide by the thyroid gland. It is secreted in response to low levels of circulating thyroid hormone.

goiter
An enlargement of the thyroid gland; this can be caused by a lack of iodide in the diet

goitrogens
Substances in food that interfere with the absorption of utilization of iodide, and therefore may cause goiter if consumed in large amounts.

Goiters are also associated with the consumption of large amounts of raw turnips and rutabagas. These vegetables contain compounds called **goitrogens,** which inhibit the function of the thyroid gland, and in turn, thyroid hormone synthesis. However, goitrogens are not an important cause of goiter, since they are destroyed by cooking and the foods they are found in do not often play an important role in human diets.

If a woman consumes an iodide-deficient diet during the early months of her pregnancy, her infant may be born with growth failure and may develop

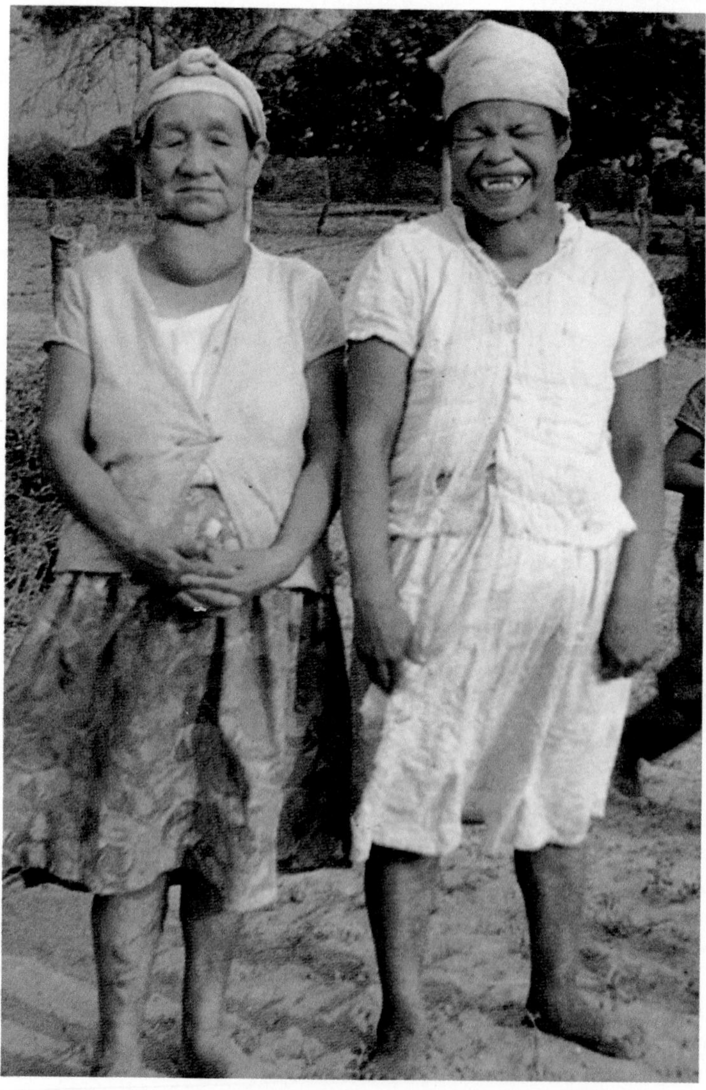

Figure 14-5

Goiter and cretinism in Bolivia. The mother on the left is goitrous, but otherwise normal. The daughter is goitrous, mentally retarded, and a deaf mute.

mental retardation (Figure 14-5). Maternal iodide needs take precedence over fetal needs. This stunted growth is referred to as **cretinism.** Cretinism appeared in North America before the program for iodide fortification of table salt began. Today, cretinism still appears in Europe, Africa, Latin America, and Asia.

cretinism
Stunting of body growth and mental development that results from inadequate maternal intake of iodide during pregnancy.

Food sources of iodide

Saltwater fish, seafood, iodized salt, molasses, and some plants contain various forms of iodide, especially plants grown near the sea. Sea salt found in health food stores, however, is not a good source, since the iodide is lost during processing. A half teaspoon of iodide-fortified salt (about 2 grams) supplies the adult RDA for iodide (the actual fortification level in the U.S. is 76 micrograms of iodide per gram of salt).

The ocean is the source of most iodide naturally present in our diets. As sea water evaporates and rains on the nearby land, iodide becomes part of the soil. Plants that grow in that soil accumulate the iodide.

RDA for iodide

The RDA for iodide for adults is 150 micrograms daily. Probably the minimum intake to prevent goiter is 50 micrograms per day. Most North Americans consume much more iodide (consumption is estimated to be at least 300 micrograms per day) than the RDA. This is because of its use: (1) as a sterilizing agent in dairies and fast-food restaurants, (2) as a dough conditioner in bakeries, (3) in food colorants, and (4) in iodized salt. So there is no need for concern about insufficient iodide intake in North America, unless dietary sodium intake must be kept below 500 milligrams per day. However, these types of low-sodium diets are rarely used today.

Toxicity of iodide

Reports in scientific literature raise concern about high-iodide intake. Levels up to 2 to 3 milligrams (13 to 20 times the RDA) per day appear to be safe. However, when very high amounts of iodide are consumed, thyroid hormone synthesis is inhibited, as in a deficiency. A "toxic goiter" results. "Toxic goiter" can appear in people who eat a lot of seaweed, since some seaweeds contain as much as 1% iodide by weight. Total iodide intake then can add up to 60 to 130 times the RDA. Manufacturers are working to reduce unnecessary iodide use in dairies, restaurants, and bakeries.

FLUORIDE

Dentists in the early 1900s noticed a lower rate of dental caries in the Southwestern United States. These areas naturally contained high amounts of fluoride (chemical symbol is F) in the water. The levels were sometimes so high that small spots on the teeth, called **mottling,** appeared. Even though these mottled teeth were quite discolored, they contained very few dental caries. After experiments showed that fluoride in the water did indeed decrease the rate of dental caries, controlled fluoridation of water in parts of the United States began in 1945.

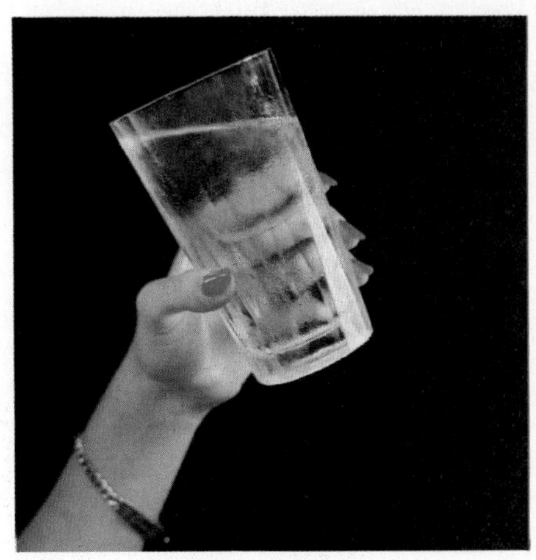

Use of flouridated tap water in childhood provides significant protection against dental caries throughout life.

Those of us who grew up drinking fluoridated water generally have 50% to 70% fewer dental caries than people who did not drink fluoridated water as children. Dentists can provide fluoride treatments, and schools can provide fluoride tablets, but it is much less expensive and more reliable to simply put fluoride in a community's drinking water. Neither all state nor all private water sources contain enough fluoride. When in doubt, contact your local water plant, or have the water in your home analyzed for fluoride content. If it doesn't supply the recommended amount—1 part per million parts of water (1 ppm)—talk to your dentist about the best means for children to obtain the needed fluoride.

mottling
Discoloration or marking of the surface of teeth due to fluorosis.

fluroapatite
A tooth crystal containing fluoride ions that make the tooth relatively acid-resistant.

Functions of fluoride

Dietary fluoride during bone and teeth development aids the synthesis of **fluroapatite** crystals, rather than hydroxyapatite crystals (see Chapter 13). Fluroapatite crystals strongly resist acid, so teeth containing fluroapatite crystals are very resistant to dental caries. Fluoride also inhibits the growth of bacteria that cause dental caries (see Chapter 4 for a review of the development of dental caries).

Fluoride has its greatest effect when bones and teeth are developing. Thus consuming fluoride during childhood is important. Dietary fluoride also improves growth rate in mice, but scientists are not sure if fluoride is actually necessary for growth in humans.

Fluoride in foods

Tea, seafoods, seaweed, and some natural water sources are the only good food sources of fluoride. Most fluoride intake of North Americans comes from water-fortification, toothpaste, and fluoride treatments performed by dentists. No evidence shows that water fluoridation at present U.S. levels is harmful.

ESADDI for fluoride

The estimated safe and adequate daily dietary intake of fluoride for adults is 1.5 to 4 milligrams daily. This range of intake provides the benefits of resistance to dental caries without causing mottling of the teeth.

Toxicity of fluoride

A fluoride intake greater than 6 milligrams daily can mottle teeth during a developmental stage. High-fluoride intake in adults does not cause mottling. In addition, when fluoride intakes reach 20 milligrams daily during tooth development, the tooth structure is weakened and can crumble. This is called fluorosis and appears in humans and other animals.

High doses of fluoride (20 or more milligrams per day) are used experimentally in adults to treat severe osteoporosis. This dose causes side effects, such as stomach upset and bone pain, and some people cannot tolerate this treatment. Scientists are not sure if fluoride will ultimately reduce osteoporosis symptoms. However, the preliminary findings are encouraging. It appears that fluoride may stimulate the osteoblast cells in the bone to synthesize more bone mass (see Chapter 13).

Concept Check

Selenium is important for the activity of glutathione peroxidase, an enzyme that reduces the concentration of peroxides, lessening the free radical load in the body. In this way, selenium spares some of the need for vitamin E. A deficiency results in muscle and heart disorders. Organ meats, eggs, fish, and grains are good selenium sources; however, the selenium content in plants depends on the selenium concentration in the soil. A high-selenium intake is potentially toxic. Iodide is vital in the synthesis of thyroid hormones. A prolonged insufficient intake will cause the thyroid gland to enlarge, resulting in a goiter. The use of iodized salt in North America has virtually eliminated this condition. Fluoride incorporated into teeth during development makes them resistant to acid and bacterial growth, in turn reducing the chance of developing dental caries. Most North Americans get adequate amounts via water fortification and toothpaste. A high-fluoride intake during tooth development may lead to spotted, or mottled, teeth.

CHROMIUM

The importance of chromium (chemical symbol is Cr) in human diets had been recognized only in the past 20 years. There is much we do not understand about this mineral, but chromium deficiency may be related to both diabetes mellitus and coronary heart disease.

Functions of chromium

The most studied function of chromium is the maintenance of normal glucose uptake into cells. Researchers are not sure how chromium does this. Early work suggested that it formed a glucose tolerance factor with the vitamin niacin, but that is no longer accepted. Our current understanding is that chromium forms a type of complex that appears to help insulin bind to cells.

In both animals and man, a chromium deficiency is characterized by impaired glucose tolerance and elevated serum cholesterol and triglyceride levels. The mechanism by which chromium influences cholesterol metabolism is not known, but may involve enzymes that control cholesterol synthesis. Chromium deficiency appears in people maintained on total parenteral nutrition not supplemented with chromium and in children with malnutrition. Since sensitive measures of chromium status are not available, marginal chromium deficiencies may go undetected.

Food sources of chromium

Overall, there is little data regarding chromium values of foods. Vegetable oils, such as corn oil, are good sources of chromium, but it is present as an impurity. Egg yolks, whole grains, and meats are also good sources. Fruits, vegetables, many seafoods, highly processed foods, and drinking water are generally poor sources. The ultimate chromium level in foods is closely tied to local soil content of chromium. To provide yourself with a good chromium intake, eat as many whole grains, rather than refined grains, as possible.

ESADDI of chromium

The estimated safe and adequate daily dietary intake of chromium is 50 to 200 micrograms daily. Marginal to low chromium intakes in the elderly may contribute to their increased risk for developing diabetes mellitus. Some research shows that an intake at the high end of the ESADDI, or slightly above, may raise HDL cholesterol levels. More studies are needed on this effect. Chromium toxicity has been reported in people exposed to industrial waste and in painters using art supplies with a very high chromium content. Liver damage and lung cancer can be the result.

MANGANESE

It is easy to confuse the mineral manganese (chemical symbol is Mn) with magnesium. Their names are similar, and in metabolic pathways they often substitute for each other.

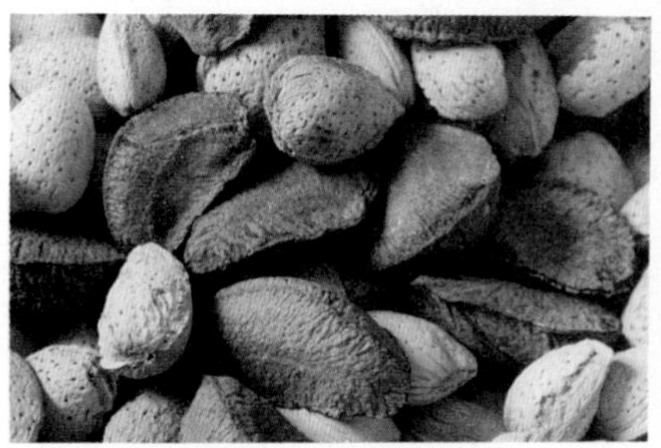

Nuts are a good source of manganese.

Functions of manganese

Manganese is a component of many different enzymes, such as pyruvate carboxylase, an important enzyme in carbohydrate metabolism. Manganese is also important in bone formation.[2]

No human deficiency symptom is associated with a low manganese intake. Animals on manganese-deficient diets suffer alterations in brain function, bone formation, reproduction, and blood glucose regulation. If human diets were low in manganese, these symptoms would probably appear in us as well. As it happens, our need for manganese is very low, and our diets tend to be quite high in manganese content.

Manganese in foods

Good food sources of manganese are nuts, rice, oats and other whole grains, beans, and leafy vegetables. The estimated safe and adequate daily dietary intake of manganese is 2 to 5 milligrams daily. Studies of young men show that 3.5 milligrams per day meets their manganese needs.[17] Manganese is toxic at high doses, as evidenced by toxicity that appears in miners of manganese.

MOLYBDENUM

Molybdenum (chemical symbol is Mo) is notable for its interactions with iron and copper, especially inhibition of copper absorption.

Functions of molybdenum

xanthine dehydrogenase An enzyme containing molybdenum and iron that functions in the formation of uric acid and the mobilization of iron from liver ferritin stores.

Several enzymes, including **xanthine dehydrogenase** and a related form, xanthine oxidase, require molybdenum. The oxidase form of the enzyme is produced from the dehydrogenase form during tissue injury. No molybdenum deficiency has been noted in a person consuming a normal diet, though deficiency symptoms have appeared in people on total parenteral nutrition. These symptoms include increased heart and respiration rates, night blindness, mental confusion, edema, and weakness.

Molybdenum in foods

Good food sources of molybdenum include beans, whole grains, and nuts. The estimated safe and adequate daily dietary intake for molybdenum is 75 to 250 micrograms per day. A minimum intake for good health is probably about 80 to 115 micrograms per day.[24] When consumed in high doses, symptoms of molybdenum toxicity in animals include weight loss and decreased growth.

OTHER TRACE MINERALS

A variety of minerals are found in the body for which researchers are still trying to justify a human need.[23] We probably consume too much of these minerals to suffer a deficiency, and they are required by so few enzymes or metabolic systems that widespread deficiency symptoms have never been noted. We briefly note them here because as more research is reported, these may achieve more importance. If you have a concept of their roles in the body, you can put new research into perspective. And you can refute the need for widespread use of supplements based on what you know now.

Boron

Boron (chemical symbol is B) is an important growth factor for plants. Research in the early 1980s suggested that boron in humans is involved in the metabolism of steroid (cholesterol-containing) hormones, such as the vitamin D hormone calcitriol and the estrogens. So boron may play a role in the disease osteoporosis, but that is merely speculation at this time. Good sources of boron include fruits, vegetables, and nuts. Meats and fish are poor sources. Adults need about 1 to 2 milligrams daily. Human intakes vary widely.[23]

Nickel

Plants and animals need nickel (chemical symbol is Ni) for the activity of certain enzymes, and perhaps for iron metabolism. Humans have never shown a deficiency of nickel when consuming a normal diet. Good food sources of nickel include nuts, beans, grains, and chocolate. Researchers estimate adults need about 35 micrograms of nickel per day. Our diets supply much more than this.

Vanadium

We need vanadium (chemical symbol is V) to regulate some enzymes, such as those involved in sodium and potassium transport in the red blood cell. To produce a vanadium deficiency in animals, researchers need to use an ultra-clean environment. Even the air must be filtered. Good food sources of vanadium include grain products and sweeteners. Researchers estimate adult vanadium needs are about 10 to 25 micrograms per day. Our dietary intakes exceed this amount, so humans do not run a risk for a vanadium deficiency.

Arsenic

While arsenic (chemical symbol is As) is a very poisonous compound, animals need it in small amounts to metabolize protein and amino acids, especially methionine and taurine. Researchers estimate adults need about 12 to 25 micrograms per day. There is no known human deficiency of arsenic.

Possible essential minerals

We can add lithium, silicon, tin, cadmium, and cobalt (chemical symbols are Li, Si, Sn, Cd, and Co, respectively) to the list of minerals that humans possibly need. Animal data suggest that human needs are possible, but this is unconfirmed. Of course, we need cobalt in the form of vitamin B-12, and there is some speculation that dietary cobalt may be synthesized into vitamin B-12 in the human intestines by bacteria. However, this is not known. For cobalt needs, food sources of vitamin B-12 should be the focus.

See Table 14-6 to review what we have covered on trace minerals.

Table 14-6

A summary of the major trace minerals

Mineral	Major functions	Deficiency symptoms	People most at risk	RDA or ESADDI	Dietary sources	Results of toxicity
Iron	Part of hemoglobin, myoglobin and cytochromes; used for immune function.	Low serum ferritin levels; small, pale red blood cells; low blood hemoglobin and hematocrit values.	Infants, preschool children, adolescents, women in child-bearing years, some endurance athletes.	Men: 10 milligrams. Women: 15 milligrams.	Meats, spinach, seafood, broccoli, peas, bran, enriched breads	Toxicity is seen when children consume 200-400 milligrams in iron pills, and in people with hemochromatosis. In this case people overabsorb iron.
Zinc	Over 200 enzymes need zinc. These include enzymes involved in growth, immunity, alcohol metabolism, sexual development, and reproduction.	Skin rash, diarrhea, decreased appetite and sense of taste, hair loss, poor growth and development, poor wound healing.	Vegetarians, and women in general, the elderly.	Men: 15 milligrams. Women: 12 milligrams.	Seafoods, meats, greens, whole grains,	Reduces iron and copper absorption; causes diarrhea, cramps, and depressed immune function.

Continued.

Table 14-6, cont'd

A summary of the major trace minerals

Mineral	Major functions	Deficiency symptoms	People most at risk	RDA or ESADDI	Dietary sources	Results of toxicity
Copper	Aids in iron metabolism; part of many enzymes, such as those involved in protein metabolism and hormone synthesis.	Anemia, low white blood cell (neutrophil) count, poor growth.	Infants recovering from malnutrition, intestinal surgery patients, and overzealous supplementation of zinc.	1.5-3 milligrams	Meats, liver, cocoa, beans, nuts, whole grains	Vomiting; nervous system disorders (Wilson's disease).
Selenium	Peroxide metabolism, as is part of glutathione peroxidase.	Muscle pain, muscle weakness, heart disease.	Unknown.	55-70 micrograms.	Meats, organ meats, eggs, fish, milk, seafoods; grains grown where selenium is high in the soil.	Nausea, vomiting, hair loss, weakness, liver disease.
Iodide	Part of thyroid hormone.	Goiter; poor growth in infancy when mother is deficient in pregnancy.	None in North America, as salt is usually fortified.	150 micrograms.	Iodized salt, white bread, saltwater fish, dairy products.	Inhibition of function of the thyroid gland.
Fluoride	Increases resistance of tooth crystal to acidic erosion.	Increased risk of dental caries.	Areas where water is not fluoridated and dental treatments do not make up for this lack of fluoride.	1.5-4 milligrams.	Fluoridated water, toothpaste, dental treatments, tea,seaweed.	Stomach upset, mottling (staining) of teeth during development.
Chromium	May increase action of the hormone insulin.	High blood glucose levels after eating.	People on total parenteral nutrition, and perhaps elderly people with adult-onset diabetes mellitus.	50-200 micrograms.	Vegetable oils, egg yolks, whole grains, pork, yeast.	Due to industrial contamination, not dietary excess.
Manganese	Part of some enzymes, such as those involved in carbohydrate metabolism.	None in humans.	Unknown.	2.0-5 milligrams.	Nuts, rice, oats, beans.	Unknown in humans.
Molybdenum	Part of enzymes, such as xanthine dehydrogenase.	None in humans.	Unknown	75-250 micrograms.	Beans, grains, and nuts.	Unknown in humans.

Concept Check

Chromium may act to increase the action of the hormone insulin. The amount of chromium found in food depends on soil content. Vegetable oils, whole grains, and egg yolks are some of the better sources. Manganese is a component of bone and many enzymes, including those involved in glucose production. Since our need for it is low, deficiencies are rare. Good food sources are nuts, rice, oats, and beans. Molybdenum is a component of enzymes. Deficiencies appear only with total parenteral nutrition. Beans, grains, and nuts are good sources. The needs for some other trace minerals, such as boron, nickel, arsenic, and vanadium, have not been fully established in humans. They are required in such small amounts that our current diets are probably adequate.

Summary

1. Some trace mineral deficiencies are difficult to detect in humans, and were first observed in small geographically isolated groups or in patients on total parenteral nutrition. Eating a variety of foods maximizes your chances of consuming adequate amounts of trace minerals. Supplementing with trace minerals is potentially harmful, since so many questions remain regarding daily needs and interactions.
2. Iron is the only nutrient for which the RDA is greater in adult women than men, due to women's iron losses that occur during menstruation. Iron absorption depends mainly on the form of iron present and the body's need for it. Heme iron from animal sources is better absorbed than the nonheme iron obtained primarily from plant sources. Consuming vitamin C simultaneously with iron will increase nonheme absorption.
3. The main function of iron is for synthesizing hemoglobin and myoglobin. It is also important in the synthesis of some enzymes, cytochromes, and in the action of the immune system. A prolonged low iron intake can lead to decreased production of red blood cells, and in turn reduced ability of the blood to carry sufficient oxygen. Such a condition is called iron-deficiency anemia, and may result in fatigue, apathy, and decreased learning ability.
4. Foods rich in iron include beef, oysters, broccoli, and liver. Other sources are spinach and enriched breads and cereals. However, iron from plant sources is not well absorbed. Iron toxicity usually results from a genetic disorder called hemochromatosis. This disease causes overabsorption and accumulation of iron, which can result in severe liver and heart damage.
5. Zinc functions as a cofactor for over 200 enzymes that are important for growth, development, immune function, wound healing, and taste sensation. A zinc deficiency results in poor growth, loss of appetite, reduced sense of taste and smell, hair loss, and a persistent rash.
6. Zinc is best absorbed from animal sources, especially when body needs are high. A mucosal block in the intestinal cells regulates zinc absorption in a manner similar to that of iron. Both iron and copper compete with zinc for absorption, especially when all are consumed as supplements. The most nutrient-dense sources of zinc are oysters, shrimp, crab, and beef. Good plant sources are whole grains, peanuts, and beans.
7. Copper is important for iron metabolism, collagen cross-bonding, nerve cell myelination, and scavenging of free-radicals. A copper deficiency can result in microcytic, hypochromic anemia and rupture of blood vessels. Copper is found mainly in meats, liver, cocoa, legumes, and whole grains. Milk is a poor source. Soil content greatly affects the copper content in plants.

8. The most important role of selenium is as a cofactor in the glutathione peroxidase system, which reduces the production of free radicals. In this way, selenium reduces the need for vitamin E, whose role is to neutralize free radicals once they are produced. Muscle pain, muscle wasting, and heart disease may result from a selenium deficiency. Meats, especially organ meats, eggs, fish, and shellfish are good animal sources of selenium. Good plant sources include grains and seeds. Selenium is potentially toxic because there is no physiological control of the amount absorbed. Symptoms of toxicity are a garlicky breath odor, hair loss, weakness, nausea, and vomiting.
9. Iodide forms part of the thyroid hormones. A lack of dietary iodide results in the development of a goiter. Iodized salt is a good food source. Fluoride incorporated into teeth during development makes them resistant to dental caries. Most North Americans receive the bulk of their fluoride from fluoridated water and toothpaste.
10. Chromium may help increase the action of insulin. Vegetable oils and whole grains are good sources of chromium. Manganese and molybdenum are components of various enzymes. Deficiencies are rarely seen for all three of these nutrients. The body's need for other trace minerals is so low that deficiencies are uncommon.

Take Action

Design a 1-day diet that supplies 100% of the RDA for an adult woman for iron and zinc. Keep in mind mineral bioavailabilty. Could you plan this diet using only plant foods?

Diet	iron (milligrams)	zinc (milligrams)	only plant foods	iron (milligrams)	zinc (milligrams)
Breakfast					
Lunch					
Dinner					
TOTAL:	iron	zinc	TOTAL:	iron	zinc

REFERENCES

1. Anonymous: Essentially of copper in humans, Nutrition Reviews 45:176, 1987.
2. Anonymous: Manganese deficiency in humans: fact or fiction? Nutrition Reviews 46:348, 1988.
3. Barrett S: Commercial hair analysis, Journal of the American Medical Association 254:1041, 1985.
4. Beard JL: Iron fortification - rationale and effects, Nutrition Today, July/August:17, 1986.
5. Black MR and others: Zinc supplements and serum lipids in young adult white males, American Journal of Clinical Nutrition 47:970, 1988.
6. Brittin HC and Nossaman CE: Iron content of food cooked in iron utensils, Journal of the American Dietetic Association 86:897, 1986.
7. Burk RF: Selenium and cancer: meaning of serum selenium levels, Journal of Nutrition 116:1584, 1986.
8. Castillo-Duran C and Uauy R: Copper deficiency impairs growth in infants recovering from malnutrition, American Journal of Clinical Nutrition 47:710, 1988.
9. Chandra RK: Excessive intakes of zinc impairs immune responses, Journal of the American Medical Association 252:1443, 1984.
10. Clydesdale FM: The relevance of mineral chemistry to bioavailability, Nutrition Today, March/April:23, 1989.
11. Cook JD and Finch CA: Assessing iron status of a population, American Journal of Clinical Nutrition 32:2115, 1979.
12. Cook JD and Lynch SR: The liabilities of iron deficiency, Blood 68:803, 1986.
13. Dallman PR: Biochemical basis for the manifestations of iron deficiency, Annual Reviews of Nutrition 6:13, 1986.
14. Danks DM: Copper deficiency in humans, Annual Reviews of Nutrition 8:235, 1988.
15. Edwards CQ and others: Prevalence of hemochromatosis among 11,065 presumably healthy blood donors, New England Journal of Medicine 318:1355, 1988.
16. Fairbanks VF: Hemochromatosis: the neglected disease, Mayo Clinic Proceedings 61:296, 1986.
17. Freeland-Graves JH and others: Metabolic balance of manganese in young men consuming diets containing five levels of dietary manganese, Journal of Nutrition 118:764, 1988.
18. Gordeuk VR and others: Iron overload: causes and consequences, Annual Reviews of Nutrition 7:485, 1987.
19. Herbert V: Recommended dietary intakes (RDI) of iron in humans, American Journal of Clinical Nutrition 45:679, 1987.
20. Keusch GT and Farthing MJG: Nutrition and infection, Annual Reviews of Nutrition 6:131, 1986.
21. Klevay LM and others: Hair analysis in clinical and experimental medicine, American Journal of Clinical Nutrition 46:233, 1987.
22. Levander OA: A global view of human selenium nutrition, Annual Reviews of Nutrition 7:227, 1987.
23. Monsen ER: Iron nutrition and absorption: dietary factors which impact iron bioavailability, Journal of the American Dietetic Association 88:786, 1988.
24. Nielsen FH: Nutritional significance of the ultratrace elements, Nutrition Reviews 46:337, 1988.
25. Pennington JAT and others: Nutritional elements in U.S. Diets, Journal of the American Dietetic Association 89:859, 1989.
26. Robinson MF: Selenium in human nutrition in New Zealand, Nutrition Reviews 47:99, 1989.
27. Sanstead HH: Discovery of zinc deficiency in patients receiving total parenteral alimentation, clinical correlations, Nutrition 5:21, 1989.
28. Simmer K and others: Nutritional rehabilitation in Bangladesh—the importance of zinc, American Journal of Clinical Nutrition 47:1036, 1988.
29. Turnlund JR: Copper nutriture, bioavailability and the influence of dietary factors, Journal of the American Dietetic Association 88:303, 1988.
30. Yip CE and others: Declining prevalence of anemia among low-income children in the United States, Journal of the American Medical Association 258:1619, 1987.
31. Younoszai HD: Clinical zinc deficiency in total parenteral nutrition: zinc supplementation, Journal of Parenteral and Enteral Nutrition 7:72, 1983.

SUGGESTED READINGS

To learn more about iron metabolism and iron deficiency, see the articles by Cook and Finch, Herbert, and Dallman. Then, look at the articles by Edwards and Fairbanks to learn more about hemochromatosis. This will allow you to see both sides of iron—its essential and toxic natures. To learn more about copper, see the article by Turnlund. Then review the article by Levander on selenium. This provides an excellent background on these two exciting trace minerals. The role of selenium in cancer prevention is reviewed by Burk. Finally, Nielsen discusses our current knowledge for some of the more misunderstood trace elements, providing a window into our needs for future nutrition research.

CHAPTER 14

Answers to the nutrition awareness inventory

1. *True.* The small amounts needed by the body make trace mineral deficiencies difficult to detect in humans. Laboratory techniques are not even available to adequately measure some trace elements in tissues, and there are gaps in our knowledge about metabolism and storage of many minerals. This hampers interpretation of laboratory results.
2. *True.* Trace minerals that have the same charge and are chemically similar or use the same carrier proteins often compete with each other during absorption and metabolism. This must be considered when setting the RDA for a trace mineral and when using mineral supplements.
3. *True.* Eating a variety of foods will ensure an intake from a variety of soil conditions and help maximize the chances of consuming an adequate amount of trace minerals.
4. *True.* The refinement process strips a food, such as flour, of many minerals. The enrichment process only replaces one: iron.
5. *True.* Women in their childbearing years have a greater need for iron due to their greater iron loss during menstruation.
6. *False.* The body has no efficient mechanism for eliminating excess iron. Excess iron intake can be very damaging. In response, iron absorption is very carefully regulated in an attempt to prevent excess absorption.
7. *True.* A main function of zinc is promoting growth and development. A zinc deficiency can cause poor growth in children, whereas a zinc supplement can help increase appetite and the rate of weight gain in children recovering from malnutrition.
8. *False.* Hair analysis is not a reliable method at this time. Too many contaminating substances such as shampoos invalidate the results.
9. *True.* Taking zinc supplements often disrupts the natural nutrient balance found in a good diet and so can do more harm than good.
10. *True.* Copper is a component of the protein ceruloplasmin. This compound converts Fe^{+2} into Fe^{+3}, the form in which iron can leave the mucosal cell and storage sites in the liver to bind with transferrin in the blood.
11. *True.* Copper and zinc compete with each other for absorption.
12. *False.* Most iodide in our diets comes from iodized salt added to foods during processing, cooking, or at the table.
13. *True.* Fluoride prevents caries in two ways. It inhibits the growth of bacteria on teeth, and it makes teeth resistant to acid during tooth development.
14. *False.* We know little about chromium metabolism, and it is likely that, as happens with other trace minerals, it is quite toxic even at moderate doses.
15. *False.* A prolonged iron deficiency can eventually lead to iron-deficiency anemia, but most people with poor iron intakes take years to develop symptoms if they remain untreated. In addition, some types of anemia are caused by conditions other than an iron deficiency.

Nutrition Perspective 14–1

Nutrients and Immunity

We have frequently mentioned the importance of good nutrition for immune function in this book. Early humans were plagued by famine, infections, and death. Many of us now, due to better nutrition, can avoid that cycle. Some of us, striving for optimum nutrition, even go too far: while adequate intakes of many nutrients are needed to maintain immune function,[19] excess quantities do not further boost immunity, and may in fact decrease it.[9] Let's review some major components of the immune system—the skin, intestinal cells, and white blood cells—and consider how nutrient intake affects each component (Figure 14-6).

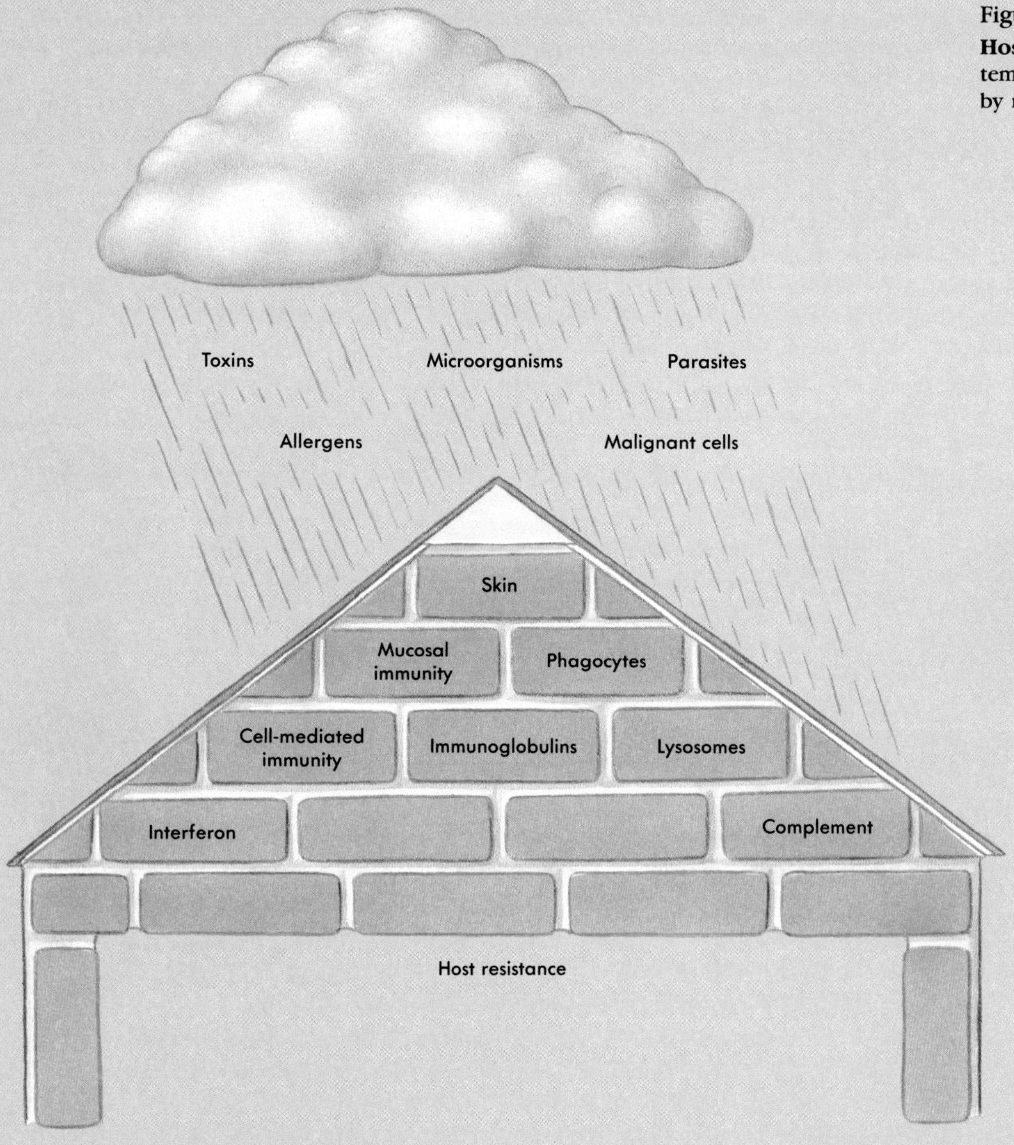

Figure 14-6

Host protective factors. The immune system has many "arms"—all are influenced by nutrient intake.

Continued.

Nutrition Perspective 14-1—cont'd

Nutrients and Immunity

In the early 1970s, physicians began feeding patients with major body burns much sooner then they had in the past. This earlier feeding dramatically reduced the number of infections (by 80%) that burned patients suffered and thus greatly improved their chances of surviving. A major reason for this improved survival is the earlier supply of nutrients to support immune function.

SKIN

The skin forms an almost continuous barrier surrounding the body. Invading microorganisms have difficulty penetrating the skin. However, if the skin is split by lesions, bacteria can easily penetrate this barrier. Nutrient deficiencies that reduce the health of the skin include those of essential fatty acids, vitamin A, niacin, and zinc. Vitamin A deficiency also decreases gland secretions in the skin, which contain enzymes that kill bacteria. Recall that in a vitamin A deficiency, a bacterial infection of the eye is often seen (see Chapter 11).

INTESTINAL CELLS

The cells of the intestines form an important barrier to invading microorganisms. Not only are the cells closely packed together, but also antibody-producing cells are scattered throughout the intestinal tract. These antibodies bind invading microorganisms, preventing them from entering the bloodstream. The production of these antibodies is low during protein and vitamin A malnutrition.

In malnutrition, the intestinal cells break down so that microorganisms more easily enter the body and cause infections. Two common results of malnutrition are diarrhea and bacterial infections of the bloodstream. To protect the health of the intestinal tract, an adequate nutrient intake is necessary, especially of protein, vitamin A, vitamin B-6, vitamin B-12, vitamin C, zinc, and other nutrients needed for intestinal cell synthesis and maintenance.

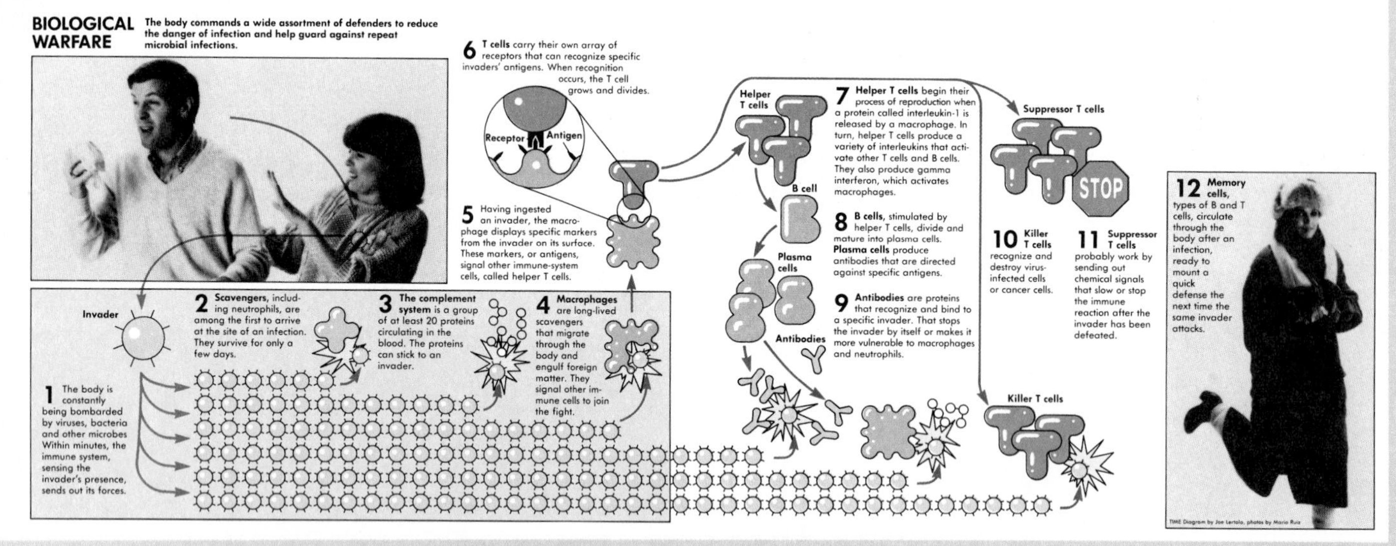

WHITE BLOOD CELLS

Once a microorganism enters the bloodstream, white blood cells attack it. A variety of white blood cells participate in this response, including **neutrophils, B-lymphocytes, T-lymphocytes,** and macrophages. As a group, together with specialized proteins called **complement,** these cells make antibodies to bind to microorganisms, engulf and digest them, and then create a template (memory) that allows future recognition of the organism. Recognition allows more rapid attacks in the future (see Figure 14-7).

Your nutrient intake affects all these white blood cells and protein factors. Some white blood cells live only a few days. Their constant resynthesis requires a steady nutrient input. The immune system needs iron to produce an important killing factor that is used, it needs copper for the synthesis of neutrophils, and it needs adequate amounts of vitamin C, protein, vitamin B-6, folate, and vitamin B-12 for general cell synthesis and, later, cell activity. Zinc and vitamin A are also needed for the overall growth and development of the immune cells.

A deficiency of any of these nutrients compromises the ability of the white blood cells and the complement protein system to seek and destroy invading microorganisms. In addition, during malnutrition, the thymus gland shrinks. This is the place where T-lymphocytes mature before they enter the bloodstream.

One proof that nutrition is important to immune status is the body's response to microorganisms: microorganisms normally present in the body usually cause disease only in severely malnourished people. A good example is measles. Your parents probably have had this viral infection and survived. (You were probably vaccinated against measles.) However, many malnourished children who contract it die. Thus the presence of a virus or microorganism in the body does not guarantee its triumph over the immune system, but if a person's health is already compromised through malnutrition, the chances of a destructive microorganism winning are greater.

The white blood cell count, especially the number of T-lymphocytes and B-lymphocytes in the blood, can predict the chances of either complications or death in hospitalized patients. When the lymphocyte count is low, disease and death are much more likely. In the future, when you see poorly nourished people in hospitals, a senior citizen center, or your neighborhood, remember that their poor nutrient intake is compromising not only the function of their liver, kidneys, and other organs, but also their immune system.

neutrophil
The major form for white blood cells, comprising 55% to 65% of their total number.

B-lymphocyte
White blood cells processed by liver and spleen tissues that are responsible for antibody production.

T-lymphocyte
White blood cells synthesized by the thymus gland and responsible for recognition of foreign substances (such as bacteria) in the body.

complement
A group of serum proteins involved in immune responses, such as phagocytosis and destruction of bacteria.

A NOTE OF CAUTION

Many studies show that a good nutritional status is associated with good immune status. However, other studies also show that an overabundance of certain nutrients can actually harm the immune system. High intakes of polyunsaturated fatty acids and vitamin E have been implicated in a decreased immune response in mice. Excess intakes of zinc (300 milligrams per day for 6 weeks) also appear to decrease immune function.[9] This decrease may be partially due to zinc's interference with copper absorption. The copper deficiency contributes to decreased synthesis of neutrophils, a class of white blood cells.

The message here is that eating a balanced diet will help you maintain the health of all components of the immune system. Your body needs this defense to continuously protect you from environmental pathogens. However, consuming nutrients in excess of needs is not going to boost the immune system to even higher abilities. In fact, this may harm certain aspects of immune function.

An infection that occurs primarily in malnourished people is called an opportunistic infection. Opportunistic infections also are characteristic of acquired immune deficiency syndrome (AIDS), a disease where the T-lymphocyte system of the body is severely compromised. Pneumonia due to an opportunistic infection by *Pneumocystis carinii* used to be rare until AIDS hampered the immune function of so many people.

Nutrition Perspective 14-2

Hair Analysis for Trace Mineral Assessment?

For the last 20 years researchers have been experimenting with hair analysis as a way of assessing trace mineral status in the body. After a clump of hair is clipped close to the scalp, the first two inches are digested in acid and trace mineral content is measured.

Hair analysis immediately encounters some problems. Hair is contaminated by air pollution and by the shampoos, conditioners, dyes, and bleaches that people use on their hair. Hair treatments can substantially change the trace mineral content of hair. In the laboratory, slight changes in the method of washing and heating the hair before analysis can even make results from different labs difficult to compare. Only trained technicians with experience can produce reliable results.

The next problem is that there are insufficient standards with which to compare the results. So, once the results of the analyses are obtained, we often don't know what they mean. There is insufficient research to show that subtle changes in trace mineral content of hair actually reflect subtle changes in trace mineral content in the body.

There are, however, some possibilities for hair analysis. It can be used to establish an environmental toxicity from arsenic and, under controlled research conditions, it may also be a good method for measuring zinc status. However, at this time, there are many questions about hair analysis, and so its place should be only in the research laboratory. There is no evidence that hair analysis is useful for routine human assessment at this time.

Commercial laboratories throughout North America perform hair analysis. For about $25 to $50 they will analyze a hair sample and some even send an impressive computer printout listing the mineral content of the hair. Some even list your vitamin status based on the hair analysis. There is *no* evidence that hair can predict vitamin status. The report may also predict the mineral status of the body and perhaps even include a few pages of health recommendations, including a catalog of supplements that will "restore" health.

A noted scientist sent samples of hair for two women to 13 commercial laboratories around the country. Reported results varied significantly from lab to lab for the same sample.[3] Considering that scientists are having a difficult time determining the role of hair analysis, it is improper for laboratories to use this as an assessment tool for the average person. You may want to read the position paper published in the American Journal of Clinical Nutrition recently on the value of hair analysis. In that paper, the scientists suggest hair analysis is still in the experimental phase and not ready for clinical applications.[20]

Part V

Nutrition Applications in the Life Cycle

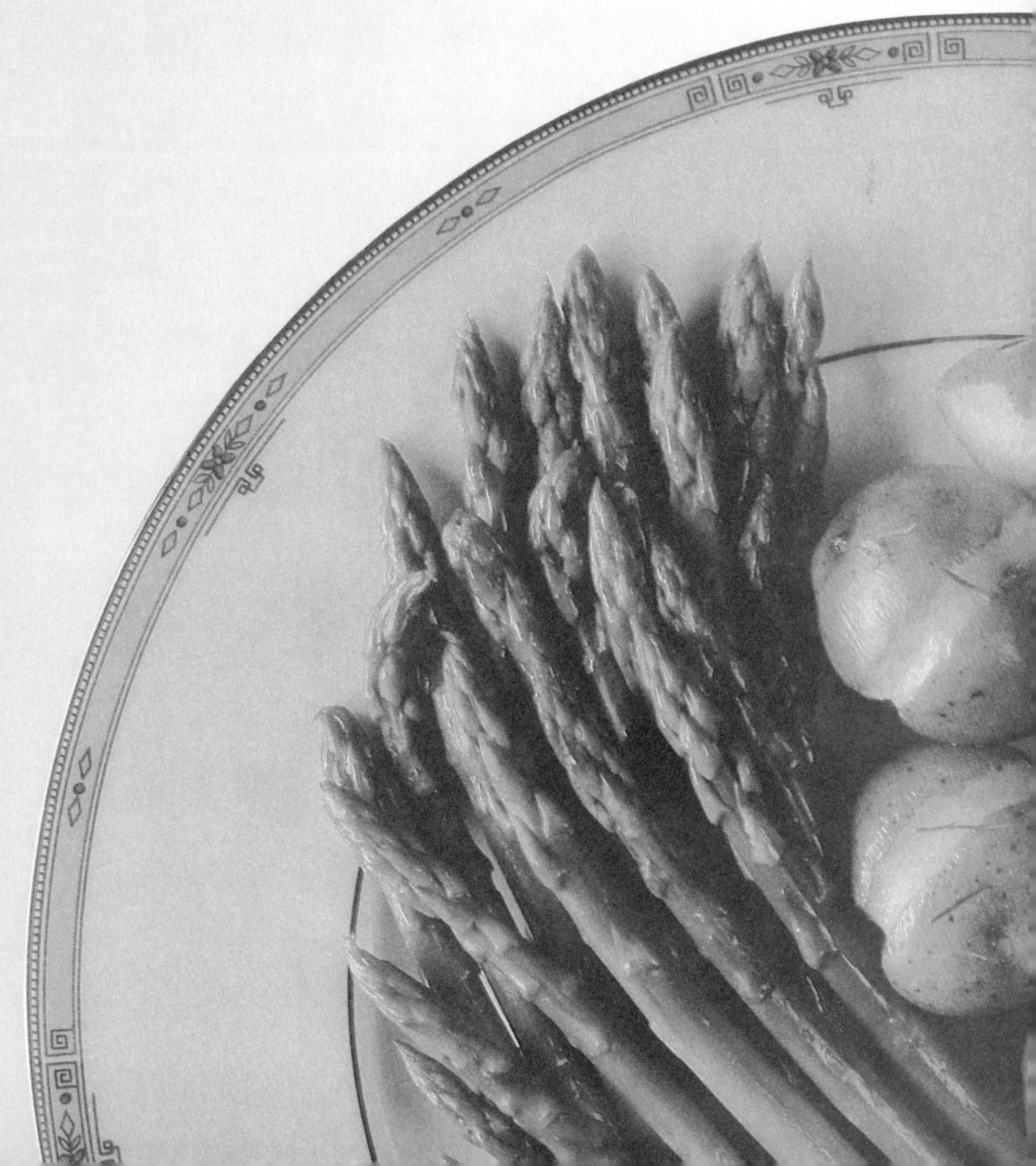

Chapter 15

Pregnancy and Lactation

Overview

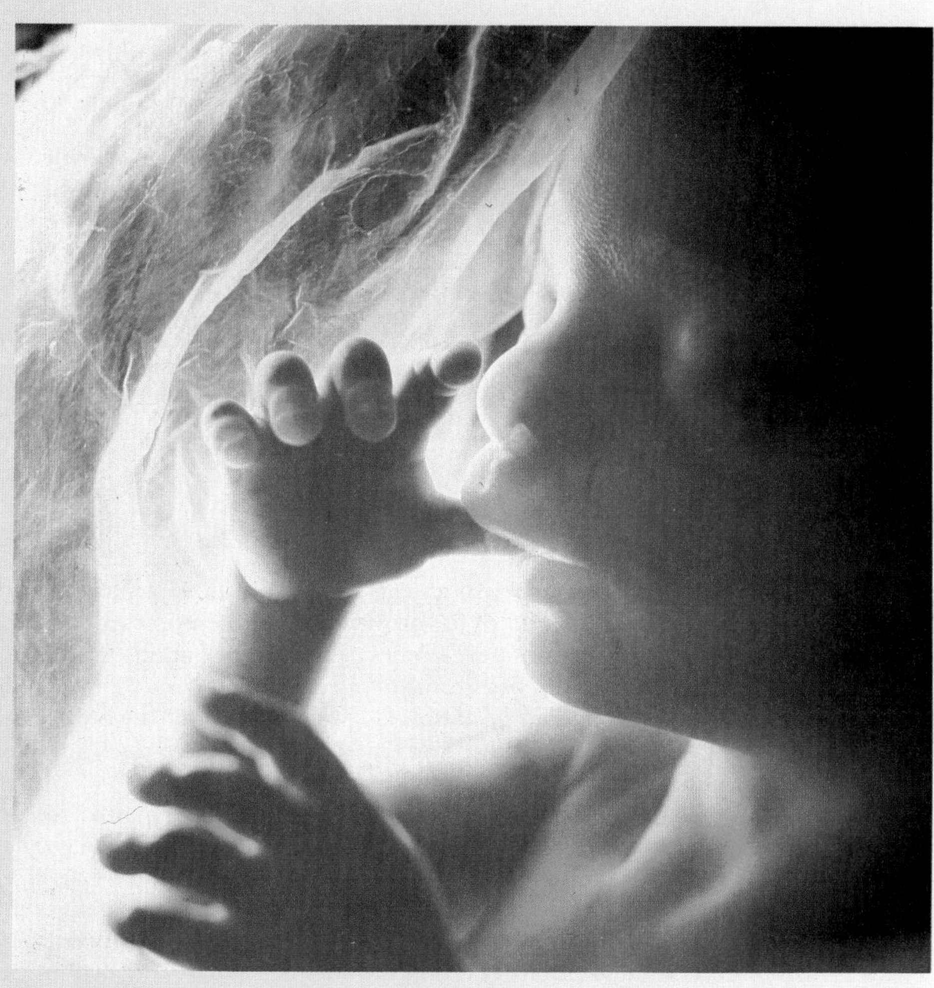

Proper nutrition is vital to both mother and child long before birth.

Pregnancy can be one of the most special times for a couple. Along with the responsibility of shaping a child's health and personality comes the exhilaration of contributing to a new life. Prospective parents often feel an overriding desire to produce a healthy baby, and that makes them very receptive to nutrition information. The parents-to-be usually want to do everything possible to maximize their chances of having a healthy baby.

Producing a healthy baby is not just a matter of luck. While some aspects of fetal and newborn health are beyond a parent's control, *conscious decisions about social, health, and nutritional factors affect the baby's health and future.* What the parents do directly relates to the likelihood of having a healthy newborn. Let's examine what contributes to helping make a healthy baby a reality.

Nutrition awareness inventory

Here are 15 statements about pregnancy and lactation. Answer them to test your current knowledge. If you think the answer is true or mostly true, circle T. If you think the answer is false or mostly false, circle F. Use the scoring key at the end of this chapter to compute your total score. Take this test again after you have read this chapter. Compare the results.

1. **T F** Infants weighing less than 5.5 pounds (2500 grams) at birth are more likely to have medical problems.
2. **T F** The most crucial time for fetal development is during the last 13 weeks of pregnancy.
3. **T F** Nutritional factors are more important than genetic factors in determining birth weight.
4. **T F** Pregnant women have increased energy needs.
5. **T F** Most women should gain about 24 to 28 pounds during pregnancy.
6. **T F** Poor food choices in pregnancy are more common than low-kcalorie intakes.
7. **T F** Pregnant women know instinctively what to eat.
8. **T F** Mineral needs increase during pregnancy.
9. **T F** Pregnancy can precipitate a form of diabetes mellitus.
10. **T F** Breast-fed infants suffer fewer respiratory infections than formula-fed infants.
11. **T F** A major barrier to breast-feeding is often a lack of information.
12. **T F** Mothers who must take medications that pass into the milk should check with their doctor before continuing to breast-feed.
13. **T F** The placenta is the site of oxygen and nutrient transfer from the mother to the fetus.
14. **T F** Most miscarriages occur during the first trimester.
15. **T F** Cow's milk can be substituted for human milk when an infant is 2 to 3 months old.

PRENATAL GROWTH AND DEVELOPMENT

The view that life begins at conception currently is a topic of much controversy and debate.

embryo
The developing human life form during the second to eighth week after conception.

gestation
The time of fetal growth from conception to birth; a period of about 40 weeks following a woman's last menstrual period.

trimester
The normal pregnancy of 38 to 42 weeks is divided into 3, 13 to 14 week periods, called trimesters.

The life of an unborn baby begins when an egg and sperm unite. A baby is born about 40 weeks later. This first form of life grows through the **embryo** stage and is known as a fetus after 8 weeks of development. The mother nourishes this offspring via a **placenta** that forms in her uterus to accommodate growth and development of the offspring throughout **gestation** (Figure 15-1). Often a woman does not suspect she is pregnant during these first few weeks, and often does not even seek medical attention during the first 3 months **(first trimester).**

Even without fanfare, the embryo grows and develops daily. For that reason, *the health and nutritional habits of a woman in the years before pregnancy and while she is trying to become pregnant—or has the potential of becoming pregnant—are particularly important.* This means that nutrition is doubly critical during a woman's childbearing years. We know that certain nutritional deficiencies, use of certain medications (even aspirin), other drugs, and alcohol can all cause detrimental effects in the growing embryo, and later in the fetus. This is true for weeks before the woman realizes she is pregnant. Some research suggests that an adequate vitamin and mineral intake in the months before conception and that first month of life may help prevent birth defects such as spina bifida. It is important for parents to be aware of this.

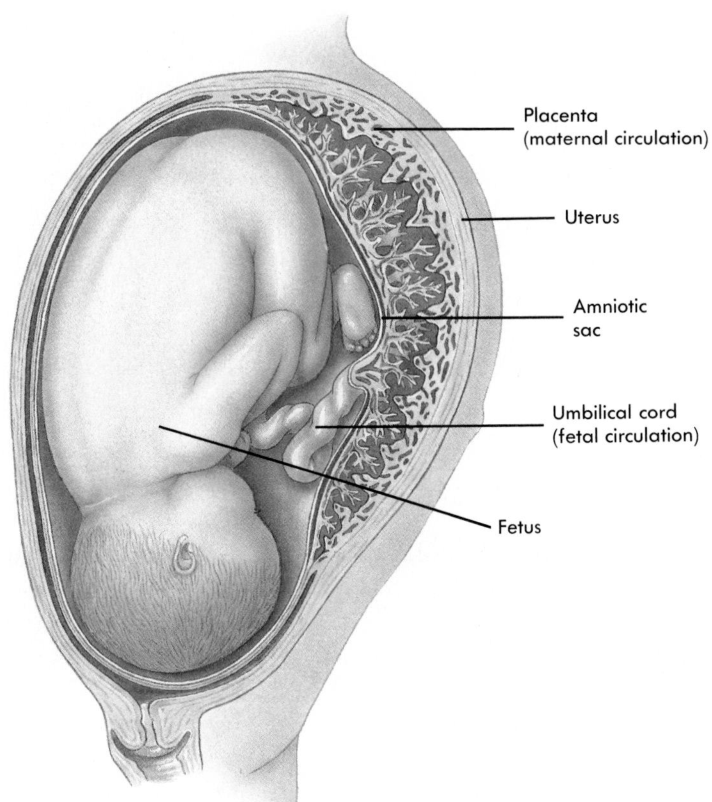

Figure 15-1

The fetus in relationship to the placenta, the organ through which nourishment flows.

The time to focus on good nutritional and other health habits, then, is before a woman becomes pregnant. These habits can then be carried into pregnancy, thereby providing optimum health and nutrition from before conception until birth (Figure 15-2).

Fetal growth

Fetal growth begins with a rapid increase in cell number (hyperplasia). This type of growth dominates fetal development. The newly formed cells then begin to grow larger (hypertrophy; see Chapter 8 to review these terms). Further growth and development of the fetus is then a combination of hyperplasia and hypertrophy. At about 3 weeks, cells begin to form specialized organs and body parts. By the end of 13 weeks, the heart is complete and beating, most organs are formed, and the fetus can move (Figure 15-3).

At any stage of development an insult (injury) to the fetus caused by nutritional deficiencies, medications and other drugs, radiation, trauma, or other factors can alter or arrest the specific phase of growth and development in progress. The effects may last a lifetime. *The most critical time for fetal development is*

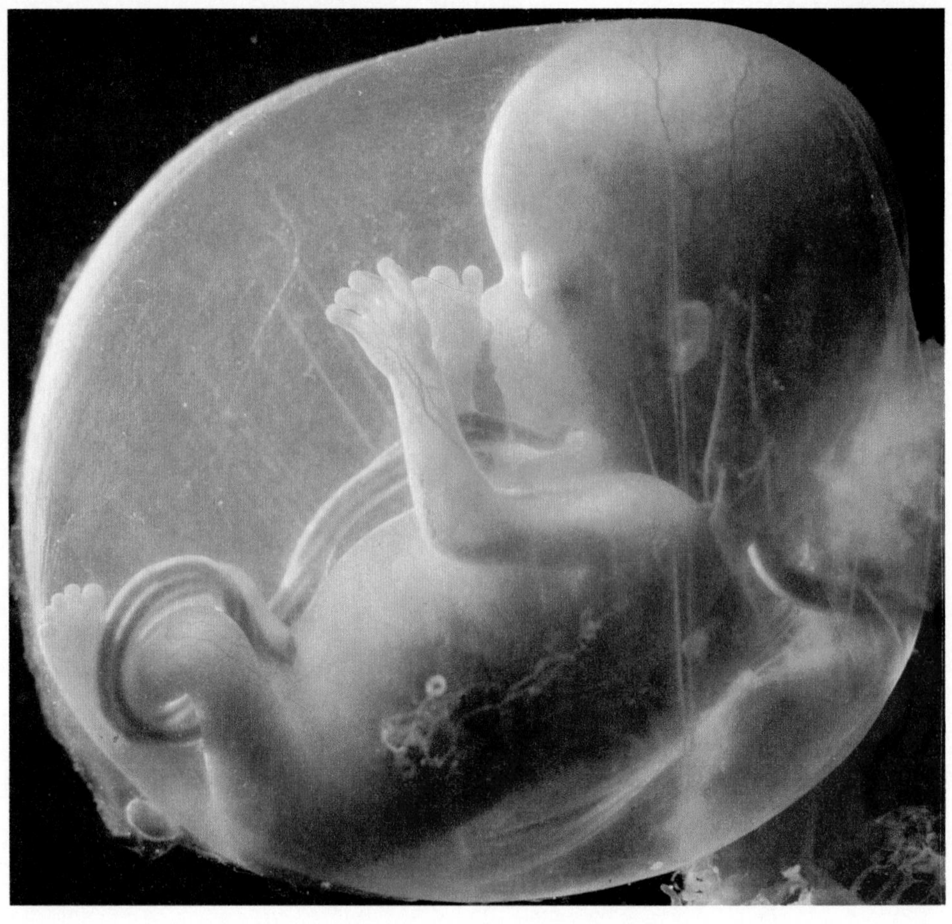

Figure 15-2

The fetus at this age is wholly dependent on the mother for nutrients.

miscarriage
Loss of pregnancy, also called spontaneous abortion, that occurs prior to 28 weeks of gestation.

the first trimester. During this period most **miscarriages** (premature termination of pregnancy) occur. Currently, about one third of all pregnancies result in miscarriage, often so early that the woman does not realize she was indeed pregnant. Early miscarriages usually result from a genetic defect or fatal error in fetal development.[28]

During this first trimester, then, a woman must be especially careful to avoid substances that may harm the developing fetus. Vitamin A, for example, when taken in large doses by the mother can result in serious infant malformations. *In addition, development is so rapid during the first trimester that if a nutrient essential to development is not sufficiently supplied, the growing fetus may be affected even before the mother shows deficiency signs.* Even though many women experience loss of appetite and nausea during the first trimester, adequate nutrition is still extremely important.

Exploring Issues and Actions

Pregnant women often become increasingly serious about nutrition as the months go by. Does this increased concern mirror the fetal developmental schedule? When should this interest begin? How could the mother's concern be encouraged to begin sooner?

The second trimester

By the beginning of the second trimester, a fetus weighs about 1 ounce. Arms, hands, fingers, legs, feet, and toes are fully formed. The fetus has ears and is beginning to form tooth sockets in its jawbone. Organs continue to grow and mature, and a physician can detect a heart beat. Eventually, the fetus begins to look more like a baby. It might suck its thumb and it may kick strongly enough to be felt by the mother. Most bones will be distinctly evident throughout the body.

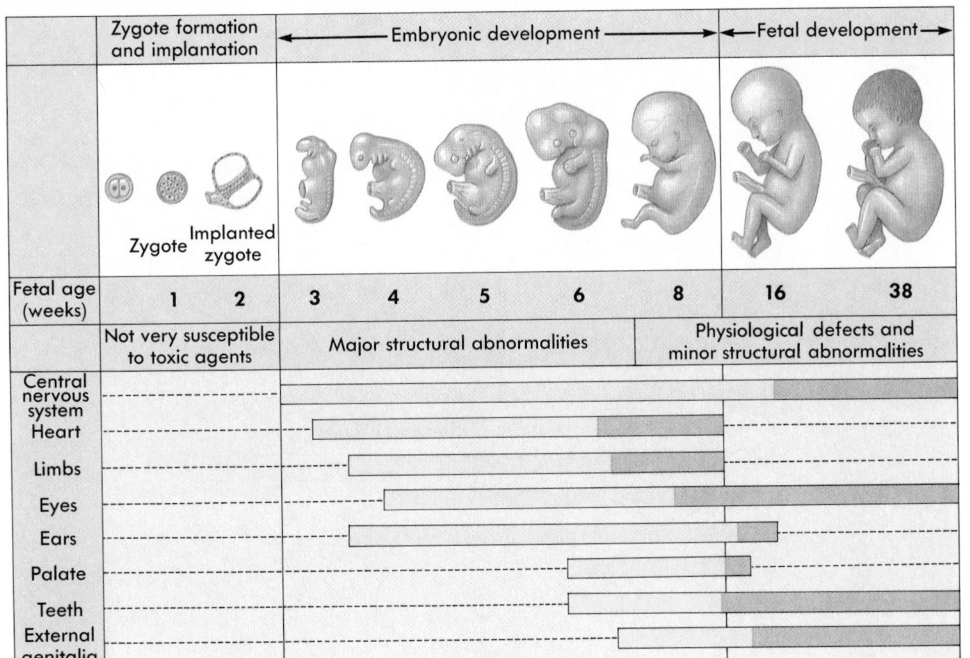

Figure 15-3

Vulnerable periods of development. The most serious damage from fetal exposure to toxins is likely to occur during the first 8 weeks after conception. As the chart shows, however, damage to vital parts of the body—including the eyes, brain, and genitals—also can occur during the last months of pregnancy.

The third trimester

By the beginning of the third trimester, a fetus weighs about 2 to 3 pounds. After about 28 to 30 weeks of gestation, there is a good chance of survival for a **premature** infant if the infant is cared for in a nursery for high-risk newborns. However, the infant will not contain the mineral and fat stores normally accumulated in the last month of gestation. This and other medical problems complicate nutritional care. At 9 months, the fetus weighs about 7 to 8 pounds (about 3.5 kilograms) and is about 20 inches long (about 50 centimeters). There is a soft spot in the forehead (fontanel) where the bones of the skull are growing together. It takes about 12 to 18 months for that soft spot to close (Figure 15-4).

premature
An infant born prior to 38 weeks of gestation.

small for gestational age (SGA)
Infants born after normal gestation length (38 weeks) but weighing less than about 5.5 pounds (2.5 kilograms).

WHAT IS A SUCCESSFUL PREGNANCY?

Defining a successful pregnancy is difficult, and no specific standards have been spelled out.[12] Protection of the mother's physical and emotional health must be a goal. *As for the infant, two goals often stated are: (1) a gestation period longer than 37 weeks and (2) a birth weight greater than 5.5 pounds (2500 grams).* The longer the gestational age, the more time for fetal lungs to develop. Sufficient lung development is critical for survival. By 37 weeks, fetal lungs are well developed, and other medical problems occur less often.

Infants born after 37 weeks, but who weigh less than 5.5 pounds, are called **small for gestational age (SGA).** These infants are more likely than normal-weight infants to have complications, such as problems with blood sugar regulation, temperature regulation, and growth and development in the early weeks after birth.

Although a mother's decisions, practices, and precautions during pregnancy contribute to the health of the fetus, she cannot guarantee the fetus good health. Some genetic and environmental factors are beyond her control. Professionals should not foster an unrealistic illusion of control.

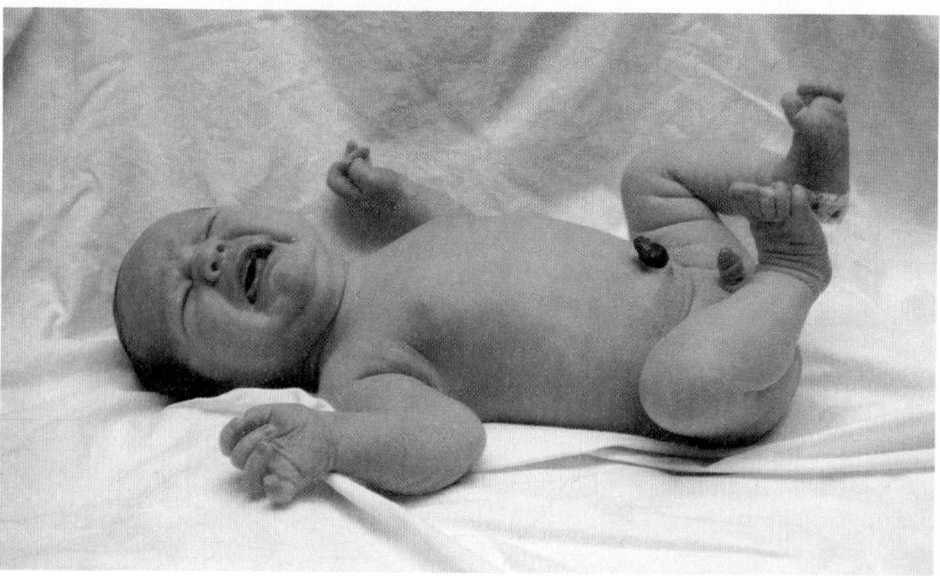

Figure 15-4
A healthy week-old baby.

A definition of a successful pregnancy must also consider the newborn's "quality of life." This consideration includes the newborn's ability to grow, develop, learn, and eventually reproduce. Parents should strive toward producing a baby who is born healthy, on time, and with the mental, physical, and physiological capabilities to take advantage of all that life offers, while also protecting the mother's health.[12]

The effect of nutrition on the success of pregnancy

The growth of the fetus and the changes in the mother's body that occur to accommodate the fetus require extra nutrients and energy. Although pregnancy is a normal process, the sizeable changes in the mother's body present nutritional stress for her. Her uterus and breasts grow, the placenta develops, her total blood volume increases, the heart and kidneys work harder, and stores of body fat increase—all in preparation for birth and milk production.[29] The nutrients needed for these "support system" changes are added to the nutrient needs of both the growing fetus and the mother's own normal physiological functions. A growing adolescent faces almost overwhelming nutritional demands during pregnancy.

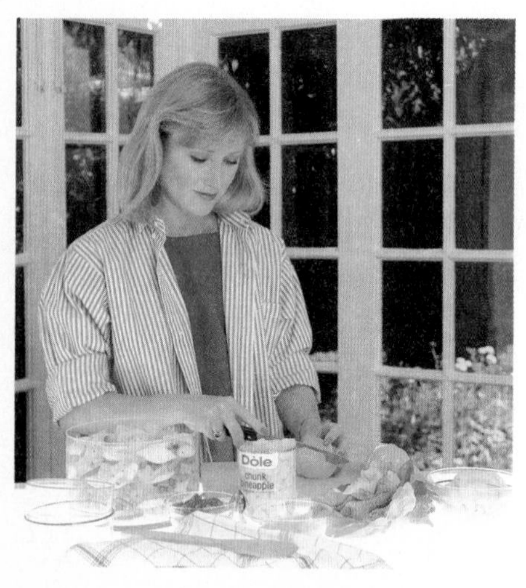

A woman contemplating pregnancy should begin good health and nutrition habits before conception.

The specific effects on fetal development of either a marginal intake of nutrients and energy during pregnancy, or marginal nutritional stores of the mother at the start of pregnancy, are difficult to establish. A diet containing only 1000 kcalories per day has been shown to greatly retard fetal growth and development. The mother's body, however, can adapt to the demands of pregnancy in a variety of ways, including increased absorption of nutrients from foods.

For some nutrients, such as iron and calcium, the fetus may also use—and deplete—the mother's stores if the diet is not adequate. However, research shows that genetic background can explain very little of the difference in birth weights of infants.[4] Both environmental factors and nutritional factors, such as the mother's weight gain, are much more important.[17] Figure 15-5 depicts many factors that influence the outcome of pregnancy.

Early research supports the importance of good nutrition in pregnancy

During World War II, parts of Russia and much of Holland were blockaded. Food supplies were quickly exhausted. The resulting malnutrition greatly affected infant birth weights of the mothers who were in their second or third trimester.

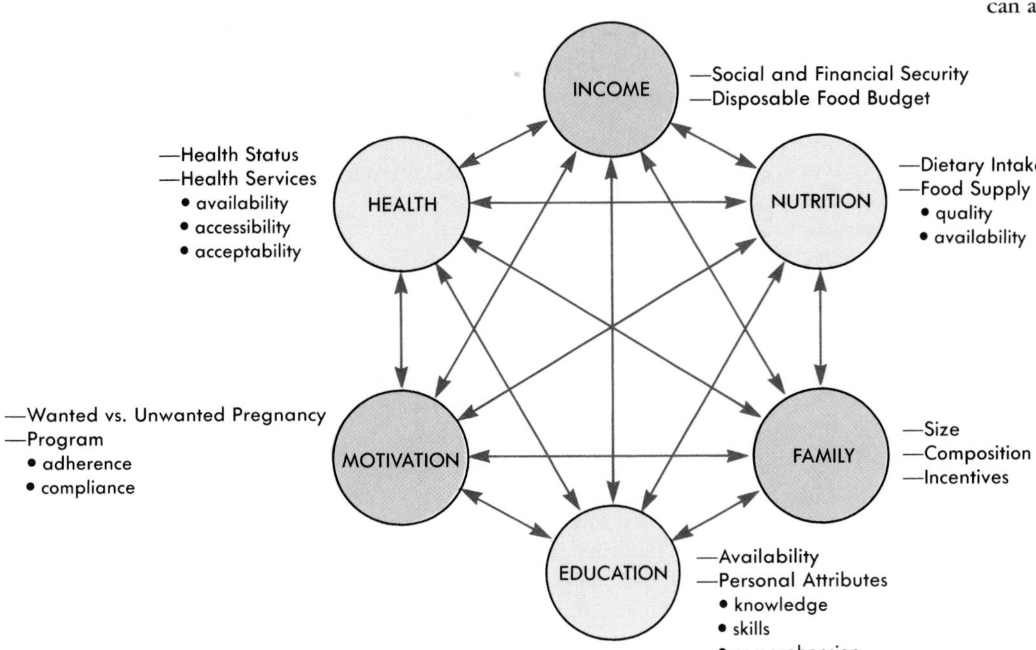

Figure 15-5

The seamless web of influences that can affect the outcome of pregnancy.

The number of new pregnancies also fell. After the blockades were lifted, birth weights and the numbers of new pregnancies quickly rose again to prewar levels.[29]

At the same time, researchers working in Boston noticed that a good protein intake was associated with a greater success of pregnancy. It appeared that the mother's diet—not only during pregnancy but also preceding conception—contributed to the health of both mother and infant. Better health care for those who could afford higher protein diets probably also contributed to the well-being of these mothers and infants. Studies in Toronto then showed that dietary supplements and nutritional counseling improved the health of the pregnant mother and yielded a healthier baby. Rates of complications also were reduced. In addition, researchers in Great Britain showed that height and social class were more important than dietary intake during pregnancy in predicting the outcome of pregnancy. *This again suggested that long-term nutritional intake may be critical to pregnancy outcome.*[29]

Later, laboratory animal studies supported the importance of diet during pregnancy. Food deprivation during pregnancy in animals resulted in decreased organ size in the pups, even in the brain, which is usually very resistant to nutritional insults. In addition, there was a decrease both in the weight of the placenta and in the number of healthy pups that survived the first weeks of life.[29]

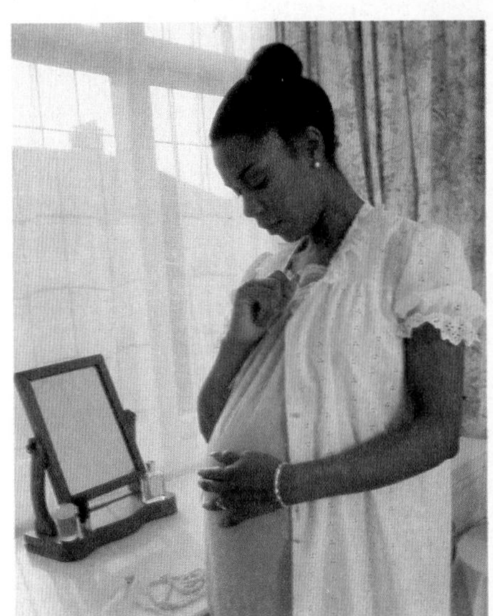

A pregnant woman experiences many physiological changes.

Concept Check

Adequate nutrition is vital during pregnancy to ensure the health of both the fetus and the mother. Fetal organs and body parts begin to develop very soon after conception. The first 13 weeks is a critical period when poor nutrition or drug use can result in birth defects. During the second and third trimesters, organs continue to mature, and very rapid growth occurs. Nutritional insults during the last 7 months of pregnancy can also interfere with fetal growth and affect the newborn infant's ability to survive.

Expert Opinion

What Do I Really Have to Give Up When I'm Pregnant?

BONNIE WORTHINGTON-ROBERTS, Ph.D., R.D.

Although a healthful life-style is recommended for everyone, it's especially important during pregnancy. The well-being of both the mother and the fetus is potentially compromised when undesirable substances enter maternal circulation and when the mother engages in overly strenuous activity. Since normal fetal growth and development depends directly on what the mother chooses to expose herself to, her awesome responsibility is obvious.

SMOKING

It's widely known that smoking during pregnancy increases the risk of both premature delivery and low birth weight. (It is also *suspected* of increasing the risk of congenital malformations, sudden infant death, and childhood cancer.) These serious problems are believed related to the physiological biochemical, and/or hormonal effects of nicotine, carbon monoxide, and possibly other compounds present in cigarette smoke. Significant dietary deficits have not been identified in pregnant women who smoke.

EXERCISE

Physical activity during pregnancy is generally advocated, especially for women who have been quite active prior to pregnancy. Not surprisingly, pregnant women who are involved in regular exercise programs have shown an improved self-image during pregnancy and higher fitness scores by their delivery date. But common sense is in order: tackle football and many gymnastic routines are hardly the best choices. In the only study to address the impact of endurance running throughout pregnancy, a marked reduction in birth weight was seen in offspring of mothers who chose to continue their rigorous training schedule until delivery. In addition, deep flexion or extension of joints—especially deep knee bends—should be avoided because connective tissue is lax during pregnancy. Activities that require jumping, jarring motions, or rapid changes in direction should be avoided because of joint instability. Clearly, what needs to be exercised in such demanding undertakings is basically moderation, especially during the last trimester.

ALCOHOL

There are very few dietary restrictions for pregnant women. Alcohol is a well-known exception. The fetal alcohol syndrome was first formally described in the early 1970s. At that time, babies of alcoholic women were reported to exhibit an array of developmental abnormalities, including growth failure, mental retardation, facial defects, cardiac anomalies, and other more minor problems. It's now appreciated that the fetal alcohol syndrome is the upper end of a spectrum of abnormalities: smaller doses of alcohol can promote more subtle defects. The term *fetal alcohol effects* is now frequently used to describe the prenatal damage done by alcohol. Although the use of small amounts of alcohol during pregnancy may not harm the fetus, an acceptable level of use has not been defined. So it's widely recommended that pregnant women play safe and *avoid* consumption of alcoholic beverages (see Nutrition Perspective 15-1).

CAFFEINE

The potential danger of caffeine use during pregnancy has been debated for quite some time. Although evidence so far doesn't justify recommending abstinence during pregnancy, several recent epidemiological studies have come up with some provocative findings. In one case, moderate-to-heavy caffeine users were found to have a significantly greater risk of spontaneous abortion during the late first and second trimesters than women who used less caffeine. Moderate caffeine use was defined as consumption of at least 150 milligrams of caffeine per day, which is equivalent to no more than about 1.5 cups of coffee daily. A second study concluded that the risk of low birth weight rose as the level of daily caffeine use increased. The risk was more than 4.5 times greater for women who consumed more than 300 milligrams of caffeine

Expert Opinion—cont'd

daily than for women who used no caffeine at all. Even though additional research is needed to confirm these observations, it seems justifiable at this point to advocate moderation in caffeine consumption during pregnancy.

FOOD ADDITIVES

Unfortunately, some pregnant women are frightened by rumors that various food additives cause abnormal fetal development. This fear is largely unjustified. True, we don't know the cause of most birth defects and, theoretically, some substances in the food supply may be problematic, but there's no proof of such relationships. Regulations currently enforced by the FDA mandate that any company proposing to introduce a new additive into the U.S. food supply must prove its safety through a series of animal studies. Proof must be provided to the federal government that the proposed new additive causes neither cancer nor birth defects. Many additives that have been used in the American food supply for years are "generally recognized as safe" (see Chapter 19). Ongoing reevaluation of many of these substances has yielded little cause for concern.

Among the additives receiving much attention in the popular press is aspartame (NutraSweet and Equal). This sweetener has now replaced sugar and saccharin in many commercially manufactured products. Many pregnant women have been led to believe that some component of aspartame may adversely affect the fetus. The phenylalanine component has been of special concern as a possible cause of fetal brain damage if maternal exposure is frequent. It is known that high levels of maternal serum phenylalanine (as seen in women with the disease called phenylketonuria) seriously interfere with the normal brain development of the fetus. But it is virtually impossible for a woman without phenylketonuria to maintain high serum levels of phenylalanine. Observations of human subjects have generated no data to support the notion that aspartame use by pregnant women adversely affects the course and outcome of pregnancy. Without such data, it's hardly warranted to recommend that pregnant women abstain from using aspartame-sweetened products.

NUTRITIONAL SUPPLEMENTS

Nutritional supplements should not be assumed to be benign. Although pregnant women with poor dietary patterns are good candidates for prenatal vitamin/mineral supplements, excessive use of supplements may harm both the mother and the fetus. This is especially true of a high intakes of vitamin A by pregnant women, which is associated with producing birth defects. Unfortunately, it is all too easy to consume megadoses of vitamin A: nutritional supplements sold over the counter in grocery and drug stores often contain doses of this vitamin far in excess of the RDA.

If vitamin A in large doses can interfere with normal fetal development, other vitamins may potentially have the same effect. Data supporting this idea, however, are not available. It makes good sense, nevertheless, to be cautious about self-supplementation. The idea that "more of a good thing is better" is foolish. If supplements are used, they should be used under medical guidance.

Unfortunately, there is still much mystery about why some babies develop abnormally or are delivered prematurely. At present, the data suggest that pregnant women should meet their nutritional needs through sensible food choices, avoid alcohol, and use caffeine-containing foods and beverages judiciously. Above all, pregnant women in North America should appreciate how lucky they are to have access to a superb food supply. They should delight in knowing that they can provide all the nutrition the fetus needs through wise food choices and, generally, without nutritional supplements.

Dr. Worthington-Roberts is professor of nutritional sciences and chief nutritionist at the Child Development Center at the University of Washington.

Maternal and infant mortality

In the United States, approximately 12 of every 100,000 live births lead to the mother's death. One thousand infant deaths occur for each 100,000 live births. Compared with other developed countries, the United States ranks poorly. Considerable efforts are being made to reduce both infant and maternal deaths. Good health care and nutritional practices can reduce both these figures (Table 15-1).[25,26] Specific nutrition-related factors that affect the health of both the mother and the fetus (infant) include:

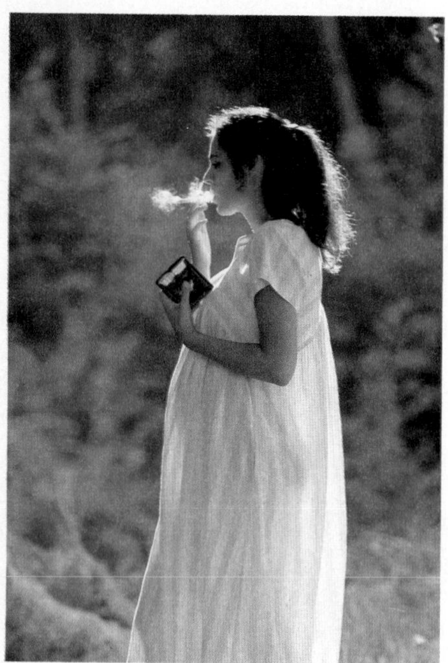

Smoking while pregnant can lead to low birth weight in the infant.

- **Socioeconomic status**—Poverty, inadequate health care, poor health practices, lack of education, and unmarried status are all related to problems in pregnancy.[5,18]
- **Obesity** leads to an increased rate of high blood pressure and diabetes during the pregnancy and to surgical and other complications during delivery.[27] These pregnancies require intense monitoring.
- **Poor, absent, or delayed prenatal care** can allow maternal nutritional deficiencies to deprive the fetus of needed nutrients or can increase the risk of fetal damage in the cases of chronic diseases, such as hypertension or diabetes mellitus. Ideally, prenatal care should start before conception.
- **Smoking, alcohol consumption, use of some medications, or illegal drug use in pregnancy**—Nutrition Perspective 15-1 reviews fetal alcohol syndrome.[16] Smoking is linked to low birth weight in the infant, probably because the fetus is denied needed oxygen when nicotine constricts the arteries, and so the blood supply.
- **Pica** is the practice of eating nonfood items such as dirt, starch, ice, or clay, especially while pregnant. Although **pica** occurs more frequently in populations that have poor iron and zinc status, this practice probably results more from habit, culture, and superstition than from a need for specific nutrients. Eating soil raises the risk of infections from parasites and can cause life-threatening blockages of the intestinal tract. Eating laundry starch should be discouraged because it contains silicons and other toxic compounds. Eating ice may break the teeth.
- **Teenage pregnancy**—Because the two years after a woman begins menstruating are basically her last years of linear growth, she needs a steady nutrient supply for adequate growth. Teen pregnancy adds fetal needs to those of the mother: mother and fetus need nutrients for their growing bodies. The resulting nutrient demand is almost overwhelming. Consequently, teen pregnancy presents a very high risk for low infant birth weights.[1]
- **Prenatal ketosis**—There is debate about the extent to which ketosis harms a growing fetus. Ketone bodies are thought to be poorly used by the fetal brain, and thus can slow fetal brain development. Researchers stress the need for a pregnant woman not to "crash" diet nor to fast for more than 12 hours. A pregnant woman can develop significant ketosis after only 20 hours of fasting.
- **Inadequate weight gain** increases the risk of having a **low– birth weight infant (LBW).**

low birth weight (LBW)
Infant weight at birth of less than 5.5 pounds 2.5 kilograms, usually because of premature birth; these infants are at higher risk for health problems.

In the United States, 7% to 10% of infants have a low birth weight, that is, they weigh less than 5.5 pounds (2.5 kilograms). *Low–birth weight infants show a greater risk for infection, illness, disabilities, and death than normal weight infants.* Premature birth, poor diet during pregnancy, some medical conditions in the mother, and the above mentioned factors influence an infant's birth weight. Reducing the number of low–birth weight infants born will help reduce infant deaths.

Education, an adequate diet, and early and consistent prenatal medical care are vital for increasing the chances for producing a healthy baby. Early prenatal

Table 15-1

A good method for predicting the risk for delivering a low–birth weight infant[12]

WIC obstetrical risk score (Massachusetts Department of Health):

Scoring components	Factor and code	Scoring standard
Maternal age, first visit this pregnancy	A. 15 years	15
	B. 16-17 years	10
	C. 18-19 years	5
	D. 20-39 years	0
	E. 40 years plus	5
Number of previous pregnancies	F. 0	15
	G. 1-5	0
	H. over 5	15
Period pregnancies	I. 2 or more ICPs* of less than 2 years	10
	J. 1 ICP of less than 2 years	5
Prepregnancy weight this pregnancy*	K. OK	0
	L. under	30
	M. over	10
Outcome, previous pregnancies		
a. spontaneous abortion or miscarriage	N.	10
b. low birth weight (LBW)	O.	30
Scoring: 50 = high risk		TOTAL SCORE
20-49 = moderate risk		
0-19 = low risk		

*Based on the following height and weight table: Height and weight table (without shoes):

Height	Weight range	Height	Weight range
4′11″	99-128 lb	5′5″	118-152 lb
5′0″	102-132 lb	5′6″	122-157 lb
5′1″	105-135 lb	5′7″	126-162 lb
5′2″	108-139 lb	5′8″	129-168 lb
5′3″	111-143 lb	5′9″	133-173 lb
5′4″	114-148 lb	5′10″	136-178 lb

*ICP stands for interconceptual period, which is the time between pregnancies.
From: Kennedy ET: A prenatal screening system for use in a community-based setting, Journal of the American Dietetic Association 86:1372, 1986.

care should include a medical examination, dietary advice, laboratory tests, and counseling. The woman should be counseled to avoid x-ray exposure, smoking, vitamin A supplements, medicines, illegal drugs, and alcohol use. If diabetes mellitus is present or developing, it must now be carefully controlled to minimize complications in the pregnancy. We will address this problem in a later section.

It is best if these examinations and counseling strategies begin before the woman becomes pregnant, but certainly they should begin early in pregnancy. Many problems can develop in pregnancy that a physician can diagnose and quickly treat.[18,20]

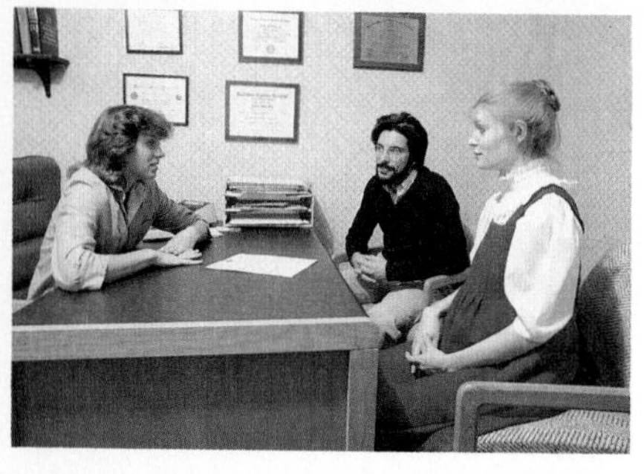

Exploring Issues and Actions

Should nutritional counseling and medical aid, as well as nutritious foods, be available free during pregnancy? Should they be mandatory? How could such a program save tax dollars?

Almost all women need prenatal nutritional counseling. *Food habits cannot be predicted from income, education, or life-style. It is important for all women to review the principles of an adequate diet for pregnancy.* While some women may already have good nutritional habits, most can benefit from nutritional advice, including warnings about habits that may harm the growing fetus, such as severe dieting or fasting. Focusing on excellent prenatal care, good nutritional intake, proper health habits, and common sense can give the fetus, and later the infant, the best chance of thriving.[12]

U.S. Government programs aim to reduce infant mortality by providing high-quality health care and foods designed to alleviate the effects of poverty and poor education. An example of such a program is a Supplemental Food Program for Women, Infants, and Children (WIC). This program offers health assessments and foods (or vouchers for foods) that supply high-quality protein, calcium, iron, vitamin A, and vitamin C to pregnant women, infants, and children (to age 5 years) from low-income populations.

Concept Check

Infants born after 37 weeks of gestation and weighing more than 5.5 pounds (2.5 kilograms) have the fewest medical problems at birth. Individual mothers and whole societies can attempt to reduce infant and maternal death and medical problems by limiting factors that increase the risk of having a premature or small-for-gestational-age (SGA) infant. Adequate nutrition helps prevent these problems. Other contributing factors are poor socioeconomic status, obesity, poor, absent or delayed prenatal care, smoking, imprudent medicine use, alcohol consumption, illegal drug use, pica, teenage pregnancy, inadequate prenatal weight gain, and prenatal ketosis.

MEETING INCREASED NUTRIENT NEEDS OF A PREGNANCY

Dietary advice given to pregnant women by the medical community has varied tremendously over the past century. In the 1950s, a common recommendation

Figure 15-6

Changes in the RDA for pregnancy. During pregnancy, many nutrients are needed in greater amounts than at other times; these include vitamin D, folate, and iron.

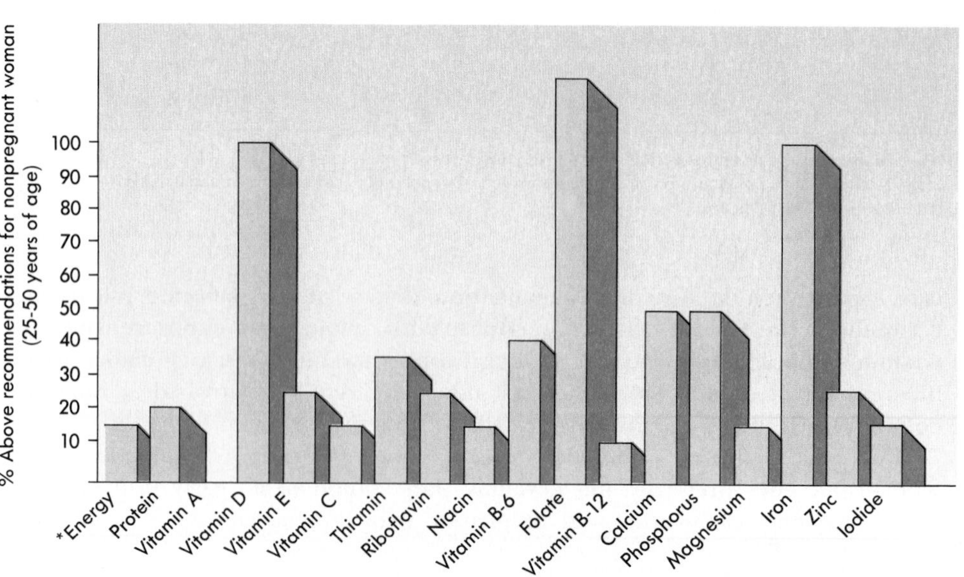

was that women restrict weight gain to between 15 and 18 pounds. Severe kcalorie and sodium restrictions were at times also recommended to keep the baby small, in hopes of easing labor and avoiding complications. Few of these practices were based on sound scientific information, and we know now that many of these recommendations are in fact harmful to the mother and fetus.

The first comprehensive scientific report about nutrition and pregnancy was issued in 1970 by The National Academy of Sciences and titled *Maternal Nutrition and the Course of Pregnancy.*[19] This document remains a landmark source of research information on the role of nutrition in human reproduction. It emphasizes the increased nutritional requirements during pregnancy (not restrictions) and the importance of individual assessment and counseling.

Increased energy needs

An average pregnancy requires 80,000 extra kcalories: divided by 280 days, *this averages approximately 300 extra kcalories daily (the equivalent of just 2 cups of low-fat milk and a piece of bread).* Most extra kcalories are actually needed in the last half of pregnancy. *Though she may "eat for two," the pregnant woman must not double her normal kcalorie intake.* She cannot afford a "Big Mac" for herself and another for the fetus. She will want to seek the best quality foods to create the best possible health for her child. Many vitamin and mineral needs are increased, but the mother doesn't have so many extra kcalories to use in meeting the extra nutrient needs (Figure 15-6).

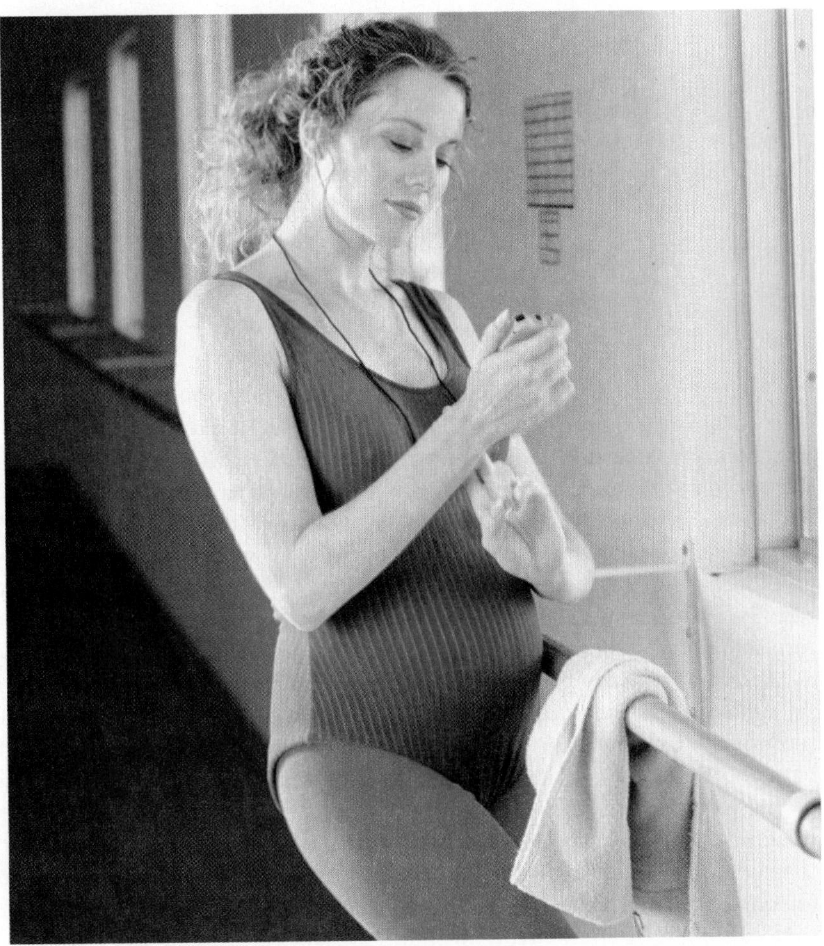

As long as a woman feels comfortable exercising, she can continue exercising during her pregnancy.

If a woman is active during pregnancy, the extra kcalories burned can be added to the 300 kcalories per day to balance her energy expenditure. The greater body weight of a pregnant woman requires a higher energy cost for activity. Physicians strongly encourage women to continue existing activities in pregnancy. However, many women find that they are quite inactive during the later months, partly because of the increased size, and so an extra 300 kcalories per day is usually enough.

Recommended weight gain

The prenatal diet should allow for approximately 2 to 4 pounds of weight gain during the first trimester, and then a subsequent weight gain of ¾ to 1 pound per week during the second and third trimesters. *The weight gain goal is about 24 to 28 pounds.*[19] This increases to about 30 pounds for underweight women and decreases to about 16 to 19 pounds for obese women. Figure 15-7 shows why the recommendation is 24 to 28 pounds. It accounts for the total weight of the baby, placenta, and amniotic fluid, the mother's increased breast tissue and increased blood supply, and the increased fat and muscle tissue she needs to support pregnancy and lactation. About 24 to 28 pounds of weight gain has been shown in many studies to yield optimum health for both mother and fetus. It should yield an infant birth weight of 8 to 9 pounds.[26]

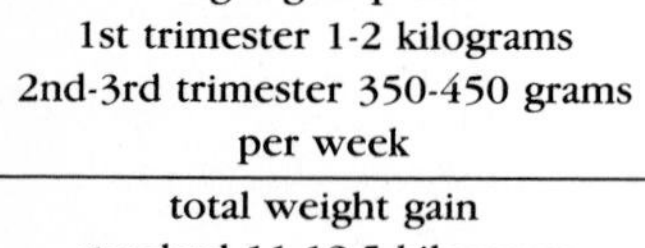

For metric units:
weight gain pattern 1st trimester 1-2 kilograms 2nd-3rd trimester 350-450 grams per week
total weight gain standard 11-12.5 kilograms underweight 13.5 kilograms obese 7-8.5 kilograms
usual birth weight 3.5-4 kilograms

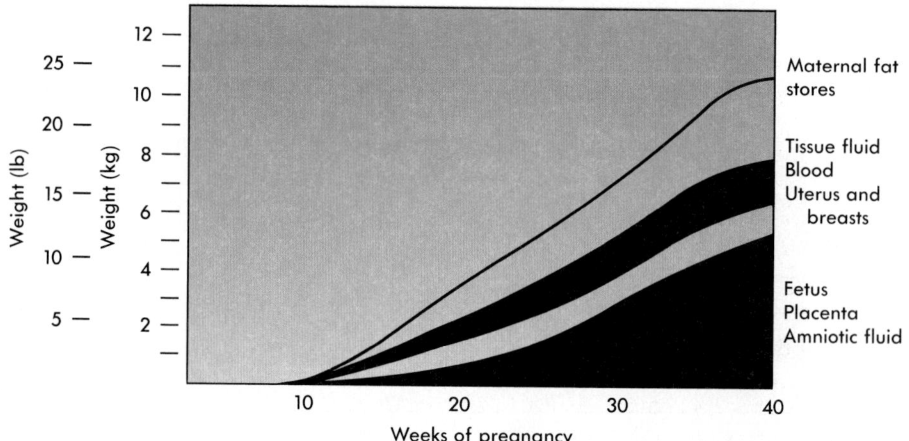

Figure 15-7
The components of weight gain in pregnancy.

Weight gain during pregnancy needs regular monitoring. A prenatal weight gain chart can be used for this (Figure 15-8).[19] If a woman deviates from the ideal weight gain pattern, she should be warned of that. If she gains too much weight, she should *not* be encouraged to lose weight in order to get back on the curve. She should simply slow the increase in weight to parallel the rise on the prenatal weight gain chart. If a woman fails to gain as much weight as she should at a given point in pregnancy, she shouldn't be encouraged to gain the needed weight rapidly: instead, she should slowly gain a little more weight than the typical pattern in order to meet the charted line by the end of pregnancy.

During pregnancy, excess weight gain and poor food choices are more common than an inadequate kcalorie intake. In North America, the problem is often how to limit weight gain appropriately—to about 24 to 28 pounds—to prevent the need for significant weight loss after pregnancy. Excessive weight gain increases risk for complications in pregnancy and encourages excess fetal growth, which can increase the risk for birth trauma. Multiple pregnancies can contribute to creeping obesity in women. Loose, accommodating maternity clothes designed for comfort do not provide the usual feedback about weight gain, and fluid retention can likewise mask "true" weight gain during pregnancy.

Extra weight gain in underweight or normal-weight women is usually not harmful, but it can set the stage for creeping obesity during the childbearing years, especially if the mother intends to have more than one child.

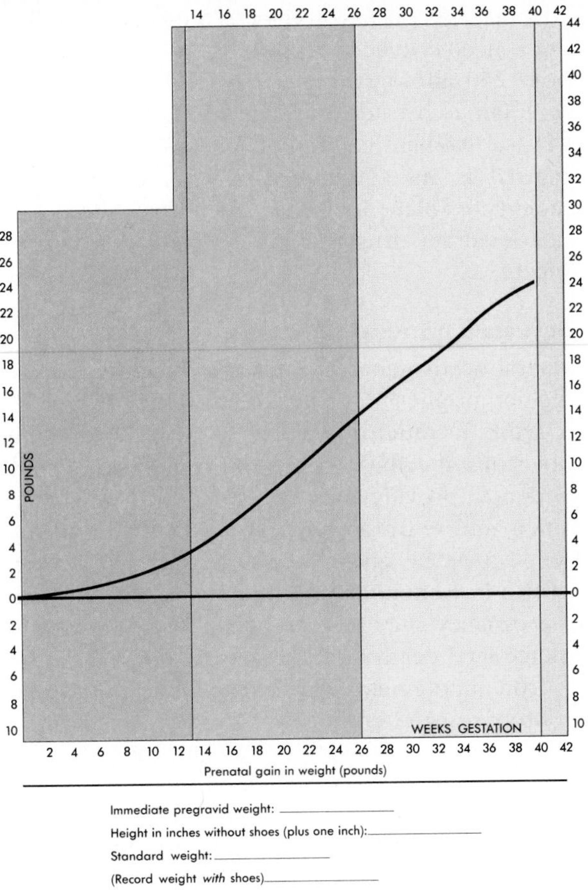

Figure 15-8

A chart for following weight gain in pregnancy. Charting weight gain is a routine, but vital, part of prenatal care.

Increased protein needs

The RDA for protein is increased by 10 grams per day. However, many women already eat the recommended 60 grams of protein per day.

Increased carbohydrate needs

Carbohydrate needs are at least 100 grams per day. This amount prevents ketosis and the interruption of fetal development and brain maturation that may result from ketosis.

Increased vitamin needs

Vitamin needs in general are increased (Figure 15-6), especially the need for vitamin D and folate.

Vitamin D. Calcium metabolism increases during pregnancy. To facilitate the absorption and distribution of calcium for forming fetal bones, the mother's need for vitamin D doubles to 10 micrograms per day. Pregnant women should get regular sunlight exposure. If that is impossible and insufficient vitamin D–fortified milk is consumed to make up the difference (1 liter [4 cups] yields 10 micrograms), a pregnant woman should consider a supplement containing 5 to 10 micrograms (200 to 400 IU). The typical prenatal supplement contains this extra amount of vitamin D.

Folate. The synthesis of DNA requires folate. This means the growth in pregnancy of the fetus and mother depends on an ample supply of folate. Red blood cell formation increases in pregnancy and that also requires folate. Serious anemia can result if folate intake is inadequate. The RDA is increased by an additional 220 micrograms of folate, for a recommended total of 400 micrograms per day.

The RDI published in 1987 reduced that total to 500 micrograms of folate per day (see Chapter 2 to review the concept of an RDI).

Some women have difficulty consuming sufficient folate to satisfy their pregnancy needs. Recent studies show that some pregnant women consume only about 250 micrograms per day. However, by choosing foods wisely—for example, folate-rich fruits and vegetables as outlined in the Daily Food Guide (Table 2-4)—a woman can meet her needs. A prenatal vitamin supplement may be used to meet the RDA for folate, especially by women with histories of inadequate folate intake, frequent or multiple births, megaloblastic anemia or anticonvulsant drug therapy.[11] Folate deficiency has been associated with birth defects.

Increased mineral needs

Mineral needs generally increase during pregnancy, especially the need for iron, calcium, magnesium, zinc, and fluoride (Figure 15-6).

The RDI for iron published in 1987 reduced this level to 15 to 30 milligrams of iron per day.

Iron. So much extra iron is needed for hemoglobin synthesis during pregnancy that the RDA increases from 15 to 30 milligrams a day. A supplement is needed to provide that much iron. In some cases, even a supplement does not suffice, and extra amounts, beyond those normally present in prenatal supplements, must be given (see Appendix O). Eating foods rich in vitamin C along with an iron supplement increases iron absorption. Severe iron-deficiency anemia in pregnancy may lead to premature delivery, low birth weight, and increased risk for fetal death in the first weeks of life.[19]

Iron supplements can cause nausea, constipation, and decreased appetite. A group of researchers recently suggested that pregnant women start with 30 to 60 milligrams of extra iron per day and then increase their intake only when laboratory tests dictate more is needed.[21]

Calcium. Calcium is needed during pregnancy to promote adequate mineralization of the fetal skeleton and teeth. Most calcium is required during the third trimester, when skeletal growth is maximum and teeth are forming, but extra intake should start immediately. The RDA in pregnancy increases by 400 milligrams for calcium for women over age 24 years. Pregnant teenage women should consume an extra 600 milligrams of calcium per day. The only practical food sources for this calcium belong to the milk and cheese group and fortified orange juice. Otherwise, calcium supplements are needed.

Zinc. Zinc is an important mineral for supporting growth and development. The RDA increases from 12 to 15 milligrams per day. The extra protein foods in the diet of a pregnant woman should supply most of this zinc. A poor zinc status in pregnancy increases the risk for having a low–birth weight infant.[15]

Fluoride. Fluoride can improve fetal tooth development. Women should ask their dentists if extra fluoride is needed, depending on the local water supply.

Is there an instinctive drive in pregnancy to eat more nutrients?

Extra needs in pregnancy for folate, iron, calcium, and zinc are the most difficult for women to satisfy. These, then, should be the focus of diet planning for pregnancy. Before we discuss diet planning, however, one very important misconception about pregnancy needs to be dispelled. Some people believe that mothers instinctively know what to eat and that their drive for pickles or ice cream is dictated by a natural desire to consume needed nutrients. However, no studies support that notion, and if it were true, one would wonder why women seek out clay, starch, ice, and other nonfood items during pregnancy. There may be a natural instinct to consume the right foods in pregnancy, but we are so far removed from living by instinct that relying on our desires is risky. Good nutritional counseling can focus food choices more reliably.

Table 15-2

A diet plan for pregnancy and lactation

Food group	Pregnant women	Lactating women
Milk and cheese:	4	4-5
Low-fat milk or yogurt, 8 ounces		
Low-fat cheese, 1½ ounces		
Meat, poultry, fish and beans:		
Animal (meat, fish, poultry, eggs), 2-3 ounces	2	2
Vegetable (beans, nuts, seeds), 1 cup	2	2
Vegetables and fruits:		
vitamin C-rich, ½ cup or ½ -1 piece	1	1
green vegetables, ¾-1 cup,	1-2	1-2
other, ½ cup	1-2	1-2
Breads and cereals	4	4
1 slice or ½ -¾ cup		

A diet for pregnancy

Table 15-2 outlines one approach to a good diet during pregnancy. It includes four servings from the milk and cheese group, four servings from the meat, poultry, fish, and beans group, four servings from the vegetable and fruit group, and four servings from the breads and cereals group. Specifically, the servings from the milk and cheese group could include low-fat milk, yogurt, and cheese. These supply extra protein, calcium, riboflavin, and magnesium. Servings from the meat, poultry, fish, and beans group should include two animal sources and two vegetable sources. Besides protein, the animal sources help provide the extra iron and zinc needed, and the vegetable sources help provide much of the extra magnesium needed.

The vegetable and fruit group provides vitamins and minerals. One serving should be a good vitamin C source, and then one serving should be a green vegetable or another rich source of folate, such as orange juice. For the breads and cereals group, four servings should be whole grains or enriched grains. Table 15-3 shows this basic diet plan can contain as little as 2200 kcalories and still meet the extra needs of pregnancy, except for iron.

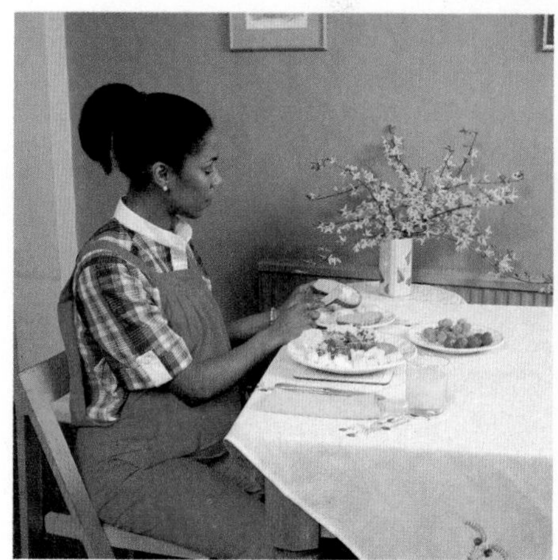

A woman should be able to receive adequate nutrition for pregnancy (except for iron) through dietary sources, but it is not always the case.

Prenatal vitamin and mineral supplements are needed

Ideally, maternal dietary changes during pregnancy should enable a woman to meet all increased nutrient needs, except perhaps for iron.[6] In reality, that doesn't always happen. Because adequate nutrition during pregnancy is crucial to the health of both mother and child, physicians routinely prescribe a specially formulated prenatal supplement (Appendix O). These include the critical nutrients for pregnancy—iron, folate, vitamin D, and calcium—and many others, as well. Not all physicians and researchers, however, agree with this practice. But despite the controversy, there is no evidence that this level of supplementation

Table 15-3

A sample diet based on recommendations in Table 15-2
Breakfast
1 cup raisin bran
6 ounces orange juice
1 cup 2% milk
Snack
2 tablespoons peanut butter
1 slice whole-wheat toast
1 cup plain low-fat yogurt
½ cup strawberries
Lunch
spinach salad with
2 tablespoons oil and vinegar dressing
1 hard-cooked egg
1 slice whole-wheat toast
1-½ ounces of provalone cheese
Snack
1 pear
4 whole-wheat crackers
1 cup 2% milk
Dinner
4 ounces lean ham
1 cup navy beans
1 cornbread muffin
¾ cup cooked broccoli
1 teaspoon corn oil margarine
iced tea or milk (if desired during lactation stage)

This diet meets the RDA for pregnancy and lactation except for iron (80% if 30 milligrams is used for comparison) for only 2200 kcalories.

Pregnancy, in particular, is not a time to self-prescribe vitamin and mineral pills.

causes problems, aside perhaps from the combined amounts of supplementary and dietary vitamin A. Under certain conditions, such as poverty, teenage pregnancy, poor maternal diet, and multiple fetuses (twins or more), the use of supplements is wise.

The pregnant vegetarian

The vegetarian woman who becomes pregnant should not necessarily have special nutritional problems if she is a lacto-ovo vegetarian or a lacto vegetarian. A total vegetarian (vegan), on the other hand, must carefully plan a diet that includes sufficient protein, vitamin B-6, iron, calcium, zinc, and a vitamin B-12 supplement. The basic vegan diet listed in Chapter 6 should be supplemented in the grain group, as well as in the beans, nuts, and seeds group to supply more needed nutrients. Since iron and calcium are poorly absorbed from most plant foods, an iron and calcium supplement is probably necessary. The levels provided by a typical prenatal supplement should suffice for iron needs but not for calcium needs.

Concept Check

Energy needs increase by an average of 300 kcalories per day during pregnancy. Actual energy needs are less in the first trimester and greater during the remainder of pregnancy. Weight gain should be slow and steady up to a total of 24 to 28 pounds for a woman of normal weight. Protein, vitamin, and mineral needs all increase during pregnancy. Vitamin D, folate, iron, calcium and zinc are nutrients of particular concern. A pregnant woman's diet should be varied and generally include more milk products and more specified fruits and vegetables than a prepregnancy diet. Prenatal supplemental vitamins and minerals are commonly prescribed, but excess intake of supplements, especially vitamin A, can be dangerous.

PHYSIOLOGICAL CHANGES AND RESULTING PROBLEMS IN PREGNANCY

During pregnancy, the fetus' needs for oxygen, nutrients, and excretion increase the burden on the mother's lungs, heart, and kidneys. Although the mother's digestion and metabolism work very efficiently, some discomfort accompanies the changes her body undergoes to accommodate the fetus.

Heartburn, constipation, and hemorrhoids

Progestins produced by the placenta relax muscles in both the uterus and the intestinal tract. This often causes heartburn as stomach acid slips up through the lower esophageal sphincter into the esophagus (see Chapter 3). When that happens, the woman should avoid lying down after eating, reduce fat consumption so that foods pass quickly from the stomach into the small intestine, and avoid spicy foods if they are not tolerated. She should also consume liquids between meals to decrease volume, and pressure in the stomach. Constipation often results from the relaxation of these muscles, especially late in pregnancy as the fetus competes for space with the GI tract. Consuming more water, dietary fiber, and dried fruits and exercising can help a pregnant woman avoid constipation[29] and an often accompanying problem, hemorrhoids. Straining can lead to hemorrhoids, which are more likely to occur during pregnancy, anyway, because of physiological changes occuring during pregnancy.

progestins
Hormones, including progesterone, that are necessary for maintaining pregnancy and lactation.

Edema

Estrogens and progestins combine to cause connective tissue to retain fluid during pregnancy. Blood volume also greatly expands during pregnancy and normally contributes some edema. There is no reason to restrict salt or use diuretics to limit mild edema. However, the edema may limit physical activity late in pregnancy and occasionally require the woman to elevate her feet to control the symptoms. Edema spells trouble only if hypertension and the appearance of protein in the urine accompany fluid retention.[27]

Morning sickness

Nausea is common in the early stages of pregnancy, possibly a reaction to pregnancy-related hormones circulating in the bloodstream. Although known as "morning sickness," nausea may occur at any time and persist all day. It is often the first signal to a woman that she is pregnant. Some women partially control mild nausea by eating soda crackers or dry cereal before getting out of bed, cooking with open windows to dissipate nauseating smells, eating smaller, more frequent meals, and avoiding foods that increase nausea.[29] Usually, nausea stops after the first trimester, but it can continue throughout the entire pregnancy. In cases of serious nausea, the preceding practices offer little relief. When appetite is severely reduced or vomiting persists, medical therapy is needed.

Gestational diabetes mellitus

gestational diabetes mellitus
A high blood glucose level that develops during pregnancy and returns to normal after birth; one cause is placental production of hormones that antagonize blood glucose regulation.

Hormones synthesized by the placenta antagonize the action of the hormone insulin, and the antagonism can precipitate **gestational diabetes mellitus,** particularly in women with family histories of diabetes mellitus. During pregnancy, it is important for women to have regular checks of their urine or blood glucose levels to detect developing diabetes. Once detected, a special diet and sometimes insulin injections are needed. Gestational diabetes often disappears after the birth. Proper control of both gestational diabetes mellitus and diabetes mellitus present in the mother prior to pregnancy is extremely important. If not treated, the fetus can grow quite large, often necessitating an early delivery. and increasing the risk of birth trauma and malformations.[8]

Anemia

physiological anemia
The normal increase in blood volume that dilutes the concentration of red blood cells, resulting in anemia; also called hemodilution.

To supply fetal needs, the mother's blood volume expands up to approximately 150% of normal. The red cell mass expands only 20% to 30% above normal, and this occurs more slowly. This leaves proportionately fewer red blood cells in a pregnant woman's bloodstream. The lower ratio of red blood cells is a condition known as **physiological anemia**, since it is a normal response to pregnancy, rather than the result of poor nutrient intake.[19] If during pregnancy, however, iron stores and/or dietary intake—particularly of iron and folate—is inadequate, resulting anemia may require medical attention.

PREGNANCY-INDUCED HYPERTENSION

pregnancy-induced hypertension
A serious disorder that can include high blood pressure, kidney failure, convulsions, and even death of the mother and fetus. Although exact cause is not known, good nutrition and prenatal care can prevent or limit its severity. Mild cases are known as preeclampsia; more severe cases are called eclampsia. Another term for this disorder is *toxemia*.

A high risk to pregnancy results from **pregnancy-induced hypertension.** This disorder, also known in mild forms as preeclampsia and in severe forms as eclampsia, and resolves once the pregnancy state ends. Early signs and symptoms include a rise in blood pressure, excess protein in the urine, and fluid retention. More severe results, including convulsions, can occur in the second and third trimesters.[29] Good nutrition, especially a good calcium intake, may prevent or lessen the disorder.[2] Mild effects can be lessened by bedrest. If not controlled, liver and kidney damage, and even death of the mother and fetus may result. Careful medical attention is needed.

Concept Check

Heartburn, constipation, nausea and vomiting, edema, gestational diabetes mellitus, and anemia are possible discomforts and complications of pregnancy. Changes in food habits can often ease these problems. Pregnancy-induced hypertension, with high blood pressure and kidney failure, can lead to severe complications, even death to both the mother and fetus, if not treated.

BREAST-FEEDING

Before the 1900s, if you were not breast-fed by your mother, a "wet nurse" may have breast-fed you. Formula feeding was fraught with complications, primarily because people did not know the importance of sterilizing formulas against bacteria nor much about the nutritional needs of infants. During the early 1900s, the technology of formula feeding improved. Then from the 1920s and especially in the 1940s, when women worked in armament factories during World War II, more and more babies were fed formulas. Throughout the 1950s and early 1960s, interest in breast-feeding further waned. In the 1970s, breast-feeding enjoyed a resurgence, which has since leveled off.

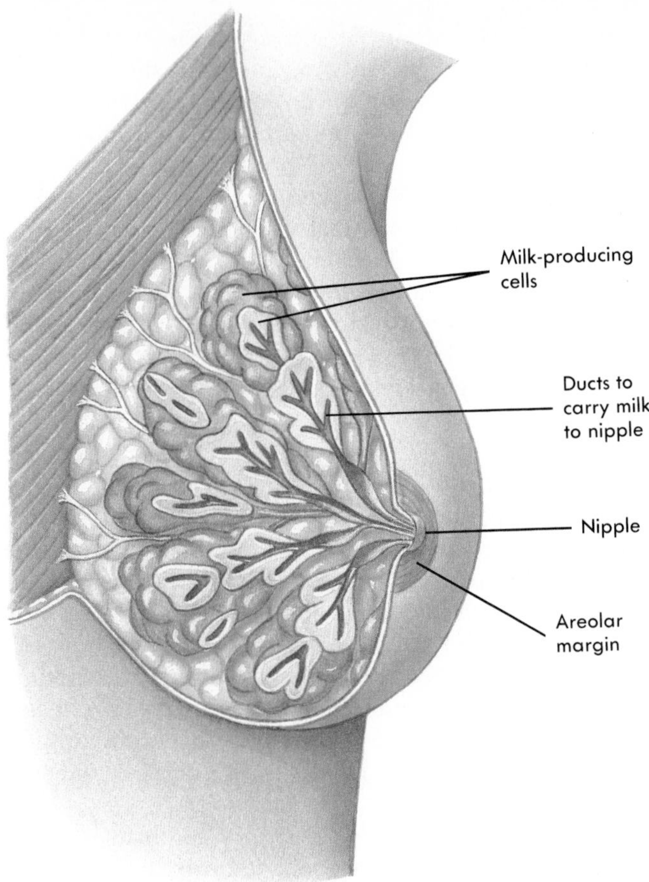

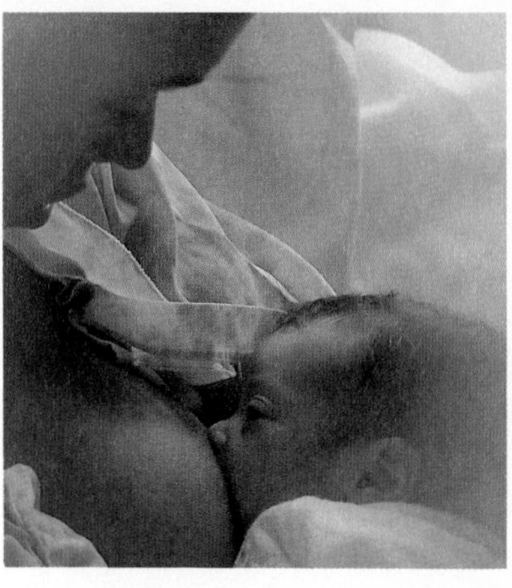

Women who choose to breast-feed often find it a pleasurable experience.

Recent statistics show that about 62% of white women nurse their babies in the hospital, and 25% of black women do so. The same approximate ratio of white to black women holds after the infant is 4 months old.[14] Those women who choose to breast-feed usually find it an enjoyable and "special" time in their lives and in the relationship with their new baby. Bottle feeding using an infant formula is also a nutritious choice, as we will discuss in the next chapter.

If the woman does not nurse her child, breast weight returns to normal very soon after birth. Medications given after delivery can speed this process.

Physiology of lactation

Almost all women can breast-feed their children. Major problems are usually due to a lack of information. Anatomic problems in breasts, such as inverted nipples, can be corrected during pregnancy. Breast size is no indication of success in breast-feeding. First-time mothers who plan to breast-feed should learn as much as they can about the process before delivering the baby (see Nutrition Perspective 15-2 to learn about the mechanics of breast-feeding). Interested women should learn the proper technique, what problems to expect, and how to respond to them. Familiarity with the process builds the confidence and knowledge necessary for success.

Producing human milk

During pregnancy, cells in the breast aggregate to form milk-producing cells called lobules (see the illustration above). Hormones from the placenta stimulate these changes in the breast. After birth, the rise in the maternal production of **prolactin** acts to maintain these changes in the breast, and therefore the ability to produce milk. During pregnancy, breast weight increases by 1 to 2 pounds.

lobules
Sac-like structures in the breast that store milk.

prolactin
A hormone secreted by the mother that stimulates the synthesis of milk.

The hormone prolactin also stimulates the synthesis of milk. Suckling stimulates prolactin release. Milk synthesis then occurs as an infant nurses. *The more the infant suckles, the more milk is produced. Milk production closely parallels infant demand.*[29] In this way, even twins can be nursed. Demand is the driving force for milk production.

Most protein found in human milk is synthesized by breast tissue. Some proteins also enter the milk directly from maternal circulation. These proteins include immune factors and enzymes. Long-chain fatty acids, found as triglycerides in human milk, come from the mother's diet. Short-chain fatty acids, also found as triglycerides in breast milk, are synthesized by breast tissue. The monosaccharide galactose is synthesized in the breast, while glucose enters from maternal circulation. Together these monosaccharides form the disaccharide lactose, the main carbohydrate in human milk.

The let-down reflex

let-down reflex
A reflex stimulated by infant suckling that causes the release (ejection) of milk from milk ducts in the mother's breasts.

An important brain-breast connection—the **let-down reflex**—is necessary for breast-feeding (Figure 15-9). The brain releases the hormone oxytocin to allow the breast tissues to "let down" or release the milk from storage sites to travel to the nipple area. A tingling sensation signals the let-down reflex shortly before milk flow begins. If the let-down reflex doesn't operate, little milk is available to the infant. The infant gets frustrated, and this can frustrate the mother.

The let-down reflex is easily inhibited by nervous tension, a lack of confidence, and fatigue. Mothers should be especially aware of the link between tension and a weak let-down reflex. They need to find a relaxed and supportive environment where they can breast-feed.

After a few weeks, the let-down reflex becomes automatic. The mother's response can be triggered just by thoughts about the baby or by seeing or hearing

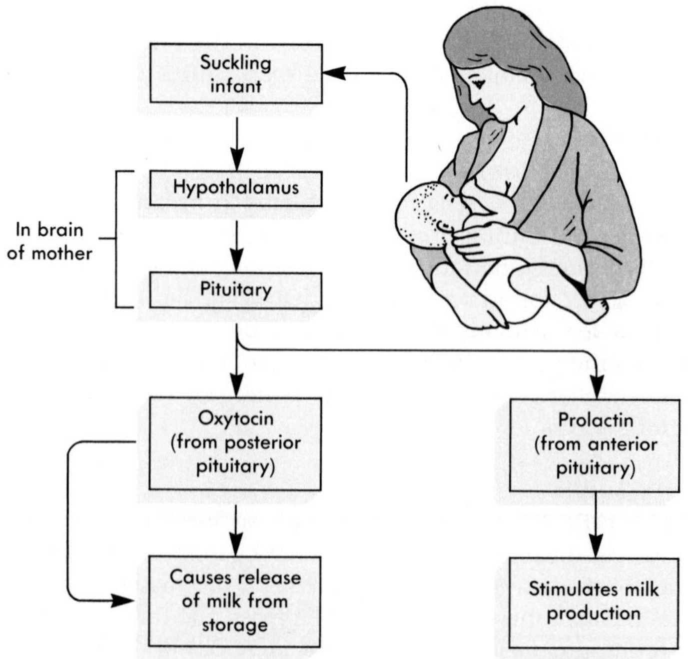

Figure 15-9

The let-down reflex. Suckling by the infant initiates hormonal changes that lead to milk production and the "let-down reflex." This reflex releases the milk from storage cells in the breast.

another baby. But at first, the process can be a bit bewildering. Because she cannot measure the amount of milk the infant takes in, a mother may fear that she is not adequately nourishing the baby. *A good standard of comparison for a breast-fed baby is that it should have 6 or more wet diapers per day and show normal growth.* The stool should also look like mustard. If so, enough milk is being consumed.

It generally takes 2 to 3 weeks to fully establish the feeding routine: infant and mother both feel comfortable, the milk supply meets infant demand, and initial nipple soreness disappears. Establishing the routine requires patience, but the rewards are great. The adjustments are easier if supplemental formula feedings are not introduced until breast-feeding is well-established, after about 2 to 3 months. However, providing water in a bottle during hot weather is fine and often desirable.

Composition of human milk

Human milk is very different in composition from cow's milk. *Unless altered, cow's milk should not be used in infant feeding until the infant is 6 to 12 months old.* Many authorities recommend against using cow's milk until the infant is at least 1 year old—*it is too high in minerals and protein and does not contain enough carbohydrate to meet infant needs.* In addition, the major protein in cow's milk, casein, is harder for an infant to digest than the major protein found in human milk, called lactalbumin.

Colostrum. The first milk made by the human breast is **colostrum.** This type of milk is produced for a few days to a week after birth. It is yellowish and thick and may appear during late pregnancy. Colostrum contains immune factors (especially immunoglobulin A, or IgA) that supply the infant immunity from some diseases. These immune factors compensate for the infant's immature immune system in its first few months of life. *One reason breast-fed infants have fewer respiratory and intestinal infections than formula-fed infants is the presence of these immune bodies in colostrum and in breast milk.*[9]

Colostrum has potent laxative properties that help the baby pass **meconium,** a stool produced during fetal life. One compound in colostrum, the ***Lactobacillus bifidus* factor,** encourages the growth of *Lactobacillus bifidus* bacteria. These bacteria limit the growth of potentially toxic bacteria in the intestine, such as *Escherichia coli,* and so promote the intestinal health of the breast-fed infant.

Mature milk. Human milk composition gradually changes until several days after delivery, when it achieves the normal composition of mature milk. Human milk looks very different from cow's milk. Human milk is thin, almost watery, in appearance and often has a slight bluish tinge. It has a number of impressive nutritional qualities:

- **Type of protein**—The lactalbumin proteins present form a soft, light curd in the infant's stomach, easing digestion. The lactoferrin proteins bind iron, reducing the growth of iron-requiring bacteria. Many of these types of bacteria cause diarrhea. The immunoglobulin proteins offer important immune protection. The amino acid composition of the protein is noted for its low concentration of phenylalanine, which the infant has a limited ability to metabolize. Human milk also has a high concentration of the amino acid taurine, which is needed for bile salt synthesis to aid lipid digestion.
- **Lipid**—Lipids in the milk are high in linoleic acid and cholesterol, which are needed for brain growth. Milk delivered near the end of a breast-feeding session, the **hind milk,** is richer in fat—and therefore energy—than the early, or **fore milk.** Lipase enzymes in the milk improve the intestinal digestion of the lipid.
- **Lactose**—The major carbohydrate in breast milk is lactose, which creates

colostrum
The first milk secreted during late pregnancy and the first few days after birth. This thick fluid is rich in immune factors and protein.

meconium
The first thick mucousy stool passed after birth.

Lactobacillus bifidus factor
A protective factor secreted in the colostrum that encourages growth of beneficial bacteria in the newborn's intestines.

an acidic environment in the intestine by stimulating the growth of acid-producing bacteria. It also provides galactose for nerve sheath synthesis.

- **Vitamin D**—An easily used form of vitamin D is present in human milk. Nevertheless, it is best to provide a vitamin D supplement for the infant if adequate sunlight exposure cannot be guaranteed.
- **Iron**—While human milk is low in iron, about 50% of it is absorbed, compared with 2% to 30% for typical foods. The infant needs another source of iron by the age of 4 to 6 months. By that time, the baby's iron stores, formed in utero, are probably depleted. Some researchers recommend iron supplements by 1 to 2 weeks after birth.

Diet for breast-feeding

Nutrient requirements for a breast-feeding mother change slightly—if at all—from those of the pregnant woman. Exceptions are decreases in folate and iron needs, and increases in vitamin A, vitamin C, niacin, and zinc. However, the diet for breast-feeding can be the same as that for pregnancy, except that the woman should add an additional serving from the milk group, especially if she is a teenager (Tables 15-2 and 15-3). It is important for the woman to drink fluids every time the baby nurses. *A high fluid intake encourages ample milk production. If a woman restricts her kcalories too severely, the quantity of milk also decreases. This is not a time to crash diet.*

Milk production requires approximately 800 kcalories per day. The RDA for energy during lactation is an extra 500 kcalories per day, though this may be too generous to allow loss of excess fat from pregnancy.[3] The difference between kcalorie needs and intake should allow for slow loss of the 3 to 5 plus pounds of fat accumulated during pregnancy. This shows how practical the link is between pregnancy and breast-feeding. If the mother continues to breast-feed beyond 4 to 6 months, or is physically active, more kcalories will be needed.

Most substances the mother ingests are secreted to some extent into the milk. For this reason, alcohol and caffeine intake should be limited or avoided, and all medications should be checked with a pediatrician. Some mothers believe that some foods, such as garlic and chocolate, flavor the breast milk and upset the infant. If a woman notices a connection between a food she eats and later fussiness in the infant, she could consider avoiding that food. However, she might want to experiment again with it later. Infants become fussy for many reasons, and the suspected ingredient may not be the cause.

Concept Check

Recognition of the importance of breast-feeding has contributed to its popularity in the last 20 years. Almost all women have the ability to breast-feed. The hormone prolactin stimulates synthesis of milk by the breast tissue. Some components of human milk come directly from the mother's bloodstream. Infant suckling triggers a let-down reflex that releases the milk. The more an infant nurses, the more milk is synthesized. The nutrient composition of human milk is very different from that of cow's milk and changes as the infant matures. The first milk, colostrum, is very rich in immune factors. The diet for breast-feeding is generally similar to that for pregnancy except that additional kcalories and fluids are recommended.

Advantages of breast-feeding

Human milk is tailored to meet infant needs for the first 4 to 6 months of life. The possible exceptions are fluoride, iron, and vitamin D. Although formula feeding can be satisfying for the infant, mother, and the rest of the family (see Chapter 16), there are many physiological and practical advantages to breast-feeding.

Fewer infections. Breast-feeding reduces the general risk of infections to the infant.[9] This is partially due to the antibodies in human milk that an infant can use. As already mentioned, these antibodies reduce the risk of respiratory and intestinal infections. Ear infections are also reduced because infants cannot sleep with a bottle in the mouth, as bottle-fed infants often do. While an infant sleeps with a bottle in its mouth, milk pools in the mouth and backs up through the throat into the **eustachian tubes** and into the ears. This creates a growth media for bacteria. Infant ear infections are a common problem that parents want to avoid to decrease discomfort for the infant and trips to the doctor and to prevent possible hearing loss.

eustachian tubes
Thin tubes in the middle ear that open into the throat.

Fewer allergies and intolerances. *Breast-feeding reduces the incidence of allergies, especially in allergy-prone infants.* Cow's milk contains a number of potentially allergy-causing proteins that are absent from human milk. Breast-feeding also avoids the possibility of infant intolerance of formulas. Formulas sometimes must be switched several times until caregivers find one the infant can tolerate.

Convenience. Breast-feeding frees the mother from time and expense involved in buying and preparing formula and washing bottles. Breast milk is already "prepared" and sterile. This allows the mother to spend more time with her baby.

On the other hand, if the child is bottle-fed, the mother may be freed to do other things while others feed the baby.

Barriers to breast-feeding

A lack of role models, widespread misinformation, fear of appearing immodest, and women working away from their children all serve as barriers to breast-feeding.

Misinformation. Probably the major barriers to breast-feeding are misinformation and lack of role models. If a woman is interested in breast-feeding, we suggest that she talk to women who have done it successfully. Experienced mothers can be an enormous help to the first-time mother. She should find a friend she can call on to ask questions. In almost every community, a group called La Leche League offers classes in breast-feeding and advises women who have problems with it.

Returning to an outside job. Working outside the home can complicate plans to breast-feed. After 1 or 2 months of breast-feeding, a mother can regularly express milk either by breast pump or by hand into a sterile plastic bottle or nursing bag to use in a disposable bottle system. Saving breastmilk requires careful sanitation and rapid chilling. There is a knack to learning how to do this, but the freedom can be worth it. Then others can feed the mother's milk to the infant.

Some women can juggle both a job and breast-feeding, but others find it too cumbersome and decide instead to formula-feed. A compromise—balancing some breast-feedings, say early morning and at night, with formula-feedings during the day—is possible. However, keep in mind that too many supplemental feedings decrease milk production. A schedule of expressing milk and using supplemental formula-feedings is most successful if not initiated until after 1 to 2 months of exclusive breast-feeding. After 2 months, the baby is well adapted to breast-feeding and probably feels enough emotional security and other benefits from nursing that it is willing to drink both ways.

The key months for breast-feeding are the first 2 to 3 months of an infant's life. A longer commitment is better, but these few months are critically important. During that time human milk provides the anti-infective properties needed until the infant begins to synthesize its own immune factors in high concentrations. Women can try to find infant day care close to the workplace so that they can visit a few times during the day for feeding. Some businesses have day-care facilities on the premises that enable women to return to work and still breast-feed their children. A combination of breast-feeding and formula-feeding may work. If a woman wants to breast-feed her baby, she has a lot of options.

Social reticence. Another barrier for some women is embarrassment when nursing a child in public. Our society historically has stressed modesty and frowned on baring breasts in public—even in so good a cause as nourishing babies. With appropriate clothing, it is possible to nurse quite discreetly.

When is breast-feeding not a good idea?

Mothers should not breast-feed their infants if they don't want to do so. There are distinct advantages to breast-feeding, but none so great that a woman who decides to bottle-feed should feel she is penalizing her infant.

Infants with the disease phenylketonuria often cannot be breast-fed, and those with galactosemia never can because of the amount of phenylalanine and galactose in human milk (see chapter 6). Mothers who take medications that pass into the milk and adversely affect the child also should not breast-feed. In addition, a woman who has a serious chronic disease, such as tuberculosis or hepatitis, or is being treated for cancer, should not breast-feed.

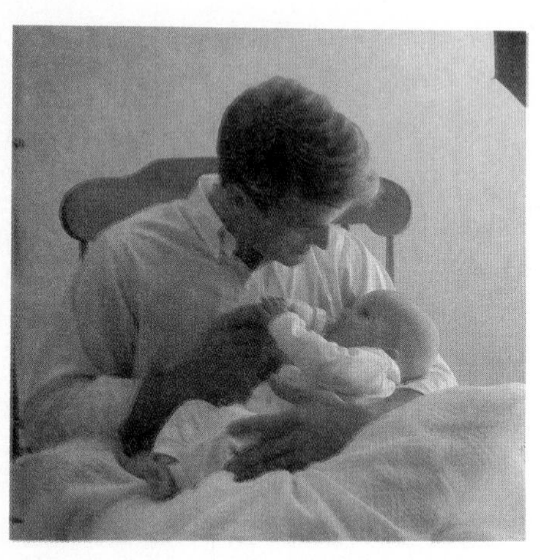

Bottlefeeding is a nutritionally acceptable alternative to breast-feeding.

What about environmental contaminants?

Some women wonder whether breast-feeding is safe. There is some legitimate concern over the levels of various environmental contaminants in human milk, but the benefits from human milk are very well established, and the risks from environmental contaminants are still largely theoretical. Thus it is probably best to operate with what we know works until sufficiently strong research data dissuade us.

A few measures a woman might take to counteract some known contaminants would be to avoid freshwater fish from polluted waters, carefully wash and peel fruits and vegetables, and remove the fatty edges of meat. In addition, a woman should not try to lose weight rapidly while nursing, because contaminants stored in fat tissue then enter the bloodstream and milk in turn. If a woman questions whether her milk is safe, especially if she has lived in an area known to have a high concentration of toxic wastes or environmental pollution, she should consult her local health department.

Can a premature infant be breast-fed?

There is no clear-cut answer to whether a woman can breast-feed a premature infant. In some cases human milk is the most desirable form of nourishment. It must usually be expressed from the breast and fed through a tube. This type of feeding demands great dedication from the mother. Fortification of the milk with nutrients such as calcium, phosphorus, sodium, and protein is often needed to match an infant's rapid growth. In other cases, special feeding problems may prevent use of human milk or necessitate some supplementation with formula. Sometimes even total parenteral nutrition is the only option.[10] Working as a team, the pediatrician, neonatal nurses and registered dietitian guide the parents in this decision.

Concept Check

Human milk provides most of an infant's nutritional needs for the first 6 months. Vitamin D, iron, and fluoride may be supplemented. The advantages of breast-feeding over formula-feeding include fewer intestinal, respiratory, and ear infections; fewer allergies and food intolerances; and convenience. Lack of role models, misinformation, and social reticence may dissuade a mother from breast-feeding. A combination of breast- and formula-feeding is possible when a mother is regularly away from the infant. Breast-feeding is not desirable if a mother has certain diseases or must take medication potentially harmful to the infant. The premature infant, depending upon its condition, may benefit from consuming human milk.

Summary

1. Adequate nutrition is vital during pregnancy to ensure the well-being of both the infant and the mother. Insults due to poor nutrition and some medications can cause birth defects, especially if they occur in the first trimester, and growth retardation and altered development if they occur later in pregnancy.
2. Infants born prematurely (before 37 weeks of gestation) or with low birth weight (less than 5.5 pounds, or 2500 grams) usually have more medical problems at birth than normal infants.
3. Teenage pregnancy requires very careful prenatal and nutritional care. Complications are more common in these pregnancies because of the very high physiological demands and often poor social and economic support.
4. Daily energy needs increase by an average of 300 kcalories during pregnancy. Weight gain should be gradual to a total 24 to 28 pounds in a normal weight mother.
5. Protein, vitamin, and mineral requirements increase during pregnancy. Extra servings from the milk and cheese group and the meat, poultry, fish, and beans group of the Daily Food Guide are recommended. Supplements of iron and folate, in particular, may be needed.
6. Pregnancy-induced hypertension, gestational diabetes mellitus, heartburn, constipation, nausea, vomiting, edema, and anemia are all possible discomforts and complications of pregnancy. Nutrition therapy can often help minimize these problems.
7. The popularity of breast-feeding has increased in the past 20 years. Almost all women have the ability to nurse their infants. The nutrient composition of human milk is very different from cow's milk. Colostrum, the first milk produced by humans, is very rich in immune factors. Mature milk is rich in the protein lactalbumin and in lactose.
8. Advantages for the infant of breast-feeding over formula-feeding include fewer intestinal, respiratory and ear infections; fewer allergies and food intolerances; and convenience. An infant can be adequately nourished with formula if the mother chooses to not breast-feed. Breast-feeding is not desirable if the mother has certain diseases or must take medication potentially harmful to the infant.

Take Action

Design a diet you would like to follow that is adequate for prenatal needs. Show it to at least one pregnant woman. What insights have you gained?

BREAKFAST ______________________________

LUNCH ______________________________

SNACK ______________________________

DINNER ______________________________

SNACK ______________________________

____

REFERENCES

1. ADA reports: Position of the American Dietetic Association: nutritional management of adolescent pregnancy, Journal of the American Dietetic Association 89:104, 1989.
2. Belizan JM and others: The relationship between calcium intake and pregnancy-induced hypertension: up-to-date evidence, American Journal of Obstetrics and Gynecology 158:898, 1988.
3. Brewer MM and others: Postpartum changes in maternal weight and body fat deposits in lactating vs nonlactating women, American Journal of Clinical Nutrition 49:259, 1989.
4. Carr-Hill R and others: Is birth weight determined genetically? British Medical Journal 295:687, 1987.
5. Clay G and others: A comprehensive nutrition case management system, Journal of the American Dietetic Association 88:196, 1988.
6. Department of Health and Welfare: Canada's national guidelines on prenatal nutrition, Nutrition Today July/August:34, 1987.
7. Eidelman AI and others: The grand multipara: is she still a risk? American Journal of Obstetrics and Gynecology 158:389, 1988.
8. Evans ER and others: Gestational diabetes, American Family Physician 36:119, 1987.
9. Habicht J and others: Mothers milk and sewage: their interactive effects on infant mortality, Pediatrics 81:456, 1988.
10. Hopkinson JM and others: Milk production by mothers of premature infants, Pediatrics 81:815, 1988.
11. Huber AM and others: Folate nutriture in pregnancy, Journal of the American Dietetic Association 88:791, 1988.
12. Jacobson HN: A healthy pregnancy, the struggle to define it, Nutrition Today, p 30, January/February, 1988.
13. Kennedy ET: A prenatal screening system in a community-based setting, Journal of the American Dietetic Association 86:1372, 1986.
14. Kurinij N and others: Breast-feeding incidents and duration in black and white women, Pediatrics 81:365, 1988.
15. Lazebnic N and others: Zinc status, pregnancy complications, and labor abnormalities, American Journal of Obstetrics and Gynecology 158:161, 1988.
16. Macgregor SN and others: Cocaine use during pregnancy: adverse perinatal outcome, American Journal of Obstetrics and Gynecology 157:686, 1987.
17. Meis PJ and others: Causes of low birth weight births in public and private patients, American Journal of Obstetrics and Gynecology 156:1 165, 1987.
18. Mitchell MC and Lerner E: Weight gain and pregnancy outcome in underweight and normal weight women, Journal of The American Dietetic Association 89:634, 1989.
19. Maternal nutrition and the course of pregnancy, Washington DC, 1970, National Academy of Sciences—National Research Council.
20. Orstead CO and others: Efficacy of prenatal nutrition counseling: weight gain, infant birth weight, and cost-effectiveness, Journal of the American Dietetic Association 85:40, 1985.
21. Reece J and others: Iron supplementation in pregnancy: testing a new clinic protocol, Journal of the American Dietetic Association 87:1682, 1987.
22. Streissguth AP and others: Teratogenic effects of alcohol in humans and laboratory animals, Science 209:353, 1980.
23. Swanson CA and King JC: Zinc and pregnancy outcome, American Journal of Clinical Nutrition 46:763, 1987.
24. Taffel SM and Keppel KG: Advice about weight gain during pregnancy and actual weight gain, American Journal of Public Health 76:13 96, 1986.
25. Thomson M and Hanley J: Factors predisposing to difficult labor in primiparas, American Journal of Obstetrics and Gynecology 158:1074, 1988.
26. Villar J and Rivera J: Nutrition supplementation during two consecutive pregnancies, and the interim lactation period: affect on birth weight, Pediatrics 81:51, 1988.
27. Whitehead RJ: Pregnancy and lactation. In Shils ME and Young VR, editors, Modern nutrition in health and disease, Philadelphia, 1988, Lea & Febiger.
28. Widdowson EM: Fetal and neonatal nutrition, Nutrition Today September/October:16, 1987.
29. Worthington-Roberts B and others: Nutrition in Pregnancy and Lactation, St. Louis, 1989, The CV Mosby Co.

SUGGESTED READINGS

For a more detailed look at nutrition and pregnancy see *Maternal Nutrition in the Course of Pregnancy* by the National Research Council of the National Academy of Sciences, and the textbook, *Nutrition in Pregnancy, and Lactation,* by Worthington-Roberts and others. Together these sources contain essentially all the information a health professional needs about nutrition in pregnancy and breast-feeding. The review of fetal and neonatal nutrition by Widdowson in *Nutrition Today* provides a look at early nutrient needs, and the article by Streissguth and others supplies the classic description of the effects of alcohol in pregnancy. The article by Evans and others details the management of gestational diabetes mellitus. Finally, read the position paper by the American Dietetic Association on the nutritional management of adolescent pregnancy. This age-group presents a great challenge to health care professionals because of the simultaneous problems of meeting nutritional needs of growth by the fetus and teenage mother.

CHAPTER 15

Answers to nutrition awareness inventory

1. *True.* Infants weighing less than 5.5 pounds (2.5 kilograms) at birth are considered to have low birth weight. The risk of sickness and death in the early months of life is much greater for these infants.
2. *False.* During the first trimester (13 weeks), when organs and body parts are forming, the potential for birth defects is greatest.
3. *True.* The quality of the mother's diet and the amount of weight she gains during pregnancy are more important than genetic background in determining birth weight.
4. *True.* During pregnancy, an average increase of 300 kcalories per day is needed. Energy demands are greatest during the second and third trimesters.
5. *True.* This range of weight gain normally allows optimal development of the fetus without an excessive increase of fat stores in the mother.
6. *True.* Gaining excessive weight from eating too many kcalories is a problem for many pregnant women.
7. *False.* Eating a healthful diet requires learning wise food choices.
8. *True.* Many mineral needs, but particularly those for iron, calcium and zinc, are increased. Iron requirements usually necessitate taking supplements in addition to changing the diet.
9. *True.* Symptoms of gestational diabetes mellitus may first occur during pregnancy and then disappear after birth. This happens more frequently in women who have a family history of diabetes mellitus.
10. *True.* Immune factors passed from mother to infant via breast milk reduce the number of respiratory and intestinal infections.
11. *True.* Almost all women are capable of breast-feeding; the size of the breasts, and even the presence of twins, pose no major barrier.
12. *True.* Many substances ingested by the mother, including medicines, are secreted into the milk.
13. *True.* The placenta is a specialized organ of pregnancy that both secretes hormones and allows for the transfer of oxygen, nutrients, and wastes between mother and fetus.
14. *True.* Good nutrition and health habits should begin early, ideally before pregnancy begins.
15. *False.* Cow's milk is too difficult for an infant to digest and fully metabolize until approximately 6 to 12 months of age.

Nutrition Perspective 15-1

Fetal Alcohol Syndrome

fetal alcohol syndrome (FAS)
A group of physical and mental abnormalities in the infant that result from the mother consuming alcohol during pregnancy.

The effect of alcohol use during pregnancy is a very important issue. Scientists do not know if alcohol must be totally eliminated from the diet, but there is no question that large amounts of alcohol harm the fetus. Women suffering from chronic alcoholism produce children with a recognizable pattern of malformations called **fetal alcohol syndrome (FAS).**[22] Figure 15-10 shows the major characteristics of FAS. A diagnosis of FAS is based mainly on poor prenatal and infant growth, physical deformities, and mental retardation. The range of abnormalities varies from severe FAS to reduced birth weight, behavioral effects, and poor learning ability in infants of women reporting only social drinking. The latter category is termed *fetal alcohol effects.* Annually, about 2000 infants are born in the United States with FAS, and about 35,000 are born with fetal alcohol effects.

Exactly how alcohol causes these defects is not known, but other factors such as poor nutrition, cigarette smoking (nicotine intake), and other drugs compound the problems. In addition, no one knows how much alcohol intake produces these problems. It is not pos-

Figure 15-10

Fetal alcohol syndrome. Milder forms of alcohol-induced changes on the fetus, and so the infant, are known as fetal alcohol effects.

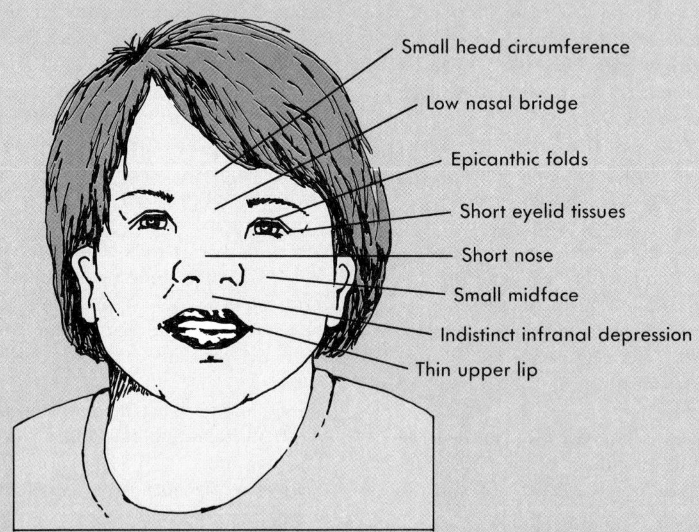

Facial features that are characteristic of FAS.

sible to scientifically measure absolute safety, and experimental evidence suggests there is no measurable risk from consuming less than 1 ounce of absolute alcohol per day. Because its safety is not proved, *many authorities, including the U.S. surgeon general and the American Medical Association, believe it is best for mothers-to-be to avoid alcohol altogether.* Alcohol reaches the fetal blood at the same concentration as is in the mother's blood within 15 minutes of her drinking. However, the effect on the fetus may be up to 10 times greater. Just one bout of binge drinking can arrest and alter cell division occurring during a critical phase of fetal development. The fetus then may develop with an irreversible defect.

Since alcohol has the capacity to adversely affect each stage of fetal development, the earlier in pregnancy that heavy drinking ceases, the greater is the potential for improved outcome. The best course is to consider alcohol an indulgence that can be eliminated until after pregnancy. Not only is it important for pregnant women to abstain from alcohol during pregnancy, but also when trying to conceive, and anytime the possibility of conception is present. Recall that many women are not aware they are pregnant until 2 to 3 months after conception, and during that time much fetal growth and development takes place. Considering that pregnancy lasts only 9 months, and that parents may spend a lifetime caring for a handicapped child, it is important for parents—especially women—to realize that avoiding alcohol completely during pregnancy is a lesser sacrifice. Although an affected child is still loved, the life that results is needlessly difficult for the child and the family.

Alcohol abuse during pregnancy is a major risk factor. Women who drink heavily often respond to supportive therapy focused on abstinence. Prenatal care providers have a unique opportunity to intervene in a cost-effective manner while providing benefits for both the mother and her newborn.

Nutrition Perspective 15-2

The Mechanics of Breast-Feeding

Each infant is unique and has a distinct personality that begins to form before birth. Some eagerly breast-feed the first time they get the chance; others may be disinterested for the first couple days. A mother should expect the unexpected. She shouldn't be discouraged if her infant doesn't act like others she's seen. *Her infant will soon become hungry and will breast-feed when ready.*

In the hospital, a mother can begin breast-feeding by asking a postpartum nurse to help her. Nurses are experienced in helping women begin the process and can suggest various positions to try—traditional, football hold, or others.

To get started, a woman should take the dark area of the nipple, the **areola,** between two fingers so the infant can get a good hold. This is especially important with very large or full breasts. The mother should then rub the infant's cheek with the nipple. The infant will naturally "root" for the nipple and latch on. The mother may have to continue to hold on to the areola so that it won't block the infant's nose.[29]

areola
The circular dark area of skin at the center of the breast.

It may take a few days for the mother and infant to get to know each other and to establish comfortable positions. The mother should not be alarmed if after the first few days or weeks breast-feeding still does not feel totally "natural." It takes time, especially with a first child.

Continued.

Nutrition Perspective 15-2—cont'd

The Mechanics of Breast Feeding

A mother should begin by nursing about 5 minutes on each side every 1 to 2 hours, eventually increasing nursing time to 10 minutes on each side spaced every 3 to 4 hours, after about one week. It is important at the start for the mother not to allow the infant to use the breast as a pacifier. This can cause nipple soreness and much pain.

To get a baby's attention, a mother may try squirting a bit of milk into its mouth or perhaps change its diapers to wake it. To stop a session the mother can break an infant's suction by inserting a finger along the breast into the child's mouth. Merely pulling the infant off her breast could be quite painful. Now she should burp the baby, and then start on the other breast. To keep nursing enjoyable, the mother should try to reduce other stresses in her life, eat a nutritious diet, and get plenty of sleep—at least 8 hours when possible.

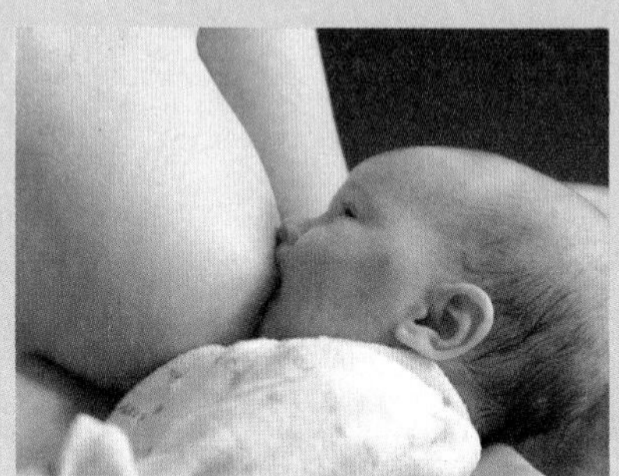

Mother and infant must learn to be comfortable with each other during breast-feeding.

WHEN BREAST-FEEDING DOES NOT GO PERFECTLY

Problems may arise while nursing a baby.[29] This is typical—there is no reason for panic. *Breast-feeding is more a skill than an instinct—it takes practice.*

Engorgement

Engorgement of milk in the breast may occur when an infant isn't an established nurser. The breasts fill with milk, but the infant does not empty them. The woman should then express milk from the breast in order to reduce the size and resulting pain. It is probably best to buy an inexpensive (about $35) breast pump and stimulate the breasts with a towel soaked in warm water. The woman can also manually express milk by squeezing gently while moving her hands from the back to the front of the breast.

Leakage

Breasts may leak between feeding sessions, especially if a let-down reflex is stimulated. Absorbent pads or a handkerchief can be worn to soak up the milk.

WHEN THE BABY IS STILL HUNGRY

When it appears an infant is not satisfied after 20 minutes of nursing, the mother should first attempt to breast-feed the infant more often, at least every 2½ to 4 hours. This will increase milk production and in turn probably satisfy the infant. Recall that even twins can be nursed. Demand drives milk production. *Foods other than breast milk or formula are rarely needed before 4 months of age.* Recall that a breast-fed baby normally wets six to eight diapers a day and shows normal growth.

Nipple soreness

If nipples become sore, using a pacifier can satisfy some suckling needs of the infant. Allowing the nipples to air-dry and using a lanolin cream should reduce tenderness in a couple of days. It is important to keep nursing sessions to 10 minutes per side until the soreness subsides and to use the sore side last. The infant suckles more vigorously on the first side.

Overall, the mother should expect that small problems will arise, but these can be easily dealt with. If the mother wants to continue to nurse, she should be encouraged to do so.

Chapter 16

Infants, Children, and Teens

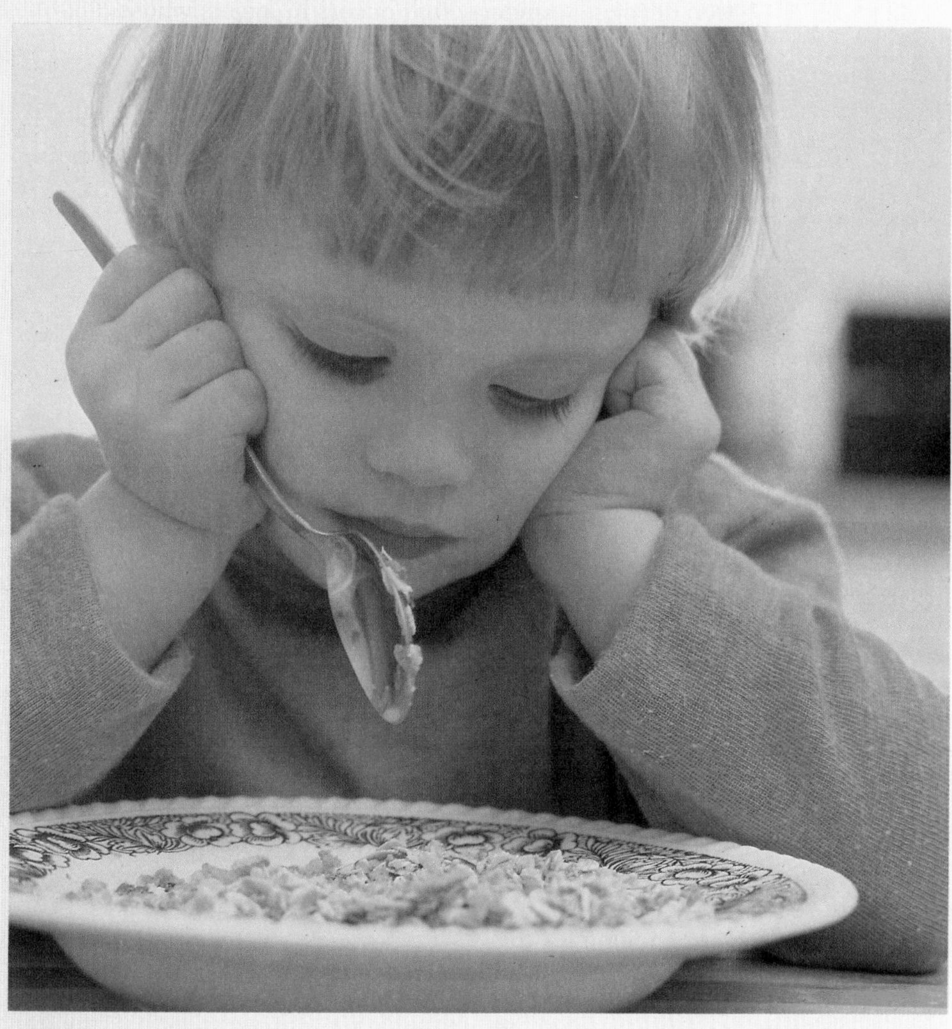

Within guidelines, offering choices to a child can encourage acceptance of many different foods.

Overview

Nutrient requirements vary as we progress through different stages of growth. Infancy is a time of tremendous body growth and development. Disproportionately large amounts of energy, protein, vitamins, and minerals are needed. As growth tapers, so do nutrient needs and appetite. During the teen years, another growth spurt occurs, and new dietary issues arise from eating habits and a lifestyle that encourages "eating on the run." Let's explore these critical stages of life and the key role nutrients play in them.

Nutrition awareness inventory

Here are 15 statements about nutrition for infants, children, and teens. Answer them to test your current knowledge. If you think the answer is true or mostly true, circle T. If you think the answer is false or mostly false, circle F. Use the scoring key at the end of this chapter to compute your total score. Take this test again after you have read this chapter. Compare the results.

1. **T F** Consuming low-protein diets in childhood can greatly affect ultimate adult height.
2. **T F** An infant's length increases by 50% in the first year.
3. **T F** Brain growth is greatest during the teen years.
4. **T F** Most obese infants become obese adults.
5. **T F** Infants have lower energy needs per pound than older children.
6. **T F** An infant's diet should be very low in fat.
7. **T F** Infants need solid food by 3 months of age.
8. **T F** Infants enjoy blander foods than do adults.
9. **T F** Colic is caused by a gas buildup in the intestinal tract.
10. **T F** Cow's milk fed during early infancy can cause allergies.
11. **T F** Iron-deficiency anemia often occurs in infants whose diets are composed mainly of cow's milk.
12. **T F** It is nutritionally important to put children on a three-meals-per-day schedule.
13. **T F** The two most common nutritional problems in childhood are obesity and anemia.
14. **T F** Parents should carefully control the amount of food their children eat.
15. **T F** Acne can be avoided by limiting certain foods in the diet.

INFANT GROWTH AND PHYSIOLOGICAL DEVELOPMENT

During infancy a child's attitudes toward foods and the whole eating process are shaped. Depending on the nutritional knowledge and flexibility of parents and other caregivers, an infant can start life with both an optimum nutritional status that accommodates brain and body growth spurts and a willingness to experiment and try new foods.

The growing infant

Rapid growth characterizes infancy. An infant's birth weight doubles in its first 4 to 6 months and triples within the first year. After that, the child grows slowly and steadily for 5 more years before fully doubling weight again. An infant's length increases by 50% in the first year and continues to increase throughout preschool and teen years. This stops when the bone ends (epiphyses) fuse together, halting further significant linear growth (Figure 16-1).

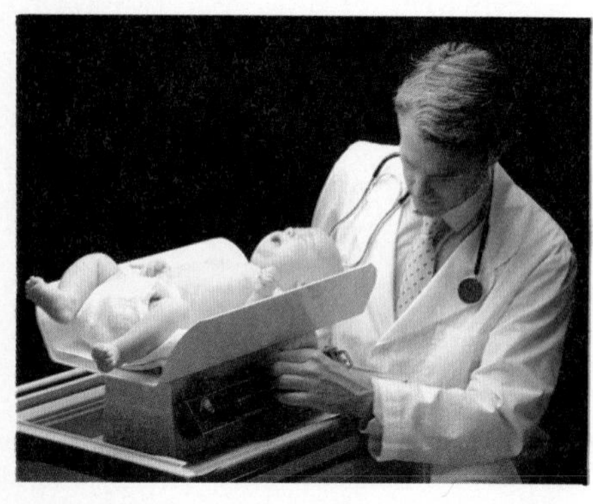

An infant's birth weight doubles in its first 4 to 6 months of age.

Growth requires a generous nutrient intake to support body needs. We know from observing Egyptian mummies that infants were about the same size in 300 BC as they are today. However, adult mummies are much smaller than adults are today. Notice from museum collections of the Middle Ages the small sizes of the suits of armor. *People of the past ate poor diets that did not supply enough nutrients for maximum growth.*

In Third World countries today, about half the children are short and underweight for their age. They are simply smaller versions of nutritionally fit children. In these countries, when breast-feeding ceases, children are often left to consume a high-carbohydrate, low-protein diet. This diet supports some growth but does

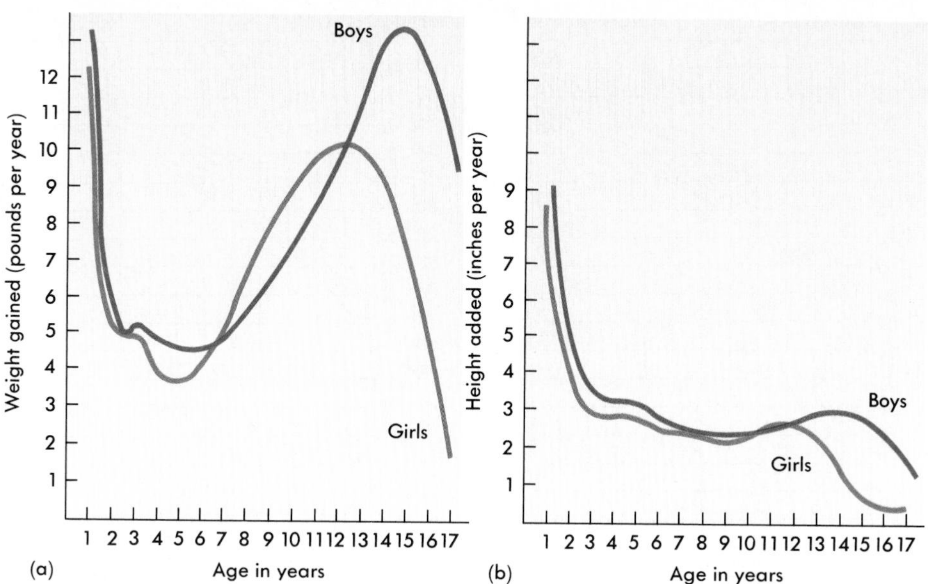

Figure 16-1

Growth rates. (A) Average gains in weight for girls and boys. (B) Average additions to height for girls and boys.

not allow them to achieve their genetic potential. Adequate protein intake is critical for growth. Weight primarily reflects current nutrient intake, while height is a better measure of long-term nutrient intake.

Infants show a pattern of physiological development in which body water is reduced from about 75% at birth to 60%, the proportion typical in adults. By 1 year of age an infant's body nitrogen content (and so, protein content) has increased from 2% of body weight at birth to 3%, indicating the infant has synthesized much new lean tissue.[17] A further indication of this lean tissue synthesis is increased potassium concentration in the body from infancy to adulthood. Recall from Chapter 13 that potassium is the major positive ion operating inside cells. As children build more cells, they accumulate more potassium.

The effect of malnutrition on growth

In Chapter 15 we described growth as a process of cell division (hyperplasia) and then of cell growth (hypertrophy). The long-term effects of nutritional problems in infancy and childhood depend on the severity, timing, and duration of the nutritional insult to these cell processes, just as they did when the fetus was **in utero.**[14] Poor hypertrophy is reversible. Organs in the process of hypertrophy during a nutritional famine can regain and restore that growth when an adequate diet is resumed.

in utero
"In the uterus," or in other words, during pregnancy.

Hyperplasia stopped by a poor diet probably cannot be reversed. If cell division is arrested, an adequate diet later probably will not help much because the appropriate hormonal environment necessary for that cell division will no longer be present. A 15-year-old Central American girl who is 4 feet 8 inches tall cannot by improving her diet attain the adult height of a typical North American. Once the time for growth ceases (in women this is about 2 years after the onset of menses), a good nutrient intake will help maintain health but will not compensate for lost growth.

Assessing infant growth and development

Health professionals monitor a child's increases in height, weight, and head circumference, and interpret the records using growth charts. All these parameters

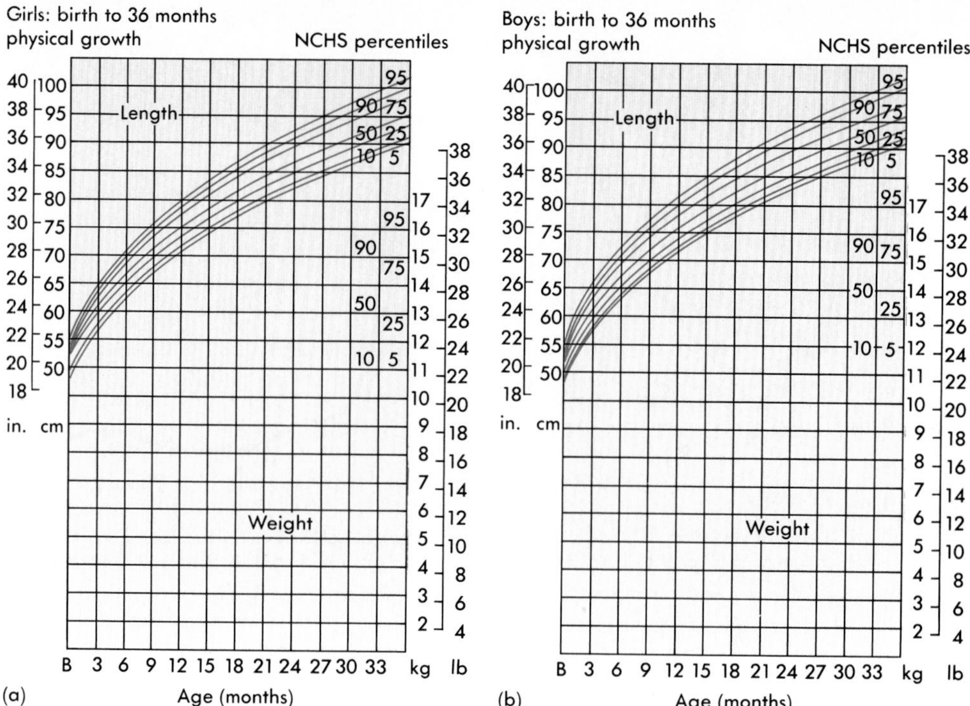

Figure 16-2

Growth charts used to assess height (length), weight, and head circumference in young boys and girls. See Appendix P for charts that apply to older children.

are useful indicators of nutritional health. The typical charts contain seven **percentile** divisions, which represent 90% of children (Figure 16-2). A percentile simply represents the rank of the person among 100 age- and gender-matched peers. If Tony, for example, is at the 90th percentile height for age, this description means that if you measure 100 children of that age 10 children will be taller than Tony, and 89 will be shorter. A child at the 50th percentile is considered average. Fifty children will be taller than this child, while 49 will be shorter.

The two growth charts that give the most useful information are height-for-age—which assesses linear growth—and weight-for-height—which assesses weight status based on height. For children under 3 years of age, head circumference for age is also a useful measure of growth. Since children under 2 to 3 years of age are measured stretched out, lying on their backs, the term length is used instead of height.

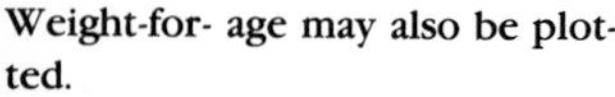
Weight-for- age may also be plotted.

Individual growth charts are available for both males and females, for ages ranging from 0 to 36 months or 2 to 18 years (see Appendix P). Growth of infants and children should be plotted regularly during their health check ups. It takes one year to three years for an infant to establish his or her "genetic" percentile. Once this figure is established, such as length- (height-) for-age, the child's measurement should then track along that percentile. If the child's growth does not keep up with his or her percentile, the physician needs to investigate whether a medical or nutritional problem is impeding the predicted growth.

Infants born prematurely may catch up in growth in 2 to 3 years. This requires that the child jump up in the percentiles. If this occurs—especially in height-for-age—it is usually no cause for alarm. On the other hand, jumping percentiles in weight-for-height can be disturbing if the child approaches the 80th to 90th percentiles. Generally a child at the 90th percentile for weight-for-height is considered "overweight." Above the 95th percentile, the child is considered obese.

Exploring Issues and Actions

Next time you visit your physician, ask to see your childhood growth records.

Brain growth

The rate of brain growth is maximal at birth. Increases in cell number (hyperplasia) cease between 12 and 15 months of age. However, different areas of the brain peak in hyperplasia at different times. When studying the effect of nutritional status on brain development and ultimate intelligence quotient (IQ), it is difficult to separate the effects of nature from nurture. However, studies from Central America suggest that IQ after age 5 years correlates more closely with the amount of schooling the child receives than with nutritional intake during childhood.

Adipose Tissue Growth

Since 1970, researchers have speculated that overfeeding during infancy may increase adipose tissue cell number (see Chapter 8 for details). This link has been difficult to establish, since researchers can neither see nor count empty adipose cells. Therefore, when analyzing an adipose sample from a thin infant, researchers are not sure if they are counting all cells present. It could be that an obese infant has just filled up more cells, while a lean infant has as many cells, but some are hidden (still not filled).

If energy intake is restricted in infancy to decrease adipose tissue hyperplasia, the growth of other organ systems may decrease as well. In addition, no evidence strongly links infant obesity with adult obesity. Most obese infants become normal-weight preschoolers. In addition, one thing *is* certain: *infants need an adequate diet so they can obtain their intended adult height.* Taller people necessarily use more energy at rest, and given the sedentary life-style of most North Americans, they probably have a greater chance of avoiding obesity than shorter people.

Concept Check

Growth occurs rapidly during infancy: birth weight doubles in 4 to 6 months, and triples within the first year. Other physiological changes during infancy include an increase in lean tissue and a reduction in the percentage of body water. Malnutrition can cause irreversible changes in growth and maturation. Infant and child growth is monitored by tracking body weight, height (or length) and head circumference over time. The most useful growth charts plot height-for-age and weight-for-height. Development of obesity is not desirable in infancy, though there is no strong evidence that an obese infant will become an obese adult.

Failure to thrive

Occasionally an infant does not grow, in spite of adequate physical health. Physical causes might include poor development of the oral cavity, presence of infections, heart problems, and constant diarrhea associated with intestinal problems. However, about half the infants who show **failure to thrive** show no disease.[10] About 40% show a combination of medical and parental neglect as the cause. In only 6% of the cases is a medical problem the main cause. Thus the problem often stems from poor child-rearing practices, which result from misinformation or lack of attention and concern for the child's welfare. The parents may also be overcommitted to maintaining a lean child in hopes of preventing future obesity. In addition, the child might be psychologically withdrawn and therefore not cry out for food when hungry.

Clinicians faced with an infant who is failing to thrive must first determine if the child is consuming enough energy: for infants that is approximately 100 kcalories per kilogram of body weight per day. For a breast-fed infant, the clinician needs to make sure that sufficient milk is being consumed. The child should be nursing about six to eight times a day for about 20 minutes a session, have six to eight wet diapers each day, and the mother should have an adequate intake of food and fluid (see Chapter 15). Failure to thrive is not often seen in children older than 2 years of age because they can often get food for themselves. Younger children are limited to what the caregivers provide.

Development of feeding skills

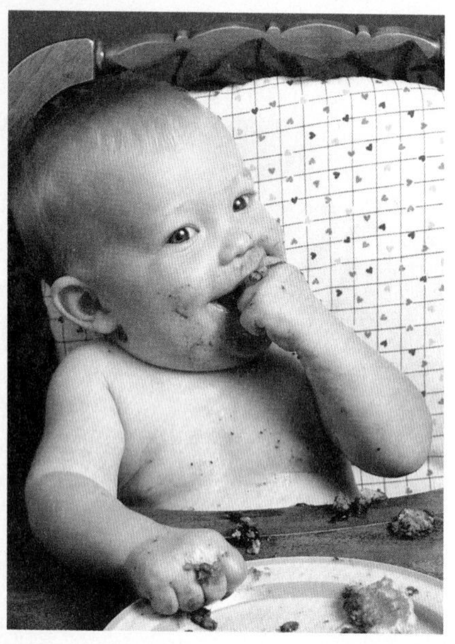

An infant first practices self-feeding at around 6-7 months of age.

By 6 to 7 months of age, the infant has learned to grab and transfer objects from one hand to the other. About this time teeth begin to appear, and the infant begins to handle "finger foods" with some dexterity. Dry toast slices offer hours of enjoyment.

By age 8 to 9 months the infant can push a plate around and play with a drinking cup. He or she can now hold a bottle and self-feed a cracker or piece of toast. This is an important time for the infant to develop self-confidence and self-esteem, so the parent must be patient and supportive with these early feeding attempts.

Around 10 months of age, the infant practices in earnest self-feeding finger foods and drinking from a cup. Feeding time may be very messy. Food is seen as something not only to eat but also to feel, smear, and drop. By the first birthday, an infant's body has developed sufficiently to accommodate crawling, probably walking, and self-feeding. While first attempts at feeding are erratic, the developing child soon takes great pride in doing more things independently. As the child drinks from a cup more frequently, fewer bottle- or breast-feedings are necessary. The mobility of walking should naturally lead to gradual weaning from the bottle or breast.

INFANT NUTRITIONAL NEEDS

An infant's nutrient needs differ from adult needs in both amount and proportion, and vary with stages of growth. Fortunately, most early needs can be met by human milk or formula. Solid foods are usually not needed to supplement these nutrient supplies until after 4 to 6 months. Even so, the basis of an infant's diet for the first year remains human milk or formula.

Energy

Daily energy needs in infancy are about 45 to 50 kcalories per pound per day (98 to 108 kcalories per kilogram per day). Based on body weight, this is proportionately 2 to 4 times the energy needs of an adult. Infants need an easy way to meet their high-energy needs. Either human milk or formula is ideal for this in the first few months. Both are high in fat and supply about 650 kcalories per 32 ounces of

Table 16-1

Composition of infant formulas per liter*

Milk or formula	Kcalories	Protein (grams)	Fat (grams)	Carbohydrate (grams)	Minerals† (grams)
Human milk	750	11	45	70	2
Casein-based formulas					
Similac	680	15.5	36	72	3.3
Enfamil	670	15	38	69	3
SMA	670	15	36	72	2.5
Gerber	670	15	36	72	2.4
Cow's milk					
Whole	670	36	36	49	7
Skim	360	36	1	51	7
Soybean protein-based formulas					
ProSobee	670	20	36	68	4
Isomil	570	20	36	68	4
Nursoy	670	20	36	68	4

* 1 liter equals about 30 fluid ounces.

† Calcium, phosphorus, and other minerals

fluid (700 kcalories per liter; Table 16-1). Later, human milk or formula, with solid foods, can provide even more energy.

The high energy needs of the infant are primarily driven by rapid growth and a high metabolic rate—the latter is in part due to the ratio of the infant's great surface area to its weight. More surface area allows more heat loss from the skin; energy metabolism is required to replace that heat.

Protein

Daily protein needs vary in infancy from 1.6 to 2.2 grams per kilogram of body weight (0.7 to 1 grams per pound per day). One liter of formula or human milk contains about 13 grams (or 12 grams per quart). About 40% of this protein should be from essential amino acids. Total protein intake should not exceed 20% of kcalorie needs. Excess nitrogen and minerals supplied by high-protein diets would overtax the infant's kidney function.[17]

In North America, a protein deficiency in infants is unlikely, except in cases of mistaken feeding practices, such as overdiluting an infant's formula. A protein deficiency may also result from allergies: the clinician needs to closely watch infants with allergies because, as foods are eliminated from their diets, they may be offered insufficient protein (see Nutrition Perspective 16-1, "Food Allergies and Intolerances").

Fat

Fat should make up about 30% to 50% of an infant's energy intake. More than that may lead to poor fat digestion. Both human milk and formula supply about 50% of energy as fat. Essential fatty acids should make up 3% of total energy. Fats are an important part of the infant's diet because they are energy-dense. This characteristic helps resolve the dilemma of high energy needs but small stomach capacity.[15]

Vitamins of special interest

Vitamin K is routinely injected into all infants at birth. This dose lasts until the infant's intestinal bacteria are established and begin to synthesize vitamin K. Formula-fed infants receive the rest of the vitamins they need from the formula. Breast-fed infants, especially dark-skinned ones, may require a vitamin D supplement if they are not exposed to much sunlight. The time needed in the sun is approximately 15 to 30 minutes per day for white infants and longer for those with dark skin. Breast-fed infants whose mothers are total vegetarians (vegans) should receive a vitamin B-12 supplement. Infants who drink goat's milk need supplements of folate and vitamin B-12 because this type of milk lacks these vitamins.

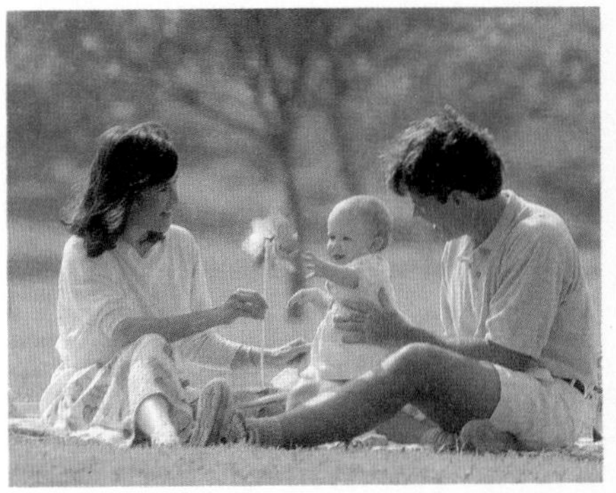

An infant should get some exposure to sunlight to ensure enough vitamin D production.

Minerals of special interest

Iron stores present at birth are generally depleted by the time birth weight doubles, which is around 4 to 6 months of age. Formula-fed infants should use an iron-fortified formula.[18] Breast-fed infants need solid foods to supply extra iron at about 6 months of age. The need for iron is a major consideration in setting the time for solid food introduction. Some researchers recommend liquid iron supplements from birth or by 1 month of age for breast-fed infants.

It is important for an infant to receive adequate amounts of iodide and zinc to support growth. Human milk and formula supply these needs if the infant's energy needs are met. In addition, fluoride supplementation may be needed for the breast-fed infant and for the bottle-fed infant where the water supply used in home formula preparation does not contain fluoride. Note that formula manufacturers use fluoride-free water in formula preparation. Parents should consult their dentist.

Water

An infant needs approximately 1.5 milliliters of water per kcalorie daily. This corresponds to about 2 ounces per pound of body weight. (150 milliliters per kilogram of body weight). The typical consumption of human milk or formula usually meets this need. In hot climates supplemental water may be necessary. In addition, diarrhea, vomiting, and fever also often lead to a need for supplemental water. It is important to remember that an infant is easily dehydrated. Dehydration can result in a rapid decrease in kidney function, and the infant may then require hospitalization for rehydration.

Concept Check

When an infant does not grow properly, this failure to thrive may be due to medical problems or inappropriate feeding practices. Most nutrient needs in the first 6 months are met by human milk or formula. Vitamin D, fluoride, and iron may need to be supplemented for breast-fed infants. Water needs are generally met by the human milk or formula consumed.

Formula-feeding for infants

We discussed breast-feeding in detail in Chapter 15. Let's now focus on formula-feeding. Recall that a major advantage of breast-feeding is providing immune bodies, which impart immune protection to the infant. That advantage is very impor-

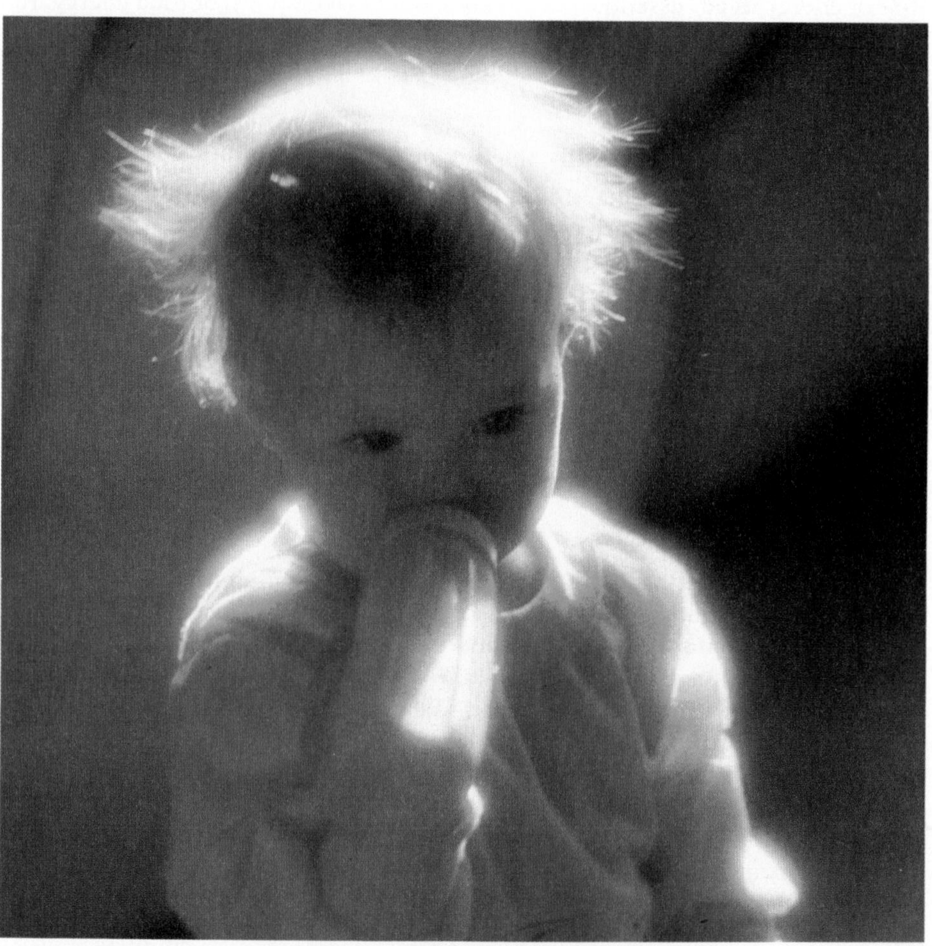

With careful preparation, formula feeding is a safe alternative to breastfeeding.

tant in the context of poverty and poor hygiene. It is less important in affluent North America, where high standards for water purity and cleanliness make formula-feeding a safe alternative for infants.

Formula composition. Cow's milk, because of its high protein and mineral content, cannot be used in early infancy. It must be altered. The altered forms, known as infant formulas, were first available commercially in 1931. Since 1980 they have been required to conform to strict guidelines for nutrient composition and quality set by federal law. They generally contain lactose or sucrose for carbohydrate needs, heat-treated **casein** and **whey** proteins from cow's milk for protein needs, and vegetable oils for fat needs (Table 16-1). Today's formulas are much improved over earlier versions because the new heat-treated casein is easier to digest than the previously used natural forms of casein. Whey proteins are naturally easy to digest, so many formulas are supplemented with extra whey protein.

casein
Proteins found in milk that form curds, and are difficult for infants to digest.

whey
Proteins, such as lactalbumin, that are found in great amounts in human milk, and are easy to digest.

Formulas contain vitamins and minerals in amounts suggested by the guidelines of the American Academy of Pediatrics. We recommend an iron-fortified formula, though some are not iron-fortified. Research shows that added iron does not lead to intestinal complaints, such as constipation, any more than nonfortified formulas do, though some people believe this misconception.[4]

A variety of specialized formulas exist. These vary in energy content; types of protein, carbohydrate, and fat used; and iron fortification. The variations are responses to the special needs of some normal term infants, premature infants, infants with allergies, infants with higher energy needs, and infants with special metabolic problems, such as those with phenylketonuria (see Chapter 6).

Formula preparation. In the 1950s, it was common to prepare a day's supply of bottles and then sterilize them in boiling water for about 30 minutes. Today, it is often more convenient to prepare bottles one at a time. All utensils should be washed before preparing the formula. Concentrated or powdered formulas are poured into a bottle to which clean water is added (follow label directions). The formula is mixed and fed immediately to the infant. Either warm or cold water can be added, depending on preference. Ready-to-feed formula is also available. *Formula for baby foods should not be heated in a microwave oven. Hot spots can develop that may burn the infant's mouth.*

If an infant does not tolerate a standard formula, the protein source is usually switched to soy beans and the carbohydrate to corn syrup or sucrose. If the soy bean-based formula is not tolerated, the next step is to try a predigested (hydrolyzed) protein source, such as Nutramigen or Alimentum.

It is very convenient when using a powdered formula to simply have bottles on hand that have the powder added. These then can be quickly diluted with water and fed to the infant. It is safe to refrigerate diluted formula for a day. However, formula left over from a feeding should be discarded because it will be contaminated by bacteria and enzymes from saliva. If well water is used, it should be boiled before making formula and should also be checked to make sure it is not too high in naturally occurring nitrates, which can bind hemoglobin in the red blood cells and lead to severe anemia.

Whether bottle-feeding or breast-feeding, it is important to burp a baby after about 10 minutes of feeding, or 1 to 2 ounces (30 to 60 milliliters), and at the end of feeding. Spitting up a bit of milk is normal at this time (be prepared). Once fed, the child should be placed on the stomach with the head to one side. If the infant spits up milk, this position will decrease the infant's tendency to inhale the milk and choke.

It is important to stop the feeding when the infant indicates he or she is full. Parents and other caregivers need to develop a sense to detect when the young infant is full, and watch for those cues: turning the head away, inattention, falling asleep, or turning playful. It is best to focus on an infant's appetite rather than the amount of milk left in the bottle. This is not a concern for breast-fed infants, because the mother cannot tell how much milk is left to consume. After about 20 minutes, the baby has probably had enough.

Solid food introduction

The time to introduce solid foods into an infant's diet hinges on a few important factors:

- **Nutritional need**—As noted, iron stores are exhausted by about 6 months of age. Either solid foods or iron supplements are then needed to supply iron if the child is breast-fed or is fed a formula not supplemented with iron. *No nutritional needs besides iron require solid foods before 6 months of age.*
- **Physiological capabilities**—Starch digestion is not very active before 3 months of age. As an infant ages, the ability to digest starch increases. In addition, kidney function is quite limited until about 4 to 6 weeks of age. Until then, waste products from high levels of dietary protein or minerals are difficult to excrete.
- **Physical ability**—Before 3 to 4 months of age, the infant practices tongue thrusting. Generally, the child quickly spits out any solid food put on the tongue. It is about 5 or 6 months before an infant can sit up, turn the head away when full, and control tongue thrusting.
- **Preventing allergies**—During the first 3 months of life, absorption of whole proteins is possible—but undesirable—through the intestinal tract. Whole-protein absorption may set up the child for future allergies, including food allergies. (See Nutrition Perspective 16-1) It is best to minimize the number of different types of foods in a child's diet during these first 3 months to limit chances of developing as allergy.

Table 16-2

One approach for the introduction of semisolid foods and table foods in infancy

Food	Age (Months) 4 to 6	6 to 8	9 to 12
Iron-fortified cereals for infants	Add		
Vegetables		Add strained	Gradually delete strained foods, introduce table foods
Fruits		Add strained	Gradually delete strained foods, introduce chopped well-cooked or canned foods
Meats*		Add strained or finely chopped table meats	Decrease the use of strained meats, increase the varieties of table meats
Finger foods such as arrowroot biscuits, oven-dried toast		Add those that can be grasped	Increase the use of small finger foods as the pincer grasp develops
Well-cooked mashed or chopped table foods, prepared without added salt or sugar			Add
Juice by cup			Add

* These can be added first, if the infant begins solid foods at 4 to 6 months of age. Adapted from: Pipes, PL: Nutrition in infancy and childhood, Times Mirror/Mosby, 1989.

Keeping these considerations in mind—nutritional need, physiological and physical readiness, and allergy prevention—*the American Academy of Pediatrics recommends that solid foods not be introduced until 4 to 6 months of age* (Table 16-2). Before that time it is difficult to get the infant to consume much solid food, anyway. This may lead to force-feeding with a feeder (a giant syringe) or to mixing infant cereal with milk and putting that in a bottle. The inconvenience of these practices alone *should* make one consider whether all the effort is worth it.

Even so, many children are already eating solids by 2 months of age. In a recent study, one half of all black infants were consuming solid foods by 2 months of age, mostly infant cereals.[16] Again, this practice is unnecessary nutritionally, tedious for parents, and possibly dangerous for the infant because it raises the risk of allergies and choking. Young infants can easily be frightened when eating with a spoon and may start crying. If feeding proceeds, the crying infant may then take a deep breath during spoon feeding and inhale that food into its lungs.

Sometimes a rapidly growing infant—one who consumes more than 32 ounces (1 liter) of formula per day—may need solid foods at 4 months of age to meet high energy needs.[15] However, most infants can easily wait until 6 months of age. By that age, the infant is ready for solid food, and feeding is much easier.

Why start solid foods before 4 to 6 months of age?

A common reason offered for introducing solid foods early—before 4 to 6 months of age—is the belief that it helps the infant sleep through the night. However, *many studies have shown that sleeping through the night is a developmental milestone for the infant: it has nothing to do with how much food an infant eats before going to bed.*[4] Infants naturally begin sleeping through the night between the ages of 1 to 3 months. Girls reach this stage before boys.[15] Filling them with cereal is not going to influence that process.

Which solid foods should be fed first?. The first solid foods for infants can be iron-fortified cereals.[15] Some pediatricians may recommend lean ground (strained) meats for a more absorbable forms of iron. If parents wait to 4 to 6 months before introducing solid foods, the type of first food may not be an issue. Before this age, infant cereal is best. Rice cereal is the best cereal to begin with because it is least likely to cause allergies. Although yogurt and cottage cheese are also well tolerated as early foods because of their consistency, they are not good sources of iron. Once a new food has been fed for 7 days without ill effects, another food can be added to the infant's diet. In the early days, this may be another type of cereal or perhaps a cooked and strained (blended) vegetable, meat, fruit, or egg yolk.

Waiting 7 days between each new food is important because it can take that long for signs of an allergy, such as a rash, asthma, or diarrhea, to develop. *It is important not to introduce mixed foods early. If an allergy or intolerance develops, the food component causing it will not be easy to identify.* Thus all components must be fed separately to find out which one is the offender.

It is probably best not to introduce common allergy-causing foods during infancy. These include egg whites, chocolate, nuts, and cow's milk. However, the American Academy of Pediatrics does condone the use of cow's milk in infancy (up to about 24 ounces or about 0.75 liters daily) if the child is consuming at least one third of total energy from solid food. This is usually the case by about 8 to 9 months of age.

A variety of strained foods is available for infant feeding. Parents should read prepared baby food labels if they are concerned about sugar or salt in the infant's diet. Single-food items are more desirable than mixed dinners and desserts, which are less nutrient dense. Most brands have no added salt, but some fruit desserts have a lot of added sugar. Alternately, one can simply grind plain foods from the table—vegetables, fruits or meats (no seasoning added)—in an inexpensive plastic baby food grinder/mill, and feed the food to the infant. Another option is to blender large amounts of food, freeze and store it as ice cubes in plastic bags, and then defrost and warm as needed. *Infant foods made at home do not need extra salt or sweeteners. The infant does not taste the difference. Introduction of a variety of foods should occur throughout this period so that by the end of the first year the infant is consuming a variety of foods listed in the Daily Food Guide.*[15]

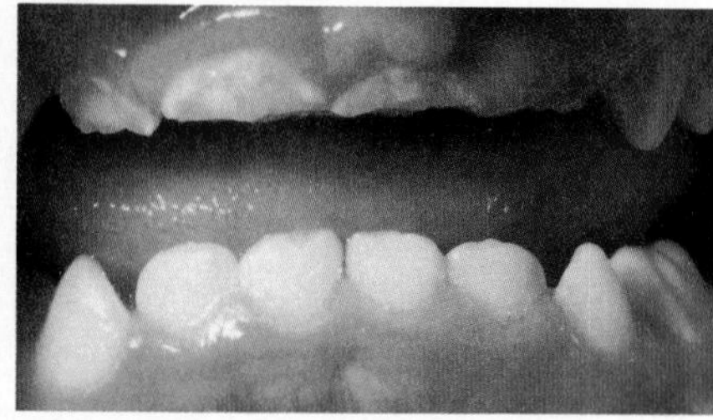

Nursing bottle syndrome—an extreme example of tooth decay. This child was probably often put to bed with a bottle. The upper teeth have decayed almost all the way to the gum line.

Juices and liquids other than water and formula are best given in a cup. Juices fed from a bottle may cause "nursing bottle syndrome." As an infant toys with a bottle, the carbohydrate-rich fluid bathes the teeth, providing an ideal growth media for bacteria. Bacteria on the teeth then make acids from the carbohydrate, and the acids dissolve tooth structure. In addition, an infant should not be put to bed with a bottle or placed in an infant seat with a bottle propped up for him. As the child lies in bed, fluid (even milk) pools around the teeth, increasing the likelihood of dental caries.

In the early months of solid food introduction, it is quite a challenge just to get the food into the infant, as opposed to on and around the child. Self-feeding skills require coordination and practice and are slow to develop. Also by 9 to 10 months of age, the infant's desire to explore, experience, and play with food further hinders feeding. It is best to relax and take this phase of infant development in stride. Sloppy, friendly mealtimes actually can make good memories about one's infant—who too quickly develops into a toddler.

By the end of the first year, finger-feeding becomes more efficient, drinking from a cup improves, and chewing is easier as more teeth erupt. The child's eating becomes neater, but experimentation and a lack of predictability still rule the day.[18]

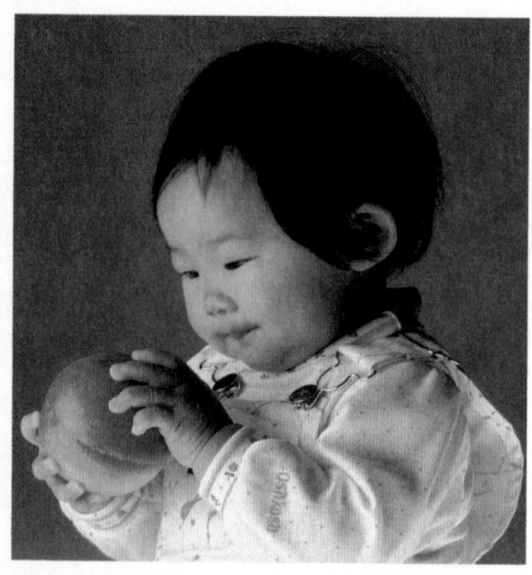

By the end of the first year self-feeding comes much easier.

What not to feed an infant

Several foods and practices to avoid when feeding an infant are:

- **Honey and corn syrup**—These products may contain spores of *Clostridium botulinum.* The spores can eventually develop into bacteria in the stomach and lead to botulism food poisoning, which is often fatal in children under 1 year old (see Chapter 19).
- **Overly salty and overly sweet foods**—Infants do not need a lot of sugar or salt added to their foods. They enjoy bland foods, much blander than do adults.
- **Feeding more than 40 ounces (1.2 liters) of formula or 32 ounces (1 liter) of milk per day**—Solid foods should play a greater role in satisfying an infant's increased appetite after 6 to 8 months of age. About 24 to 32 ounces (¾ to 1 liter) of human milk or formula per day is ideal after 6 months of age, with food supplying the rest of energy needs. This is mainly because foods can contain much iron, whereas human milk, cow's milk, and low-iron formulas do not.
- **Certain foods that tend to cause choking**—These foods include hot dogs (unless finely cut into sticks, not coin shapes), candy, nuts, grapes, coarsely cut meats, raw carrots, and popcorn.
- **Low-fat or nonfat cow's milk**—After 2 years of age, children can use 2% or 1% fat milk because they are then consuming enough solid foods to meet energy needs. The use of low-fat milk in infancy would yield too many minerals as the infant attempts to meet its energy needs. This would overtax the kidneys. Cow's milk is approximately 3 times higher in protein and minerals than human milk.

- **Excessive apple or pear juice**—The sorbitol contained in these juices can lead to diarrhea because sorbitol is a poorly absorbed sugar alcohol (see Chapter 4).

Will infants instinctively eat a diet that meets their nutritional needs?

In the 1920s, Dr. Clara Davis investigated this question. She studied a small number of infants and allowed them to choose their own diet from a number of foods, such as milk, eggs, bananas, apples, oranges, and oatmeal. Her work showed that, given a variety of nutritious food choices, infants could choose a healthy diet. She also showed that solid foods were well digested during the ages of 6 months to 1 year. At the turn of the century, it was common to wait at least a full year before feeding solid foods to infants.

Other investigators misinterpreted that research, stating that "infants naturally knew what foods to eat." It is probably better stated that *given nutritious food choices, infants instinctively chose a balance of foods to meet their needs.*[26] We do not know if an infant would act like a mouse or a rat when faced with doughnuts, cookies, cake, and ice cream and gobble them up. Recall from Chapter 8 that when given these food options, rats and mice quickly become obese.

Concept Check

Infant formulas generally contain lactose or sucrose, heat-treated casein and whey proteins from cow's milk, and vegetable oil. Formulas may or may not be fortified with iron. Sanitation is very important in preparing and storing formula. Solid food should not be added to an infant's diet until the child is ready for solid food, which is usually between 4 and 6 months of age. The first solid food given can be iron-fortified infant cereals with very gradual additions of other foods, one at a time each week. Some foods to avoid giving infants in the first year include honey, low-fat cow's milk, overly salty or sweet foods, and foods that may cause choking.

NUTRITION-RELATED PROBLEMS IN INFANCY

Parents, other caregivers, and clinicians should be aware of a variety of potential problems related to infant nutrition.

Possible feeding problems

Feeding problems to watch out for in infancy include:

- Insufficient iron in the diet.
- Avoidance of an entire food group.
- Use of raw cow's or goat's milk. Raw cow's milk raises the possibility of viral and bacterial contamination (see Chapter 19). Goat's milk is low in folate and vitamin B-12.
- No progression to using a cup by 1 year of age.
- Bottle- feeding past 18 months of age.
- Supplemental vitamin use beyond 150% of an infant's or child's U.S. RDA.

Colic

There is a lot we don't know about **colic.** It appears to be caused by a painful building of gas in the gastrointestinal (GI) tract. A child typically cries during episodes of colic. However, episodic crying during the first 3 months is not uncommon and is not always related to feeding. Infant nervous systems are immature, and fussy periods may reflect this or may merely be a means of dissipating tension and energy.

colic
Periodic crying in a healthy infant, apparently due to GI gas buildup.

A recent study showed that the best way for parents to minimize colic-related problems was to learn how to respond to an infant's cries. Infants cry when they are wet, cold, hungry, or lonely (need to be held) and when they want to suckle. When parents appropriately read an infant's cries and responded to her needs, the total amount of crying time was reduced, even when the infant experienced colic. Determining the cause of an infant's crying succeeded better than switching from cow's-milk, protein-based formula to a soy-based one.[28]

Positioning a colicky baby upright during feeding allows him to more easily expel trapped air by burping. In addition, the infant should be burped regularly during feeding, and fed for not more than 30 minutes. As a child suckles longer and longer at the bottle or the breast, he takes in additional air.

Diarrhea

Diarrhea results from various causes in infancy, including bacterial and viral infections. In the United States, about 500 infants per year die of simple dehydration resulting from diarrhea. To prevent dehydration, infants with diarrhea should be given plenty of fluids. Specialized fluids, such as Pedialyte, are available. This contains glucose, sodium, potassium, chloride, and water. It is best to have a pediatrician's recommendations concerning fluid replacement.

Diarrhea is less common with breast-fed infants. The natural immunity provided by human milk reduces the risk of developing diarrheal disease.

Once diarrhea subsides, a bottle-fed infant may be switched to a soy-based, lactose-free formula for 2 weeks. This allows time for the lactase enzyme to again reach a high enough production rate in the intestine to digest the large amount of lactose found in a typical formula.

Milk allergy

Over 25 proteins in milk can lead to allergies. Some of these are **heat-labile** and so are inactivated sufficiently by scalding milk. However, some proteins are very heat stable. A "true" milk allergy is actually quite rare and develops in less than 1% of formula-fed infants. However, many infants are switched to soy-based formulas in an attempt to decrease their crying and spitting up. Just because a child thrives better on a soy-based formula does not mean he has a true milk allergy (see Nutrition Perspective 16-1 to learn more about what causes allergies).

Iron-deficiency anemia

Iron-deficiency anemia typically occurs in infants who consume few solid foods and whose diets are dominated by cow's milk, which has little iron.[18] Iron stores are then quickly depleted by the daily demand for the synthesis of new red blood cells. To prevent iron deficiency anemia, it is best to start an infant at about 6 months of age on iron-fortified cereals and meats and limit formula or cow's milk to 16 to 25 ounces (500 to 750 milliliters) per day. The infant *should* also avoid cow's milk for the first year of life because it tends to cause intestinal bleeding, especially before 3 months of age. If anemia does develop, medicinal iron supplements are advised. Infants are given about 1 milligram of iron per kilogram of body weight per day under a physician's guidance.

The premature infant

The premature infant is fed either a specially designed formula or human milk. As noted in Chapter 15, nutrients may be added to human milk to increase its protein, mineral, and energy content. Two amino acids not normally needed in the diet—tyrosine and cysteine—may be essential amino acids for the premature infant. In addition, some vitamins—such as vitamin E—and vitamin-like compounds—such as taurine and carnitine—may be helpful additions to this infant's diet (see Chapters 11 and 12).

Because many bacteria require iron to thrive, iron supplementation may be delayed for the premature infant to limit the tendency for bacterial infections (see Chapter 14). The premature infant must be fed immediately because he has little fat or glycogen storage. Body composition of the full-term infant includes about 12% fat, while the composition of the premature infant may include only about 2% fat, depending on gestational age.

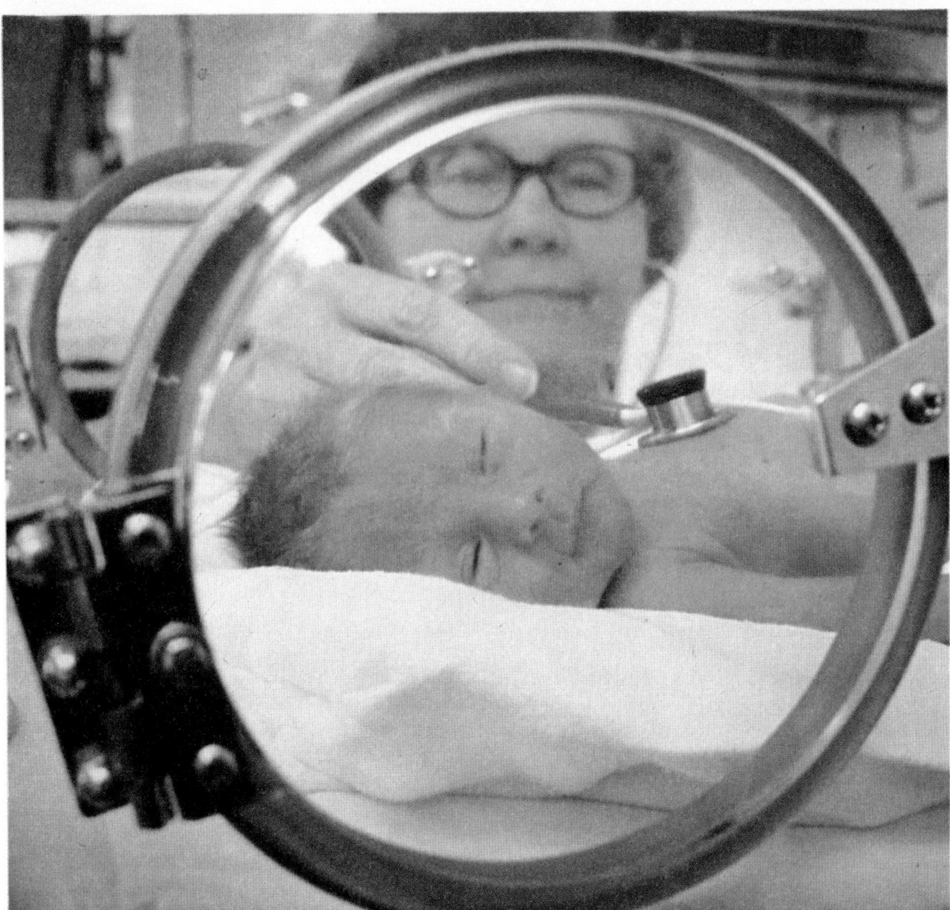

Premature infants need special nutritional care.

Obesity in infancy

Infant obesity does not necessarily result in childhood obesity, so parents need not worry about it too much. But if an infant is over the ninetieth percentile weight for length and is still gaining weight—it is time to reevaluate the infant's diet and activity patterns. A quick dietary assessment can detect if the infant is consuming about 105 to 115 kcalories per kilogram of body weight per day, the amount recommended for an infant.

The infant can be encouraged to crawl and climb more often, and parents might decrease confinement in playpens and walkers. If the infant tends to cry for a bottle, water can be given. It may also be time to switch from a bottle to a cup. Finally, if this infant is still less than 6 months old, decreasing the use of solid foods (if already given) is a good idea. Severe restriction of food or milk is not desirable. Instead, the infant's height should be allowed to catch up to his or her present weight.

The overall goal is to moderate weight gain so that the infant is satisfied and yet remains below the 95th percentile of weight-for-height. See Nutrition Perspective 16-2, "Obesity in the Growing Years" for a more detailed discussion of this problem.

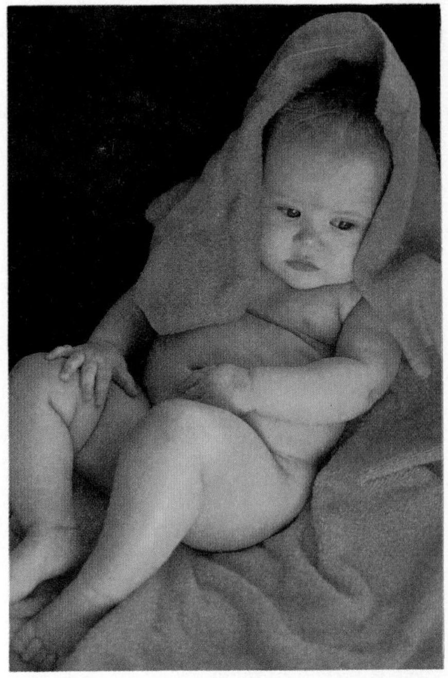

Obesity in infancy often does not result in obesity in childhood.

Dietary guidelines for infant feeding

In response to various controversies surrounding infant feeding, experts have written dietary guidelines for infants.[15]

- Build to a variety of foods.
- Listen to your baby's appetite to avoid over-feeding or under-feeding.

- Don't restrict fat and cholesterol too much.
- Don't overdo high-fiber foods.
- Sugar is OK, but in moderation.
- Sodium is OK, but in moderation.
- Babies need more iron, pound for pound, than adults.

These guidelines have been accepted by the American Academy of Pediatrics and the American Dietetic Association. The recommendations in this chapter are also consistent with these guidelines. In essence, the evidence supporting a positive effect of dietary restrictions during infancy is equivocal, while the hazards of this approach are well documented.

Concept Check

Colic appears to be caused by gas buildup in the GI tract, and may be reduced by regular burping during feeding. Switching formulas is rarely needed to treat colic. Diarrhea requires additional fluids to prevent dehydration. Allergy to milk proteins is rare, but may require switching to soy-based formula. Introducing iron-containing solid foods at an appropriate time and avoiding cow's milk can generally prevent iron deficiency anemia in infancy. Infant obesity does not necessarily result in adult obesity, but unnecessary use of solid foods in the diet can be decreased and an infant can be encouraged toward increased activity.

CHILDHOOD

The rapid growth rate of infancy quickly tapers during the next few years. The average weight gain is only 5 pounds during the second year of life (Figure 16-1). The toddler shows conformational changes however the percentage of body water and fat decreases, while the percentage of lean tissue increases.[14]

As a toddler's growth rate tapers, food habits may change, and feeding problems can appear. One major cause of potential feeding problems stems from the slower growth and accompanying decrease in appetite that characterizes the preschool years. *Preschoolers normally have less hunger than they did as infants.*

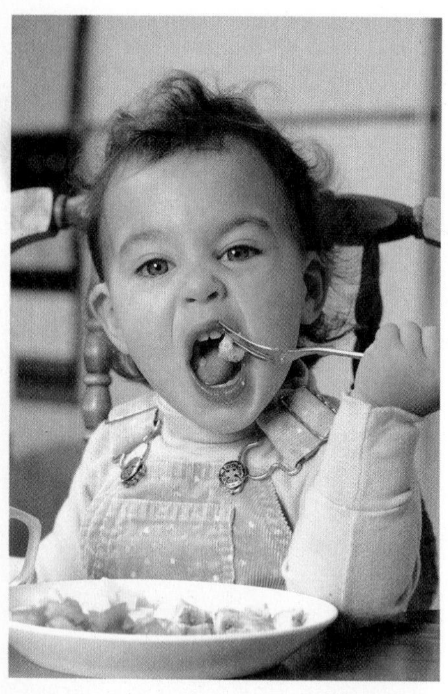

Within reason, toddlers will often eat whatever is served to them.

One nutritional challenge at this age is to adapt food choices to the new growth rate. When little food is consumed, the nutrient density of each food choice should be carefully considered. This usually means watching fat intake while increasing intake of whole grains and vegetables. There is no need to decrease fat intake severely, but fatty food choices should not overwhelm more nutritious ones.

Surprisingly, children eat what they are exposed to. At this age, children can eat a well-rounded and healthy diet if one is served to them. If offered whole-grain breakfast cereals, whole-wheat bread, vegetables, salad, and fresh fruits regularly, young children accept most of these foods and eat them. Only a lack of imagination limits—and possibly deprives—a child's diet.

The preschool years are the best time for a child to start a healthful pattern of living and eating. Self-esteem and successful eating are closely tied. *Parents and other caregivers are role models: if they eat a variety of foods, the children will eat a variety of foods. A good policy is the "1- bite" policy: children should take at least 1 bite of the foods presented to them.* For snacks, parents should decide the options. Children should then be allowed to choose; responsibility for food choice should start early.

How to help a child choose nutritious foods

One way adults can encourage young children to eat nutritiously well-balanced meals is to repeat exposure to new foods. If a child sees a food over and over again, there is a good chance it will be accepted eventually, especially if adults and older children are seen eating the food and enjoying it. Above all, one needs to feed the preschool child affectionately. This is a time for children to experience new foods. It is also a time for them to develop their own likes and dislikes.

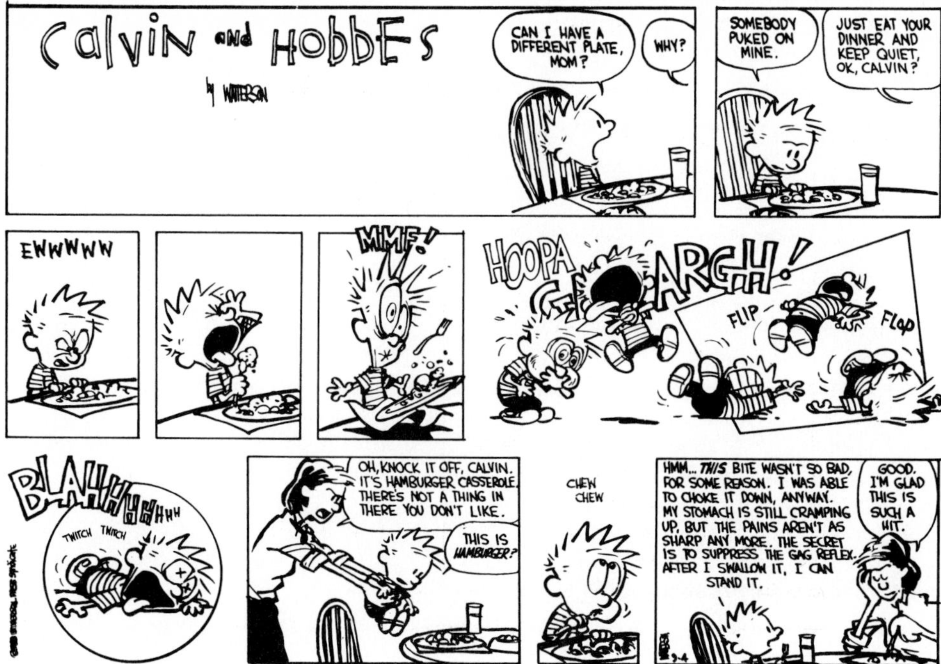

Figure 16-3

Preschool children are very unpredictable. Be ready for setbacks. If adults can be patient and persevere, children eventually build good food habits (Figure 16-3).

Perseverance is critical because it takes quite a commitment to introduce children to a variety of foods. If left to their own devices, preschool children would find a few foods they like and eat them every day. *But by constantly being introduced to new foods, children this age can expand their nutritional choices, develop an experimental approach, and learn to tolerate a variety of foods.*

Research shows that children like certain foods, especially those with crisp textures and mild flavors, and familiar foods. Young children are especially sensitive to and reject hot-temperature foods.

If children see good table manners, they more readily learn good table manners. Using good table manners leads to harmony and a positive environment for learning good nutrition habits. Preschoolers eventually develop skill with spoons and forks and can even use dull knives. But it is also a good idea to allow some finger foods.

Childhood feeding problems

Tensions between parents, or between parents and children, often contribute to eating problems. Getting to the root of family problems and creating a more harmonious family atmosphere is an important part of resolving many childhood feeding problems. In addition, parents must often be educated to know what to expect of a preschool child and what goals to set. Following are a few typical problems, their causes, and suggestions for correcting the problem.

"My child won't eat as much, or as regularly, as he did as an infant." This is to be expected. The growth rate slows from that of infancy, so the child does not need as much food. Parents must often be reminded that they shouldn't expect a 3-year-old to eat as voraciously as an infant, nor to eat adult- sized portions (Table 16-3). In addition, appetite varies depending on a child's activity level and how the child feels—whether well or sick.

Parents should also be reminded that food likes and dislikes change rapidly in childhood and are influenced by food temperature, appearance, texture, and taste. Children usually prefer mild flavors, but there are exceptions to this rule.[20]

Battling with a child to get him to eat more is rarely worth the effort.[21] There is little reason to beg or bribe a child to eat. Parents should present the food, eat it themselves, and let their child decide. In addition, they should recognize that

Table 16-3

Daily food guide for children.

Foods included in this group are:	1 year	2-3 years	4-5 years
	Serving sizes*		
Milk and cheese			
4 servings daily in the amounts recommended from a variety of foods listed in this group:			
Milk, yogurt, and milkbase soups	¼-½ cups	½-¾ cup	¾ cup
Cottage cheese	2-4 tablespoons	4-6 tablespoons	6 tablespoons
custard, milk pudding, and ice cream (served only after a meal)			
Cheese (1 oz = 1 slice or a 1″ cube) (limit due to saturated fat)	⅓-⅔ ounces	⅔-1 ounces	1 ounce
Meat, poultry, fish, and beans			
4 servings daily in the amounts recommended from a variety of foods listed in this group:			
Beef, pork, lamb, veal, and fish	1 ounce	1 ½ ounces	4 tablespoons or 2 ounces
Eggs	½	¾	1
Peanut butter	2 tablespoons	3 tablespoons	3 tablespoons
Cooked legumes, dried beans, or peas	¼ cups	⅜ cup	½ cup
Nuts	†	†	†
Fruits and vegetables			
4 servings daily in the amounts recommended from a variety of foods listed in this group:			
citrus fruits, berries, melons, tomatoes peppers, cabbage, cauliflower, broccoli, and chilies	¼ cups	¼ cup	¼ cup
Melons, peaches, apricots, carrots, spinach, broccoli, orange squash, pumpkin, sweet potatoes, peas, beans (green, yellow and lima) and Brussels sprouts	1-2 tablespoons	3-4 tablespoons	4-5 tablespoons
Other	⅛ cup	¼ cup	½ cup
Other	1-2 tablespoons	3-4 tablespoons	4-5 tablespoons
Breads and cereals			
4 servings daily in the amounts recommended from a variety of foods listed in this group:			
Whole grain or enriched breads	½ slice	¾ slice	¾-1 slice
Cooked cereals, rice and pasta	¼ cup	⅓ cup	½ cup
Whole-grain or fortified ready-to-eat cereals	½ ounce	¾ ounce	1 ounce
Fats/oils			
Margarine, oils, mayonnaise and salad dressings	1 teaspoon	1 teaspoon	1 teaspoon
Other foods			
Jams, jellies, soft drinks, candy, sweet desserts, salty snacks, gravies, pickles and catsup		USE IN MODERATION	

* Basically 1 tablespoon per year of age; up to ½ cup (or 2 oz for meat or meat alternatives)
† not recommended for children under 5 years of age because they can cause choking

Adapted from Endres J and Rockwell R: Food, nutrition and the young child, St. Louis, 1980, C.V. Mosby Co.

this is an important age for children to explore the world around them. *Even "good" eaters are sometimes more interested in exploring than in a meal.*

"My child is always snacking, yet she never finishes her meal." Children have small stomachs. Offering many small meals succeeds better than limiting children to 3 meals per day. Actually, 3 meals per day is just a social custom. There is nothing nutritionally important about that type of plan. Snacking is fine as long as good dental care is practiced. *It is really not when one eats, but what one eats, that is important.* Nutritious snacks should be readily available (see Table 16-4). Then, when the child becomes hungry in mid-morning or mid-afternoon, there are good foods to offer.

Table 16-4

Serving Nutritious Snacks and Beverages

Snack suggestions:	
Fresh raw vegetables	Serve with a dip of cottage cheese or yogurt blended with dried buttermilk dressing
Celery	Spread with peanut butter and sprinkle on raisins, shredded carrots or nuts finely chopped
Bananas	Dip in sweetened yogurt or spread with peanut butter and roll in coconut, chopped nuts or granola
Sliced apples or crackers	Serve with a dip of peanut butter, honey, nuts, raisins and coconut mixed together
Bagels	Spread with cream cheese or peanut butter and top with chopped bananas, crushed pineapple or shredded carrots
Quick bread or muffins	Make with carrots, zucchini, pumpkin, bananas, nuts, dates, raisins, lemons, squash, and berries
Flour tortillas	Spread with refried beans or canned chili, sprinkle with grated cheese and broil; top with chili sauce
Ready-to-eat cereals	Use brands low in sugar and containing fiber. Serve with raisins.
Pita loaf	Place sliced meat, cheese, lettuce and tomato in open pocket
English muffins or pita bread	Top with spaghetti sauce, grated cheese and meats; broil or bake and cut in fourths
Potato skins	Sprinkle with shredded cheese, broil and top with yogurt and bacon bits
Canned chili	Heat and top with onions, lettuce and tomato; use as dip for Italian or French bread, biscuits or corn bread
Kabobs	Make with any combination of the following: fruit, vegetables and sliced or cubed cooked meat (remove toothpicks before serving)
Popcorn	Serve plain or make three quarts and sprinkle with ¼ c grated cheese and ½ t garlic or onion salt
Parfait	Make with yogurt, fruit and granola
Gelatin	Add fruit or vegetable juice, vegetables, fruits, or cottage cheese
Frozen fruit cubes	Freeze pureed applesauce or fruit juice into cubes
Fruit fizz	Add club soda to juice instead of serving soft drinks
Fruit shake	Blend milk with fresh fruit (bananas, berries or a peach) and a dash of cinnamon or nutmeg
Yogurt frost	Combine fruit juice and yogurt; add fresh fruit if desired
Hot chocolate	Make hot chocolate or cocoa with milk chocolate and a dash of cinnamon
Seeds	Shelled sunflower seeds

From: A food guide for the first five years, National Meat and Livestock Board/444 North Michigan Avenue/Chicago, ILL 60611.

"My child never eats his vegetables." Everyone dislikes certain foods. Again, the "1- bite" policy can be encouraged and guidelines can be set to discourage fussing over unfamiliar foods. Children eventually learn that they can eat foods they don't particularly like without first gagging, choking, and yelling "Oh gross!" It takes time for a child to become enthusiastic about a new food, but with continual exposure and a positive role model, chances are the child may even grow to like it.

Hunger is still the best sauce. It may work to feed a child vegetables at the start of a meal, when he is hungriest. Offer new foods with familiar ones. A platter of raw or blanched (lightly cooked to soften) carrots, broccoli, green and red peppers, cabbage, and mushrooms eaten as a snack with friends can do a lot to remedy a vegetable problem. Nutritious dips sell vegetables to many children. Using heroes as role models may be an effective tool. Finally, letting a child help prepare vegetables may increase their appeal (Figure 16-4). When a child reaches the age at which he can safely handle raw vegetables without fear of choking (about 4 or 5 years), offer thin carrot sticks or broccoli flowers as an option to cooked ones. The child may find the taste and texture more pleasing.

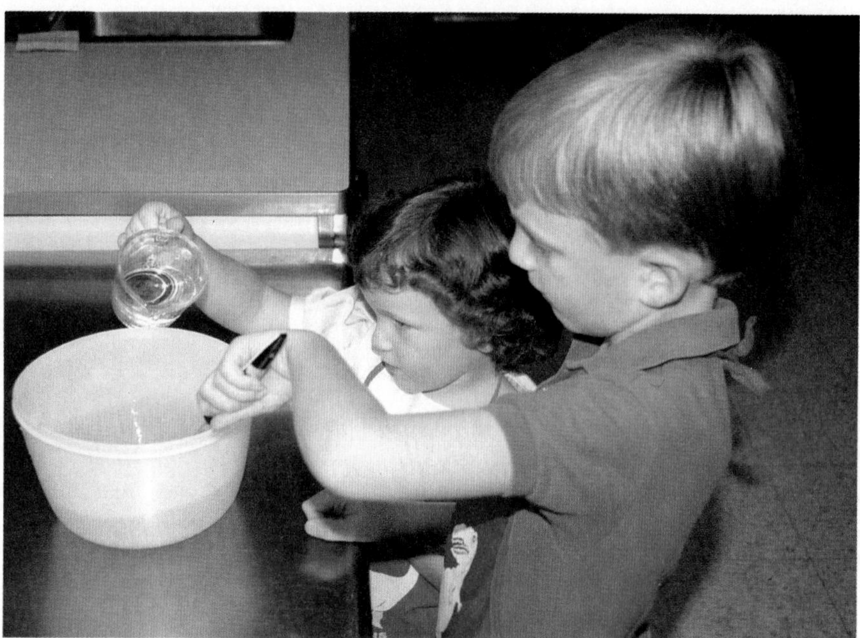

Figure 16-4
Parents can involve children in meal preparation. This helps children develop an interest in new foods.

"How do I know if my child is eating healthfully?" The Daily Food Guide listed in Table 16-3 forms the basis for a healthy diet in childhood. If a child eats from those food groups and shows regular increments in height and weight, that is evidence of a good diet. Some nutrients that deserve special attention during childhood are calcium, iron, and vitamins A, B-6, and C.[11] These nutrients need not be deficient in a child's diet if it includes foods from all the food groups—milk and cheese group; meat, poultry, fish, and beans group; fruits and vegetables group; and breads and cereals group.

Major scientific groups, such as the American Dietetic Association and the American Society for Clinical Nutrition, believe that giving vitamin and mineral supplements is unnecessary for healthy children (see Chapter 11).[2] It is better to focus on good foods, rather than on nutrient supplements. However, a nutrient supplement at the RDA level may be needed when a child is ill, especially if the illness is prolonged. If the child is a total vegetarian, special consideration should be given to the intake of protein, vitamin B-12, iron, and zinc.

Exploring Issues and Actions

Think back about your childhood and your food likes and dislikes. What particular memories pop up? How do your early food habits relate to your food habits today?

Nutritional problems in childhood

The two most common nutritional problems in childhood are obesity and iron-deficiency anemia. Childhood obesity is the focus for Nutrition Perspectives 16-2, "Obesity in the Growing Years."

Iron-deficiency anemia

Childhood iron deficiency anemia is most likely to occur in children between 6 and 24 months of age. It can lead to poor stamina and learning ability because the oxygen supply to cells is decreased. However, the incidence of childhood anemia is decreasing. In 1970, about 12% of children ages 18 to 23 months were diagnosed anemic in the United States. In 1984, the figure had dropped to 4%. Probably this decrease is due to the increased use of iron-fortified formulas and increased iron fortification of breakfast cereals that began in the early 1970s.[29] In addition, the Supplemental Food Program for Women, Infant, and Children (WIC) Program sponsored by the federal government, which also began in the early 1970s emphasizes the importance of iron-fortified formulas and cereals and distributes these items to infants and preschool children.

Prevention of iron-deficiency anemia in children should center on regular consumption of adequate sources of iron. Iron-fortified breakfast cereals and a few ounces of lean meat are convenient means for incorporating more iron into a child's diet. The high proportion of heme-iron in many animal foods allows it to be more readily absorbed than iron from plant foods. In addition, consuming a vitamin C source with any plant or supplemental source of iron aids absorption (see Chapter 14).

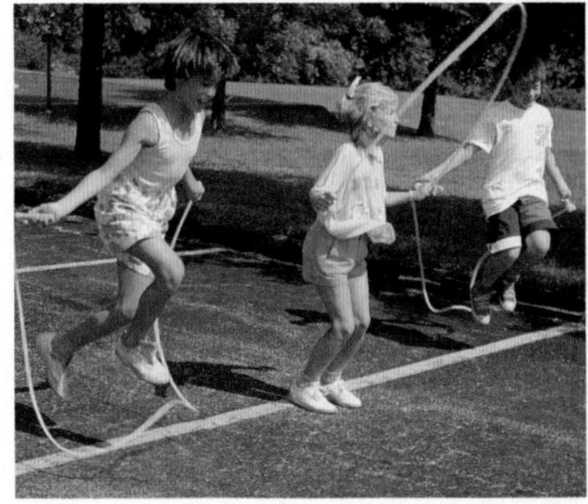

Girls grow rapidly between the ages of 10 and 13.

Is childhood the time to start a diet designed to limit the risk for heart disease?

Parents may wonder whether it is important to limit children's cholesterol and fat intake to minimize future risk of heart disease. The American Academy of Pediatrics does not recommend low-fat diets for young children.[8] It does recommend screening children for blood cholesterol levels in families in which early heart disease is common, and then treating children with high blood cholesterol levels with appropriate diet and drug therapy (see Chapter 5).

Although there may be no reason to put children on low-fat diets at this time, parents can introduce "heart-healthy" habits by limiting a child's exposure to saturated fats. Heart disease appears to start in childhood. Autopsies of young military men who died in Korea and Vietnam showed the early signs of plaque buildup in their blood vessels. It is best to encourage foods that have a higher proportion of monounsaturated and polyunsaturated fat. Moderation is the best strategy: overly restrictive diets can be detrimental to overall growth. The child needs to consume enough energy while also building good health habits that can be practiced into the teen years. One strategy is to have them consume milk that is 2% or 1% fat after 2 years of age and to limit the intake of high-fat cheese and butter.

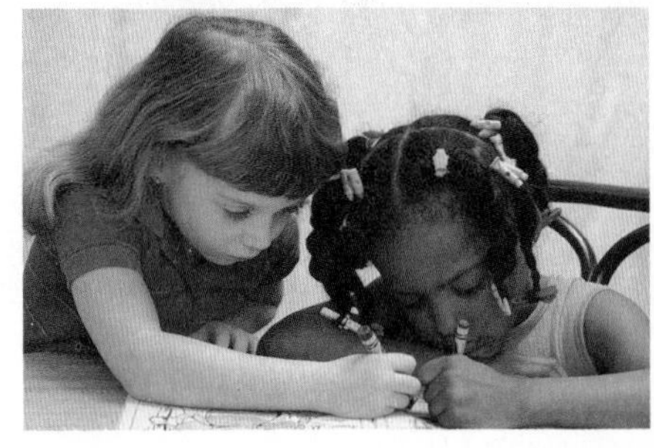

School-age children should have a healthy breakfast to help them perform well in school.

How about low-sodium diets for children?

Scientific data neither confirm nor refute that a reduction in sodium intake reduces the risk of future high blood pressure. Moderation in sodium consumption does help build good health habits for the future—especially if the person later develops hypertension, and needs to control sodium intake even more.

The importance of breakfast

Many school-age children skip breakfast. This may reduce their attention span and performance during school, as well as performance in sports. Breakfast provides children fuel for the morning hours and helps rebuild glycogen stores de-

Expert Opinion

Helping Children to Eat Well

ELLYN SATTER, M.S., R.D.

Parents want their children to eat well and be healthy. They worry that their children eat too much—or too little—or won't eat their vegetables or drink their milk. They feel guilty and responsible when children leave the table without eating—and angry when they come back 10 minutes later wanting a snack.

In some families, the dinner table becomes a battleground. Parents turn into reluctant food hustlers, insisting that children eat a regulation "four bites of broccoli before you can have dessert." Children gag. Adults feel pity. They know as one sensitive mother observed, that "when you don't want to eat something, it feels as if it grows in your mouth." Nonetheless, this perceptive mother feels obligated to insist that her son eat his vegetables.

How many bites of broccoli *does* it take to earn dessert? How do you get yourself out of the position where you have to make such ridiculous rules?

RESPECT THE CHILD'S CAPABILITY

Children have built-in motivators to eat. They get hungry, they are interested in eating, they have hearty appetites for good food, and they are interested in survival. But the way they operate with eating can fool you.

Children are wary of new food. Studies by child psychologist LL Birch at the University of Illinois indicate that children are *neophobic* about food: if it's new, they don't like it.

But children work to master new foods and new eating skills in the same way that they work to master other skills. Birch found that children *do* learn to like new foods. They see new foods, taste them (as many as 15 or 20 times), and eventually learn to like them. Keep in mind that a taste is just a *taste* and not a *swallow.* Toddlers put foods into their mouths, sample them for flavor and texture, and take them out again.

Unfortunately, to adults, these attempts at mastery look very much like rejection. While children are learning to like the new foods, the adults get anxious and try to hurry them along. It doesn't work. Bribing backfires: Birch found that preschoolers who were rewarded for eating a new food were less likely to go back to it later than were preschoolers who were allowed to approach the food on their own. In addition, food rewards produce a negative side effect: children who get dessert for eating their vegetables learn to like the dessert more and the vegetables less. Giving a reward for eating a new food is not a good idea: it gives the child the clearest of messages that you don't expect her to learn to like the new food. So she won't.

Some parents try to pressure children into trying new foods. Pressure tactics might get children to eat, but these methods won't teach long-term eating skills. As soon as the pressure is off, children revert to eating the foods they like.

It's important for adults to find that delicate balance between being helpful and supportive and being controlling. Children do need adults to help them with their eating. But what helps the most is just being there with your child while he or she eats. Children can do more and dare more when a supportive adult is nearby.

Children naturally eat a variety of foods. An internal process called *sensory specific satiety* ensures that they will tire of even favorite foods and eat something different. Adults have the same tendency, but they ignore it. They override their appetites and eat because the food is good for them, or because they paid for it, or to keep from getting hungry later.

Children know *how much* they need to eat. They respond to their internal sense of hunger and fullness more strongly than adults do, and they eat the right amount of foods for proper growth. Unlike most adults, they stop when they are

Expert Opinion—cont'd

full rather than when the food is gone. Their food intake fluctuates considerably from meal to meal and day to day. This is alarming to parents, who often try to train this sensitivity out of their children by encouraging them to eat past satiety or restraining them when they eat heavily.

Whether these tactics succeed depends on the determination of the parent—and the child. Some children submit to parental controls. Others fight back. Children whose parents attempt to overfeed them may be revolted by food and may tend to undereat when they get the chance. Children whose parents attempt to underfeed them may become preoccupied with food and then overeat when they get the chance.

Attempts at underfeeding often grow out of parents' or health professionals' concerns about obesity. Vehement tactics for obesity prevention are unnecessary and may cause the very problem they are intended to prevent. In a 16-year longitudinal study in the San Francisco Bay area, Dr. L. Shapiro and colleagues found that the obese infant or toddler does not have an increased risk of obesity in later life. But parents' attempts to restrict a child's food intake can increase a child's risk of later obesity, if, as is highly likely, those tactics lead to problematic eating. Shapiro's study found that early eating problems are associated with increased risk of obesity in later life. Psychologists at Duke University found that obese freshman women have a consistent pattern of restrained feeding early in life. They also found that parents are more sensitive to fatness in their daughters than in their sons. They are inclined to struggle with their daughters about eating but indulge their sons.

PROVIDE APPROPRIATE SUPPORT

So what's a parent to do? They can only provide a variety of attractive, wholesome foods in pleasant surroundings and approach feeding in a positive way. One can't force children to eat.

Maintaining structure is important. Children eat best and are more likely to learn to like a variety of foods if they have regular meals and snacks at predictable times and aren't allowed to panhandle between times. Consistent eating times help children to come to the table hungry and, therefore, more likely to accept the food.

Don't limit the menu to foods the child readily accepts, and don't be a short-order cook. Prepare a variety of foods: a main dish, a fruit or vegetable, and a starchy food such as potato or rice. Also serve milk and bread. Then let the child pick and choose from what's available.

Let the child learn from mistakes. If a toddler gets down from the table having eaten nothing and comes around 5 minutes later begging for a cookie, tell him, "Nothing until snack time." He may feel frustrated, but if you hold firm, the next time he may take his meal more seriously.

MAINTAIN A DIVISION OF RESPONSIBILITY IN FEEDING

It all boils down to what I call a "division of responsibility in feeding." The parents are responsible for what their child is offered to eat and for setting up a pleasant eating environment. The child is responsible for deciding how much or even whether he eats. Children master their eating when adults provide opportunities to learn, give support for exploration, and limit inappropriate behavior.

But kids have their own ways of learning—and eating—so over the short term, it can *look* as if they are doing poorly. But children *will* eat, and they *will* learn to like a variety of foods, and they *will* grow appropriately. Just don't hold your breath.

Ellyn Satter, M.S., R.D., A.C.S.W., is a family therapist and specialist in eating disorders at Family Therapy Center of Madison, Wisconsin. The information in this article was taken from her new book, How to Get Your Kid to Eat...But Not Too Much, Palo Alto, CA 1987, Bull Publishing Co.

pleted during the night's fast. *Children should be encouraged to find foods they like to eat for breakfast.* These do not have to be traditional foods. Instead, they might be pizza, spaghetti, soups, yogurt with trail mix on top, chili, sandwiches, and shish kebab. Food composition, not social tradition, is the key.

Concept Check

The rapid growth rate of the first year of life slows during the toddler and preschool years. Appetite decreases, necessitating selection of nutrient-dense foods. Adults should select the foods served, but allow the child to decide the amount to eat. Snacking is appropriate if there is careful selection of foods and attention to dental hygiene. Vitamin and mineral supplementation is usually not needed. In childhood, prevention of iron-deficiency anemia should center on regular consumption of good sources of iron. Developing "heart-healthy" habits at this age is good health insurance.

THE TEENAGE YEARS

A rapid growth spurt begins in most girls between the ages of 10 and 13 years, and in most boys between the ages of 12 and 15 years. These growth spurts last about 3 years. Early maturing girls may begin their growth spurt as early as 7 to 8 years of age, while early maturing boys may begin it by 9 to 10 years of age. During this growth spurt, girls gain about 10 inches (25 centimeters) in height and boys gain about 12 inches (30 centimeters). Girls also tend to lay down both lean and fat tissue, whereas boys tend to lay down mostly lean tissue. This growth spurt provides about 42% to 51% of ultimate adult weight, and 15% to 25% of ultimate adult height (Figure 16-1).[12]

The growth spurt in girls surrounds the onset of menses, called **menarche.** Little further increase in height occurs beyond 2 years after menarche. Because the time for the growth spurt varies during the teen years, it would be ideal to base the RDA at this age on the presence or absence of the growth spurt, rather than on chronological age.

Fortunately, as the growth spurt begins, so does an increase in food intake. If teens choose nutritious food, they can take advantage of their increased hunger and easily satisfy their nutrient needs.

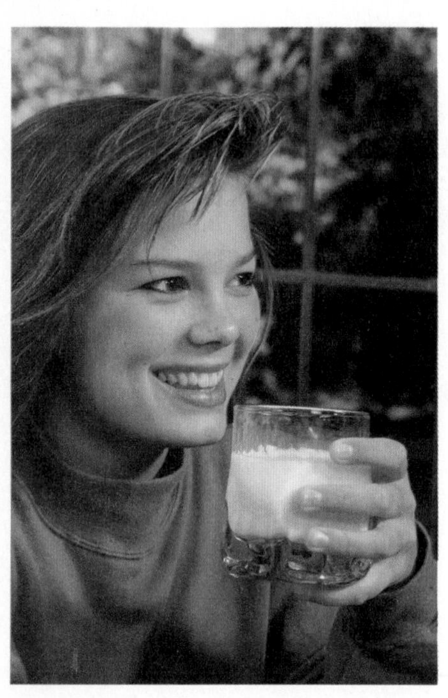

Three to four servings of milk per day are recommended for teenage girls.

Nutritional problems of teens

We covered anorexia nervosa and bulimia in Chapter 10. Other nutritional problems are more common during the teen years. A major concern is that many teenage girls stop drinking milk, and so they may not consume sufficient calcium to allow bones maximum mineralization through their early twenties. Although this issue is still being researched, many investigators are concerned that *young women who do not drink milk are sowing the seeds for future osteoporosis* (see Chapter 13). Depending on age, 3 to 4 servings of milk per day are recommended (Table 16-5). The RDA increases between ages 11 and 24 years from 800 to 1200 milligrams for males and females. Only about 1 in 6 teenage girls consume that amount.

Another concern is iron deficiency. Iron-deficiency anemia appears in girls after the onset of menses, and in boys during their growth spurt. About 12% to 14% of teenagers show low iron stores.[12] It is important that teenagers choose good food sources of iron, such as lean meats, whole grains, and enriched cereals. In addition, it is always a good idea to consume a vitamin C source with any plant or supplemental source of iron.

Adolescent and teenage girls especially need to eat good sources of iron (or regularly consume an iron supplement), particularly girls with heavy menstrual flows. Iron-deficiency anemia is not a desirable state for a teen. It can produce an

Table 16-5

Daily food guide for adolescents and teens*

	Include at least this many servings daily	
	Child 9-12 years	**Teen†**
Milk and cheese		
(preferably low-fat or nonfat)	3	3-4‡
Meats, poultry, fish, and beans	2	2
Fruits and vegetables		
Vitamin A-rich	1	1
Vitamin C- rich	1	1
Others to make a group total of . . .	4	4
Breads and cereals		
(preferably whole grain; otherwise enriched or fortified	4	4

* Use serving sizes from Adult Daily Food Guide.
† Here we define "teen" as a person who has added height in the past year, and is at least 12 years old.
‡ Through age 24 years.

increased tendency for fatigue and decreased ability to concentrate and learn. School performance may falter.

Another potential problem primarily involves boys during their growth spurt, when food consumption is great. Their great energy needs can accommodate large intakes of saturated fat and cholesterol, especially if they regularly consume hamburgers, French fries, fried chicken, and milk shakes. This high intake of saturated fat and cholesterol may pave the arteries for early coronary heart disease. We know of no specific research in this area to support this fear, but we believe it is prudent for boys to begin to choose "heart-healthy" foods, especially during the high energy intake years associated with the teen growth spurt (see Chapter 5).

Acne, diet, and vitamin A

Diet appears not to affect acne. Though one hears that eating nuts, chocolate, and pizza can make acne worse,. scientific studies have been unable to show a strong link between any dietary factor and acne. Acne naturally waxes and wanes, and so it falls easy prey to notions about relationships to dietary factors. Acne may be more dormant in summer, since sunlight appears to improve acne. The effect of artificial ultraviolet light is not so pronounced.

androgen
A general term for hormones that stimulate development in male sex organs; testosterone is an example.

The main culprit promoting acne is overactivity by the **sebaceous glands** in the skin. They respond to testosterone, which is mainly a male hormone. This is why men tend to have more serious cases of acne and to a greater extent than do women. Women also secrete testosterone and other **androgen** (testosterone-like) compounds. And if something, such as high doses of birth control pills, pushes this testosterone off the proteins in the bloodstream that it normally binds to, a woman may experience serious acne.

The sebaceous glands surround hair follicles on the face, ears, back, chest, eyelids, and other areas. In these glands are cells that secrete triglycerides, very long-chain fatty acids (waxes), and other lipids. Collectively, these substances are known as sebum. If the sebum blocks a duct in the gland, this can lead to an infection and local pressure, resulting in an acne lesion.

The most exciting news about acne is probably the introduction of Accutane (13-cis retinoic acid, or isotretinoin). This medication, a derivative of vitamin A, appears to change the nature of sebaceous gland development, as vitamin A might

sebum
Secretion of the sebaceous glands consisting of lipids, waxes, and other triglycerides.

be expected to do. It decreases the production of **sebum** and in turn reduces the number of acne lesions. The medication is especially helpful in treating cases resistant to antibiotic therapy (see Chapter 11 for more information about Accutane).

A closer look at the diets of teenage girls

Teenage girls have been found to consume inadequate amounts of nutrients other than calcium and iron: vitamin A, vitamin B-6, vitamin C, and zinc. Fear of excessive weight gain may cause young girls to limit their energy intake, and this limits their food choices.[11] If their limited food choices then consist of French fries, soft drinks, and pastries, little room is left for foods that are good nutrient sources. These nutrients are easy to obtain through nutrient-dense food choices based on the Daily Food Guide.

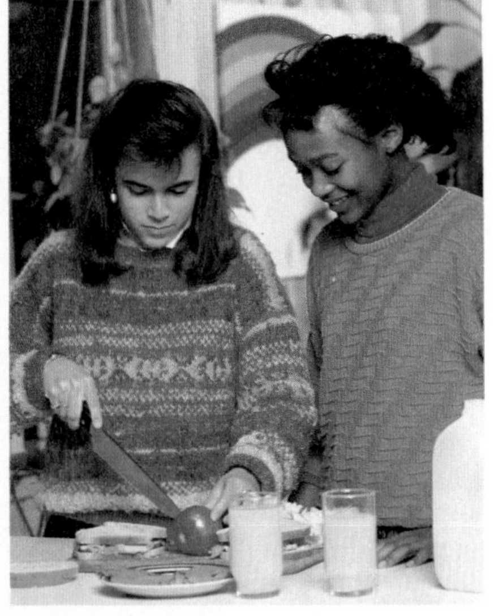

Teen girls should eat a variety of foods.

Helping teens eat more nutritious foods

Teenagers face a variety of upheavals in their lives. They pursue their independence, experience identity crises, seek peer acceptance, and worry about physical appearance. All these factors affect food choice.

Teens often do not think well in abstractions. They have a hard time relating today's actions to tomorrow's health outcomes. Physicians face this problem in counseling teenagers with diabetes mellitus. If diabetes mellitus is not controlled in the teenage years, the ultimate life span of a person can be significantly reduced, because serious complications tend to happen at a much earlier age. Still, it is hard for clinicians to convince teenagers of this because they often lack a future orientation.

Overcoming the teenage "mind set"

One strategy for working with teenage boys is to stress the importance of nutrition for physical development—especially muscular development—and for fitness, vigor, and health. With teenage girls, one approach is to help them under-

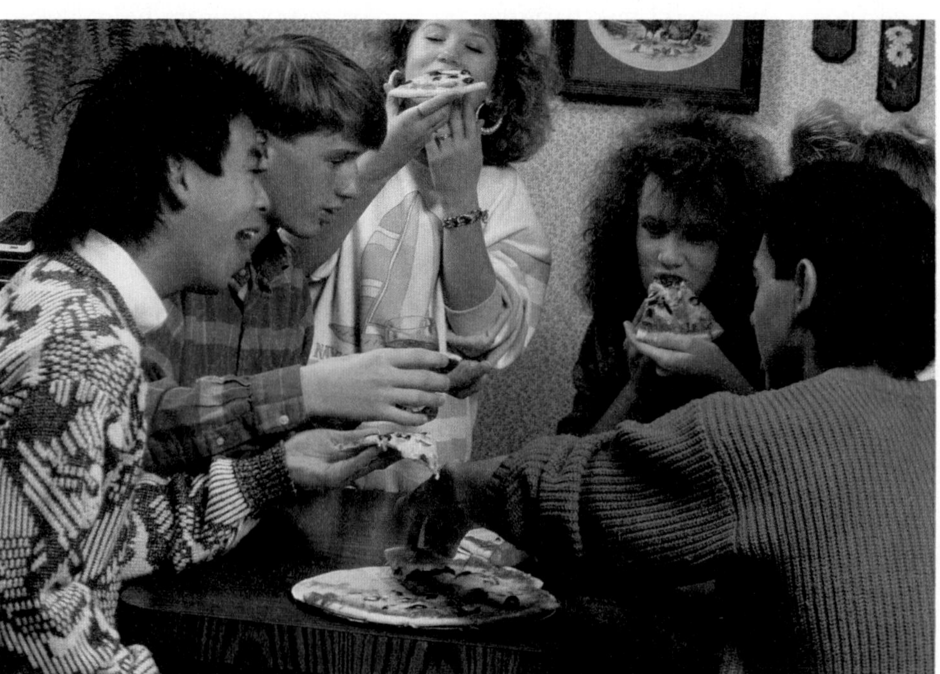

Figure 16-5 **Nutritional problems associated with teenagers' eating fast food** are due more to food choice than the foods available. *What* one eats, rather than where or when, is the key.

stand how to make nutrient-dense food choices that lead to better health while maintaining appropriate weight. It can be explained that beauty is based on the glow of health, and that sick people wither unappealingly.

Are teenage snacking practices harmful?

As we discussed concerning children, *the major focus with snacks should be what one eats.* Teens often obtain one fourth to one third of all their energy and major nutrients from snacks (Figure 16-5). Teenagers can obtain many nutrients from snacking. Even fast food restaurants offer some good food choices. By choosing wisely, teens can eat at fast food restaurants and still consume a very good diet (see Chapter 17). *Snacks and fast food restaurants in and of themselves are not the problem: poor food choices are.*

Clinicians—whether physicians, registered dietitians, or nurses—need to hone their skills when working with teenagers. Topics such as sports nutrition, eating disorders, and drugs and alcohol are typical issues that the clinician may face. These topics, except for drugs and alcohol, are usually not the concern of older adult clients.

Concept Check

Another period of rapid growth occurs during the teen years. Girls generally start this earlier than boys. Common nutritional problems in these years arise from poor food choices, and include poor calcium intake in girls, iron-deficiency anemia, and sometimes excessive saturated-fat intake. Acne is common among teens but not directly linked to diet. The importance of nutrition may be difficult to impress upon this age group. Clinicians must be aware of the implications of the social, psychological, and physical changes that occur during these years.

Summary

1. Growth is very rapid during infancy: birth weight doubles in 4 to 6 months, and length increases by 50% in a year. An adequate diet, especially protein intake, is very important to support normal growth. Malnutrition can cause irreversible changes in growth and development.
2. Growth in an infant and child is monitored by measuring body weight, height (or length) and head circumference over time. The most useful growth charts measure height-for-age and weight-for-height.
3. Nutrient needs in the first 6 months can be met by human milk or formula. Supplementary vitamin D and iron may be needed in the first 6 months for breast-fed infants, and supplemental fluoride may be needed by all infants.
4. Infant formulas generally contain lactose or sucrose, heat-treated casein and whey proteins from cow's milk, and vegetable oil. Formulas may or may not be fortified with iron. Sanitation is very important when preparing and storing formula.
5. Solid food should not be added to an infant's diet until there is a nutritional need, the GI tract can digest these complex foods, the infant has the physical ability to swallow voluntarily and control tongue thrusting, and the risk of developing food allergies decreases. For most infants, this readiness for solid food occurs between 4 and 6 months of age.
6. The first solid food given should be iron-fortified infant cereals or ground meats with very gradual addition of single other foods, perhaps adding one per week. Some foods to avoid giving infants in the first year include honey, low-fat cow's milk, overly salty or sweet foods, or foods that may cause choking.
7. Introduction of iron-containing solid food at the appropriate time and avoidance of cow's milk can generally prevent iron-deficiency anemia in later infancy.
8. A slower growth rate in preschool years makes the choice of nutrient-dense foods and a reduction in serving size important. Iron-rich foods, such as lean red meats, are an important part of the Daily Food Guide at this age. In the teen and young adult years, a focus on adequate iron and calcium in the diet is important, especially for girls.

Take Action

Suppose you are given the responsibility of feeding a 3-year-old for a weekend who refuses all foods except bananas and Cocoa Puffs cereal. How would you approach this problem? Write out a day's menu that you will encourage this child to eat.

Breakfast ______

Snack ______

Lunch ______

Snack ______

Dinner ______

Snack ______

Strategies to help the child eat your meal plan

1. ______
2. ______
3. ______
4. ______
5. ______

REFERENCES

1. The American Dietetic Association: Diet and criminal behavior, Journal of The American Dietetic Association 85:361,1985.
2. The American Dietetic Association: Child nutrition services, Journal of The American Dietetic Association 87:217, 1987.
3. Anonymous: Gastrointestinal permeability in food-allergic children, Nutrition Reviews 43:233, 1985.
4. Barness LA: Infant feeding: formula, solids, Pediatric Clinics of North America 32:355, 1985.
5. Barrett S: Unproven allergies: an epidemic of nonsense, Nutrition Today, p. 6, March/April, 1989.
6. Behrman RE and others: Nelson Textbook of Pediatrics ed 13, p. 64-67, Philadelphia, 1987, WB Saunders Co.
7. Butkus SN and Mahan LK: Food allergies: immunological reactions to food, Journal of The American Dietetic Association 86:601, 1986.
8. Committee on Nutrition, American Academy of Pediatrics: Prudent life-style for children, dietary fat and cholesterol, Pediatrics 78:521, 1986.
9. Epstein LH and others: Childhood obesity, Pediatric Clinics of North America 32:363, 1985.
10. Fauson A and Wilson J: Family interactions surrounding feeding of infants with nonorganic failure to thrive, Clinical Pediatrics 26:518, 1988.
11. Frank GC and others: Sodium, potassium, calcium, magnesium, and phosphorus intakes of infants and children, Bogalusa Heart Study, Journal of The American Dietetic Association 88:801, 1988.
12. Gong EJ and Spear BA: Adolescent growth and development: implications for nutritional needs, Journal of Nutrition Education, 20;273, 1988.
13. Gortmaker SL and others: Increasing pediatric obesity in the United States, American Journal of Diseases of Children 141:535, 1987.
14. Guthrie GM: Six to eighteen - the perilous months, Nutrition Today p. 4, May/June 1988.
15. Johnson GH: Dietary guidelines for infants, Fremont, MI, 1989, Gerber Products Co.
16. Parraga, IM and others: Feeding patterns of urban black infants, Journal of The American Dietetic Association 88:796, 1988.
17. Pipes PL: Nutrition in infancy and childhood, St. Louis, 1989, The CV Mosby Co.
18. Ritchey AK: Iron deficiency in children, Postgraduate Medicine 82:59, 1987.
19. Roberts SB and others: Energy expenditure and intake in infants born to lean and overweight mothers, New England Journal of Medicine 318:461, 1988.
20. Rozin P and Zollemecke TA: Food likes and dislikes, Annual Reviews of Nutrition 6:433, 1986.
21. Satter EM: Childhood eating disorders, Journal of The American Dietetic Association 86:357, 1986.
22. Schwab EK and Conners CK: Nutrient-behavior research with children: methods, considerations, and evaluation, Journal of The American Dietetic Association 86:319, 1986.
23. Serafin WE and Austen KF: Mediators of immediate hypersensitivity reactions, New England Journal of Medicine 317:30, 1987.
24. Stern M and Walker WA: Food allergy and intolerance, Pediatric Clinics of North America 32:471, 1985.
25. Story M and others: Adolescent nutrition: self-perceived deficiencies and needs of practitioners working with youth, Journal of The American Dietetic Association 88:591, 1988.
26. Story M and Brown JE: Do young children instinctively know what to eat? New England Journal of Medicine 316:103, 1987.
27. Taras HL and others: Early childhood diet: recommendations of pediatric health care providers, Journal of the American Dietetic Association 88:1417, 1988.
28. Taubman B: Parental counseling prepared with the elimination of cow's milk or soy milk protein for the treatment of infant colic syndrome: a randomized trial, Pediatrics 81:756, 1988.
29. Yip R: Declining prevalence of anemia among low-income children in the United States, Journal of The American Medical Association 258:1619, 1987.
30. Wolraich ML and others: Dietary characteristic of hyperactive and controlled boys, Journal of The American Dietetic Association 86:500, 1986.

SUGGESTED READINGS

The textbook by Pipes entitled "Nutrition in Infancy and Childhood" is an excellent source for more details on nutrition issues during the growing years. The article by Story and Brown summarizes the work by Dr. Clara Davis, and further explores whether children instinctively know what to eat. The booklet recently produced for health professionals by Gerber Products Company outlines dietary guidelines for infants developed by experts on infant feeding and nutrition. Call the Gerber Products Company in Fremont, Michigan (1-800-4-Gerber). A pamphlet designed by parents is also available. Gong and Spear summarize many important points regarding the role of nutrition in supporting adolescent growth and development. Ritchey outlines in very practical terms the diagnosis and treatment of iron-deficiency in children. Finally, the American Dietetic Association has published a position paper on diet and criminal behavior.

CHAPTER 16

Answers to nutrition awareness inventory

1. *True.* Although all nutrients and an adequate kcalorie intake are needed for growth, protein is particularly important for reaching one's genetic potential.
2. *True.* Infancy is a period of very rapid growth.
3. *False.* Brain growth rate is maximal at birth and continues through 12 to 15 months of age.
4. *False.* No evidence strongly links infant obesity to obesity in childhood or adulthood.
5. *False.* Infant energy needs are higher per pound.
6. *False.* Infants need relatively high-fat diets to support brain growth and supply enough energy for other growth with a small volume of food.
7. *False.* Infants are not usually developmentally or nutritionally ready for solid food until 4 to 6 months of age.
8. *True.* It is not necessary to add salt, sugar, or spices to infant foods.
9. *True.* However, little besides patience helps deal with colic.
10. *True.* Cow's milk should not be fed a child until about 6 months of age at the earliest, and preferably not until 12 months of age.
11. *True.* Cow's milk is low in iron, and the protein is more difficult to digest than that in human milk. This may cause intestinal irritation that contributes to iron losses.
12. *False.* *What* is eaten is most important—not when.
13. *True.* Anemia and obesity are the nutritional problems clinicians need to focus on.
14. *False.* Parents should control what food is available, but let children decide the amount to eat. With good foods available, children can reliably decide on serving size.
15. *False.* Scientific studies have never shown a very strong link between any dietary factor and acne.

Nutrition Perspective 16-1

Food Allergies and Intolerances

Adverse reactions to food are commonly reported, in some cases approaching 8% to 33% of people. They occur more frequently in women. The most common ages for adverse food reactions are in infancy and young adulthood. Types of reactions associated with food ingestion are:

- **Classical allergic**—Symptoms include shock, itching, redness of the skin, asthma, and a runny nose.
- **Gastrointestinal**—Symptoms include nausea, vomiting, diarrhea, intestinal gas, bloating, pain, constipation, and indigestion.
- **General**—Symptoms include headache, skin reactions, tension and fatigue, tremor, and psychological dysfunction.

Foods frequently identified with adverse reactions include milk, alcohol, meat and meat products, vegetables, sugars, cereals, fish and seafood products, fats and oils, eggs, fruits, chocolate, and cheese. About 90% of food allergies are caused by milk, eggs, nuts, and wheat. A family history of allergies greatly increases the risk.

FOOD ALLERGIES

A food allergy is caused by an immune response to a food substance. **Food Sensitivity** is a term often used today to describe milder reactions. The word **allergy** specifies a disorder of the immune system. Allergens are usually acid-like proteins with a specific configuration. Their typical molecular weight is between 18,000 and 40,000.[23] The actual allergy-producing part of the protein is thought to be present in a series of amino acids that are able to bind to the immunoglobulin IgE.[24]

Normally, proteins foreign to the body—also called antigens—are met by special immune proteins of the immunoglobulin G, A, and M types. These are important factors for immune protection. However, in most people susceptible to allergies, immunoglobulin E also has a major role. This immunoglobulin is normally found in low concentrations in the body, except when functioning as a natural defense mechanism against parasitic invasions.

When an antigen enters an allergic-prone host for the first time, specific antibodies of the IgE class are formed. These attach to specialized cells, called **mast cells,** which are located primarily in the GI tract. No reaction occurs at the first encounter. However, on subsequent exposures the antigen attaches to the specific IgE proteins on the mast cell. This joining of the mast cell and the antigen leads to a combination of chemical reactions and changes that cause the mast cell to release **histamine,** serotonin, and other chemical factors. These factors then cause the symptoms associated with an allergy.

Histamine, in particular, excites various receptors on cells, in turn causing contraction of smooth muscle, increased permeability and relaxation of blood vessels, nasal secretions, itching, and changes in dilation of the airways.

food sensitivity
A mild reaction to a substance in a food that might be expressed as slight itching or redness of the skin.

allergy
An immune response that occurs when antibodies react with a foreign substance (antigen).

mast cells
Cells that contain histamine and are responsible for some aspects of allergic and inflammatory reactions.

histamine
A chemical that causes a variety of effects on the body, such as contraction of smooth muscles, increased nasal secretions, relaxation of blood vessels, and changes in relaxation of airways.

WHY DO ALLERGIES OCCUR?

A big question concerning food allergies is how intact food proteins (antigens) can cross the natural barriers of the GI tract to interact with the immune system. Considering the thoroughness of the digestive system, it seems that these particles would break down into amino acids that the body could then metabolize with no adverse effects. Evidence now shows that large particles, however, can gain access to the immune system through gaps between intestinal cells.[3] These large particles can enter the lymph system or the capillaries, and eventually be transported via the bloodstream to various body sites. Now they can cause a reaction, as is the case when they join specific IgE sites on mast cells.

In a nonallergic person, the immunoglobulin IgA synthesized by intestinal cells acts as a natural barrier against absorption and transportation of large molecules into circulation. This protection doesn't seem to function efficiently for a person with food allergies.

Nutrition Perspective 16-1, cont'd

Food Allergies and Intolerances

TESTING FOR A FOOD ALLERGY

The first step in determining whether a food allergy is present is to record in detail a history of symptoms, time from ingestion to onset of symptoms, most recent reaction, quantity of food needed to produce a reaction, and the food suspected of causing a reaction. A family history of allergic disease can also help. The physician can look for signs of allergy, such as inflammation in the nasal cavity, skin diseases, and asthma.

Perhaps the best laboratory test for determining what compounds a person is allergic to is the RAST test. This test estimates the amount of IgE present in a person's blood that binds certain food-borne antigens. Skin tests may also be used, where a drop of the antigen is placed on skin that has been scratched or punctured. However, skin tests are often unreliable because they sometimes overdiagnose the presence of a food allergy.

The next step is to eliminate from the diet all tested compounds that appear to cause allergic symptoms plus all other foods the person's history suggests may cause an allergy. If symptoms are still present, the person can even more severely restrict the diet, or even use special formulas that are hypoallergenic.

elimination diet
A restrictive diet that systematically tests foods that may cause an allergic response by first eliminating, and then adding them back, one at a time.

anaphylactic shock
A severe allergic response that results in lowered blood pressure and respiratory and GI distress. This can be fatal.

cytotoxic test
An unreliable test to define food allergies that involves mixing whole blood with food proteins.

Once the **elimination diet** yields no symptoms, then cautious introduction of foods—those which don't cause **anaphylactic shock**—can begin after 2 to 4 weeks. Doses of ½ to 1 teaspoon (2.5 to 5 milliliters) are given first. The amount is increased until the dose approximates usual intake. This may be done using a double-blind approach (see Chapter 1), especially when there is a psychological component to the reaction, or when symptoms are vague or ill-defined. Dried foods can be encapsulated and then given to the person.

A bogus method to test for food allergies is the **cytotoxic test.** In this case, food proteins are mixed with whole blood or serum, and then the number of white blood cells broken during the subsequent reaction between the proteins and the blood are counted. This method is quite unreliable in predicting food allergies. We recommend exploring the possibility of food allergies with a physician-allergist instead of relying on a pseudoscientific method such as cytotoxic testing.[5]

TREATMENT OF FOOD ALLERGIES

Once potential allergens are identified, the best treatment is to avoid them, especially for people with zero tolerance. Cromolyn sodium may also be prescribed. This medication limits activity of mast cells.

The American Academy of Allergy and Immunology has a 24-hour toll-free hot line (1-800-822-ASMA) to answer questions about food allergy and to help direct people to specialists who treat the problem.

If a woman is pregnant or breast-feeding, she should avoid the offending foods because antigens can cross the placenta, and will be secreted in her milk. Moreover, when food allergies run in the family, women are advised to breast-feed their infants. Formula-fed infants have a greater risk of developing allergies. Breast-feeding should continue for as long as possible, preferably at least 1 year, and early introduction of cow's milk should be avoided. If breast- feeding is not possible, special formulas that contain altered forms of cow's milk proteins are available (such as Nutramigen and Alimentum). These are especially valuable when treating an infant with an allergy to cow's milk.

A major challenge for the clinician treating a person with a food allergy is to make sure that what remains in the diet can still provide the essential nutrients needed. Especially great care should be taken when removing many potentially offending foods from a child's diet.

WILL A CHILD ALWAYS HAVE THE FOOD ALLERGY?

prognosis
A forecast of a disease's problem course.

The **prognosis** for IgE-related food allergies that occur before 3 years of age is good. About 40% of children outgrow a food allergy. Food allergies diagnosed after age 3 years often are more long-lived. Adults have reported reactions that still will appear even after 15 or more years of the first episode.

Except in cases where shock (anaphylaxis) is possible, foods causing allergies may be reintroduced every 6 months or so to see whether the allergy symptoms have decreased, but not before 1 year of age. If so, it indicates that tolerance to a food has developed. People with mild or moderate allergies to several foods may benefit from a diet in which an offending food is eaten every 5 days to encourage a tolerance. If cow's milk sensitivity starts in infancy, the child usually outgrows this sensitivity by 2 to 3 years of age.

FOOD INTOLERANCES

Besides food allergies, there can be other causes of adverse food reactions known as **food intolerances.** These do not involve the immune system, and so it is important to separate them from typical food allergies. These cases have a higher threshold for the offending food before symptoms occur, and the treatment differs from that for food allergies. Causes of food intolerances can be categorized as:

food intolerance
An adverse reaction to food that does not involve an immune response.

- Substances that produce pharmacological (drug) activity, such as tomatoes or pineapples.
- Toxic contaminants, such as bacterial toxins; synthetic compounds such as tartrazine (F, D, & C yellow no. 5); antibiotics; and insect parts.
- Deficiencies in digestive enzymes, such as lactase.
- Food poisoning because of improper handling or cooking, as in *Clostridium botulinum* food poisoning (see Chapter 19).
- Viral and bacterial infections, as in *Salmonella* food poisoning.

All these conditions can lead to GI symptoms. In addition, anyone can expect to be sensitive to one or more of these causes—not only people with specific changes in their immune system.

Four very common food intolerances are induced by the presence of sulfites, monosodium glutamate, tartrazine, and tyramine in food. A sulfite reaction causes flushing, spasms of the airways, and a loss of blood pressure. Evidence of reaction to monosodium glutamate might be an increase in blood pressure, sweating, vomiting, headache, and facial pressure. A reaction to tartrazine includes spasm of the airways, itching, and redness of the skin. About 8% to 15% of people with aspirin intolerance are also intolerant to tartrazine. A final compound, tyramine, can cause high blood pressure in people taking monoamine-oxidase inhibitor medications (for depression). Tyramines are commonly found in "aged" foods, such as cheeses and red wines.

The basic treatment for food intolerances is to avoid specific offending components. However, this usually does not require total elimination. *Again, we need to emphasize that most people are generally less sensitive to factors that cause food intolerances than are allergic people to their offending food components.* For instance, a slight amount of sulfites in a glass of wine may be tolerable, whereas a large dose from a chef's salad may cause a reaction. See Chapter 19 on food safety for more details about toxic reactions from foods.

DOES SUCROSE HAVE ILL EFFECTS ON CHILDREN?

Some researchers have suggested that sucrose affects behavior, especially in children. They claim sucrose creates an excited, even antisocial, state, which may lead to violence and disruptive behavior. However, most researchers find that sucrose itself is not the villain.[1] No adequate evidence supports the hypothesis that reactive hypoglycemia caused by sugar consumption commonly causes violent behavior (see Chapter 4). If there is a villain, it is probably the excitement or tension surrounding high-sucrose foods (such as is seen at parties and during Halloween), or the extra attention a child receives when put on a relatively sucrose-free diet.[30]

Continued.

Nutrition Perspective 16-1—cont'd

Food Allergies and Intolerances

HOW MANY CHILDREN ARE SENSITIVE TO FOOD ADDITIVES?

In 1973, Dr. R. Benjamin Feingold suggested that food additives caused **hyperactivity** (now known as a part of the attention deficit disorder) in children. He theorized that because some children are allergic to aspirin-like compounds, and some food additives have aspirin-like structures, such children would also be allergic to certain food additives. Much research followed this proposal: generally, the research has not supported a strong or predictable association between the consumption of food additives and hyperactivity in children.[22]

The incidence of attention deficit disorder with hyperactivity is approximately 5% to 10% of school-age children; boys are affected 4 to 6 times more than girls. The initial identification of hyperactivity in children commonly occurs as they enter nursery or elementary school. Teachers report that these students are uncontrollable, unable to sit still, bother other children, and, especially, intrude into other children's activities.[6]

There are many pitfalls in studying this diet-behavior relationship. If parents put a "hyperactive" child on an additive-free diet, it will tend to be a more nutrient-rich diet because it will contain more whole, unadulterated foods. In addition, the child will receive much more attention from the parents, which alone can decrease disruptive behavior.

The only definitive way to study this relationship is to use a double-blind protocol. A child would be given an additive-free food and then later one full of additives. Both the parents and the child must not know what is in the food. Then researchers would have to score the child's behavior after consuming these foods, again not knowing which foods the child had consumed.

This procedure is much too cumbersome to be used in a school system or by a private pediatrician. Thus many suspected cases of food additive-linked hyperactivity are not tested in a definitive scientific manner. This is problematic since some diets used for hyperactive children are limited, and eliminate more than food additives. Some popular "defined diets" eliminate dietary essentials such as milk, fruit, and some grain products. The more limited the diet, the greater the risk of nutrient deficiency and poor growth.

If an additive-free diet follows the Daily food Guide and actually improves a child's attention span and behavior, there is no reason not to employ it. About 5% to 10% of cases may be helped by this treatment.[6] This does not mean the diet free of additives is the key factor; more attention and other changes could still be the major reason for the behavioral change. *Parents must ensure they do not leave the child with a sense of deprivation, nor should they make peer interactions more difficult for their child, without agreement from medical advisors that the special diet and restrictions are worth the effort.* In addition, the child should not see behavior as more directed by diet than by how one feels. Hyperactivity tends to decrease as a child ages. In addition, parents of children whose hyperactivity contributes to an attention deficit disorder syndrome need to be reminded that important behavior therapies can be used to treat this problem. The advice of a pediatrician skilled in this disease should be sought.

Nutrition Perspective 16- 2

Obesity in the Growing Years

About 40% of obese children become obese adults, and about 70% of obese adolescents become obese adults. *The time to strike against obesity is in childhood because there is such a high likelihood that an obese school-age child will become an obese adult.* In North America, 15% to 25% of children are overweight.[13] About 15% of adolescents in North America are obese. This incidence of overweight children and adolescents leads not only to an increased chance of later obesity, but also to a decrease in physical fitness, and sooner or later to other aspects of ill health, as well.

The first way to evaluate obesity in childhood is to plot weight-for-height on a growth chart. Children over the 90th percentile are considered overweight, and those over the 95th percentile are considered obese. Skinfold thickness can also be measured to assess obesity (see Chapter 8).

WHAT CAUSES CHILDHOOD OBESITY?

Current research indicates that there are many potential causes for childhood obesity. Recall the nature versus nurture comparison discussed in Chapter 8. Some infants are born with lower metabolic rates: they use energy more efficiently, and in turn have an easier time saving kcalories for fat storage.[19] Some infants are less active than others, and so use fewer kcalories per day. Research shows a moderate relationship between the amount of hours a child spends watching television and obesity. Obesity also tends to run in families. We can also expect further environmental influences, such as snacking, decreased physical activity, and high-fat/high-kcalorie food choices to contribute to childhood obesity.

TREATING CHILDHOOD OBESITY

A first approach to treating childhood obesity is assessing the child's activity level. If a child spends much free time in sedentary activities (such as watching television), more physical activities should be encouraged. These do not necessarily have to be competitive

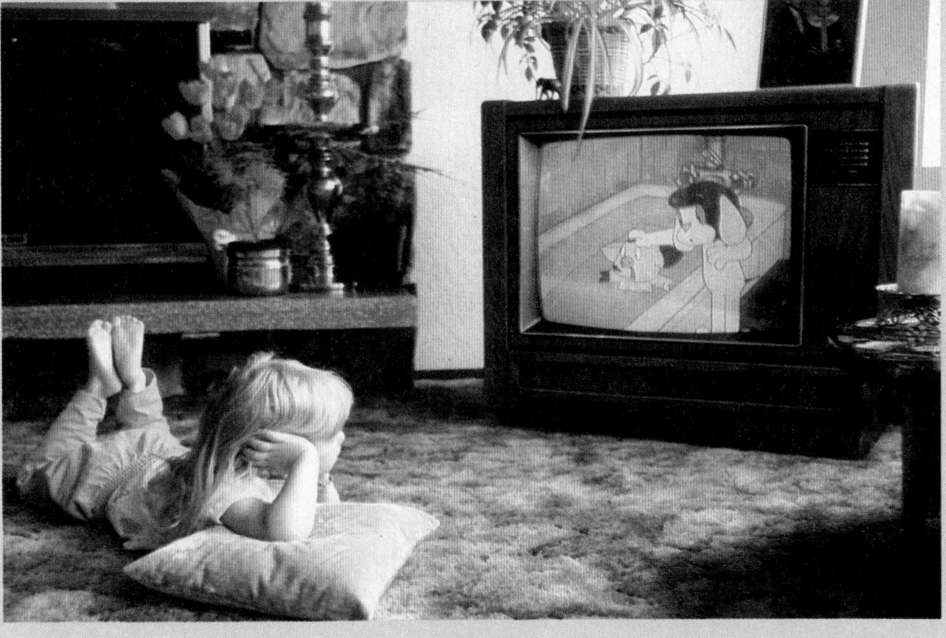

Some children spend too much time in sedentary activities.

Continued.

Nutrition Perspective 16-2—cont'd

Obesity in the Growing Years

sports. Children should be given opportunities to enjoy activities that they like, such as walking, cycling, swimming, and jazz dancing, and then encouraged to do these often.

Moderation in kcalorie intake, especially high-fat/high-kcalorie food choices, is important. Resorting to a weight-loss diet is usually unnecessary. Children have an advantage over adults in losing weight—some stored kcalories can be used by growth. *If weight gain can be moderated, height gains may soon catch-up.* This is one reason why treating obesity in childhood is so desirable. Further growth can contribute to success.[9]

Sometimes weight loss is necessary if a child will still be obese after attaining ultimate adult height. Then weight loss should be gradual, perhaps ½ pound per week. The child should be closely monitored to ensure that during this weight loss the rate of growth is normal. It is important that the child's kcalorie intake is not so compromised that height gains diminish.

Behavior modification adds a third important component to treating childhood obesity. Children often need to find a new way to relate to foods, especially snack foods. It may be important for children to eat only at the kitchen table. This could stop endless hours of snacking in front of the television.

Parents play a key role in treating childhood obesity. After all, they select and bring the food home. One goal is to keep healthy, nutrient-rich but kcalorie-light snacks on hand. The parents also must help a child turn his interest from food consumption toward other interests, such as sports, hobbies, and school. Any management plan for treating childhood obesity must involve the parents.

The self-esteem of a child is quite fragile. Humiliation does not work: it only makes the child feel worse. *Support, admiration, and encouragement—these are offerings to be emphasized.*

With young children, a counselor can stress the advantages of weight loss, including peer acceptance and better sports ability. With adolescents, a counselor might stress the relationship of weight loss to dating and other interactions with the opposite sex. With the parents, the importance of weight loss for the child's long-term physical health should be the key point. The clinician can clarify for the parent that by denying a child favorite foods, they do not necessarily deny love. In treating the family, a counselor often must help the parents and child develop new ways of relating—that do not involve food and obesity.

CAN INFANT FEEDING PRACTICES PREVENT OBESITY?

Studies conducted over the last 20 years have shown no clear relationship between later obesity and either breast-feeding or the age that solid food was introduced. Parents should allow an infant to eat as much as desired while not encouraging overeating. Infants should be masters of their food intake.

This probably should also be the rule for children. Researchers feel that denying children enough food may spur further obesity and overeating: in such cases, children lose confidence that they will always be able to meet their food needs (see the Expert Opinion by Ellyn Satter). Restrained eating may lead to overeating when a child gets the chance, which in turn encourages a greater restraint by the parents and then even further overeating by the child. Parents need to realize that a child is really the best judge of how much food is needed. *It is the parent's job to provide a healthy food environment, and the child's job to determine proper portion size.*

Chapter 17

Nutrition for Adult and Elderly Years

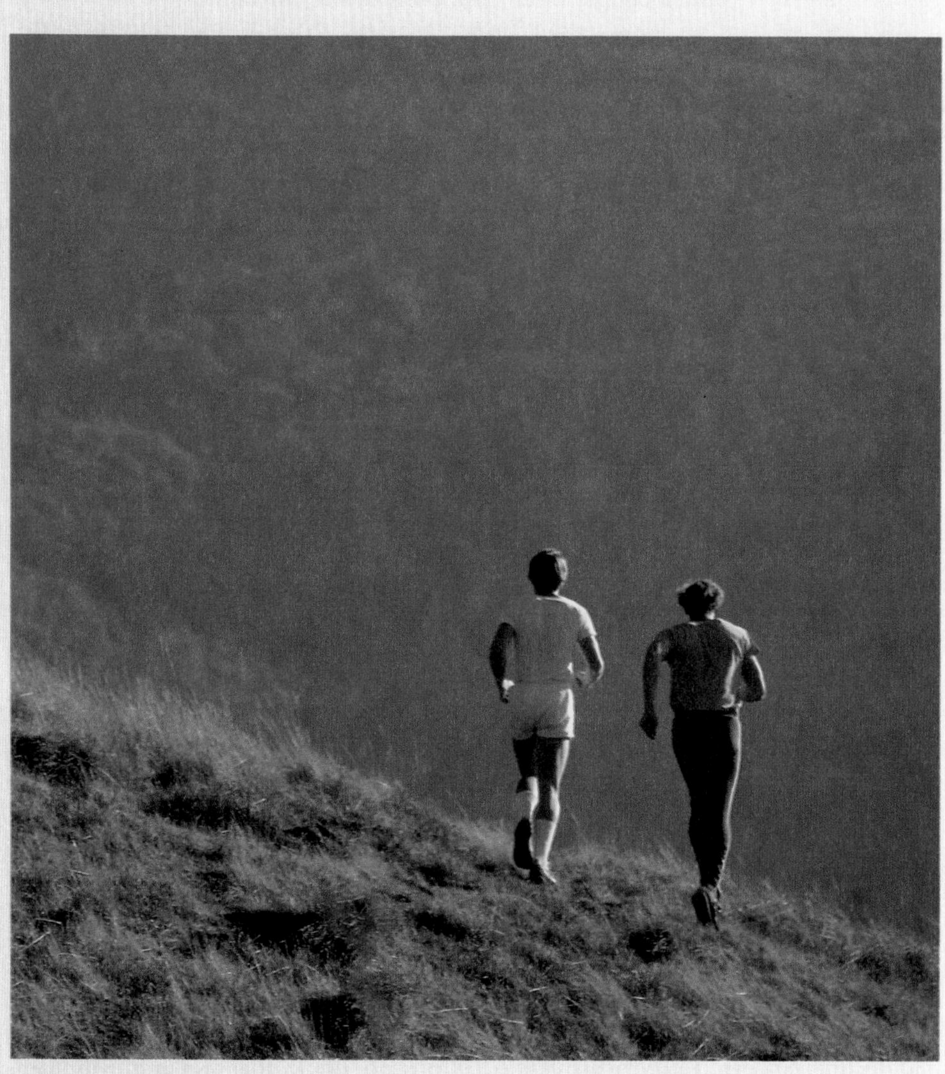

The need for regular exercise continues throughout adulthood.

Overview

We can now review some major nutrition concepts. A review may help you focus and tailor information from the previous chapters into a personal nutrition and overall health plan. Chapter 18, "How To Improve Your Diet," will then help you implement your plan.

We have noted many times that *nutritional recommendations should be individualized because responses to foods are often idiosyncratic.* Some of us are very sensitive to the amounts of cholesterol or sodium in our diets, and some have family histories of heart disease, cancer, diabetes mellitus, alcoholism, and osteoporosis that may make us more susceptible than others to major chronic diseases. Assuming that you know your serum cholesterol level, your blood pressure values, your blood glucose level, and your family history for major diseases among North Americans, you are now ready to formulate your personal nutrition and health plan.

In this chapter we want to extend your nutrition knowledge to the special needs of the elderly. Keep in mind that *the choices you make now in your younger adult years concerning food intake and overall health practices can significantly influence your health during your elderly years.*

Nutrition awareness inventory

Here are 15 statements about nutrition for adults and the elderly. Answer them to test your current knowledge. If you think the answer is true or mostly true, circle T. If you think the answer is false or mostly false, circle F. Use the scoring key at the end of this chapter to compute your total score. Take this test again after you have read this chapter. Compare the results.

1. **T F** The maximum age at which people die has increased dramatically.
2. **T F** Adults should aim to expend about 2000 kcalories per week exercising.
3. **T F** Medications taken by the elderly can cause nutritional problems.
4. **T F** The greatest nutritional problem for many North Americans is overeating.
5. **T F** People over age 65 years account for more than half the health care costs in the United States.
6. **T F** Optimal diets can stop the aging process.
7. **T F** The senses of taste and smell usually increase with age.
8. **T F** Older people often lose their desire for liquids.
9. **T F** Vitamin B-12 absorption often decreases in elderly people.
10. **T F** The most frequently occurring intestinal problem in the elderly is constipation.
11. **T F** An excessive intake of vitamin A supplements in the elderly can cause bone pain and hair loss.
12. **T F** Poor wound healing should alert a clinician to examine the protein, zinc, and vitamin C intake of an elderly person.
13. **T F** An active life-style tends to maintain muscle mass.
14. **T F** Dietary recommendations made by the American Heart Association could, if followed, substantially reduce blood cholesterol in all people.
15. **T F** People over 65 years of age are quite similar in physical capabilities.

YOUR ADULT YEARS

While most of us wish for long life, we do not like the thought of poor health in old age. And rightfully so! A long life can be enjoyable if it is productive and free of illness. Rather than suffer the ravages of heart disease, strokes, diabetes mellitus, osteoporosis, and other chronic diseases from age 50 or 60 years until death, we should strive to be as free of disease as possible and to enjoy vitality even in the last several years of life.

compression of morbidity Maintaining good health practices to delay the onset of disabilities due to chronic disease.

The goal of striving to have the greatest number of healthy years and the fewest years of illness is referred to as **compression of morbidity.** An example of this concept is illustrated in Figure 17-1 for heart disease.[9] Of the three lines shown, the line on the left shows rapid deterioration in health status, where symptoms of heart disease appear by about age 40 and death occurs at about age 60. In addition, between the ages of 40 and 60 years, symptoms of heart disease—and therefore disability—are present. A healthier life-style follows the middle line pattern. Here, heart disease is postponed so that the first symptoms are not apparent until age 60, severe symptoms until age 80, with death following a few years later. The line on the right is the ideal: *the disease progresses at such a slow rate that symptoms do not appear throughout a person's lifetime, and therefore the disease does not hamper a person's activities.*

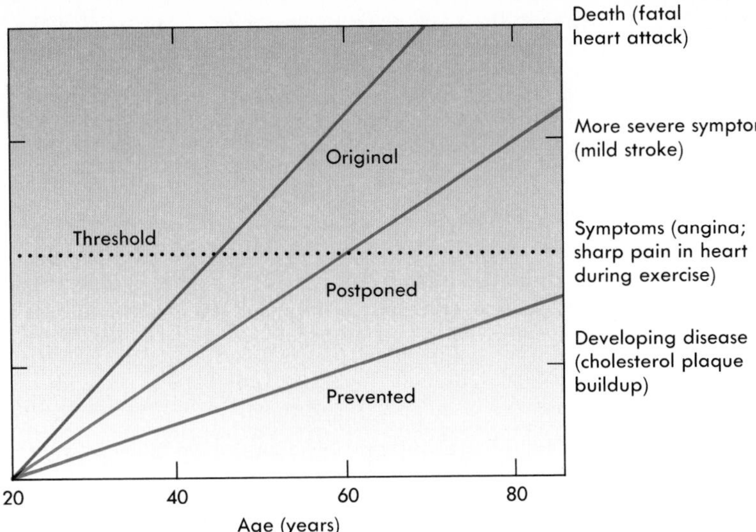

Figure 17-1

"Compression of morbidity." The goal is to postpone sickness in life until one's final days and, in turn, lead a life as disease-free as possible.

Aging is a natural process: body cells age no matter what health practices we follow. But to a considerable extent you can choose how fast you age throughout your adult years. You have some say in the matter (Table 17-1). "Successful" aging is the goal. Dr. Kenneth Cooper says: "Age fast or age slow—you choose."

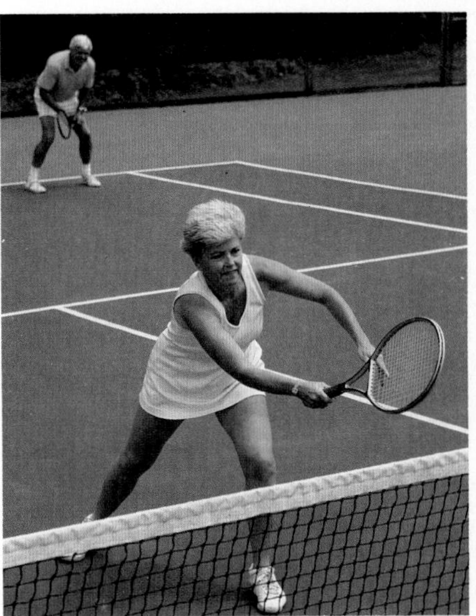

Cardiovascular stimulation is important to maintain the health of the heart.

A basic plan for health promotion and disease prevention

Adults can best promote health and prevent disease by practicing the following behaviors:

- **Consume a proper diet**—A varied diet that maintains a desirable weight should be a priority. The Daily Food Guide in Chapter 2 is a great place to start. Especially emphasize plant proteins, whole grains, plant oils, and dark green or leafy vegetables.
- **Exercise**—Research suggests that about 2000 kcalories per week should be spent in brisk walking, jogging, swimming, stair climbing, and other activities that stimulate the cardiovascular system.
- **Abstain from smoking**—Lung cancer, which is primarily due to smoking cigarettes, is the only form of cancer whose rates still increase every year.
- **Limit alcohol intake**—Limit alcohol consumption to not more than 1 to 2 ounces per day. Blacks are especially sensitive to the effects of alcohol on blood pressure. Furthermore, women shouldn't consume alcohol during pregnancy.
- **Limit stress, or adjust to the causes of stress**—Practice better time management, relax, listen to music, have a massage, exercise regularly—do your favorite things to reduce stress.

The key to maximizing health is to establish harmony between the physical, mental, psychological, and social states. There is no general formula for achieving this ideal; each of us must juggle and balance personal goals with opportunities and obstacles encountered. In addition, people who practice health promotion and disease prevention may not live longer—because of heredity, accidents, or other things outside their control—but they probably live healthier lives. It is especially important for health care professionals to develop and follow a plan that emphasizes wellness for themselves. By taking this initiative, they act as positive models for others to follow.

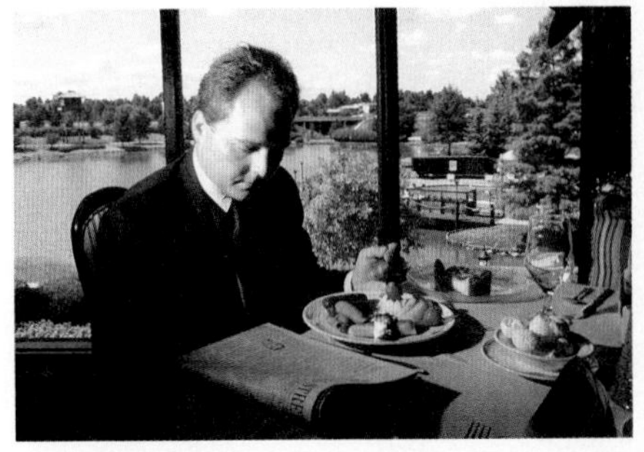

We all struggle to maintain harmony in the different aspects of our lives.

The 1990 health objectives for the United States

Health promotion and disease prevention became a public health strategy in the United States in the late 1970s. In 1979, a variety of health-related areas were

Table 17-1

What can we expect from good nutrition and health habits?

- Meeting our needs for protein, kcalories, and other essential nutrients helps prevent:
  Birth defects and low birthweight in pregnancy
- Poor growth and poor resistance to disease in infancy and childhood
  Poor resistance to disease in adult years
  Deficiency diseases, such as cretinism, scurvy, and anemia due to iron or folate deficiency
- Meeting our needs for calcium intake helps prevent:
  Some adult bone loss
- Obtaining adequate fluoride and minimizing sugar intake helps prevent:
  Dental caries
- Eating enough dietary fiber helps prevent:
  Digestive problems such as constipation and diverticulosis, and possibly colon cancer
- Enough vitamin A and beta-carotene intake in the diet may help reduce:
  Susceptibility to some cancers, especially in smokers
- An adequate, regular exercise helps prevent:
  Obesity
  Non–insulin-dependent (adult-onset) diabetes mellitus
  Heart disease
  Some adult bone loss
  Loss of muscle tone
- Moderation in kcalorie intake helps prevent:
  Obesity and related diseases, such as diabetes mellitus, hypertension, cancer, and heart disease
- Limiting sodium intake helps prevent:
  Hypertension and related disease of the heart and kidney in susceptible people
- Avoiding saturated fat intake helps prevent:
  Heart disease
- Minimizing alcohol intake helps prevent:
  Liver disease
  Fetal alcohol syndrome
  Accidents
- Moderation in intake of essential nutrients by using supplements wisely, if at all, prevents:
  Most chances for nutrient toxicities

The latest Surgeon General's report states that "for most of us, the more likely problems are overeating—too many calories for our activity levels—and an imbalance in the nutrients consumed." The report recommends diets lower in fat, especially saturated fat; diets lower in sodium, with an increase in the amount of whole grains, calcium, and iron; and regular exposure to fluoride. See the Expert Opinion by Dr. Frank E. Young, Commissioner of the FDA, for the specific recommendations.

highlighted as goals for national efforts in the document *Healthy People: The U.S. Surgeon General's Report on Health Promotion and Disease Prevention.* Some goals in this document became the 1990 Health Objectives for the nation.[15]

This document's nutrition-related objectives addressed iron-deficiency anemia, poor growth in infants and children, obesity, high serum cholesterol levels, high sodium intake, a relative lack of breast-feeding, poor general nutrition knowledge, the need for more food labeling information, and the need for a comprehensive, nationwide, nutritional monitoring system both in clinical and consumer settings.

In addition to these objectives, the American Dietetic Association also recommends addressing the risks of developing diabetes mellitus and osteoporosis. Implementing any objectives that apply to you could be part of your personal nutrition and health plan.[1]

Dietary recommendations for adults

The American Heart Association (AHA) began recommending that adults consume a nutritious diet for maintaining a healthy heart in 1957. Some scientists believe the recommendations should apply to all people over 2 years of age. Table 5-4 lists the latest recommendations by the AHA. Then, in 1977, the Senate Select Committee on Nutrition issued dietary goals for the United States. (We discussed this in Chapter 2.) These goals—actually the revised version published soon after the first edition—are listed in Table 2-6. The goals generated controversy in the United States, primarily because they set such specific dietary recommendations for consumption of kcalories, fats, cholesterol, sucrose, sodium, and other dietary factors.

Table 17-2

Diet and health recommendations by the National Academy of Sciences

1. Reduce total fat intake to 30% or less of calories.
   Reduce saturated fatty acid intake to less than 10% of calories, and the intake of cholesterol to less than 300 milligrams daily. The intake of fat and cholesterol can be reduced by substituting fish, poultry without skin, lean meats, and low-fat or nonfat dairy products for fatty meats and whole-milk dairy products; by choosing more vegetables, fruits, cereals, and legumes; and by limiting oils, fats, egg yolks, and fried and other fatty foods.
2. Every day eat five or more servings (an average serving is equal to a half cup of most fresh or cooked vegetables, fruits, dry or cooked cereals and legumes, one medium piece of fresh fruit, one slice of bread, or one roll or muffin) of a combination of vegetables and fruits, especially green and yellow vegetables and citrus fruits. Also, increase intake of starches and other complex carbohydrates by eating six or more daily servings of a combination of breads, cereals, and legumes.
3. Maintain protein intake at moderate levels.
4. Balance food intake and physical activity to maintain appropriate body weight.
5. The Committee does not recommend alcohol consumption. For those who drink alcoholic beverages, the committee recommends limiting consumption to the equivalent of less than 1 ounce of pure alcohol in a single day. This is equivalent to two cans of beer, two small glasses of wine, or two average cocktails. Pregnant women should not consume alcoholic beverages.
6. Limit total daily intake of salt (sodium chloride) to 6 grams or less. Limit the use of salt in cooking and avoid adding it to food at the table. Salty, highly processed, salt-preserved, and salt-pickled foods should be consumed sparingly.
7. Maintain an adequate calcium intake.
8. Avoid taking dietary supplements in excess of the RDA in any one day.
9. Maintain an optimum intake of fluoride, particularly during the years of primary and secondary tooth formation and growth.

From: National Academy of Sciences report on diet and health, Nutrition Reviews 47:142, 1989.

More general dietary guidelines for Americans were published in 1980 (and revised in 1985) by a joint commission of the U.S. Department of Agriculture (USDA) and the U.S. Department of Health and Human Services (DHHS). The National Cancer Institute (NCI), the Surgeon General's Office,[26] and most recently, the National Academy of Sciences (NAS)[17] (Table 17-2) have added to or clarified these dietary guidelines. We reviewed the current dietary guidelines issued by USDA and DHHS in Chapter 2. We list them here with clarifying statements by the other organizations just mentioned:

1. **Eat a variety of foods**—Focus on the Daily Food Guide outlined in Chapter 2. The NAS report suggests limiting protein intake to twice the RDA and not taking a nutrient supplement in quantities greater than the RDA in any one day. Both the NAS and surgeon general's reports encourage everyone to meet their RDA for calcium, especially adolescent girls and women.
2. **Maintain desirable weight**—The midranges of the Metropolitan Life Tables can serve as a standard, or one can use a body mass index range of 19 to 24 (see Chapter 8). Both the NAS and the surgeon general's reports emphasize balancing food intake with regular physical activity.
3. **Avoid too much fat, saturated fat, and cholesterol**—The NAS, AHA, and NCI suggest limiting fat intake to 30% of total kcalories. The NAS report and AHA recommend limiting saturated fat to one third of total fat intake (10% of total kcalories) and dietary cholesterol to 300 milligrams per day.
4. **Eat foods with adequate starch and fiber**—Emphasize complex rather than simple carbohydrates. The NAS report suggests five or more servings of vegetables and fruits daily and six or more servings of breads, cereals, and legumes daily. The NCI intends this intake to yield 20 to 35 grams of dietary fiber per day.
5. **Avoid too much sugar.**
6. **Avoid too much sodium**—The NAS report suggests limiting salt intake to 6 grams per day, which would yield 2.4 grams of sodium. A restriction of this magnitude would require a great change in food habits for many people, such as eliminating processed meats, salted snack foods, most canned and prepared soups, regular cheese, and many tomato-based products (see Chapter 13).
7. **If you drink alcoholic beverages, do so in moderation**—Both the NAS and surgeon general's reports recommend not more than two drinks daily and no alcohol use during pregnancy.

See Chapter 2 to review the Canadian Dietary Goals.

The NCI further recommends moderation in consuming salt-cured, smoked, and nitrate-cured foods. The NAS and surgeon general's reports add a recommendation for obtaining an optimum fluoride intake, particularly during the growing years. Finally, the Surgeon General's Report recommends that children, adolescents, and women of child bearing age consume iron-rich foods.

These guidelines do not apply equally to everyone. We vary in susceptibility to high serum cholesterol levels, high blood pressure, obesity, and other health problems these guidelines seek to counteract. For instance, in people who have a low energy output, a high sugar intake may be a problem, since they need to consume a nutrient-dense diet. However, for adolescents who have very active lifestyles and practice good dental hygiene, dietary sugar causes no apparent health problems (see Chapters 4 and 16). The same argument applies to sodium: no scientific data show that typical North American sodium intakes necessarily produce high blood pressure later in a person who presently has normal blood pressure (see Chapter 13), although the NAS report cautions this may be true. *You must consider your own health status to apply these guidelines appropriately.*

A note of caution

Not all nutrition and health researchers agree with the nutrition guidelines set by our major health and science institutions. *Most researchers agree on the need for varying the diet, controlling body weight, reducing dietary total fat and saturated fat for adults, eating more fruits, vegetables, and cereals, and moderating alcohol intake.* However, many scientists do not think that general recommendations for the public can be justified for consuming sugar, complex carbohydrate, fiber, salt, specific vitamins, and cholesterol. Rather, they believe these recommendations need to be individualized.[12]

It can be argued that while individualized dietary recommendations are best, that approach is too costly and therefore impractical. If that is indeed the case, general recommendations can be made that benefit the health of most people while not hampering the health of others. Not all people would benefit equally from following the general recommendations—for example, a reduction in sodium intake—but no one would be harmed. The dietary change could, however, cause some inconvenience, and perhaps for some people require new eating habits.

Nevertheless, *we should all consider some of the general dietary recommendations, such as emphasizing low-fat dairy products, lean meats and plant proteins, fruits and vegetables, and ample breads and cereals.* These recommendations are consistent with the Daily Food Guide and form the best approach to optimizing health, based on current scientific knowledge. See the Expert Opinions in this chapter by Dr. Frank Young of the FDA and by Dr. David Klurfeld of the Wistar Institute. These scientists have different opinions about the extent to which dietary guidelines should be applied.

Exploring Issues and Actions

Throughout the last 20 years, the American Heart Association has issued general diet and health recommendations. The American Medical Association has countered with the argument that recommendations should be made on a person-by-person basis. What do you think is the proper approach?

Concept Check

Compression of morbidity is the goal of delaying symptoms and disabilities primarily due to chronic diseases for as many years as possible. A basic plan to promote health and prevent disease includes eating a proper diet, exercising, abstaining from smoking, limiting alcohol intake, and limiting stress. More specific dietary guidelines direct people to eat a variety of foods; maintain desirable weight; avoid too much fat, saturated fat, and cholesterol; eat foods with adequate starch and fiber; avoid too much sugar; avoid too much sodium; and, if you drink alcoholic beverages, do so in moderation. Recommendations to pay particular attention to fluoride, iron, and calcium intake during certain life stages are also included. Some scientists believe these guidelines do not necessarily constitute an individual "prescription."

Are we following these nutrition and health recommendations?

North Americans generally are trying to follow many recommendations listed above. In the United States, saturated fat intake in the form of whole milk and cream has decreased since the mid-1950s. Skim and low-fat milk have replaced them. However, cheese consumption has increased, and that is usually a concentrated form of saturated fat. Since 1963, butter, egg, and animal fat consumption have fallen, while use of vegetable fats and oils and fish consumption have increased.[10] All these changes, except the increased cheese consumption, are generally consistent with recommendations to reduce saturated animal fat intake and to increase the intake of monounsaturated and polyunsaturated plant fats.

Animal breeders are raising much leaner cows and hogs today than in 1950. The demand for chicken has skyrocketed. In fact, a major fast food chain recently had to delay introducing a new chicken product for several months until enough chickens were available for the day of introduction.

Other aspects of the U.S. diet are more mixed. The NHANES II survey showed that white bread, rolls, and crackers; doughnuts, cakes, and cookies; alcoholic beverages; whole milk and whole milk beverages; and hamburgers, cheeseburgers, and meatloaf are the five major contributors of kcalories to the U.S. diet. If the new thrust in diets truly is toward a decrease in alcohol, sugar, and saturated fat intakes, along with increased consumption of fiber, the foods listed above are not the types we would expect to top the list. In terms of sheer frequency, coffee and tea; white bread, rolls and crackers; margarine; whole milk and whole milk beverages; doughnuts, cakes and cookies; and sugar are still the top six food categories most commonly consumed. (The overall U.S. diet may have improved

Text continued on p. 528

Expert Opinion

Prescription for a Healthy Diet

FRANK E. YOUNG, M.D., Ph.D.

We Americans are continually bombarded with information about diet and health. Almost daily, it seems, the media bring us reports of new studies showing how what we eat affects our well-being. Bookstores display shelves of volumes telling us what to eat and what not to eat to keep our bodies healthy. Food manufacturers and industry associations tell us that their products will make our bones strong, keep our bowels in good order, and keep our bodies slim and trim. But what is advanced as a preventative for one ill this week all too often is denounced as the cause of another the next. With all the conflicting messages we receive, it is no wonder that we are often tempted to throw up our hands in exasperation.

As a physician, I've witnessed this confusion and frustration among patients. And as a physician and former educator, I believe the public needs to know that what we eat *does* make a difference in our health. Evidence identifies diet as a risk factor for 5 of the 10 leading causes of death: heart disease, stroke, atherosclerosis (commonly known as hardening of the arteries), diabetes, and some types of cancer. These disorders together now account for more than two thirds of all deaths in the United States. Also among the leading causes of death in Americans are three associated with excessive alcohol consumption—cirrhosis of the liver, accidents, and suicides.

Indeed, the recently published *Surgeon General's Report on Nutrition and Health* states that "for the two out of three adult Americans who do not smoke and do not drink excessively, one personal choice seems to influence long-term health prospects more than any other: what we eat."

Whereas in years past our main nutrition concerns focused on nutrient *deficiencies* that produced diseases such as rickets (vitamin D deficiency), scurvy (vitamin C deficiency), and pellagra (niacin deficiency), the problem for most of us nowadays has shifted to *overconsumption* of certain dietary components—particularly fat. Americans tend to eat foods high in fat, often at the expense of others high in complex carbohydrates and fiber—such as vegetables, fruits, and whole-grain products—that may promote better health. Dietary fat accounts for about 37% of the total caloric intake of Americans—well above the 30% maximum recommended by the American Heart Association and the American Cancer Society. In light of the evidence linking fat and cholesterol consumption to heart and circulatory diseases, the old saying "The way to a man's heart is through his stomach" takes on a different, more ominous, meaning—for men and women alike.

Because various other factors—for example, genetics and environment—also influence disease development, we cannot say exactly to what extent diet contributes to a particular illness. However, substantial laboratory, animal, clinical, and epidemiologic research data suggest that dietary habits can influence our risk of developing chronic diseases. Most people can reduce their risk of getting these diseases by following these five guidelines:

- ***Reduce consumption of fat (especially saturated fat) and cholesterol.*** High fat intake is associated with a greater risk for obesity, some cancers, and possibly gallbladder disease. There is also strong evidence of a link between saturated fat intake, high amounts of cholesterol in the blood, and coronary heart disease. (Fats in food are mixtures of saturated and unsaturated fatty acids. Foods high in saturated fat include, for example, butter, cream, shortenings, and fatty meats. Most vegetable oils, such as corn and safflower oils, contain mostly unsaturated fat. Cholesterol is a fat-like substance found in foods derived from animals).

To reduce the amount of fat you eat, choose foods relatively low in saturated fat and cholesterol. Trim the fat on meats, and add more fruits, vegetables, whole-grain products, and cereals to your diet. Include fish, poultry prepared without the skin, lean meats, and low-fat dairy products. Prepare foods using as little fat as possible. Broil, bake or boil foods rather than frying them. When you do use fat in cooking, use unsaturated vegetable oils.

- ***Keep your weight at a desirable level.*** Overweight people are at greater risk of diabetes mellitus, high blood pressure, stroke, coronary heart disease, possibly some types of cancer—especially uterine and breast cancer—and other chronic diseases.

To achieve and maintain proper weight, eat a variety of foods relatively low in kcalories, fat and sugar, and minimize your alcohol consumption. Keep up a routine exercise program. Walking daily or jogging, bicycling, or swimming three times a week for at least 20 minutes will help expend kcalories and maintain fitness.

Expert Opinion—cont'd

▪ ***Eat more foods with complex carbohydrates and fiber.*** Diets high in complex carbohydrates and fiber are associated with lower rates of diverticulosis and may decrease the risk of colon cancer. Eating foods high in fiber can also alleviate chronic constipation. There is some evidence, too, that frequent consumption of fruits and vegetables, especially dark green and deep yellow vegetables, may lower the risk of cancers of the lung and bladder and some cancers of the digestive tract. And the more kcalories you derive from whole-grain foods, vegetables, and fruits, the fewer fatty foods you will tend to eat, which is a benefit in itself.

▪ ***Reduce sodium intake.*** High sodium intake is related to high blood pressure and stroke in some individuals. Because Americans generally consume more sodium than they need, it would be wise for most of us to cut down our use of salt, which is the major source of sodium in our diets. Average daily sodium intake for adults in the United States is 4 to 6 grams—far above the 1.1 to 3.3 grams found safe and adequate by the National Research Council. Blacks and people with a family history of high blood pressure are at a particular risk of this "silent killer."

So, choose foods relatively low in sodium, and add little or no salt to cooking and at the table.

▪ ***If you drink alcoholic beverages, do so in moderation*** (no more than two drinks a day).

Susceptible individuals can become addicted to alcohol. Heavy drinkers often develop nutritional deficiencies, partly because of decreased appetite and impaired absorption of nutrients. Liver disease, some types of cancer, high blood pressure, stroke, and heart disease are also associated with excessive alcohol consumption. Alcohol can cause impaired judgment and impaired ability to operate machinery and to drive vehicles. Alcohol abuse has also been associated with severe family problems, suicides, and homicides. Because a threshold of safety for alcohol intake during pregnancy has not been established, pregnant women should avoid drinking alcoholic beverages.

While following these five guidelines can benefit almost everyone, other nutritional issues are of particular importance to certain groups:

▪ ***Fluoride:*** People who live in areas without sufficient fluoride in the drinking water should consult their dentists about supplementary fluoride sources for their children to help reduce cavities.

▪ ***Sugar:*** People who are particularly prone to cavities, especially children, should limit their consumption of high-sugar foods. Sticky sweets that cling to the teeth are more harmful in producing cavities than those that wash off quickly. Development of cavities depends not only on how much, but also on how often, these foods are eaten.

▪ ***Calcium:*** Adolescent girls and adult women especially should eat more foods high in calcium, including low-fat dairy products. Sufficient calcium intake in the first 30 to 40 years of life helps build peak bone mass and may decrease the risk of developing osteoporosis (a progressive loss of bone mass) later in life.

▪ ***Iron:*** Foods rich in iron are important for children, adolescents, and women of childbearing age. Lean red meats, fish, certain kinds of beans, iron-enriched cereals, and whole-grain products are good sources of iron.

For some time now, the food industry has expressed interest in marketing and promoting products for their possible health benefits in lowering the risk for some diseases. In the past, the FDA prohibited any such health claims on food product labels because of the potential for abuse. Fraudulent, misleading, and unproved statements could, at the worst, damage rather than improve public health. The authority to prohibit such claims stems from provisions of the Federal Food, Drug, and Cosmetic (FD&C) Act that spell out how industry must present nutrition information on food labels and rule out certain types of claims.

However, believing it important for the public to be better informed about the benefits of sound nutrition, the agency in August 1987 proposed a regulation that would allow manufacturers to include health messages on product labels, so long as they meet specific criteria developed to protect the public. The criteria would not change the agency's basic interpretation of the requirements of the FD&C Act. We are now in the process of preparing a final rule, based on review of public comments we have received.

Almost to a man—and woman—we can agree that enjoyment of good food is one of life's great pleasures. If we remember to use common sense and moderation in what we eat and drink, we can hope to enjoy improved health as well.

Dr. Young is the Commissioner of Food and Drugs.

For a contrasting opinion, see the next Expert Opinion.

Expert Opinion

What Should I Eat to Live Longer?

DAVID KLURFELD, Ph.D.

The fountain of youth emanates, according to popular culture, from a proper diet. This rosy view stems, in part, from the dietary recommendations made by many scientific groups to reduce the risk of heart disease, cancer, and other chronic illnesses. The most recent, and arguably the most definitive, are the *Surgeon General's Report on Nutrition and Health* and the National Academy of Sciences' *Diet and Health: Implications for Reducing Chronic Disease Risk.* Implicit in proposed dietary recommendations is the promise of longer life—but how long and for whom?

Cardiovascular disease and cancer account for almost three-fourths of all deaths in affluent societies. One reason for this is that many causes of premature death—infections, poor sanitation, and accidents—have been dramatically allayed. This change translates into a life expectancy at birth in the United States of 71 years for men and 78 years for women. In only a few other countries is this life span exceeded—but by no more than a few years—and in most of them the diet is similar to that in the United States. In spite of our highly publicized "killer diet," deaths from heart disease, stroke, and cancer unrelated to tobacco use have all declined significantly over the last 20 years. We don't know for sure why this drop occurred, but it has been attributed, in part, to less use of tobacco and reductions in hypertension and in serum cholesterol, along with better medical care. These changes in risk factors point to the multifaceted causes of both heart disease and cancer. In addition, since many environmental factors interact with genetic predisposition to a disease, it is incorrect to attribute most of the risk for chronic diseases to diet alone.

Many of the estimates of dietary contribution to the risk of cancer are made by default; that is, cancers that are not traceable to other risk factors are often lumped as being caused by diet. The National Academy of Science's report concluded that "the data are not sufficient, however, to quantitate the contribution of the diet to overall cancer risk or to determine the amount of reduction in risk that might be achieved by dietary modification." Nevertheless, this committee and others have proposed a low-fat, high–complex-carbohydrate diet to reduce cancer risk. They point out that in Mediterranean countries the death rates for diet-associated cancers are half those in the United States. But do these people live longer or enjoy better health? There is a conspicuous lack of good data to decide this.

One troubling point is that there is a strong inverse correlation between rates of stomach and colon cancer. Most affluent countries with high-fat diets have high colon-cancer rates but fairly low stomach-cancer rates. By contrast, in countries where people eat low-fat diets, there is not much colon cancer but the rates of stomach cancer are higher than the U.S. rates of stomach, colon, and breast cancer combined. This relationship is unexplained and has been attributed to differences in refrigeration of foods, an uncontaminated food supply, and consumption of specific foods.

So we cannot reliably estimate the quantitative impact of diet on cancer. Can we, though, reduce cardiovascular disease by dietary means with some degree of certainty? Probably, according to epidemiologic and animal data. But epidemiology offers only leads—it cannot demonstrate cause and effect.

Today, there's little controversy over increased risk of heart disease with elevated levels of serum cholesterol. What is debated is at what point dietary treatment should be supplemented with drugs. And although the consensus recommendation is to reduce cholesterol below 200 milligrams per deciliter (mg/dl), some argue that this is too modest a target, while others contend that it's an unnecessary one.

Advocates of reducing the population's serum cholesterol via diet often cite the Lipid Research Clinic trial, which found that a 1% drop in serum cholesterol leads to a 2% decline in heart disease. There are at least three crucial reasons for not jumping the gun and applying this finding to the general population. First, this study was concerned with effects of medications; it excluded men whose serum cholesterol was normalized by diet. Second, the slope of heart disease versus serum

Expert Opinion—cont'd

cholesterol is quite steep at the upper levels (over 250 milligrams per deciliter) but very shallow near 220 milligrams per deciliter. So much less benefit, if any, is derived from lowering average cholesterol values. Finally, although heart disease was reduced, all-cause mortality was the same in treated and untreated men.

These results (and those from other studies) indicate that a reduction in high serum cholesterol levels is of benefit in preventing heart disease but not in prolonging life. There is no indication of what would happen at lower cholesterol levels. The Multiple Risk Factor Intervention Trial (MRFIT) data show that at average serum cholesterol levels, there's the least mortality; at higher levels, heart disease increases; and at the lowest levels, there's excess mortality from cancer and other causes. The relationship of low-fat diets or low serum cholesterol to increased mortality from cancer is baffling. It's likely that early disease accounts for some of the excess mortality with low cholesterol levels, but some studies have shown low cholesterol existed many years before diagnosis indicated excess cancer risk. A potential explanation is that carotenes (yellow to red pigments found especially in yellow and green vegetables), as well as other potential anticarcinogens, are transported with lipoproteins, which carry cholesterol in the blood.

Both epidemiologic and experimental studies point to specific nutrients that are associated with the incidence of chronic disease. Generally, these nutrients are found in a high-fat, low-fiber diet—a diet that is also an indicator of affluence. There's a strong statistical correlation between gross national product, telephones, flush toilets, and other signs of wealth and the incidence of cancer and heart disease because life expectancy is longer in more affluent countries. Populations that can afford to eat a lot of fat, sugar, and salt do so because these three dietary components are what make—or what people think make—food taste good. Poor people who eat a lot of starch do so because they cannot afford more nutritious foods. Americans tend to eat far more protein than they need, yet there's little debate over this indulgence as a contributor to essential hypertension—even though it is known that high protein intake increases renal blood flow. Instead, everyone in the country has been told to follow a low-sodium diet when only a minority are hypertensive and a few of those are salt sensitive.

A potential explanation for the lack of uniformity in response to dietary factors is that perhaps only some of the population shows elevated serum cholesterol from eating saturated fat, only some people are genetically predisposed to cancer of the colon, while a fortunate few are destined to live long healthy lives no matter what rules they violate. This observation does not necessarily discount the importance of nutrition but suggests that recommendations for dietary modification should not be blanket public health policies, but instead recommendations need to be made on individualized bases—that is, only for those who are at increased risk for killer diseases via family history or the presence of other risk factors. The ability of diet to alter the risk of disease needs to be kept in perspective. Although data suggest that consumption of dark green vegetables reduces the risk of lung cancer in smokers (but not the risk to nonsmokers), it makes far more sense to avoid tobacco because it is probably the strongest environmental risk factor for both cancer and heart disease.

There is little firm evidence that the general population will benefit from any of the low-fat, high-fiber diets proposed to reduce heart disease and cancer. The explanation that such diets wouldn't hurt may satisfy some, but it's certainly not scientific. The burden of proof should fall on those who suggest major dietary changes rather than on those who question the efficacy of those changes. Although what is written today will surely be outdated in the future, there are two general nutritional rules that will probably make sense over time: (1) eat a variety of foods, and (2) consume all foods in moderation. Boring, perhaps, but advice one can take to heart.

Dr. Klurfeld is associate professor at the University of Pennsylvania School of Medicine and The Wistar Institute.

since that study was completed in 1980.) Our suggestions for improvement would stress low-fat milk; whole-wheat bread and whole-grain cereals; lean meat and tuna; and oranges and broccoli. What would your list look like?

Is there an ideal diet?

There probably is an ideal diet for you, based on your particular nutritional and health status, but there is no single type of diet that provides optimal health for everyone. The Japanese diet is often promoted as a healthful alternative for North Americans. At the same time, it has been associated with one of the highest rates of stomach cancer in the world, which offsets its low risk for colon or breast cancer. Death from heart disease is about seven times lower in Japan than in the United States, but life expectancy is quite similar.[12]

Many cultural dietary patterns encompass the practices recommended by nutrition experts: eating a variety of foods, maintaining a desirable body weight, and maintaining a physically active life-style. (See Nutrition Perspective 17-1 on the need for physical activity and Nutrition Perspective 17-2 on diets for our generally rushed life-styles.) For you, the key is to focus on the likely causes of morbidity and mortality in your life, and to make specific changes to address those. Whether these changes include switching to bran cereal, rice, pasta, fish, chicken, broccoli, and bok choy and walking 2 miles four times a week is up to you. These practices all provide a means to further and maintain nutritional and overall health, but are not the only path to health. Your overriding consideration should be the overall quality and length of life and how they can be enhanced by dietary changes. Now is the time to design this plan. Chapter 18, How to Improve Your Diet, will help you put it into practice.

Concept Check

Surveys show that North Americans are beginning to follow general health recommendations. Some health promotion goals, however, are far from being met. Scientists do not agree as to the best dietary recommendations for the public. Genetic background, medical conditions, and other life-style practices influence an individual's optimal diet. Many scientists support general dietary recommendations that benefit the health of most people, while not hampering the health of others, but individual plans should be developed when possible.

NUTRITION IN THE ELDERLY YEARS

life span
The potential oldest age to which a person can survive.

The human **life span** is approximately 120 years. This is about as long as anyone can expect to live. In comparison, the domestic dog has a life span of 20 years, while a rat has a life span of 5 years.

Life expectancy

life expectancy
The average length of life for a given group of people.

Life expectancy is the time an average person can expect to live. In 1988 life expectancy in North America was 71 years for men and 78 years for women. It hasn't always been this long. Life expectancy for primitive humans was about 30 to 35 years. It had increased to 49 years by medieval England, and remained so until the turn of this century in the United States. During the last 80 years, life expectancy for nearly all people has lengthened, mainly because of changes in the principal causes of death.

Note that although life expectancy has increased since 1900, the maximum life span of a human has remained constant.

At the turn of this century, infectious diseases were a common cause of death. *Now the principal causes of death in Western societies are related to heart disease and cancer* (Figure 17-2). The decline in infant and childhood deaths and better diets and health care have allowed more people to age into their elderly years. Because of all these changes, life expectancy has increased.

1900

Rank	Cause of death	Percent mortality
1	Pneumonia and influenza	11.8
2	Tuberculosis	11.3
3	Diarrhea and enteritis	8.3
4	Heart disease	8.0
5	Cerebrovascular disease	6.2
6	Nephritis	5.2
7	Accidents	4.2
8	Cancer	3.7
9	Diphtheria	2.3
10	Meningitis	2.0

1988

Cause of death	Percent mortality
Heart disease	35.7
Cancer	22.4
Cerebrovascular disease	7.0
Accidents	4.4
Pneumonia and influenza	7.1
Digestive and liver disease	3.6
Endocrine, metabolic, and immune disease (diabetes)	2.3
Genitourinary disease	1.6
Diseases of the nervous system	1.3
Infections and parasitic disease	1.1

Figure 17-2

Changes in the causes of death during this century. Chronic diseases, rather than the infectious diseases, are now the major "killers."

In 1900, half of all whites died before reaching age 55. In 1940, half were still alive at age 68. Today, half are alive at ages exceeding 70 years. In the year 2035 there will be twice as many people older than age 65 years than today (Figure 17-3). This is the first time in history a society will need to deal with such a large elderly population.

The "graying" of North America

The "graying" of North America poses some problems. Today, while people older than age 65 account for 11% of the U.S. population, they account for 25% of all prescription drugs used, 40% of acute care hospital stays, and one half the federal health budget. Of the elderly, 85% have nutrition-related problems, such as heart disease, diabetes mellitus, hypertension, osteoporosis, and obesity (Table 17-3).

Compression of morbidity, as suggested at the beginning of this chapter, is an important goal for controlling health care costs, since merely by increasing our numbers we will require more total health care services as we age. The more independent, healthy years we live, the less we burden our health care system, which will increasingly have to scramble to accommodate our burgeoning elderly population.

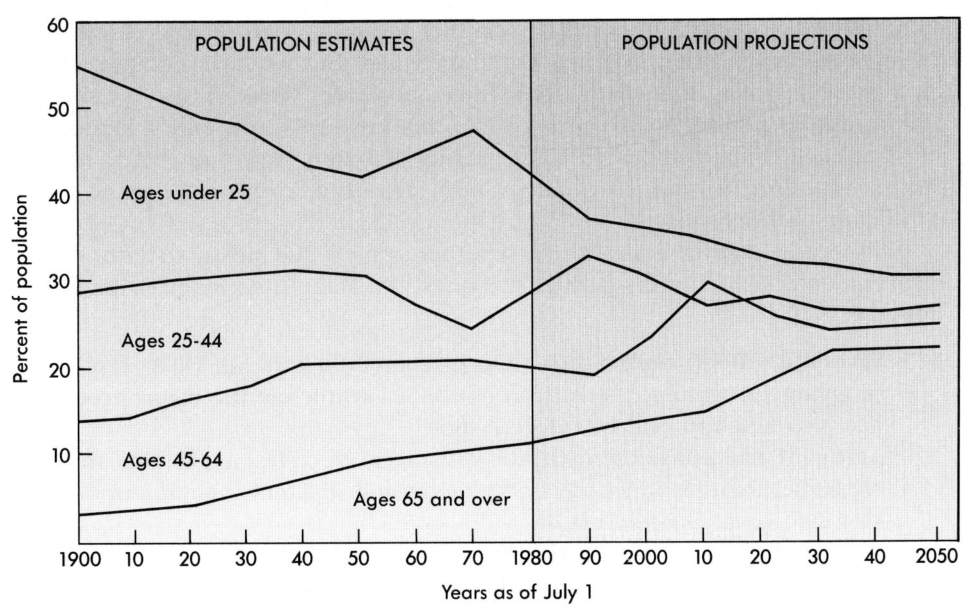

Figure 17-3

Trend in age distribution of U.S. population (including Armed Forces overseas), 1900-2050. The United States has never had a population with so many elderly people as it will soon have.

Table 17-3

Selected disease conditions associated with aging

Chronic condition	Rate of occurrence per 1000 persons		
	Total	**45-64 years**	**65+ years**
Arthritis	121	247	465
Hypertension	113	244	379
Hearing impairments	83	143	284
Heart conditions	76	123	277
Visual impairments	40	55	137
Arteriosclerosis	—	—	—
Deformities or orthopedic impairments	82	118	128
Diabetes	24	57	83
Diseases of urinary system	25	32	56
Asthma	32	34	29

From: Hegarty V: Decisions in nutrition, St. Louis, 1988, The CV Mosby Co.

reserve capacity
The extent to which an organ can preserve essentially normal function, despite decreasing cell number or cell activity.

kidney nephrons
Unit of kidney cells that filter wastes from the bloodstream.

A good example of this aging process is lactase deficiency. For some people, lactase enzyme activity may decline during childhood but, generally, clear symptoms of gas and bloating after milk consumption do not appear until adulthood. Although lactase output decreases in these cases, perhaps from birth, enough enzyme is present to maintain sufficient lactose digestion until adulthood.

What causes aging?

One view of aging describes it as processes beginning soon after fertilization. When we are young, aging is not apparent because the major metabolic activities are geared toward growth and maturation. We produce plenty of active cells to meet physiological needs. During adolescence and early adulthood, maintenance and homeostasis become the body's major tasks. Eventually, as more cells age and die, homeostatic mechanisms cannot totally adjust to meet physiological demands. Physiological functioning begins to decrease, but organs usually retain enough **reserve capacity** so that for a long time they show no disease. While no symptoms appear, subclinical disease may develop, and if allowed to progress for years and years, organ function noticeably deteriorates.

Cell aging probably results from both automatic cellular changes and environmental influences. Throughout the animal kingdom, aging is predictable. Eventually, cells lose their ability to regenerate needed components, and they die. As more and more cells in an organ system die, organ function decreases. After age 14 months, human brain cells are continually lost, but we have enough reserve capacity to maintain mental function throughout life. There is also a continual loss of **kidney nephrons.** In some people this loss leads to eventual kidney failure, but most of us maintain sufficient kidney function. Again, *in aging, there is first a reduction in reserve capacity. Only after that is exhausted does actual organ function decrease.*

Why cells age remains a mystery. Whether aging is due mostly to automatic or environmental influences is part of the question. Many theories have been promoted:[13,30]

- **Errors in DNA replication**—Once enough errors in DNA replication (copying) accumulate, a cell can no longer synthesize the major proteins it needs to function, and therefore it dies.
- **Aging of the connective tissue**—Changes in collagen proteins may decrease flexibility in key body components and so alter organ function. Wrinkled skin is an apparent result.
- **Build-up of toxic products**—Breakdown products of lipids, such as **lipofuscin,** may hamper normal metabolic processes by clogging cells. You

can think of lipofuscin as intracellular "sludge."

lipofuscin (ceroid pigments)
Signs of accumulation of lipid breakdown products in cells often seen as brown spots on the skin.

- **Free radical damage**—Free radicals attack cells and damage cell membranes and proteins. One way to prevent some damage from free radicals is to consume adequate (but not excessive) vitamin E. In contrast, consuming cellular enzymes that are designed to break down free radicals and other highly oxidative compounds does not help: ingested enzymes are dismantled during digestion—before they can act in the body. For example, the enzyme **superoxide dismutase,** which is sold by some health food stores, is made by cells to destroy super oxide negative free radicals (O_2^-). *Adding superoxide dismutase to a diet does not help, because digestion in the intestine breaks it into amino acids along with other proteins in the diet.*

superoxide dismutase
An enzyme that can neutralize a superoxide negative free radical.

- **Changes in hormone function**—The hormone dehydroepiandrosterone (DHEA), produced by the adrenal glands, is present in extremely high levels in the blood of young adults and falls sharply with age. This has led to speculation that it may play a role in aging. Long-term effects of using products containing this hormone are unknown. The FDA has not approved use of DHEA so any marketing of this drug in the United States is illegal.
- **Changes in the efficiency of the immune system**—The thymus gland, located in the upper chest, is a major component of the immune system. Present at birth, it reaches maximum size during adolescence and is barely visible by age 50. The immune system itself runs along a somewhat parallel track: it is most efficient during childhood and young adulthood, but with advancing age, it is less able to recognize and counteract foreign substances, such as viruses, that enter the body.
- **Autoimmune effects—Autoimmune** reactions occur when white blood cells and antibodies fail to distinguish between you and foreign compounds invading your body. White blood cells and antibodies then begin to attack body tissues, as well as foreign compounds. Many diseases, including some forms of diabetes mellitus and arthritis, involve an autoimmune response.

autoimmune
Immune reactions against normal body cells; self against self.

- **Programmed death**—Each cell can divide only a limited number of times, about 50. Once this number of divisions occurs, the cell automatically succumbs.

Most likely, the actual cause of aging is a combination of these events and changes.

Can diet stop the aging process?

No diet can stop aging, but research in this century shows that raising laboratory animals after weaning on low-energy diets—about two thirds the energy they normally consume—greatly slows aging. Animals on these Spartan rations live about 50% longer than control groups allowed to feed "ad libitum" (at their pleasure).[29]

The key is to restrict only kcalories, not other nutrients. Humans living in semistarvation conditions do not live longer than our typical "western" life expectancy: their diets are low in kcalories, but also low in proteins, many vitamins, and many minerals.

It is not clear how a low-kcalorie diet increases the life span of animals. Hormonal or immune system changes may be involved, as suggested in Chapter 5. Delaying puberty may also play a key role. Researchers doubt that a decreased metabolic rate is the reason.[16] It is clear that the animals grow more slowly, and this may affect their tendency to develop disease. How to apply the findings from these animal studies to humans is unknown. Severe kcalorie restriction, especially for infants, can be dangerous. We must wait for further research.

Concept Check

While life span has not changed, life expectancy has increased dramatically over the past century. For societies, this means an increasing proportion of the population is, and will be, over 65 years of age. Continually rising health care costs make compression of morbidity very important. Aging may begin prior to birth and probably results from both automatic cellular changes and environmental influences. Some popular theories about why we age raise these possibilities: errors in DNA replication accumulate and cause cell death; aging of the connective tissue; buildup of lipid by-products, such as lipofuscin; free-radical damage; hormonal and immune system dysfunction; and autoimmune damage. Diet can play a role in slowing some of these processes.

THE EFFECTS OF AGING ON THE NUTRITIONAL HEALTH OF THE ELDERLY

Elderly people vary more in health status among themselves than do any other age-group. ***Physiological age is much more important than chronological age in the elderly years.*** To predict the nutritional problems of an elderly person, it is necessary to know to what extent physiological capabilities have been affected by aging (Figure 17-4), as well as the extent to which the person shows early warning signs for malnutrition (Table 17-4).[4] Let's examine how aging affects some major body systems and how these changes contribute to malnutrition, and then note which changes in nutrient intake are needed to counteract problem conditions.[4,30]

Taste and smell

Sensitivity to taste and smell usually decreases with aging. About one third to one half of a person's taste buds die by age 70 years. Food companies are carving a niche in the marketplace by capitalizing on this change: by using a variety of flavor enhancers they simply make foods tastier for the elderly. But for this group, a poor diet and possibly zinc deficiency can also contribute to a loss of taste.[28] So a poor appetite should never be dismissed as a characteristic of old age. Many causes can be remedied.[3]

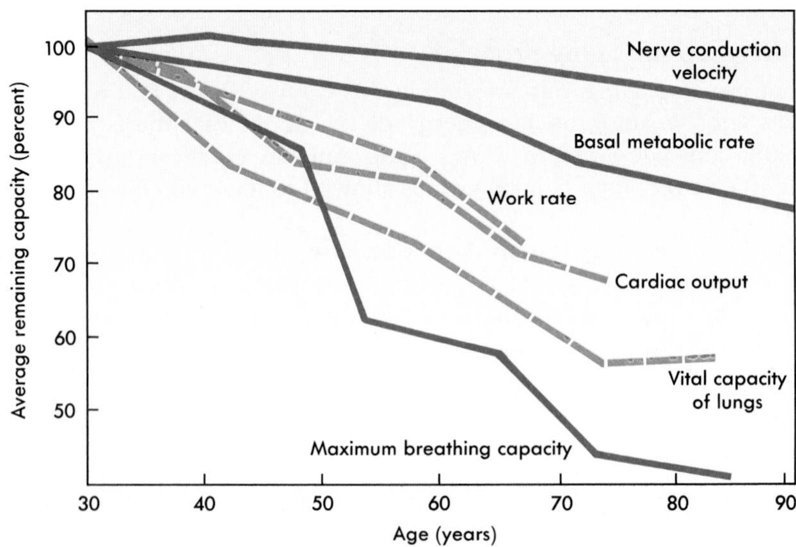

Figure 17-4

The declines in physiological function. Some decline is seen in aging, especially in primarily sedentary people.

Table 17-4

Potential, easily recognizable warning signals for malnutrition	
Recent weight change of ±3 kg (7 lb)	High alcohol intake
Chewing/swallowing difficulties	Side effects of medication
After stomach surgery	Missing meals or drinks
Physical disability	No food stores
Lack of sunlight	Food wastage/rejection
Depression/loneliness	Lack of fruit, fruit juices, raw or freshly cooked vegetables
Mental confusion	Low budget for food
	Poor nutritional knowledge

From: Davies L: Practical nutrition for the elderly, Nutrition Reviews 46:83, 1988.

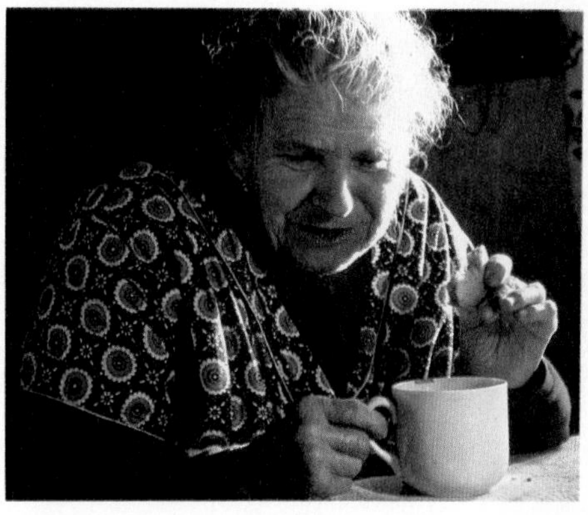

Older people should be careful to maintain an adequate fluid intake.

Dentition

About 50% of people over age 50 years have lost all their teeth. Replacement dentures enable some to chew normally, but many elderly people, especially men, have denture problems. A pureed diet is not necessarily the remedy, but the elderly do require some individual dietary problem-solving to identify which foods need to be modified in consistency and which can be eaten in a typical state.

Thirst

Elderly people often partially lose their sense of thirst. They are then more likely to suffer from dehydration, which can lead to confusion. It is important for them to consume enough fluids, and if necessary, they should sometimes be monitored to ensure they do so. An approximate fluid recommendation is the same for younger adults, 1 milliliter per kcalorie. This amount must be adjusted to reflect increased urination due to the use of diuretics, or loss of fluid through other routes, such as from an **ostomy.**

Some important signs of dehydration, other than confusion, include dry lips, sunken eyes, increased body temperature, decreased blood pressure, constipation, decreased urine output, and nausea.

ostomy
A surgically created short circuit in intestinal flow where the end point usually opens from the abdominal cavity rather than the anus, as in the case with a colostomy.

The intestinal tract

The main intestinal problem for the elderly is constipation. Elderly people generally need to consume more dietary fiber than they did in their youth, approximately 35 grams a day. Fluid intake should also increase to avoid intestinal obstruction resulting from a high fiber intake. However, all age-groups should avoid using mineral oil as a laxative at mealtimes because it binds fat-soluble vitamins.

Lactase synthesis frequently slows in elderly people. The options for people with lactose intolerance are listed in Nutrition Perspective 3-2. A decrease in stomach acid production in the elderly is usually accompanied by decreased intrinsic factor synthesis. These last two changes can lead to poor absorption of vitamin B-12, and in turn, to pernicious anemia. Elderly people should be watched by their physicians for signs of pernicious anemia (see Chapter 12).

The reduced synthesis of stomach acid may also hamper iron absorption. Factors that further interfere with iron status in the body include: regular use of aspirin, which causes blood loss in the stomach; use of antacids, which may bind iron; and ulcers and hemorrhoids, which also cause blood loss.

Liver, gallbladder, and pancreas

The liver functions less efficiently in the elderly years. Some decline results from a fat buildup if there is long-standing alcohol consumption. If actual cirrhosis develops, the liver functions even less efficiently (see Chapter 7). This drop in liver function decreases the ability to detoxify many medications, and also increases the possibility for vitamin A toxicity. *Elderly people should be warned not to take excessive amounts of vitamin A.* Recall that vitamin A toxicity causes hair loss, malaise, headache, bone pain, liver dysfunction, and a decrease in white blood cell count (see Chapter 11).

Gallstones may cause problems for the liver by damming the fluids intended for secretion through the gallbladder. The fluids pool and back up into the liver. Gallstones can also hamper fat digestion because less bile is secreted into the small intestine. A low-fat diet may be necessary.

The digestive function of the pancreas may decline in the elderly years, but the pancreas has a large reserve capacity. A sign of a failing pancreas is high blood glucose due to decreased insulin secretion. High blood glucose levels in the elderly can also be caused by insulin resistance, a common result of obesity (see Chapter 4), or by a poor intake or absorption of chromium (see Chapter 14). *Where appropriate, improved nutrient intake and weight loss may improve insulin action.*

Kidney function

Kidneys eventually filter wastes more slowly as they lose nephrons (filters). Kidneys deteriorate in aging partly because of excess dietary protein and, in some cases, excess kcalories. The deterioration significantly decreases their ability to excrete the products of protein breakdown. While an increase in protein intake to 1 gram per kilogram of desirable body weight has generally been recommended for physically active elderly people, that does not apply to cases where decreased kidney function causes urea, the by-product of protein metabolism, to build up in the bloodstream.

Immune function

With age, the immune system often operates less efficiently. Adequate protein and zinc intakes are necessary to maximize the health of the immune system. Recurrent sicknesses and poor wound healing are warning signs of deficient protein and zinc intakes. They may be due to insufficient total food or to too few animal proteins in the diet, possibly because meats are difficult to chew. *Recall that animal proteins are an excellent source of zinc.*

Lung function

alveoli
Small air sacs in the lung.

Lung efficiency declines somewhat, but especially in elderly people who have smoked tobacco products and continue to smoke. Breathing becomes shallower and faster and more difficult as the number of **alveoli** decreases. Smoking often leads to emphysema and/or lung cancer. The decrease in lung efficiency accompanies a general downward spiral in body function: it leads to decreased physical activity and endurance and frequently to decreased food intake. These eventually hamper the ability to maintain overall health.

Hearing and vision

Vision and hearing both decline in the elderly years, though hearing impairment occurs mainly in industrial societies with urban traffic, aircraft, loud music, and pile drivers. People differ as to when or if these losses become disabling. Vision and hearing losses can make food shopping difficult. Elderly people may be unable to drive or read food labels. They may also avoid social contacts as much as possible because they can't hear and respond to others. Poor vision may make them afraid to walk for fear of falling. They may need assistance in shopping.

Decrease in lean tissue

Some muscle cells shrink and others are lost as muscles age; some muscles lose their ability to contract as they accumulate fat and collagen. Life-style partially determines the rate of muscle mass deterioration: an active life-style tends to maintain muscle mass, whereas a very inactive one causes a loss of muscle mass.

As lean tissue decreases with age, less energy is used while a person is resting. Accompanying the loss in lean body mass is a continual decline in basal metabolism of about 2% every 10 years from age 30 years. This requires elderly people to choose foods wisely, because while their energy needs decrease, their needs for most vitamin and minerals do not.

Physical activity is desirable for elderly people because it allows them to eat more food, thereby increasing their chances of consuming an adequate diet. Another advisable practice is to decrease sugar and fat consumption as energy needs fall to increase the diet's nutrient density. An elderly person may need to take a multivitamin and mineral supplement with a physician's guidance if energy intake falls below 1500 kcalories (see Nutrition Perspective 11-1).

Cardiovascular health

Cardiac output often drops in elderly people. The decline is usually due to inactivity and consequent poor heart conditioning, which allow fatty and connective tissues to infiltrate the heart's muscular wall. If an elderly person remains physically active, **cardiac output** does not fall, so the decline is not due to an aging process per se.[13]

cardiac output
The amount of blood pumped by the heart.

The dramatic problems of the cardiovascular system associated with aging—heart attack and stroke—are caused primarily by atherosclerosis and high blood pressure. Atherosclerotic plaque accumulates in the arteries, reducing their elasticity and constricting blood flow, which then elevates blood pressure.[11] You already know the main way to limit the build up of atherosclerotic plaque: keep the serum cholesterol level below 200 milligrams per 100 milliliters. As for high blood pressure, while a severe sodium restriction works for most people, a mild sodium restriction (4 grams of sodium daily) is not as helpful for people who are not sensitive to salt; it is more effective for "salt sensitive" people. A limit of 2 grams of sodium helps almost all people with hypertension, but that is a difficult diet to plan and follow (see Nutrition Perspective 13-2). *We can do much to prevent heart attack and stroke just by eating nutritiously, walking briskly or exercising regularly, controlling blood pressure, and avoiding smoking.*

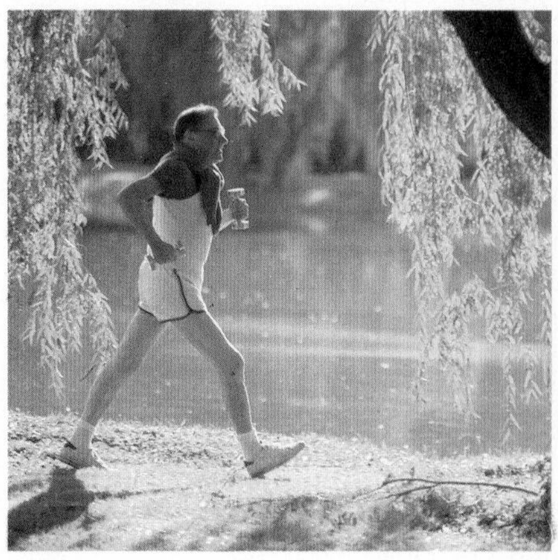

Regular exercise forms one step toward preventing heart attack and stroke.

Bone health

We discussed the decline in bone density with aging in Nutrition Perspective 13-2 on calcium and osteoporosis. Recall that bone loss in women occurs especially after menopause. Bone loss in men is slow and steady from middle age throughout the elderly years. For women, increasing one's calcium intake to 1500 milligrams per day can help maintain density in the cortical-type bones, but this does not predictably prevent bone loss in the more trabecular bony parts throughout the body. Presently, only estrogen replacement therapy, calcitriol therapy, calcitonin therapy, and possibly high doses of fluoride—administered with a physician's guidance—can claim that. Practicing weight-bearing exercises is also a good idea.

If osteoporosis becomes very severe, it limits the ability of elderly people to exercise, shop, prepare food, and live normally. Thus a further decrease in nutrient intake will likely result. There is concern that much hidden osteomalacia (vitamin D deficiency) may be present in the elderly.[8,14] Osteomalacia occurs primarily from a lack of sun exposure and possibly poor vitamin D synthesis in the skin. If predictable sun exposure is not available, as when the person is homebound, then a source for 10 micrograms of vitamin D per day should be found: fortified milk products or a vitamin supplement.

It is important to encourage elderly women to continue consuming the RDA for calcium and to seriously consider estrogen replacement therapy if they are still within 10 years of menopause.

OTHER FACTORS THAT INFLUENCE NUTRIENT NEEDS IN THE ELDERLY

Use of certain medications can profoundly affect nutrient needs in the elderly (Table 17-5).[20] Often at this age several medications must be taken for long peri-

Table 17-5

Potential drug-nutrient interactions for some commonly used drugs

Drug	Use	Nutrient	Potential side effect
Alcohol	—	Thiamin, vitamin B-6, folate, and zinc	Poor absorption/poor utilization
Antacids	Reduce stomach acidity	Calcium, vitamin B-12 and iron	Decreased absorption due to altered gastrointestinal pH
Anticoagulants	Prevention of blood clots	Vitamin K	Poor utilization
Antihistamines	Treatment of allergies and nausea; as local anesthetic	—	Weight gain
Beta-blocker (propanolol)	Decrease hypertension	(Cholesterol)	Some can increase serum cholesterol levels
Aspirin	Anti-inflammatory, pain reduction	Iron	Anemia from blood loss
Cathartics (laxatives)	To induce bowel movements	Calcium, potassium	Poor absorption
Cholestyramine	Reducing blood cholesterol	Vitamins A, D, E, K	Poor absorption
Cimetidine	Treatment of ulcers	Vitamin B-12	Poor absorption
Colchicine	Treatment of gout	Vitamin B-12, carotenes, and magnesium	Decreased absorption due to damaged intestinal mucosa
Corticosteroids	Anti-inflammatory	Zinc Calcium	Poor absorption Poor utilization
Furosemide	Potassium-wasting diuretic	Potassium and sodium	Increased loss
Isoniazid	Tuberculosis	Vitamin B-6	Poor utilization
Neomycin	Antibiotic	Fat, protein, sodium, potassium, calcium, iron, and vitamin B-12	Decreases pancreatic lipase, binds bile salts, and so interferes with absorption
MAO inhibitors	Antidepressant	Tyramine in aged foods	Hypertension caused by poor tyramine metabolism
Phenobarbital	Sedative; treatment of epilepsy	Vitamin D and folate	Reduced metabolism and utilization
Phenytoin	Treatment of epilepsy	Vitamin D and folate	Reduced metabolism and utilization
Tricyclic antidepressants	Antidepressant	—	Weight gain due to appetite stimulation

ods of time. Drug-related nutritional problems can be significant. The most notable ones are an increased need for potassium when consuming some types of diuretics, and changes in appetite when taking some types of antidepressant agents or antibiotics.

About 12% to 14% of elderly people experience significant depression. That, combined with isolation and loneliness as family and friends die, move away, or become less mobile frequently contributes to disinterest in eating and so to weight loss. Depression can descend into poor appetite, weakness, and then in to

Figure 17-5

The descent of poor health in the elderly. This decline needs to be prevented.

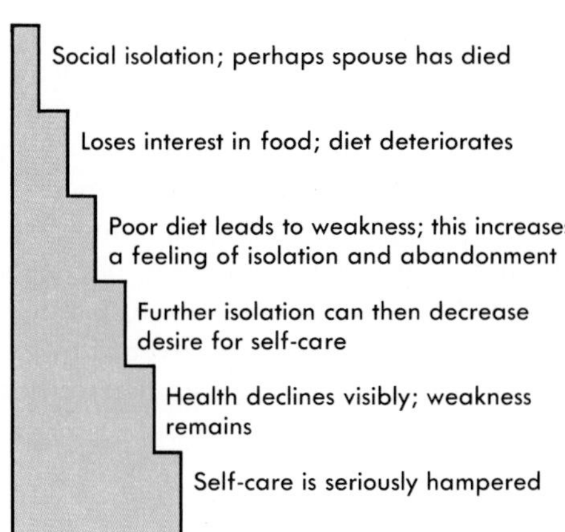

an even poorer appetite. In the elderly, the resulting poor nutritional state can lead to further mental confusion and increased isolation and loneliness (Figure 17-5).

The role of nutrition in preserving mental function in the elderly remains unclear. Specific nutritional deficiencies of thiamin, niacin, vitamin B-6, and vitamin B-12, as well as excessive alcohol use, cause well-recognized central nervous system disorders. However, the subtle effects of a low kcalorie intake that leads to semi-starvation are often overlooked. In addition, as mentioned earlier, a poor fluid intake may lead to dehydration and in turn to confusion.

We know mental illness can lead to a poor nutritional state, but the extent to which subtle nutritional deficiencies can lead to a poor mental state is not clear. It is important to prevent overt nutrient deficiencies, especially the ones mentioned above. Whether extra intake of specific amino acids, such as tryptophan, tyrosine, or choline, can increase brain neurotransmitter synthesis and therefore alter behavior is still unknown.

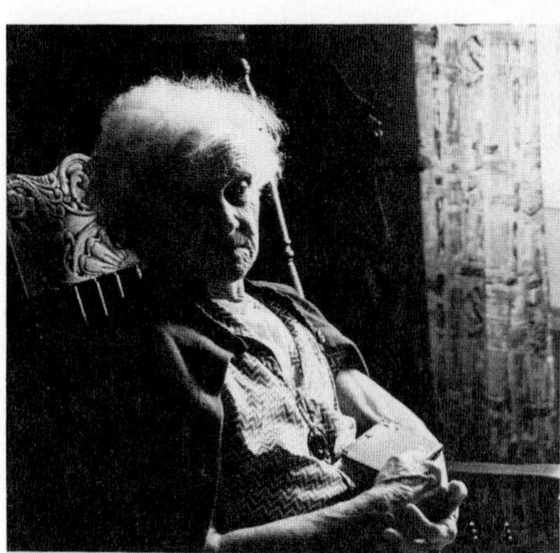

Loneliness and depression often contribute to a lack of appetite.

Concept Check

Nutritional problems of the elderly are related to the both presence of chronic diseases and to the normal decreases in organ function that occur with time. All these organ systems and functions decrease as we age: senses of taste, smell, thirst, hearing, and sight; digestion and absorption; liver, gallbladder, pancreas, kidneys, lungs, heart; and the immune system. In addition, muscle mass (largely due to inactivity) and bone mass gradually decrease. Diet changes can often help reduce the impact of these results of aging.

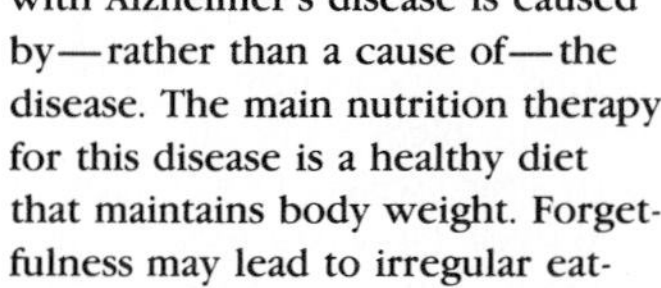

Scientists think that high aluminum retention in the brain of a person with Alzheimer's disease is caused by—rather than a cause of—the disease. The main nutrition therapy for this disease is a healthy diet that maintains body weight. Forgetfulness may lead to irregular eating habits and in turn to weight loss.[5,21]

DO THE RDA INCREASE IN THE ELDERLY YEARS?

Currently, the RDA for nutrients and kcalories includes one category for both men and women who are 51 years of age and older. Scientists know very little about the nutrient needs of the elderly, especially for those over age 75 years.[16,23,27] Only during the last few years has much research focussed on this. Our lack of information is reflected in the lack of changes in the RDA for nutrients for people older than 51 years.

Recently, a noted research team suggested that the current RDA for the elderly is probably too high for vitamin A and too low in protein (for active elderly people), for vitamins D, B-6, and B-12, and "about right" for the other nutrients.[27] In this case, the "about right" label may reflect either that studies suggest the RDA is adequate, or that we lack sufficient data to make a more definitive statement.

There is a concern that the RDA for calcium should be increased to help stem the acceleration of bone loss suffered by elderly women (see Chapter 13). Iron needs do not increase, since elderly women have no menstrual periods. However, chronic ulcers, hemorrhoids, and aspirin use may necessitate an increased iron intake. Recall, though, that the RDA applies only to healthy people. Elderly people with ulcers and heavy aspirin use are not covered by the RDA.

If an elderly person decides, with a physician's guidance, to use vitamin and mineral supplements, the focus should be on these nutrients.

Overall, nutrient needs for the elderly are similar to those for younger adults, but individual modifications are necessary to compensate for specific diseases present.[22]

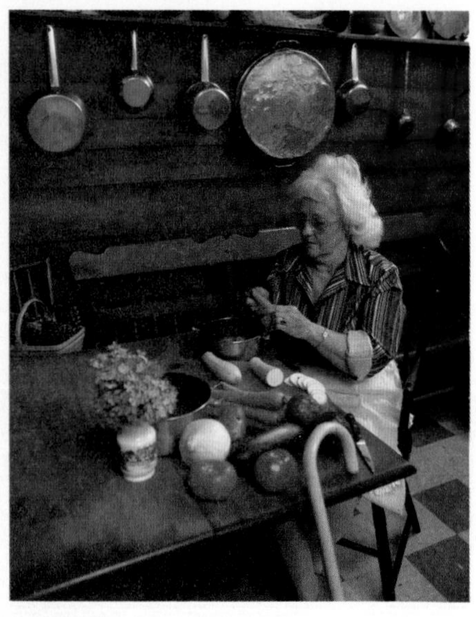

Vegetables continue to be a welcome food choice for the elderly.

Planning a diet for the elderly

Diet plans for the elderly should focus on vitamin D (and sun exposure), vitamins E, B-6, B-12, C, and thiamin and the minerals iron, calcium, and zinc.[7] It is best if the elderly can increase physical activity level so that they can safely increase food intake. This expands nutrient sources, simplifying the planning of an adequate diet. Also, as mentioned earlier, protein needs are approximately 1 gram per kilogram of desirable body weight (for physically active people), and fluid needs are 1 milliliter per kcalorie. A high-fiber diet can decrease constipation, but fiber intake should be slowly increased to about 35 grams, making sure a glass of water (or other fluid) follows each dose of fiber (see Chapter 4).

The majority of elderly people like most vegetables. There is no need to follow stereotypes suggesting that they do not like broccoli because it forms gas or tomatoes because they are too acidic. Eating habits at that age are individualistic, reflecting region, social class, ethnic group, and life experiences. Individual patterns need to be respected and explored.

The benefits of good nutrition in the elderly are many. It delays disease progression, improves management of existing diseases, hastens recovery from illnesses, increases mental, physical, and social well-being, and decreases the need for and length of hospitalization. Overall, a good nutritional intake should be a vital part of the health maintenance program for elderly people. Table 17-6 lists a

In the early elderly years, weight gain is the major problem, while in the later elderly years, weight loss is more of a concern. (It is best to compare an elderly person's weight with their previous year's weight.) Weight loss in elderly people often means increased risk of death. It may also indicate increased sickness and poor tolerance of medications.

Table 17-6

Guidelines for promoting healthful eating in later years

- Eat regularly. Small frequent meals may be best.
- Find out which convenience foods and labor-saving devices can be of help.
- Try new foods, new seasonings, and new ways of preparing foods. Don't just use convenience foods and canned goods.
- Keep some easy-to-prepare foods on hand for times when tired.
- Have a treat occasionally, perhaps an expensive cut of meat or a favorite fresh fruit.
- Eat in a well-lit or sunny area; arrange the table or tray attractively.
- Arrange things so food preparation and clean-up are easier.
- Eat when possible with friends, relatives, or at a senior citizen center.
- Share cooking responsibilities with a neighbor.
- Use community resources for help in shopping and other daily care needs.
- Stay physically active.

variety of ideas to promote healthful eating in the elderly years. These should focus on presenting nutritious, tasty food in a pleasant, friendly environment.

COMMUNITY NUTRITION SERVICES FOR THE ELDERLY

Health care advice and services can come from clinics, private practitioners, hospitals, and health maintenance organizations. Hospice centers, home health care agencies, adult day-care programs, and adult overnight-care programs can supply day-to-day care.

Nutrition programs for the elderly include congregate meal programs, for which elderly people gather for lunch; meals-on-wheels, which delivers meals to homes; food cooperatives; and a variety of clubs and social organizations. The congregate meal programs and meals-on-wheels are funded partially by the U.S. government under Title III of the Older Americans Act (Figure 17-6) and through volunteer community efforts. The U.S. government also sets specific standards for home-served meals and for those served in congregate feeding centers.[2] The meals are constructed so they include one-third of the RDA. The basic meal pattern is 3 ounces of meat or meat alternative, 1 cup of vegetables (2 or more servings), 1 slice of bread or alternative, 1 teaspoon of butter, 1 cup of milk, and ½ cup of dessert. The social aspect often improves an eldery person's appetite and general outlook.

Feeding sick, infirm, and/or mentally confused elderly people is time-consuming and demanding work that requires special training. It is important to look for a poor nutrient intake, even in those who live in nursing home settings.

To help elderly people shop for food, special transportation arrangements may be available through a local transit company or taxi service. Elderly people need to be aware of opportunities available to them in their community. In this way, they can be assisted in their day-to-day health and nutrition care and, ideally, remain as healthy and free to conduct their own lives independently for as long as possible.

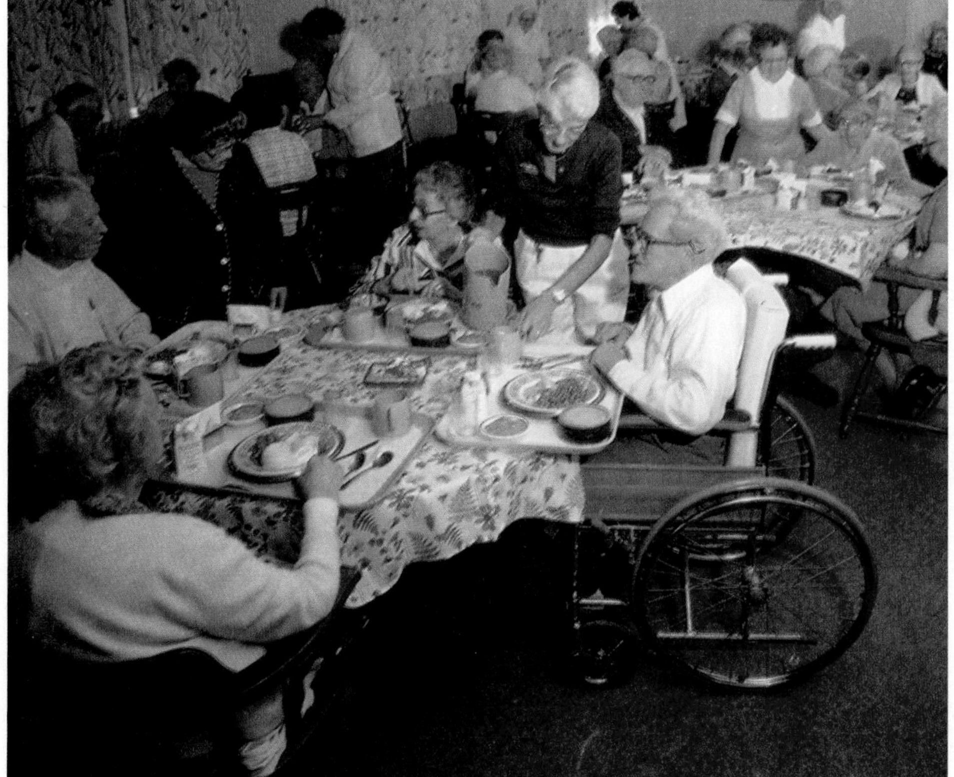

Figure 17-6

Congregate meals for the elderly. Sites in many communities in the United States provide nutritious meals and an opportunity to socialize for elderly people.

Concept Check

Specific nutrient requirements for the elderly are only now being extensively studied. Diet plans for the elderly should consider decreased physical abilities, presence of drug-nutrient interactions, possible depression, and economic constraints. Particular attention should be paid to sun exposure and intake of the vitamins D, E, B-6, B-12, thiamin, and C and the minerals iron, calcium, and zinc. Many services such as congregate meals and meals-on-wheels are available to assist the elderly population in the United States obtain a healthy diet.

Take Action

This is the time to make a thorough nutrition assessment of your diet and analyze your intake, or redo this if you did this earlier in the course. You know so much more now. A main barrier to understanding your diet is forgetting or overlooking what you consume. You can achieve surprising insights by keeping an accurate record of what you eat. Appendix Q has complete directions for recording your food intake and degree of physical activity, as well as analyzing both.

Now that you have calculated a single day's (or multiple day's) dietary intake and energy output:

1. Compare your intake to your RDA and ESADDI. Consider the adequacy of your day's diet and areas where you might improve your diet.
2. Pay special attention to those nutrients that affect your particular health status and are important to your health goals. If you have high blood pressure, for example, look closely at your sodium consumption. Or, if you don't drink milk, consider whether your calcium intake is adequate.
3. Now, let's examine some aspects of your diet in more depth.

Carbohydrate

What was your carbohydrate intake? ______________ grams/day

Is this enough to prevent ketosis? (see Chapter 4)

What percentage of your average daily total kcalorie intake is derived from carbohydrate? ______________%
([grams of carbohydrate × 4] ÷ kcalories) × 100

How does this percentage compare with the guideline of about 55% to 60% total kcalories? ______________

What was your daily intake of dietary fiber? ______________

What was your daily dietary fiber intake per 1000 kcalories? ______________

Does this intake meet the goal of 10 to 13 grams of dietary fiber per 1000 kcalories?

In what ways do you think you need to change your diet to better meet the carbohydrate and fiber recommendations listed above?

Take Action—cont'd

Fat

What was your fat intake? ________________ grams/day

What percentage of your total daily fat intake was from saturated fat? ________________% ([grams saturated fat ÷ total grams fat] × 100)

What percentage of your total daily fat intake was from polyunsaturated fat? ________________% ([grams polyunsaturated fat ÷ total grams fat] × 100)

What was your cholesterol intake? ________________ mg/day

What percentage of your total daily kcalorie intake was from fat? ________________% ([grams fat × 9] ÷ kcalories) × 100 ________________%

Identify two changes in your diet, if necessary, that are needed to allow you to meet the guideline of less then 10% of kcalories from saturated fat.

Protein

What was your protein intake? ________________ grams/day

What percentage of your daily total kcalorie intake is from protein? ([grams protein × 4] ÷ kcalories) × 100

How does this percentage compare with the general recommendations from dietary protein of 10% to 15% of total kcalories?
________________ Above ________________ Recommended ________________ Below

What is your approximate desirable body weight (see Table 8-5) ________________ pounds. Pounds ÷ 2.2 = ________________ kilograms

Calculate your RDA for protein:
0.8 grams × ________________ kilograms desirable body weight = ________________ grams/day

Compare your daily protein intake with your RDA. Are you consuming more or less protein than recommended? How much more or less? If less, what changes in your diet can you make so that you may more closely meet your RDA?

List: Total kcalories eaten = ________________ kcalories

Total kcalorie output = ________________ kcalories

Energy balance (input − output) = ________________ kcalories

Briefly discuss your energy balance, or lack of it.

Summary

1. "Compression of morbidity" is the goal of delaying symptoms of and disabilities from chronic diseases for as many years as possible. Good nutritional habits—especially following the Daily Food Guide—play a role in this process.
2. A basic plan for health promotion and disease prevention includes eating a proper diet, exercising regularly, abstaining from smoking, limiting alcohol intake, and limiting stress.
3. The 1985 Dietary Guidelines for Americans recommend that individuals eat a variety of foods; maintain desirable weight; avoid too much fat, saturated fat, and cholesterol; eat foods with adequate starch and fiber; avoid too much sugar; avoid too much sodium; and, for those who drink alcoholic beverages, do so in moderation. In addition, specific recommendations to reduce cancer risk emphasize moderation in use of cured and smoked meats. Fluoride use can also minimize dental caries.
4. Scientists disagree as to the best diet recommendations for the general public. Genetic background, medical conditions, and other life-style practices influence a person's optimal diet. An overall emphasis on variety in the diet, control of body weight, moderation in total fat and saturated fat intake, eating ample fruits and vegetables, and moderation in alcohol intake has wide support.
5. While life span has not changed, life expectancy has increased dramatically over the past century. For societies this means an increasing proportion of the population is over 65 years of age. Health care costs are increasing, making the goal of compression of morbidity very important.
6. Aging begins prior to birth. Cells aging probably results from automatic cellular changes and environmental influences, such as DNA damage, free radical reactions, hormonal changes, and alterations in the immune system.
7. Nutritional problems of the elderly are related to the presence of chronic diseases and to the normal decreases in organ function that occur with time. These include loss of teeth, a reduction in senses of taste and smell, changes in gastrointestinal tract function, and deterioration in cardiac and bone health.
8. Specific nutrient requirements for the elderly are only now extensively being studied. Diet plans should be based on the Daily Food Guide, with consideration for present health problems, decreased physical abilities, presence of drug-nutrient interactions, possible depression, and economic constraints. Specific nutrients, such as vitamins D, E, thiamin, B-6, C, B-12, iron, zinc and calcium, often deserve special attention in diet planning.

REFERENCES

1. The American Dietetic Association: Nutrition, aging, and the continuum of health care: technical support paper, Journal of the American Dietetic Association 87:345, 1987.
2. Asp EH and Darling ME: Home-delivered meal: food quality, nutrient quality, and characteristics of recipients, Journal of the American Dietetic Association 88:55, 1988.
3. Chauhan J and others: Age-related olfactory and taste changes and interrelationships between taste and nutrition, Journal of the American Dietetic Association 87:1543, 1987.
4. Chernoff R: Aging and nutrition, Nutrition Today, p 4, March/April 1987.
5. Claggett MS: Nutritional factors relevant to Alzheimer's disease, Journal of the American Dietetic Association 89:392, 1989.
6. Cronin FJ and Shaw AE: Summary of dietary recommendations for healthy Americans, Nutrition Today, p 26, November/December 1988.
7. Davies L: Practical nutrition for the elderly, Nutrition Reviews 46:83, 1988.
8. Delvin EE: Vitamin D nutritional status and related biochemical indices in autonomous elderly population, American Journal of Clinical Nutrition 48:373, 1988.
9. Fries JF and Crapo LM: Vitality and aging: implications of the rectangular curve 1981, WH Freeman and Co Publishers.
10. James P and others: Summary on elderly nutrition symposium, Nutrition Reviews 46:109, 1988.
11. Kannel WB: Nutrition and the occurrence and prevention of cardiovascular disease in the elderly, Nutrition Reviews 46:68, 1988.
12. Klurfeld DM and Kritchevsky D: The western diet: an examination of its relationship with chronic disease, Journal of the American College of Nutrition 5:477, 1986.
13. Leaf A: The aging process: lessons from observations in man, Nutrition Reviews 26:40, 1988.
14. Lips P and others: Determinants of vitamin D status in patients with hip fracture and in elderly control subjects, American Journal of Clinical Nutrition 46:1005, 1987.
15. Miller SA and Stephenson MG: The 1990 national nutrition objectives: lessons for the future, Journal of the American Dietetic Association 87:1665, 1987.
16. Munro HN and others: Nutritional requirements of the elderly, Annual Reviews of Nutrition 7:23, 1987.
17. National Academy of Sciences report on diet and health, Nutrition Reviews 47:142, 1989.
18. Paffenbarger RS and others: Physical activity, all-cause mortality, and longevity of college alumni, The New England Journal of Medicine 314:605, 1986.
19. Rippe JM: 29 tips for staying with it, American Health, p 43, June 1988.
20. Roe DA: Therapeutic affects of drug-nutrient interactions in the elderly, Journal of the American Dietetic Association 85:174, 1985.
21. Root EJ and Longenecker JV: Nutrition, the brain, and Alzheimer's disease, Nutrition Today, p 11, July/August 1988.
22. Sahyoun NR and others: Dietary intakes and biochemical indicators of nutritional status in an elderly, institutionalized population, American Journal of Clinical Nutrition 47:524, 1988.
23. Schneider EL and others: Recommended dietary allowances and the health of the elderly, The New England Journal of Medicine 314:157, 1986.
24. Simopoulos AP: Conference on diet and health: scientific concepts and principles, Nutrition Today, p 4, January/February 1987.
25. Smith EL and others: Diet, exercise, and chronic disease patterns in older adults, Nutrition Reviews 46:52, 1988.
26. Surgeon general's report on nutrition and health: summary and recommendations, Nutrition Today, p 22, September/October 1988.
27. Suter BM and Russell RM: Vitamin requirements of the elderly, American Journal of Clinical Nutrition 45:501, 1987.
28. Swanson CA and others: Zinc status of healthy elderly adults; response to supplementation, American Journal of Clinical Nutrition 48:34 3, 1988.
29. Walford RL and others: Dietary restriction and aging: historical phases, mechanisms and current directions, Journal of Nutrition 117:1650, 1987.
30. Zoller DP: The physiology of aging, American Family Physician 36:112, 1987.

SUGGESTED READINGS

The summary of the surgeon general's report on nutrition and health published in *Nutrition Today,* and the summary of the National Academy of Sciences report on diet and health in *Nutrition Reviews* underscore the importance of diet to health maintenance. See Zoller's article on the physiology of aging to learn more about how body functions deteriorate over time. The article by Suter and Russell and that by Schneider and others review how nutrient needs change in response to aging. The article by Paffenbarger and others shows the importance of regular physical activity for the maintenance of health. Finally, Rippe's article provides numerous tips for sticking with an exercise program.

CHAPTER 17

Answers to nutrition awareness inventory

1. *False.* The average length of time North Americans live has increased during the last century, but not the age of the oldest people.
2. *True.* This amount of exercise is thought to adequately stimulate the cardiovascular system and help reduce stress and obesity.
3. *True.* Drug-nutrient interactions can be a problem at any age, but because the elderly generally take more and different combinations of drugs over a long period, nutritional status is more likely to be affected.
4. *True.* Being overweight contributes to almost all the chronic diseases common in our society.
5. *True.* In addition, because the elderly population is rapidly growing, society will need to continue dealing with this concern.
6. *False.* Good nutrition can delay some symptoms of aging, but no diet can magically prevent aging; aging probably begins at conception.
7. *False.* The senses of smell and taste tend to decrease with age. Adding seasonings can enhance food appeal.
8. *True.* The sense of thirst may diminish with age, but not the need for fluids.
9. *True.* Stomach secretions that promote absorption of vitamin B-12 decrease with age.
10. *True.* Increasing fiber and fluid intakes can help reduce constipation.
11. *True.* Excessive intake of vitamin A supplements results in many toxicity problems. These are only a few examples (see Chapter 11).
12. *True.* Be aware of these nutrients if you are involved in the health care of elderly people or have the chance to advise elderly relatives.
13. *True.* Exercise is an important part of body maintenance.
14. *False.* People differ in genetic backgrounds, abilities to regulate cholesterol metabolism, and responsiveness to diets aimed at lowering blood cholesterol. There is, however, no way to know how much a diet will help until a person tries it.
15. *False.* This age-group varies more in physical ability than any other.

Nutrition Perspective 17-1

The Importance of Regular Physical Activity

A common practice of healthy people throughout the world is regular physical activity.[25] People confined to bed quickly lose muscle tone and, eventually, health. Once they are back on their feet and active, physical stamina can be rebuilt.

Physical activity throughout life helps maintain the health of the cardiovascular system and bones. It maintains proper blood glucose levels both by minimizing chances of obesity and by encouraging glucose use by active muscles. Physical activity is also an important component of mental well-being. *People who exercise often derive a great sense of satisfaction and enjoyment from knowing they are doing something important for their overall health.* We also secrete more endorphins during exercise, and they serve as natural tranquilizers.

Recent research shows that while serum cholesterol levels may be higher among farmers than nonfarmers, farmers exercise more and end up with a lower expected mortality from heart disease. A study of Harvard University alumni found that those who expended 2000 kcalories per week in walking, climbing, and sports play showed a 25% lower mortality rate compared to the less active alumni.[16] Other researchers, responding to that finding, noted that people should choose exercise they enjoy because the average increase in longevity is about the same amount of time spent in physical activity.

GETTING STARTED

If you are younger than 35 years and in good health, it is not necessary to see a physician before beginning an exercise program. If you are over 35 and have been inactive for many years, consider seeing a physician first. Existing health problems that indicate a possible need for medical clearance are heart disease, high blood pressure, shortness of breath after

Table 17-7

The beginning of an exercise program
Warmup—5-10 minutes of exercises such as walking, slow jogging, knee lifts, arm circles or trunk rotations. Low-intensity movements that simulate movements to be used in the activity can also be included in the warmup.
Muscular strength—A minimum of two 20-minute sessions per week that include exercises for all the major muscle groups. Lifting weights is the most effective way to increase strength.
Muscular endurance—At least three 30-minute sessions each week that include exercises, such as calisthenics, pushups, situps, pullups, and weight training, for all the major muscle groups.
Cardiorespiratory endurance—At least three 20-minute bouts of continuous aerobic (activity requiring oxygen) rhythmic exercise each week. Popular aerobic conditioning activities include brisk walking, jogging, swimming, cycling, rope-jumping, rowing, cross-country skiing, and some continuous action games like racquetball and handball.
Flexibility—10-12 minutes of daily stretching exercises performed slowly, without a bouncing motion. This can be included after a warmup or during a cool-down.
Cool down—A minimum of 5-10 minutes of slow walking, low-level exercise, combined with stretching.

From: Fitness fundamentals, USDHHS, 1985; U.S. Government Printing Office.

Continued.

Nutrition Perspective 17-1—cont'd

The Importance of Regular Physical Activity

Lifelong health and fitness through exercise can allow a person to do the activities he or she wants to do throughout life. This may be world traveling at age 60, camping with grandchildren, or building a retirement home. Exercise is important for people who want to continue taking full advantage of life's opportunities.

mild exertion, arthritis, and other chronic disease. Although vigorous exercise does involve minimal health risks for those in good health, far greater risks accumulate with long-term inactivity and obesity.

A basic activity program should consist of a warm-up, activities to increase muscular strength and endurance, activities designed to increase flexibility, and a cool-down. Setting a target exercise heart rate for cardiovascular fitness was covered in Figure 9-3. Table 17-7 outlines recent recommendations for a program of this type. Table 17-8 adds some motivational tips.[19]

Table 17-8

Tips for staying with an exercise program

1. Chart a specific, realistic plan.
   When you decide to begin exercising, consider mapping out an exercise agenda with a doctor or fitness instructor.
2. Find a bench mark for an exercise prescription.
   The Rockport Fitness Walking Test is an easy way to determine your present level of conditioning. All you have to do is walk a mile. You then follow a program specially designed for your needs. For a free copy, send an SASE to: The Rockport Walking Institute, 72 Howe Street, Marlboro, MA 01752.
3. Start easy.
   Don't plunge into unfamiliar movements that leave you aching, but realize that some soreness should be expected.
4. Go for low injury potential, and consider past injuries.
   Walking and stationary cycling are safe, low-impact sports. Injuries are the death knell of exercise programs.
5. Choose exercises you enjoy and vary activities.
   This is especially important during the change of seasons. Plan ahead for activities you can do indoors during the winter. Variety will also help prevent injuries and boredom.
6. Exercise for about 30 minutes a day. You can find this much time in a busy day.
7. Exercise with, or simply use the support of other family members or friends.
   Music with a beat similar to the pace of a heart beat is comfortable to exercise to.
8. Give yourself frequent self-tests.
   We tend to notice the bad things (sore muscles), but not the good things. After exercise, ask yourself: Do I feel less tired? Am I in a better mood? If your body and mind tell you the benefits are already there, you're on the way to the next workout.
9. Consider other habits: it may be time for a life-style change.
   If you smoke, try to stop. Studies show that people who start to exercise begin to eat more fruit and vegetables and make other healthy changes.
10. Notice the long-term benefits.
    Research has shown that once you exercise for about 20 weeks, even if you quit for a while, you will probably return to it again.
11. Take lessons to increase your aerobic efficiency and reduce frustrations, and use quality, comfortable equipment.

From: Rippe JM: 29 tips for staying with it, American Health, p 43, June 1988.

WHEN TO EXERCISE AND HOW MUCH IS ENOUGH?

The time between work and the evening meal is a popular time to exercise. After the evening meal is another good time, as long as you wait an hour or so afterward for digestion. Some people like to exercise early in the morning, but for those who can't get out of bed, try it later in the day. Rather than giving up the whole idea when obstacles impede the exercise program, try adjusting your schedule. Aim for 30 to 60 minutes of exercise at 60% to 75% your maximum heart rate for 3 to 5 times per week.Keep trying new types and times of programs until you find several pleasurable alternative ways to exercise in a weekly agenda: combine walking and swimming, tennis with jogging and maybe aerobic class, each several times a week. Lots of variety keeps it interesting. Finding an exercise partner may help. Hang in there!

Table 17-9

Approximate energy costs of activity for a 150 pound (68 kilogram) person

Activity	Expenditure (kcal/kg/min)
In bed (resting, sleeping)	1.0
Sitting (desk work)	1.7-2.0
Driving	1.7
Standing quietly	1.7
Dressing	1.8
Playing the piano	2.7
Cooking	3.1
Cleaning	4.2
Golf	5.8
Dancing or Aerobics	3.5-7.0
Calisthenics	4.5
Walking (4 mph)	5.4
Cycling (10 mph)	6.8
Working with a shovel	9.9
Weight Lifting	9.9
Tennis (singles)	7.4-10
Jogging (5 mph)	9.2
Swimming	10.0
Cycling (12 mph)	8.0
Basketball	9.4
Running (7 mph)	13.5
Handball or Raquetball	14.4
Running (10 mph)	17.3

Nutrition Perspective 17-2

Food for Fast Times

Choosing healthy foods is not so difficult in many of today's fast-food restaurants. Some restaurants have evolved beyond hamburgers, French fries, and milk shakes to include a variety of vegetables, salad bars, and ethnic foods. In addition, some restaurants are trying to cater to their more health-conscious clientele. What follows is a list of suggestions for a good nutritional path among food choices in fast food restaurants.

BREAKFAST

Before entering a local fast-food restaurant for breakfast, decide whether you can fix this meal at home. Can breakfast be prepared the night before so that it is ready for the next morning? The effort might be as simple as putting bread next to the toaster or cereal on the counter with a bowl. Breakfast can be a relaxing time, and many of us need time away from the fast pace of daily life. If you have abandoned breakfast at home, think again. *Breakfast at home is usually faster than a visit to a fast-food restaurant.*

If you still prefer breakfast out, we suggest a plain scrambled egg, or an English muffin with not more than 1 teaspoon of margarine. Add orange juice for a tasty breakfast. Substitute pancakes without the butter and minimal syrup instead of the egg and English muffin. Either way, you consume a lot less fat and kcalories than if you choose the typical meat, egg, and cheese-laden muffin or croissant. Be especially wary of croissants: they are loaded with fat. If you still want meat, consider Canadian bacon, the leanest of all breakfast meats.

LUNCH

A good choice for lunch is a sandwich made of whole-wheat bread and some lean meat or tuna. Pizza is a good idea once or twice a week. If ordered with vegetable toppings—mushrooms, green peppers, and onions—pizza provides a very nutritious lunch for a moderate amount of kcalories. The cheese used primarily is a low-fat variety. The next best choice is probably a hamburger, but not the king-size model. Consider buying the basic hamburger. Ideally, choose a restaurant that provides a plain hamburger on a bun and then allows you to create a masterpiece. At that point, emphasize lettuce, tomatoes, mustard, and a little ketchup. Be especially wary of mayonnaise, sauces, melted cheese, fried onions, or other sources of added fat. Chili is another alternative. It is lower in fat than a king-size hamburger, and the beans supply additional dietary fiber.

If you want chicken, bite-size pieces should be made from chicken breast only, and not from processed chicken that can include ground chicken skin. Ask the restaurant manager from which parts of the chicken the entree is made. Let him or her know your nutrition and health interests. Broiled or baked chicken is healthiest; however, it is usually fried. To minimize fat intake, remove the coating. The same applies to fish: remove the coating. Actually, chicken and fish start out as low-fat protein sources, but by the time they are deep-fat fried, they resemble the protein:fat ratio of a hamburger. You do not save that many kcalories.

For side dishes, consider portion sizes. Order a small rather than a large portion of French fries. Order a baked potato, and to spice it up, put on plenty of chives but not more than a pat of margarine. Stay away from sour cream, cheese, and other toppings. Some stuffed broccoli and cheese baked potatoes contain as much as 500 kcalories, while the plain baked potato, with a little margarine added, has only about 200 kcalories.

At the salad bar, watch the addition of cheese, bacon bits, and dressing. Mayonnaise-based salads, such as macaroni and potato salad, are relatively high in kcalories. To minimize saturated fat intake, try the oil and vinegar and French dressings, rather than the blue cheese dressings. Some people even find fresh squeezed lemon juice is a satisfying alternative to dressing. Some fast food restaurants do supply low-kcalorie dressings. Try these, or otherwise, add as little regular dressing as possible. You can always take your own with you too.

For beverages, consider low-fat (nonfat) milk, water, diet soft drinks, or ice tea. *A typical milk shake contains about 350 to 400 kcalories. A cup of low-fat milk has only 120 kcalories.*

DINNER

In more formal restaurants, it is important to be your own advocate. Restaurants are responsive to customer demand. If you want lower-fat, healthier food, ask for it. Request low-fat milk, margarine, broiled meats and fish, low-kcalorie salad dressings, or whatever else you want. Ask even if you know it is not available. It will become available when enough requests are made.

For appetizers, choose fruit juice or a fruit cup instead of creamed soup. Vegetable juice and broth-based soups are good choices as well, but can be high in sodium (if that is a nutrient you are trying to avoid).

For salads, use limited amounts of cheese, chopped meats, bacon bits, marinated vegetables, potato salad, macaroni salad, and salad dressing. You can build a creative and tasty salad without relying on these products.

Discover how the main dish is prepared. Find an entree that is not fried, coated, or hidden in a sauce, so you can tell what happened to it.

Ask for baked or mashed potatoes rather than French fries: even with a small amount of butter or gravy added, both baked and mashed potatoes contain far fewer kcalories. Consider whole-grain breads, pita bread, bread sticks, Italian bread, or French bread. Avoid biscuits, croissants, and other kcalorie-rich dinner rolls. Use margarine sparingly—each pat contains 45 kcalories.

Choose among fresh fruit, fruit ices, frozen yogurt, gelatin, sherbet, and cake without frosting for dessert. Remove frosting from pastries to reduce kcalorie and fat intake. For fruit pie, eat only the filling.

For beverages, if you drink alcoholic beverages, drink them in moderation. Alcohol can melt away many good intentions and add numerous kcalories. Use low-fat or skim milk in coffee or tea, instead of cream. When drinking milk, choose low-fat or skim milk instead of whole milk.

In all, focus on fat. It will be easier to do that in some restaurants than in others. Mexican and French cuisine are noted for their high fat content, while Italian and Oriental cuisine offers many more low-fat alternatives.

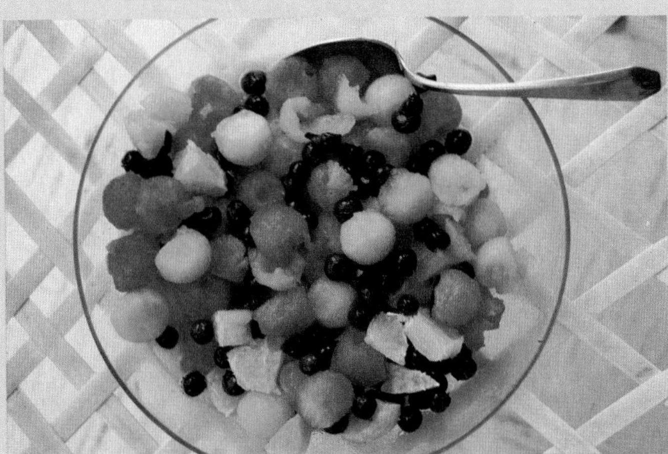

Fresh fruit makes a tasty and healthful dessert.

Part VI

Putting Nutrition Knowledge to Practice

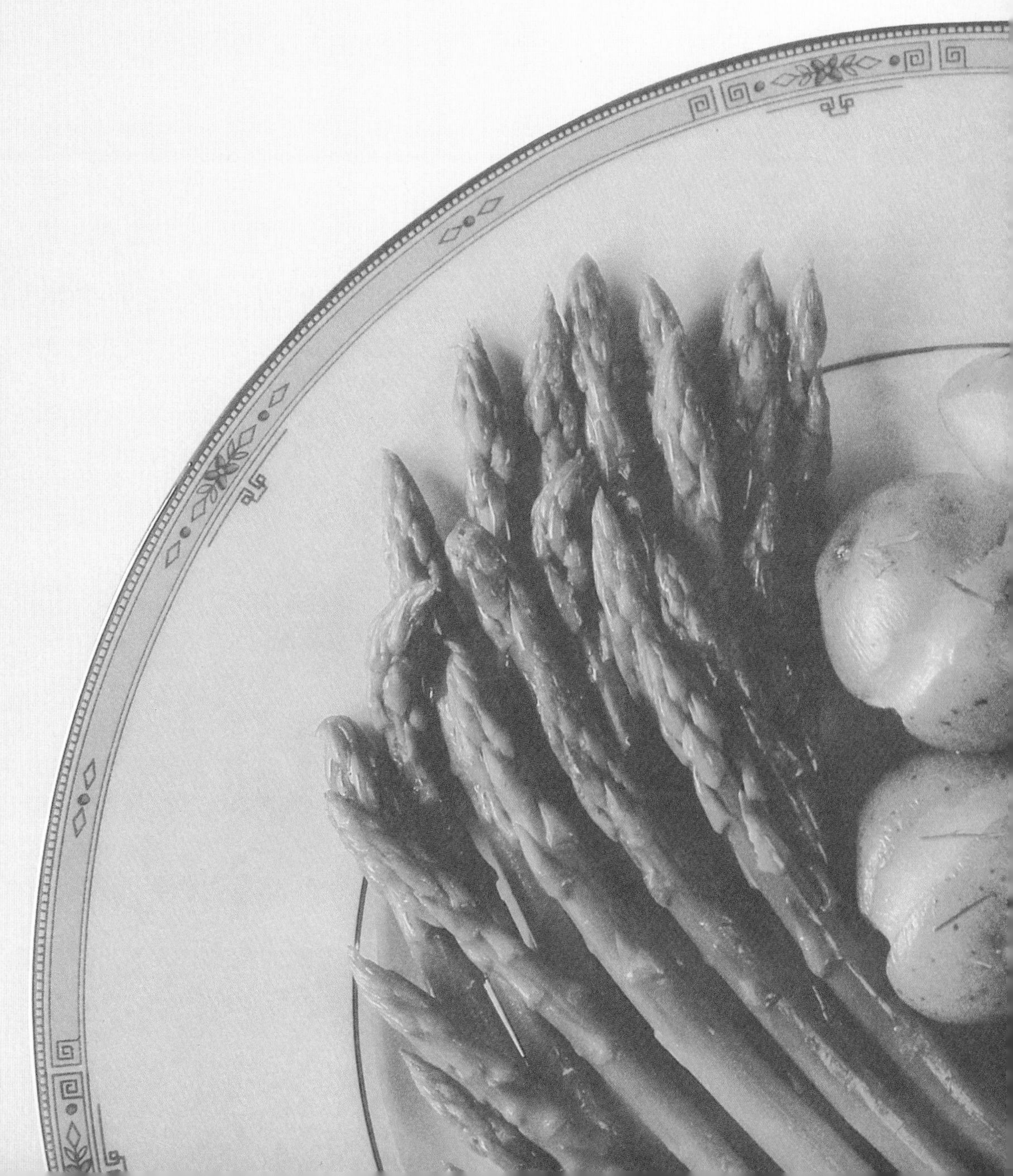

Chapter 18

How to Improve Your Diet

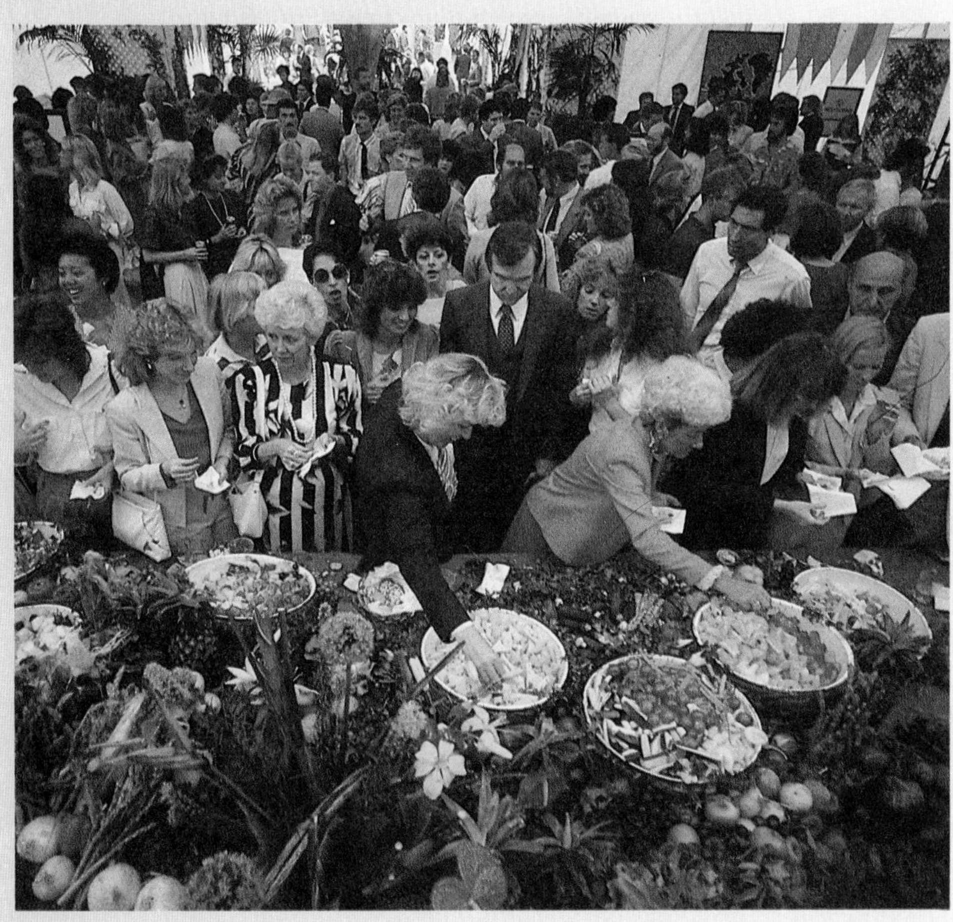

Behavior changes, such as choosing healthful food at a party, are one part of a successful weight loss plan.

Overview

In the last chapter, we suggested goals for a personal nutrition and health plan. Once you know what you want to accomplish, it is time to act. This chapter will help you put a plan into practice.

The path to nutritional health should be tailored to a person's particular needs. It must consider current health status, family history, occupation, stress factors, budget, time considerations, and any other elements of daily living that affect health. Some behavior changes to consider include improving your overall diet (see Chapter 2), decreasing saturated fat intake (see Chapter 5), decreasing kcalorie intake (see Chapter 9), decreasing salt intake (see Chapter 13), and decreasing food costs (see Nutrition Perspective 18-1, "What does it cost to have a healthy diet?"). Adapting some elements of diets of other countries to your tastes can be useful and fun (Nutrition Perspective 18-2, "Is there a best ethnic diet?").

Overall, your plan should provide external and internal environments that support the body's natural ability to heal itself. In general, health changes should move you toward eating a variety of foods, striving to maintain a desirable body weight, and participating in regular physical activity.

Nutrition awareness inventory

Here are 15 statements about improving your diet. Answer them to test your current knowledge. If you think the answer is true or mostly true, circle T. If you think the answer is false or mostly false, circle F. Use the scoring key at the end of this chapter to compute your total score. Take this test again after you have read this chapter. Compare the results.

1. **T F** Behavior change is mostly a matter of willpower.
2. **T F** People have different food preferences depending on their moods.
3. **T F** If a goal is sufficiently worthwhile, a person will usually achieve it even when the commitment is weak.
4. **T F** If you lapse while attempting to change your eating behavior, it is best to abandon that plan and try something else.
5. **T F** Eating habits are difficult to overcome because people eat for pleasure.
6. **T F** If you aim for the best and try to attain a body type you most admire, you are more likely to achieve it.
7. **T F** Behavior change involves measuring progress.
8. **T F** For changing behavior, punishment works more effectively than reward.
9. **T F** Midafternoon is the toughest time for most dieters.
10. **T F** To achieve a diet change it is best to keep as little food as possible in the refrigerator.
11. **T F** People can improve their diets without eating foods they don't like.
12. **T F** When beginning to change behavior, one should seek potential problem situations to test personal strength.
13. **T F** Behavior changes are more successful if they simultaneously address all facets of a problem.
14. **T F** Changes in dietary habits may meet opposition or sabotage from friends and relatives.
15. **T F** Rewards should be given only when the final goal has been accomplished.

THE BEHAVIOR CHANGE PROCESS

Health-related behavior patterns rarely change instantaneously. Changes occur progressively when a person realizes he or she is responsible for his or her own health. First, a person becomes *aware* of a problem—such as being overweight enough to incur health risks. The person may notice the problem, or someone, perhaps a health professional, may point it out. In this chapter, we single out the problem of being overweight as an example of the overall process of behavior change. With minor modifications, the process can be applied to any other nutrition goal.

After recognizing a problem, an interested person develops a **receptive framework for learning** more about the problem. This might involve evaluating the costs and benefits of changing behaviors: perhaps balancing the time and effort exercising requires plus sacrificing some favorite foods against the benefits of lowering weight, decreasing health risks, and feeling and looking better.

Receptive framework for learning The process by which a person opens and responds to learning more about a problem—it usually involves seeking more information about the issue from books and people.

Considering earlier experiences, the would-be changer must decide whether the change is feasible. Can his or her life-style accommodate the new goal? Can the person continue the new behaviors for the rest of his or her life? By reading about and speaking with others who have worked on similar health projects, a person might find the changes less threatening. Here the credibility of a health professional can be critical. Where the change may at first appear to demand too much sacrifice or seem impossible, a health professional can possibly provide the information and encouragement necessary to start the change process.[6]

Once a decision to attempt a change is made, the *trial* for change begins. The person tries new behaviors and experiences both rewards and difficulties: maybe hunger, weight loss, discomfort, and compliments. Some experiences may be perceived as positive, but some will be perceived as negative—otherwise, the old practices would not have been cherished. Familiar foods now missing from the diet may leave a void. At this time, *positive reinforcement* is critical and should be built into the plan: the changer is attempting behaviors that are difficult and deserves credit for that. The person needs rewards for hard work, in whatever form is appropriate for the defined goals—such as enjoying a night at the movies, buying a favorite compact disc, fishing with friends, or sleeping late. *During this trial period, it is good to capitalize on success and learn how to derive psychological nourishment from the victory over poor habits.*

Finally, the person adopts the new behaviors into his overall life-style. He comes full circle from awareness of the problem to adopting behaviors designed to correct it. In doing that, he has taken charge of his health. Now the possibilities for other improvements can be investigated, and the cycle repeated.[8]

BECOMING AWARE

W.L. is a 20-year-old male college student who has been gaining weight since high school. At the YMCA, a bioelectrical impedance analysis (see Chapter 8) indicated that he has 32% body fat and the registered dietitian suggests W.L. is 140% of his desirable body weight. W.L. remembers from a health education class that obesity often leads to other more serious health problems. He is concerned about his long-term health, and wants to correct this weight problem before it leads to more problems. Having seen his father change his diet and lose weight after a heart attack, W.L. thinks that he too can make dietary changes with success.

CHARTING A PLAN FOR CHANGE

A good plan evolves. It is based on rational, deliberate decisions and trial and error methods. It is built after considering and evaluating many options. While a person can't know all possible strategies and tactics before beginning, a good plan incorporates the information at hand. Revisions are necessary and expected.

In planning to control weight, for example, a person needs to know that the typical restrictive diet not only fails to produce the desired results for most people but also can produce undesired results, such as fatigue and depression. More effective weight control programs lead people away from severe dieting and toward raising their activity levels. So it's best to know the following before choosing a program: what programs are available, how up-to-date is their information, and how effective are their methods.[1] Useful information about programs can be found by visiting clinic programs, reading health and nutrition books on weight control, and speaking with registered dieticians, physicians, and other health professionals.

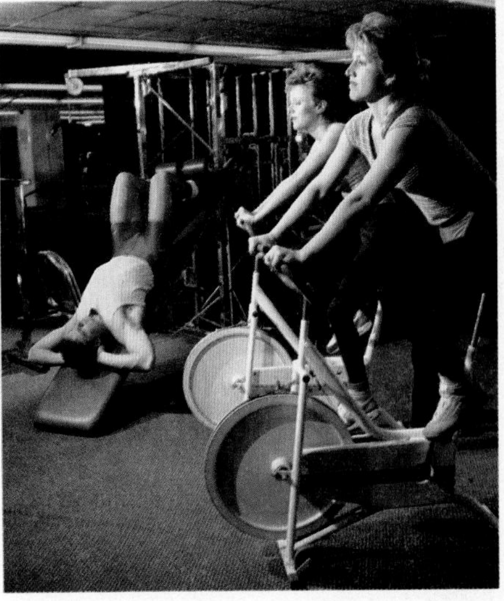

Effective weight control programs should include regular physical activities and moderation in food intake.

Gathering baseline data

A next step in creating a personal plan for dietary change is to observe present eating behavior, noting strengths and weaknesses. Monitoring eating behaviors is

Expert Opinion

Breaking the Chains That Lead to Overweight

JAMES FERGUSON, M.D.

We are creatures of habit. All our behaviors are linked, one to the next. Much like the chain that holds a boat to its anchor, our behavior chains can anchor us to relatively fixed conditions, like obesity. The chains can be simple or complicated, emotional or situation-specific.

An emotional chain might be formed by a stressful relationship, a disappointing date, or an unpleasant conversation after a movie. Once the goodbyes are said, the distressed person, despite having dined out and had a couple of drinks, begins to snack.

Also, there's the simple habit pattern. Consider the man who has established a routine throughout the years after shopping for food: he comes in the front door, carries the groceries to the kitchen, puts them in the cupboards and refrigerator—and then snacks. Soon, every time he comes in the front door and goes to the kitchen, he reaches for a snack.

Or consider the businesswoman who comes home after a hard day at work. She puts down her briefcase, picks up the paper, turns on the TV, sits down, gets up and looks in the refrigerator, grabs a snack, again sits in front of the TV, snacks while reading the paper and/or watching TV, and, afterward, eats a meal. After dinner, she sits down to watch TV, gets bored, walks into the kitchen, browses through the refrigerator, eats a piece of cheesecake, wanders back to the TV, feels guilty about the snack, and assuages her guilt with another piece of cheesecake.

The specifics vary, but the patterns are similar. The behavior chain is a series of interconnected habitual behaviors (Figure 18-2). The initial event, such as stress or boredom can seem innocuous, but the ending is always the same: extra kcalories.

How many eating situations in your life can you describe with a behavior-chain diagram? A study of the series of linked events suggests a strategy for eliminating extra habitual eating or snacking. Break the chain! It's hard to just say no. The easy way to break the chain is to substitute an alternate activity. The earlier the chain is broken, the better and the easier it is to cut kcalories. Once the snack touches your taste buds, it's too late. When that cheesecake is only a gleam in your eye or, even better, a "pregleam," the awareness that you are headed for something to eat makes it easier to break the chain.

The way to cast off your chains is to identify them, pinpoint the weak links, and substitute another behavior. Using alternate activities sounds easy, but it's hard to do on the spur of the moment.

If your behavior chain is broken at any point, it will probably not continue. (The businesswoman's final behavior—eating, feeling guilty, eating—probably won't occur.) The earlier in the chain you substitute a nonfood link, the easier it is to intervene.

Four types of behavior can be substituted in an ongoing behavior chain:

1. Fun activities (grabbing your mate, taking a walk, reading a book)
2. Necessary activities (cleaning a room, balancing your checkbook)
3. Incompatible activities (taking a shower)
4. Time-consuming activities (setting a kitchen timer for 20 minutes before allowing yourself to eat)

Using activities to interrupt behavior patterns that lead to inappropriate eating can be a powerful means of changing eating habits. This technique can also be useful when you are eating in response to environmental as well as to internal cues for eating: for example, a TV ad for food or a hunger pang that you feel at an odd time after a meal or before going to bed. If it's pushing you to eat, substitute!

Several conditions have to be met before you succeed at chain-breaking. First, you must identify the chain, pay attention to your habitual eating patterns, and note which patterns relentlessly recur daily. Write down the behavior chain, starting with the eating or final behavior in the chain, and work backward to the beginning. The earliest behavior in the chain, for example, might be a boring TV show.

Second, you must have a list of alternative activities at hand. It's hard to remember what's fun, exciting, necessary, or even sexy when that piece of apple pie is warming in the microwave. Have a list available of each kind of chain breaker so that you won't have to spend time thinking about alternatives. Include at least three necessary, three pleasant, three incompatible, and three time-consuming alternatives in your list to use at any time.

Third, remember that hunger pangs triggered by your head rather than by your stomach are short-lived. (You'll gradually discern the crucial difference between the imagined, emotional need and the real, physical need to eat.) If you delay eating for 10 to 15 minutes, usually the urge to eat will diminish or disappear.

Finally, keep track of when you are successful. Pat yourself on the back for counteracting the snacking reflex with some novel, nonkcaloric activity. With enough effort, snacking—which can add a colossal amount of calories—might not even be fun anymore.

Dr. Ferguson is a nationally prominent psychiatrist who specializes in weight control. He is the author of the book Habits, Not Diets.

a good beginning exercise—recording meals and snacks in a diary may reveal eating patterns previously unnoticed. Let's assume that you want to adjust habits to control weight and are working to lower your fat intake as one means of doing that. In a diary, you might want to list some—or all—of the following: foods eaten and portion sizes, percentage of fat in the food eaten, intensity of hunger, the time, location, any concomitant activity (such as watching TV), perhaps whether you were influenced by the social aspects of eating with others, and your feelings at the time (Table 9-4). We have included a blank facsimile for your use in Appendix Q.

A review of the diary might reveal how the external environment and internal cues work together to affect nutrition and health habits. This is the time to look for patterns, identifying positive decisions and needed changes. You might classify food choices as "can't give up," "desirable," and "neutral." Patterns might suggest which food habits should be easy to change and which may be difficult to change. Eating habits may be paired with another activity: you may find that you eat mostly while visiting with friends, while in an angry mood, or perhaps after 6 PM. Subtle associations can influence eating habits and be the starting point for behavior changes.

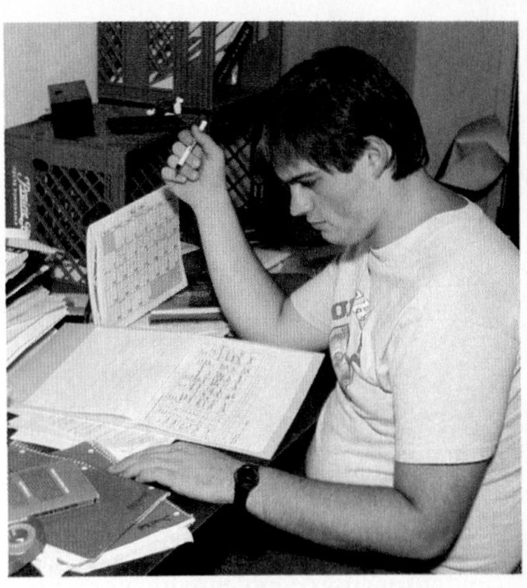

A diary can help to point out weaknesses and strengths in eating behavior.

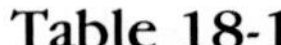

Table 18-1

Food Choice Quiz

Rate the factors listed as 3 (very important), 2 (somewhat important), 1 (seldom important), and 0 (never important).

Influence of background and other people

a. Culture or religion
b. Parents
c. Friends
d. Spouse
e. Children

Personal considerations

f. Weight
g. Health
h. Food appeal

Practical considerations

i. Food costs
j. Availability
k. Convenience

The news media

l. Advertisements (television, radio, magazines, newspapers)
m. Television/radio talk shows or specials dealing with food or nutrition
n. Food, nutrition, or health articles in magazines or newspapers
o. Public affairs announcements in the media dealing with nutrition, research, or food safety

Self-selected sources of information

p. Courses dealing with food and nutrition
q. Articles in scientific journals
r. Government bulletins
s. Professional advice—physician, registered dietician, dentist, cooperative extension agent
t. The health food store

From: Snook JT: Nutrition: a guide to decision-making, Englewood Cliff, NJ, 1984, Prentice Hall Inc.

BASELINE

To better understand his eating habits, W.L. keeps a food diary. In it, he tracks what and how much he eats, how quickly he eats, the hour, the situation, and his feelings at the time. From this diary, he sees a previously unnoticed pattern—he starts snacking after his 2 PM class and does not stop until dinner. He is alarmed that he consumes so many kcalories unconsciously. In addition, W.L. notes that his lunches usually are high in fat and that his days lack much physical activity.

Exploring Issues and Actions

Diary information coupled with an evaluation of your current health status should help pinpoint behaviors you need to change for establishing better nutrition and health practices. Discuss these impressions with a professional if you feel unsure about proceeding further.

Sensory appeal—flavor, appearance, and odor—and habit usually drive both our intended and actual food choices. Of secondary significance in choosing foods to eat are health value, expediency, social influence, energy value, and cost. Complete the assessment in Table 18-1 to understand more about the factors that affect food choices most.[8] See how this agrees with your Take Action assignment in Chapter 1.

Concept Check

In the behavior change process, a person first becomes aware of the problem. Then, the person studies the problem and develops a receptive frame of mind for making a change. She attempts a trial change of behavior. If she receives positive reinforcement, the change may eventually become part of her life-style—it is adopted. Because behavior change is most successful when tailored to personal needs, it is important for people to carefully study their own behaviors, such as snacking habits, and then make changes based on specific habits rather than general guidelines.

Setting attainable goals

Whatever one's mission, the first decisions in the plan for change should narrow the focus to specific goals, in terms of both time and what can be accomplished. You might set a goal of 4 to 6 months, at which time you will reevaluate your program. If one goal is to improve iron status, for example, planning an iron-rich diet and taking iron supplements can increase blood hematocrit and hemoglobin values within a few months. Progress toward other types of goals, such as weight loss, might be apparent within several days and progress from week to week. Seeing week-to-week progress may be the impetus needed to continue moving ahead with a program.[4]

If the aim is to control a disease, such as hypertension, diabetes mellitus, or heart disease, specific behavior goals are already well-defined, and feedback from a physical examination will confirm your degree of success. If the goal is broader, for example, to maintain and improve overall nutritional health, it is best to choose and practice a few specific behavior changes first—possibly lowering fat and refined flour intake and not eating after 7 PM—for several months before trying others. By attempting only several small and perhaps easier dietary changes, a big problem is generally easier to tackle, and the success rate is usually greater.

Measuring commitment

Success at changing behavior is strongly tied to a person's commitment: the greater the personal commitment, the greater the chances of success. Examine the goals you set. Are they worth pursuing? Are health benefits greater than the sacrifices to be made? Some people can ignore persistent arthritis in the knees—which is magnified through the condition of overweight—because they derive great pleasure from eating. Others may love eating ice cream and chips and dips but finally realize that the price is too high: they realize the benefits of losing the weight added from immoderate snacking would eventually be greater than the momentary pleasure of continuing their present behavioral patterns. They understand that in changing their eating habits, they would feel better about themselves, could move around more easily, would feel less anxious in public, and would limit some future health problems.

One way to measure commitment is to list the costs and benefits of changing behavior. Some costs and benefits are immediate, others delayed. Immediate costs might include monetary expenditures, inconvenience, reduced enjoyment, time and effort, and physical discomforts.[7] Conversely, you might want to list the costs of continuing your present health habits. They might involve loss of health and vitality, poor professional image, poor self-image, and perhaps even criticism from others. Then, benefits of changing can be contrasted with continuing the present practices (Figure 18-1). *If a person is not strongly committed to pursue a behavior change goal, the attempt will probably fail and further discourage the person.*

BENEFITS AND COSTS ANALYSIS

1 Benefits of losing weight?
What do you expect to get, now or later, that you want? What do you get to avoid that would be unpleasant?

- better job possibilities
- feel better physically
- look better
- people pay more attention to me

3 Costs involved in losing weight?
What do you have to do that you don't want to do? What do you have to stop doing that you would rather continue doing?

- give up some fast food
- cut down on alcohol
- take time to exercise

2 Benefits of not losing weight?
What do you get to do that you enjoy doing? What do you avoid having to do?

- eat whatever I want

4 Costs of not losing weight?
What unpleasant or undesirable effects are you likely to experience now or in the future? What are you likely to lose?

- criticism from others
- low self esteem
- poor health

Figure 18-1
Benefit and cost analysis applied to weight loss.

Usually, the more profound benefits of changing health and nutrition behaviors take time to achieve. It is easier to be influenced by immediate feelings and urges. Working toward long-term goals, such as fitness, lowering blood pressure, and losing weight is more difficult. Long-term goals require a life-long commitment. Only the person who wants to change can determine whether the value of good nutrition and good health is worth the price. Can your life-style accommodate your goals?

Working out the details

Once goals are established and the changer discovers personal strengths and weaknesses in pursuing them, it is time to set details of the plan. Some nutrition

Table 18-2

Tactics for managing eating behavior

Many things can trigger inappropriate eating behavior. But effective tactics can be used to gain control of eating. Here is a list of tactics, organized by problem area, that have proved effective for many people. These add to the suggestions in Table 9-3. Decide which tactics might be most effective in helping you gain control of your eating behavior. Then, make them part of a behavior change strategy.

Buying and storing food

Avoid aisles of problem foods
Don't pretend it's for the children or company
Store problem food so it is out of sight and hard to get
Inventory the kitchen and pantry, then give away or discard problem foods

Cooking, preparing, and serving food

Broil, bake, or poach—don't fry
Substitute low-fat and low-kcalorie ingredients
Don't sample while cooking
Plan menus
Measure portions
Let others get their own snacks, desserts, and second helpings

Eating food

Drink plenty of water
Drink little or no alcohol
Eat more complex carbohydrates (vegetables, grains, legumes)
Avoid high-fat foods
Eat three meals a day
Replace impulse snacking with planned, healthy snacks

Coping with problem food

Make problem food temporarily off-limits, but not permanently illegal or forbidden
Plan to eat a little of a problem food under "safe" conditions (where you can't binge)

Eating out in restaurants

Choose a restaurant that allows healthy food choices
Ask the waitress not to put bread and butter on the table before the meal
Request no butter and no sauce on vegetables or entree
Choose a broiled entree
Request water with a meal
Request salad dressing on the side or bring your own
Don't look at the dessert list or dessert tray

Coping with others

Ask co-workers not to offer food
Instead of eating to be polite, thank the person offering food and decline firmly
Just say "No, thank you, I've had enough. It was delicious, and I'm full."

Coping with emotions

Avoid people and situations that upset you
Go for a walk or use other exercise to unwind
Lighten up, don't take it all so seriously
Join a support group or seek counseling

Managing your body

Exercise regularly
Get adequate rest

Adapted from Nash JD: Maximize your body potential, Palo Alto, Calif., 1986, Bull Publishing Co.

cathy® **by Cathy Guisewite**

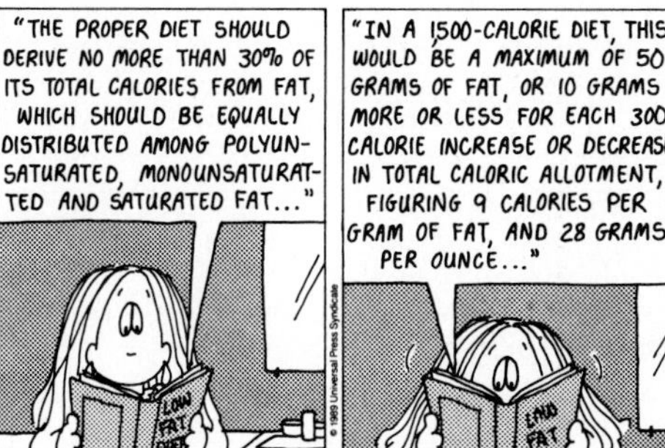

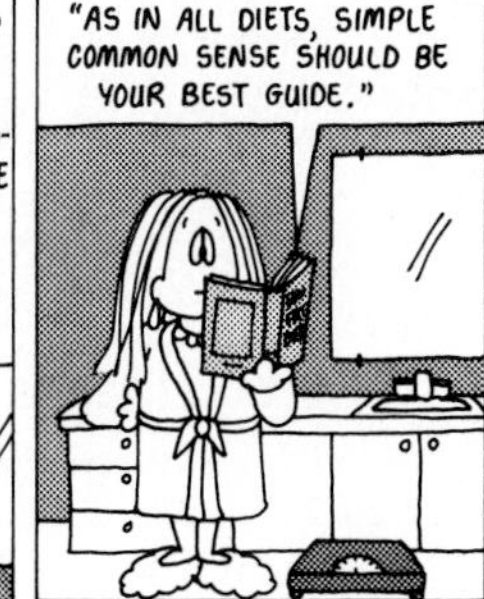

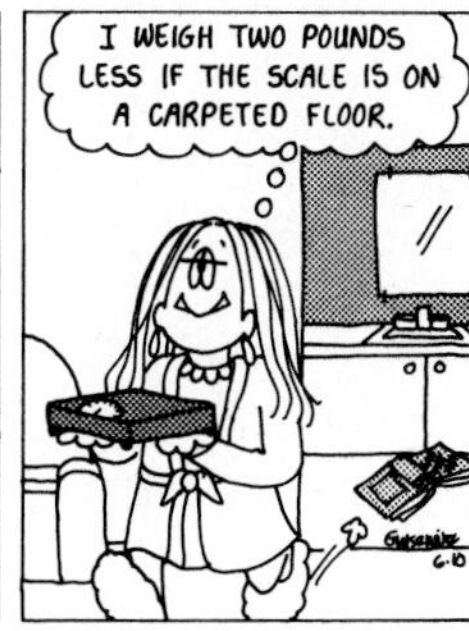

knowledge is necessary, and the information contained in this book is a good place to start. If you feel unable to work out a plan, professional help is also available (see Chapter 20).

One goal may be to reduce saturated fat intake. There are several means of doing this. You can reduce high-fat meat consumption by cutting either portion sizes or frequency of use. You might cut high-fat meats from daily consumption to twice a week. You could also search for new recipes and methods of preparation that use leaner meats and less meat—stir frying, for example, or broiling to reduce fat content. Further tactics for managing eating behavior are listed in Table 18-2. Once you take control of high-fat meat use, you can try other changes to help reach your goal.

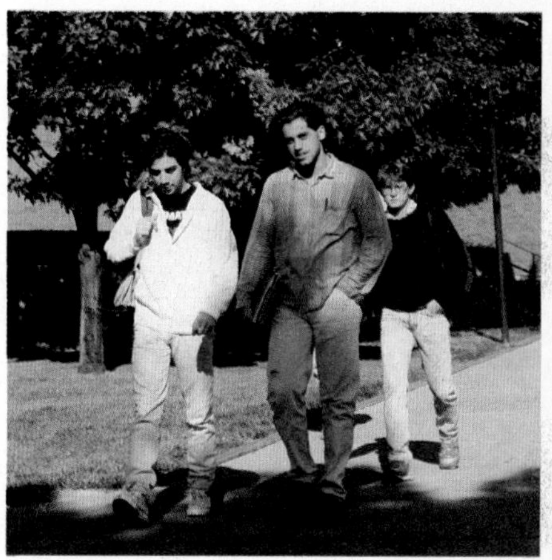

One way to increase your activity is to walk to class.

PLANNING THE DETAILS

W.L. addresses his overall weight problem in small steps. He plans to eat a better breakfast and lunch everyday so he won't feel ravenous by mid-afternoon. He will keep low-kcalorie snack foods, such as oranges, handy in the apartment—instead of the usual bag of chips or box of cookies. He will start packing his lunch and limit visits to fast food restaurants to twice a week. In addition, at fast food restaurants he will make wiser selections from the menu, opting for such choices as the "create your own hamburger bar." He will use lots of tomato slices for juiciness and have a diet soda, instead of a double cheeseburger, fries, and a milkshake. Finally, he plans to increase activity by walking to class instead of driving, and purchasing an exercise bike to ride each night while watching sports on TV.

Making it official

You might want to develop a behavior contract to encourage yourself to follow through. The contract could list goal behaviors and objectives, mileposts for measuring progress, and regular rewards for meeting the terms of the contract. Positive reinforcement contributes more to successful behavior change than negative reinforcement. Initially, the focus should be on positive behaviors, then on positive results. Positive behaviors, such as regular exercise, eventually lead to positive outcomes.[2] It may take months to see the effects. Look at the example of a behavior contract for weight loss in Table 9-5. Table 18-3 is a simplified version. When you have finished your contract, sign it in the presence of some friends.

Table 18-3

Behavioral contract

Name____

Goal

I agree to ____

(specify behavior)

____

under the following circumstances: ____________________

(specify where, when, how much, etc.)

____

Substitute behavior and/or reinforcement schedule ____________________

____

Environmental planning

In order to help me do this, I am going to (1) arrange my physical and social environment by ____________________

____

and (2) control my internal environment (thoughts, images) by ____________________

____

Reinforcements

Reinforcements provided by me daily or weekly (if contract is kept):

____

____

Reinforcements provided by others daily or weekly (if contract is kept):

____

____

Social support

Behavior change is more likely to take place when other people support you. During the quarter/semester please meet with the other person at least three times to discuss your progress.

The name of my "significant helper" is: ____________________

This contract should include:

1. Baseline data (one week)
2. Well-defined goal
3. Simple method for charting progress (diary, counters, charts, etc.)
4. Reinforcements (immediate and long-term)
5. Evaluation method (summary of experiences, success, and/or new learnings about self).

From Davis TM: Instructor's Resource Guide to accompany *Core concepts in health* by PM Insel and WT Roth, Mountain View, Calif, 1988, Mayfield Publishing Co.

DRAFTING A CONTRACT

To motivate himself, W.L. drafts his plan into contract form. In it, he outlines his behavior changes and his choice of positive reinforcement for carrying out the plan: a weekend film with his roommates. He introduces his roommates to the plan, and one of them even wants to join him, knowing that he too will benefit from exercise and weight loss. W.L. posts a chart on the dresser to record the amount of time spent on the exercise bike each night and his weekly body weight.

Concept Check

Successful plans for behavior change focus on small steps with positive reinforcement built in. At first, it is important to reinforce positive behaviors. Later, the focus can switch to positive changes, such as a loss of body weight or a lower blood cholesterol level. Before beginning a plan, the person should determine the degree of commitment to it. Behavior change, no matter how necessary, is ill-advised if one is not committed to that change.

PSYCHING YOURSELF UP

When you wish to change yourself, you are likely to get feedback from people who may support the planned changes, but some may prefer to keep things the way they are. They may try to dissuade you from your plan. Even you may have days or moments when you try to talk yourself out of your plan. We all respond to others' opinions, especially about ourselves.[5] We like approval, generally, and are influenced by others to behave in certain ways. One problem in undertaking behavior change is to be strong enough to behave in a chosen manner when others encourage—unconsciously or not—behavior inappropriate to the desired goal.

A certain amount of "psyching yourself up" is sometimes necessary to enable you to pursue your goals—*in spite of* others' expectations. Almost everyone benefits from some assertiveness training when it comes to changing behaviors.[6] Here are a few things you might consider.

- No one's feelings should be hurt if you say, "No, thank you," firmly and repeatedly, when others try to dissuade you from a plan. Rather, ask them—and yourself—why they want you to eat their way. Your needs are as important as someone else's.
- You don't have to order "big" to accommodate anyone—your mother, business clients, or the chef. Ordering "big" just because someone else is paying for the meal is a trap.
- When entertaining, you can serve lighter, more healthful low-fat meals.[10] You might have to try some new recipes, but that will be a useful step en route to changing your overall approach to cooking.
- Dealing with parties and social occasions built around food is possible but difficult. You can plan celebrations around a hike or a tennis court, rather than around cake and ice cream. When you must attend parties where food is everywhere, you can eat before you go, take low-kcalorie foods with you, and converse far from the food table.
- Learn ways to handle "put-downs"—inadvertent or conscious. The most effective response may be to communicate feelings honestly, without hostility. Tell criticizers that they have hurt your feelings; that you are working to change your habits, and that you would really like understanding and support from them.
- Fostering feelings of self-worth will facilitate the ability to change behavior. Getting rid of the habit of self-criticism requires strong self-retraining. Create and memorize lists of strengths, giving credit where deserved. Practice forgiving yourself. Lower unrealistic expectations. Practice stopping negative thoughts about yourself. Purposely switch to positive thoughts.
- Coerce the cook to change the family diet. The best situation is when the whole family wants to eat healthfully. The cook can influence that a great deal. There is extra effort involved in finding and developing new recipes and learning substitutions and shortcuts to cutting fat or kcalories. But the information exists in good cookbooks and recipes and is becoming more widespread as people get more excited about health and good nutrition.

PRACTICING THE PLAN

Once you determine your nutrition and health plan and, perhaps, write a contract, it is time to implement the plan. To begin, plan a trial of at least 6 to 8 weeks. Thinking of a lifetime commitment can be overwhelming. Remember that you win the game one point at a time. *Aim for a total duration of 6 months of new activities before giving up.* It is difficult to overcome the inertia of 20, 30, 40 or more years. More than once you may have to persuade yourself of the value of continuing the behavior change program. You may even backslide. That is not totally disastrous, if you can learn to manage your thinking. Following are a variety of suggestions that may help you keep your plan on track:

- **Focus on reducing, but not necessarily extinguishing, undesirable behaviors**—It is usually unrealistic to say you will never eat chocolate ice cream again. Better to say you will not eat chocolate ice cream as regularly as before.
- **Monitor progress**—Note your progress in a diary and refer to it often.[1] Reward yourself according to your contract. Prove to yourself regularly that you are succeeding in following your plan, and so are on the road to better health. As you conquer some habits and see yourself improve, and as the

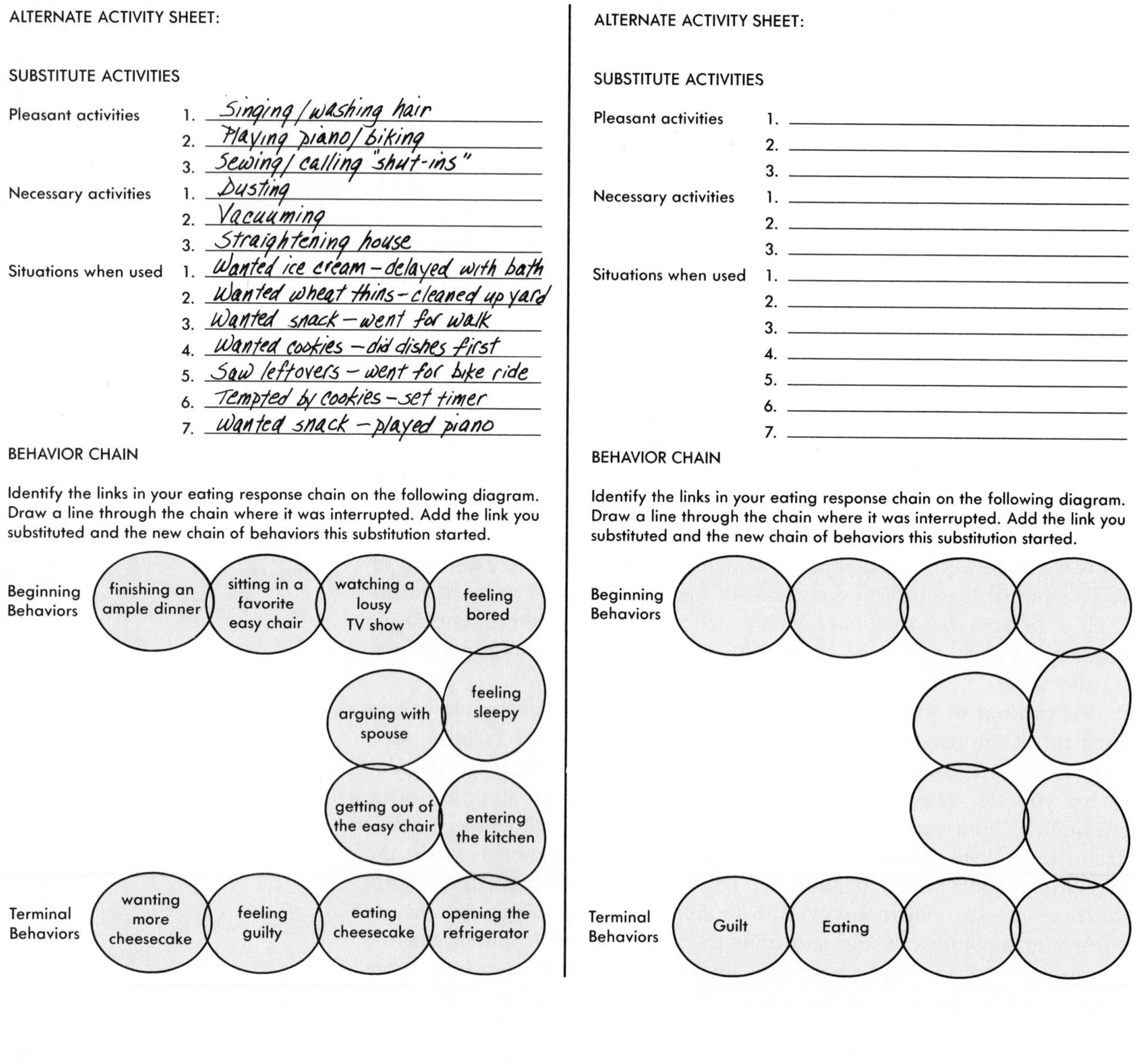

Figure 18-2

Identifying behavior chains is a good tool for understanding more about your habits and pinpointing ways to change unwanted habits.

ALTERNATE ACTIVITY SHEET:

SUBSTITUTE ACTIVITIES

Pleasant activities
1. Singing/washing hair
2. Playing piano/biking
3. Sewing/calling "shut-ins"

Necessary activities
1. Dusting
2. Vacuuming
3. Straightening house

Situations when used
1. Wanted ice cream—delayed with bath
2. Wanted wheat thins—cleaned up yard
3. Wanted snack—went for walk
4. Wanted cookies—did dishes first
5. Saw leftovers—went for bike ride
6. Tempted by cookies—set timer
7. Wanted snack—played piano

BEHAVIOR CHAIN

Identify the links in your eating response chain on the following diagram. Draw a line through the chain where it was interrupted. Add the link you substituted and the new chain of behaviors this substitution started.

Beginning Behaviors: finishing an ample dinner → sitting in a favorite easy chair → watching a lousy TV show → feeling bored → feeling sleepy → arguing with spouse → getting out of the easy chair → entering the kitchen → opening the refrigerator → eating cheesecake → feeling guilty → wanting more cheesecake (Terminal Behaviors)

ALTERNATE ACTIVITY SHEET:

SUBSTITUTE ACTIVITIES

Pleasant activities
1. ______
2. ______
3. ______

Necessary activities
1. ______
2. ______
3. ______

Situations when used
1. ______
2. ______
3. ______
4. ______
5. ______
6. ______
7. ______

BEHAVIOR CHAIN

Identify the links in your eating response chain on the following diagram. Draw a line through the chain where it was interrupted. Add the link you substituted and the new chain of behaviors this substitution started.

Beginning Behaviors

Terminal Behaviors: Guilt, Eating

new practices become more natural to you, you may find yourself quite encouraged—even enthusiastic—about your plan of action. That can be the impetus to move ahead with the program.

- **Control environments**—In the early phases of behavior change, it is best to avoid problem situations, such as parties, coffee breaks, and favorite restaurants.[3] Once new habits are firmly established, you can probably better resist the temptations in these environments.
- **Control related behaviors**—These are known as *behavior chains.* If one goal is to reduce snacking, control linked behaviors that encourage snacking, such as skipping meals and watching television (see Figure 18-2 and the Expert Opinion by Dr. James Ferguson).
- **Plan for failures**—This is often called contingency management (see Chapter 9). When faced with a situation or mood that may disrupt your plan, decide in advance what to do. If all else fails . . .
- **Forgive and forget**—Cultivate a long-term vision for a nutrition and health plan. Forgive occasional indiscretions. Focus on behaviors that have been established and performed day after day. An occasional lapse does not justify a relapse, and certainly not a collapse.
- **Recruit support from others**—from family members, roommates, and friends. Let some of them witness your contract; educate them about the program and your needs. Have the people around you help prevent problem situations that encourage you to deviate from your plan.
- **Watch for rationalization, the attempt to fool oneself**—Distorting information and denying facts to support wishful thinking are ways to rationalize. Trying to justify backsliding by saying "I can't do it"—when you have done it for 4 months already—is rationalizing. You don't fool even yourself.
- **Be realistic**—We cannot control every facet of our overall health. Genetic makeup and environment affect health. If you yearn for the body build of a sports hero or a movie star but have inherited other tendencies, then you probably cannot achieve the shape you want, even though you maintain an ideal body weight. Accept and like yourself for who you are.
- **Focus on the big picture**—Remember that we eat for pleasure, and that some habits we enjoy do not necessarily maximize health—watching the "Late Show" instead of sleeping, for example. A nutrition and health plan does not need to dominate all waking hours. Nutrition and health are part of a larger plan for satisfaction in life, one that includes a feeling of safety, reducing stress, and seeking the friendship and love of others, and seeking greater knowledge.

We must accept and like ourselves for who we are.

IMPLEMENTATION

As W.L. follows his new practices, unexpected obstacles arise. Friday night parties are a challenge with their abundance of "munchies" and alcoholic beverages. W.L. does not enjoy waking up earlier in the morning to pack his lunch, and he has to shop at the grocery store every few days for things he needs.

Entering the workforce often brings big changes in our life-style.

REEVALUATING THE PLAN

After you have practiced a program for several months, reevaluating it may clarify some issues. Does the plan of action actually take you to your goals? Are your goals in line with an overall nutrition and health plan? Reevaluation is especially in order if one's general life-style changes.

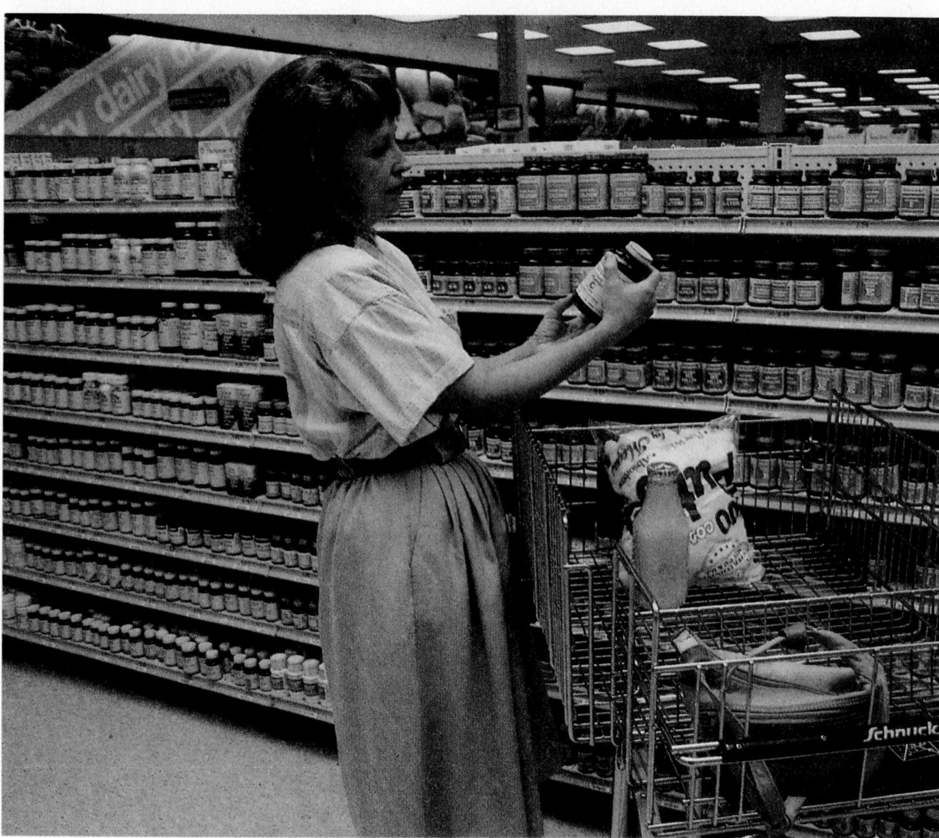

Figure 18-3
Supplements. Should this be the first step in improving a diet?

For example, as a person switches from a student life-style to that of a full-time worker, that person's level of physical activity may change drastically. A student may walk to classes and participate on intramural sports teams. But a job may require long hours at a desk. Though life-styles change, the need for physical activity doesn't.[9] Therefore we need to reevaluate plans for physical activity and adapt plans of action to new situations.

Changing habits for a few days or a few months is easy. Changing forever is tough, unless you learn somehow to enjoy it and identify the new habits as your own, not another's (Figure 18-3).

REEVALUATION

W.L. evaluates the obstacles he has encountered, and brainstorms with his roommates to find ways to overcome them. He decides to cut back slightly on kcalories during the day on Fridays, and at the parties allow himself a limited number of alcoholic drinks. He begins packing his lunch at night so he can grab it on the way to class and writes a complete grocery list that enables him to shop and stock up only once per week.

He begins to notice how much more energy he has and plans to continue the exercise program. He is beginning to really enjoy it. He also realizes that he should try a variety of foods so he doesn't get bored with his cooking and revert to a reliance on fast food restaurants. After a month, he has not reached his desirable body weight, but friends are commenting on changes they see in him. This encouragement helps him to remain patient with his progress and focus on the ultimate goal rather than the time needed to achieve it.

Concept Check

To implement a behavior change plan, write a contract that identifies behaviors to practice, desirable reinforcements, and a time frame for accomplishing the plan. While trying to change behaviors, it is important to control the environment (to discourage deviation from the plan), get support from others, and expect problems. A problem should not be an excuse for a relapse. Problems may require reconsideration of the behavior plan—this is to be expected. Reevaluating and refocusing naturally accompanies long-term behavior changes.

Preventing relapse

Relapse often starts with a high-risk situation. Most people don't recognize when they are at high risk for relapse, and just "one slip" becomes a series of lapses that lead to complete relapse into "old behaviors." The first "lapse" should be a signal to the person that she is stressed, having interpersonal conflicts, and is not coping adequately with everyday events. This is a high-risk situation. One or two slips is not fatal. Healthful behavior can be recovered if the potential for relapse is planned in advance and even expected. Here's how to do it.

- **Identify high-risk situations**—If and when you backslide, ask yourself if you are in a high-risk situation. This should help you to focus on the event rather than feel guilty about backsliding.
- **Mentally rehearse a response to a backsliding behavior**— Imagine yourself backsliding and see yourself taking positive action to recover. Rehearse a response to as many potential lapses as you can think of.
- **Remember your goals**—Remind yourself of the reasons for making the commitment to change your behavior and of the hard work that has gone into achieving progress.

Summary

1. Behavior change occurs progressively. First, a person becomes *aware* of a problem. Then the person openly receives new information about it, evolving a *receptive framework for learning.* He or she then undertakes a *trial* period for the change, in which *positive reinforcement* is critical. If an initial trial is successful, the person may permanently *adopt* new behaviors.
2. Before charting a behavior plan, it is important for a person to discover personal strengths and weaknesses regarding the behavior. A diary can be kept for a week or more. This may show patterns of eating and other behaviors that will either contribute to or discourage new behaviors. The diary can reveal areas of the external environment that need altering to reduce temptation.
3. When setting goals for a behavior plan, it is best to focus on small steps that lead to an intended result. Building positive reinforcement into the plan to reward achievements helps maintain momentum.
4. After setting a plan of action, it is often helpful to develop a contract that lists the actions intended to occur, the positive reinforcement to be received, and the time frame for the behavior change. The contract should at first reward positive behaviors, and later reward ultimate objectives.
5. Before embarking on a behavior-change program, the person should evaluate personal commitment. A plan, no matter how skillfully developed, will not succeed unless a person has a strong commitment to achieving the goals.
6. To implement a plan, it is important to monitor progress and provide rewards. Controlling the environment can reduce temptations to deviate from the plan. Small failures should be expected—not seen as an excuse to abandon change. A forgive-and-forget attitude can prevent collapse of the whole strategy.

7. Plan for the possibility of relapse. Most people revert to old behaviors during periods of stress or interpersonal conflict. Strategies to recover from relapse include identifying high-risk situations and mentally rehearsing a coping response.

Take Action

How physically active are you? Here are five activity levels: (1) sedentary, (2) mostly inactive (3) moderately active, (4) active, and (5) superactive. Each category is defined below. Your task is to track your activities for 3 weeks (even if this class ends before 3 weeks). Assign yourself an activity level each week.

Activity Levels

(5) **Superactive**—One hour of vigorous activity at least 5 days per week. Examples are competitive sports, full-court basketball, mountain climbing, weight training, treadmill work, soccer, and other similar activities.

(4) **Active**—Twenty minutes of sustained activity at least 5 days per week. Examples are swimming, tennis singles, jogging, cross-country skiing, or walking continuously for 45 minutes.

(3) **Moderately Active**—Twenty minutes of sustained activity at least 3 days per week or 10 to 15 minutes of sustained activity at least 4 days a week. Examples include tennis, downhill skiing, skating, aerobic dancing, golf or similar activities.

(2) **Mostly Inactive**—Sustained activity fewer than 3 days per week that usually involves mostly walking. Examples include fishing, bowling, or sporadic jogging.

(1) **Sendentary**—Most activities are limited to sitting or walking.

Start on a Monday, for example, and estimate your activity level for the previous week. After 3 weeks, average the numbers by adding them and then dividing the answer by 3. This should result in a number between 1 and 5. Find your location on the physical activity ladder. What kind of program would allow you to move up the ladder, if appropriate?

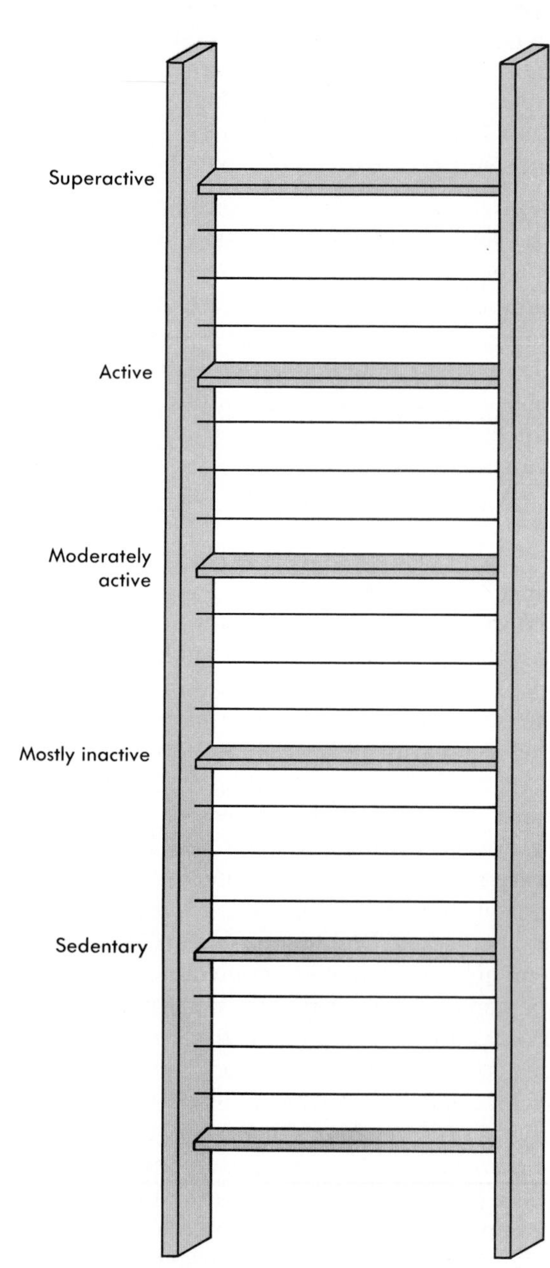

REFERENCES

1. Brownell KD: The LEARN program for weight control, Philadelphia, 1989.
2. Ferguson J and Taylor C Barr: A change for heart: your family and the food you eat, Palo Alto, Calif, 1978, Bull Publishing Co.
3. Ferguson J: Habits, not diets: the secret to lifetime weight control, Palo Alto, Calif, 1988, Bull Publishing Co.
4. Frankle RT and Yang M: Obesity and weight control, Rockville, Md, 1988, Aspen Publishers Inc.
5. Gifft HH and others: Nutrition, behavior, and health change, Englewood Cliffs, NJ, 1972, Prentice-Hall, Inc.
6. Insel PM and Roth WT: Core concepts in Health, Fifth Edition, Mountain View, Calif, 1988, Mayfield Publishing Co.
7. Nash JD: Maximize your body potential, Palo Alto, Calif, 1986, Bull Publishing Co.
8. Snook JT: Nutrition: A guide to decision-making, Englewood Cliffs, NJ, 1984, Prentice-Hall Inc.
9. Wood P: California diet and exercise program, Mountain View, Calif, 1983, Anderson World Books Inc.
10. Weinstock CP: The grazing of America: a guide to healthy snacking, FDA Consumer, p 8, March 1989.

SUGGESTED READINGS

Two excellent manuals that chronical the path to behavior change are the books by Ferguson and Brownell. They focus primarily on the treatment of overeating, but the general principles could be applied to other diet changes. To learn more about a variety of health issues and how total life-style influences health, see the book by Insel and Roth. For a very technical treatment of obesity, consult the book by Frankle and Yang.

CHAPTER 18

Answers to nutrition awareness inventory

1. *False.* It is commonly believed that people who cannot change their behaviors are weak-willed. This destructive misconception perpetuates unsuccessful attempts to change. Instead, changing one's environment is a key to behavior change.
2. *True.* For some people, food preferences vary with emotional state. For example, eating chocolate may reduce stress for some people, while pizza may be considered solely a party food.
3. *False.* Commitment to a goal is the best predictor of success. Realistic goal setting includes scrutiny of commitment.
4. *False.* Occasional backsliding is expected when undertaking behavioral change but is not reason to abandon a goal.
5. *True.* Food is more than nourishment for most people. By identifying the roles food plays in a person's life and finding appropriate substitutes for food, food habits are more easily changed.
6. *False.* Body types are partially genetically determined. Striving for an unrealistic, unattainable body type deprives a person of the success deserved for maximizing personal potential.
7. *True.* Monitoring progress from a beginning baseline yields tangible reinforcement and encouragement to a changer.
8. *False.* Positive reinforcement helps instill self-confidence, maintain enthusiasm, and foster the self-worth that facilitates behavior change.
9. *False.* Some dieters restrict themselves during the day so that, by late evening, hunger and feelings of deprivation encourage overeating.
10. *False.* Diet changes need not be so restrictive. Long-term change results from practical, possible routines that can be continued throughout life—not from starvation.
11. *True.* Even the most finicky eaters, with the guidance of nutrition experts, can have healthier diets consisting of foods they enjoy.
12. *False.* It is wiser to avoid tempting situations when initiating behavior change. Once a person is comfortable with new behaviors, it will be easier to confront and cope with problem situations.
13. *False.* Separating final behavior goals into smaller steps that are more easily and quickly achieved can give a person the confidence and motivation needed to reach the ultimate goal. It is also a key to understanding that behaviors require daily decisions, not magic pills or a once-in-a-lifetime change.
14. *True.* Even friends and relatives do not always understand a person's choices or motivations. A strong commitment to change and honesty with friends can enable one to continue a plan, even if support from others is lacking.
15. *False.* Rewarding oneself in constructive ways along each step of the plan can motivate a person to continue following the plan. Every step made toward the final goal is worth recognition.

Nutrition Perspective 18-1

What Does It Cost to Have a Healthy Diet?

Serving nutritious meals on a limited income takes careful planning. In 1985, the USDA published a food plan designed to meet the nutrient needs of two adults. In January 1989, this plan's monthly cost was about $185. A slightly revised menu plan is given in Table 18-4. Of importance are the basic guidelines from which these plans were developed that encourage nutritious eating at a minimum cost. Some are listed here:

- Choose low-cost varieties of foods
- Feature grain products
- Use smaller amounts of meat, poultry, and fish
- Avoid waste; plan for leftovers
- Make your own convenience mixes

Let's now investigate each of these suggestions in more detail.

CHOOSE LOW-COST FOODS

The first step is to develop a menu plan for a week. When preparing for a weekly shopping trip, consult a calendar, recipe books, coupons, and the grocer's weekly flier. Write each dinner plan on the calendar. Consider ingredients that are not on hand and list your needs. If you check the weekly store specials at this time, you can take advantage of bargains.

Nonfat dry milk and skim milk are usually the best buys for dairy products. Large containers are usually less expensive. Higher cost dairy products are cheese, yogurt, ice cream, and ice milk; these can be included in the diet for variety, but need not be a major focus. Grate your own cheese: packages of shredded cheese cost more than the same amount of cheese in blocks and lose freshness faster.

When in season, fresh fruits and vegetables are usually good buys. At other times, frozen and canned fruits and vegetables may cost less. Large bags of frozen vegetables can be bargains, and you can pour out the exact amount needed.

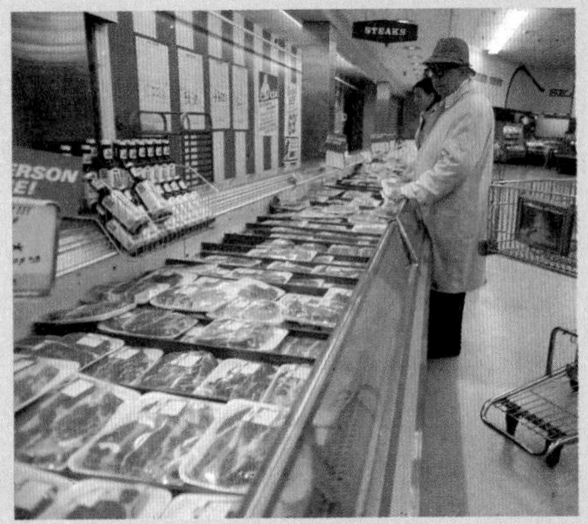

Meat is often the most expensive food item we buy.

Dried beans, peas, and peanut butter are less expensive than many varieties of meat, poultry, and fish. Using peanut butter, dried beans, and peas also adds variety to meals. Pay special attention to meat, poultry, and fish purchases. They are usually the more expensive foods in meals. Careful selection can mean food dollars saved. Buying sale cuts and "family pack" sizes can yield big savings. Cut up meats and chickens yourself. Chicken parts often cost more than whole chickens, and stew meat often costs more than a chuck roast. Some higher priced meats may fit into a budget when they are on sale.

Whole-grain breads that carry store labels are often much less expensive than national brands. Convenience foods, such as cookies, pies, and other bakery products, often cost more than similar ones you can make at home.

In addition to those already mentioned, it is especially important to minimize purchases of soft drinks, candy, alcohol, coffee, and tea; frozen vegetables in seasonings and sauces; sugar-coated cereals; and potato, corn, or cheese chips and puffs. This doesn't mean that a person should never have these foods but, rather, should use these items sparingly.

FEATURE GRAIN PRODUCTS

Enriched and whole-grain products are among the most economical sources for many vitamins and minerals. Economical meal plans count heavily on foods from the breads and cereals group. A person should plan to feature them at every meal and snack. To stretch food dollars, a person can use grain products as side dishes or combine them with small portions of meat, poultry, or fish in main dishes. Recall from Chapter 2 that the Daily Food Guide requires only 1200 to 1500 kcalories. Many people need more kcalories than that to meet energy needs. Adding grain products, especially whole-grain products, can make up for the missing kcalories economically and healthfully.

Table 18-4

Thrifty meals for two*

Sunday	Monday	Tuesday	Wednesday	Thursday	Friday	Saturday
Orange (1) Ready-to-eat cereal (3 oz) Toast (3 sl) Milk (2 c)	Grapefruit juice (1 c) Eggs (2) Toast (4 sl) Ham (¼ lb)	Banana (1) Oatmeal (1 c dry) Toasted drop biscuits (3) Milk (2 c)	Grapefruit juice (1 c) Cornmeal pancakes Syrup (4 T)	Banana (1) Oatmeal (1 c dry) Muffins (3) Milk (2 c)	Orange (1) Ready-to-eat cereal (3 oz) Quick bread (4 sl) Milk (2 c)	Grapefruit juice (1 c) Scrambled eggs (2) on toasted hamburger rolls (2)
Braised turkey (6 oz) with gravy Baked potatoes (2 med) Spinach (½ 10-oz pkg) Drop biscuits (2) Chocolate pudding	Turkey-potato salad on lettuce leaves (2) Drop biscuits (3)	Grilled cheese (4 oz) sandwich (2) Carrot sticks (about 1 carrot)	Taco salad Toasted peanut butter snack loaf (4 sl)	Split pea soup (2-⅔ c) Cottage cheese (1 c) on lettuce leaves (2) Crackers (24)	Hamburger (½ lb) on roll (2) Hot potato salad	Split pea soup (2-⅔ c) Tomato (1), Ham (¼ lb), and lettuce (2 leaves) sandwich (2)
Cheeseburger on hamburger roll (2 oz cheese, ½ lb ground beef, 2 rolls) Banana (2)	Bean tamale pie Lettuce (⅓ lb) wedge with dressing (2 T) Crackers (24) Peanut butter snack loaf (4 sl)	Turkey Spanish rice Spinach (½ 10-oz pkg) Apple (1) wedges Toast (2 sl) Peanut butter snack loaf (4 sl)	Salted chicken (6 ounces) Noodles (2 c dry) Lettuce (⅓ lb) wedge with dressing (2 T) Toasted hamburger rolls (2)	Stir-fried beef and peppers Rice (⅓ c dry) Chopped broccoli (½ 10-oz pkg) Apple cobbler (half)	Pork chops with stuffing Mashed potatoes (2 med) Lettuce (⅓ lb) wedge with dressing (2 T) Muffins (3)	Braised beef with noodles Chopped broccoli (½ 10-oz pkg) Apple (1) wedges Quick bread (4 sl)
Toast (4 sl) with peanut butter (2 T)	Ready-to-eat cereal (3 oz) Milk (2 c)	Cornmeal chips (22)	Muffins (2) Milk (2 c)	Quick bread (4 sl)	Apple cobbler (half)	Ready-to-eat cereal (3 oz) Milk (2 c)

*Amounts to serve two healthy people are shown in parentheses after most of the foods on the menu.
This meal plan was revised slightly from one developed by the USDA. Recipes can be found in the original publication, available from county Home Economics Extension agents in the United States. We suggest further modifying the plan by including, when possible, whole-wheat breads and whole-grain crackers and cereals; making the baked goods with vegetable oils or tub margarines (as appropriate); and using low-fat or nonfat milk.

From: Thrifty Meals for Two, USDA Home and Garden Bulletin 244, December, 1985.

Continued.

Nutrition Perspective 18-1—cont'd

What Does It Cost to Have a Healthy Diet?

USE SMALLER AMOUNTS OF MEAT, POULTRY, AND FISH

Meats are good sources of several nutrients, but most meats are more expensive than other foods. Smaller amounts of lower priced meat, poultry, and fish should be combined in hearty main dishes with bread, cereal, rice, pasta, or potatoes. Dried beans, dried peas, and peanut butter can often be used in casseroles, soups, salads, and snacks. They provide many of the same nutrients as meats, and at a lower cost.

AVOID WASTE: PLAN FOR LEFTOVERS

To avoid waste, consider leftovers as part of a meal plan. For example, consider preparing a recipe for four, and serving it twice. Or cook a large cut of meat or whole chicken, eat some, and save the rest for use in other main dishes. Planning for leftovers necessitates having a weekly meal plan and knowing ahead of time how leftovers will be used. To save time, consider cooking for the week on just 1 or 2 days, and then freeze or store most of the food. Then, you can enjoy just heating and eating the food for the rest of the week.

MAKE YOUR OWN CONVENIENCE MIXES

Recipes available from local Home Economist Extension agents are available for making biscuit mixes, pudding mixes, and hamburger extenders. Many mixes keep in the refrigerator for months and cost much less than their commercial counterparts.

If you want more information about low-cost meal plans, in the United States, contact the local Home Economist Extension agent for your county. A library may have catalogs listing available government pamphlets. Those pertaining to low-cost food purchasing are inexpensive and contain numerous recipes and weekly menu plans. Otherwise, the general suggestions listed at the beginning of this Nutrition Perspective can apply to other low-cost menus you may want to develop.

Nutrition Perspective 18-2

Is There One Best Ethnic Diet?

Based on research begun in the 1940s and 1950s, some scientists have developed a formula for a diet they consider one of the best overall for our bodies. The key is to eat simple foods, not elite treats. In many countries, scientists discovered that an especially healthy diet is the inexpensive, traditional fare—precisely the diet people abandon as they move into affluence.

The simple healthful diet—perhaps at one time a peasant diet—is the traditional cuisine of relatively agrarian societies, such as Mexico and China. It is usually based on a grain (rice, wheat, and corn), fruits and vegetables, small amounts of dairy products or meat, fish, and eggs, and a legume. The advantages are that they are low in fat and high in fiber, and most kcalories come from grains and legumes.

Few people would choose the African !Kung diet—wild-growing roots, beans, nuts, fibrous tubers and fruits, and wild game animals—or a simple peasant diet from eastern Europe. In an affluent society, which has an abundance of rich foods, a person must exercise willpower to keep fat intake down. When a country reaches a certain level of affluence, as have the United States and Canada throughout the past century and, recently, Japan, consumption of grains and beans gives way to marbled meats and cheeses—both high in kcalories and saturated fat. The trick to finding healthy food is to look carefully at each dish. No single cuisine is all good or all bad.

JAPANESE FOODS

The Japanese diet highlights soybeans, rice, vegetables, and fish. This cuisine appears to embrace the best and worst of diets. The core of the traditional diet is low in fat: protein-rich soybean products (tofu and miso, made of fermented soybeans), fish, vegetables, noodles, and rice. Meat is used sparingly, more as a garnish than as a main course. Seaweed—the Japanese "lettuce"—is high in nutrients. These are the staples that have helped keep heart disease rates low in Japan.

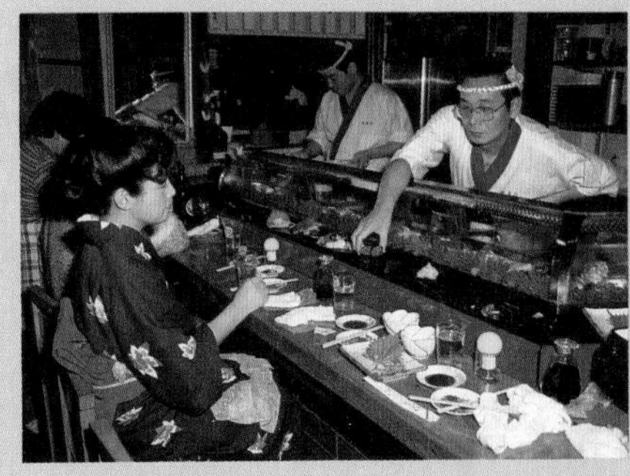

The Japanese diet is low in fat but high in salted, smoked, and pickled foods.

But another aspect of traditional Japanese cuisine is reliance on salty, smoked, and pickled foods. They combine to create Japan's two most serious public health problems: stroke and stomach cancer. Sodium (in salted fish, salty pickled foods, and soy sauce) is linked to hypertension and risk of stroke. And salt plus smoked foods rich in nitrates contributes to Japan's rate of stomach cancer—one of the world's highest.

The Japanese diet is changing—for better and worse. Widespread refrigerator ownership during the last 30 years has allowed use of more fresh foods and fewer preserved (salted, pickled, and soaked) ones. It also allows more dairy products to be used. Both changes may be related to the decline in stomach cancer, a decrease of roughly one third, between 1950 and 1982. (The benefits of dairy products are supported by a controlled Japanese study showing less stomach cancer in men and women who drink milk daily.)

The *bad* news is that fat intake has doubled since the 1950s, when it accounted for only 10% to 15% of kcalories consumed in the Japanese diet. Current Japanese fat consumption still is only about half that of the United States, probably too low to create real heart disease problems. But fat intake among Japanese teens—thanks partly to French fries, fried chicken, and other fast food imports—almost matches that of U.S. teens. And there is some evidence that the Japanese rate of breast cancer—a disease that may be linked to high fat intake—is rising.

MEXICAN FOODS

The Mexican diet is built around corn, beans, fish, chicken, and vegetables. Mexican fare eaten in the United States is not the same as that eaten in Mexico. The familiar fatty dishes—beef burritos swimming in melted cheese—aren't a staple in Mexico. Rich meat dishes are generally reserved for holiday fiestas. Instead, corn and beans are the core of the diet. The corn is steeped in lime water, adding to its calcium and free niacin content. It is

Continued.

Nutrition Perspective 18-2—cont'd

Is There One Best Ethnic Diet?

part of every meal—used in tortillas, steamed in corn husks to make tamales, or served as hot gruel. Beans provide complementary protein so that when corn and beans are eaten together, the body can synthesize any protein it needs. It is best if lard is not used in the preparation of the beans: read the label of any commercially prepared refried beans.

Guacamole is likewise good for health-conscious diners, if they can handle the kcalories: most fat in avocado is monounsaturated, like the fat in olive and canola oils. And seviche—fish marinated in lime juice—is generally low in fat content, as are some chicken dishes, such as tostadas, if they're not fried. Hot chili peppers, excellent sources of vitamins A and C, can be good for the body, if you can "take the heat."

TRADITIONAL ESKIMO FOODS

You may not find any Eskimo restaurants around, but studies of some of their extreme food habits have led to a new dietary recommendation: eat fish regularly.[6] Throughout the first half of this century, some Eskimo groups existed almost solely on seal, whale, and fish, much of it raw, with some caribou, berries, and other plant foods thrown in.

In studying the Eskimos, scientists were amazed to find that fish oil helps prevent heart disease by lowering blood pressure, blood triglycerides, and the blood's capacity to clot (see Chapter 5). The benefits of fish, especially the cold-water species—mackerel, salmon, herring, smelts, and sardines—are now well accepted.

THE CHINESE DIET

Known for its variety, the average Chinese diet consists of about 69% carbohydrate, 10% protein, and 21% fat—similar to proportions some Western nutritionists and cancer experts recommend. There is a richness and variety in Chinese cuisine, evidenced by the use of over 2000 different vegetables. In the southeastern coastal area around Canton, estimates of the number of dishes range up to 50,000.

Rice is the core of the diet in the south; wheat in the temperate north is made into noodles, bread, and dumplings. Common preparations are hot pots—stews containing dozens of ingredients—and stir-fried vegetables, meats, and fish, which are cooked almost instantaneously in a lightly oiled, very hot wok. Bok choy and other forms of Chinese cabbage—perhaps the most widely consumed vegetables in the world—are cruciferous, high in vitamin C, and contribute to general good health.

North American restaurant versions of Chinese cooking, regrettably, usually emphasize the meats and the sauces. Chinese cooks usually use less of many of the basic sauces—oyster, hoisin, soy, and black bean. But you can still order a healthful meal in a Chinese restaurant here by substituting vegetable dishes for some main dishes. The average Chinese consumes the same amount of salt as an American. Health authorities in China are calling for a cut in salt intake, and a switch from saturated to unsaturated fats.

SOUTHERN ITALIAN CUISINE

Southern Italy thrives on pasta, bread, olive oil, fruits, and vegetables. Compared with northern Italians of the same economic class, southern Italians consume only two-thirds as much beef and veal, less than half the chicken, and one-fifth the butter. Southern Italians also eat one-fifth more bread, pasta, vegetables, and fruit, and twice the fish.

Pasta is the heart of the Italian diet: Italians still eat six times as much of this simple wheat and water concoction as do North Americans. People in Mediterranean cultures eat at least three times as much bread as Americans. But it's rarely buttered. A healthful, delicious alternative is *bruschetto,* a slice of hot Italian-bread toast brushed with olive oil and rubbed with raw garlic.

Chapter 19

Food Safety

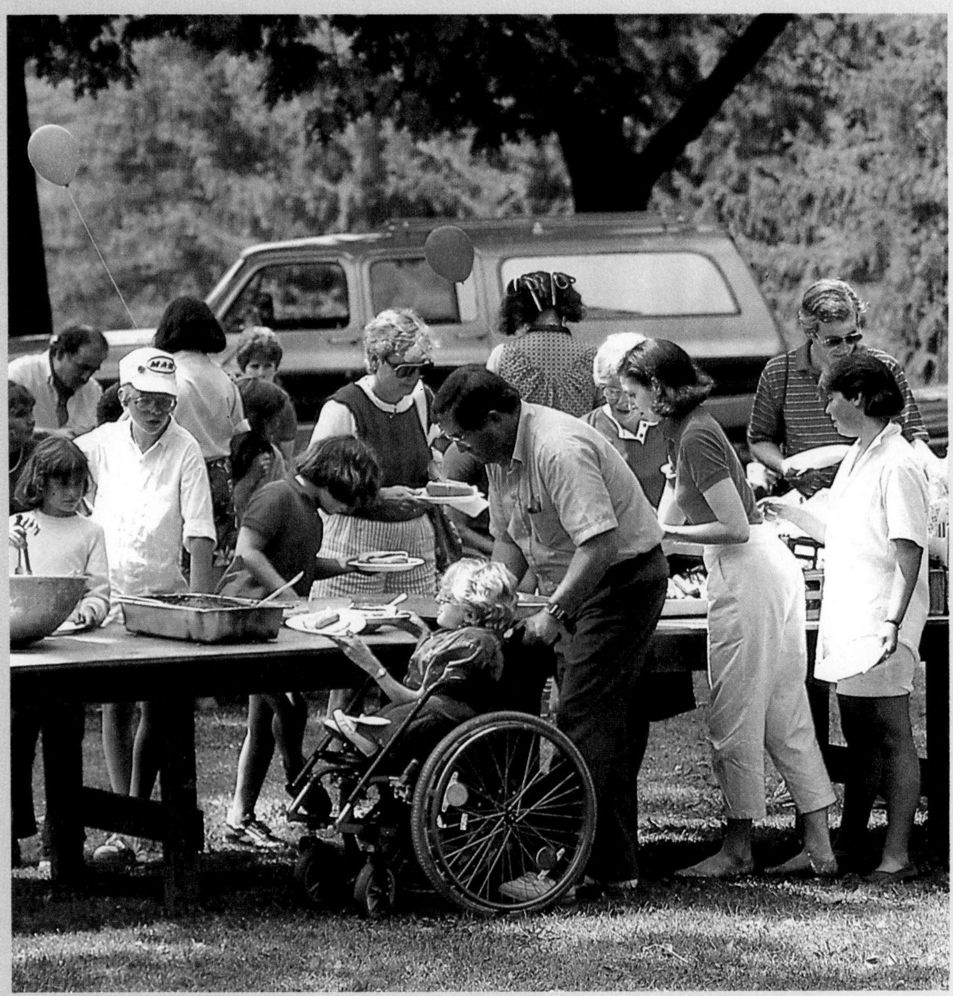

Many cases of food poisoning happen at events like this family picnic, as foods may be out in the warm air for hours at a time.

Overview

How safe is our food? Scientists and health authorities, whether working independently or for the government, agree that North Americans enjoy the safest, most wholesome food supply in the world. Yet, they also acknowledge that despite making tremendous progress in food safety throughout the past half century, a health risk from microbes and chemicals is still present in foods.

The greatest health risk from food is microbial contamination from bacteria and, to a lesser extent, from molds, fungi, and viruses. These microbes in foods can cause food poisoning.[23] However, regardless of evidence that microbial contamination is by far the major cause of food-related illness in North America and throughout the world, North Americans seem more concerned about health risks from chemicals in foods.[8] Fully 75% of consumers surveyed in a recent Gallup poll said that pesticide contamination was a major concern to them.

Let's first explore some general issues involved in food safety. Then, we'll discuss food poisoning and the use and safety of food additives.

Nutrition awareness inventory

Here are 15 statements about food safety. Answer them to test your current knowledge. If you think the answer is true or mostly true, circle T. If you think the answer is false or mostly false, circle F. Use the scoring key at the end of this chapter to compute your total score. Take this test again after you have read this chapter. Compare the results.

1.	**T**	**F**	In North America, 1 of every 10 people suffers a bout of diarrhea from food poisoning each year.
2.	**T**	**F**	You can usually tell from a food's taste, odor, or appearance if that food poses a risk for food poisoning.
3.	**T**	**F**	Imported food does not pose a risk for food poisoning because of careful inspection on entry into this country.
4.	**T**	**F**	Synthetic (man-made) chemicals are necessarily more harmful than those that occur in nature.
5.	**T**	**F**	Exposure to oxygen causes some foods to spoil.
6.	**T**	**F**	Food can be preserved by reducing its water content.
7.	**T**	**F**	Most kinds of bacteria can cause food poisoning.
8.	**T**	**F**	Most food-poisoning microbes thrive on temperatures between 40°F and 140°F (4°C and 60°C).
9.	**T**	**F**	Symptoms of food poisoning resemble flu symptoms.
10.	**T**	**F**	Food-poisoning victims receive some immunity against future attacks.
11.	**T**	**F**	Chickens are a common source of Salmonella food poisoning.
12.	**T**	**F**	Botulism is the deadliest form of food poisoning, and the bacteria that cause it are present in soil.
13.	**T**	**F**	*Clostridium botulinum,* the bacteria that cause botulism, grows only in the absence of air.
14.	**T**	**F**	Eating raw fish can cause serious health problems.
15.	**T**	**F**	Alcoholic beverages are free of toxic compounds.

FOOD POISONING

About one third to one half of all diarrhea cases in North America—upward of 20 million per year in the United States alone—are due to food-borne organisms. Estimates of the yearly incidence of diarrhea caused by food poisoning in North America vary from about 1 of every 10 persons to 1 of every 36 persons. Either way, the presence of microbes in food poses a health risk.[13,19]

Food poisoning is not always a brief—although distressing—episode of diarrhea, also known as *Montezuma's revenge.* Some people, especially children, the elderly, people with alcoholism, and people with underlying health problems, such as cancer, can suffer greatly from illnesses caused by certain food-borne microbes. Some bouts of food poisoning are lengthy and lead to rheumatic diseases, food allergies, seizures and other nervous disorders, blood poisoning, or other ills.[15,16]

It is usually not possible to tell from taste, smell, or sight that eating a particular food poses a risk for food poisoning. The main exception to this rule is the uncommon *Bacillus subtilis,* which causes "off flavors" in pastry items. So the last case of the "flu" you had actually may have been due to food poisoning. The symptoms of both disorders are often the same: diarrhea, vomiting, fever, and weakness.

Why is food poisoning so common?

The risk of having food poisoning is rising, partly because of efforts by the food industry to increase the shelf life of products. Longer shelf life allows foods to remain at room temperatures long enough for bacteria to multiply sufficiently to cause food poisoning. Some bacteria can grow even at refrigeration temperatures. Partially cooked—and some fully cooked—products pose a special risk because refrigerated storage many only slow—not prevent—bacterial growth. This is an area of great concern to the FDA.

Another factor increasing food poisoning risk is a change in dietary practices.[3,6] Supermarkets, in becoming major food processors during the past decade, now offer a variety of prepared foods from specialty meat shops, salad bars, and bakeries. The foods are usually prepared in central kitchens and shipped to individual stores, often across state lines. If a food product is contaminated in the central kitchen, patrons of stores across the country can suffer an attack (Figure 19-1). A malfunction in a dairy plant in 1985 resulted in 16,284 confirmed cases of *Salmonella* bacteria infections and at least two deaths from contaminated low-fat milk.

Still another cause of increased food-poisoning incidents in North America is greater consumption of ready-to-eat foods imported from foreign countries. In the past, food imports were mostly raw products processed here under strict sanitation standards. Now, however, imports of processed foods, such as cheese from France and seafood from Asia—some of which are contaminated—are on the rise.

Finally, reported cases of food-borne disease have increased because of our greater awareness of food as a vehicle for microorganisms, not only those that grow in food but also those merely transmitted by food. For example, it was not

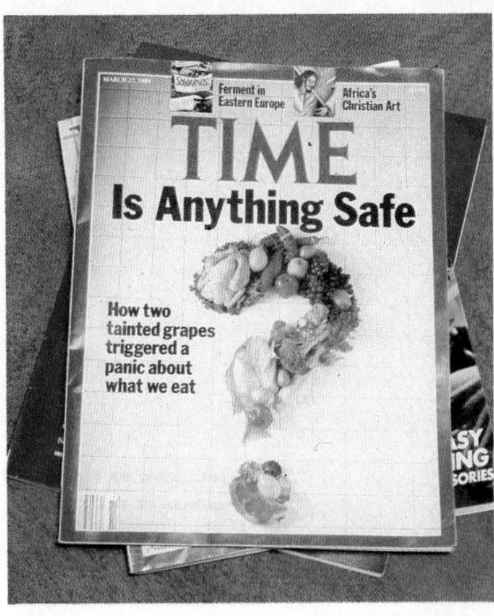

Food safety should be an issue that all of us pay attention to.

Figure 19-1

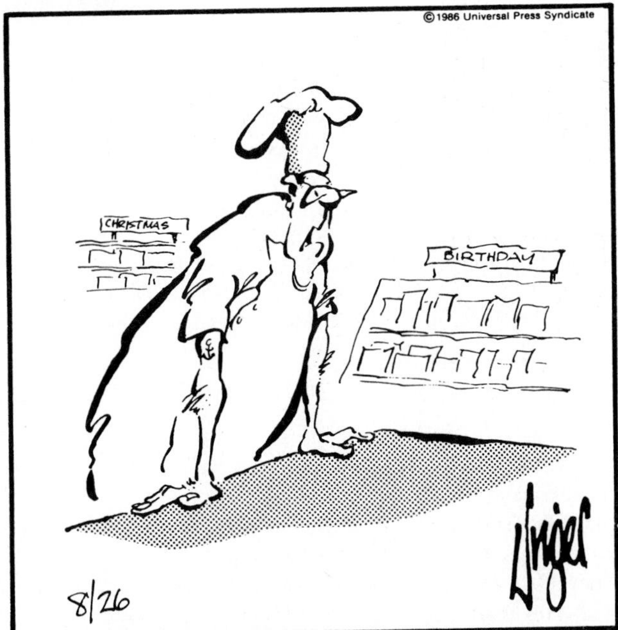

"I need 148 get-well cards."

Table 19-1

Organisms that cause foodborne illness: their source, symptoms, and prevention

Organism: bacteria	Source of illness	Symptoms	Prevention methods
Staphylococcus aureus	Live in nasal passages and in cuts on skin. Toxin is produced when food contaminated by bacteria is left for extended time at room temperature. Meats, poultry, egg products, tuna, potato, and macaroni salads, and cream-filled pastries are good environments for these bacteria to produce toxin.	Onset: 2-6 hours after eating. Diarrhea, vomiting, nausea, and abdominal cramps. Mimics flu. Lasts 24-48 hours. Rarely fatal.	▪ Sanitary food-handling practices ▪ Prompt and proper refrigeration of foods ▪ Keep cuts on skin covered
Salmonella	Found in raw meats, poultry, eggs, fish, milk, and products made with these items. Multiplies rapidly at room temperature. The bacteria themselves are toxic.	Onset: 5-72 hours after eating. Nausea, fever, headache, abdominal cramps, diarrhea, and vomiting. Can be fatal in infants, the elderly, and the sick.	▪ Handling food in a sanitary manner ▪ Thorough cooking of foods ▪ Prompt and proper refrigeration of foods ▪ Watch cross-contamination
Clostridium perfringens	Widespread in environment. Generally found in meat and poultry dishes. Multiply rapidly when foods are left for extended time at room temperature. The bacteria themselves are toxic.	Onset: 8-24 hours after eating (usually 12 hours). Abdominal pain and diarrhea. Symptoms last a day or less, usually mild. Can be more serious in older or debilitated people.	▪ Sanitary handling of foods, especially meat and meat dishes, gravies, and leftovers ▪ Thorough cooking and reheating of foods ▪ Prompt and proper refrigeration
Clostridium botulinum	Widespread in the environment. However, bacteria produce toxin only in low-acid, anaerobic (oxygen-free) environments, such as in canned green beans, mushrooms, spinach, olives, and beef. Honey may carry spores.	Onset: 12-36 hours after eating. Neurotoxic symptoms include double vision, inability to swallow, speech difficulty, and progressive paralysis of the respiratory system. OBTAIN MEDICAL HELP IMMEDIATELY. BOTULISM CAN BE FATAL.	▪ Using proper methods for canning low acid foods ▪ Avoiding commercial cans of low acid foods that have leaky seals or are bent, bulging, or broken ▪ Toxin can be destroyed after can or jar is opened by boiling contents hard for 20 minutes, but discard if suspect toxin is present because of off-odors
Campylobacter jejuni	Found on poultry, cattle, and sheep, and can contaminate their meat and milk. Chief food sources are raw poultry and meat and unpasteurized milk.	Onset: 3-5 days after eating, or longer. Diarrhea, abdominal cramping, fever, and sometimes bloody stools. Lasts 2-7 days.	▪ Thorough cooking of foods ▪ Handling food in a sanitary manner ▪ Avoiding unpasteurized milk

Organisms that cause foodborne illness: their source, symptoms, and prevention

Organism: bacteria	Source of illness	Symptoms	Prevention methods
Listeria monocytogenes	Found in soft cheeses and unpasteurized milk. Resists acid, heat, salt, and nitrate well.	Onset: 4-21 days. Fever, headache, vomiting, and sometimes even more severe symptoms. May be fatal.	▪ Thorough cooking of foods ▪ Handling food in a sanitary manner ▪ Avoiding unpasteurized milk
Yersinia enterocolitica	Ubiquitous in nature; carried in food and water. They multiply rapidly at both room and refrigerator temperatures. Generally found in raw vegetables, meats, water, and unpasteurized milk.	Onset: 2-3 days after eating. Fever, headache, nausea, diarrhea, and general malaise. Mimics flu and appendicitis. An important cause of gastroenteritis in children.	▪ Thorough cooking of foods ▪ Sanitizing cutting instruments and cutting boards before preparing foods that are eaten raw ▪ Avoidance of unpasteurized milk and unchlorinated water.
Organism: viruses			
Hepatitis A virus	Chief food sources: shellfish harvested from contaminated areas and foods that are handled a lot during preparation and then eaten raw (such as vegetables).	Onset: 30 days. Jaundice, fatigue. May cause liver damage and death.	▪ Sanitary handling of foods ▪ Use of pure drinking water ▪ Adequate sewage disposal ▪ Adequate cooking of foods
Norwalk, Human Rotavirus	Found in the human intestinal tract and expelled in feces. Contamination of foods occurs: 1) when sewage is used to enrich garden/farm soil 2) by direct hand-to-food contact during the preparation of meals, and 3) when shellfish-growing waters are contaminated by sewage.	Onset: 1-3 days. Severe diarrhea, nausea and vomiting. Respiratory symptoms. Usually lasts 4-5 days, but may last for weeks.	▪ Sanitary handling of foods ▪ Use of pure drinking water ▪ Adequate sewage disposal ▪ Adequate cooking of foods
Organism: parasites			
Trichinella spiralis	Found in pork and wild game.	Onset: weeks-months. Muscle weakness, fluid retention in face, fever, flu-like symptoms.	▪ Thoroughly cook pork and wild game
Anisakis	Found in raw fish.	Onset: 12 hours. Stomach infection, severe stomach pain.	▪ Thoroughly cook fish.
Organism: mycotoxins			
A group of toxic compounds produced by molds, such as aflatoxin B-1 and ergot.	Produced in foods that are relatively high in moisture. Chief food sources: beans and grains that have been stored in a moist place.	May cause liver and/or kidney disease.	▪ Checking foods for visible mold and discarding those that are contaminated. ▪ Proper storage of susceptible foods.

Foods	Water Activity
fruits and vegetables	0.97
eggs	0.96
meats	0.96
cheese, bread	0.96
jam	0.85
honey	0.75
dried fruit	0.70

pasteurization
The process of heating food products to kill pathogenic microorganisms. One method heats milk at 161° F for 20 seconds at least.

irradiation
A process whereby radiation energy is applied to foods, creating compounds (free radicals) within the food that destroy cell membranes, break down DNA, link proteins together, limit enzyme activity, and alter a variety of other proteins and cell functions that can lead to food spoilage.

aseptic processing
A method by which both food and container are simultaneously sterilized; it allows manufacturers to produce boxes of milk that can be stored at room temperature. Variations of this process are also known as ultra high temperature (UHT) packaging.

until 1982 that experts suspected soft cheeses were vehicles for the bacteria *Listeria.* Every decade the list of microorganisms suspected of causing food poisoning expands.

Food preservation—past, present, and future

For centuries, salt, sugar, smoke, fermentation, and drying have been used to preserve food. Ancient Romans used sulfites to disinfect wine containers and preserve wine. European travelers to the New World stored meat in salt to preserve it. Many preserving methods work on the principle of reducing the amount of free water—the water not bound to other components in the food. Salts and sugar reduce free water by binding it, and drying drives off free water. A measure of free water in a food is known as its **water activity.** Most bacteria need a water activity greater than 0.9 to grow. Yeasts can grow at water activity above 0.8, and molds grow at water activity above 0.6. The water activities of typical foods are listed in the margin. Using this list, you can now predict why bacteria are a problem in eggs and meat, but not in jam or honey. You can also see that, unless properly treated and stored, dried fruits can still support the growth of molds.

Some foods with high water activity would be greatly altered by decreasing their free-water content. In these cases, selected bacteria are used to ferment (pickle) or "spoil" the food. Pickles, sauerkraut, yogurt, and wine are all examples of this type of processing. The fermenting bacteria make acids and alcohol, which minimize the growth of other microbes. The acid produced is especially helpful in preventing the growth of *Clostridium botulinum.*

Today, we can add **pasteurization,** sterilization, refrigeration, freezing, **irradiation,** canning, and chemical preservatives to the list of food preservation techniques. A new method for food preservation—**aseptic processing**—simultaneously sterilizes the food and package separately before the food enters the package. Liquid foods, such as fruit juices, are especially easy to process in this manner. With aseptic packaging, boxes of sterile milk and juices can remain untainted on supermarket shelves, free of microbial growth, for many years. This method often also allows the advantages of a lower price, lighter weight, and excellent flavor qualities.

Food poisoning—when undesirable microbes alter foods

In 1871, an Italian toxicologist named Selmi proposed that food poisoning was caused by ptomaines, protein by-products found only after significant bacterial spoilage of food. Although people speak of ptomaine poisoning today, this idea has been rejected for a long time because ptomaines are not really so poisonous. And, as noted earlier, a food that causes poisoning usually looks and tastes unspoiled.

Today, research shows that specific toxin-producing bacteria and other microbes cause food poisoning. *These organisms do so either directly, by invading the intestinal wall, as do Salmonella organisms, or indirectly, by producing a toxin, as does the Staphylococcus bacterium.* Many different types of bacteria cause food poisoning, such as *Bacillus, Campylobacter, Clostridium, Escherichia, Listeria, Vibrio, Yersinia, Salmonella,* and *Staphylococcus.*[19] Because each teaspoon of soil contains about two billion bacteria, we are constantly at risk for food poisoning. Luckily, only a small number of all bacteria actually pose a threat. Determining which microbe has caused a food-poisoning incident depends on identifying the clinical features of the poisoning, the incubation period for symptoms, and the food source (Table 19-1).

General rules for preventing food poisoning

Following a few important rules greatly minimizes the risk for food poisoning:

- **Thoroughly wash hands with hot, soapy water before handling food.** Always wash hands after handling raw meat, fish, poultry, or eggs.

- **Don't let groceries sit in a warm car: this allows bacteria to grow.** Get the food home to refrigerate or freeze promptly.
- **Don't buy or use food from flawed containers that leak, bulge, or are severely dented, nor buy or use food from jars that are cracked or have loose or bulging lids.** Do not taste or use food that has a foul odor or any food that spurts liquid when the can is opened.
- **Make sure counters, cutting boards, dishes, and other equipment are thoroughly cleaned and rinsed before being used.** Be especially careful to use hot, soapy water to wash countertops, cutting boards, utensils, and other pieces of equipment that have come in contact with raw meat, fish, poultry, and eggs as soon as possible.
- **Carefully wash fresh fruit and vegetables to remove dirt.**
- **If possible, cut foods to be eaten raw on a clean, plastic cutting board reserved for that purpose.** If the same board must be used for both meat and other foods, cut the raw items *before* cutting any potentially contaminated items.
- **Cook foods thoroughly, especially beef (160° F, 71° C), poultry (180° F, 82° C), fish and pork (170° F, 77° C), and eggs (until the yolk and white are hard).** A good general precaution is to eat no raw animal products. We will discuss the reason later. Once a food is cooked, cool it rapidly (to 40° F, 4° C within 4 hours) if it is not to be eaten immediately. Do this by separating the foods into as many pans as needed to provide a large surface area. Be careful not to recontaminate cooked food by contact with raw meat or juices via hands, cutting boards, dirty utensils, or in other ways. Then reheat leftovers to 165° F, 74° C; reheat gravy to a rolling boil.
- **Avoid time and temperature abuses.** Store food below 40° F (4°C) or above 140° F (60° C) (Figure 19-2). Food poisoning microbes thrive in more moderate temperatures (60° to 90° F, 16° to 32° C).[12] Keep hot foods hot and cold foods cold. Observe timelines for safe food storage (see Appendix S). This is important because some food-poisoning microbes can grow in the refrigerator. Do not leave cooked or refrigerated foods, such as meat and salads, at room temperature for more than 2 hours because that provides microbes an opportunity to grow. Store dry food at 60° F to 70° F (16° C to 21° C).
- **Avoid coughing or sneezing over foods, even when you are healthy.** Cover cuts on hands.
- **Make sure the refrigerator stays below 40° F (4° C).**
- **Cook stuffing separately from poultry (or wash poultry thoroughly, stuff immediately before cooking, and then transfer the stuffing to a clean bowl immediately after cooking).** Make sure the stuffing obtains a temperature of 165°F (74° C).
- **Consume only pasteurized milk.**

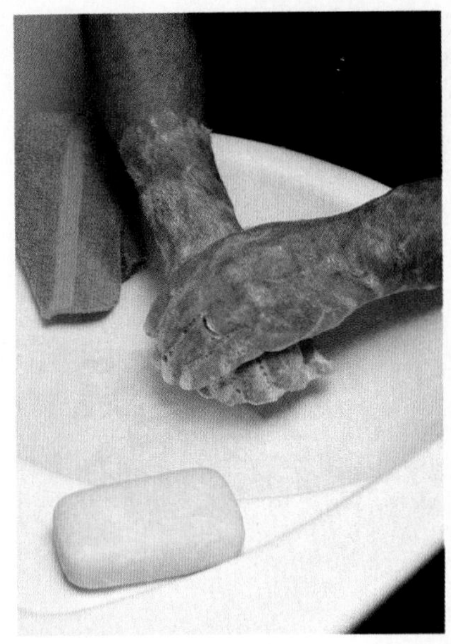

Washing hands should be a first step in preparing food.

Microbes that cause food poisoning commonly enter food through cross-contamination and grow because they are allowed to thrive in temperatures favorable to them. Many foods contain problem microbes. It is important to practice sanitary food-handling procedures when preparing any food.

Treatment for food poisoning

To offset the effects of diarrhea, drink a lot of fluids. To prevent further contamination, thoroughly wash hands and avoid food handling until the diarrhea disappears. Bedrest speeds recovery. A fever of 102° F (39° C) or greater, blood in the stool, and dehydration from frequent vomiting or diarrhea (a sign of dehydration is dizziness when standing) deserve a physician's evaluation, especially if symptoms persist for more than 2 or 3 days. In cases of suspected botulism poisoning, consult a physician immediately because use of an antitoxin may speed recovery (see page 584).

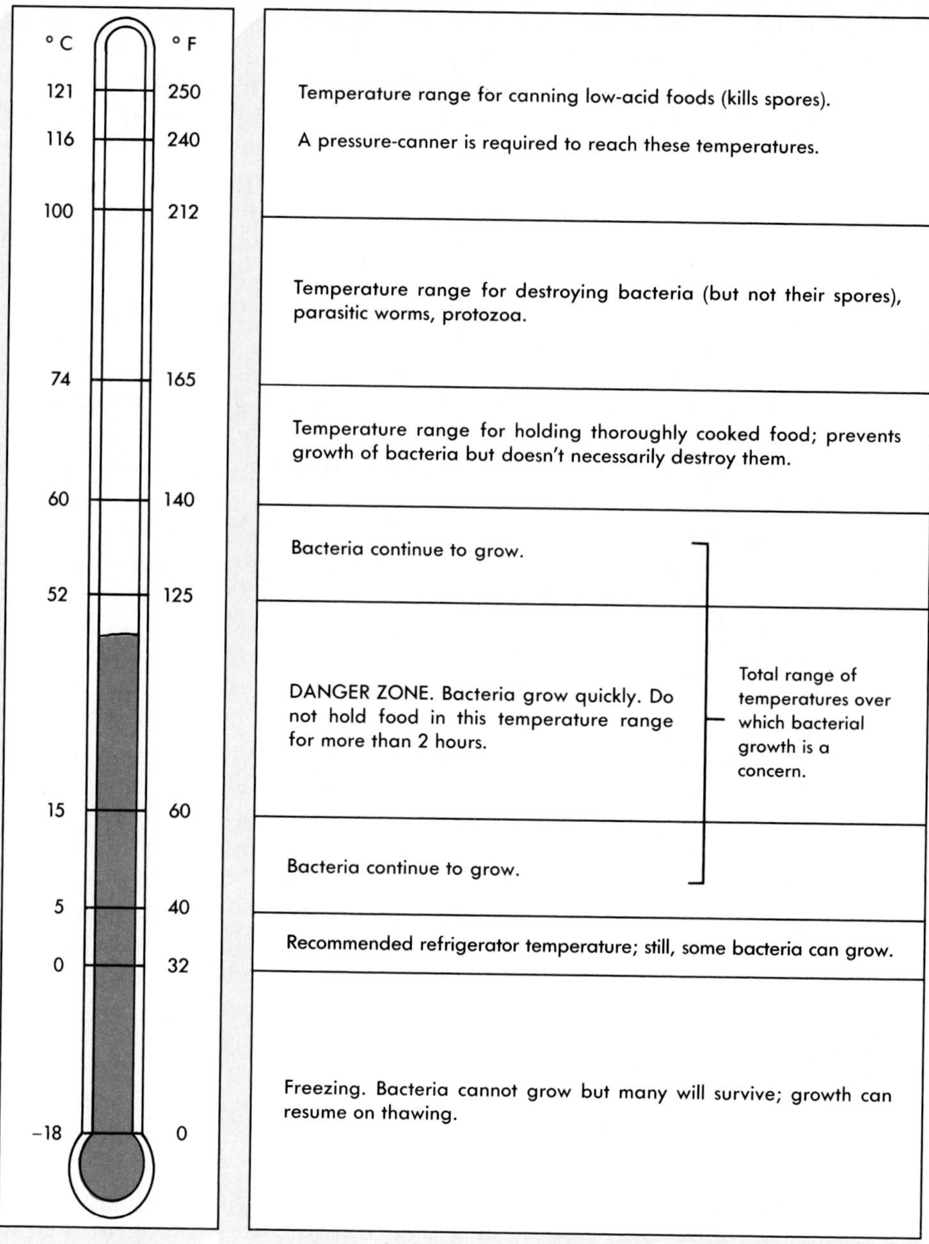

Figure 19-2

Effects of temperature on organisms that cause food-borne illness. (Adapted from Temperature guide to food safety: Food and Home Notes, No. 25, Washington, USDA, June 20, 1977.)

Concept Check

The presence of bacteria and the toxins they produce pose the greatest risk for food poisoning. In the past, the addition to foods of sugar, salt, and smoke, as well as drying, were used to prevent the growth of microorganisms. Today, we know that cleanliness, keeping hot foods hot and cold foods cold, and cooking foods thoroughly offer additional protection from food poisoning. Treat all raw animal products, any cooked food, and raw bean sprouts as potential food poisoners. Symptoms of an attack are similar to those of flu: diarrhea, vomiting, abdominal bloating, and headache. Treatment generally requires only bedrest and extra fluids.

A CLOSER LOOK AT MICROBES THAT CAUSE FOOD POISONING

We noted that finding a food-poisoning agent requires some detective skills. Determining the agent depends on knowing the food source, the incubation time for symptoms, the types of symptoms, and the duration of illness associated with an outbreak. Let's begin by looking at the characteristics of the major "problem" microbes individually. One general rule: when you exhaust the possibilities, the cause of the illness is probably a virus.

Staphylococcus aureus

The organism *S. aureus* causes 20% to 40% of food-poisoning cases each year. While growing in food, this microbe produces toxins that, once ingested, cause nausea, vomiting, diarrhea, headaches, and abdominal cramps. Symptoms usually develop within 2 to 6 hours of eating the contaminated food. The person rarely dies, but develops no immunity against future attacks. Bed rest and fluids are generally the only treatment, and recovery takes place usually within 2 to 3 days.

S. aureus bacteria live mainly in the nasal passages and in sores on the skin. *These microbes enter food when people sneeze and cough over food or handle food with open skin sores.* Once present in significant numbers in a food, they can make enough toxin to cause illness in about 4 hours if the temperature stays near 100° F (38° C). The toxin is undetectable by flavor, odor, and appearance and can even withstand prolonged cooking.

Common foods associated with S. aureus food poisoning are custard, ham, egg salad, cheese, seafood, cream-filled pastries, and milk. Whipped cream standing at room temperature for hours is a typical source. Keeping these and other foods above 140° F (60° C) or below 40° F (4°) prevents the bacterium's growth, preventing production of its toxin. It is especially important to never leave susceptible foods inside this temperature range for more than 2 hours. To further prevent this type of food poisoning, hand cleanliness and sanitation are important, as are directing coughs and sneezes away from food and covering skin cuts when in contact with food.

Salmonella food poisoning

A variety of *Salmonella* bacteria causes food poisoning. Ingesting live bacteria causes the symptoms. These bacteria are commonly found in animal and human feces and enter food via infected water, contaminated cutting boards, contaminated meat products, cracked eggs, and actual bits of feces in food. The FDA calculates that medical care and illness in the United States for Salmonella food poisoning costs more than $10 billion a year. In 1985, an incident of contaminated milk in Chicago may have caused 200,000 cases in six states.

Symptoms of Salmonella food poisoning are the same as those of Staphylococcus food poisoning, but they take 5 to 72 hours to develop. Again, bed rest and fluids are the only treatment, and recovery usually occurs within 2 to 3 days. Fatalities are rare. Salmonella food poisoning occurs most frequently from consuming eggs, chicken, meat, meat products, custard made with infected eggs, raw milk, and inadequately refrigerated and reheated leftovers. *About 40% of raw chickens are contaminated. Undercooked foods pose a special risk, but thorough cooking kills Salmonella bacteria.*

To be safe, eggs should be boiled 7 minutes, poached 5 minutes, or fried 3 minutes on each side until the yolk is not runny and the white is firm. No raw eggs should be used in salads or sauces. Hollandaise sauce, often warmed at low heat, is a significant threat. Recent research indicates that not only are cracked eggs at risk for *Salmonella* bacteria infections but also strains of the bacteria may exist inside an intact egg, especially if it has been left at room temperature for a few hours.[1]

Most outbreaks of Salmonella food poisoning can be traced to mistakes in

Recently, the FDA warned people to not consume homemade ice cream, eggnog, and mayonnaise because of the risk of Salmonella food poisoning. Follow professional journals and the *FDA Consumer* for further information. Commercial forms of these products are safe because they have been pasteurized. This process kills *Salmonella* bacteria. In addition, commercial mayonnaise has enough acid to prevent bacterial growth.

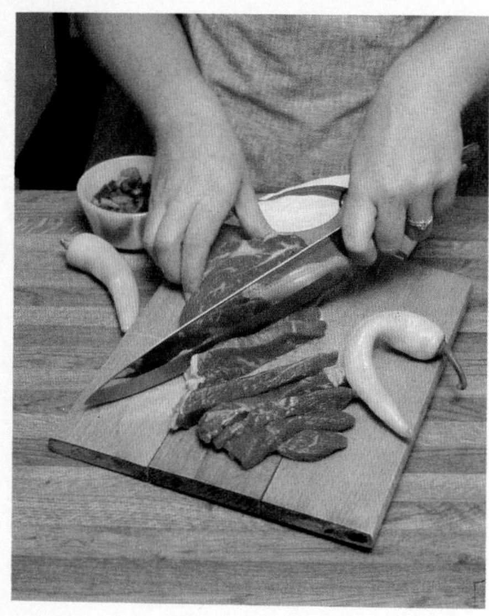

Wooden cutting boards are difficult to sanitize.

food handling in either food establishments or homes. *Salmonella* bacteria need about 8 hours to produce quantities sufficient to cause illness. Observing the temperature precautions for *Staphylococcus* organisms also prevents *Salmonella* bacteria growth.

Salmonella food poisoning poses a great risk for cross-contamination of foods. Keep hands and utensils clean when preparing foods; scrub the cutting board with a chlorinated cleanser after contact with raw meat or poultry, and store foods in temperatures either hot or cold enough to prevent bacterial growth. Wooden cutting boards pose a special risk because they are difficult to sanitize. Plastic cutting boards are recommended. Do not allow susceptible foods to stand for more than 2 hours at room temperature and marinate meats in the refrigerator. While acid in a marinade slows bacterial growth, it does not stop it. Finally, thaw foods in the refrigerator, in a microwave oven, or under a stream of cold water—not on the kitchen counter.

Clostridium perfringens

The bacterium *C. perfringens,* another major cause of food poisoning, is present throughout the environment, especially in soil, the intestines of animals and humans, and sewage. It is called the cafeteria germ because most food-borne outbreaks by this organism are associated with the foodservice industry or with events where large quantities of food are prepared and served. Symptoms of an infection resemble those of Salmonella food poisoning, but the victim usually doesn't vomit. Symptoms are seen within 8 to 24 hours after consuming enough live bacteria. Again, bed rest and fluids are the only treatment, and recovery occurs usually within a few days.

C. perfringens is an anaerobic bacterium that can form a spore quite resistant to heat. At temperatures between 70° F and 120° F (21° C to 49° C) these spores germinate and become bacteria, multiplying quickly to disease-causing levels. Foods stored in deep serving dishes are especially fertile media for bacterial growth because the centers are isolated from air and stay warm.

C. perfringens organisms are often found in cooked beef, turkey, gravy, dressing, stews, and casseroles. *The best insurance against promoting their growth is to maintain proper holding temperatures and to divide large "leftover" portions into smaller ones.* The latter treatment exposes more food to air, reducing the anaerobic conditions. Be especially careful to cook meats completely and cool them rapidly in small containers. Thoroughly reheat leftover meat to 165° F (74° C) before serving. Always bring leftover gravy to a rolling boil. Store cold cuts and sliced meats below 40° F (4° C) and serve them cold.

Clostridium botulinum

C. botulinum bacteria can cause fatal food poisoning. This anaerobic microbe is present in the soil, and is therefore probably present as a bacterium or spore in all foods. The bacteria release a deadly toxin as they grow in food. The death rate, which depends on the amount of toxin consumed, is about 60%.[2]

Symptoms of botulism appear within 12 to 36 hours of contaminated food consumption. The toxin blocks nerve function, causing vomiting, abdominal pain, double vision, dizziness, and acute respiratory failure. Diarrhea does not occur. If the person survives, recovery is within 10 days. Normally, bed rest is the only therapy. With quick diagnosis, treatment with an antiserum is possible. Still, ultimate recovery may be slow. Although botulism receives much public attention, few cases are reported each year in the United States.

Since *C. botulinum* grows only in the absence of air, it thrives primarily in canned food, especially improperly home-canned low-acid foods, such as string beans, corn, mushrooms, beets, and asparagus. *Recently, other foods with "anaerobic centers," such as potato salad, sauteed onions, stew, and chopped garlic have caused botulism.* Cured meats also pose a risk for botulism; however, the nitrates and vitamin C used to preserve the meats are potent inhibitors of its growth.

Canned foods are a major problem because, while the canning process kills all bacteria present and the heat used drives out all oxygen, if insufficient heat is used, spores of *C. botulinum* remain in the food. When the can or jar cools, the spores germinate into bacteria and the bacteria produce toxin.

Following canning directions explicitly is essential when food is canned at home. Boiling home-canned foods for 10 to 20 minutes before serving is an excellent idea because that destroys any toxin present. In the first few minutes of boiling, smell the food. Heat often brings out the tell-tale sign of botulism odors. If no odor is detected, lower the heat and continue boiling the food for 10 minutes for high-acid foods and 20 minutes for low-acid foods, such as meat and poultry products, peas, beans, and corn.

Commercially canned foods may also harbor botulism. Always check cans carefully. Look for rust on the seams, holes, and swollen sides or tops. Make sure the can sucks in air when opened and the liquid inside is clear, not milky, and does not smell bad. If there are any signs of spoilage, return the can to the store or to the nearest public health department. Whatever you do, DON'T TASTE THE FOOD. ONE STRING BEAN CAN CONTAIN ENOUGH TOXIN TO KILL YOU.

Recently, researchers have noted that botulism poisoning may develop in vivo (inside the body). Infants between 2 and 6 months of age are at special risk, as are people with poor stomach acid production. Bacteria spores germinate in the stomach and produce toxin. For this reason, honey should not be given to young infants because it can contain the spores of this bacteria.

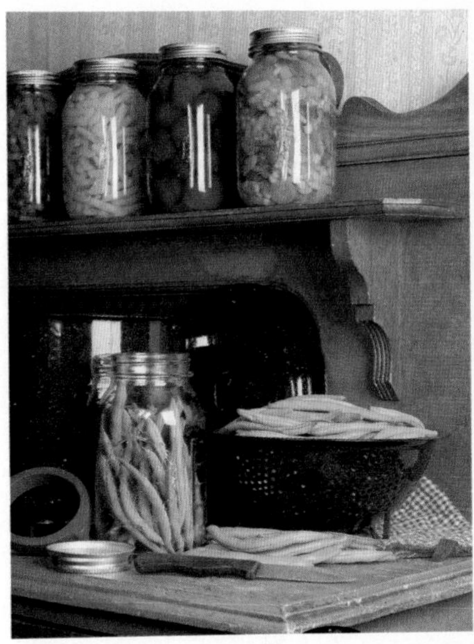

The USDA publishes several inexpensive booklets on canning and freezing. For a catalog and order form, write to the Superintendent of Documents, U.S. Government Printing Office, Washington, D.C. 20402.

Campylobacter jejuni

Few cases of food poisoning are currently linked to *Campylobacter* organisms, but this bacterium is thought to be a common food-poisoning microbe. It was established as a human pathogen as recently as 1971. Probably an enormous number of cases of food-borne illness caused by *Campylobacter* organisms are unreported because they are difficult to detect in foods.[19] A 1985 USDA study found that 30% of chickens contained *Campylobacter* organisms.

Nearly all outbreaks of Campylobacter illness result in acute intestinal pain, fever, headache, and diarrhea. *These cases are associated with raw or inadequately cooked animal foods, including raw milk.* Because this organism grows slowly, the onset of symptoms is delayed, occurring 3 to 5 days after intake of contaminated food, although it may take weeks. Most people recover in less than 1 week, and death is rare. Recently, the nerve disorder Guillain-Barre syndrome has been linked to food-poisoning incidents from *C. jejuni* organisms. In addition, one form of this microbe, *Campylobacter pylori,* may be an important cause of stomach ulcers.

Luckily, *Campylobacter* organisms are very sensitive to heat. This trait probably saves us from numerous attacks. Complete cooking of food and careful storage of leftovers at cold temperatures are important ways to prevent its growth.

Listeria monocytogenes

L. monocytogenes is a very tough microbe.[24] It resists heat, salt, nitrate, and acidity much better than many other microorganisms. It survives and even grows below refrigeration temperatures of 40° F (4° C).[17] The first documented report of food-borne illness caused by *Listeria* organisms in North America occurred in 1981 in Canada. It was linked to commercially prepared coleslaw. Later, incidents that involved 47 deaths were associated with soft "Mexican style" cheeses. Since pasteurization destroys *Listeria* organisms, reports of milk and cheese products contaminated by *Listeria* organisms suggest that contamination occurs following pasteurization, probably from addition of raw milk. Although the incidence of listeriosis in the United States is unknown, it appears to be relatively rare, with about 1600 cases occurring each year.

Listeria bacteria infections cause mild flu-like symptoms, such as fever, headache, and vomiting, about 7 to 30 days after exposure. However, newborn infants, pregnant women, and people with depressed immune function may suffer severe symptoms, including meningitis, spontaneous abortion, and serious blood infections. In high-risk people, 25% of infections may be fatal. *Because unpasteurized milk and soft cheeses can be a source of Listeria, it is especially important that pregnant women and other people at high risk avoid these products.*[19]

Recently, raw hot dogs and undercooked chicken have been suspected to be a major source of *Listeria* infections. Even vegetables can carry *Listeria* organisms, and once cut, support its growth. Wash fresh produce thoroughly to remove contaminants.

We advise not consuming unpasteurized milk and cooking meat, poultry, and seafood thoroughly to kill this organism. The USDA recommends cooking meat to an internal temperature of 160° F (71° C) at the thickest part, and poultry to 180° F (82° C). Avoid eating raw meats; even their juices can contaminate cooked foods. Although *Listeria* organisms can grow at low temperatures, it is still important to keep food refrigerated to slow its growth.

Yersinia enterocolitica

Y. enterocolitica was recognized as a human pathogen in 1939. Food-poisoning incidents have been noted since 1976. Foods implicated include chocolate milk, reconstituted dry milk, and tofu. Usually the microbe enters the food after pasteurization. Symptoms of an infection occur 24 to 36 hours after eating contaminated foods and include diarrhea, fever, headache, and severe abdominal pain that mimics appendicitis. There are cases where unnecessary appendictomies have been performed after *Yersinia* infections. An infection may also trigger arthritis, inflammation of heart tissue, and widespread blood infections.

Yersinia organisms grow at cold temperatures, so refrigerated storage does not control its growth in food. Therefore sterilization methods, such as sufficient cooking or pasteurization, must occur to destroy this microbe.[19] It is fortunate that the strains of *Yersinia* bacteria primarily associated with human illness do not commonly occur in foods at this time.

Other food-poisoning bacteria

Escherichia coli is commonly found in the intestinal tract of humans and animals. Certain strains are now recognized as food-poisoning microbes. Symptoms include severe abdominal cramps, bloody diarrhea, and kidney failure. Thoroughly cooking meat and avoiding recontamination of meat should protect against illness. The bacteria *Shigella* recently infected 407 people who ate at one restaurant, causing symptoms of diarrhea, vomiting, and headaches.

Infections from *Vibrio vulnificus,* a newly identified bacterium, have been linked to eating raw seafood.[9] It causes a serious infection that can be fatal. *Eating raw shellfish poses a high risk, as does eating any raw or lightly (partially) cooked seafood.* Symptoms include diarrhea, blood infections, and other serious health problems.

Viruses

The hepatitis A virus can be transmitted in food, although this route accounts for only a small percentage of the total number of hepatitis A infections. This foodborne agent most often thrives because of unsanitary food handling in restaurants. People have also contracted hepatitis from eating raw or undercooked shellfish—clams, oysters, muscles—harvested from contaminated waters. Symptoms include intestinal problems, weakness, fatigue, jaundice, and sometimes even development of serious liver disease requiring hospitalization. Because symptoms do not usually occur until about 1 month after eating contaminated food, the source is difficult to identify. The only effective cure for this illness is the body's own immune defenses.

Raw clams and oysters are especially risky to eat because they are filter feeders, a process that concentrates viruses and toxins present in the water as it is filtered for food. It is important to buy oysters and clams only from the most reliable sources. By law, shellfish to be sold must come from licensed beds, but often they do not. So be careful when you either purchase these foods or harvest them yourself. Check with the local health department if you question the safety of waters in an area.

Norwalk viral infections usually cause mild illness with nausea, vomiting, diarrhea, weakness, abdominal pain, loss of appetite, headache, and fever. Because the virus is found in water and foods, shellfish and salads are most often implicated. Norwalk viruses are probably responsible for about 30% to 40% of all cases of viral intestinal flu in adults. Recently, an outbreak from contaminated ice occurred in Pennsylvania and Delaware.

Human rotavirus is another important cause of diarrhea; it is a main cause in children. Symptoms appear in 1 to 7 days. Day-care centers are common sites for infections. Thorough, regular hand-washing is a necessary, important practice at these sites.

Parasites

Parasites that enter the body through the intestinal tract include some protozoans, flukes, nematodes, roundworms, and tapeworms. In North America, the parasite most apt to be in the food supply is *Trichinella spiralis.* This tiny organism may be present in raw and undercooked pork and pork products, such as sausage. Trichinosis is rare today, probably because people realize that pork must be cooked thoroughly to kill the nematode worm that causes it and modern sanitary feeding practices have reduced trichina in hogs. About a hundred cases of trichinosis per year are reported in the United States. However, other cases may be unreported. Besides pork, bear meat and other raw meats are potential sources. The worm is seldom found in commercial meat.

In its early stages, trichinosis is difficult to diagnose. The symptoms in mild cases develop over weeks to months and are usually thought to be flu. If enough **larvae** are present, muscle weakness, fever, and fluid retention in the face may eventually result. Greater numbers of larvae usually mean more severe symptoms. *Thoroughly cooking meat, especially pork, to 170° F (77° C) destroys the larvae.* Ideally, irradiation is the best method for destroying this worm in contaminated meats (see Nutrition Perspective 19-2, "Food Irradiation").

larvae
An early developmental stage in the life history of some microorganisms, such as parasites.

Anisakis is a roundworm parasite found in larval form in raw fish.[11] They invade the stomach or intestinal tract, causing mild or serious effects. The infection is difficult to diagnose and cannot be treated. A stomach infection is characterized by sudden onset of violent pain within 12 hours of eating raw fish. The larvae may penetrate the stomach lining. Serious stomach pain can continue until the larvae are surgically removed. The fresher the fish, the less likely this disease will occur because larvae move from the fish's stomach to the tissues only after the fish is dead. Thoroughly cooking fish or freezing it for at least 72 hours are reliable methods for eliminating the threat of *Anisakis* disease. Consumption of raw or slightly cooked fish increases the risk for infection, especially from Japanese-style sushi and sashimi.[27]

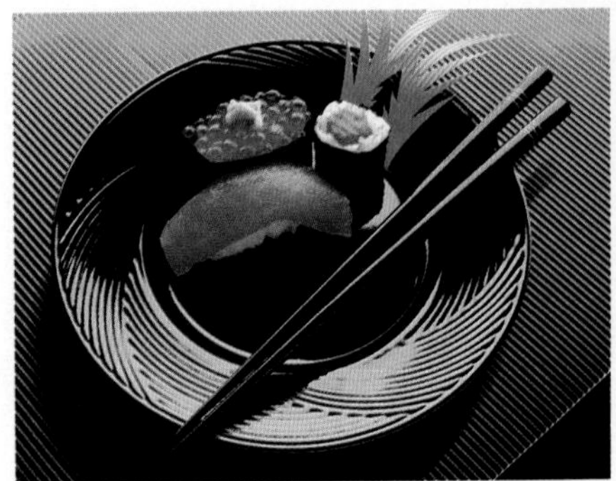

Sushi, like all raw fish dishes, is a high-risk food.

Other risks from fish and shellfish

Scombroidosis results from an acute allergic reaction to eating spoiled fish. Fish typically implicated are tuna, mackerel, and mahimahi. An affected person develops facial flushing, itching, intestinal upset, and headache within 10 to 60 minutes of consumption. The illness is caused by a toxin found in the muscle of the spoiled fish. Improperly refrigerated fish pose a special problem, and cooking does not destroy the toxin. So it is important to carefully refrigerate and use fresh fish soon after purchasing, especially those mentioned above.

Paralytic shellfish poisoning occurs when toxins produced by microscopic algae, called dinoflagellates, are consumed. These toxins are associated with a red tide, which is actually an explosive growth of the dinoflagellates in water. Symptoms, such as respiratory difficulty, appear within 4 hours. It is important that shellfish are harvested in clean waters, uncontaminated by sewage, industrial waste, and high levels of toxic dinoflagellates. An outbreak in Guatemala in 1985 killed 26 people.

Mycotoxins

mycotoxins
A group of toxic compounds produced by molds, such as aflatoxin B-1, found on moldy grains.

Mycotoxins are a group of compounds produced by molds growing on food. The best known are the aflatoxins. Aflatoxin B-1 causes cancer in animals and is thought to be a potent carcinogen in humans. The mold that produces it is *Aspergillus flavus.* The foods most often contaminated with aflatoxins are tree nuts, peanuts, corn, wheat, and oil seeds, such as cottonseed. The FDA considers aflatoxins unavoidable contaminants on foods and therefore has set practical limits for aflatoxins in foods and animal feeds.

Ergot is a toxin produced by a fungus that also grows on grains, especially rye. The toxin can cause hallucinations because ergot is a natural source of lysergic acid dimethylamine (LSD).

Cooking and freezing halts mold growth but does not eliminate mycotoxins already produced. Moldy food should not be eaten, or at least not without discarding the moldy portion. When in doubt, throw the food out. Mold growth is prevented by properly storing foods at cold temperatures and using them within a reasonable length of time.

Concept Check

To prevent food poisoning from *Staphylococcus* organisms, cover cuts on hands and avoid sneezing on foods. To avoid *Salmonella* food poisoning, separate raw meats, especially poultry products, from cooked foods. Thoroughly cook meat and poultry products to destroy any *Salmonella* bacteria present. To avoid poisoning from *Clostridum perfringens,* rapidly cool leftover foods and thoroughly reheat them. To avoid botulism from *Clostridium botulinum,* carefully examine canned foods and don't allow cooked foods to stand for more than 2 hours at room temperature. For other less frequent causes of food poisoning, carefully handle raw animal products so that their juices do not contaminate other foods; thoroughly cook all foods, especially fish and other seafood; and consume only pasteurized dairy products.

FOOD ADDITIVES

Food additives are used to maintain or increase a food's nutritional value, preserve freshness, enhance flavor or appearance, or aid in processing and/or preparation.

Do we need to use food additives?

Limiting food spoilage is the major impetus for using additives. Foods spoil in two ways. The first and potentially most serious is the spoilage already discussed, that caused by bacteria, molds, fungi, and yeast. This may lead to food poisoning and changes in food texture and flavor. Food additives, such as potassium sorbate, are used to maintain the safety and acceptability of foods by retarding microbial growth (Appendix R provides a comprehensive list of food additives and their purposes in foods).

Today, sugar, salt, corn syrup, and citric acid still constitute 98% of all additives by weight.

Table 19-2

Food additive categories		
Anticaking	Formulation aids: carriers, binders, fillers, plasticizers	Processing aids: clarifying, clouding, catalyst, floculants, filter aids, crystallization inhibitors
Antimicrobial	Fumigants	Propellants
Antioxidants	Humectants	Sequestrants
Color, and adjuncts	Leavening	Solvents and vehicles
Conditioners	Lubricants and release agents	Stabilizers and thickeners
Curing and pickling	Nonnutritive sweeteners	Surface active agents
Dough strengtheners	Nutritive sweeteners	Surface-finishing agents
Drying agents	Oxidizing and reducing	Synergists
Emulsifiers	pH control	Texturizers
Enzymes		
Firming agents		
Flavor enhancers		
Flavoring agents		
Flour treating		

See appendix R for examples of compounds that fall within these categories.

Hegarty V: Decisions in Nutrition, St. Louis, 1988, The CV Mosby Co.

The second and less serious means of food spoilage is through oxygen exposure, which causes undesirable changes in color and flavor. The rust color that appears when apple and peach slices are exposed to air is a good example of this reaction. Antioxidants, which are a group of preservatives, retard the action of oxygen on food surfaces. These preservatives are not necessarily novel chemicals—they include vitamin E, vitamin C, and a variety of sulfites.

Without the use of some food additives, it would be impossible to safely produce massive quantities of foods and distribute them nationwide or worldwide, as is now done. Despite consumer concerns about the safety of food additives, many have been extensively studied and proven safe when FDA guidelines for use are followed.

intentional food additives
Additives knowingly (directly) incorporated into food products by manufacturers.

Intentional versus incidental food additives

Food additives are classified as those that are either **intentionally** (directly) added to foods or **incidentally** (indirectly) enter foods. Both are regulated by the FDA. The latter group includes substances that may be reasonably expected to become components of food through surface contact with equipment or packaging materials. This includes substances that may be formed during processing; for example, various compounds formed when a food is irradiated. Currently over 2800 different substances are intentionally added to our foods. As many as 10,000 other substances incidentally enter our foods.

incidental food additives
Additives that gain access to food products indirectly from environmental contamination of food ingredients, or during the manufacturing process.

The GRAS list

In 1958, all food additives used in the United States and considered safe were put on a **generally recognized as safe (GRAS)** list. The U.S. Congress established the GRAS category because it felt manufacturers did not need to prove the safety of substances already generally regarded as safe by knowledgeable scientists. As is still the case, the FDA was assigned responsibility for proving that a substance did not belong on the GRAS list. Since 1958, some substances on the list have been reviewed. A few, such as cyclamates, failed the review process and were removed from the list. Largely because of expense, many chemicals on the GRAS list have not been rigorously tested. These chemicals have received a low priority for test-

generally recognized as safe (GRAS)
A group of food additives that in 1958 were considered safe, and therefore manufacturers were allowed to use them from then on when needed in food products. The FDA bears responsibility for proving they are not safe.

Table 19-3

What you can do
The FDA's sampling and testing show that pesticide residues in foods do not pose a health hazard. Nevertheless, if you want to reduce dietary exposure to pesticides, follow this advice from the Environmental Protection Agency: ▪ Thoroughly rinse and scrub (with a brush, if possible) fruits and vegetables. Peel them, if appropriate—though some nutrients will be peeled away. ▪ Remove outer leaves of leafy vegetables, such as lettuce and cabbage. ▪ Trim fat from meat and poultry and skin (which contains most of the fat) from poultry and fish, and discard fats and oils in broths and pan drippings. Residues of some pesticides in feed concentrate in the animals' fat. Trim skin and fatty deposits from fish. ▪ Throw back the big fish—the little ones have less time to take up and concentrate pesticides and other harmful residues.

Adapted from: Food and Drug Administration: Safety first: protecting America's food supply, p. 26, November 1988.

See the discussion on naturally occurring and environmental toxins in foods beginning on page 595.

ing mostly because they have long histories of use without evidence of harm and/ or because their chemical structures do not suggest they are harmful.

Are synthetic chemicals always bad?

Nothing about a natural product makes it inherently safer than a synthetic (man-made) product. Many synthetic products are simply chemicals that also occur in nature. In addition, although humans are responsible for some toxins in foods—synthetic pesticides and industrial chemicals, for example—nature's poisons are often even more potent and prevalent. Dr. Bruce Ames, a noted cancer researcher, suggests that we ingest at least 10,000 times more (by weight) natural toxins produced by plants than we do man-made pesticide residues. This comparison doesn't make man-made chemicals any less harmful, but it does lend perspective.

Some definitions here might help you:
toxicology — The scientific study of harmful substances.
safety — The relative certainty that a substance won't cause injury.
hazard — The chances that injury will result from use of a substance.
toxicity — The capacity of a substance to produce injury at some level of intake.

Consider the familiar food additive baking powder, which is used to make batter rise for cakes, pancakes, and other "quick breads." When manufacturers list potassium acid tartrate, sodium aluminum phosphate, or monocalcium phosphate on the labels of cake mixes, they are referring to baking powder by its chemical names. Baking soda could be listed by its proper name sodium bicarbonate, just as ordinary table salt could be called sodium chloride. *The question should not be whether a food additive, such as salt, is a chemical, but rather whether the chemical additive is safe to use.*

Vitamin E is often added to food additives to prevent rancidity of fats. This chemical is safe when used within certain limits. However, high doses have been associated with health problems (see Chapter 11). Thus even well-known chemicals we are comfortable using can be toxic in certain circumstances. We see again that an old adage often applies: "The dose determines the poison."

Testing food additives for safety

Food additives are tested for safety on at least two animal species, usually rats and mice. Scientists determine the highest dose of the additive that produces no deleterious health effects in the animals. This is called the **no observable effect level (NOEL).** The NOEL is then divided by a number between 100 and 1000 to establish a margin of safety for human use. The 100-fold safety factor is most often used. *Thus the highest level of an additive found in a food should be at least 100 times less than the highest level that produced no apparent deleterious health effects in animals.*

no observable effect level (NOEL) This corresponds to the highest dose of an additive that produces no deleterious health effect in animals.

One important exception appears in to this schema for testing food additives. If an additive is shown to cause cancer, no margin of safety is allowed. The food additive **cannot** be used because it would violate the **Delaney clause** in the 1958 Food Additive Amendments. This clause prohibits the intentional use of cancer-causing compounds in food introduced after that date. Evidence for cancer could come from either laboratory animal or human studies.

However, incidental food additives are difficult to control. The FDA cannot simply ban pesticide residues, various industrial chemicals, and mold toxins from foods, even though they cause cancer. These products are not purposely added to foods—they are present whether we like it or not. The FDA sets an acceptable level for these substances.[5] Basically, it establishes a safety margin of one million, which means that during the entire lifetimes of one million people, cancer cases can theoretically increase by no more than one case (see Chapter 5).

In the last few years, the FDA has argued that this one million safety factor could also be applied to **all** food additives that cause cancer. However, the U.S. Supreme Court recently ruled against the FDA and insisted the Delaney clause be followed.

Delaney clause
This clause to the 1958 Food Additives Amendment of the Pure Food and Drug Act in the United States prevents the intentional (direct) addition to foods of a compound introduced after that date, which has been also been shown to cause cancer in animals or man.

Note that the margin of safety for some vitamins and trace minerals is only 1:5 or 1:10. So food additives are subjected to much stricter limits than are essential nutrients, such as selenium and vitamin A.

Obtaining approval for a new food additive

Today, a new substance to be added to foods must undergo strict testing to establish its safety. Manufacturers present information to the FDA in the form of a petition that identifies the new additive, its chemical composition, how it is manufactured, and laboratory methods used to measure its presence in the food supply at levels of intended use. The petition must establish that the proposed laboratory method can actually detect the substance so that the FDA can later monitor whether food manufacturers are complying with regulations.

There also must be proof that the additive will accomplish the intended result in a food and that the level sought for use is no higher than is reasonably necessary to do the job intended. Finally, information must prove that the additive is safe for its intended use.

Additives cannot be used to hide defective food ingredients, deceive customers, or replace good manufacturing practices. A petitioner must establish that the ingredient is really necessary for producing a specific food product.

Common food additives

A list of food additive categories appears in Table 19-2. Let's look at some of the major categories to understand exactly why food additives are used and to learn more about the specific chemicals that are used as food additives.[20]

Acidic or alkaline agents. Acids, such as calcium lactate, have many uses in foods. They serve as flavor-enhancing agents, preservatives inhibiting microbial growth, antioxidants preventing discoloration or rancidity, and adjustors of pH. Acids impart a tart taste to soft drinks, sherbets, and cheese spreads. Acids also increase the safety of naturally low-acid vegetables, such as beets.

Alkaline products, such as sodium hydroxide, are used to alter the texture and flavor of foods, including chocolate. In processing, alkaline products are sometimes used to produce a milder flavor by neutralizing the acids produced during fermentation.

Anticaking agents. By absorbing moisture, compounds such as calcium silicate, ammonium citrate, magnesium stearate, and silicon dioxide keep table salt, baking powder, powdered sugar, and other powdered food products free-flowing. These chemicals prevent the caking, lumping, and clustering that would make powdered or crystalline products inconvenient to use.

Antioxidants. These preservatives help delay discoloration of foods, such as cut potatoes. They also help keep fats from turning rancid. Two widely used antioxidants are BHA (butylated hydroxyanisole) and BHT (butylated hydroxytoluene). Vitamin E and related compounds also serve as antioxidants.

Sulfites have been widely used as antioxidants in foods and drugs for centuries.[10,25] Sulfites are actually a group of sulfur-based chemicals—sulfur dioxide, sodium sulfide, sodium and potassium bisulfite, and sodium and potassium metabisulfite. Sulfites inhibit the action of the enzyme polyphenyl oxidase, thus preventing the browning reaction that this enzyme encourages.

Since August 8, 1986, the FDA has prohibited use of sulfites on raw fruits and vegetables—an action directed mainly at salad bars. Potatoes were not covered by that regulation. As of January 9, 1987, the FDA also requires manufacturers to declare the presence of sulfites on labels of packaged foods containing at least 10 parts per million of sulfites. Labels on wine bottles often list a sulfite warning, and drug companies are required to produce a warning statement on prescription drugs containing sulfites. *Some people are very sensitive to sulfites and suffer difficulty in breathing, wheezing, hives, diarrhea, vomiting, abdominal pain, cramps, and dizziness after exposure.*

The term *coal-tar* color often refers to food colors. Early food colors were derived from by-products of the manufacture of illuminating gas from coal. Today, the raw materials of colors are obtained from petroleum and other synthetic products. So it is more appropriate to refer to food colors today as synthetic or organic dyes rather than coal-tar derivatives.

Colors. This special class of additives is distinct by law from intentional or unintentional food additive classes. Color additives do not improve eating or nutritional qualities, but they do make foods appear more appetizing. No food coloring can be used if it promotes deception of the consumer. They cannot be used to cover a blemish, conceal inferiority, or mislead the consumer in any way.

Controversy has surrounded the use of some of the red food colors. Currently, the safety of using the color additive tartrazine (FD&C yellow No. 5) is disputed.[22] It is known to cause allergic symptoms, such as hives, itching, and nasal discharge in sensitive individuals. Sensitivity is especially common in people allergic to aspirin (see Chapter 16). The number of North Americans sensitive to tartrazine is small. Nevertheless, the FDA requires manufacturers to list yellow dye No. 5 on labels of any food products containing it.

Exploring Issues and Actions

You are asked by a consumer group to vote for banning color additives, since they have no real importance. What is your response?

Emulsifiers. These products suspend and distribute fat in water, and so improve the uniformity, smoothness, and body of foods such as bakery goods, ice cream, and candies. Emulsifiers also stabilize fat-and-water mixtures so that they do not separate. In mayonnaise, for example, egg yolks act as emulsifiers to prevent the oil from separating from the acids. Lecithin, derived from soybeans, acts as an emulsifier in chocolate and margarine. Monoglycerides and diglycerides, found also as by-products of lipid digestion, are used as emulsifiers in cake mixes.

Flavors and flavoring agents. Naturally occurring and artificial agents can impart more flavor to foods. These agents include extracts from spices and herbs and man-made agents. You are probably familiar with flavors of some spices and of liquid derivatives of onion, garlic, cloves, and peppermint. To meet the demand of industry, manufacturers have developed synthetic flavors that not only accurately resemble natural flavors, but also have the advantage of stability. Often artificial flavors, such as butter or banana flavors, are the components of the natural flavor.

Flavor enhancers. These substances—monosodium glutamate (MSG), for example—help bring out the natural flavors of foods. *Some people are sensitive to MSG and suffer flushing, chest pain, facial pressure, dizziness, sweating, rapid heart rate, nausea, vomiting, and high blood pressure after exposure.*[21] MSG is often used in Chinese food, and thus reactions to it have acquired the name "Chinese restaurant syndrome." The onset of symptoms occurs about 10 to 20 minutes after ingestion and may last from 2 to 3 hours. People who find themselves sensitive to MSG should avoid it.

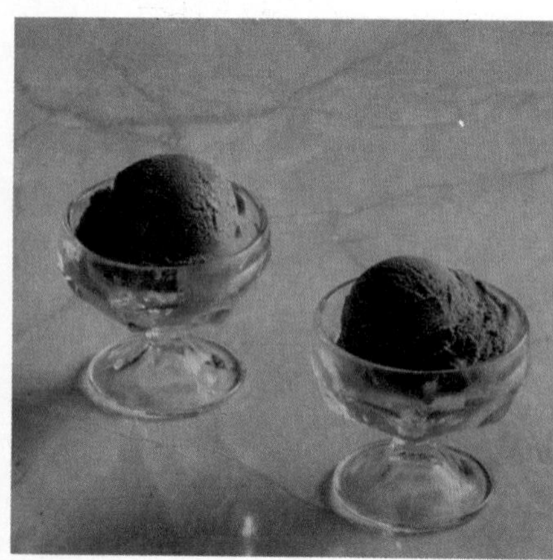

Ice cream often contains added emulsifiers.

Humectants. These chemicals, such as glycerol, propylene glycol, and sorbitol, are added to foods to help retain proper moisture, fresh flavor, and texture. They are often used in candies, shredded coconut, and marshmallows.

Leavening agents. Air and steam can be used to create a light texture in breads and cakes; however, carbon dioxide is much more reliable for this purpose. Common leavening agents that produce carbon dioxide include yeast, baking powder, and baking soda. Baking soda must be used in the presence of acid, and baking powder can be used in either acidic or alkaline conditions.

Maturing and bleaching agents. By hastening the aging process of flour, these compounds enable its early use in bread products. Freshly milled flour makes very poor bread because it lacks the qualities necessary to make a stable, elastic dough. When aged for several months, flour gradually whitens and matures to become useful for baking. Compounds, such as bromates, peroxides, and ammonium chloride, enhance the natural aging and whitening processes.

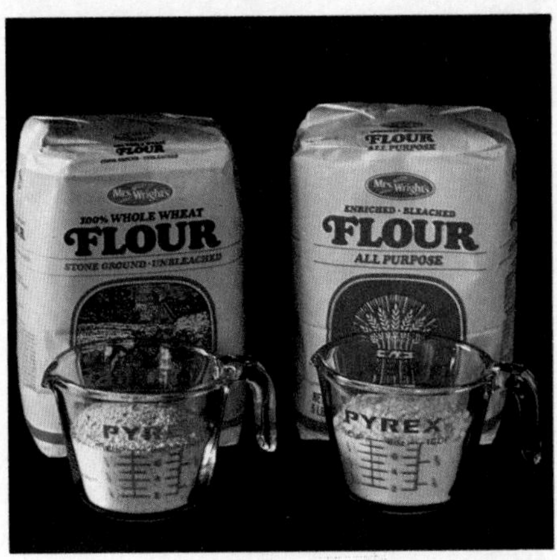

Flour is available with or without bleaching agents such as bromates or peroxides.

Nutrient supplements. Vitamin and mineral supplements are added to foods to improve their nutritional quality, and sometimes to replace nutrients lost in processing, as in the case of enriched flour. Vitamin A is added to margarine and to some forms of milk; vitamin D is added to some dairy products. Potassium iodide is added to salt.

Preservatives. There are many types of **preservatives.** Some function as antioxidants, inhibitors of microbial growth, or **sequestrants** (see later category). Sodium benzoate, sorbic acid, and calcium proprionate are common preservatives. Sorbic acid is a potent inhibitor of molds and fungal growth. Calcium proprionate is a natural part of some cheeses.

preservatives
Compounds that extend the shelf life of foods by inhibiting microbial growth or minimizing the destructive effect of oxygen and metals.

sequestrants
Compounds that bind free metal ions. By so doing, they reduce the ability of ions to cause rancidity in compounds containing fat.

Nitrates—and the related form, nitrites—are used as preservatives, especially to prevent growth of *C. botulinum.* Sodium and potassium nitrates and nitrites are used to preserve meats such as bacon, ham, salami, and hot dogs. Nitrates and nitrites have been used for centuries—in conjunction with salt—to preserve meat. An added effect of nitrates is their reaction with myoglobin pigments in meat to form a bright pink color. This gives the characteristic appearance to ham, hot dogs, and other cured meats.

Nitrate consumption from both cured foods and natural vegetables has been associated with the synthesis of nitrosamines in the stomach. These are potent cancer-causing agents, particularly in the stomach and esophagus. However, actual risk appears to be low, except for people with low stomach acid output (some elderly people, for example). The FDA also feels that consumers "take for granted" a margin of microbial safety from nitrite use in cured meats. People often serve them cold or at least underheated. Consequently government agencies have chosen not to ban nitrate or nitrite use in foods, but rather to change manufacturing practices to lower amounts of preformed nitrosamines.

If nitrates and nitrites form chemical substances that can cause cancer, why aren't they banned? In the United States, the USDA regulates the use of these chemicals in meats, and the governing laws are not part of the 1938 Federal Food, Drug, and Cosmetic Act. Therefore the Delaney clause, an amendment to the 1938 law, does not apply. Currently, the USDA sees no clear threat to public safety from the regulated use of nitrates or nitrites in meats, and so no action appears warranted.

The addition of vitamin C to cured meats, such as bacon, is one way to reduce the amount of nitrosamines formed in foods. This is a common practice today. Other antioxidants, such as vitamin E, also reduce synthesis of nitrosamines.

About 35% of the nitrite in the U.S. food supply is added in manufacturing, as is about 13% of nitrates. The rest is found naturally in foods, mostly in vegetables and baked goods.

Nonnutritive sweeteners. Currently, saccharin and acesulfame (Sunette) are the only nonnutritive sweeteners used in foods. Recall that aspartame (Nutrasweet) yields energy (see Chapter 4). Saccharin has been found to be a carcinogen only in rats and only if administered over two generations. The cancers are found primarily in the bladder of these animals. Recall that the U.S. Congress has prevented the FDA from banning saccharin, but a warning label must accompany any use.

Epidemiological studies of humans have not found an increased risk of developing bladder cancer from exposure to saccharin. It is estimated that in the United States, approximately 80 million to 100 million people consume saccharin in foods. In comparison, approximately 25,000 to 30,000 people develop bladder cancer each year in the United States. The question for society is whether the risk of developing cancer from saccharin consumption is worth the benefit of using this sweetener.

The Delaney clause has not been applied to saccharin because the U.S. Congress exempted it from the rule (see Chapter 4).

Stabilizers and thickeners. These give a smooth texture and uniform color

How Safe Is the American Food Supply?

JOHN N. HATHCOCK, PH.D.

Today, those who take too seriously every scary headline about pesticides, food additives, and bacterial contamination are apt to feel that practically anything they eat may lead to dire consequences. On one hand, we are told to eat more fruits, vegetables, fish, and poultry, and on the other, we are warned that these foods may contain dangerous substances. Within a recent short period, we were alarmed by reports that poisons in apples, grapes, fish, poultry, and eggs could make us ill, even violently so. Often one set of claims contradicted another, leading to widespread confusion. How can we distinguish between extremist claims and the truth?

THE CONCEPT OF SAFETY

What is a safe food supply? To a nutritionist, it is a food supply available in quantity and at prices allowing easy selection of a variety of diets that provide good nutrition without excessive intakes of specific food components, such as fats. To a toxicologist, it is a food supply that allows easy selection of a variety of diets that doesn't generate significant hazard because of toxic components.

Absolute safety is the total absence of hazard. Because of the logic and statistical nature of the evidence, proof of absolute safety would require proof of a negative—that something cannot occur. The science of toxicology never allows such a proof. It does provide evidence that supports the conclusion that almost all foods in the American food supply provide usually adequate safety. "Usually" and "adequately" may seem like hedge words, but really they are not; they simply recognize that proof of absolute safety is not possible and that, occasionally, some particular foods may not be adequately safe. Why don't we strive for "always" in safety? There are three reasons: (1) it's not possible; (2) there are trade offs that make it unwise, that is, actions taken to decrease one type of risk may generate another; and (3) maximum reduction in many types of risk would be prohibitively expensive.

TRADE OFFS IN FOOD SAFETY

Cooking improves food safety. Safety is improved because microbes are killed, reducing food spoilage and food-borne infections. On the other hand, cooking may produce mutagenic and carcinogenic chemicals in very small quantities, usually through heat destruction of fat or protein. Although these chemicals are produced in only trace quantities, some of them may cause more risk of cancer than the worrisome pesticides and food additives.

The safety of food additives, such as sodium nitrite, has been widely questioned in the popular press and by some scientists. Nitrite has antibacterial properties that help protect against the growth of the bacteria that cause botulism, a disease that quickly causes death. Nitrite also contributes color and flavor to some foods. No responsible scientist will tell you that the use of nitrite is perfectly safe. It can react with naturally present amines and other essential substances to produce nitrosamines. Many nitrosamines have some potential to cause cancer in experimental animals. With only this in mind, it may seem logical to avoid all nitrite-containing foods, but that is not the case. The first reason relates to the protective action of nitrite against botulism. The second is that such avoidance would have little effect on exposure to nitrite. Most nitrite in the human body does not come from food additives. Instead, nitrates normally present in vegetables are converted by bacteria in the mouth and intestine to nitrite. This vegetable source provides most of the nitrite to which most people are exposed (approximately 75%, depending on the particular dietary pattern).

Many foods, especially those containing polyunsaturated oils, have synthetic antioxidants (such as BHA, BHT, and propyl gallate) added to prevent rancidity. Some products formed when fats undergo oxidative rancidity have toxic effects, possibly including risk of cancer and accelerated aging. The safety of these synthetic antioxidant food additives has been questioned in relation to reports that BHT can have cancer-enhancing effects under some experimental conditions. These reports indicate that bladder cancer increases but liver cancer decreases in experimental animals also treated with certain chemical carcinogens. Under other experimental conditions, treatment with synthetic antioxidants decreases the effects of chemical carcinogens. Overall, the evidence indicates that the antioxidants are more likely to decrease risk of cancer in humans than to increase it. Nevertheless, if synthetic antioxidants have any adverse effects, why not replace them with a natural antioxidant, such as vitamin E? The answer relates to comparative effectiveness and to avoidance of excessive intakes of any one substance—including vitamin E.

The replacement of all other antioxidants by vitamin E is not desirable for several reasons. Such replacement would dramatically increase intakes of vitamin E, and if intakes become high enough, questions of the safety of high intakes of vitamin E would arise. Furthermore, vitamin E as a food antioxidant is more expensive than synthetic antioxidants.

CONCLUSIONS

The familiar advice to eat a variety of foods to ensure nutritional adequacy also makes sense for avoiding excessive intakes of any particular substance. Certainly, eating a variety of foods increases the probability that a variety of contaminating chemicals will be consumed in small quantities. The common fear that such multiple exposure will dramatically enhance toxicity of those substances is not well founded. Actually, just the opposite is likely. Often one substance will enhance our ability to metabolize and detoxify others, thereby decreasing risk of toxicity rather than increasing it.

Overall, the American food supply is outstandingly safe. Occasional exceptions, such as contamination with microbes or their toxins can make certain foods unsafe. Absolute safety of food is impossible, but the greatest dietary risks are associated with too much food, too much fat, and too much sodium rather than with chemical contaminants.

Dr. Hathcock is a senior scientist with the FDA. No official support or endorsement by the Food and Drug Administration is intended or should be inferred.

and flavor to candies, ice creams, and other frozen deserts, chocolate milk, and artificially sweetened beverages. Commonly used substances are pectins, vegetable gums (such as guar gum and carrageenan), gelatins, and agars. These compounds work by absorbing water. Without stabilizers and thickeners, ice crystals form in ice cream and other frozen desserts, and particles of chocolate separate from chocolate milk. These stabilizers are also used to prevent evaporation and deterioration of the volatile flavor oils used in cakes, puddings, and gelatin mixes.

Sequestrants. These compounds include EDTA and citric acid. They bind free ions, and by doing so, they reduce the ability of ions to cause rancidity in products containing fat.

Exploring Issues and Actions

If this list of compounds seems bewildering, you can easily avoid most of them. By emphasizing unprocessed whole foods, you can essentially eliminate most them from your diet. However, no evidence shows that this will necessarily make you healthier. It amounts to a personal decision. Do you have enough faith in the FDA and food manufacturers to protect your health and welfare, or would you like to minimize your intake of compounds not naturally found in foods? Choose the path that seems best to you. If you will be preparing your own dinner tonight, make a point of reading each label to discover more about what you *are* eating.

Concept Check

Food additives are used to reduce spoilage from microbial growth, oxygen, metals, and other compounds. Additives are also used to adjust pH, improve flavor and color, leaven, provide nutritional fortification, thicken, and emulsify food components. Additives are classified as intentional (direct), which are those purposefully added to foods, and incidental (indirect), which are those that end up in foods due to environmental contamination or manufacturing practices. The addition of an additive to a food is limited to 1/100 of the highest amount that has no observable effect when fed to animals. The Delaney clause further limits intentional addition of any cancer-causing compounds introduced after 1958 to food in the United States. Carcinogens that incidentally enter foods have maximum levels set for their presence in foods.

NATURALLY OCCURRING AND ENVIRONMENTAL TOXINS IN FOODS

Foods contain a variety of naturally occurring toxic substances.[14] Following are some of the more important examples:

- **Safrole**—found in sassafras, mace, and nutmeg; causes cancer.
- **Solanine**—found in potato shoots and green spots on potato skins; inhibits the action of neurotransmitters.
- **Aflatoxin**—found on moldy grains (especially corn and wheat); causes cancer.
- **Avidin**—found in raw egg whites; binds biotin, preventing its absorption.
- **Goitrogens**—found in brussels sprouts, broccoli, kale, and soybeans; inhibit thyroid hormone metabolism.
- **Thiaminase**—found in raw clams and mussels; destroys the vitamin thiamin.
- **Glycyrrhizic acid**—found in pure licorice extracts; causes hypertension.
- **Tetrodotoxin**—found in puffer fish; causes respiratory paralysis.
- **Protease inhibitor**—found in raw soybeans; inhibits digestive enzymes.
- **Saponins**—found in alfalfa sprouts; destroys red blood cell membranes.
- **Tannins**—found in tea; binds calcium and iron.
- **Oxalic acid**—found in spinach; binds calcium.
- **Herbal teas**—containing senna or comfrey; can cause diarrhea and liver damage.
- **Nitrates**—found in spinach, lettuce, and beets; can be converted into the carcinogen nitrosamine.
- **Browning products**—found in toasted grains; can cause DNA mutations.

People have coexisted for centuries with these naturally occurring toxins and have learned to avoid some of them. Farmers know potatoes must be stored in the dark so that solanine won't be synthesized. Operators of grain elevators check grain deliveries for the presence of aflatoxins. (Aflatoxins fluoresce under ultraviolet light.) And we have naturally limited our consumption of other toxins or developed cooking and food preparation methods to limit their potency. *Nevertheless, it is important to understand that some potentially harmful chemicals in foods occur naturally.*

Environmental contaminants in food

A variety of environmental contaminants may be found in foods. We mention some of them here:[4]

Lead. This metal can cause anemia, kidney disease, and damage to the nervous system. Lead toxicity is especially a problem for children and is related to poor learning ability. It is important to not store food in a can with a lead solder joint after the can has been opened. Contact with air speeds degradation of the solder joint and the release of lead into the food product. This is especially important for acidic food products, such as tomatoes. Many cans today are lead free if used for acidic products, like soft drinks. In addition, never store acidic products, such as fruit juice, sauerkraut, or pickled vegetables, in galvanized or other metal containers, except stainless steel. Acid can dissolve the metal, and lead will then leach into the food product. Lead can also leak out of solder joints in copper pipes, so let tap water run a minute or more before drinking it or cooking with it, especially first thing in the morning.

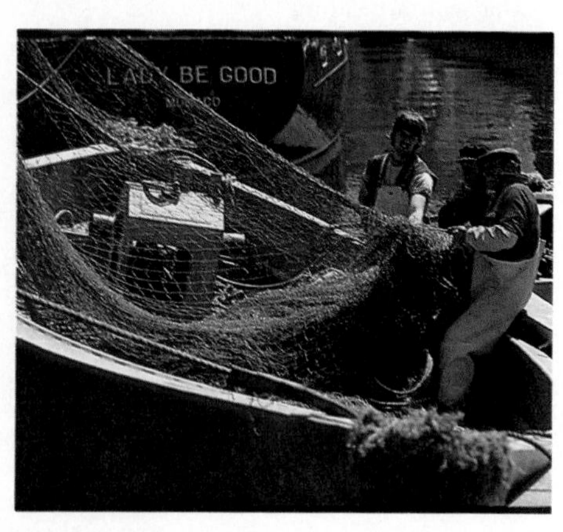

Eating a variety of fish is a key to avoiding high doses of environmental toxins from fish.

Lead can enter the food supply via pottery glazes. Lead is no longer used in glazes on commercially produced dishes in the United States because of this hazard. However, there is no way to ensure the safety of homemade or imported pottery items. It is important not to use antiques or collectibles for food or beverage storage because of the potential presence of lead.

Dioxin. This is an abbreviated name for a complex chemical defoliant. Dioxin is believed to cause cancer and other harmful effects in animals, even in small doses. For North Americans, major food sources of dioxin are bottom fish from the Great Lakes—an area with a great deal of industrial activity and chemical production. *Dioxin is primarily a problem for people who frequently consume fish caught locally.* People who eat commercial fish normally eat a variety, and even people who stick to one type of fish do not usually have a problem because fish in interstate commerce generally come from different waters, only a few of which may contain dioxin.

Mercury. The FDA first limited mercury in foods in 1969 after 120 people in Japan became ill from eating fish contaminated with high amounts. Birth defects in offspring of some of those people were also blamed on the mercury poisoning. The fish most often contaminated was swordfish. Currently, swordfish shipments are automatically detained until they are shown to meet mercury standards.

Urethane in alcoholic beverages. This chemical forms during fermentation of alcoholic beverages. If the fermented product is heated, as in the production of sherry and bourbon, urethane levels increase even more. Although urethane causes cancer in animals, it is unclear whether it causes cancer in humans. FDA research on urethane in food products is now a high priority.

Polychlorinated biphenyls (PCBs). These chemicals were widely used for years in a variety of industrial products, but because they are linked to liver tumors and reproductive problems in animals, they are no longer produced. The FDA has banned their use in machinery associated with food and animal feed and has established limits for PCBs in susceptible foods and in paper used for food-packaging material.

The most significant food source of PCB residues is fish, primarily freshwater fish such as Coho and Chinook salmon from the Great Lakes and bottom-feeding fresh water species from waters in other industrial areas. A key point in fish consumption is variety and moderation when local sources have the potential for contamination.

Protecting yourself from environmental hazards

To avoid toxins that naturally occur in food, find out which foods pose a risk. We have reviewed some of them. In addition, *emphasize variety and moderation in your food selection.* The presence of mercury in swordfish may concern you, but it is a health risk only if your diet is dominated by swordfish. The small amount of mercury in most swordfish is not harmful if you are exposed to it infrequently. Table 19-3 on page 590 provides some other practical tips for limiting the amount of pesticides in your diet.

Concept Check

You can avoid many food additives by consuming unprocessed foods. This is a personal choice. No evidence suggests avoidance is necessary. A general program to minimize exposure to environmental contaminants includes thoroughly rinsing and scrubbing fruits and vegetables, removing outer leaves of leafy vegetables, and trimming fat from meat and poultry, including the skin, and discarding any fat that is rendered from meat or fish during cooking.

Summary

1. Bacteria and other microbes in foods pose the greatest risk for food poisoning. In the past, salt, sugar, smoke, fermentation, and drying were used mostly to protect against food poisoning. Today, careful cooking, pasteurization, and keeping hot foods hot and cold foods cold provide additional insurance.
2. Cross-contamination commonly causes food poisoning. It occurs when bacteria on raw animal products contact foods that can support bacterial growth. Because of the risk of cross-contamination, no food should be kept at room temperature for more than 2 hours if there is a possibility that it has come in contact with raw animal products and can support bacterial growth.
3. Treatment for food poisoning usually requires drinking a lot of fluids, avoiding food-handling while diarrhea is present, thorough hand washing, and bedrest.
4. The three major causes of food poisoning today are the bacteria *Salmonella, Staphylococcus,* and *Clostridium perfringens.* To protect against these agents of food poisoning, cover cuts on the hands, do not sneeze on foods, avoid contact between raw meat or poultry products and other food products, and rapidly cool and then thoroughly reheat leftovers. Thorough cooking of foods and the use of pasteurized dairy products further protects against other bacteria and viruses that scientists are only now beginning to understand.
5. Food additives are used primarily to extend shelf life by preventing microbial growth and destruction of food components by oxygen, metals, and other substances. Food additives are classed as those intentionally added to foods and those that incidentally end up in foods. An additive to a food is limited to $1/100$ to $1/1000$of the greatest amount that causes no observable symptoms in animals. In most cases, the Delaney clause bans use of any intentional food additive in the United States if it causes cancer.
6. Antioxidants, such as vitamin E and sulfites, prevent oxygen and enzyme destruction of food products. Emulsifiers suspend fat in water, improving the uniformity, smoothness, and body of foods, such as ice cream. Common preservatives include sodium benzoate and sorbic acid, which prevent bacterial growth. Sequestrants bind metals, and so prevent spoilage of food from metal contamination.
7. Toxic substances occur naturally in a variety of foods, such as green potatoes, moldy grains, raw fish, raw soy beans, and raw egg whites. Cooking foods limits their toxic effects. Over the centuries, people have purposely avoided some of these foods, such as moldy grains and the green parts of potatoes.

8. A variety of environmental contaminants can be found in food. Because most of them are fat soluble, trimming fat from meats and discarding fat that is rendered during cooking of meats, fish, and poultry are good steps to minimize exposure. In addition, washing fruits and vegetables thoroughly and discarding the outer leaves of leafy vegetables are also helpful.

Take Action

1. Evaluate the food labels of 3 commercial products. Start with the ice cream product listed here. Identify all food additives and their functions and comment on the "necessity" of each additive (such as for consumer appeal, to maintain safety). Use Appendix R for help.

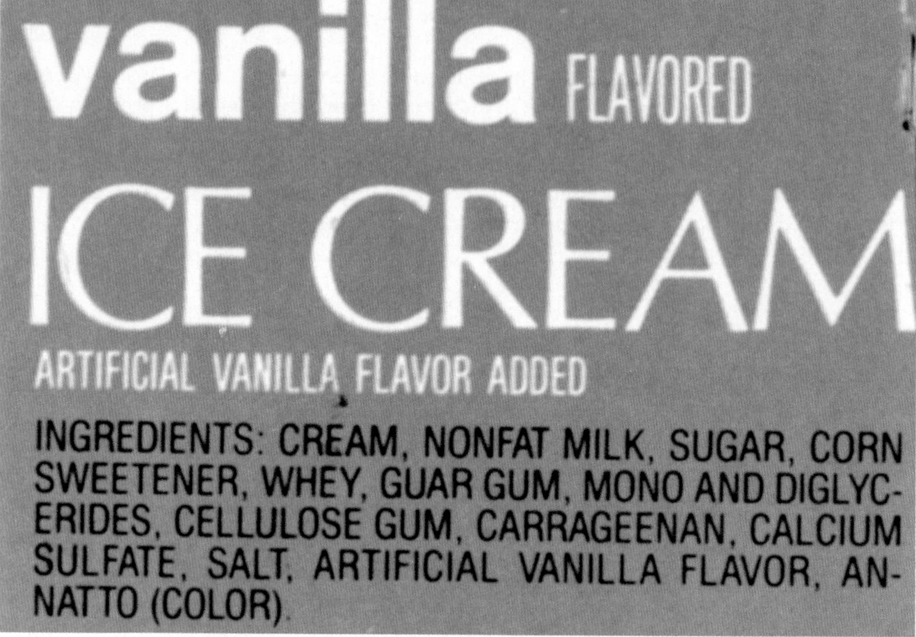

Food additive	Function	Could the product be produced without it?

REFERENCES

1. Anonymous: Eggs-ercise care, FDA Consumer, p3, December 1988.
2. Chia JK and others: Botulism in an adult associated with food-borne intestinal infection with *Clostridium botulinum,* New England Journal of Medicine 315:239, 1986.
3. Cohen SM: Saccharin: past, present, and future, Journal of The American Dietetic Association 86:929, 1986.
4. Farley D: Chemicals we'd rather dine without, FDA Consumer, p 10, September 1988.
5. Farley D: Setting safe limits on pesticide residues, FDA Consumer, p 8, October 1988.
6. Fennema OR: Food additives—an unending controversy, American Journal of Clinical Nutrition 46:201, 1987.
7. Flieger K: The Delaney dilemma, FDA Consumer, p 19, September 1988.
8. Gas LL: A response to today's food safety concerns, Nutrition News 48:9, 1985.
9. Klontz KC and others: Syndromes of *Vibrio vulnificus* infections, Annals of Internal Medicine 109:318, 1988.
10. Leikos CW: An order of fries—hold the sulfites, FDA Consumer, p 10, March 1988.
11. McKerrow JH and Sakanari J: Anisakiasis: revenge of the sushi parasite, New England Journal of Medicine 319:1228, 1988.
12. Miller RW: Mother nature's regulations on food safety, FDA Consumer, p 32, April 1988.
13. Mitchell JE and Skelton MM: Diarrheal infections, American Family Physician 37:195, 1988.
14. Newberne PM: Naturally occurring foodborne toxicants. In Schills ME and Young VR, eds: *Modern Nutrition in Health and Disease,* Philadelphia, 1988, Lea & Febiger.
15. Nightingale SL: Foodborne disease: an increasing problem, American Family Physician 35:353, 1987.
16. Noah ND: Food poisoning, British Medical Journal 291:879, 1985.
17. Palumbo SA: Is refrigeration enough to restrain foodborne pathogens? Journal of Food Protection 49:1003, 1986.
18. Rogan A and Glaros G: Food irradiation: the process and implications for dietitians, Journal of The American Dietetic Association 88:833, 1988.
19. Ryser ET and Marth EH: New food-borne pathogens of public health significance, Journal of the American Dietetic Association 89:949, 1989.
20. Schweigert BS: Food irradiation: What is it? Where is it now? Where is it Going? Nutrition Today, p 13, November/December 1987.
21. Senti FR: Food additives and contaminants. In Schills ME and Young VR eds: *Modern Nutrition in Health and Disease,* Philadelphia, 1988, Lea & Febiger.
22. Settipane GA: The restaurant syndromes, Archives of Internal Medicine 146:1258, 1986.
23. Segal M: Invisible villians—tiny microbes, our biggest food hazard, FDA Consumer, p 9, July/August 1988.
24. Skinner KJ: *Listeria* —battling back against one tough bug, FDA Consumer, p 13, July/August 1988.
25. Taylor SL and Bush RK: Sulfites as food ingredients, Contemporary Nutrition 11:20, 1986.
26. Weiss R: The gamma-ray gourmet, Science News 132:398, 1987.
27. Wittner MW and others: Eustrongylidiasis—a parasitic infection acquired by eating sushi, New England Journal of Medicine 320:1124, 1989.

SUGGESTED READINGS

An excellent source of information about food poisoning and food additive safety is the *FDA Consumer.* See the articles by Farley, Segal, and Skinner published there in 1988 to learn more about microbial food poisoning. The articles by Klontz and others and Ryser and Marth discuss "new" food-poisoning bacteria, including *Vibrio vulnificus.* For a review of parasites in seafood, see the article by McKerrow and Sakanari. To review the potential for food irradiation as a method of food preservation, see the article by Schweigert and the article by Rogan and Glaros. These articles plus the material in this chapter will enable you to evaluate the safety of your daily food intake.

CHAPTER 19

Answers to nutrition awareness inventory

1. *True.* We do not realize food poisoning is so common because the symptoms mimic other disorders, such as flu.
2. *False.* Foods having the potential to cause food poisoning often show no signs of it in taste, smell, or appearance.
3. *False.* Imported foods, such as soft cheeses from Mexico, have been implicated in food-poisoning incidents. While foods are inspected when they enter from foreign countries, there is not enough manpower to inspect all foods carefully.
4. *False.* Chemical structure—not origin—is the key to evaluating chemicals: whether a chemical is made in a laboratory or found in nature is irrelevant to its harmfulness to humans. Some naturally occurring toxins in foods, such as solanine in green potatoes, are much more toxic than synthetic food additives.
5. *True.* When the pulp of an apple is exposed to oxygen, a "browning" reaction occurs. Antioxidants, such as vitamin C, can prevent this browning.
6. *True.* The growth of bacteria and fungi in foods requires sufficient free water, that is, water not bound by other food compounds. If the water content of a food is reduced considerably, the lack of free water curtails growth of bacteria and fungi.
7. *False.* Only a few of the many bacteria, fungi, viruses, and other earthly microbes are known to cause food poisoning.
8. *True.* And for this reason, foods generally should be kept cold (below 40° F or 4° C) or hot (above 140° F or 60° C).
9. *True.* The symptoms of food poisoning are abdominal bloating, gas, diarrhea, vomiting, and headache, all of which are also symptoms of flu.
10. *False.* One food-poisoning incident provides no immunity against future attacks.
11. *True. Salmonella* bacteria are commonly associated with chickens, especially raw chicken carcasses. Raw chicken should be handled very carefully so that juices do not contaminate other foods, thereby spreading *Salmonella* bacteria to other foods.
12. *True.* The bacterium that produces the very deadly botulism food poisoning is present in all soil.
13. *True. Clostridium botulinum* grows only in the absence of air. Thus it may be found in improperly canned foods and in thick foods where air is excluded from the center. Chili is an example.
14. *True.* Many viruses and parasites that may be present in raw fish are destroyed by cooking. Consuming raw fish poses a significant health risk for hepatitis, parasite infections, and other health problems.
15. *False.* Aside from the alcohol present in high amounts (which over time can lead to cirrhosis of the liver), alcoholic beverages contain urethanes, which the FDA is now studying carefully to assess the degree of health risk these agents pose.

Nutrition Perspective 19-1

Protecting the U.S. Food Supply

A variety of federal, state, and local agencies in the United States monitors food safety. The history of the food laws they enforce is listed below with some of the agencies involved:

- **The U.S. Department of Agriculture (USDA).** This agency enforces standards for wholesomeness and quality of meat, poultry, milk, and eggs produced in the United States. Its activities include inspection of production plants and of grains, fruits, vegetables, meat, poultry, and dairy products. This agency also routinely monitors animal foods for antibiotic residues.
- **Bureau of Alcohol, Tobacco, and Firearms.** This agency is responsible for enforcing laws that cover the production, distribution, and labeling of alcoholic beverages—except wine beverages that contain less than 7% alcohol (those are the responsibility of the FDA).
- **Environmental Protection Agency (EPA).** This agency regulates pesticides. In the United States alone, pests destroy nearly $20 billion of food crops yearly despite extensive pesticide use. But while pest control is necessary to ensure an adequate food supply, the presence of pesticide residues in foods raises concerns. Some of these chemicals, for example, have caused birth defects, sterility, tumors, organ damage, and injury to the central nervous system in laboratory animals. Some persist in the environment for many years.

  The EPA must approve all pesticides before they are sold in the United States. It determines the safety of new pesticide products and sets allowable limits (tolerances) for pesticide residue in foods. For agricultural use, the EPA tolerances specify residue limits for about 10,000 pesticide/food combinations involving about 300 active pesticide ingredients. A tolerance is not necessarily the maximum safe level of a pesticide in a food. The EPA sets tolerances no higher than needed for a product's intended use. These limits are then enforced by the FDA. The EPA also establishes water quality standards, including those for drinking water.

Key U.S. Food Laws

1906: **Pure Food and Drug Act**—This most importantly defined adulterated foods: those foods containing "any added poisons or other added deleterious ingredient which may render such article injurious to health".

1938: **Federal Food, Drug, and Cosmetic Act**—This provided for exemptions and safe tolerances for substances that, although not that desirable in foods, were either necessary in production or unavoidable.

1958: **Food Additives Amendment (and the Color Additives Amendment of 1960)**—These made it necessary for manufacturers to demonstrate the safety of a new food additive before approval by the FDA. The 1958 Act also included the Delaney clause: "no additive shall be deemed to be safe if it is found to produce cancer when ingested by man or animals, or if it is found after tests which are appropriate for the evaluation of the safety of the food additives to induce cancer in man or animals."

Nutrition Perspective 19-1—cont'd

See Chapter 2 to review the FDA's role in regulating both the terms used and health claims made on food labels.

Traditionally, the FDA does not regularly inspect food-processing plants. It relies instead on its "Good Manufacturers Procedures" plan that food processors and manufacturers are expected to follow. The FDA inspectors may visit a specific food processing establishment only infrequently. The agency relies on consumer complaints to alert it to potential dangers—then it researches these in greater detail.

Protecting the U.S. Food Supply

- **Food and Drug Administration (FDA).** This agency is responsible for ensuring the safety and wholesomeness of all foods sold in interstate commerce (except for meat and poultry, which are primarily under USDA jurisdiction). The FDA also sets standards for specific foods and enforces federal regulations for labeling, food and color additives, food sanitation, and the safety of foods. The agency inspects food plants, imported food products, and mills that make feeds containing medications or nutritional supplements for animals destined for human consumption.

  The FDA acts primarily when the public health is endangered or when proper medical care is being discouraged. It regulates products, not people. *The FDA cannot control what people say, just what is on the label and how a product is promoted.* The FDA gives low priority to simple economic deception by products.

  To monitor foods for contaminants, the FDA routinely samples items that are of dietary importance, such as produce. Foods suspected of illegal residues receive a more intensive evaluation. An important part of the FDA's safety sampling is a "market basket" study of foods that typify the American diet. Four times a year, identical purchases of 234 foods, including processed foods, are analyzed for pesticide residues, radioactive elements, toxic metals, and other undesirable substances. Of the few samples found containing illegal pesticide residues, most involve pesticides approved for use on other foods, but not on that particular food.

  Imported foods with illegal residues can be refused entry into the country by the FDA. In the case of domestic foods, the FDA can impose the sanctions of seizure, injunction, and prosecution.
- **National Marine Fishery Service.** This agency is part of the Department of Commerce. It is responsible for seafood quality and other aspects of fisheries management. It has a voluntary inspection program for fish products, but no mandatory program. This is probably one reason why one fourth of all food poisoning incidents in the United States involve eating fish, according to the Centers for Disease Control in Atlanta, Georgia. The FDA does inspect seafood processing plants and spotchecks imported fish and seafood.
- **State and local government.** States inspect restaurants, retail food establishments, dairies, grain mills, and other food-related establishments within their borders. States have the primary responsibility for milk safety. The FDA provides guidelines to state and local governments for regulating dairy products and restaurants.
- **Foreign governments.** Governments of at least 40 nations are now partners with the United States in ensuring food safety through agreements that cover 24 food products, including shellfish. International cooperation is expanding in terms of food inspection and regulatory standards.

Nutrition Perspective 19-2

Food Irradiation

Food irradiation was added to the permissible methods for food preservation in the United States by the FDA in 1983. In 1986, the FDA approved the use of food irradiation for the preservation of spices, potatoes, and grains.

Food irradiation causes "ionizing" radiation by creating ions, or free radicals, in foods.[18,26] These highly reactive agents can destroy cell membranes, break down DNA, and link proteins. The gamma radiation used does not make the food radioactive; however, the energy is strong enough to break chemical bonds. *By altering DNA, enzymes, and a variety of proteins, irradiation can prevent the growth of microorganisms, parasites, and insects.* It can do this without creating much heat in the food product. Thus it is referred to as "cold sterilization."

A few problems still hamper the widespread use of irradiation for food preservation. A variety of "radiolytic" products are produced in the process, and there is concern that some of them may be harmful. At present, scientists cannot tell whether they are harmful because there is no way to concentrate these products to feed them in high doses to animals. Scientists cannot coax test animals to eat 100 times a normal intake of irradiated potatoes, for example, as they can with chemical food additives, such as colors, flavors, and preservatives.

Another problem stems from the fact that the FDA views food irradiation as an additive. This classification makes it crucial for processors to establish the level of radiation that a food receives. Recall that to have a food additive approved, the manufacturer must show the FDA that the additive can be measured at the levels ultimately found in foods. This is not possible with food irradiation. The "radiolytic" products are in too low a concentration to be easily measured. Critics of this method argue that a food can be irradiated in an early step of processing and then needlessly re-irradiated by another manufacturer because no method exists to determine how much prior radiation the food received.

Proponents claim that food irradiation is a safe and effective means of preservation that extends the shelf life of foods, destroys microorganisms, slows the rapid ripening of harvested produce, and reduces the need for pesticides, some of which are harmful.[20] However, researchers have also shown that irradiation can cause unpleasant flavors, off colors, and changes in texture. In addition, decreases in thiamin, vitamin A, and vitamin E content of foods have been detected after irradiation.

To date, consumer acceptance of food irradiation in the United States remains very low. Recent attempts to sell irradiated papayas failed. Some people are concerned about this form of food preservation. Still, the FDA condones it.

Worldwide, countries such as Japan, France, the Soviet Union, Italy, and Mexico use food irradiation technology. When food is irradiated, it must carry the label shown in the margin. However, note that if irradiated spices are incorporated into another food, there is no requirements that the "second-generation" food carry the irradiation label.

Chapter 20

Your Future in Nutrition

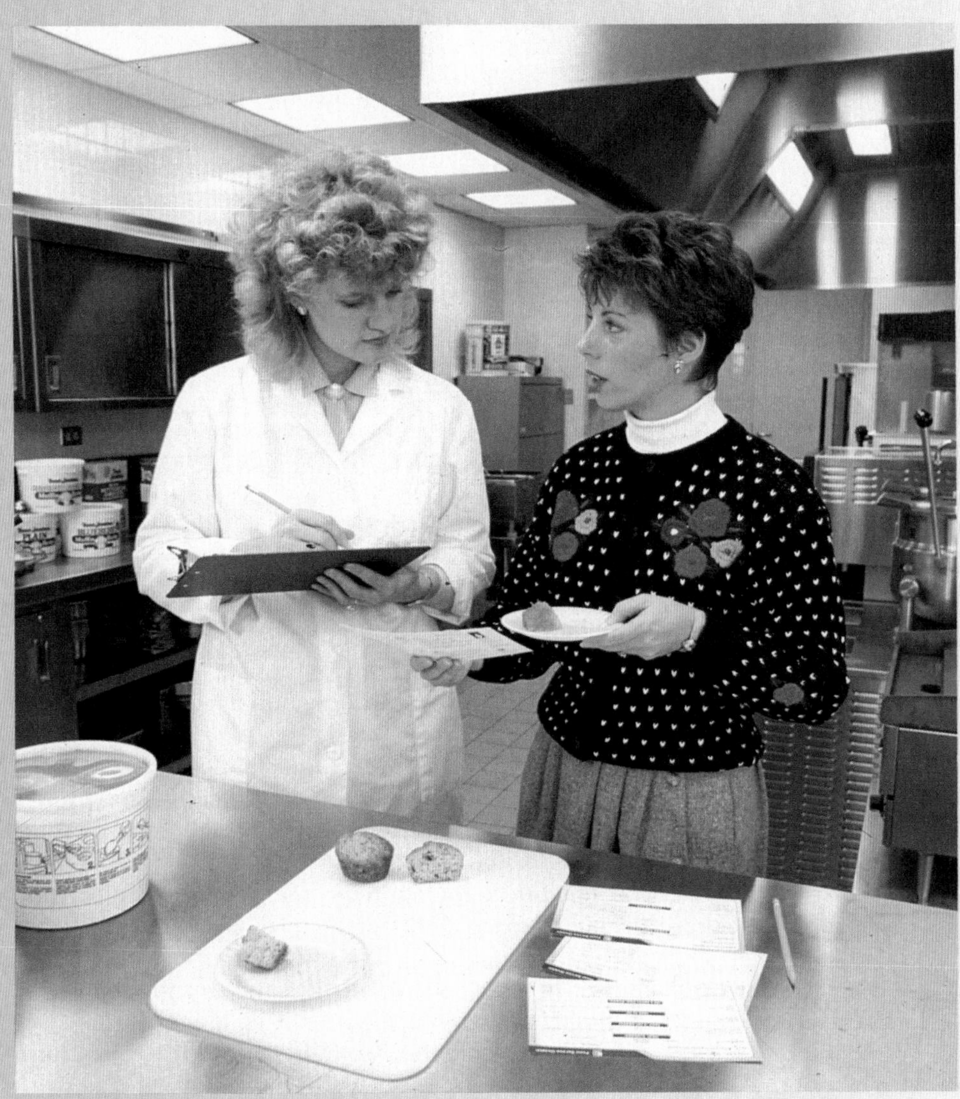

Registered Dietitians are no longer confined to the traditional hospital workplace; consulting, private practice, and research are just a few of the exciting areas open to RDs.

Overview

Nutrition studies are increasingly in the news, alerting us to new findings.[4,17] Also, the public is more willing to hear about health issues, because people are realizing that good nutrition and health habits can help control and even prevent many diseases.

Our eagerness for more information is creating opportunities for professionals who want to influence the food habits and health of others throughout the life cycle.[9] This makes nutrition a rapidly growing field. Currently, the U.S. government predicts a need for 30% more registered dietitians by the year 2000. Most current federal health strategies include the need for dietetic expertise.[14]

If these types of activities sound good to you, consider majoring in Nutrition and Dietetics. You already have some basic knowledge necessary for understanding nutrition issues and giving health advice. However, you need more detailed study and clinical and laboratory experience to help hone your skills. If the field of food and nutrition interests you, consider a program leading to a Registered Dietitian (RD) credential. In the future, many states will allow only RDs to give nutrition advice or even call themselves dietitians or nutritionists.

Nutrition awareness inventory

Here are 15 statements about your future in the field of nutrition. Answer them to test your current knowledge. If you think the answer is true or mostly true, circle T. If you think the answer is false or mostly false, circle F. Use the scoring key at the end of this chapter to compute your total score. Take this test again after you have read this chapter. Compare the results.

1. T F Many Registered Dietitians (RDs) are licensed.
2. T F RDs spend most of their time preparing menus.
3. T F All RDs are required to have a college degree.
4. T F DTRs are dietetic technicians.
5. T F DTRs are required to have a college degree.
6. T F Clinical experience is required to become an RD.
7. T F Anyone can offer nutrition advice for a fee.
8. T F Health food stores are often run by nutritionists.
9. T F Hospitals employ the greatest number of RDs.
10. T F RDs can be commissioned as officers in the military.
11. T F Nutrition is a subspecialty of nursing.
12. T F Nutrition as a career has been growing in popularity.
13. T F There are no popular magazines devoted entirely to nutrition.
14. T F All RDs are nutritionists, but not all nutritionists are RDs.
15. T F In a coordinated program leading to an RD credential, classroom and clinical experience are combined in the college degree program.

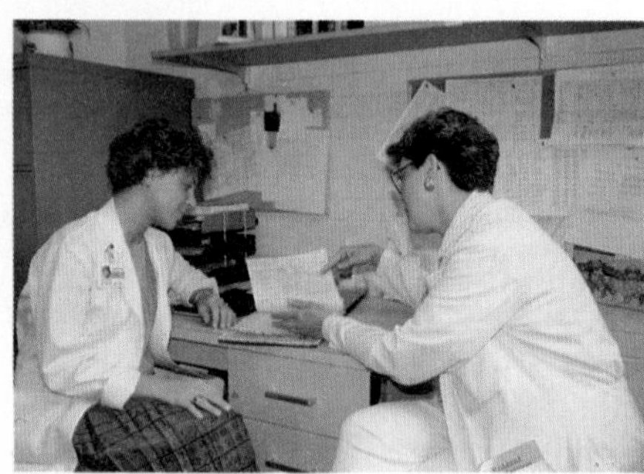

An RD discusses research findings with her colleague.

THE FIELD OF NUTRITION

If you choose nutrition science as your career path, where could that lead? As a nutrition professional, you might find yourself doing a variety of the following tasks:[6,13]

- Directing a study in a university hospital to determine the relationship between dietary fiber and cancer of the colon
- Counseling a client with adult-onset diabetes mellitus in your own private practice to control the disease by attaining an appropriate weight
- Directing a multimillion dollar foodservice program in a public school district or hospital
- Participating on a health-care team with doctors, nurses, pharmacists, social workers, physical therapists, and other health professionals to map out a complete rehabilitation and health maintenance program for a hospital patient
- Overseeing foodservice operations or studying the acceptability of food products for either wartime or space flight personnel as an officer in military service
- Teaching university courses in basic and advanced nutrition and foodservice management
- Serving as a consultant to a restaurant chain to help improve the nutritional quality of its meals
- Participating on a committee with economists, food scientists, physicians, agricultural scientists, anthropologists, and others to help devise strategies for alleviating world hunger

The key concepts of nutrition science covered in this textbook can be of great value whether you major in nutrition, premedicine, predental, nursing, pharmacy, home economics, physical education, or almost any other professional area. A dual degree in nutrition and any other professional area could pose exciting opportunities: it is becoming quite clear that nutrition knowledge is vital in most areas associated with human health, and certainly in careers of medicine, pharmacy, nursing, dentistry, and home economics.

- Helping a day-care center set up a feeding program for poorly nourished children
- Overseeing a company's research, evaluation, and marketing of food products.

Today, 36% of RDs work primarily in hospitals and clinics providing nutrition care, while 24% function in foodservice capacities. Consultation in both foodservice management and nutrition care as part of a private practice account for another 20%, while 12% work in the community. RDs in education and research round out the last 8%.[7]

This list of jobs could stretch on and on. Nutrition professionals are employed today in a variety of professional activities. *Some of these are open only to people who are registered dietitians.* We will point those out in the next sections. In addition, for positions opened to people who do not need to have the RD, qualifications are enhanced by the training an RD receives.

Who am I?

If a career as a registered dietitian or other nutrition professional seems exciting, ask yourself if you have these characteristics:[11,12]

- Do I enjoy working with other people? Am I a skilled communicator?
- Do I maintain good health and nutrition habits?
- Am I self-confident? Can others look to me for help?
- Am I responsible and conscientious about following through with commitments? Do I have a strong work ethic?
- Can I be discreet about other people's secrets?
- Can I tolerate frustration, such as substituting for an employee who fails to come to work when it's my day off?
- Am I adaptable and flexible? Can I mold my career to the changes dictated by new methods of health care delivery?
- Do I have good organizational skills?
- Am I creative at solving problems?
- Do I have a real interest in the food, health, and/or medical field?
- Do I feel comfortable with overall concepts of chemistry, biochemistry, and management? How are my math skills, including the metric system, weights, measures, fractions, and simple arithmetic calculations?

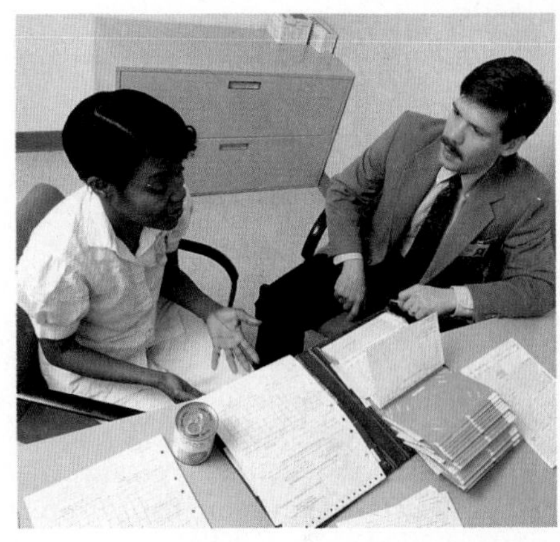

An RD counseling a client in private practice.

Not all of these are necessary characteristics for every nutrition professional, and some can be developed and nurtured. But, overall, one should have a basic curiosity about food and nutrition issues and a desire to work with others—clients, staff members, employees, or the public—to improve the nutrition health of people.

Dietitian or nutritionist: is there a difference?

Nutrition professionals who work in hospitals or health-care clinics and give nutrition advice usually call themselves dietitians. Nutrition professionals who work in the community for a university department, government program, business, or private agency, such as the American Heart Association or National Dairy Council, often call themselves **nutritionists.** In this chapter we will use this terminology to represent those distinctions—hospital versus community practice. The major issue, however, is not the title, but the responsibilities of a person.

nutritionist
A person who advises about nutrition and/or works in the field of food and nutrition. In many of the United States, a person does not need formal training to use this title; some other states protect this title, allowing only holders of the RD credential to use it.

In a hospital or other health-care setting where nutrition counseling or care is given, the nutrition professional usually must have an RD credential. *In some states—not all—anyone using the title dietitian must have the RD credential.* However, in a community or business setting the RD credential is sometimes unnecessary. When applying for a job, the important consideration is whether the RD credential is necessary (Table 20-1). *Use of the job title nutritionist is no indication that the employer does or does not require applicants to have an RD credential.*

Future sections review the routes for obtaining an RD credential and list where these titles may be used only by RDs.

Without an RD credential, the title nutritionist often reveals nothing about a

Table 20-1

Do any of these advertisements sound like you—after you become an RD?

Clinical dietitian

Rehabilitation Institute, a 120-bed physical medicine and rehabilitation facility, has an opening for a full-time registered dietitian. Responsibilities include nutrition assessment; enteral feeding evaluation; patient, family, and staff education; and participation in health-care team. Registered or registration-eligible* required.

Public health nutritionist

Responsibilities include nutrition counseling and patient education, with emphasis in maternal and child health. Must be RD or registration-eligible.

Assistant director of patient care

Hospital & Medical Center, a 378-bed acute-care facility is searching for an Assistant Director of Patient Care. Responsibilities include computerized nutrition office, quality assurance, clinical and trayline areas. Clinical services include cardiology, renal, diabetes, and TPN among general medical surgical areas. Must be RD or registration-eligible.

Assistant director: food systems management

A 436-bed hospital is seeking a highly motivated individual who is goal oriented and works well in a rapidly expanding and progressive foodservice operation. This is a challenging opportunity for an enthusiastic individual wanting to become a part of our dynamic management team. Areas of responsibility include overseeing the operations of the cafeteria, coffee shop, in-house catering, computerized food procurement and inventory control, sanitation, and food production. The individual we are seeking should possess high standards related to quality of foodservice operations, good communication skills, initiative and judgment in planning and delegating responsibility, and strong interpersonal and supervisory skills. Must possess demonstrated skills and knowledge in foodservice management, including budget preparation and control, financial management and fiscal accountability, long-range planning, and computerization of a foodservice operation. Must be RD or registration-eligible.

Program specialist

Challenging full-time position available immediately for registered dietitian to organize the professional and personnel components of our multidisciplinary weight-loss program. Successful candidate will be highly motivated and flexible. Sensitivity in working with the obese is required. Registered or registration-eligible required.

Registered dietitian

Needed to develop nutritional standards of care for dietetic services. Plan regular modified menus for patient foodservice and develop the hospital diet manual in accordance with recognized standards. Direct and participate in all areas of nutrition care for acute- and long-term care patients, coordinating with medical, nursing, and paramedical staff. Direct and participate in nutritional educational efforts. Contribute to department planning, in-service education, and management. Registered or registration-eligible.

Clinical dietitian, pediatric specialty

Developmental disabilities program has an immediate opening for a pediatric dietitian. Responsibilities include assessment and care plan development for infants and young children with developmental disabilities, training activities, and clinical investigations. Must be RD or registration-eligible.

Dietitian

Excellent opportunity for a clinical dietitian. Areas of practice shall include nutrition support for adults and neonates, maternal/child nutrition, diabetes, heart disease, skilled care, acute rehabilitation, and inpatient and outpatient education. Registered or registration-eligible required.

Faculty position

Assistant Professor in Foods and Nutrition with emphasis in Food Service Systems Management. Master's degree required. Registered dietitian (RD) or registration-eligible. Professional experience necessary. Teaching and research experience desirable. Primary teaching in foodservice management courses to undergraduate majors in dietetics (Coordinated Program) and restaurant management. Participate in departmental/university activities, committee work, and professional development. Nine-month appointment.

*Registration-eligible indicates all college course work and supervised professional practice has been completed; only successful completion of the registration examination remains

person's training. It could be used appropriately in some states by a highly qualified M.D. or Ph.D. but inappropriately in some states by a salesperson for bogus cures in a health food store. One must investigate the person's credentials. On the other hand, the title registered dietitian indicates that the holder has completed college or university courses in food and nutrition science—and 900 hours of supervised professional practice to ensure basic competency in assessing nutrient needs, providing nutrition advice, and directing a foodservice operation.

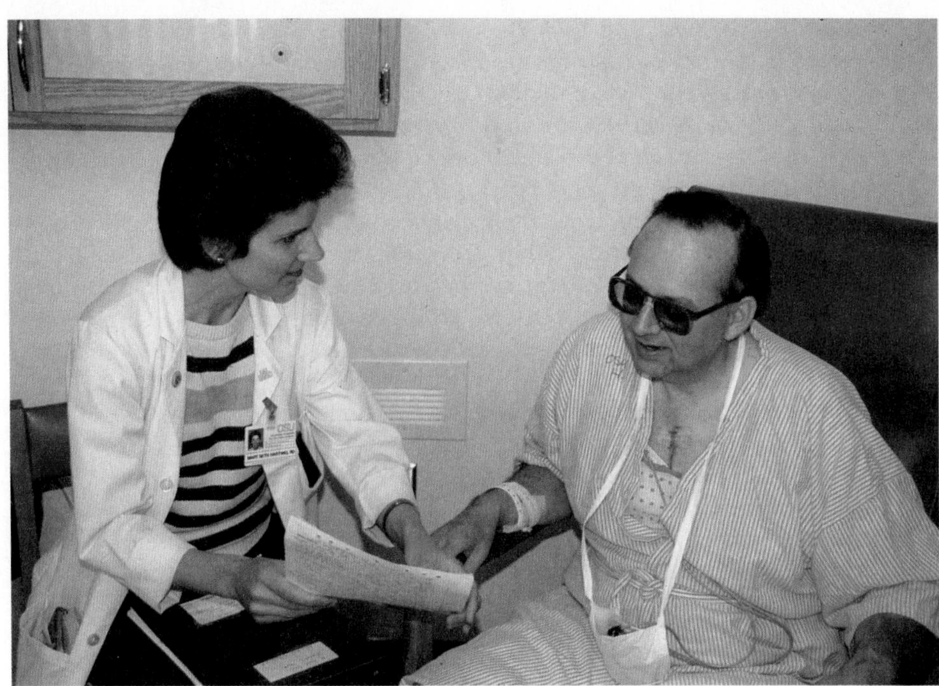

The nutrition advice provided by RDs often plays a vital part in a patient's medical care.

What are the different branches of professional nutrition practice?

As mentioned above, a variety of professional activities are open to nutrition professionals today. Let's focus on some general areas of professional nutrition practice.

Clinical practice. Clinical practice usually requires an RD credential and involves providing food and nutrition services in health-care settings. Nutrition care is a pivotal service in medical care provided by hospitals, outpatient clinics, clinical research centers, and private-practice settings.[9] In clinical practice, dietitians team with physicians, nurses, pharmacists, and other health-care providers to chart the best course for individual treatments. Dietitians evaluate eating habits of individual patients and attempt to change eating behavior where necessary to remedy specific health problems. Clinical practice also involves developing and teaching classes for people with diseases that require specific dietary plans. Dietitians sometimes concentrate on a particular area of nutrition care, such as diabetes mellitus, kidney (renal) disease, organ transplant, infant care, and intensive nutritional support, among others.[9]

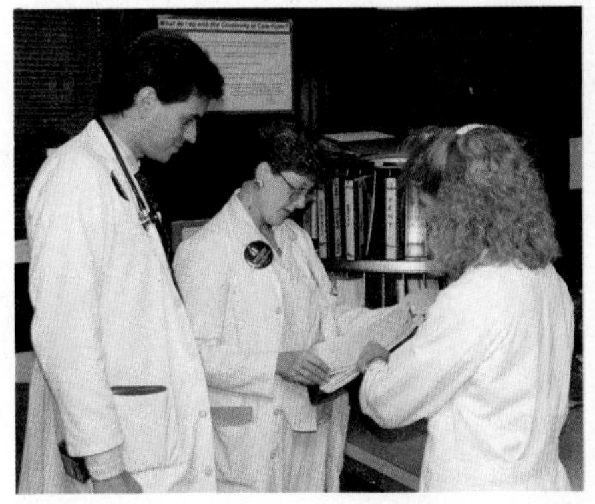

Clinical dietitians often participate with a health care team.

A recent study showed that dietitians in clinical practice spend about 50% of their time in client-related activities. Of this time, they spent 16% documenting nutrition care, 11% in preliminary nutrition screening, 10% in health team conferences, 10% in evaluation and reassessment of nutritional care, 8% in comprehensive nutrition assessments, 7% in menu preparation for individual clients, and 7% in nutrition counseling and education. For the 50% of time not related to client care, delays and transit time between work responsibilities required 35%, and administrative activities took most of the remainder.[16]

The importance of a clinical nutrition expert on the health-care team is acknowledged by the Joint Commission for the Accreditation of Hospitals. This commission evaluates U.S. hospitals that qualify for federal funds. Their examiners look for specific evidence that dietitians are assessing the nutritional needs of the people served, developing nutritional goals and plans to meet those needs, and assessing the effects of the nutritional therapy.

Clinical practice is changing. The focus in today's health-care settings is switching from hospitals to outpatient clinics. There is strong motivation to trim costs in health care, since the U.S. government now reimburses hospitals based on the disease state rather than on the length of a client's stay in the hospital.[5] This change has reduced the length of hospitalization. In response, *many services once offered only in hospitals are now offered in the community, creating a large home-health–care industry* and allowing for the greater demand for hospital-level care in nursing homes.

The activities of dietitians are evolving to accommodate these recent changes in the health-care environment.[15] While their roles are not yet clearly established in all these newer settings, dietitians are beginning to define how they can best serve. The new ambulatory care centers, extended care centers, nursing homes, hospices, and health maintenance organizations all need the expertise of clinically oriented nutrition professionals. If the nutritional care of people interests you, but hospital work does not, *there are many opportunities outside the hospital to practice nutrition care and still provide great benefit to people.*[9]

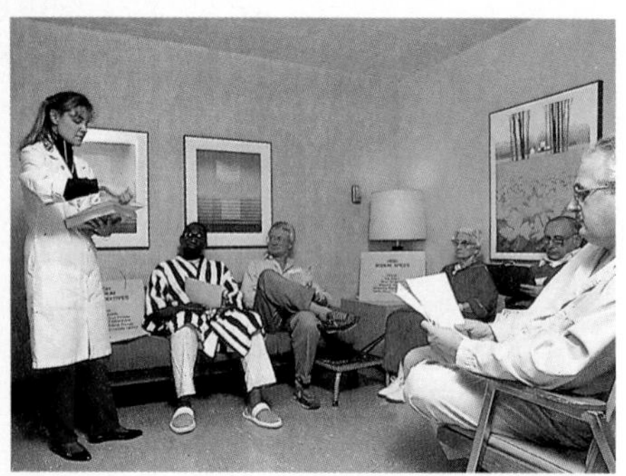

Many ambulatory care centers, extended care centers, and hospices need the expertise of a nutrition professional.

Tools used in clinical nutrition practice. We have already introduced many tools used in clinical nutrition practice. In Chapter 2, we discussed nutrition assessment based on analysis of a person's diet, height, weight, and other anthropometric measures; measurements of enzyme function in red blood cells; and, finally, a physical examination to detect clinical signs of malnutrition. Once a nutritional diagnosis is made in consultation with a physician, a specific course of diet therapy might be planned. Some possible approaches from Chapter 5 include reducing total fat, saturated fat, and cholesterol intake. Chapter 4 reviewed controlling the intake of simple sugars or increasing fiber intake, and Chapter 9 focused on reducing total kcalorie intake. All these diet therapies can use the exchange system to ease the task of planning actual food consumption.

In the future, more and more differentiated roles and functions will open to dietitians. As these roles become more specialized, they will increasingly require delegation of some present tasks and responsibilities to other less highly trained workers.[4,10]

Many problems associated with poor nutrition that clinical practice may need to address already have been discussed in this book. People who have high blood cholesterol levels, are overweight or underweight, suffer from constipation, or have diabetes mellitus can benefit from information covered in Chapters 4, 5, 8, and 9. Questions also often arise in clinical practice about a proper overall diet, the dangers of sodium, the relationship between osteoporosis and calcium intake, a proper diet during pregnancy, what to feed children, inadequacies in teenage diets, or choosing between breast- and bottle-feeding—you already know much about these issues.

If these challenges interest you, and you would like to design diets or to advise others how to eat to maximize health, seriously consider following an education program that leads to an RD credential. That is the key to many career paths in clinical nutrition care.

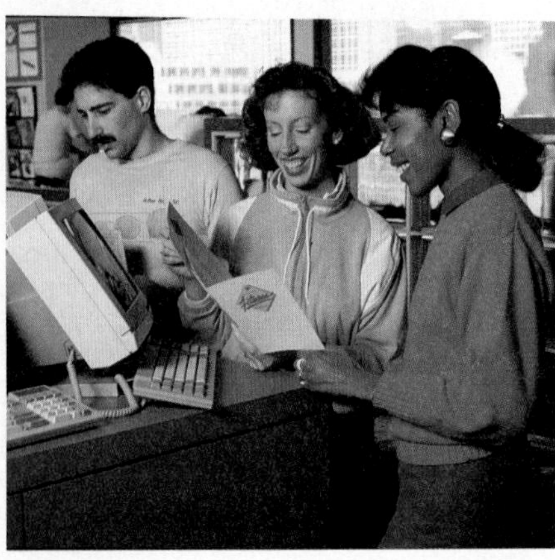

An RD may work as a consultant, devising fitness programs for athletes.

Private consulting. Dietitians in clinical practice may also be self-employed consultants. A consultant who concentrates on counseling clients and designing nutrition programs for them functions much the same as the dietitian in a medical center. Consulting dietitians may also provide nutrition advice for the food and pharmaceutical industries; represent food companies at professional seminars and meetings; develop work site nutrition programs; write food, nutrition, and diet books; and tailor nutrition regimens to fitness programs for athletes, dancers, and others.

Many dietitians are consultants for small nursing homes, small hospitals, and other agencies that need foodservice management and clinical nutrition expertise but can't afford a full-time dietitian. For the most part, these consulting jobs are not available to nutrition professionals who lack an RD credential.

Community practice. Nutritionists practicing in the community work primarily with healthy clients, rather than with the sick. These nutritionists develop nutrition and health programs, teach nutrition classes, and counsel those who need to maintain or improve their health. Health and wellness education has become a major emphasis for community nutritionists.[8] Employment or consultation in the fitness area has expanded in recent years. In addition, opportunities in work site nutrition programs are increasing. U.S. government programs, such as the Women, Infants, and Children Program (WIC) and the Head Start Program, city and county health departments, and various state agencies employ nutrition professionals. An RD credential is often necessary for employment in these areas.

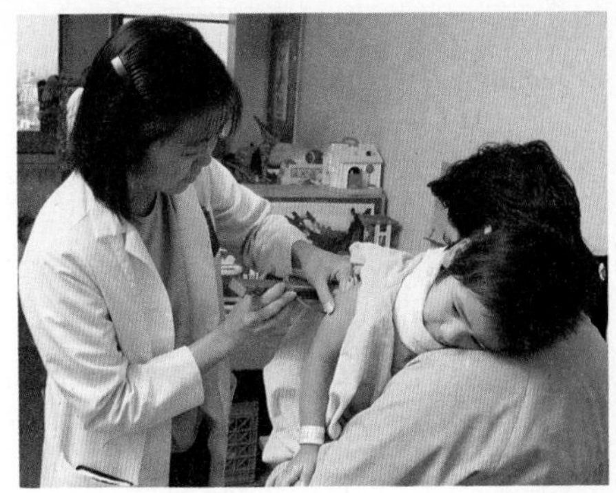

Community health care can be rewarding for a nutritionist.

Foodservice management. Foodservice management in hospitals and nursing homes includes overseeing kitchens, employee cafeterias, and patient foodservice. Efficient management of a department of dietetics assumes a critical importance in the overall management of a medical center. In a hospital, dietetics is often the second largest department after the nursing department. A department of dietetics might have 150 to 200 employees and a $4 million budget, tied mainly to foodservice operations. Foodservice managers also direct school lunch operations and foodservice activities in restaurants, businesses, and industries.

In all these settings, foodservice managers administer personnel, design and implement employee training programs, plan food systems, and develop and administer department budgets. While they are primarily concerned with the operation of foodservice departments, the nutritional intake of the people they serve remains an important consideration.

Foodservice managers in business and industry may assume broad administrative responsibilities and high management positions. Some are also involved in the development of computer programs for foodservice systems, while others streamline foodservice operations.[9] Not all foodservice management positions require an RD credential, but many do, and the extra status it brings never hurts.

Nutrition educators and researchers. Educators usually teach college and university courses in foods, nutrition, and foodservice management in departments of food and nutrition, dietetics, and home economics, and in hospital nutrition and dietetics departments. They conduct research in food, nutrition, or foodservice systems issues, and publish articles and books. Schools of nursing, medicine, and dentistry provide additional employment opportunities for educators.[9] Most of these jobs require advanced academic degrees beyond baccalaureate training, such as the master's and doctorate degrees.

Nutrition educators form the backbone of nutrition research in North America: they expand and refine our nutrition knowledge through experiments and analysis of data. Other nutrition researchers work for industrial institutions. The chance to expand nutrition knowledge and refine nutrition practice can be part of an exciting career.

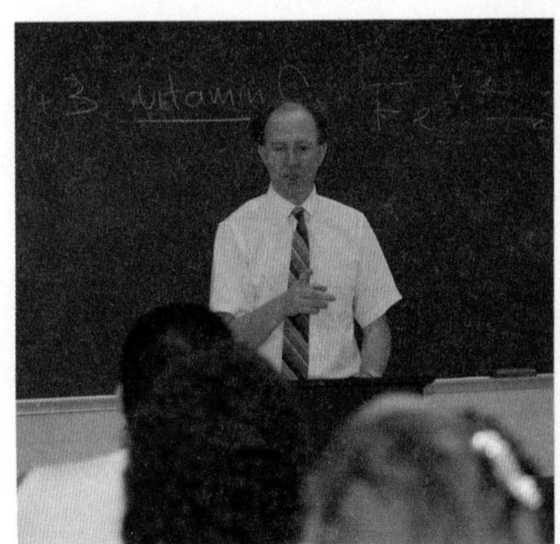

Nutrition educators expand knowledge of nutrition through both instruction and research.

Some nutrition educators and researchers are not RDs. These people hold advanced degrees in nutrition and/or foods but did not complete requirements for an RD credential. While they may be excellent scientists, the lack of an RD credential can limit chances of finding an academic position. In addition, educators who are not RDs are prohibited from assessing the nutritional status of individuals and designing nutrition therapy protocols in many states. If you are considering a career as a nutrition educator or researcher, we encourage you to follow a program that provides the required skills and background while allowing you to gain the RD credential.

Food and nutrition careers in business and industry. Nutrition professionals in business and industry may work for equipment manufacturers, food companies, supermarket chains, and pharmaceutical companies.[9] Besides basic nutrition research, their activities often include food product development, menu design, sales and promotion, purchasing, marketing, and public relations and media. Opportunities in business for nutrition professionals are expanding rapidly.[12] (See Nutrition Perspective 20-2, "An RD credential is just the start.") An RD credential is unessential for some of these jobs but is often the added bonus a company seeks.

Public relations and the media are rapidly expanding career areas for RDs.

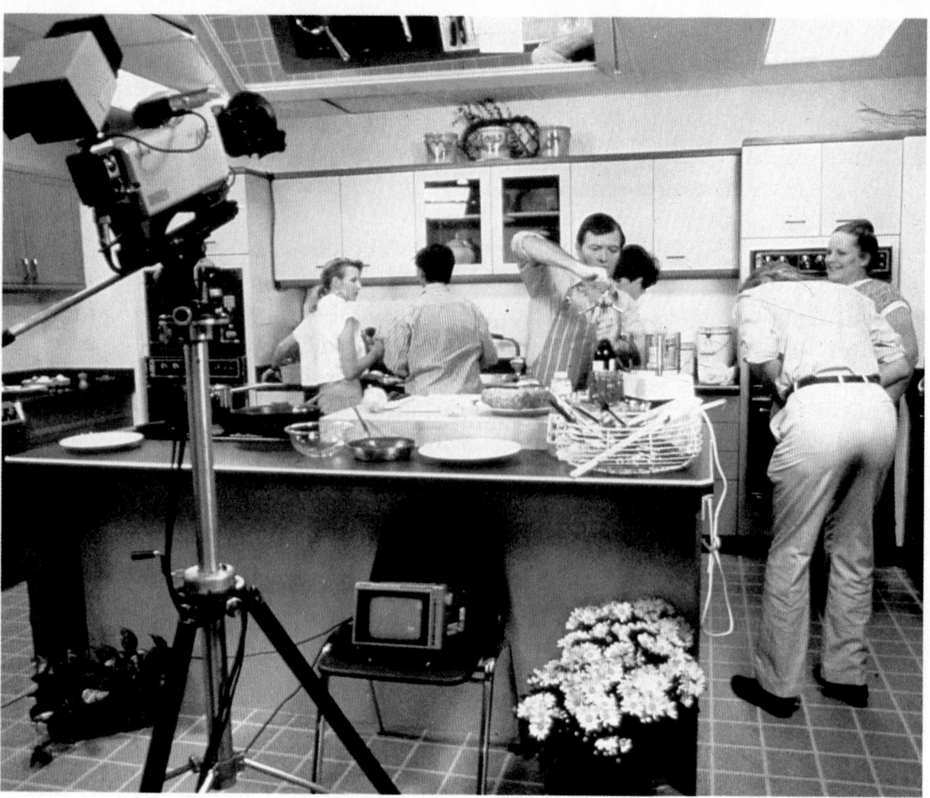

Concept Check

The term *dietitian* usually refers to a person who has the RD credential and works in a hospital or clinical setting. The term *nutritionist* can refer to nutrition professionals who work outside the hospital or clinical setting—but in many states this title gives no guarantee of a person's training in nutrition. Nutrition professionals work in a variety of settings, such as hospitals, community programs, foodservice operations, universities, and business and industry. An RD credential is usually necessary for clinical practice in hospitals or dietetic consulting for health-care institutions, such as nursing homes. In other settings, such as foodservice management or industry, the RD credential is desirable, but often not necessary.

ROUTES TO AN RD CREDENTIAL

Program requirements and titles for dietitians and nutritionists have some similarities in Canada and the United States, but may also vary significantly. We consider them separately here.

Obtaining and maintaining the RD credential in the United States

All RDs in the United States have earned college baccalaureate degrees and completed a total of 900 hours of supervised professional practice in hospitals, community agencies, nursing homes, school systems, and other sites. All colleges, universities, and health-care institutions that offer either courses or supervised practice programs must be approved or accredited by the American Dietetic Association. Graduates of these programs receive solid training in basic science, communications, nutrition, foods, foodservice management, health and wellness, diet therapy, and business. This foundation allows them to understand the complex issues and problems they face in daily practice.

The traditional route to an RD credential includes a four-year plan of specific coursework at a college or university. The student then applies for an **internship** to acquire the necessary 900 hours of supervised practice. The internship may be offered by a hospital or other nutrition-related agency, and is usually completed in 9 to 24 months, depending on the program. After completing the internship, the student is eligible to take the national registration examination to obtain the RD credential.

internship
A program offered by a hospital or other health organizations that provides 900 hours of supervised professional practice.

Since 1962, **coordinated programs in dietetics** have been available at colleges and universities. These programs incorporate the 900 hours of supervised practice in hospitals and/or other health-related organizations into the junior and senior years of college. Thus, upon graduating from college, a student is eligible to take the registration examination. These coordinated programs have the advantage of providing all the supervised practice and courses needed to gain the RD credential, and thus save students the concern of gaining acceptance into an internship. Although many internships are available throughout the United States there are always more applicants than opportunities.

coordinated program in dietetics
A baccalaureate program that integrates 900 hours of supervised professional practice with the junior and senior years' curriculum needed for the RD credential exam.

On the other hand, a disadvantage of a coordinated program is that the student may have little free time to pursue other college activities. The student essentially adds 6 months of supervised practice to an already full junior and senior year academic program. This type of program turns out to be very intensive and can require more work than the typical junior and senior years demand from most college students.

Another route to becoming an RD is to enter an Approved Preprofessional Practice Program (AP4). First, the student completes academic courses approved by The American Dietetic Association and obtains a college degree. Then completion of the necessary 900 hours of supervised practice must occur within a maximum of 2 years, at a rate of at least 20 hours per week. This allows the possibility of doing a part-time internship. The student can then take the registration examination.

Today, all U.S. undergraduate work in dietetics follows (or will by 1995) essentially the same curriculum pattern. This pattern supplies each entry-level RD with a common foundation of knowledge, skills, and values that contributes to high quality practice. In the past, students could specialize in clinical dietetics, community dietetics, or foodservice management, but this is no longer possible. Specialization today is done at the graduate level as a student pursues a master's degree or via conferring of specialty credentials through a professional organization (see below).

The registration examination

Once all courses and professional practice are completed, the student is eligible for registration; only the registration examination remains to be passed. In the United States, the registration examination is given in April and October of each year. Once passed, the RD maintains registered status by accumulating every 5 years at least 75 hours of continuing education approved by the American Dietetic Association and by paying an annual registration maintenance fee (currently $25).

Canadian programs

Dietitians in Canada perform roles similar to those in the United States: clinicians, foodservice managers, community nutritionists, consultants, educators, and researchers. To become a dietitian, a person must complete a four-year program in foods and nutrition approved by the Canadian Dietetic Association. Currently, 19 colleges and universities in Canada offer such programs. The student then completes an internship of 12 months or an alternate plan of 24 months of work experience. It is possible to integrate the internship with the last 2 years of college.

Expert Opinion

Whither Goest Thou?—Career Development in Nutrition and Dietetics

M. ROSITA SCHILLER, Ph.D., R.D.

Soldiers of ancient Rome would often greet strangers and other travelers with the words, "Quo vadis?"—"Where are you going?" These same words can aptly be addressed to students in the field of nutrition and dietetics. With so many career options, such as those presented in this chapter, it is important to plot a course—to decide where you are going.

A successful career requires two basic elements: a place to work and a plan of action. Before you begin, recognize the difference between a "job" and a "career." One definition of a job is "a piece of work undertaken for a fixed price." Many nutritionists and dietitians are satisfied with a "job;" they either give priority to other interests, such as a family, or they lack the motivation necessary for career development. These individuals often move from one position to another without a plan for professional growth or advancement. They may have poorly defined career goals, and they often lack a clear picture of skills needed for the next step. They may participate in professional activities, but they usually do not prepare themselves to preside over major committees.

Those who decide to make nutrition and dietetics a *career* (instead of a "job") make a more exciting choice. They seek positions for a defined purpose. They have a general plan that will lead them toward self-fulfillment and the achievement of professional success. Their goals are focused on activities rather than the actual workplace; they think of accomplishments more than time spent in routine tasks.

How does one plan career development? A few easy steps and some realistic expectations are all you need. First, accept the fact that the only people who start at the top are grave diggers. Getting to the top of most fields requires hard work and clear direction. On occasion, people find themselves in the right place at the right time; luck then catapults them rapidly to the top. For most people though, reaching the zenith professionally takes years of calculated effort. By the time they earn credentials, most dietitians know whether they want to work in clinical nutrition or foodservice management. These two basic areas outline the focus for opportunities in health care settings, private consulting, research, teaching, community agencies, and industry. Some dietitians begin in clinical nutrition and, later, switch to foodservice management but most select an area of practice and remain in it throughout their careers. Thus the nature of one's first position usually sets the stage for future advancements.

The first job then, is important, not so much for what or where it is, but for where it can lead. Entry-level practitioners should spend their first 2 to 3 years learning the fundamentals of the profession. Skills that were adequate for graduation now must be both refined through repetition and enhanced through greater complexity of challenges. During this first job, new professionals develop an awareness of professional expectations, policies, procedures, and standards of practice. They expand their ability to think conceptually and creatively, and they begin to initiate new projects, solve problems, and contribute toward organizational growth. With a little experience, these new professionals begin to focus more clearly on a career path.

The next phase of professional maturation lasts 3 to 5 years. During this time, professionals take a broader view of dietetic practice; they take on increased responsibility and begin to see the relationship between personal growth and career advancement. Many career- minded dietitians and nutritionists seek new positions at this point to gain broader experiences and to create a new environment for further development. This is the time to select a specialization and, if it were not completed earlier, pursue a master's degree.

About 5 to 8 years after graduation, a dietitian would be ready to launch an independent practice or become a consultant. Numerous advanced positions in business and industry require not only a master's degree but also the several years of experience that are needed to fine-tune skills.

Finally, one reaches the last phase of development: professional mastery, marked by self-direction and extensive professional involvement in committees or projects. Work is punctuated with continuing education and activities that bring enrichment and stimulation. This is the time that many professionals shift toward research or university teaching. Others find true fulfillment in advanced dietetic practice. A few use their nutrition backgrounds as springboards for positions in such areas as marketing, sales, health-care administration, communication, and consultation. Some of these opportunities require an MBA degree; for others, a doctorate is essential. Either way, self-motivation provides the impetus for obtaining the needed knowledge, skills, and credentials.

Successful people regularly practice three virtues: they always present themselves in a positive light, they are continually poised for advancement, and they diligently **network** with people who can help them connect with the right opportunities. These are good habits for anyone at every phase of career development.

Where are you going in life? How can a career in nutrition and dietetics help you get there? Remember, most individuals require several "passages" or stages to reach their long-term goals. You'll be more successful if you create a general plan for growth and professional development. Then, in every phase of your career, sell yourself, position yourself for growth and advancement, and create networks that can help you up the ladder of self-fulfillment.

Dr. Schiller is Professor and Director of Medical Dietetics at Ohio State University.

Individual provinces set standards for practice and legal definitions for the use of the title dietitian. It is best to consult each province to find out specific regulations.

How to find a program that leads to an RD credential

To select a college or university that offers an approved or accredited program for RDs in the United States, look in the *Directory of Dietetic Programs* published annually by the American Dietetic Association. This book lists both undergraduate and graduate programs. Your college nutrition and dietetics department may have a copy, and copies may also be found in college libraries or in offices of career guidance counselors. You can also purchase a copy directly from the American Dietetic Association. This book also lists all internships.

For other information about programs or careers in dietetics, write the American Dietetic Association, Department 12, 216 West Jackson Boulevard, Suite 800, Chicago, Illinois 60606. You can also contact them by telephone at 1-800-877-1600 for more information.

Information about Canadian programs is available from the Canadian Dietetic Association, 480 University Avenue, Suite 601 Toronto, Ontario, M5G IV2.

Exploring Issues and Actions

For answers to your initial questions about a career in nutrition, you may want to contact a dietitian at a hospital or through the state dietetic association. Your professor for this class may be an RD or know an RD you can talk to. Consider shadowing a dietitian or other nutrition professional for a day or two to see what the job entails and whether that career looks like the right step for you.

LICENSURE FOR RDS

Initial interest in licensing RDs in the United States began in the early 1970s. A **license** in this case defines the practice capabilities of a person who has earned the RD credential. It may also specifically exclude untrained people from practicing in the nutrition care field. By the late 1980s, most states and U.S. territories were actively involved in licensure and 25 had already passed laws (Table 20-2). Licensure laws may, however, exempt from its jurisdiction certain professionals, such as physicians, pharmacists, teachers of nutrition, and people who were in clinical nutrition practice before passage of the law.

license
Established by a state legislature, a professional license confers on its owner the right to use specific titles or practice specific activities. In some instances, people who are not licensed are prevented from using certain titles and/or practicing some activities.

Some states, like Ohio, have mandatory licensure. The law limits the assessment of nutritional status, nutrition counseling, and setting nutrition standards to licensed dietitians. An RD credential provides automatic licensure. In Ohio, collecting data for nutrition assessment does not require a license, nor does reporting the progress of a person adhering to an established plan of care if the results are consistent with anticipated goals initially written by a dietitian. However, the ultimate responsibility for all nutrition care services lies with the licensed RD in states with mandatory licensure. Nonlicensed persons can be reported to the State Board of Dietetics if found practicing skills that fall within the scope of practice dictated by the licensure law. Appropriate legal action can then be taken.

Other states, such as California, have title acts or voluntary licensure. These protect the use of the titles such as dietitian and/or nutritionist for those people who have met predetermined qualifications set by the state, specifically, earning an RD credential. The laws do not restrict who may offer nutrition advice and services. If you become an RD and practice in a state with a licensure law, contact the local license board in the state capital to find out more details.

Proponents of licensure argue that these laws protect the nutrition field and individuals in the community from people who use the title dietitian or nutritionist but who, nevertheless, practice without qualifications. Without licensure, anyone can practice as a nutritionist and dispense nutrition advice. In many cases, people not qualified to provide nutrition advice have given totally erroneous advice that has led to serious disease and death.

Today we must be wary of people who gain diplomas from correspondence or purchase mail-order certificates to masquerade as nutritionists or other health professionals, despite having little or no training in the field.[1] Licensure for nutrition professionals protects the public, since it requires that people who call themselves dietitians or nutritionists possess the knowledge and skills needed to practice competently.

Table 20-2

Laws that regulate nutrition practice

State/Territory	Type of Regulation*
Alabama	Title Act
Arkansas	Mandatory
California	Title Act
District of Columbia	Mandatory
Florida	Mandatory
Georgia	Voluntary
Iowa	Mandatory
Kansas	Mandatory
Kentucky	Voluntary
Louisiana	Mandatory
Maine	Mandatory
Maryland	Mandatory
Mississippi	Mandatory
Montana	Mandatory
Nebraska	Voluntary
New Mexico	Mandatory
North Dakota	Voluntary
Ohio	Mandatory
Oklahoma	Mandatory
Puerto Rico	Mandatory
Rhode Island	Mandatory
Tennessee	Mandatory
Texas	Voluntary
Utah	Voluntary†
Washington	Voluntary

**Mandatory licensure* (practice act) establishes a state board to protect the scope of practice and professional titles.
Voluntary licensure regulates use of professional titles through a state board.
Title act (entitlement) protects use of professional titles.
†Utah's certification law is similar to voluntary licensure.
Note that the title dietitian is covered by the law, however, the title nutritionist is often not covered by the law.
Adapted from: Minskoff JB and Oudekerk LM: Dietetic currents, Ross Laboratories 14:21, 1987.

SPECIALIZATION IN DIETETIC PRACTICE

Presently there is no formal identification of specialty areas in the field of dietetics, although physicians and nurses can be certified in specialty practice areas. Specialty certifications carry prestige, and many RDs feel that because of the complex cases they deal with, special certification should be established in areas such as renal nutrition and nutrition support in trauma cases, among other areas.[3] These areas require in-depth knowledge and specific advanced practice skills. When specializations are recognized, these areas will most likely be the first ones established.

To qualify for specialty certification, an RD will probably have to complete several years of experience in the area, pass a rigorous specialty exam, and meet other requirements of the specialty board.

DIETETIC TECHNICIANS

Dietetic technicians are another group of nutrition professionals. They graduate from associate degree programs approved by the American Dietetic Association that may require 2 to 4 years of study. Dietetic technicians must also complete a minimum of 450 hours of supervised professional practice. Then, they may elect to take a special registration examination. Once they pass the examination, they can use the DTR credential to signify their level of competence. They are then required to complete 50 hours of approved continuing education classes every 5 years to maintain their DTR status. However, dietetic technicians can practice without this certification if their employers allow them to do so.

Dietetic technicians are employed by hospitals, public health nutrition programs, long-term care facilities, child feeding programs, and food management companies. They usually work under the supervision of an RD. Dietetic technicians in clinical practice often teach normal nutrition and food preparation classes to clients. They may also prepare special diet menus, shopping lists, and budgets for families. They can also assist in performing dietary interviews, screening patients for nutritional problems, calculating special diets, and checking menus to ensure that appropriate foods are chosen.

Dietetic technicians in foodservice are primarily supervised by dietitians in large institutions. In smaller units, such as those in nursing homes and small hospitals, dietetic technicians may work autonomously on a day-to-day basis, but under the direction of an RD who consults for the institution.[9]

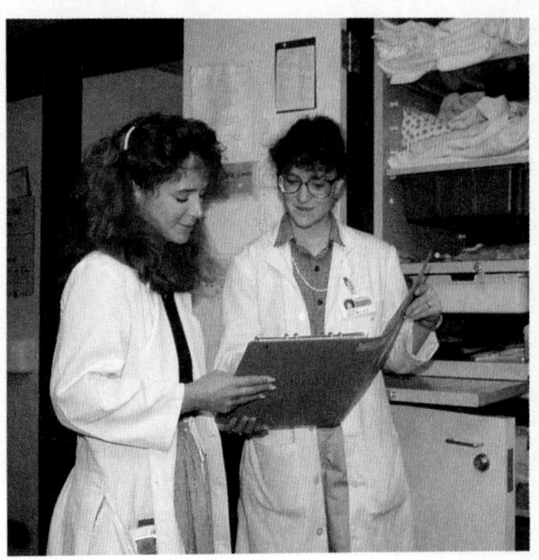

A dietetic technician works under RD supervision, must complete two to four years of college and a minimum of 450 hours of supervised professional practice.

DIETETIC CODE OF ETHICS FOR PRACTICE

Once a nutrition professional accepts the RD or DTR credential, he or she must then abide by the code of ethics for the profession of dietetics adopted by the American Dietetic Association.[2] This code of ethics includes providing professional services that respect the uniqueness of each individual without discriminating on the basis of race, creed, religion, sex, age, or national origin. The person must also fulfill professional commitments in good faith, conduct nutrition practice with honesty and integrity, remain free of conflict of interest, maintain confidentiality of information, provide the most sound and current information available, and comply with all applicable laws and regulations concerning the profession.

Dietetic technicians can become members of the American Dietetic Association.

Concept Check

To obtain an RD credential, a person must complete a specific baccalaureate program that includes courses in foods and nutrition, complete 900 hours of supervised professional practice, and pass a registration examination. The 900 hours of supervised professional practice may be integrated into the junior and senior years of college in some universities or may be obtained after graduation by completing a dietetic internship or an approved pre-professional practice program. A dietetic technician must complete a college program 2 to 4 years in length and have 450 hours of supervised professional practice. Dietetic technicians can elect to take a special registration examination, and if successful, can use the title DTR.

IDENTIFYING A NUTRITION PROFESSIONAL TO HELP YOU

In many states with licensure laws it is easy to identify a nutrition professional, since the titles dietitian and nutritionist are protected. Otherwise, an RD certificate is evidence of competence because all RDs have met and continue to meet rigorous standards set by the American Dietetic Association.

In the absence of these credentials, certain behaviors are expected of a professional nutritionist. In most cases the professional should:

- Ask questions about a client's medical history, life-style, and current eating habits. The professional may request a detailed diet diary be kept to establish a baseline before making major diet changes or recommendations.
- Formulate an individual diet plan—not simply tear a form sheet from a tablet that could apply to almost anyone.

- Schedule follow-up visits to monitor progress, answer any questions, and help keep enthusiasm high.
- When appropriate, involve family members in the diet plan.
- Consult directly with a client's physician, and readily refer one back to the physician for health problems beyond the scope of nutrition practice.

People sometimes try to disguise themselves as nutrition professionals by flaunting a Ph.D. degree from an unrelated field (or correspondence university). Some people may be capable of giving sound advice, while others may promise results that sound too good to be true, such as making weight loss appear easy. They may encourage the use of bogus tests, such as cytotoxic allergy tests or hair analyses. They may promote pills, gimmicks, and gadgets, boast success with numerous testimonials, and generally either refuse to consult a doctor or try to convince the client that a doctor does not have the answer for the ailment.[1]

In essence, a true nutrition professional will provide you much of the advice given in this book, while the con artist will provide numerous other options not considered here. Use this guide to evaluate nutrition credentials. If there were major areas in nutrition science that could contribute to your health, be confident that we would have brought them to your attention. Aside from specific diet therapies for certain health disorders, you already know a lot about the science of nutrition.

Concept Check

To find a nutrition professional, look for the RD credential. It is evidence that a person has completed a rigorous program of coursework, supervised professional practice experience, and passed an examination to verify entry level competence in nutrition practice. If a nutrition advisor does not have an RD credential, the advisor can be gauged by whether he or she formulates an individual plan that includes the client's physician and provides advice consistent with that given in this book.

Summary

1. The title registered dietitian refers to a person who has completed a specific baccalaureate degree program that includes courses in foods and nutrition, at least 900 hours of supervised professional practice, and passed a registration examination. Generally, nutrition professionals in hospitals are known as dietitians and nutrition professionals outside the hospital often use the term nutritionist. In many states, the term nutritionist has no legal meaning. The person may be well-trained in nutrition or have no training at all.
2. The 900 hours of supervised professional practice needed to obtain an RD credential may be integrated into the junior and senior years of college, or be completed through a dietetic internship or an approved preprofessional practice program after graduation.
3. Some states in the United States license dietetic practice. This licensure varies from simply protecting the titles dietitian and nutritionist for those people with specific nutrition training, to excluding anyone without nutrition training from assessing nutritional health or providing nutrition counseling.
4. Dietetic technicians are support personnel for dietitians. Dietetic technician programs are 2 to 4 years in length and contain at least 450 hours of supervised professional practice. Dietetic technicians may elect to take a special registration examination. Once they pass this examination, they can use the credential DTR.
5. The RD credential guarantees that the holder has (1) trained in classroom and practice settings approved by the American Dietetic Association and (2) has

passed a registration examination that assesses the ability to perform as a nutrition professional at entry level. Nutrition professionals without the RD credential should be questioned about their training, and the nutrition advice offered should be consistent with that outlined in this book.

Take Action

POSITIONS AVAILABLE

CLINICAL DIETITIAN
The Indiana Department of Mental Health is seeking clinical dietitians for openings in our JCAHO-accredited facilities at Richmond, Logansport, and Evansville. Responsibilities include direct client services, treatment planning, nutrition assessment, staff supervision, and participation on interdisciplinary treat-

DIETITIAN/SPEAKER, NORTHEAST/WESTERN U.S.
Noncommercial scientific corporation needs dietitians to speak about nutrition. Must have master's/doctoral degree in nutrition, clinical experience, and excellent speaking skills. Audience: health professionals. Excellent pay. Send resumé to: INR Corp., 2425-B Channing Way, Suite 457, Berkeley, CA 94704. We cannot acknowledge all applications.

Assume you decide to pursue a career in nutrition. What kind of setting would you choose? Find advertisements for nutrition positions in journals such as the *Journal of the American Dietetic Association* or *FASEB Journal* (see also Table 20-1). How many positions can you find that might interest you? Are there unanswered questions about the position? Write a letter of inquiry to a prospective employer asking for more details.

REFERENCES

1. ADA Reports: Position of the American Dietetic Association: identifying food and nutrition misinformation, Journal of the American Dietetic Association 89:1589, 1988.
2. ADA Reports: Code of ethics for the profession of dietetics, Journal of the American Dietetic Association 88:1592, 1988.
3. ADA Reports: President's Page: Specialization in dietetics, the time has come, Journal of the American Dietetic Association 86:1072, 1986.
4. ADA Reports: President's Page: The strategic plan: the vision. Journal of the American Dietetic Association 89:110, 1989.
5. Adamow LL and Clipper AJ: Is prospective payment inhibiting the use of nutrition support services? Journal of the American Dietetic Association 85:1616, 1985.
6. American Dietetic Association: A new look at the profession of dietetics, Chicago, 1985 The Association.
7. Bryk JA: Report on the 1986 census of The American Dietetic Association, Journal of the American Dietetic Association 87:1080, 1987.
8. Cantlon AT and Lillios IT: The role of dietitians in a work-site health promotion program, Journal of the American Dietetic Association 86:367, 1986.
9. Finan R: Careers in nutrition and dietetics, Dietetic Educators of Practitioners, The American Dietetic Association (slide-tape series).
10. Hess MA: Reflections on the hundredth monkey: the new consciousness in dietetics, Journal of the American Dietetic Association 88:659, 1988.
11. Kane JK: Exploring careers in dietetics and nutrition, New York, 1987 The Rosen Publishing Group Inc.
12. Kirk D and others: Attributes and qualifications that employers seek when hiring dietitians in business and industry, Journal of the American Dietetic Association 89:494, 1989.
13. Lanz SJ: Introduction to the profession of dietetics, Philadelphia, 1983, Lea & Febiger.
14. Nestle M and Porter D: Federal nutrition policies: impact on dietetic practice, Journal of the American Dietetic Association 89:944, 1989.
15. Ryan AS and others: The role of the clinical dietitian: I. Present professional image and recent image changes, Journal of the American Dietetic Association 88:671, 1988.
16. Shanklin CW and others: Documentation of time expenditures of clinical dietitians: results of a statewide time study in Texas, Journal of the American Dietetic Association 88:38, 1988.
17. Visoccan BJ and Lazin B: Use of a consultant to assist a dietetic association in its media and public relations effort, Journal of the American Dietetic Association 89:513, 1989.

SUGGESTED READINGS

Reading current issues of the *Journal of the American Dietetic Association* will give you a good picture of the diversity and depth of the field of dietetics. The ADA Report on the code of ethics provides valuable information, and the article by Kirk and others about what employers are seeking in a dietician in business and industry is quite practical. The ADA Report on the Strategic Plan: the Vision outlines one view of the future of the field of dietetics, and the article by Hess comments further on how this field should develop. You may see your place in that development.

CHAPTER 20

Answer to nutrition awareness inventory

1. *True.* Currently, many states in the United States license dietitians to practice nutrition care.
2. *False.* RDs in a hospital generally delegate menu writing to support staff, such as dietetic technicians.
3. *True.* All RDs have a baccalaureate degree.
4. *True.* DTR stands for registered dietetic technician. Many, though not all, dietetic technicians are registered.
5. *True.* DTRs must have an associate (2-year) degree.
6. *True.* To obtain the RD credential, 900 hours of supervised professional practice are required.
7. *False.* In some states, nutrition advice can be offered only if a person has earned an RD credential. In other states, however, anyone can offer nutrition advice: no nutrition training is necessary.
8. *False.* Health food stores generally do not employ trained nutrition professionals. Some states allow anyone to label himself a nutritionist.
9. *True.* Hospitals still employ the greatest number of RDs, but the trend is toward employment outside the hospital setting.
10. *True.* RDs can be commissioned as officers in the military, and even advance to a high rank, such as colonel.
11. *False.* Although dietitians and nurses often work together on medical teams, each group has its own separate duties and types of training.
12. *True.* Opportunities for nutrition professionals are increasing because of federal programs in the United States, such as the Women, Infant, and Children program, and because expanding nursing home and home-health–care markets need their expertise.
13. *False. Nutrition Today* is an excellent nutrition magazine. In addition, a variety of newsletters is devoted entirely to nutrition issues.
14. *True.* Any RD may use the term *nutritionist.* However, some states permit only nutrition professionals with an RD credential to use the term *dietitian* or *nutritionist.*
15. *True.* A coordinated program leading to an RD credential combines 900 hours of supervised professional practice with classwork completed in the last 2 years of a baccalaureate degree program. After completing required classwork and practice hours, a graduating student qualifies to take the registration examination for an RD credential.

Nutrition Perspective 20-1

Nutrition and Dietetics—Past and Present

The earliest known written dietary prescriptions were found on stone tablets from Babylonia dated about 2500 BC. As early as 250 BC, references to the measurement of energy needs and specific dietary treatments can be found. The oldest known cookbook originates from approximately 100 BC.

The Chinese left written observations about diabetes mellitus that date to the third century. A Chinese medical book from the seventh century mentions night blindness and its correct dietary cure. A medical book published in Florence in 1478 referred to dietetics—the treatment of disease by diet—as a branch of medicine. The term *diet* was derived from the Greek *diaita,* which means "mode of life."[13]

THE ROOTS OF HOSPITAL DIETETICS

The first authentic record of a hospital menu dates from 1123. From the Middle Ages to the eighteenth century, bread formed the basis of the hospital diet. Scurvy, caused by a lack of vitamin C, was rampant among patients on these diets. During the Crimean War (1853 to 1856), Florence Nightingale organized the food service for troops as part of her job as superintendant of the Female Nursing Corps. By improving the food supply and sanitary conditions, she reduced mortality in the last 5 months of the campaign.

NUTRITION BECOMES A SCIENCE IN THE 1800s

Advances in chemistry and physics made possible a series of experiments in the eighteenth century that granted nutrition its scientific status. Frenchman Antoine Lavoisier is often credited with the first modern nutrition experiments in his studies of digestion and respiration. During this time, Osborn and Mendel, Liebig, and other scientists began to understand more about the composition of living tissues. By 1846, scientists knew that tissues contained carbohydrates, fats, and proteins.

THE DIETETICS PROFESSION EMERGES

The American Medical Association formed a committee on dietetics in 1877 and asked a graduate of a Philadelphia cooking school, Sarah Tyson Rorer, to edit a section in their new publication. She is recognized as the first American dietitian, a term that the 1899 Conference on Home Economics in Lake Placid, New York, stated should apply to persons who specialize in the knowledge of food, and who can meet the demands of the medical profession for diet therapy advice.[13] The term *nutritionist* did not appear until the 1920s, and came into use particularly among community nutrition workers associated with the American Red Cross. Previously, practitioners in the community were called Social Service Dietitians, Social Dietitians, Home Economists, Visiting Housekeepers, and Nutrition Workers.

VITAMINS ARE DISCOVERED IN THE EARLY 1900S

In the early 1900s, nutrition science began to flourish. Casimer Funk isolated a chemical substance he called a "vitamine," which later became the *vitamin,* the term we use today. In 1896, the U.S. Department of Agriculture published Bulletin 28 by W.O. Atwater and A.P. Bryant. It provided detailed food composition tables that dietitians used for many years. Atwater is often credited as the "father" of nutrition science in the United States.

EDUCATION FOR DIETITIANS IS DEFINED

In 1890, John Hopkins University became the first university to offer courses in nutrition and dietetics. The first course enabling students to become dietitians began in 1903. It lasted 3 months and was the forerunner of the dietetic internship. Dietitians of this era fought food fads and fallacies among the general public, much the same as today. One popular notion was "fletcherizing," chewing each mouthful of food 32 times (once for each

Continued.

Nutrition Perspective 20-1—cont'd

Nurition and Dietetics—Past and Present

tooth) before swallowing. This method allowed Horace Fletcher to lose a massive amount of weight but it still was considered an ineffective nutritional measure in its time. This was also the time of John Harvey Kellogg and other proponents of whole grains and natural foods who provided the many "battles" in Battle Creek described in Chapter 4.

THE AMERICAN DIETETIC ASSOCIATION IS ESTABLISHED

The American Dietetic Association as we know it today began in 1917 when Lenna Cooper and Lula Graves brought together a group of professionals employed in hospital foodservice to discuss means by which dietitians could best serve hospitals and the war needs of World War I. The following year, 1918, they held the first official meeting of The American Dietetic Association. E.V. McCollum was the first speaker, probably America's most eminent nutrition scientist. He presented a paper on his recent findings with the new vitamins called "A," "B," and "C". By 1922, established custom required all professionals entering the dietetics field to have completed 4 years of academic courses plus an intensive period of internship. In 1924, The American Dietetic Association was legally incorporated and, in 1925, the first *Journal of The American Dietetic Association* was mailed to its members. By 1945, the U.S. Congress gave full military status to dietitians and, in 1947, dietitians in the Woman's Medical Specialist Corps obtained permanent military status as commissioned officers.

NUTRITION KNOWLEDGE EXPANDS

In the 1930s and 1940s, nutrition knowledge expanded rapidly. Symptoms of an essential fatty acid deficiency were described in 1929, vitamin C was extracted from lemon juice in 1932, zinc was determined to be essential in the diets of rats in 1934, and thiamin was synthesized in 1936. The first RDA were published in 1943.

After World War II, a "health team" concept gained momentum, and the dietitian was an important member of it. The American Dietetic Association published its first edition of the *Handbook of Diet Therapy* in 1946. A major study to identify risk factors for heart disease started in Framingham, Massachusetts in 1949 and, in the 1950s, many studies extended examinations of complex nutrition and health issues, such as coronary heart disease and cancer.

In the 1960s, researchers first suggested the importance of non-nutrient components in the diet, such as fiber. The effects of human deficiencies of zinc and vitamin B-6 were first described. In 1968, the possibility of providing total parenteral nutrition to a young child was demonstrated. This ushered in a new era of dietetic practice—intensive nutrition support.

HEALTH AND NUTRITION ARE LINKED IN A COMPREHENSIVE VIEW

In the 1960s and 1970s, government groups surveyed the nutritional status of populations in Canada and the United States. In addition, the U.S. Congress initiated and/or expanded the USDA's food assistance programs to low-income families. These programs include the Food Stamp Program, School Lunch and Breakfast Programs, and supplemental feeding programs for women, infants, children, and the elderly. In 1977, the Senate Select Committee on Nutrition and Human Needs focused on the role of diet in the cause and prevention of chronic disease. The first registration examination for dietitians was administered in 1970.

NEW VIEWS DICTATED BY THE 1980S

The 1980s are notable for the first description of prostaglandin substances, as well as the potential importance of omega-3 fatty acids, found in high concentration in fish oils. The 1980s also are known for innovations in health promotion. Finally, the switch to determining medical reimbursement based on disease type rather than on length of hospital stay caused great upheaval in the delivery of medical care. That development encouraged the RD to look outside the hospital for practice settings.

WHAT WILL THE FUTURE HOLD?

The role of nutrition and dietetics in the future could depend on you.[10] Many research questions remain unanswered. Smarter and more effective methods for the delivery of nutrition services need to be developed. If you enjoy working with people, enjoy science and business, and have an internal drive to make things better, then you may have what it takes to be a successful registered dietitian, food scientist, educator, researcher, or other food and nutrition professional. *Within this group of professionals are some of the most educated, committed, and personable people found anywhere.*

Nutritional Perspective 20-2

An RD Credential is Just the Start

BY DONNA HAVERSTOCK, MS, RD

The employment opportunities for dietitians are diverse and exciting. Some newer, nontraditional roles for dietitians include working in business and industry and in the media. These career paths require some specific skills and attributes that should be developed as soon as possible in an undergraduate curriculum.

Food and nutrition used to have a therapeutic connection. Now, we look at food and nutrition as a route to health promotion and disease prevention. This new perspective provides an ideal climate for dietitians to market their expertise to business and industry and to the consumer.

Because of the increasing competitive business environment, business and industry employers view dietitians as a means to increasing the credibility of their organization, their understanding of consumers' nutrition needs and interests, and, ultimately, their business, particularly in the health-care sector.

Good communication skills, both verbal and written, are essential to a position in business and industry. Major responsibilities of dietitians include providing technical information, participating in food and trade shows, developing marketing and sales strategies, and conducting seminars. These responsibilities all require the ability to write clearly and concisely and to speak with self confidence. Dietetic students should develop these skills by taking writing, journalism and public speaking classes.

Other requirements include registration status, knowledge of the food business, and a varied background. Prior work experience in a subject area, whether professional or volunteer, is important. For those making the transition from a clinical position or newly entering the job market, get some marketing or public relations experience. Volunteer to write press releases for a local chapter of a health promotion organization, such as the American Heart Association. Offer to do a nutrition and health segment on a local radio station. These activities will strengthen your skills, confidence and your resume. In addition, an MBA degree is becoming increasingly important as more dietitians enter the industry.

Continued.

Nutrition Perspective 20-2—cont'd

An RD Credential is Just the Start

Although one can gain work experience through several avenues, some attributes you must develop for yourself. Some key attributes include a pleasant personality, professional appearance, creativeness, planning and implementation skills, a strong work drive, sales skills, and perseverance. In many instances, you will be creating a new position for yourself within a company. Selling yourself with aggressive confidence is important.

There is also much to be said for being in the right place at the right time. Thus making contacts in the industry through professional "networking" is essential. Attend meetings where you are likely to meet potential employers.

Join professional organizations, such as Dietitians in Business and Industry, a practice group of the American Dietetic Association, to keep in touch with new job openings and opportunities. There are many challenging positions out there for dietitians if you're prepared and persistent. Here are some typical job positions for dietitians in business and industry:

- Account managers for advertising and public relations firms
- Brand managers for food product companies
- Equipment specialists for retail and foodservice businesses
- Editors and writers for magazines, newspapers, and publishers
- Foodservice directors and multi-unit managers of nursing homes, hospitals, schools, and executive dining rooms
- Food standard directors for restaurant chains
- Consumer affairs specialists for supermarket chains
- Food stylists
- Purchasing managers for restaurant and hospital groups
- Market research managers for food and equipment companies
- Sales representatives and sales managers for food brokers, distributors, and manufacturers
- Software specialists
- Test kitchen managers and directors
- Association executives for food and health-care promotion organizations
- Self-employed consultant to the food, pharmaceutical, and health industries
- Television/radio consumer reporters and producers
- Media spokesperson for the food, pharmaceutical, and health industries

A CASE IN POINT: ONE DIETITIAN'S CLIMB UP THE NONTRADITIONAL LADDER

A nontraditional career in dietetics can begin right after college or after having had more a traditional experience. With a BS degree in foods and nutrition, I entered the U.S. Army Medical Corp, as a second lieutenant, to do my internship training. After 2 years and a promotion to first lieutenant, I wasn't satisfied with hospital dietetics. I thought perhaps it was military dietetics I didn't care for, so I gave it another try. After 6 months as a clinical dietitian in a mid-size community hospital, I knew I had to change directions. My beginning work experiences were structured and traditional and it wasn't for me.

Although I wanted to be in business, industry, or communications, I had no skills to help me compete in that world. I attended a unique graduate program at Boston University and received a master's degree in nutrition communications. It wasn't the answer to a new career, but it gave me some new skills and the confidence that there were other jobs out there for a dietitian. While attending graduate school, I worked part-time at an advertising agency, which serviced foodservice clients, and also did consumer reporting—for no pay—at a local cable television station. I knew good writing skills and television experience would come in handy.

It took almost 10 months to land a job in business after graduate school, but I accepted a sales position, covering 7 states, for a manufacturer of foodservice frozen entrees. My accounts included all types of foodservice establishments but particularly health-care accounts.

After this experience "out on the street," I took a position as promotion manager at an advertising agency for several of their food accounts. It didn't have much to do with nutrition, but after all, I'm a dietitian, and it was related to food. Learning how the creative and business side of an agency works was valuable experience.

Ready for more responsibility, I spent the next 4 years at the Campbell Soup Company as manager of the consumer nutrition center. This was a public relations/marketing function that included acting as a corporate spokesperson (the media experience was handy), writing brochures, developing direct mail programs to doctors and dietitians, speaking to professional and consumer groups, providing nutrition guidance on new products, and a variety of other marketing-related tasks. I learned all facets of the food business and made lots of contacts in the industry. Industry knowledge and networking contacts gave me the confidence to then go into business for myself.

I've been an entrepreneur for over 2 years now. It means constantly selling yourself and your expertise, as well as actually doing the work. My clients are food companies, and I provide many different services to them—everything from recipe development to nutrition labeling. I also write freelance articles for consumer and trade magazines and speak at health professional conferences whenever possible. These activities help increase my visibility and credibility. I'm interested in developing my business internationally; I have a client in France and also do work for a U.S. client in Canada and Puerto Rico.

It's definitely not a 9 to 5 job, and there's no guaranteed paycheck. The responsibility is all mine and I make all the decisions. Yet I wouldn't want it any other way.

Appendixes

Appendix A
Food Composition Tables

Nutritive Components for Baby Foods

Food Name	Serving	Gm wt	KCAL Kc	PROT Gm	CARB Gm	FAT Gm	CHOL Mg	SAFA Gm	SOD Mg	POT Mg	MAG Mg
BABY-TEETHING BISCUITS	1 item	11.0	43.00	1.200	8.400	0.500	—	—	40.00	35.00	4.000
BABY-MIXED CEREAL/MILK	1 srvg	28.4	32.00	1.300	4.500	1.000	—	—	13.00	56.00	8.000
BABY-OATMEAL CEREAL/MILK	1 srvg	28.4	33.00	1.400	4.300	1.200	—	—	13.00	58.00	10.00
BABY-RICE CEREAL/MILK	1 srvg	28.4	33.00	1.100	4.700	1.000	—	—	13.00	54.00	13.00
BABY-CEREAL & EGG YOLKS	1 srvg	28.4	15.00	0.500	2.000	0.500	18.00	0.170	9.000	11.00	1.000
BABY-COOKIE-ARROWROOT	1 item	6.0	24.00	0.400	4.300	0.900	—	0.200	22.00	9.000	1.000
BABY-APPLE BETTY	1 srvg	28.4	20.00	0.100	5.600	0.000	—	—	3.000	14.00	—
BABY-BEEF & EGG NOODLES	1 srvg	28.4	15.00	0.600	2.000	0.500	—	—	8.000	13.00	2.000
BABY-BEEF LASAGNA	1 srvg	28.4	22.00	1.200	2.800	0.600	—	—	129.0	35.00	3.000
BABY-BEEF STEW	1 srvg	28.4	14.00	1.400	1.500	0.300	3.550	0.160	98.00	40.00	3.000
BABY-MIXED VEGETABLES	1 srvg	28.4	11.00	0.300	2.700	0.000	—	—	2.000	34.00	—
BABY-TURKEY & RICE	1 srvg	28.4	14.00	0.500	2.100	0.400	2.840	0.120	5.000	12.00	—
BABY-VEAL & VEGETABLES	1 srvg	28.4	20.00	1.700	1.700	0.800	—	—	7.000	43.00	2.000
BABY-ORANGE JUICE	1 fl oz	31.0	14.00	0.200	3.200	0.100	—	—	0.000	57.00	3.000
BABY-EGG YOLKS	1 srvg	28.4	58.00	2.800	0.300	4.900	223.0	1.470	11.00	22.00	2.000
BABY-APPLE BLUEBERRY	1 srvg	28.4	17.00	0.100	4.600	0.100	0.000	—	0.000	20.00	—
BABY-APPLESAUCE	1 srvg	28.4	12.00	0.100	3.100	0.000	0.000	0.000	1.000	20.00	1.000
BABY-PEACHES	1 srvg	28.4	20.00	0.100	5.400	0.000	0.000	0.000	2.000	46.00	2.000
BABY-PEARS	1 srvg	28.4	12.00	0.100	3.100	0.000	0.000	0.000	1.000	37.00	2.000
BABY-APPLE JUICE	1 fl oz	31.0	14.00	0.000	3.600	0.000	0.000	0.000	1.000	28.00	1.000
BABY-APPLE PEACH JUICE	1 fl oz	31.0	13.00	0.000	3.200	0.000	0.000	0.000	—	30.00	1.000
BABY-BEEF	1 srvg	28.4	30.00	3.900	0.000	1.500	—	0.730	23.00	62.00	5.000
BABY-CHICKEN	1 srvg	28.4	37.00	3.900	0.000	2.200	—	0.580	13.00	40.00	4.000
BABY-HAM	1 srvg	28.4	32.00	3.900	0.000	1.600	—	0.550	12.00	58.00	4.000
BABY-LAMB	1 srvg	28.4	29.00	4.000	0.000	1.300	—	0.660	18.00	58.00	4.000
BABY-PORK	1 srvg	28.4	35.00	4.000	0.000	2.000	—	0.680	12.00	63.00	3.000
BABY-TURKEY	1 srvg	28.4	32.00	4.000	0.000	1.700	—	0.540	16.00	65.00	4.000
BABY-PRETZELS	1 item	6.0	24.00	0.700	4.900	0.100	—	—	16.00	8.000	2.000
BABY-BEANS-GREEN	1 srvg	28.4	7.000	0.400	1.700	0.000	0.000	0.000	1.000	45.00	7.000
BABY-BEETS	1 srvg	28.4	10.00	0.400	2.200	0.000	0.000	0.000	24.00	52.00	4.000
BABY-CARROTS	1 srvg	28.4	8.000	0.200	1.700	0.000	0.000	0.000	11.00	56.00	3.000
BABY-CORN-CREAMED	1 srvg	28.4	16.00	0.400	4.000	0.100	—	—	12.00	26.00	2.000
BABY-GARDEN VEGETABLES	1 srvg	28.4	11.00	0.700	1.900	0.100	—	—	10.00	48.00	6.000
BABY-PEAS-CREAMED	1 srvg	28.4	15.00	0.600	2.500	0.500	—	—	4.000	25.00	—
BABY-PEAS	1 srvg	28.4	11.00	1.000	2.300	0.100	—	—	1.000	32.00	4.000
BABY-SPINACH-CREAMED	1 srvg	28.4	11.00	0.700	1.600	0.400	—	—	14.00	54.00	16.00
BABY-SQUASH	1 srvg	28.4	7.000	0.200	1.600	0.100	—	—	1.000	51.00	3.000
BABY-SWEET POTATOES	1 srvg	28.4	16.00	0.300	3.700	0.000	—	0.000	6.000	75.00	4.000
BABY-ZWIEBACK	1 piece	29.5	30.00	0.700	5.200	0.700	1.460	0.280	16.00	21.00	1.000
BABY-BEANS-GREEN-BUTTERED	1 srvg	28.4	9.000	0.300	1.900	0.200	—	—	1.000	45.00	—
BABY-LIVER	1 srvg	28.4	29.00	4.100	0.400	1.100	52.00	0.390	21.00	64.00	4.000

Key To Abbreviations:

V-A, vitamin A
V-ET, vitamin ET
V-C, Vitamin C
THIA, thiamine
RIBO, riboflavin
NIAC, niacin
V-B6, Vitamin B6
FOL, folate
V-B12, Vitamin B-12
CALC, Calcium
PHOS, phosphorus
SEL, selenium
FIBD,
Mg, milligrams
Gm, grams
IU, International units
Ug, micrograms

IRON Mg	ZINC Mg	V-A IU	V-ET Mg	V-C Mg	THIA Mg	RIBO Mg	NIAC Mg	V-B6 Mg	FOL Ug	V-B12 Ug	CALC Mg	PHOS Mg	SEL Mg	FIBD Gm
0.390	0.102	13.00	—	1.000	0.026	0.059	0.476	0.012	—	0.008	29.00	18.00	—	—
2.960	0.202	30.00	0.287	0.300	0.122	0.165	1.640	0.019	3.200	—	62.00	40.00	—	0.000
3.440	0.262	30.00	0.241	0.400	0.143	0.160	1.700	0.017	2.800	—	62.00	45.00	0.001	—
3.460	0.182	30.00	0.236	0.300	0.132	0.142	1.480	0.032	2.300	—	68.00	50.00	0.001	0.000
0.130	0.081	40.00	0.111	0.200	0.003	0.012	0.014	0.006	0.900	0.020	7.000	11.00	—	0.000
0.180	0.032	—	0.014	0.300	0.030	0.026	0.344	0.002	—	0.004	2.000	7.000	—	0.000
0.050	—	5.000	0.065	9.800	0.004	0.010	0.013	—	0.100	—	5.000	—	—	0.000
0.120	0.106	233.0	0.088	0.300	0.010	0.012	0.205	0.014	1.400	0.026	3.000	8.000	0.003	—
0.250	0.198	330.0	0.088	0.500	0.020	0.025	0.384	0.020	—	—	5.000	11.00	—	—
0.200	0.247	467.0	0.088	0.900	0.004	0.018	0.372	0.021	—	—	3.000	12.00	0.003	0.340
0.090	—	773.0	0.207	0.800	0.004	0.009	0.142	—	2.300	—	6.000	—	0.000	—
0.070	—	173.0	0.088	0.300	0.001	0.006	0.087	0.009	0.900	—	6.000	6.000	—	0.000
0.170	0.284	77.00	0.088	0.500	0.006	0.021	0.457	0.024	—	0.128	3.000	15.00	—	—
0.050	0.017	17.00	0.211	19.40	0.014	0.009	0.074	0.017	8.200	—	4.000	3.000	0.000	—
0.780	0.543	355.0	0.471	0.400	0.020	0.075	0.007	0.045	26.10	0.437	22.00	81.00	0.005	0.000
0.060	—	6.000	0.193	7.900	0.005	0.010	0.034	0.010	1.000	—	1.000	2.000	0.000	—
0.060	0.007	5.000	0.193	10.90	0.003	0.008	0.017	0.009	0.500	—	1.000	2.000	0.000	—
0.070	0.024	46.00	0.193	8.900	0.003	0.009	0.173	0.004	1.100	—	2.000	3.000	0.000	—
0.070	0.021	9.000	0.193	7.000	0.004	0.008	0.054	0.002	1.000	—	2.000	3.000	0.000	—
0.180	0.009	6.000	0.211	18.00	0.002	0.005	0.026	0.009	0.000	—	1.000	2.000	0.000	—
0.170	0.008	19.00	0.211	18.10	0.002	0.003	0.066	0.007	0.400	—	1.000	1.000	0.000	—
0.420	0.696	52.00	0.119	0.600	0.003	0.040	0.808	0.040	1.600	0.403	2.000	24.00	0.003	0.000
0.400	0.343	38.00	0.119	0.500	0.004	0.043	0.923	0.057	2.900	—	18.00	27.00	0.003	0.000
0.290	0.637	11.00	0.119	0.600	0.039	0.044	0.746	0.071	0.600	—	2.000	23.00	0.003	0.000
0.420	0.781	24.00	0.119	0.300	0.005	0.057	0.829	0.043	0.600	0.621	2.000	27.00	0.004	0.000
0.280	0.644	11.00	0.119	0.500	0.041	0.058	0.643	0.058	0.500	0.281	1.000	27.00	0.004	0.000
0.340	0.519	159.0	0.119	0.600	0.005	0.059	1.040	0.051	3.200	0.284	7.000	36.00	0.003	0.000
0.230	0.047	0.000	0.046	0.200	0.028	0.021	0.214	0.005	—	—	1.000	7.000	—	0.000
0.210	0.058	127.0	0.207	1.500	0.007	0.024	0.098	0.011	9.800	—	11.00	6.000	0.000	—
0.090	0.034	9.000	0.207	0.700	0.003	0.012	0.037	0.007	8.700	—	4.000	4.000	—	—
0.100	0.043	3249	0.204	1.600	0.007	0.011	0.131	0.021	4.200	—	6.000	6.000	0.000	—
0.080	0.054	21.00	0.207	0.600	0.004	0.013	0.145	0.012	3.200	0.005	6.000	9.000	—	—
0.240	0.074	1720	0.207	1.600	0.017	0.020	0.221	0.028	11.40	—	8.000	8.000	0.000	—
0.160	0.110	24.00	0.207	0.500	0.025	0.016	0.230	0.013	6.400	0.023	4.000	9.000	—	—
0.270	0.099	160.0	0.207	1.900	0.023	0.017	0.289	0.020	7.400	—	6.000	12.00	0.000	—
0.180	0.088	1182	0.207	2.500	0.004	0.029	0.061	0.021	17.20	—	25.00	15.00	—	—
0.080	0.040	574.0	0.207	2.200	0.003	0.016	0.100	0.018	4.400	—	7.000	4.000	0.000	—
0.100	0.058	1825	0.207	2.800	0.008	0.009	0.101	0.026	2.800	—	4.000	7.000	0.000	—
0.040	0.038	4.000	—	0.400	0.015	0.017	0.092	0.006	—	—	1.000	4.000	—	0.000
0.360	—	129.0	0.207	2.300	0.005	0.030	0.096	—	8.100	—	18.00	—	0.170	—
1.500	0.844	10810	0.119	5.500	0.014	0.514	2.360	0.097	95.70	0.612	1.000	58.00	0.007	0.000

Nutritive Components for Beverages

Food Name	Serving	Gm wt	KCAL Kc	PROT Gm	CARB Gm	FAT Gm	CHOL Mg	SAFA Gm	SOD Mg	POT Mg	MAG Mg
BEER-LIGHT	1 fl oz	29.5	8.000	0.100	0.400	0.000	0.000	0.000	1.000	5.000	1.000
BEER-REGULAR	1 fl oz	29.7	12.00	0.100	1.100	0.000	0.000	0.000	2.000	7.000	2.000
CARN INST BREAK-CHOC-ENV	1 item	36.0	130.0	7.000	23.00	1.000	—	—	136.0	422.0	80.00
BRANDY/COGNAC-PONY	1 item	30.0	73.00	—	—	—	—	—	—	—	—
CHAMPAGNE-DOMESTIC-GLASS	1 item	120.0	84.00	0.200	3.000	—	—	—	—	—	—
CHOC BEV DRINK-NO MILK-DRY	1 srvg	28.0	97.70	0.924	25.30	0.868	0.000	0.513	58.80	165.0	27.40
CIDER-FERMENTED	1 fl oz	30.0	11.80	—	0.300	—	—	—	0.000	—	—
CLUB SODA	1 fl oz	29.6	0.000	0.000	0.000	0.000	0.000	0.000	6.000	0.000	0.000
COFFEE-BREWED	1 fl oz	30.0	1.000	0.000	0.100	0.000	0.000	0.000	1.000	16.00	2.000
COFFEE-INSTANT-PREPARED	1 fl oz	30.3	0.610	0.000	0.121	0.000	0.000	0.000	0.910	10.90	1.210
COFFEE SUBSTITUTE-PREPARED	1 fl oz	30.3	1.520	0.030	0.192	0.000	0.000	0.000	1.210	7.270	1.210
COLA-TYPE-SODA	1 fl oz	30.8	13.30	0.000	3.200	0.000	0.000	0.000	1.000	0.000	0.000
SANKA-DECAF-PREPARED	1 fl oz	29.8	0.364	0.000	0.182	0.000	—	—	0.000	10.00	—
CORDIALS/LIQUEUR-54-PROOF	1 fl oz	34.0	97.00	—	11.50	0.000	—	0.000	1.000	1.000	0.000
CREAM SODA	1 fl oz	30.9	16.00	0.000	4.100	0.000	0.000	0.000	4.000	0.000	0.000
DIET SOFT DRINK	1 fl oz	29.6	0.000	0.000	0.000	0.000	0.000	0.000	2.000	0.000	0.000
FRUIT PUNCH DRINK-CAN	1 fl oz	31.0	14.00	0.000	3.700	0.000	0.000	0.000	7.000	8.000	1.000
GINGER ALE-SODA	1 fl oz	30.5	10.00	0.000	2.700	0.000	0.000	0.000	2.000	0.000	0.000
HOT COCOA-PREP/MILK-HOME	1 cup	250.0	218.0	9.100	25.80	9.050	33.00	5.610	123.0	480.0	56.00
KOOL AID-CHERRY-MIX-DRY	1 srvg	28.4	107.0	0.000	27.00	0.000	0.000	0.000	39.80	17.00	—
LEMON LIME SODA-7UP	1 fl oz	30.7	12.00	0.000	3.200	0.000	0.000	0.000	3.000	0.000	0.000
OVALTINE-CHOC-PREP/MILK	1 cup	265.0	227.0	9.530	29.20	8.790	—	—	228.0	600.0	52.00
PERRIER-MINERAL WATER	1 cup	237.0	0.000	0.000	0.000	0.000	0.000	0.000	3.000	0.000	1.000
POSTUM-INST GRAIN BEV-DRY	1 srvg	28.4	103.0	1.930	24.10	0.028	0.000	0.000	28.40	896.0	—
ROOT BEER-SODA	1 fl oz	30.8	13.60	0.000	3.300	0.000	0.000	0.000	4.000	0.000	0.000
TANG-INST DRINK-ORANGE-DRY	1 srvg	28.4	104.0	0.000	26.10	0.000	0.000	0.000	12.80	80.90	—
TEA-BREWED	1 fl oz	29.6	0.000	0.000	0.100	0.000	0.000	0.000	1.000	11.00	1.000
TEA-HERB-BREWED	1 fl oz	29.6	1.000	0.000	0.100	0.000	0.000	0.000	0.000	3.000	0.000
TEA-INSTANT-PREP-SWEETENED	1 cup	259.0	87.00	0.100	22.10	0.100	0.000	0.008	—	50.00	5.000
TEA-INSTANT-PREP-UNSWEET	1 cup	237.0	2.000	0.100	0.400	0.000	0.000	0.000	8.000	47.00	5.000
TONIC WATER-QUININE SODA	1 fl oz	30.5	10.00	0.000	2.700	0.000	0.000	0.000	1.000	0.000	0.000
WATER	1 cup	237.0	0.000	0.000	0.000	0.000	0.000	0.000	7.000	1.000	2.000
WHIS/GIN/RUM/VOD-80 PROOF	1 fl oz	27.8	64.00	0.000	0.000	0.000	0.000	0.000	0.000	1.000	0.000
WHIS/GIN/RUM/VOD-86 PROOF	1 fl oz	27.8	69.00	0.000	0.000	0.000	0.000	0.000	0.000	1.000	0.000
WHIS/GIN/RUM/VOD-90 PROOF	1 fl oz	27.7	73.00	0.000	0.000	0.000	0.000	0.000	1.000	0.000	0.000
WHIS/GIN/RUM/VOD-94 PROOF	1 fl oz	27.8	76.50	0.000	0.000	0.000	0.000	0.000	0.000	0.000	0.000
WHIS/GIN/RUM/VOD-100 PROOF	1 fl oz	27.8	82.00	0.000	0.000	0.000	0.000	0.000	0.000	0.000	0.000
WINE-DESSERT	1 fl oz	30.0	46.00	0.100	3.500	0.000	0.000	0.000	3.000	28.00	3.000
WINE-RED-TABLE	1 fl oz	29.5	21.00	0.100	0.500	0.000	0.000	0.000	19.00	40.70	4.000
WINE-ROSE-TABLE	1 fl oz	29.5	21.00	0.000	0.400	0.000	0.000	0.000	1.000	29.00	3.000
WINE-VERMOUTH-DRY-GLASS	1 item	100.0	105.0	0.000	1.000	0.000	0.000	0.000	4.000	75.00	—
WINE-VERMOUTH-SWEET-GLASS	1 item	100.0	167.0	0.000	12.00	0.000	0.000	0.000	—	—	—
WINE-WHITE-TABLE	1 fl oz	29.5	20.00	0.000	0.200	0.000	0.000	0.000	18.00	33.30	3.000
WINE COOLER-WHITE WINE/7UP	1 srvg	102.0	54.90	0.050	5.720	0.000	0.000	0.000	7.480	41.00	5.000
GATORADE-THIRST QUENCHER	1 fl oz	30.1	7.000	0.000	1.900	0.000	0.000	0.000	12.00	3.000	0.000

Nutritive Components for Breads

Food Name	Serving	Gm wt	KCAL Kc	PROT Gm	CARB Gm	FAT Gm	CHOL Mg	SAFA Gm	SOD Mg	POT Mg	MAG Mg
BAGEL-EGG	1 item	55.0	163.0	6.020	30.90	1.410	8.000	0.500	198.0	40.70	11.00
BAGEL-WATER	1 item	55.0	163.0	6.020	30.90	1.410	—	0.200	198.0	40.70	11.00
BISCUITS-PREPARED/MIX	1 item	28.0	93.20	2.070	13.60	3.320	—	0.600	262.0	56.00	6.720
BREAD-CORN-HOME REC	1 slice	45.0	108.0	2.210	15.60	3.940	0.000	—	126.0	42.30	8.100
BREAD-CRACKED WHEAT	1 slice	25.0	65.50	2.320	12.50	0.868	0.000	0.100	108.0	33.30	8.750

Continued.

IRON Mg	ZINC Mg	V-A IU	V-ET Mg	V-C Mg	THIA Mg	RIBO Mg	NIAC Mg	V-B6 Mg	FOL Ug	VB12 Ug	CALC Mg	PHOS Mg	SEL Mg	FIBD Gm
0.010	0.010	0.000	—	0.000	0.003	0.009	0.116	0.010	1.200	0.000	1.000	4.000	0.000	—
0.010	0.000	0.000	—	0.000	0.002	0.008	0.135	0.015	1.800	0.010	1.000	4.000	—	—
4.500	3.000	1750	5.000	27.00	0.300	0.070	5.000	0.400	0.000	0.600	100.0	150.0	—	—
—	—	—	—	—	—	—	—	—	—	—	—	—	—	—
—	—	—	—	—	—	—	—	—	—	—	—	—	—	—
0.879	0.434	5.600	0.630	0.196	0.010	0.041	0.143	0.003	—	0.000	10.40	35.80	—	—
—	—	—	—	—	—	—	—	—	—	—	—	—	—	—
—	0.030	0.000	—	0.000	0.000	0.000	0.000	0.000	0.000	0.000	1.000	0.000	—	0.000
0.120	0.000	0.000	—	0.000	0.000	0.000	0.066	0.000	0.000	0.000	1.000	0.000	0.000	0.000
0.015	0.009	0.000	—	0.000	0.000	0.000	0.088	0.000	0.000	0.000	0.910	0.910	0.000	0.000
0.018	0.009	—	—	—	—	0.000	0.065	—	—	0.000	0.910	2.120	—	0.000
0.010	0.000	0.000	—	0.000	0.000	0.000	0.000	0.000	0.000	0.000	1.000	4.000	—	0.000
—	—	—	—	—	—	—	—	—	—	—	—	—	—	—
0.020	0.020	—	—	0.000	—	—	—	—	—	—	0.000	0.000	—	—
0.020	0.022	0.000	—	0.000	0.000	0.000	0.000	0.000	0.000	0.000	2.000	0.000	—	0.000
0.010	0.020	0.000	—	0.000	0.001	0.007	0.000	0.000	0.000	0.000	1.000	3.000	—	0.000
0.060	0.040	4.000	—	9.200	0.007	0.007	0.007	0.000	0.400	0.000	2.000	0.000	0.000	0.000
0.050	0.020	0.000	—	0.000	0.000	0.000	0.000	0.000	0.000	0.000	1.000	0.000	—	0.000
0.780	1.220	318.0	—	2.400	0.102	0.435	0.365	0.107	12.00	0.870	298.0	270.0	—	0.300
0.028	—	0.000	—	10.80	0.000	0.000	0.000	—	—	—	47.40	0.000	—	—
0.020	0.020	0.000	0.000	0.000	0.000	0.000	0.005	0.000	0.000	0.000	1.000	0.000	—	0.000
4.770	1.130	2343	—	29.00	0.630	0.970	12.70	0.766	29.00	0.871	392.0	302.0	—	—
0.000	0.000	0.000	—	0.000	0.000	0.000	0.000	0.000	0.000	0.000	32.00	0.000	—	0.000
1.870	—	0.000	—	0.000	0.165	0.076	6.760	—	—	—	76.70	189.0	—	0.000
0.015	0.020	0.000	—	0.000	0.000	0.000	0.000	0.000	0.000	0.000	2.000	0.000	—	0.000
0.028	—	1782	—	107.0	0.000	0.000	0.000	—	—	—	71.00	75.80	—	—
0.010	0.010	0.000	—	0.000	0.000	0.004	0.000	0.000	1.500	0.000	0.000	0.000	0.000	0.000
0.020	0.010	0.000	0.000	0.000	0.003	0.001	0.000	0.000	0.200	0.000	1.000	0.000	—	0.000
0.050	0.080	0.000	—	0.000	0.000	0.047	0.093	—	9.600	0.000	6.000	3.000	0.000	—
0.040	0.080	0.000	—	0.000	0.000	0.005	0.088	0.005	0.700	0.000	5.000	3.000	0.000	0.000
—	—	0.000	0.000	0.000	0.000	0.000	0.000	0.000	0.000	0.000	0.000	0.000	—	0.000
0.010	0.060	0.000	—	0.000	0.000	0.000	0.000	0.000	0.000	0.000	5.000	0.000	—	0.000
0.030	0.020	0.000	0.000	0.000	0.002	0.000	0.000	0.000	0.000	0.000	0.000	1.000	0.000	0.000
0.010	0.010	0.000	0.000	0.000	0.002	0.000	0.014	0.000	0.000	0.000	0.000	2.000	0.000	0.000
0.000	0.000	0.000	0.000	0.000	0.000	0.000	0.000	0.000	0.000	0.000	0.000	0.000	0.000	0.000
0.010	0.010	0.000	0.000	0.000	0.002	0.001	0.004	0.000	0.000	0.000	0.000	1.000	—	0.000
0.010	0.010	0.000	0.000	0.000	0.002	0.001	0.004	0.000	0.000	0.000	0.000	1.000	—	0.000
0.070	0.020	—	—	0.000	0.005	0.005	0.064	0.000	0.100	0.000	2.000	3.000	—	0.000
0.130	0.030	0.000	—	0.000	0.001	0.008	0.024	0.010	0.600	0.000	2.000	4.000	—	0.000
0.110	0.020	—	—	0.000	0.001	0.005	0.022	0.007	0.300	0.000	2.000	4.000	—	0.000
—	—	—	—	—	0.010	0.010	0.200	—	—	—	8.000	—	0.005	0.000
—	—	—	—	—	—	—	—	—	—	—	—	—	—	0.000
0.090	0.020	0.000	—	0.000	0.001	0.001	0.020	0.004	0.100	0.000	3.000	4.000	—	0.000
0.193	0.063	—	—	—	0.002	0.003	0.043	0.007	0.100	0.000	6.110	6.950	—	—
0.020	0.010	0.000	0.000	0.000	0.002	0.000	0.000	0.000	0.000	0.000	0.000	3.000	—	0.000

IRON Mg	ZINC Mg	V-A IU	V-ET Mg	V-C Mg	THIA Mg	RIBO Mg	NIAC Mg	V-B6 Mg	FOL Ug	VB12 Ug	CALC Mg	PHOS Mg	SEL Mg	FIBD Gm
1.460	0.286	17.60	—	0.000	0.209	0.160	1.940	0.024	13.20	0.052	23.10	36.90	—	0.506
1.460	0.286	0.000	—	0.000	0.209	0.160	1.940	0.024	13.20	0.000	23.10	36.90	—	0.506
0.574	0.176	15.70	0.694	0.000	0.120	0.106	0.840	0.013	1.680	0.045	58.20	128.0	—	—
0.671	0.212	61.70	—	0.000	0.081	0.081	0.675	0.032	4.500	0.077	48.60	43.70	—	—
0.665	—	0.000	0.225	0.000	0.095	0.095	0.840	0.023	—	0.000	16.30	31.80	0.011	1.000

Continued.

Nutritive Components for Bread—cont'd

Food Name	Serving	Gm wt	KCAL Kc	PROT Gm	CARB Gm	FAT Gm	CHOL Mg	SAFA Gm	SOD Mg	POT Mg	MAG Mg
BREAD-FRENCH-ENRICHED	1 slice	35.0	98.00	3.330	17.70	1.360	0.000	0.200	193.0	30.10	7.000
BREAD-MIXED GRAIN	1 slice	25.0	64.30	2.490	11.70	0.930	0.000	—	103.0	54.50	12.30
BREAD-PITA	1 item	38.0	105.0	3.950	20.60	0.570	—	—	215.0	44.80	—
BREAD-PUMPERNICKEL	1 slice	32.0	81.60	2.930	15.40	1.100	0.000	0.100	173.0	139.0	21.80
BREAD-RAISIN-ENRICHED	1 slice	25.0	69.50	2.050	13.20	0.990	—	0.200	94.00	60.00	6.250
BREAD-RYE-AMERICAN-LIGHT	1 slice	25.0	65.50	2.120	12.00	0.913	0.000	0.000	174.0	51.00	6.000
BREAD STICK-VIENNA TYPE	1 item	35.0	106.0	3.300	20.30	1.100	—	—	548.0	33.00	—
BREAD-WHITE-FIRM	1 slice	23.0	61.40	1.900	11.20	0.902	0.000	0.200	118.0	25.80	4.830
BREAD-WHITE-FIRM-TOASTED	1 slice	20.0	65.00	2.000	12.00	1.000	0.000	0.200	117.0	28.00	4.800
BREAD-WHOLE WHEAT-HOME REC	1 slice	25.0	66.50	2.250	11.60	1.610	0.000	—	89.00	85.00	23.30
BREAD-WHOLE WHEAT-FIRM	1 slice	25.0	61.30	2.410	11.30	1.090	0.000	0.100	159.0	44.00	23.30
BREAD-WHEAT-FIRM-TOASTED	1 slice	21.0	59.00	2.310	10.90	1.050	—	0.100	153.0	42.40	22.50
BREADCRUMBS-DRY-GRATED	1 cup	100.0	390.0	13.00	73.00	5.000	0.000	1.000	736.0	152.0	32.00
MUFFIN-BLUEBERRY-HOME REC	1 item	40.0	110.0	3.000	17.00	4.000	21.00	1.100	252.0	46.00	10.00
MUFFIN-BRAN-HOME REC	1 item	40.0	112.0	2.960	16.70	5.080	21.00	1.200	168.0	98.80	35.20
MUFFIN-CORN-HOME REC	1 item	40.0	125.0	3.000	19.00	4.000	21.00	1.200	192.0	54.00	18.40
MUFFIN-ENGLISH-PLAIN	1 item	56.0	133.0	4.430	25.70	1.090	—	—	358.0	314.0	10.60
MUFFIN-ENGLISH-PLAIN-TOAST	1 item	53.0	154.0	5.130	29.80	1.260	—	—	414.0	364.0	12.20
MUFFIN-PLAIN-HOME REC	1 item	40.0	120.0	3.000	17.00	4.000	21.00	1.000	176.0	50.00	10.80
ROLL-BROWN & SERVE-ENR	1 item	26.0	85.00	2.000	14.00	2.000	—	0.400	144.0	25.00	5.460
CROISSANT-ROLL-SARA LEE	1 item	26.0	109.0	2.300	11.20	6.100	—	—	140.0	40.00	7.000
ROLL-HAMBURGER/HOTDOG	1 item	40.0	114.0	3.430	20.10	2.090	—	0.500	241.0	36.80	7.600
ROLL-HARD-ENRICHED	1 item	50.0	155.0	5.000	30.00	2.000	—	0.400	312.0	49.00	11.50
ROLL-SUBMARINE/HOAGIE-ENR	1 item	135.0	390.0	12.00	75.00	4.000	0.000	0.900	761.0	122.0	—
ROLL-WHOLE WHEAT-HOMEMADE	1 item	35.0	90.00	3.500	18.30	1.000	—	—	197.0	102.0	40.00

Nutritive Components for Breakfast Cereals

Food Name	Serving	Gm wt	KCAL Kc	PROT Gm	CARB Gm	FAT Gm	CHOL Mg	SAFA Gm	SOD Mg	POT Mg	MAG Mg
CEREAL-ALL BRAN	1 cup	85.2	212.0	12.20	63.40	1.530	0.000	—	961.0	1051	318.0
CEREAL-ALPHA BITS	1 cup	28.4	111.0	2.200	24.60	0.600	—	—	219.0	110.0	17.00
CEREAL-BRAN BUDS	1 cup	85.2	220.0	11.80	64.80	2.040	—	—	523.0	1425	271.0
CEREAL-BRAN CHEX	1 cup	49.0	156.0	5.100	39.00	1.400	0.000	—	455.0	394.0	126.0
CEREAL-C.W. POST-PLAIN	1 cup	97.0	432.0	8.700	69.40	15.20	0.000	11.30	167.0	198.0	67.00
CEREAL-CHEERIOS	1 cup	22.7	88.80	3.420	15.70	1.450	0.000	0.270	246.0	81.00	31.30
CEREAL-CORN-SHREDDED-SUGAR	1 cup	25.0	95.00	2.000	22.00	0.000	0.000	—	247.0	—	3.500
CEREAL-CORN BRAN	1 cup	36.0	124.0	2.500	30.40	1.300	0.000	—	310.0	70.00	18.00
CEREAL-CORN CHEX	1 cup	28.4	111.0	2.000	24.90	0.100	—	—	271.0	23.00	4.000
CEREAL-CORN FLAKES-KELLOGG	1 cup	22.7	88.30	1.840	19.50	0.068	0.000	0.000	281.0	20.90	2.720
CEREAL-CRACKLIN BRAN	1 cup	60.0	229.0	5.500	41.10	8.800	0.000	—	487.0	355.0	116.0
CEREAL-CRISPY RICE	1 cup	28.0	111.0	1.800	24.80	0.100	0.000	0.000	205.0	27.00	12.00
CEREAL-FORTIFIED OAT FLAKE	1 cup	48.0	177.0	9.000	34.70	0.700	0.000	0.000	429.0	343.0	58.00
CEREAL-BRAN FLAKES-KELLOGG	1 cup	39.0	127.0	4.900	30.50	0.700	0.000	0.000	363.0	248.0	71.00
CEREAL-FROSTED MINI WHEATS	1 item	7.1	25.50	0.731	5.860	0.071	0.000	0.000	2.060	24.20	55.80
CEREAL-FRUIT LOOPS	1 cup	28.4	111.0	1.700	25.00	0.500	0.000	0.000	145.0	26.00	7.000
CEREAL-GRANOLA-HOMEMADE	1 cup	122.0	595.0	15.00	67.30	33.10	0.000	5.840	12.00	612.0	141.0
CEREAL-GRAPE NUTS	1 cup	114.0	407.0	13.30	93.50	0.456	0.000	0.000	792.0	381.0	76.30
CEREAL-GRAPE NUTS FLAKES	1 cup	32.5	116.0	3.480	26.60	0.358	0.000	0.000	250.0	113.0	35.80
CEREAL-HEARTLAND NATURAL	1 cup	115.0	499.0	11.60	78.60	17.70	0.000	—	294.0	385.0	147.0
CEREAL-HONEY BRAN	1 cup	35.0	119.0	3.100	28.60	0.700	0.000	0.000	202.0	151.0	46.00
CEREAL-HONEY NUT CHEERIOS	1 cup	33.0	125.0	3.600	26.50	0.800	0.000	0.130	299.0	115.0	39.00
CEREAL-LIFE-PLAIN/CINNAMON	1 cup	44.0	162.0	8.100	31.50	0.800	0.000	0.000	229.0	197.0	14.00
CEREAL-LUCKY CHARMS	1 cup	32.0	125.0	2.900	26.10	1.200	0.000	0.220	227.0	66.00	27.00
CEREAL-GRANOLA-NATURE VAL	1 cup	113.0	503.0	11.50	75.50	19.60	0.000	13.00	232.0	389.0	116.0

Continued.

IRON Mg	ZINC Mg	V-A IU	V-ET Mg	V-C Mg	THIA Mg	RIBO Mg	NIAC Mg	V-B6 Mg	FOL Ug	VB12 Ug	CALC Mg	PHOS Mg	SEL Mg	FIBD Gm
1.080	0.221	0.000	0.417	0.000	0.161	0.123	1.400	0.019	13.00	0.000	38.50	28.40	0.010	0.546
0.815	0.300	0.000	0.225	0.000	0.098	0.095	1.040	0.026	16.30	0.000	26.00	53.00	0.011	1.000
0.916	—	0.000	—	0.000	0.171	0.076	1.400	—	—	—	30.80	38.00	—	0.357
0.877	0.365	0.000	0.288	0.000	0.109	0.166	1.060	0.049	—	0.000	22.70	69.80	0.014	1.160
0.775	0.155	0.000	—	0.000	0.083	0.155	1.020	0.009	8.750	0.000	25.50	22.50	—	0.550
0.680	0.318	0.000	—	0.000	0.103	0.080	0.828	0.023	9.750	0.000	20.00	36.30	0.007	1.650
0.300	—	0.000	—	0.000	0.020	0.030	0.300	—	—	—	16.00	31.00	—	—
0.653	0.143	0.000	0.274	0.000	0.108	0.071	0.863	0.008	8.050	0.000	29.00	24.80	0.006	0.621
0.600	0.142	0.000	0.238	0.000	0.070	0.060	0.800	0.008	8.000	0.000	22.00	23.00	0.006	0.540
0.670	0.562	10.80	0.225	0.000	0.068	0.038	0.798	0.050	12.30	0.027	19.80	63.30	0.011	2.830
0.855	0.420	0.000	0.225	0.000	0.088	0.053	0.958	0.047	13.80	0.000	18.00	65.00	0.011	2.830
0.823	0.403	0.000	0.189	0.000	0.067	0.050	0.920	0.045	13.20	0.000	17.20	63.00	0.011	2.380
3.600	—	0.000	—	0.000	0.350	0.350	4.800	—	—	—	122.0	141.0	0.020	—
0.600	—	90.00	—	0.000	0.090	0.100	0.700	—	—	—	34.00	53.00	—	—
1.260	1.080	206.0	—	2.480	0.100	0.112	1.260	0.111	16.80	0.092	53.60	111.0	—	2.520
0.700	—	120.0	—	0.000	0.100	0.100	0.700	—	—	—	42.00	68.00	—	—
1.580	0.403	0.000	—	0.000	0.258	0.179	2.100	0.022	17.90	0.000	90.70	62.70	0.015	—
1.830	0.466	0.000	—	0.000	0.239	0.207	2.430	0.026	20.70	0.000	105.0	72.60	0.015	—
0.600	—	40.00	—	0.000	0.090	0.120	0.900	—	—	—	42.00	60.00	—	—
0.800	0.190	0.000	1.730	0.000	0.100	0.060	0.900	0.016	9.880	—	20.00	23.00	0.008	—
1.040	—	41.00	—	0.000	0.280	0.100	1.200	—	—	—	12.00	32.00	—	—
1.190	0.248	0.000	0.212	0.000	0.196	0.132	1.580	0.014	14.80	—	53.60	32.80	0.012	—
1.200	0.300	0.000	0.265	0.000	0.200	0.120	1.700	0.018	29.50	0.000	24.00	46.00	0.015	—
3.000	—	0.000	0.716	0.000	0.540	0.320	4.500	0.047	—	—	58.00	115.0	0.041	—
0.800	—	0.000	0.315	0.000	0.120	0.050	1.100	—	—	—	34.00	98.00	0.016	—

IRON Mg	ZINC Mg	V-A IU	V-ET Mg	V-C Mg	THIA Mg	RIBO Mg	NIAC Mg	V-B6 Mg	FOL Ug	VB12 Ug	CALC Mg	PHOS Mg	SEL Mg	FIBD Gm
13.50	11.20	3756	7.780	45.20	1.110	1.280	15.00	1.530	301.0	—	69.00	794.0	0.025	25.50
1.800	1.500	1250	—	—	0.400	0.400	5.000	0.500	100.0	1.500	8.000	51.00	—	0.300
13.50	11.20	3756	3.450	45.20	1.110	1.280	15.00	1.530	301.0	—	57.10	740.0	0.025	23.60
7.800	2.140	107.0	—	26.00	0.600	0.260	8.600	0.900	173.0	2.600	29.00	327.0	0.010	7.900
15.40	1.640	4277	—	—	1.300	1.500	17.10	1.700	342.0	5.100	47.00	224.0	—	2.200
3.610	0.629	1001	—	12.00	0.295	0.341	4.000	0.409	4.990	1.200	38.80	107.0	0.010	0.863
0.600	0.088	0.000	0.538	13.00	0.330	0.050	4.400	0.450	88.30	1.330	1.000	10.00	0.002	—
12.20	4.000	—	—	—	0.380	0.700	10.90	0.858	232.0	1.390	41.00	52.00	0.002	6.840
1.800	0.100	143.0	—	15.00	0.400	0.070	5.000	0.500	100.0	1.500	3.000	11.00	0.002	0.500
1.430	0.064	1001	—	12.00	0.295	0.341	4.000	0.409	80.10	—	0.681	14.30	0.001	0.250
3.800	3.200	2645	—	32.00	0.800	0.900	10.60	1.100	212.0	—	40.00	241.0	0.010	9.100
0.700	0.460	—	—	1.000	0.100	0.000	2.000	0.044	3.000	0.082	5.000	31.00	0.004	1.000
13.70	1.500	2116	—	—	0.600	0.700	8.400	0.900	169.0	2.500	68.00	176.0	0.010	1.200
11.20	5.100	1720	0.823	—	0.500	0.600	6.900	0.700	138.0	2.100	19.00	192.0	0.004	5.500
0.447	0.376	313.0	0.153	3.760	0.092	0.107	1.250	0.128	25.10	—	2.340	18.50	—	0.540
4.500	3.700	1250	—	15.00	0.400	0.400	5.000	0.500	100.0	—	3.000	24.00	—	0.200
4.840	4.470	43.00	—	1.000	0.730	0.310	2.140	0.428	99.00	—	76.00	494.0	0.040	4.360
4.950	2.510	5026	—	—	1.480	1.710	20.10	2.050	402.0	6.040	43.30	286.0	0.034	5.470
5.170	0.650	1433	0.686	—	0.423	0.488	5.720	0.585	115.0	1.720	13.00	96.90	0.010	2.080
4.330	3.040	—	—	—	0.360	0.160	1.610	—	64.00	—	75.00	416.0	—	5.400
5.600	0.900	1543	—	19.00	0.500	0.500	6.200	0.600	23.00	1.900	16.00	132.0	—	3.900
5.200	0.870	1455	—	17.00	0.400	0.500	5.800	0.600	—	1.700	23.00	122.0	—	1.300
11.60	1.450	—	—	—	0.950	1.000	11.60	—	37.00	—	154.0	238.0	—	1.400
5.100	0.560	1411	—	17.00	0.400	0.500	5.600	0.600	—	1.700	36.00	88.00	—	0.600
3.780	2.190	—	—	—	0.390	0.190	0.830	—	85.00	—	71.00	354.0	0.037	4.200

Continued.

Nutritive Components for Breakfast Cereals—cont'd

Food Name	Serving	Gm wt	KCAL Kc	PROT Gm	CARB Gm	FAT Gm	CHOL Mg	SAFA Gm	SOD Mg	POT Mg	MAG Mg
CEREAL-NUTRI GRAIN-BARLEY	1 cup	41.0	153.0	4.500	33.90	0.300	0.000	0.000	277.0	108.0	32.00
CEREAL-NUTRI GRAIN-CORN	1 cup	42.0	160.0	3.400	35.50	1.000	0.000	—	276.0	98.00	27.00
CEREAL-NUTRI GRAIN-RYE	1 cup	40.0	144.0	3.500	33.90	0.300	0.000	0.000	272.0	72.00	31.00
CEREAL-NUTRI GRAIN-WHEAT	1 cup	44.0	158.0	3.800	37.20	0.500	0.000	0.000	299.0	120.0	34.00
CEREAL-OATS-PUFFED-SUGAR	1 cup	25.0	100.0	3.000	19.00	1.000	0.000	—	294.0	—	28.00
CEREAL-100% BRAN	1 cup	66.0	178.0	8.300	48.10	3.300	0.000	0.590	457.0	824.0	312.0
CEREAL-PRODUCT 19	1 cup	33.0	126.0	3.200	27.40	0.200	0.000	0.000	378.0	51.00	12.00
CEREAL-RAISIN BRAN-KELLOGG	1 cup	49.2	154.0	5.300	37.10	0.984	0.000	—	359.0	256.0	63.50
CEREAL-RICE-PUFFED-SUGAR	1 cup	28.0	115.0	1.000	26.00	0.000	0.000	—	21.00	43.00	7.560
CEREAL-RICE-PUFFED-PLAIN	1 cup	14.0	56.00	0.900	12.60	0.100	0.000	0.000	0.000	16.00	3.000
CEREAL-RICE KRISPIES	1 cup	28.4	112.0	1.900	24.80	0.200	0.000	0.000	340.0	30.00	10.00
CEREAL-SPECIAL K	1 cup	21.3	83.10	4.200	16.00	0.085	0.000	0.000	199.0	36.80	11.70
CEREAL-SUGAR CORN POPS	1 cup	28.4	108.0	1.400	25.60	0.100	0.000	0.000	103.0	17.00	2.000
CEREAL-SUGAR SMACKS	1 cup	37.9	141.0	2.650	33.00	0.720	0.000	0.000	100.0	56.10	18.20
CEREAL-TEAM	1 cup	42.0	164.0	2.700	36.00	0.700	0.000	0.000	259.0	71.00	19.00
CEREAL-TOASTIES	1 cup	22.7	87.80	1.840	19.50	0.045	0.000	0.000	238.0	26.30	3.410
CEREAL-TRIX	1 cup	28.0	108.0	1.500	24.90	0.400	0.000	0.000	179.0	26.00	6.000
CEREAL-WHEAT-PUFFED-SUGAR	1 cup	38.0	140.0	3.000	33.00	0.000	0.000	—	57.00	63.00	22.80
CEREAL-TOTAL	1 cup	33.0	116.0	3.300	26.00	0.700	0.000	0.100	409.0	123.0	37.00
CEREAL-WHEAT-PUFFED-PLAIN	1 cup	12.0	44.00	1.800	9.500	0.100	0.000	—	0.480	42.00	17.00
CEREAL-WHEAT CHEX	1 cup	46.0	169.0	4.500	37.80	1.100	0.000	—	308.0	174.0	58.00
CEREAL-WHEAT FLAKES-SUGAR	1 cup	30.0	105.0	3.000	24.00	0.000	0.000	—	368.0	81.00	32.70
CEREAL-WHEAT GERM-TOASTED	1 cup	113.0	431.0	32.90	56.10	12.10	0.000	2.090	4.000	1070	362.0
CEREAL-WHEAT GERM-SUGAR	1 cup	113.0	426.0	24.70	68.70	9.100	0.000	1.570	3.000	803.0	272.0
CEREAL-WHEATIES	1 cup	29.0	101.0	2.800	23.10	0.500	0.000	0.070	363.0	108.0	32.00
CEREAL-CORN GRITS-ENRICHED	1 cup	242.0	146.0	3.500	31.40	0.500	0.000	0.000	0.000	54.00	11.00
CEREAL-CREAM/WHEAT-PACKET	1 item	150.0	132.0	2.500	28.90	0.400	0.000	0.000	241.0	55.00	9.000
CEREAL-CREAM/WHEAT-INSTANT	1 cup	241.0	153.0	4.400	31.60	0.600	0.000	0.000	6.000	48.00	14.00
CEREAL-CREAM/WHEAT-REG-HOT	1 cup	251.0	134.0	3.800	27.70	0.500	0.000	0.000	2.000	43.00	10.00
CEREAL-FARINA-COOK-ENR	1 cup	233.0	116.0	3.400	24.60	0.200	0.000	0.000	1.000	30.00	4.000
CEREAL-MALT O MEAL-COOK	1 cup	240.0	122.0	3.500	25.80	0.300	0.000	0.000	2.000	—	—
CEREAL-MAYPO-COOK-HOT	1 cup	240.0	170.0	5.800	31.80	2.400	0.000	—	9.000	211.0	51.00
CEREAL-OATMEAL-RAW	1 cup	81.0	311.0	13.00	54.20	5.100	—	0.940	3.000	284.0	120.0
CEREAL-OATMEAL-INST-PACKET	1 item	177.0	104.0	4.400	18.10	1.700	0.000	—	286.0	100.0	—
CEREAL-RALSTON-COOKED	1 cup	253.0	134.0	5.500	28.20	0.800	0.000	0.000	4.000	153.0	59.00
CEREAL-ROMAN MEAL-COOKED	1 cup	241.0	147.0	6.600	33.00	1.000	0.000	—	3.000	302.0	109.0
CEREAL-WHEAT-ROLLED-COOKED	1 cup	240.0	180.0	5.000	41.00	1.000	0.000	—	535.0	202.0	52.80
CEREAL-WHEAT-WHOLE MEAL	1 cup	245.0	110.0	4.000	23.00	1.000	0.000	—	535.0	118.0	53.90
CEREAL-WHEATENA-COOKED	1 cup	243.0	135.0	5.000	28.70	1.100	0.000	—	5.000	187.0	49.00
CEREAL-WHOLE WHEAT NATURAL	1 cup	242.0	151.0	4.900	33.20	0.900	0.000	—	1.000	171.0	54.00
CEREAL-RICE CHEX	1 cup	25.2	99.50	1.340	22.50	0.101	0.000	0.000	211.0	29.20	6.300
CEREAL-FROST FLAKE-KELLOGG	1 cup	35.0	133.0	1.800	31.70	0.100	0.000	0.000	284.0	22.00	3.000
CEREAL-WHEAT-SHRED-BISCUIT	1 item	23.6	83.00	2.600	18.80	0.300	0.000	0.000	0.472	77.00	40.00

Nutritive Components for Combination Foods

Food Name	Serving	Gm wt	KCAL Kc	PROT Gm	CARB Gm	FAT Gm	CHOL Mg	SAFA Gm	SOD Mg	POT Mg	MAG Mg
BEEF-RAVIOLIOS-CANNED	1 srvg	28.4	27.50	1.140	4.260	0.568	—	—	131.0	45.70	—
BEEF & VEGETABLE STEW	1 cup	245.0	220.0	16.00	15.00	11.00	72.00	4.900	1006	613.0	—
CHICKEN A LA KING-HOME REC	1 cup	245.0	470.0	27.00	12.00	34.00	186.0	12.90	759.0	404.0	—
CHICKEN CHOW MEIN-CANNED	1 cup	250.0	95.00	7.000	18.00	0.000	98.00	0.000	722.0	418.0	—
CHICKEN POTPIE-BAKED-HOME	1 slice	232.0	545.0	23.00	42.00	31.00	72.00	11.00	593.0	343.0	—
CHILI CON CARNE/BEANS-CAN	1 cup	255.0	340.0	19.00	31.00	16.00	38.00	7.500	1354	594.0	—
CHILI WITH BEANS-CANNED	1 cup	255.0	286.0	14.60	30.40	14.00	43.00	6.000	1330	932.0	115.0

Continued.

IRON Mg	ZINC Mg	V-A IU	V-ET Mg	V-C Mg	THIA Mg	RIBO Mg	NIAC Mg	V-B6 Mg	FOL Ug	VB12 Ug	CALC Mg	PHOS Mg	SEL Mg	FIBD Gm
1.450	5.400	1808	—	22.00	0.500	0.600	7.200	0.700	145.0	2.200	11.00	126.0	0.027	2.400
0.890	5.500	1852	—	22.00	0.500	0.600	7.400	0.800	148.0	2.200	1.000	120.0	0.003	2.600
1.130	5.300	1764	—	21.00	0.500	0.600	7.000	0.700	141.0	2.100	8.000	104.0	—	2.560
1.240	5.800	1940	—	23.00	0.600	0.700	7.700	0.800	155.0	2.300	12.00	164.0	0.007	2.800
4.000	0.693	1100	—	13.00	0.330	0.380	4.400	0.450	5.500	1.330	44.00	102.0	0.006	0.125
8.120	5.740	—	—	63.00	1.600	1.800	20.90	2.100	—	6.300	46.00	801.0	0.020	19.50
21.00	0.500	5820	—	70.00	1.700	2.000	23.30	2.300	466.0	7.000	4.000	47.00	—	0.400
6.000	5.020	1667	—	—	0.492	0.590	6.690	0.689	133.0	2.020	17.20	183.0	0.005	5.310
0.000	1.480	1240	—	15.00	0.000	0.000	0.000	0.504	98.80	1.480	3.000	14.00	0.002	0.200
0.150	0.140	0.000	—	0.000	0.020	0.010	0.420	0.011	3.000	—	1.000	14.00	0.001	0.100
1.800	0.480	1250	0.080	15.00	0.400	0.400	5.000	0.500	100.0	—	4.000	34.00	0.004	0.100
3.390	2.810	939.0	—	11.30	0.277	0.320	3.750	0.383	75.20	—	6.180	41.30	—	0.170
1.800	1.500	1250	—	15.00	0.400	0.400	5.000	0.500	100.0	—	1.000	28.00	—	0.200
2.390	0.379	1671	—	20.10	0.493	0.569	6.670	0.682	134.0	—	4.170	41.30	—	0.531
2.570	0.580	1852	—	22.00	0.500	0.600	7.400	0.800	—	2.200	6.000	65.00	0.007	0.400
0.597	0.066	1001	—	—	0.295	0.341	4.000	0.409	80.10	1.200	0.908	10.00	—	0.386
4.500	0.130	1235	—	15.00	0.400	0.400	4.900	0.500	—	1.500	6.000	19.00	—	0.100
0.000	2.010	1680	—	20.00	0.500	0.570	6.700	0.684	134.0	2.010	7.000	52.00	—	0.400
21.00	0.780	5820	—	70.00	1.700	2.000	23.30	2.300	466.0	7.000	56.00	137.0	—	2.400
0.570	0.280	0.000	—	0.000	0.020	0.030	1.300	0.020	4.000	—	3.000	43.00	—	0.400
7.300	1.230	—	0.971	24.00	0.600	0.170	8.100	0.800	162.0	2.400	18.00	182.0	—	3.400
4.800	0.669	1320	0.633	16.00	0.400	0.450	5.300	0.540	9.000	1.590	12.00	83.00	0.003	2.000
10.30	18.80	188.0	31.10	7.000	1.890	0.930	6.310	1.110	398.0	—	50.00	1294	—	7.800
7.710	14.10	—	—	—	1.410	0.700	4.730	0.829	298.0	—	38.00	971.0	—	5.700
4.600	0.650	1279	0.612	15.00	0.400	0.400	5.100	0.500	9.000	1.500	44.00	100.0	0.003	2.000
1.560	0.170	—	3.340	—	0.240	0.150	1.960	0.058	1.000	—	1.000	29.00	—	0.600
8.100	0.230	1250	1.410	—	0.400	0.200	5.000	0.500	100.0	—	40.00	20.00	—	—
12.00	0.410	—	—	—	0.200	0.100	1.800	—	11.00	—	59.00	43.00	—	—
10.30	0.330	—	—	—	0.200	0.100	1.500	—	9.000	—	51.00	42.00	—	—
1.170	0.160	—	2.190	—	0.190	0.120	1.280	0.023	6.000	—	4.000	28.00	—	0.400
9.500	0.170	—	—	—	0.400	0.300	5.900	0.019	6.000	—	5.000	23.00	—	0.600
8.400	1.490	2339	—	28.00	0.700	0.800	9.400	0.900	9.000	2.800	125.0	248.0	—	1.200
3.410	2.480	82.00	—	—	0.590	0.110	0.630	0.097	26.00	—	42.00	384.0	—	4.600
6.320	—	1514	2.710	—	0.530	0.290	5.490	0.742	150.0	—	163.0	133.0	—	1.620
1.640	1.420	—	2.380	—	0.200	0.180	2.050	0.114	18.00	0.109	14.00	148.0	—	4.200
2.120	1.780	—	—	—	0.240	0.120	3.080	0.113	24.00	—	30.00	215.0	—	—
1.700	1.150	0.000	9.720	0.000	0.170	0.070	2.200	—	26.40	—	19.00	182.0	—	—
1.200	1.180	0.000	9.920	0.000	0.150	0.050	1.500	—	27.00	—	17.00	127.0	—	—
1.360	1.680	—	—	—	0.020	0.050	1.340	0.046	17.00	—	11.00	146.0	0.058	2.600
1.500	1.160	—	9.800	—	0.170	0.120	2.150	—	26.00	—	17.00	167.0	0.058	2.700
1.590	0.348	15.10	0.071	13.40	0.328	—	4.440	0.454	89.00	1.340	3.530	24.70	0.004	0.151
2.200	0.050	1543	—	19.00	0.500	0.500	6.200	0.600	124.0	—	1.000	26.00	—	2.200
0.740	0.590	0.000	0.508	0.000	0.070	0.060	1.080	0.060	12.00	—	10.00	86.00	—	2.200

IRON Mg	ZINC Mg	V-A IU	V-ET Mg	V-C Mg	THIA Mg	RIBO Mg	NIAC Mg	V-B6 Mg	FOL Ug	VB12 Ug	CALC Mg	PHOS Mg	SEL Mg	FIBD Gm
0.312	—	262.0	0.136	0.426	0.026	0.023	0.398	—	—	—	4.540	—	—	0.230
2.900	—	2400	1.350	17.00	0.150	0.170	4.700	—	—	0.002	29.00	184.0	—	3.190
2.500	—	1130	—	12.00	0.100	0.420	5.400	—	—	—	127.0	358.0	—	—
1.300	—	150.0	0.125	13.00	0.050	0.100	1.000	—	—	—	45.00	85.00	—	—
3.000	—	3090	—	5.000	0.340	0.310	5.500	—	—	—	70.00	232.0	—	—
4.300	—	150.0	—	—	0.080	0.180	3.300	0.263	—	—	82.00	321.0	—	5.000
8.750	5.100	860.0	—	4.300	0.122	0.268	0.913	0.337	—	0.030	119.0	393.0	—	—

Continued.

Nutritive Components for Combination Foods—cont'd

Food Name	Serving	Gm wt	KCAL Kc	PROT Gm	CARB Gm	FAT Gm	CHOL Mg	SAFA Gm	SOD Mg	POT Mg	MAG Mg
ENCHILADA	1 item	230.0	396.0	17.30	34.70	20.90	—	—	1332	653.0	75.90
HOT DOG/BUN	1 item	82.0	214.0	9.100	13.60	13.70	36.90	—	636.0	140.0	13.10
MACARONI & CHEESE-ENR-CAN	1 cup	240.0	230.0	9.000	26.00	10.00	42.00	4.200	729.0	139.0	—
MACARONI & CHEESE-ENR-HOME	1 cup	200.0	430.0	17.00	40.00	22.00	42.00	8.900	1086	240.0	52.00
MEAT LOAF-CELERY/ONIONS	1 srvg	87.6	213.0	15.80	5.230	13.90	107.0	5.290	103.0	182.0	13.60
PIZZA-CHEESE-BAKED	1 slice	120.0	290.0	14.60	39.10	8.640	56.40	3.400	698.0	230.0	31.20
PIZZA-PEPPERONI-BAKED	1 slice	120.0	306.0	13.00	36.70	11.50	—	—	817.0	216.0	—
BEANS/PORK/FRANKFURTER-CAN	1 cup	257.0	366.0	17.30	39.60	16.90	15.00	6.050	1105	604.0	71.00
BEANS/PORK/TOM SAUCE-CAN	1 cup	253.0	247.0	13.00	49.00	2.600	17.00	1.000	1113	759.0	88.00
BEANS/PORK/SWEET SAUCE-CAN	1 cup	253.0	282.0	13.40	53.10	3.690	17.00	1.420	849.0	673.0	87.00
SALAD-CARROT RAISIN-HOME	1 cup	268.0	306.0	3.800	55.80	11.60	—	—	—	—	—
SALAD-CHEF SALAD-HAM/CHEES	1 srvg	200.0	196.0	13.40	7.420	12.70	46.00	6.980	567.0	415.0	28.40
SALAD-CHICKEN	1 cup	205.0	502.0	26.00	17.40	36.20	—	—	1395	521.0	—
SALAD-COLESLAW	1 tbsp	8.0	6.000	0.100	0.990	0.210	1.000	0.031	2.000	14.00	1.000
SALAD-FRUIT-CAN/JUICE	1 cup	249.0	125.0	1.280	32.50	0.060	0.000	0.010	13.00	288.0	21.00
SALAD-GREEN SALAD-TOSSED	1 srvg	130.0	25.00	1.310	5.190	0.291	0.000	0.040	12.80	279.0	14.00
SALAD-MACARONI	1 srvg	28.4	50.70	0.700	5.300	3.000	—	—	148.0	21.00	—
SALAD-MANDARIN ORANGE GEL	1 srvg	28.4	22.70	0.400	5.700	0.000	—	0.000	14.00	9.000	—
SALAD-POTATO	1 cup	250.0	358.0	6.700	27.90	20.50	171.0	3.570	1323	635.0	39.00
SALAD-THREE BEAN-DEL MONTE	1 srvg	28.4	22.40	0.710	5.060	0.056	0.000	0.000	101.0	38.30	6.250
SALAD-TUNA	1 cup	205.0	350.0	30.00	7.000	22.00	68.00	4.300	434.0	—	—
SAND-BAC/LET/TOM/MAYO	1 item	148.0	282.0	6.800	28.80	15.60	—	—	—	—	—
SANDWICH-CLUB	1 item	315.0	590.0	35.60	41.70	20.80	—	—	—	—	—
SPAGHETTI/TOM/CHE-HOME REC	1 cup	250.0	260.0	9.000	37.00	9.000	4.000	2.000	955.0	408.0	—
SPAGHETTI/TOM/CHE-CAN	1 cup	250.0	190.0	6.000	39.00	2.000	4.000	0.500	955.0	303.0	28.00
SPAGHETTI/TOM/MEAT-HOME	1 cup	248.0	330.0	19.00	39.00	12.00	75.00	3.300	1009	665.0	—
SPAGHETTI/TOM/MEAT-CAN	1 cup	250.0	260.0	12.00	29.00	10.00	39.00	2.200	1220	245.0	28.00
TACO	1 item	81.0	187.0	10.60	12.70	10.40	21.10	—	456.0	263.0	36.50
VEGETABLES-MIXED-FROZ-BOIL	1 cup	182.0	108.0	5.220	23.80	0.280	0.000	0.056	64.00	308.0	40.00
BEEF POTPIE-HOME RECIPE	1 slice	210.0	515.0	21.00	39.00	30.00	44.00	7.900	596.0	334.0	—

Nutritive Components for Dairy Products

Food Name	Serving	Gm wt	KCAL Kc	PROT Gm	CARB Gm	FAT Gm	CHOL Mg	SAFA Gm	SOD Mg	POT Mg	MAG Mg
CHEESE-AMERICAN-PROCESSED	1 piece	28.0	106.0	6.280	0.450	8.860	27.00	5.580	406.0	46.00	6.000
CHEESE-BLUE	1 piece	28.0	100.0	6.070	0.660	8.150	21.00	5.300	396.0	73.00	7.000
CHEESE-CAMEMBERT-WEDGE	1 item	38.0	114.0	7.520	0.180	9.220	27.00	5.800	320.0	71.00	8.000
CHEESE-CHEDDAR-SHREDDED	1 cup	113.0	455.0	28.10	1.450	37.50	119.0	23.80	701.0	111.0	31.00
CHEESE-COTTAGE-4% LAR CURD	1 cup	225.0	232.0	28.10	6.030	10.10	33.80	6.410	911.0	189.0	11.30
CHEESE-CREAM	1 srvg	28.0	99.00	2.140	0.750	9.890	31.00	6.230	84.00	34.00	2.000
CHEESE-FETA	1 srvg	28.0	75.00	4.030	1.160	6.030	25.00	4.240	316.0	18.00	5.000
CHEESE-GOUDA	1 piece	28.0	101.0	7.070	0.630	7.780	32.00	4.990	232.0	34.00	8.000
CHEESE-LIMBURGER	1 piece	28.0	93.00	5.680	0.140	7.720	26.00	4.750	227.0	36.00	6.000
CHEESE-MONTEREY	1 piece	28.0	106.0	6.940	0.190	8.580	—	—	152.0	23.00	8.000
CHEESE-MOZZARELLA-SKIM MLK	1 piece	28.0	72.00	6.880	0.780	4.510	16.00	2.870	132.0	24.00	7.000
CHEESE-PARMESAN-GRATED	1 cup	100.0	456.0	41.60	3.740	30.00	79.00	19.10	1862	107.0	51.00
CHEESE-PROVOLONE	1 piece	28.0	100.0	7.250	0.610	7.550	20.00	4.840	248.0	39.00	8.000
CHEESE-RICOTTA-SKIM MILK	1 cup	246.0	340.0	28.00	12.60	19.50	76.00	12.10	307.0	308.0	36.00
CHEESE-ROMANO	1 piece	28.0	110.0	9.020	1.030	7.640	29.00	—	340.0	—	—
CHEESE-ROQUEFORT	1 srvg	28.0	105.0	6.110	0.570	8.690	26.00	5.460	513.0	26.00	8.000
CHEESE-SWISS	1 piece	28.0	107.0	8.060	0.960	7.780	26.00	5.040	74.00	31.00	10.10
CHEESE-SWISS-PROCESSED	1 piece	28.0	95.00	7.010	0.600	7.090	24.00	4.550	388.0	61.00	8.000
CHEESE FOOD-AMERICAN-PROC	1 srvg	28.0	93.00	5.560	2.070	6.970	18.00	4.380	337.0	79.00	9.000
CHEESE SPREAD-PROCESSED	1 srvg	28.0	82.00	4.650	2.480	6.020	16.00	3.780	381.0	69.00	8.000

Continued.

IRON Mg	ZINC Mg	V-A IU	V-ET Mg	V-C Mg	THIA Mg	RIBO Mg	NIAC Mg	V-B6 Mg	FOL Ug	VB12 Ug	CALC Mg	PHOS Mg	SEL Mg	FIBD Gm
3.290	1.290	—	—	—	0.184	0.253	—	0.253	—	2.070	96.60	198.0	—	—
1.530	2.050	—	0.115	0.000	0.197	0.230	3.050	—	—	—	27.10	84.50	0.019	—
1.000	—	260.0	—	0.000	0.120	0.240	1.000	—	—	—	199.0	182.0	—	1.440
1.800	—	860.0	—	0.000	0.200	0.400	1.800	—	—	—	362.0	322.0	—	1.200
1.910	3.080	61.50	0.068	0.725	0.052	0.148	3.160	0.162	10.90	1.520	22.80	112.0	0.001	0.110
1.610	1.670	750.0	—	2.400	0.336	0.288	4.210	0.120	55.20	0.480	220.0	216.0	—	1.900
2.520	—	532.0	—	2.400	0.324	0.288	5.150	0.096	78.00	0.360	196.0	—	—	2.160
4.450	4.790	395.0	2.750	5.900	0.149	0.144	2.320	0.118	77.10	0.870	123.0	267.0	—	12.80
8.300	14.80	313.0	2.750	7.800	0.132	0.116	1.260	0.175	56.80	0.030	141.0	297.0	—	13.80
4.200	3.800	289.0	2.750	7.700	0.119	0.154	0.888	0.215	94.50	0.060	155.0	266.0	—	14.00
3.000	—	9400	—	12.00	0.160	0.160	1.000	—	—	—	96.00	130.0	—	—
1.170	1.730	7048	0.995	24.00	0.337	0.240	2.210	0.206	46.00	0.474	227.0	251.0	0.019	2.390
—	—	—	—	—	—	—	—	—	—	—	—	—	—	—
0.050	0.020	51.00	—	2.600	0.005	0.005	0.022	0.010	2.100	0.002	4.000	3.000	—	—
0.620	0.360	1494	—	8.300	0.027	0.035	0.886	—	—	0.000	28.00	36.00	0.001	1.640
0.885	0.211	3315	0.785	18.60	0.074	0.069	0.632	0.069	61.20	0.000	30.70	31.10	0.001	2.110
—	—	—	—	—	—	—	—	—	—	—	—	—	—	0.290
—	—	—	—	—	—	—	—	—	—	—	—	—	—	0.000
1.630	0.780	523.0	—	24.90	0.193	0.150	2.230	0.353	16.80	0.385	48.00	130.0	—	5.250
0.284	0.093	39.80	—	0.852	0.014	0.014	0.085	—	—	—	9.660	16.20	—	—
2.700	—	590.0	3.050	2.000	0.080	0.230	10.30	—	—	—	41.00	291.0	—	1.030
1.500	—	870.0	—	13.00	0.160	0.140	1.600	—	—	—	53.00	89.00	—	—
4.300	—	1705	—	27.00	0.380	0.410	10.20	—	—	—	103.0	394.0	—	—
2.300	—	1080	—	13.00	0.250	0.180	2.300	—	—	—	80.00	135.0	—	2.500
2.800	—	930.0	—	10.00	0.350	0.280	4.500	—	—	—	40.00	88.00	—	2.500
3.700	—	1590	—	22.00	0.250	0.300	4.000	—	—	—	124.0	236.0	—	2.730
3.300	—	1000	—	5.000	0.150	0.180	2.300	—	—	—	53.00	113.0	—	2.750
1.150	1.560	420.0	—	0.810	0.089	0.065	1.410	0.122	11.30	0.405	109.0	134.0	—	—
1.500	0.900	7784	—	5.800	0.130	0.218	1.550	0.134	34.60	0.000	44.00	92.00	0.001	4.190
3.800	—	1720	—	6.000	0.300	0.300	5.500	—	—	—	29.00	149.0	—	—

IRON Mg	ZINC Mg	V-A IU	V-ET Mg	V-C Mg	THIA Mg	RIBO Mg	NIAC Mg	V-B6 Mg	FOL Ug	VB12 Ug	CALC Mg	PHOS Mg	SEL Mg	FIBD Gm
0.110	0.850	343.0	0.280	0.000	0.008	0.100	0.020	0.020	2.000	0.197	174.0	211.0	0.003	0.000
0.090	0.750	204.0	—	0.000	0.008	0.108	0.288	0.047	10.00	0.345	150.0	110.0	0.006	0.000
0.120	0.900	351.0	—	0.000	0.011	0.185	0.239	0.086	24.00	0.492	147.0	132.0	0.008	0.000
0.770	3.510	1197	—	0.000	0.031	0.424	0.090	0.084	21.00	0.935	815.0	579.0	0.018	0.000
0.315	0.833	367.0	—	0.000	0.047	0.367	0.284	0.151	27.00	1.400	135.0	297.0	0.052	0.000
0.340	0.150	405.0	—	0.000	0.005	0.056	0.029	0.013	4.000	0.120	23.00	30.00	0.001	0.000
0.180	0.820	—	—	0.000	—	—	—	—	—	—	140.0	96.00	—	0.000
0.070	1.110	183.0	—	0.000	0.009	0.095	0.018	0.023	6.000	—	198.0	155.0	—	0.000
0.040	0.600	363.0	—	0.000	0.023	0.143	0.045	0.024	16.00	0.295	141.0	111.0	—	0.000
0.200	0.850	269.0	—	0.000	—	0.111	—	—	—	—	212.0	126.0	—	0.000
0.060	0.780	166.0	—	0.000	0.005	0.086	0.030	0.020	2.000	0.232	183.0	131.0	0.003	0.000
0.950	3.190	701.0	—	0.000	0.045	0.386	0.315	0.105	8.000	—	1376	807.0	0.024	0.000
0.150	0.920	231.0	—	0.000	0.005	0.091	0.044	0.021	3.000	0.415	214.0	141.0	—	0.000
1.080	3.300	1063	—	0.000	0.052	0.455	0.192	0.049	—	0.716	669.0	449.0	—	0.000
—	—	162.0	—	0.000	—	0.105	0.022	—	2.000	—	302.0	215.0	—	0.000
0.160	0.590	297.0	—	0.000	0.011	0.166	0.208	0.035	14.00	0.182	188.0	111.0	—	0.000
0.050	1.110	240.0	0.200	0.000	0.006	0.103	0.026	0.024	2.000	0.475	272.0	171.0	0.003	0.000
0.170	1.020	229.0	—	0.000	0.004	0.078	0.011	0.010	—	0.348	219.0	216.0	0.003	0.000
0.240	0.850	259.0	—	0.000	0.008	0.125	0.040	—	—	0.317	163.0	130.0	0.006	0.000
0.090	0.730	223.0	—	0.000	0.014	0.122	0.037	0.033	2.000	0.113	159.0	202.0	0.006	0.000

Continued.

Nutritive Components for Dairy Products—cont'd

Food Name	Serving	Gm wt	KCAL Kc	PROT Gm	CARB Gm	FAT Gm	CHOL Mg	SAFA Gm	SOD Mg	POT Mg	MAG Mg
CREAM-HALF & HALF-FLUID	1 cup	242.0	315.0	7.160	10.40	27.80	89.00	17.30	98.00	314.0	25.00
CREAM-WHIPPING-HEAVY	1 cup	238.0	821.0	4.880	6.640	88.10	326.0	54.80	89.00	179.0	17.00
CREAM-COFFEE-TABLE-LIGHT	1 cup	240.0	469.0	6.480	8.780	46.30	159.0	28.90	95.00	292.0	21.00
CREAM-SOUR-CULTURED	1 cup	230.0	493.0	7.270	9.820	48.20	102.0	30.00	123.0	331.0	26.00
CREAM-SOUR-IMITATION	1 srvg	28.0	59.00	0.680	1.880	5.530	0.000	5.040	29.00	46.00	—
CREAM-SOUR-HALF & HALF	1 tbsp	15.0	20.00	0.440	0.640	1.800	6.000	1.120	6.000	19.00	2.000
CREAM-WHIP-IMIT-FROZ	1 cup	75.0	239.0	0.940	17.30	19.00	0.000	16.30	19.00	14.00	1.000
CREAM-WHIP-IMIT-PRESSURIZE	1 cup	70.0	184.0	0.690	11.30	15.60	0.000	13.20	43.00	13.00	1.000
CREAM-WHIP-PRESSURIZED	1 cup	60.0	154.0	1.920	7.490	13.30	46.00	8.300	78.00	88.00	6.000
MILK-BUTTERMILK-FLUID	1 cup	245.0	99.00	8.110	11.70	2.160	9.000	1.340	257.0	371.0	27.00
MILK-CHOCOLATE-WHOLE	1 cup	250.0	208.0	7.920	25.90	8.480	30.00	5.260	149.0	417.0	33.00
MILK-CONDENSED-SWEET-CAN	1 cup	306.0	982.0	24.20	166.0	26.60	104.0	16.80	389.0	1136	78.00
MILK-EGGNOG-COMMERCIAL	1 cup	254.0	342.0	9.680	34.40	19.00	149.0	11.30	138.0	420.0	47.00
MILK-EVAPORATED-SKIM-CAN	1 cup	255.0	199.0	19.30	28.90	0.510	10.20	0.309	293.0	847.0	68.90
MILK-EVAPORATED-WHOLE-CAN	1 cup	252.0	338.0	17.20	25.30	19.10	73.10	11.60	267.0	764.0	60.50
MILK-HUMAN-WHOLE-MATURE	1 cup	246.0	171.0	2.530	17.00	10.80	34.00	4.940	42.00	126.0	8.000
MILK-1% FAT-LOWFAT-FLUID	1 cup	244.0	102.0	8.030	11.70	2.590	10.00	1.610	123.0	381.0	34.00
MILK-2% FAT-LOWFAT-FLUID	1 cup	244.0	121.0	8.120	11.70	4.680	18.00	2.920	122.0	377.0	33.00
MILK-2% MILK SOLIDS ADDED	1 cup	245.0	125.0	8.530	12.20	4.700	18.00	2.450	128.0	397.0	35.00
MILK-NONFAT-INSTANT-DRIED	1 cup	68.0	244.0	23.90	35.50	0.490	12.00	0.320	373.0	1160	80.00
MILK-NONFAT-FLUID	1 cup	245.0	86.00	8.350	11.90	0.440	4.000	0.287	126.0	406.0	28.00
MILK-WHOLE-LOW SODIUM	1 cup	244.0	149.0	7.560	10.90	8.440	33.00	5.260	6.000	617.0	12.00
MILK-WHOLE-3.3% FAT-FLUID	1 cup	244.0	150.0	8.030	11.40	8.150	33.00	5.070	120.0	370.0	33.00
MILKSHAKE-CHOCOLATE-THICK	1 item	300.0	356.0	9.150	63.50	8.100	32.00	5.040	333.0	672.0	48.00
MILKSHAKE-VANILLA-THICK	1 item	313.0	350.0	12.10	55.60	9.480	37.00	5.900	299.0	572.0	37.00
YOGURT-FRUIT FLAVOR-LOWFAT	1 cup	227.0	231.0	9.920	43.20	2.450	10.00	1.580	133.0	442.0	33.00
YOGURT-PLAIN-LOWFAT	1 cup	227.0	144.0	11.90	16.00	3.520	14.00	2.270	159.0	531.0	40.00
YOGURT-PLAIN-WHOLE	1 cup	227.0	139.0	7.880	10.60	7.380	29.00	4.760	105.0	351.0	26.00
YOGURT-PLAIN-NONFAT	1 cup	227.0	127.0	13.00	17.40	0.410	4.000	0.264	174.0	579.0	43.00

Nutritive Components for Desserts

Food Name	Serving	Gm wt	KCAL Kc	PROT Gm	CARB Gm	FAT Gm	CHOL Mg	SAFA Gm	SOD Mg	POT Mg	MAG Mg
BROWNIES/NUTS-MIX/PREP	1 item	20.0	85.00	1.000	13.00	4.000	0.000	0.900	50.00	34.00	—
CAKE-ANGELFOOD-MIX/PREP	1 slice	53.0	142.0	4.200	31.50	0.122	0.000	—	142.0	51.90	5.830
CAKE-CHEESECAKE-COMMERCIAL	1 slice	85.0	257.0	4.610	24.30	16.30	—	—	189.0	83.30	8.500
CAKE-FRUIT-DARK-HOME REC	1 slice	15.0	55.00	1.000	9.000	2.000	7.000	0.500	23.00	74.00	—
CAKE-GINGERBREAD-MIX/PREP	1 slice	63.0	175.0	2.000	32.00	4.000	1.000	1.100	90.00	173.0	14.00
CAKE-POUND-HOME RECIPE	1 slice	33.0	160.0	2.000	16.00	10.00	68.00	5.900	58.00	20.00	—
CAKE-SHEET-NO ICING-HOME	1 slice	86.0	315.0	4.000	48.00	12.00	1.000	3.300	382.0	68.00	12.00
CAKE-SPONGE-HOME RECIPE	1 slice	66.0	188.0	4.820	35.70	3.140	162.0	1.100	164.0	59.40	7.260
CAKE-STRAWBERRY SHORTCAKE	1 srvg	175.0	344.0	4.800	61.20	8.900	—	—	—	—	—
CAKE-YELLOW/ICING-HOME REC	1 slice	69.0	268.0	2.900	40.30	11.40	36.00	3.000	191.0	72.50	13.10
COOKIE-CHOCOLATE CHIP-MIX	1 item	10.5	50.00	0.500	6.960	2.420	5.520	0.700	37.80	13.50	2.520
COOKIE-CHOC CHIP-HOME REC	1 item	10.0	46.30	0.500	6.410	2.680	5.250	0.600	20.60	20.50	3.500
COOKIE-MACAROON	1 item	19.0	90.00	1.000	12.50	4.500	0.000	—	6.000	88.00	—
COOKIE-OATMEAL/RAISIN-MIX	1 item	13.0	61.50	0.732	8.930	2.600	0.000	0.500	37.10	22.60	3.640
COOKIE-PEANUT BUTTER-MIX	1 item	10.0	50.00	0.800	5.870	2.640	—	—	56.60	19.40	3.900
COOKIE-SANDWICH-CHOC/VAN	1 item	10.0	50.00	0.500	7.000	2.250	0.000	0.550	63.00	3.750	5.100
COOKIE-SUGAR-MIX	1 item	20.0	98.80	0.908	13.10	4.790	—	—	109.0	13.60	1.600
COOKIE-VANILLA WAFER	1 item	4.0	18.50	0.200	3.000	0.600	2.500	0.100	10.00	2.900	0.680
CUPCAKE/CHOCOLATE ICING	1 item	36.0	130.0	2.000	21.00	5.000	15.00	2.000	120.0	42.00	—
CUSTARD-BAKED	1 cup	265.0	305.0	14.00	29.00	15.00	278.0	6.800	209.0	387.0	—
DANISH PASTRY-PLAIN	1 item	65.0	250.0	4.060	29.10	13.60	0.000	4.700	249.0	60.50	9.750

Continued.

IRON Mg	ZINC Mg	V-A IU	V-ET Mg	V-C Mg	THIA Mg	RIBO Mg	NIAC Mg	V-B6 Mg	FOL Ug	VB12 Ug	CALC Mg	PHOS Mg	SEL Mg	FIBD Gm
0.170	1.230	1050	1.520	2.080	0.085	0.361	0.189	0.094	6.000	0.796	254.0	230.0	0.001	0.000
0.070	0.550	3499	1.500	1.380	0.052	0.262	0.093	0.062	9.000	0.428	154.0	149.0	—	0.000
0.100	0.650	1728	1.510	1.820	0.077	0.355	0.137	0.077	6.000	0.528	231.0	192.0	0.001	0.000
0.140	0.620	1817	—	1.980	0.081	0.343	0.154	0.037	25.00	0.690	268.0	195.0	—	0.000
—	—	0.000	—	0.000	0.000	0.000	0.000	0.000	0.000	0.000	1.000	13.00	—	0.000
0.010	0.080	68.00	—	0.130	0.005	0.022	0.010	0.002	2.000	0.045	16.00	14.00	—	0.000
0.090	0.020	646.0	—	0.000	0.000	0.000	0.000	0.000	0.000	0.000	5.000	6.000	—	0.000
0.010	0.010	331.0	—	0.000	0.000	0.000	0.000	0.000	0.000	0.000	4.000	13.00	—	0.000
0.030	0.220	548.0	—	0.000	0.022	0.039	0.042	0.025	—	0.175	61.00	54.00	—	0.000
0.120	1.030	81.00	0.980	2.400	0.083	0.377	0.142	0.083	—	0.537	285.0	219.0	0.003	0.000
0.600	1.020	302.0	—	2.280	0.092	0.405	0.313	0.100	12.00	0.835	280.0	251.0	0.003	0.300
0.580	2.880	1004	0.337	7.960	0.275	1.270	0.643	0.156	34.00	1.360	868.0	775.0	0.003	0.000
0.510	1.170	894.0	—	3.810	0.086	0.483	0.267	0.127	2.000	1.140	330.0	278.0	0.003	0.000
0.740	2.300	1000	0.459	3.160	0.115	0.788	0.444	0.140	23.00	0.609	740.0	497.0	0.003	0.000
0.479	1.940	612.0	0.454	4.740	0.118	0.796	0.489	0.126	20.20	0.411	658.0	509.0	0.003	0.000
0.070	0.420	593.0	2.440	12.30	0.034	0.089	0.435	0.027	13.00	0.111	79.00	34.00	0.004	0.000
0.120	0.950	500.0	0.220	2.370	0.095	0.407	0.212	0.105	12.00	0.898	300.0	235.0	0.003	0.000
0.120	0.950	500.0	0.220	2.320	0.095	0.403	0.210	0.105	12.00	0.888	297.0	232.0	0.003	0.000
0.120	0.980	500.0	0.220	2.450	0.098	0.424	0.220	0.110	13.00	0.936	313.0	245.0	0.003	0.000
0.210	3.000	1612	—	3.790	0.281	1.190	0.606	0.235	34.00	2.720	837.0	670.0	—	0.000
0.100	0.980	500.0	0.221	2.400	0.088	0.343	0.216	0.098	13.00	0.926	302.0	247.0	0.003	0.000
—	—	317.0	0.220	—	0.049	0.256	0.105	0.083	—	0.876	246.0	209.0	0.003	0.000
0.120	0.930	307.0	0.220	2.290	0.093	0.395	0.205	0.102	12.00	0.871	291.0	228.0	0.003	0.000
0.930	1.440	258.0	—	0.000	0.141	0.666	0.372	0.075	15.00	0.945	396.0	378.0	0.005	0.900
0.310	1.220	357.0	—	0.000	0.094	0.610	0.457	0.131	21.00	1.630	457.0	361.0	0.005	0.200
0.160	1.680	104.0	—	1.500	0.084	0.404	0.216	0.091	21.00	1.060	345.0	271.0	—	0.800
0.180	2.020	150.0	—	1.820	0.100	0.486	0.259	0.111	25.00	1.280	415.0	326.0	—	0.000
0.110	1.340	279.0	—	1.200	0.066	0.322	0.170	0.073	17.00	0.844	274.0	215.0	—	0.000
0.200	2.200	16.00	—	1.980	0.109	0.531	0.281	0.120	28.00	1.390	452.0	355.0	—	0.000

IRON Mg	ZINC Mg	V-A IU	V-ET Mg	V-C Mg	THIA Mg	RIBO Mg	NIAC Mg	V-B6 Mg	FOL Ug	VB12 Ug	CALC Mg	PHOS Mg	SEL Mg	FIBD Gm
0.400	—	20.00	1.090	0.000	0.030	0.020	0.200	—	—	—	9.000	27.00	0.001	—
0.451	0.106	0.000	4.500	0.000	0.064	0.122	0.594	0.007	4.770	0.015	50.00	63.00	0.003	0.000
0.408	0.357	216.0	—	4.250	0.026	0.111	0.391	0.054	15.30	0.421	47.60	74.80	—	—
0.400	—	20.00	—	0.000	0.020	0.020	0.200	—	—	—	11.00	17.00	0.001	—
0.900	0.284	0.000	—	0.000	0.090	0.110	0.800	0.048	5.000	0.066	57.00	63.00	0.004	0.000
0.500	—	80.00	2.800	0.000	0.050	0.060	0.400	—	1.980	—	6.000	24.00	0.002	0.080
0.900	0.301	150.0	7.300	0.000	0.130	0.150	1.100	0.024	6.020	0.087	55.00	88.00	0.006	—
1.110	0.799	125.0	5.600	0.000	0.092	0.132	0.726	0.037	14.50	0.332	25.10	65.30	0.004	0.000
2.000	—	429.0	—	89.00	0.170	0.210	1.300	—	—	—	73.00	84.00	—	—
0.787	0.338	47.60	5.860	0.000	0.076	0.097	0.656	0.023	5.520	0.123	57.30	60.70	0.004	—
0.228	0.053	6.090	0.573	0.000	0.014	0.022	0.195	0.002	0.945	—	2.940	7.460	0.001	0.040
0.249	0.044	4.300	0.545	0.000	0.015	0.015	0.146	0.002	0.900	0.010	3.300	8.400	0.001	0.080
0.150	—	0.000	1.040	0.000	0.010	0.030	0.100	—	—	—	5.000	16.00	0.001	—
0.285	0.085	10.40	0.708	0.000	0.022	0.021	0.241	0.006	1.560	—	4.420	14.40	0.001	—
0.190	0.750	15.20	0.545	0.000	0.019	0.016	0.381	0.008	2.400	—	11.50	23.50	—	—
0.175	0.086	0.000	0.545	0.000	0.015	0.025	0.175	0.004	0.300	0.000	2.500	24.00	0.001	—
0.386	0.054	14.80	1.090	0.000	0.036	0.024	0.466	0.011	1.800	—	20.80	37.80	0.001	—
0.060	—	5.000	0.218	0.000	0.010	0.009	0.080	—	—	—	1.600	2.500	0.000	0.010
0.400	—	60.00	0.720	0.000	0.050	0.060	0.400	—	—	—	47.00	71.00	0.003	—
1.100	—	930.0	—	1.000	0.110	0.500	0.300	—	—	—	297.0	310.0	0.003	—
1.200	0.546	69.60	—	0.000	0.156	0.150	1.470	—	—	—	68.90	66.30	—	—

Continued.

Nutritive Components for Desserts—cont'd

Food Name	Serving	Gm wt	KCAL Kc	PROT Gm	CARB Gm	FAT Gm	CHOL Mg	SAFA Gm	SOD Mg	POT Mg	MAG Mg
DOUGHNUTS-CAKE-PLAIN	1 item	25.0	104.0	1.280	12.20	5.770	10.00	1.200	139.0	27.30	5.750
DOUGHNUTS-YEAST-GLAZED	1 item	50.0	205.0	3.000	22.00	11.20	13.00	3.000	117.0	34.00	9.500
FROZ YOGURT-FRUIT VARIETY	1 cup	226.0	216.0	7.000	41.80	2.000	—	—	—	—	24.00
GRANOLA BAR	1 item	24.0	109.0	2.350	16.00	4.230	—	—	66.70	78.20	—
ICE CREAM-VAN-SOFT SERVE	1 cup	173.0	377.0	7.040	38.30	22.50	153.0	13.50	153.0	338.0	25.00
ICE CREAM-VAN-HARD-10% FAT	1 cup	133.0	269.0	4.800	31.70	14.30	59.00	8.920	116.0	257.0	18.00
ICE CREAM SUNDAE-HOT FUDGE	1 item	165.0	312.0	7.260	46.50	10.90	18.20	—	177.0	413.0	34.70
ICE MILK-VAN-SOFT-2.6% FAT	1 cup	175.0	223.0	8.030	38.40	4.620	13.00	2.880	163.0	412.0	29.00
PIE-APPLE-HOME REC	1 slice	135.0	323.0	2.750	49.10	13.60	0.000	3.900	207.0	115.0	10.80
PIE-BANANA CREAM-HOME REC	1 slice	130.0	285.0	6.000	40.00	12.00	40.00	3.800	252.0	264.0	—
PIE-CHERRY-HOME REC	1 slice	135.0	350.0	4.000	52.00	15.00	0.000	4.000	410.0	142.0	9.450
PIE-CUSTARD-HOME REC	1 slice	130.0	285.0	8.000	30.00	14.00	—	4.800	373.0	178.0	—
PIE-LEMON MERINGUE-HOME	1 slice	120.0	300.0	3.860	47.30	11.20	0.000	3.700	223.0	52.80	7.200
PIE-MINCE-HOME REC	1 slice	135.0	365.0	3.000	56.00	16.00	0.000	4.000	604.0	240.0	24.30
PIE-PEACH-HOME REC	1 slice	135.0	345.0	3.000	52.00	14.00	0.000	3.500	361.0	21.00	9.450
PIE-PECAN-HOME REC	1 slice	118.0	495.0	6.000	61.00	27.00	0.000	4.000	260.0	145.0	—
PIE-PUMPKIN-HOME REC	1 slice	130.0	275.0	5.000	32.00	15.00	0.000	5.400	278.0	208.0	16.90
PUDD-CHOC-COOKED-MIX/MILK	1 cup	260.0	320.0	9.000	59.00	8.000	32.00	4.300	335.0	354.0	—
PUDD-CHOC-INST-MIX/MILK	1 cup	260.0	325.0	8.000	63.00	7.000	28.00	3.600	322.0	335.0	—
PUDD-RICE/RAISINS	1 cup	265.0	387.0	9.500	70.80	8.200	—	—	188.0	469.0	—
PUDD-TAPIOCA CREAM-HOME	1 cup	165.0	220.0	8.000	28.00	8.000	80.00	4.100	257.0	223.0	—
SHERBET-ORANGE-2% FAT	1 cup	193.0	270.0	2.160	58.70	3.820	14.00	2.380	88.00	198.0	15.00
TOASTER PASTRIES	1 item	50.0	196.0	1.930	35.20	5.750	0.000	—	230.0	84.50	9.000
TURNOVER-APPLE	1 srvg	28.8	85.20	0.738	10.50	4.710	1.420	—	109.0	13.90	2.560
TWINKIE-HOSTESS	1 item	42.0	143.0	1.250	25.60	4.200	21.00	—	189.0	—	—
PIECRUST-MIX/PREP-BAKED	1 item	160.0	743.0	10.00	70.50	46.50	0.000	11.40	1300	89.50	—

Nutritive Components for Eggs

Food Name	Serving	Gm wt	KCAL Kc	PROT Gm	CARB Gm	FAT Gm	CHOL Mg	SAFA Gm	SOD Mg	POT Mg	MAG Mg
EGG-FRIED IN BUTTER-LARGE	1 item	46.0	83.00	5.370	0.530	6.410	246.0	2.410	144.0	58.00	5.000
EGG-HARD-LARGE-NO SHELL	1 item	50.0	79.00	6.070	0.600	5.580	274.0	1.670	69.00	65.00	6.000
OMELET-HAM AND CHEESE	1 item	118.0	255.0	17.10	6.730	17.70	446.0	—	399.0	189.0	18.90
EGG-POACHED-WHOLE-LARGE	1 item	50.0	79.00	6.040	0.600	5.550	273.0	1.670	146.0	65.00	6.000
EGG-SCRAMBLED-MILK/BUTTER	1 item	64.0	95.00	5.960	1.370	7.080	248.0	2.820	155.0	85.00	8.000
EGG-WHITE-RAW-LARGE	1 item	33.0	16.00	3.350	0.410	0.000	0.000	0.000	50.00	45.00	3.000
EGG-WHOLE-RAW-LARGE	1 item	50.0	79.00	6.070	0.600	5.580	274.0	1.670	69.00	65.00	6.000
EGG-YOLK-RAW-LARGE	1 item	17.0	63.00	2.790	0.040	5.600	272.0	1.680	8.000	15.00	3.000
EGG-SUBSTITUTE-LIQUID	1 cup	251.0	211.0	30.10	1.610	8.310	3.000	1.660	444.0	828.0	—

Nutritive Components for Fast Foods

Food Name	Serving	Gm wt	KCAL Kc	PROT Gm	CARB Gm	FAT Gm	CHOL Mg	SAFA Gm	SOD Mg	POT Mg	MAG Mg
ARBYS-BEEF/CHEESE SANDWICH	1 item	168.0	450.0	27.00	36.00	22.00	55.00	—	1220	—	—
ARBYS-CLUB SANDWICH	1 item	252.0	560.0	30.00	43.00	30.00	100.0	—	1610	—	—
ARBYS-HAM/CHEESE SANDWICH	1 item	154.0	380.0	23.00	33.00	17.00	60.00	—	1350	—	—
ARBYS-ROAST BEEF SANDWICH	1 item	140.0	350.0	22.00	32.00	15.00	45.00	—	880.0	—	—
ARTHUR TREACHER-CHICK SAND	1 item	156.0	413.0	16.20	44.00	19.20	—	—	708.0	279.0	27.00
BURGER KING-WHOP HAMBURGER	1 item	261.0	630.0	26.00	50.00	36.00	—	—	990.0	520.0	—

Continued.

IRON Mg	ZINC Mg	V-A IU	V-ET Mg	V-C Mg	THIA Mg	RIBO Mg	NIAC Mg	V-B6 Mg	FOL Ug	VB12 Ug	CALC Mg	PHOS Mg	SEL Mg	FIBD Gm
0.365	0.128	14.30	1.010	0.000	0.060	0.050	0.428	0.009	2.000	—	11.00	55.00	—	0.090
0.600	—	25.00	2.030	0.000	0.100	0.100	0.800	—	11.00	—	16.00	33.00	—	0.300
0.000	—	0.000	—	0.000	0.010	0.260	0.000	—	—	—	200.0	200.0	—	—
0.763	—	—	—	—	0.067	0.026	—	—	—	0.000	14.40	66.50	—	—
0.430	1.990	794.0	0.606	0.920	0.080	0.448	0.178	0.095	9.000	0.996	236.0	199.0	0.003	0.000
0.120	1.410	543.0	0.466	0.700	0.052	0.329	0.134	0.061	3.000	0.625	176.0	134.0	0.002	0.000
0.611	0.990	231.0	0.577	3.300	0.066	0.314	1.120	0.132	9.900	0.660	216.0	238.0	—	—
0.280	0.860	175.0	0.610	1.170	0.117	0.541	0.184	0.133	5.000	1.370	274.0	202.0	0.003	0.000
1.220	0.230	25.70	9.840	2.000	0.149	0.108	1.240	0.035	6.750	0.000	12.20	31.10	0.015	—
1.000	—	330.0	—	1.000	0.110	0.220	1.000	—	—	—	86.00	107.0	0.015	—
0.900	—	590.0	9.840	0.000	0.160	0.120	1.400	—	—	0.000	19.00	34.00	0.015	—
1.200	—	300.0	9.480	0.000	0.110	0.270	0.800	—	—	—	125.0	147.0	0.015	0.000
0.900	0.336	167.0	8.750	3.660	0.096	0.120	0.720	0.029	10.80	0.191	15.60	48.00	0.013	0.000
1.900	—	0.000	9.840	1.000	0.140	0.120	1.400	—	—	—	38.00	51.00	0.015	—
1.200	—	990.0	9.840	4.000	0.150	0.140	2.000	—	—	0.000	14.00	39.00	0.015	—
3.700	—	190.0	—	0.000	0.260	0.140	1.000	—	—	—	55.00	122.0	0.012	—
1.000	—	3210	9.480	0.000	0.110	0.180	1.000	—	—	—	66.00	90.00	0.015	—
0.800	—	340.0	—	2.000	0.050	0.390	0.300	—	—	—	265.0	247.0	—	0.000
1.300	—	340.0	—	2.000	0.080	0.390	0.300	—	—	—	374.0	237.0	—	0.000
1.100	—	290.0	—	0.000	0.080	0.370	0.500	—	—	—	260.0	249.0	—	—
0.700	—	480.0	—	2.000	0.070	0.300	0.200	—	—	—	173.0	180.0	—	0.000
0.310	1.330	185.0	—	3.860	0.033	0.089	0.131	0.025	14.00	0.158	103.0	74.00	—	0.000
2.000	0.290	482.0	—	0.000	0.160	0.170	2.100	0.190	40.00	0.000	96.50	96.50	—	—
0.312	0.054	11.40	2.070	0.284	0.028	0.020	0.332	0.011	1.140	0.028	3.980	11.40	—	—
0.545	—	40.50	—	0.000	0.055	0.060	0.500	—	—	—	19.00	—	—	—
3.050	—	0.000	1.390	0.000	0.535	0.395	4.950	—	—	—	65.50	136.0	—	—

IRON Mg	ZINC Mg	V-A IU	V-ET Mg	V-C Mg	THIA Mg	RIBO Mg	NIAC Mg	V-B6 Mg	FOL Ug	VB12 Ug	CALC Mg	PHOS Mg	SEL Mg	FIBD Gm
0.920	0.640	286.0	—	0.000	0.033	0.126	0.026	0.050	22.00	0.581	26.00	80.00	—	0.000
1.040	0.720	260.0	—	0.000	0.037	0.143	0.030	0.057	24.00	0.657	28.00	90.00	—	0.000
2.940	2.170	743.0	—	5.900	0.142	0.555	0.696	0.189	41.30	1.180	116.0	287.0	—	—
1.040	0.720	259.0	—	0.000	0.035	0.127	0.026	0.051	24.00	0.616	28.00	90.00	—	0.000
0.930	0.700	311.0	—	0.130	0.039	0.156	0.042	0.058	22.00	0.638	47.00	97.00	—	0.000
0.010	0.010	0.000	—	0.000	0.002	0.094	0.029	0.001	5.000	0.021	4.000	4.000	0.002	0.000
1.040	0.720	260.0	0.530	0.000	0.044	0.150	0.031	0.060	32.00	0.773	28.00	90.00	0.012	0.000
0.950	0.580	313.0	0.530	0.000	0.043	0.074	0.012	0.053	26.00	0.647	26.00	86.00	0.003	0.000
5.270	3.260	5422	—	0.000	0.276	0.753	0.276	—	—	0.748	133.0	304.0	—	0.000

IRON Mg	ZINC Mg	V-A IU	V-ET Mg	V-C Mg	THIA Mg	RIBO Mg	NIAC Mg	V-B6 Mg	FOL Ug	VB12 Ug	CALC Mg	PHOS Mg	SEL Mg	FIBD Gm
4.500	—	—	—	—	0.380	0.430	6.000	—	—	—	200.0	—	—	—
3.600	—	—	—	—	0.680	0.430	7.000	—	—	—	200.0	—	—	—
2.700	—	—	—	—	0.750	0.340	5.000	—	—	—	200.0	—	—	—
3.600	—	—	—	—	0.300	0.340	5.000	—	—	—	80.00	—	—	—
1.700	—	123.0	—	19.00	0.170	0.240	8.100	—	—	—	59.00	147.0	—	—
6.000	—	641.0	—	13.00	0.020	0.030	5.200	—	—	—	37.00	—	—	—

Continued.

Nutritive Components for Fast Foods—cont'd

Food Name	Serving	Gm wt	KCAL Kc	PROT Gm	CARB Gm	FAT Gm	CHOL Mg	SAFA Gm	SOD Mg	POT Mg	MAG Mg
CHURCHS CHICK-WHITE MEAT	1 item	100.0	327.0	21.00	10.00	23.00	—	—	498.0	186.0	—
DAIRY QUEEN-BANANA SPLIT	1 item	383.0	540.0	10.00	91.00	15.00	30.00	—	—	—	—
DAIRY QUEEN-DIP CONE-REG	1 item	156.0	300.0	7.000	40.00	13.00	20.00	—	—	—	—
DAIRY QUEEN-FLOAT	1 item	397.0	330.0	6.000	59.00	8.000	20.00	—	—	—	—
DAIRY QUEEN-CONE-REGULAR	1 item	142.0	230.0	6.000	35.00	7.000	20.00	—	—	—	—
DAIRY QUEEN-MALT-REGULAR	1 item	418.0	600.0	15.00	89.00	20.00	50.00	—	—	—	—
DAIRY QUEEN-SUNDAE-REGULAR	1 item	177.0	290.0	6.000	51.00	7.000	20.00	—	—	—	—
JACK/BOX-BREAK JACK SAND	1 item	121.0	301.0	18.00	28.00	13.00	182.0	—	1037	190.0	24.00
JACK/BOX-JUMBO JACK HAMBUR	1 item	246.0	551.0	28.00	45.00	29.00	80.00	—	1134	492.0	44.00
JACK/BOX-JUMBO JACK/CHEESE	1 item	272.0	628.0	32.00	45.00	35.00	110.0	—	1666	499.0	49.00
JACK/BOX-MOBY JACK	1 item	141.0	455.0	17.00	38.00	26.00	56.00	—	837.0	246.0	30.00
JACK/BOX-ONION RINGS-BAG	1 item	85.0	351.0	5.000	32.00	23.00	24.00	—	318.0	109.0	16.00
KENTUCKY FRIED-EXTRA CRISP	1 srvg	375.0	765.0	38.30	54.70	44.00	183.0	10.50	1480	776.0	70.00
KENTUCKY FRIED-CHICKEN DIN	1 item	346.0	643.0	35.00	46.00	35.00	180.0	7.800	1441	720.0	66.00
MCDONALD-BIG MAC HAMBURGER	1 item	204.0	563.0	26.00	41.00	33.00	86.00	—	1010	237.0	38.00
MCDONALDS-CHEESEBURGER	1 item	115.0	307.0	15.00	30.00	14.00	37.00	—	767.0	156.0	23.00
MCDONALD'S-CHICK MCNUGGETS	1 srvg	111.0	314.0	20.30	15.40	19.00	76.00	—	525.0	—	—
MCDONALDS-EGG MCMUFFIN	1 item	138.0	327.0	19.00	31.00	15.00	229.0	—	885.0	168.0	26.00
MCDONALDS-FILET O FISH	1 item	139.0	432.0	14.00	37.00	25.00	47.00	—	781.0	150.0	27.00
MCDONALD'S-FRENCH FRIES	1 srvg	68.0	220.0	3.000	26.10	11.50	9.000	—	109.0	564.0	27.00
MCDONALDS-HAMBURGER	1 item	102.0	255.0	12.00	30.00	10.00	25.00	—	520.0	142.0	19.00
MCDONALD'S-HOT CAKES-SYRUP	1 srvg	214.0	500.0	7.900	93.90	10.30	47.00	—	1070	187.0	28.00
MCDONALDS-QP HAMBURGER	1 item	166.0	424.0	24.00	33.00	22.00	67.00	—	735.0	322.0	37.00
MCDONALD-QP HAMBURGER W/ CH	1 item	194.0	524.0	30.00	32.00	31.00	96.00	—	1236	341.0	41.00
TACO BELL-BEAN BURRITO	1 item	166.0	343.0	11.00	48.00	12.00	—	—	272.0	235.0	78.00
TACO BELL-BEEF BURRITO	1 item	184.0	466.0	30.00	37.00	21.00	—	—	327.0	320.0	—
TACO BELL-BEEFY TOSTADA	1 item	184.0	291.0	19.00	21.00	15.00	—	—	138.0	277.0	—
TACO BELL-BURRITO SUPREME	1 item	255.0	457.0	21.00	43.00	22.00	—	—	367.0	350.0	—
TACO BELL-TACO-REGULAR	1 item	83.0	186.0	15.00	14.00	8.000	—	—	79.00	143.0	40.70
TACO BELL-TOSTADA-REGULAR	1 item	138.0	179.0	9.000	25.00	6.000	—	—	101.0	172.0	—
WENDYS-SINGLE HAMBURGER	1 item	200.0	470.0	26.00	34.00	26.00	70.00	—	774.0	—	—
WENDYS-DOUBLE HAMBURGER	1 item	285.0	670.0	44.00	34.00	40.00	125.0	—	980.0	—	—
WENDYS-TRIPLE HAMBURGER	1 item	360.0	850.0	65.00	33.00	51.00	205.0	—	1217	—	—

Nutritive Components for Fats & Oils

Food Name	Serving	Gm wt	KCAL Kc	PROT Gm	CARB Gm	FAT Gm	CHOL Mg	SAFA Gm	SOD Mg	POT Mg	MAG Mg
ANIMAL FAT-COOKING-CHICKEN	1 tbsp	12.8	115.0	0.000	0.000	12.80	11.00	3.800	—	—	—
BUTTER-REGULAR-TABLESPOON	1 tbsp	14.0	100.0	0.119	0.008	11.40	30.70	7.070	116.0	3.640	0.280
MARGARINE-CORN-REG-HARD	1 tsp	4.7	33.80	0.000	0.000	3.800	0.000	0.600	44.30	1.990	0.120
MARGARINE-DIET-MAZOLA	1 tbsp	14.0	50.00	0.000	0.000	5.700	0.000	1.000	130.0	—	—
MARGARINE-VEG SPRAY-MAZOLA	1 srvg	0.7	6.000	0.000	0.000	0.720	0.000	0.080	0.000	—	—
MARGARINE-CORN-REG-SOFT	1 tsp	4.7	33.70	0.000	0.000	3.800	0.000	0.700	50.70	1.770	0.110
MARGARINE-REG-HARD-STICK	1 item	113.0	815.0	1.000	1.000	91.30	0.000	17.90	1070	48.10	2.950
MAYONNAISE-IMITATION-SOY	1 tbsp	15.0	34.70	0.000	2.400	2.900	4.000	0.500	74.60	—	—
MAYONNAISE-LIGHT-LOW CAL	1 tbsp	14.0	40.00	0.000	1.000	4.000	5.000	—	—	—	—
MIRACLE WHIP-LIGHT-LOW CAL	1 tbsp	14.0	45.00	0.000	2.000	4.000	5.000	—	95.00	—	—
SAL DRESS-BLUE CHEESE	1 tbsp	15.3	77.10	0.700	1.100	8.000	9.000	1.500	167.0	6.120	—
SAL DRESS-BLUE CHE-LOW CAL	1 tbsp	16.0	10.00	0.000	1.000	1.000	4.000	0.500	177.0	5.000	—
SAL DRESS-CAESAR	1 tbsp	15.0	70.00	0.000	1.000	7.000	—	—	—	—	—
SAL DRESS-FRENCH	1 tbsp	15.6	67.00	0.100	2.700	6.400	1.950	1.500	214.0	12.30	—
SAL DRESS-FRENCH-LOW CAL	1 tbsp	16.3	21.90	0.000	3.500	0.900	1.000	0.100	128.0	13.00	—
SAL DRESS-ITALIAN	1 tbsp	14.7	68.70	0.000	1.500	7.100	0.000	1.000	116.0	2.000	—

Continued.

IRON Mg	ZINC Mg	V-A IU	V-ET Mg	V-C Mg	THIA Mg	RIBO Mg	NIAC Mg	V-B6 Mg	FOL Ug	VB12 Ug	CALC Mg	PHOS Mg	SEL Mg	FIBD Gm
1.000	—	160.0	—	1.000	0.100	0.180	7.200	—	—	—	94.00	—	—	—
1.800	—	750.0	—	18.00	0.600	0.600	0.800	—	—	0.900	350.0	250.0	—	—
0.400	—	300.0	—	0.000	0.090	0.340	0.000	—	—	0.600	200.0	150.0	—	—
0.000	—	100.0	—	0.000	0.120	0.170	0.000	—	—	0.600	200.0	200.0	—	—
0.000	—	300.0	—	0.000	0.090	0.260	0.000	—	—	0.600	200.0	150.0	—	—
3.600	—	750.0	—	3.600	0.120	0.600	0.800	—	—	1.800	500.0	400.0	—	—
1.100	—	300.0	—	0.000	0.060	0.260	0.000	—	—	0.600	200.0	150.0	—	—
2.500	1.800	442.0	—	3.000	0.410	0.470	5.100	0.140	—	1.100	177.0	310.0	—	—
4.500	4.200	246.0	—	3.700	0.470	0.340	11.60	0.300	—	2.680	134.0	261.0	—	—
4.600	4.800	734.0	—	4.900	0.520	0.380	11.30	0.310	—	3.050	273.0	411.0	—	—
1.700	1.100	240.0	—	1.000	0.300	0.210	4.500	0.120	—	1.100	167.0	263.0	—	—
1.400	0.400	—	5.360	1.200	0.240	0.120	3.100	0.070	—	0.260	26.00	69.00	—	—
4.090	3.580	255.0	—	37.00	0.320	0.380	10.40	0.540	46.00	1.560	130.0	383.0	—	—
3.900	3.470	255.0	—	37.00	0.250	0.320	8.500	0.460	42.00	1.530	116.0	363.0	—	—
4.000	4.700	530.0	—	2.200	0.390	0.370	6.500	0.270	21.00	1.800	157.0	314.0	—	—
2.400	2.600	345.0	—	2.000	0.250	0.230	3.800	0.120	21.00	0.910	132.0	205.0	—	—
1.070	—	—	—	2.000	0.120	0.160	8.600	—	—	—	11.00	—	—	—
2.900	1.900	97.00	—	1.400	0.470	0.440	3.800	0.210	29.00	0.750	226.0	322.0	—	—
1.700	0.900	42.00	—	1.400	0.260	0.200	2.600	0.100	20.00	0.820	93.00	229.0	—	1.110
0.600	0.300	17.00	—	13.00	0.120	0.020	2.300	0.220	19.00	0.030	9.000	101.0	—	—
2.300	2.100	82.00	—	1.700	0.250	0.180	4.000	0.120	17.00	0.810	51.00	126.0	—	—
2.200	0.700	257.0	—	5.000	0.260	0.360	2.300	0.120	9.000	0.190	103.0	501.0	—	—
4.100	5.100	133.0	—	1.700	0.320	0.280	6.500	0.270	23.00	1.880	63.00	249.0	—	—
4.300	5.700	660.0	—	2.700	0.310	0.370	7.400	0.230	23.00	2.150	219.0	382.0	—	—
2.800	1.400	1657	—	15.20	0.370	0.220	2.200	—	—	—	98.00	173.0	—	—
4.600	—	1675	—	15.20	0.300	0.390	7.000	—	—	—	83.00	288.0	—	—
3.400	—	3450	—	12.70	0.160	0.270	3.300	—	—	—	208.0	265.0	—	—
3.800	—	3462	—	16.00	0.330	0.350	4.700	—	—	—	121.0	245.0	—	—
2.500	2.200	120.0	—	0.200	0.090	0.160	2.900	—	—	—	120.0	175.0	—	—
2.300	—	3152	—	9.700	0.180	0.150	0.800	—	—	—	191.0	186.0	—	—
5.300	4.800	94.00	—	0.600	0.240	0.360	5.800	—	—	—	84.00	239.0	—	—
8.200	8.400	128.0	—	1.500	0.430	0.540	10.60	—	—	—	138.0	364.0	—	—
10.70	13.50	220.0	—	2.000	0.470	0.680	14.70	—	—	—	104.0	525.0	—	—

IRON Mg	ZINC Mg	V-A IU	V-ET Mg	V-C Mg	THIA Mg	RIBO Mg	NIAC Mg	V-B6 Mg	FOL Ug	VB12 Ug	CALC Mg	PHOS Mg	SEL Mg	FIBD Gm
—	—	—	0.300	—	—	—	—	—	—	—	—	—	—	0.000
0.022	0.007	428.0	0.221	0.000	0.001	0.005	0.006	0.000	0.420	—	3.360	3.220	—	0.000
—	—	155.0	2.710	0.008	0.000	0.002	0.001	0.000	0.060	0.004	1.410	1.080	—	0.000
0.000	—	500.0	1.350	0.000	0.000	0.000	0.000	—	—	—	0.000	—	—	0.000
0.000	—	0.000	—	0.000	0.000	0.000	0.000	—	—	—	0.000	0.000	—	0.000
—	—	155.0	2.000	0.007	0.000	0.002	0.001	0.000	0.050	0.004	1.250	0.950	—	0.000
0.070	—	3750	65.10	0.181	0.011	0.042	0.026	0.010	1.340	0.108	33.90	26.00	—	0.000
—	0.020	—	—	—	—	—	—	—	—	—	—	—	—	0.000
—	—	—	8.120	—	—	—	—	—	—	—	—	—	—	0.000
—	—	—	4.200	—	—	—	—	—	—	—	—	—	—	—
0.000	—	32.10	7.260	0.300	0.000	0.020	0.000	—	—	—	12.40	11.30	—	0.050
0.000	—	30.00	7.600	0.000	0.000	0.010	0.000	—	—	—	10.00	8.000	—	0.000
—	—	—	7.130	—	—	—	—	—	—	—	—	—	—	—
0.100	0.010	—	7.410	—	—	—	—	—	—	—	1.700	2.200	—	0.000
0.100	0.030	—	7.750	—	—	—	—	—	—	—	2.000	2.000	—	0.090
0.000	0.020	—	6.990	—	0.000	0.000	0.000	—	—	—	1.000	1.000	—	0.050

Continued.

Nutritive Components for Fats & Oils—cont'd

Food Name	Serving	Gm wt	KCAL Kc	PROT Gm	CARB Gm	FAT Gm	CHOL Mg	SAFA Gm	SOD Mg	POT Mg	MAG Mg
SAL DRESS-ITALIAN-LOW CAL	1 tbsp	15.0	15.80	0.000	0.700	1.500	1.000	0.200	118.0	2.000	—
SAL DRESS-MAYONNAISE TYPE	1 tbsp	14.7	57.30	0.000	3.500	4.900	4.000	0.700	104.0	1.000	0.290
SAL DRESS-MAYO-LOW CAL	1 tbsp	16.0	20.00	0.000	2.000	2.000	2.000	0.400	44.00	1.000	—
SAL DRESS-RANCH STYLE	1 tbsp	15.0	54.00	0.400	0.600	5.700	—	—	97.00	—	—
SAL DRESS-RUSSIAN-LOW CAL	1 tbsp	16.3	23.10	0.100	4.500	0.700	1.000	0.100	141.0	26.00	—
SAL DRESS-RUSSIAN	1 tbsp	15.3	76.00	0.200	1.600	7.800	0.000	1.100	133.0	24.00	—
SAL DRESS-THOUSAND ISLAND	1 tbsp	15.6	58.90	0.000	2.400	5.600	4.900	0.900	109.0	18.00	—
SAL DRESS-THOU ISL-LOW CAL	1 tbsp	15.3	24.30	0.100	2.500	1.600	2.000	0.200	153.0	17.00	—
SAL DRESS-VINEGAR/OIL-HOME	1 tbsp	15.6	71.80	0.000	0.400	8.000	0.000	1.500	0.100	1.200	—
SANDWICH SPREAD-COMMERCIAL	1 tbsp	15.3	59.50	0.100	3.400	5.200	12.00	0.800	—	—	—
SHORTENING-VEGETABLE-SOY	1 cup	205.0	1812	0.000	0.000	205.0	0.000	51.20	—	—	—
VEGETABLE OIL-CORN	1 cup	218.0	1927	0.000	0.000	218.0	0.000	27.70	0.000	0.000	0.000
VEGETABLE OIL-OLIVE	1 cup	216.0	1909	0.000	0.000	216.0	0.000	30.70	0.080	0.000	0.020
SAUCE-TARTAR-REGULAR	1 tbsp	14.0	75.00	0.000	1.000	8.000	9.000	1.500	98.00	11.00	—
BUTTER-WHIPPED-TABLESPOON	1 tbsp	9.0	64.50	0.077	0.005	7.300	19.70	4.540	74.30	2.340	0.180

Nutritive Components for Fish

Food Name	Serving	Gm wt	KCAL Kc	PROT Gm	CARB Gm	FAT Gm	CHOL Mg	SAFA Gm	SOD Mg	POT Mg	MAG Mg
FISH-ANCHOVY-FILLET-CAN	1 item	4.0	8.400	1.160	0.000	0.388	—	0.088	147.0	21.80	2.800
FISH-BASS-STRIPED-BROILED	1 srvg	100.0	228.0	20.20	7.900	12.80	0.000	—	67.10	—	43.00
FISH-BLUEFISH-BAKED/BUTTER	1 item	155.0	246.0	40.60	0.000	8.100	108.0	—	161.0	—	43.30
FISH-BLUEFISH-BROILED	1 piece	122.0	192.0	32.00	0.000	6.300	—	—	127.0	—	—
FISH-CARP-COOKED-DRY HEAT	1 srvg	85.0	138.0	19.40	0.000	6.100	72.00	1.180	54.00	363.0	32.00
FISH-CATFISH-FRIED-BREADED	1 srvg	85.0	194.0	15.40	6.830	11.30	69.00	2.800	238.0	289.0	23.00
FISH-CLAMS-BREADED-FRIED	1 srvg	85.0	171.0	12.10	8.780	9.480	52.00	2.280	309.0	277.0	12.00
FISH-CLAM-CAN-SOLID/LIQUID	1 srvg	28.4	15.00	2.330	0.667	0.333	17.70	0.067	14.70	39.70	—
FISH-CLAMS-CKD-MOIST HEAT	1 srvg	85.0	126.0	21.70	4.360	1.650	57.00	0.160	95.00	534.0	16.00
FISH-CLAMS-RAW-MEAT ONLY	1 srvg	85.0	63.00	10.90	2.180	0.830	29.00	0.080	47.00	267.0	8.000
FISH-COD-COOKED-DRY HEAT	1 piece	180.0	189.0	41.10	0.000	1.550	99.00	0.302	141.0	440.0	76.00
FISH-CRAB-IMITATION-SURIMI	1 srvg	85.0	87.00	10.20	8.690	1.110	17.00	—	715.0	77.00	—
FISH-CRAB-STEAMED-PIECES	1 cup	155.0	150.0	30.00	0.000	2.390	82.20	0.206	1662	406.0	52.70
FISH-CRAB CAKE	1 item	60.0	93.00	12.10	0.290	4.510	90.00	0.890	198.0	195.0	20.00
FISH-CRAB MEAT-KING-CAN	1 cup	135.0	135.0	24.00	1.000	3.200	135.0	0.600	675.0	149.0	29.00
FISH-CRAYFISH-CKD-MOIST	1 srvg	85.0	97.00	20.30	0.000	1.150	151.0	0.197	58.00	298.0	27.00
FISH-STICK-BREAD-FROZ-COOK	1 item	28.0	76.00	4.380	6.650	3.420	31.00	0.882	163.0	73.00	7.000
FISH-FLATFISH-CKD-DRY HEAT	1 srvg	85.0	99.00	20.50	0.000	1.300	58.00	0.309	89.00	292.0	50.00
FISH-GROUPER-CKD-DRY HEAT	1 srvg	85.0	100.0	21.10	0.000	1.110	40.00	0.254	45.00	403.0	32.00
FISH-HADDOCK-COOK-DRY HEAT	1 srvg	85.0	95.00	20.60	0.000	0.790	63.00	0.142	74.00	339.0	43.00
FISH-HALIBUT-BROILED-DRY	1 srvg	85.0	119.0	22.70	0.000	2.490	35.00	0.354	59.00	490.0	91.00
FISH-HERRING-BROIL	1 item	85.0	172.0	19.60	0.000	9.850	65.00	2.220	98.00	356.0	35.00
FISH-HERRING-CAN-PLAIN	1 srvg	100.0	208.0	19.90	0.000	13.60	98.00	—	—	—	—
FISH-LOBSTER-CKD-MOIST	1 cup	145.0	142.0	29.70	1.860	0.860	104.0	0.155	551.0	510.0	51.00
FISH-MACKEREL-BROIL/BUTTER	1 piece	130.0	300.0	28.30	0.000	20.50	4.000	—	61.20	—	—
FISH-MACKEREL-ATLANTIC-CAN	1 cup	190.0	296.0	44.00	0.000	12.00	150.0	3.390	720.0	369.0	70.00
FISH-MACKEREL-CKD-DRY HEAT	1 srvg	85.0	223.0	20.30	0.000	15.10	64.00	3.550	71.00	341.0	83.00
FISH-MUSSEL-BLUE-CKD-MOIST	1 srvg	85.0	147.0	20.20	6.280	3.810	48.00	0.723	313.0	228.0	32.00
FISH-PERCH-BREADED-FRIED	1 piece	85.0	195.0	16.00	6.000	11.00	32.00	2.700	128.0	242.0	—
FISH-OCEAN PERCH-CKD-DRY	1 srvg	85.0	103.0	20.30	0.000	1.780	46.00	0.266	82.00	298.0	33.00
FISH-OYSTER-EASTERN-CANNED	1 cup	248.0	170.0	17.50	9.700	6.140	136.0	1.570	277.0	568.0	135.0
FISH-OYSTER-EAST-CKD-MOIST	1 srvg	85.0	117.0	12.00	6.650	4.210	93.00	1.070	190.0	389.0	92.00
FISH-OYSTERS-RAW-MEAT ONLY	1 cup	248.0	170.0	17.50	9.700	6.140	136.0	1.570	277.0	568.0	135.0
FISH-OYSTERS-FRIED	1 srvg	85.0	167.0	7.460	9.880	10.70	69.00	2.720	355.0	208.0	49.00
FISH-OYSTERS-PACIFIC-RAW	1 srvg	85.0	69.00	8.030	4.210	1.960	—	0.434	90.00	143.0	19.00

Continued.

IRON Mg	ZINC Mg	V-A IU	V-ET Mg	V-C Mg	THIA Mg	RIBO Mg	NIAC Mg	V-B6 Mg	FOL Ug	VB12 Ug	CALC Mg	PHOS Mg	SEL Mg	FIBD Gm
0.000	—	—	7.130	—	0.000	0.000	0.000	—	—	—	0.000	1.000	—	0.090
0.000	—	32.00	4.400	—	0.000	0.000	0.000	—	—	—	2.000	4.000	—	0.000
0.000	—	40.00	4.800	—	0.000	0.000	0.000	—	—	—	3.000	4.000	—	0.000
—	—	—	4.500	—	—	—	—	—	—	—	—	—	—	0.000
0.100	—	—	7.740	—	—	—	—	—	—	—	3.000	6.000	—	0.200
0.100	0.070	106.0	7.270	1.000	0.010	0.010	0.100	—	—	—	3.000	6.000	—	0.000
0.100	0.020	50.00	7.450	0.000	0.000	0.000	0.000	—	—	—	2.000	3.000	—	0.600
0.100	—	49.00	6.990	0.000	0.000	0.000	0.000	—	—	—	2.000	3.000	—	0.300
—	—	—	7.410	—	—	—	—	—	—	—	—	—	—	0.000
—	—	—	5.280	—	—	—	—	—	—	—	—	—	—	—
—	—	—	197.0	—	—	—	—	—	—	—	—	—	—	0.000
0.000	0.000	—	181.0	0.000	0.000	0.000	0.000	0.000	0.000	0.000	0.000	0.000	—	0.000
0.830	0.130	—	27.30	0.000	0.000	0.000	0.000	0.000	0.000	0.000	0.380	2.630	—	0.000
0.100	—	30.00	7.210	0.000	0.000	0.000	0.000	—	—	—	3.000	4.000	—	—
0.014	0.005	275.0	0.142	0.000	0.000	0.003	0.004	0.000	0.270	—	2.160	2.070	—	0.000

IRON Mg	ZINC Mg	V-A IU	V-ET Mg	V-C Mg	THIA Mg	RIBO Mg	NIAC Mg	V-B6 Mg	FOL Ug	VB12 Ug	CALC Mg	PHOS Mg	SEL Mg	FIBD Gm
0.186	0.098	—	—	—	0.003	0.015	0.796	0.008	—	0.035	9.200	10.00	0.002	0.000
1.900	—	116.0	—	0.000	0.150	0.140	2.900	—	—	—	47.00	230.0	0.039	0.000
1.100	—	80.00	—	—	0.170	0.160	2.900	—	—	1.640	44.60	445.0	0.047	0.000
0.800	—	61.00	—	—	0.130	0.120	2.300	—	—	—	35.00	350.0	0.038	0.000
1.350	1.620	27.00	—	1.400	—	—	—	0.186	—	1.250	44.00	452.0	—	0.000
1.220	0.730	24.00	—	0.000	0.062	0.113	1.940	—	—	—	37.00	183.0	—	0.800
11.80	1.240	257.0	—	—	—	0.207	1.750	—	—	34.20	54.00	160.0	—	0.320
1.170	0.347	—	—	—	0.003	0.030	0.300	—	—	5.400	15.70	38.70	0.046	0.000
23.80	2.320	484.0	—	—	—	0.362	2.850	—	—	84.10	78.00	287.0	—	0.000
11.90	1.160	255.0	—	—	—	0.181	1.500	—	—	42.00	39.00	144.0	0.016	0.000
0.880	1.040	83.00	—	1.800	0.158	0.142	4.520	0.509	—	1.890	25.00	248.0	—	—
0.330	—	—	—	—	0.027	0.023	0.153	—	—	—	11.00	—	—	0.000
1.180	11.80	45.00	1.890	—	0.082	0.085	2.080	—	—	—	91.50	434.0	0.076	0.000
0.650	2.460	—	—	—	—	—	—	—	—	3.560	63.00	128.0	—	0.028
1.100	5.830	—	—	—	0.110	0.110	2.600	—	—	13.50	61.00	246.0	0.072	0.000
2.670	1.420	—	—	2.800	—	0.065	2.500	—	—	2.940	26.00	280.0	—	0.000
0.210	0.190	30.00	—	—	0.036	0.050	0.596	0.017	5.100	0.503	6.000	51.00	0.003	0.300
0.280	0.530	32.00	—	—	0.068	0.097	1.850	0.204	—	2.130	16.00	246.0	—	0.000
0.960	0.430	—	—	—	0.069	0.005	0.324	—	—	0.588	18.00	121.0	—	0.000
1.140	0.410	54.00	1.020	—	0.034	0.038	3.940	0.294	—	1.180	36.00	205.0	0.025	0.000
0.910	0.450	152.0	—	—	0.059	0.077	6.060	0.337	—	1.160	51.00	242.0	—	0.000
1.200	1.080	87.00	—	0.600	0.095	0.254	3.500	0.296	—	11.20	63.00	258.0	0.052	0.000
1.800	—	—	—	—	0.180	—	—	—	—	—	147.0	297.0	0.058	0.000
0.570	4.230	126.0	—	—	0.010	0.096	1.550	0.112	16.10	4.510	88.00	268.0	—	0.000
1.610	—	694.0	—	—	0.198	0.347	9.920	—	—	—	7.440	365.0	0.046	0.000
3.880	1.940	825.0	2.520	1.700	0.076	0.403	11.70	0.399	10.20	13.20	458.0	572.0	0.089	0.000
1.330	0.800	153.0	—	0.300	0.135	0.350	5.820	0.391	—	16.20	13.00	236.0	—	0.000
5.710	2.270	—	—	—	—	—	—	—	—	—	28.00	242.0	—	0.000
1.100	—	—	—	—	0.100	0.100	1.600	—	—	0.850	28.00	192.0	0.020	0.050
1.000	0.520	39.00	—	—	—	0.114	2.070	—	—	0.981	117.0	235.0	—	0.000
16.60	226.0	—	—	—	—	0.412	3.090	0.236	22.10	47.50	111.0	344.0	—	0.000
11.40	155.0	—	—	—	—	0.282	2.120	0.081	15.20	32.50	76.00	236.0	—	0.000
16.60	226.0	740.0	—	—	0.340	0.412	3.250	0.124	24.60	47.50	111.0	344.0	0.156	0.000
5.910	74.10	—	—	—	—	0.172	1.400	0.054	11.60	13.30	53.00	135.0	—	0.000
4.340	14.10	—	—	—	0.057	0.198	1.710	—	—	—	7.000	138.0	—	0.000

Continued.

Nutritive Components for Fish—cont'd

Food Name	Serving	Gm wt	KCAL Kc	PROT Gm	CARB Gm	FAT Gm	CHOL Mg	SAFA Gm	SOD Mg	POT Mg	MAG Mg
FISH-PERCH-COOKED-DRY HEAT	1 srvg	85.0	99.00	21.10	0.000	1.000	98.00	0.201	67.00	293.0	33.00
FISH-POLLOCK-ATLANTIC-RAW	1 srvg	85.0	78.00	16.50	0.000	0.830	60.00	0.115	73.00	302.0	57.00
FISH-POLLOCK-CKD-DRY HEAT	1 srvg	85.0	96.00	20.00	0.000	0.950	82.00	0.196	98.00	329.0	—
FISH-POMPANO-CKD-DRY HEAT	1 srvg	85.0	179.0	20.10	0.000	10.30	54.00	3.820	65.00	541.0	27.00
FISH-RED SNAPPER-CKD-DRY	1 srvg	85.0	109.0	22.40	0.000	1.460	40.00	0.310	48.00	444.0	31.00
FISH-ROCKFISH-CKD-DRY HEAT	1 srvg	100.0	121.0	24.00	0.000	2.010	44.00	0.474	77.00	520.0	34.00
FISH-ROE-RAW-EGGS	1 srvg	28.4	39.00	6.250	0.420	1.800	105.0	0.408	—	—	—
FISH-SALMON-BROIL/BUTTER	1 srvg	100.0	182.0	27.00	0.000	7.400	47.00	—	116.0	443.0	—
FISH-SALMON-CKD-MOIST HEAT	1 srvg	85.0	157.0	23.30	0.000	6.400	42.00	1.190	50.00	454.0	—
FISH-SALMON-PINK-CAN	1 srvg	85.0	118.0	16.80	0.000	5.140	—	1.310	471.0	277.0	29.00
FISH-SALMON-SMOKED	1 srvg	100.0	117.0	18.30	0.000	4.320	23.00	0.929	784.0	175.0	18.00
FISH-SARDINES-CAN/OIL	1 item	12.0	25.00	2.960	0.000	1.380	17.00	0.184	60.50	47.50	4.500
FISH-SCALLOPS-STEAMED	1 srvg	28.4	31.80	6.590	0.511	0.398	15.10	—	75.20	135.0	—
FISH-SCALLOPS-BREAD-FRIED	1 item	15.0	33.50	2.800	1.570	1.700	9.500	0.414	72.00	51.50	9.000
FISH-SEA BASS-CKD-DRY HEAT	1 srvg	85.0	105.0	20.10	0.000	2.180	45.00	0.557	74.00	279.0	45.00
FISH-SHAD-BAKE/MARG/BACON	1 srvg	100.0	201.0	23.20	0.000	11.30	69.40	—	79.00	377.0	—
FISH-SHRIMP-MEAT-CAN	1 cup	128.0	154.0	29.60	1.320	2.510	222.0	0.477	216.0	269.0	53.00
FISH-SHRIMP-CKD-MOIST HEAT	1 srvg	85.0	84.00	17.80	0.000	0.920	166.0	0.246	190.0	154.0	29.00
FISH-SHRIMP-FRENCH FRIED	1 srvg	85.0	206.0	18.20	9.750	10.40	150.0	1.770	292.0	191.0	34.00
FISH-SMELT-COOKED-DRY HEAT	1 srvg	85.0	106.0	19.20	0.000	2.640	76.00	0.492	65.00	316.0	33.00
FISH-SOLE/FLOUNDER-BAKED	1 srvg	127.0	148.0	30.70	0.000	1.940	86.00	0.461	133.0	436.0	74.00
FISH-SQUID-COOKED-FRIED	1 srvg	85.0	149.0	15.30	6.620	6.360	221.0	1.600	260.0	237.0	33.00
FISH-STURGEON-COOKED	1 srvg	100.0	135.0	20.70	0.000	5.180	—	1.170	108.0	364.0	—
FISH-SURIMI	1 srvg	85.0	84.00	12.90	5.820	0.770	25.00	—	122.0	95.00	—
FISH-SWORDFISH-BROIL/MARG	1 srvg	100.0	174.0	28.00	0.000	6.000	4.000	—	25.00	—	—
FISH-SWORDFISH-COOKED-DRY	1 srvg	85.0	132.0	21.60	0.000	4.370	43.00	1.200	98.00	314.0	29.00
FISH-TROUT-BROOK-COOKED	1 srvg	100.0	196.0	23.50	0.400	11.20	—	—	78.80	—	35.00
FISH-TROUT-RAINBOW-CKD-DRY	1 srvg	85.0	129.0	22.40	0.000	3.660	62.00	0.707	29.00	539.0	33.00
FISH-TUNA-CAN/OIL-DRAINED	1 srvg	85.0	169.0	24.80	0.000	6.980	15.00	1.300	301.0	176.0	26.00
FISH-TUNA-DIET-LOW SODIUM	1 srvg	28.4	35.50	7.670	0.011	0.540	9.940	—	11.40	73.80	9.090
FISH-TUNA-LIGHT-CAN/WATER	1 srvg	85.0	111.0	25.10	0.000	0.430	—	0.136	303.0	267.0	25.00
FISH-TUNA-WHITE-CAN/WATER	1 srvg	85.0	116.0	22.70	0.000	2.090	35.00	0.556	333.0	241.0	—
FISH-TUNA-YELLOWFIN-RAW	1 srvg	85.0	92.00	19.90	0.000	0.810	38.00	0.200	31.00	—	—
FISH-WHITEFISH-BAKE/STUFF	1 srvg	100.0	215.0	15.20	5.800	14.00	—	—	195.0	291.0	—
FISH-WHITE PERCH-FRI-FILET	1 item	65.0	108.0	12.50	0.000	5.300	0.000	—	—	—	—
FISH-WHITING-CKD-DRY HEAT	1 srvg	85.0	98.00	20.00	0.000	1.430	71.00	0.269	113.0	369.0	23.00

Nutritive Components for Frozen Dinners

Food Name	Serving	Gm wt	KCAL Kc	PROT Gm	CARB Gm	FAT Gm	CHOL Mg	SAFA Gm	SOD Mg	POT Mg	MAG Mg
BEEF DINNER-SWANSON	1 item	326.0	320.0	25.00	34.00	9.000	—	—	1085	—	—
BEEF SIRLOIN TIPS-LE MENU	1 item	326.0	390.0	32.00	24.00	18.00	—	—	1100	—	—
CHE CANNELLONI-LEAN CUIS	1 item	259.0	270.0	22.00	24.00	10.00	45.00	—	900.0	270.0	—
CHICKEN DINNER-SWANSON	1 item	326.0	660.0	26.00	64.00	33.00	—	—	1610	—	—
CHICKEN PARMIGIANA-LE MENU	1 item	326.0	400.0	27.00	27.00	20.00	—	—	895.0	—	—
EGG ROLL-BEEF/SHRIMP-FROZ	1 item	12.0	27.00	0.900	3.500	1.000	—	—	80.50	—	—
FETTUCINI ALFREDO-STOUFFER	1 item	142.0	270.0	8.000	19.00	18.00	—	—	1195	240.0	—
FISH DIVAN-LEAN CUISINE	1 item	351.0	270.0	31.00	16.00	10.00	85.00	—	780.0	850.0	—
FISH & CHIPS-VAN DE KAMPS	1 item	224.0	500.0	16.00	45.00	30.00	—	—	551.0	—	—
HAM-FROZ DIN-BANQUET	1 item	284.0	369.0	16.80	47.70	12.20	—	—	1590	125.0	—
MANICOTTI-CHEESE-LE MENU	1 item	241.0	310.0	18.00	29.00	13.00	—	—	840.0	—	—
MEATLOAF-FROZ DIN-BANQUET	1 item	312.0	412.0	20.90	29.00	23.70	—	—	1991	468.0	—
MEXICAN DINNER-SWANSON	1 item	454.0	590.0	20.00	64.00	29.00	—	—	1865	—	—
SALISBURY STEAK DIN-BANQ	1 item	312.0	390.0	18.10	24.00	24.60	—	—	2059	387.0	—

Continued.

IRON Mg	ZINC Mg	V-A IU	V-ET Mg	V-C Mg	THIA Mg	RIBO Mg	NIAC Mg	V-B6 Mg	FOL Ug	VB12 Ug	CALC Mg	PHOS Mg	SEL Mg	FIBD Gm
0.980	1.210	—	—	—	—	—	—	—	—	—	87.00	218.0	—	0.000
0.390	0.400	30.00	—	—	0.040	0.157	2.780	0.244	—	2.710	51.00	188.0	—	0.000
0.240	0.510	65.00	—	—	0.063	0.065	1.400	0.059	3.000	3.570	5.000	—	—	0.000
0.570	0.590	—	—	—	—	—	—	—	—	—	36.00	290.0	—	0.000
0.200	0.370	—	—	—	0.045	0.003	0.294	—	—	—	34.00	171.0	—	0.000
0.530	0.530	219.0	—	0.870	0.044	0.084	3.920	—	—	—	12.00	228.0	0.039	0.000
0.170	—	—	—	3.980	0.028	0.216	0.398	—	—	—	4.250	98.10	—	0.000
1.200	—	160.0	1.810	—	0.160	0.060	9.800	—	—	—	414.0	418.0	0.048	0.000
0.760	0.440	—	—	0.900	—	—	—	—	—	—	—	—	—	0.000
0.720	0.780	47.00	1.540	0.000	0.020	0.158	5.560	0.255	13.10	5.850	—	279.0	0.045	0.000
0.850	0.310	88.00	—	—	0.023	0.101	4.720	0.278	1.900	3.260	11.00	164.0	0.061	0.000
0.350	0.155	27.00	—	—	0.010	0.027	0.630	0.020	1.400	1.070	46.00	59.00	—	0.000
0.852	—	—	—	—	—	—	—	—	—	—	32.70	96.00	0.015	0.000
0.125	0.165	—	—	—	0.007	0.017	0.234	—	2.400	0.205	6.500	36.50	0.012	—
0.320	0.440	181.0	—	—	—	—	—	—	—	—	11.00	211.0	—	0.000
0.600	—	30.00	2.000	—	0.130	0.260	8.600	—	—	—	24.00	313.0	—	0.000
3.500	1.610	75.30	—	—	0.035	0.047	3.530	0.142	2.300	1.440	75.00	299.0	0.041	0.000
2.620	1.330	—	—	—	0.026	0.027	2.200	0.108	2.900	1.270	33.00	116.0	—	0.000
1.070	1.170	—	—	—	0.110	0.116	2.610	0.083	6.900	1.590	57.00	185.0	0.027	0.480
0.980	1.800	—	—	—	—	0.124	1.500	—	—	3.370	65.00	251.0	—	0.000
0.430	0.800	48.00	—	—	0.102	0.145	2.770	0.305	—	3.190	23.00	368.0	—	0.000
0.860	1.480	—	—	3.500	0.048	0.389	2.210	0.049	—	1.040	33.00	213.0	—	0.300
2.000	0.540	808.0	—	—	—	—	—	—	—	—	40.00	263.0	0.049	0.000
0.220	—	—	—	—	0.017	0.018	0.187	—	—	—	7.000	—	—	0.000
1.300	—	2050	—	—	0.040	0.050	10.90	—	—	—	27.00	275.0	0.047	0.000
0.880	1.250	117.0	—	0.900	0.037	0.099	10.00	0.324	—	1.720	5.000	287.0	—	0.000
1.100	—	319.0	0.200	1.000	0.120	0.060	2.500	—	—	—	218.0	272.0	—	0.000
2.070	1.180	63.00	—	3.100	0.072	0.191	—	—	—	—	73.00	272.0	—	0.000
1.180	0.770	66.00	—	—	0.032	—	—	0.094	4.500	—	11.00	265.0	—	0.000
0.341	0.142	23.00	0.800	—	0.009	0.014	3.520	0.105	0.000	0.398	1.420	62.50	0.033	0.000
2.720	0.370	—	—	—	—	—	—	0.321	4.000	—	10.00	158.0	—	0.000
0.510	—	—	—	—	0.003	0.039	4.930	—	3.500	—	—	—	—	0.000
0.620	0.450	50.00	—	—	0.369	0.040	8.330	—	—	—	14.00	163.0	—	0.000
0.500	—	2000	—	0.000	0.110	0.110	2.300	—	—	—	—	246.0	—	—
0.700	—	0.000	—	0.000	0.040	0.050	2.700	—	—	—	9.000	113.0	0.016	0.000
0.360	0.450	97.00	—	—	0.058	0.051	1.420	0.153	12.80	2.210	53.00	242.0	—	0.000

IRON Mg	ZINC Mg	V-A IU	V-ET Mg	V-C Mg	THIA Mg	RIBO Mg	NIAC Mg	V-B6 Mg	FOL Ug	VB12 Ug	CALC Mg	PHOS Mg	SEL Mg	FIBD Gm
—	—	—	—	—	—	—	—	—	—	—	—	—	—	—
—	—	—	—	—	—	—	—	—	—	—	—	—	—	—
—	—	—	—	—	—	—	—	—	—	—	—	—	—	—
—	—	—	—	—	—	—	—	—	—	—	—	—	—	—
—	—	—	—	—	—	—	—	—	—	—	—	—	—	—
—	—	—	—	—	—	—	—	—	—	—	—	—	—	0.120
—	—	—	—	—	—	—	—	—	—	—	—	—	—	—
—	—	—	—	—	—	—	—	—	—	—	—	—	—	—
—	—	—	—	—	—	—	—	—	—	—	—	—	—	—
2.500	—	6555	—	57.00	0.570	0.230	3.400	—	—	—	151.0	278.0	—	—
—	—	—	—	—	—	—	—	—	—	—	—	—	—	—
4.300	—	2134	—	8.000	0.160	0.220	4.200	—	—	—	84.00	243.0	—	—
—	—	—	—	—	—	—	—	—	—	—	—	—	—	—
3.500	—	3956	—	7.000	0.160	0.190	3.600	—	—	—	90.00	206.0	—	—

Continued.

Nutritive Components for Frozen Dinners—cont'd

Food Name	Serving	Gm wt	KCAL Kc	PROT Gm	CARB Gm	FAT Gm	CHOL Mg	SAFA Gm	SOD Mg	POT Mg	MAG Mg
SOLE-LIGHT-VAN DE KAMP'S	1 item	142.0	293.0	16.00	17.00	18.00	—	—	412.0	—	—
TURKEY DINNER-SWANSON	1 item	326.0	340.0	20.00	42.00	10.00	—	—	1295	—	—
TURKEY PIE-STOUFFER	1 item	284.0	460.0	20.00	35.00	26.00	—	—	1735	270.0	—
VEGETABLE LASAGNA-LE MENU	1 item	312.0	400.0	15.00	30.00	24.00	—	—	1135	—	—
MEATBALLS/NOODLES-STOUFFER	1 item	312.0	475.0	25.00	33.00	27.00	—	—	1620	395.0	—
BEEF/GREEN PEPPERS-STOUF	1 item	220.0	225.0	10.00	18.00	11.00	—	—	960.0	420.0	—
LASAGNA-STOUFFER	1 item	298.0	385.0	28.00	36.00	14.00	—	—	1200	580.0	—
CHICKEN CACCIATORE-STOUF	1 item	319.0	310.0	25.00	29.00	11.00	—	—	1135	300.0	—
CHICKEN KIEV-LE MENU	1 item	234.0	500.0	21.00	35.00	30.00	—	—	745.0	—	—
CABBAGE ROLL/TOM SAUC-HORM	1 srvg	28.4	23.00	1.100	3.200	0.700	3.000	0.281	127.0	87.00	4.000
VEAL PARMIGIANA-FROZ DIN	1 item	213.0	296.0	24.00	17.00	14.00	—	—	973.0	466.0	—

Nutritive Components for Fruits

Food Name	Serving	Gm wt	KCAL Kc	PROT Gm	CARB Gm	FAT Gm	CHOL Mg	SAFA Gm	SOD Mg	POT Mg	MAG Mg
APPLES-RAW-PEELED-BOILED	1 cup	171.0	91.00	0.450	23.30	0.610	0.000	0.099	1.000	150.0	5.000
APPLES-RAW-UNPEELED	1 item	138.0	81.00	0.270	21.10	0.490	0.000	0.080	1.000	159.0	6.000
APPLE JUICE-CANNED/BOTTLED	1 cup	248.0	116.0	0.150	29.00	0.280	0.000	0.047	7.000	296.0	8.000
APPLE JUICE-FROZEN-DILUTED	1 cup	239.0	111.0	0.340	27.60	0.250	0.000	0.043	17.00	301.0	12.00
APPLESAUCE-CAN-SWEETENED	1 cup	255.0	194.0	0.470	50.80	0.470	0.000	0.077	8.000	156.0	7.000
APPLESAUCE-CAN-UNSWEETENED	1 cup	244.0	106.0	0.400	27.60	0.120	0.000	0.020	5.000	183.0	7.000
APRICOTS-CAN/JUICE	1 cup	248.0	119.0	1.560	30.60	0.090	0.000	0.007	9.000	409.0	24.00
APRICOTS-DRIED-COOKED-UNSW	1 cup	250.0	211.0	3.240	54.80	0.410	0.000	0.028	9.000	1222	42.00
APRICOTS-DRIED-UNCOOKED	1 cup	130.0	310.0	4.750	80.30	0.600	0.000	0.042	13.00	1791	61.00
APRICOT-RAW-WITHOUT PIT	1 item	35.3	16.90	0.494	3.930	0.138	0.000	0.010	0.353	104.0	2.820
AVOCADO-RAW-CALIFORNIA	1 item	173.0	306.0	3.640	12.00	30.00	0.000	4.480	21.00	1097	70.00
BANANAS-RAW-PEELED	1 item	114.0	105.0	1.180	26.70	0.550	0.000	0.211	1.000	451.0	33.00
BLACKBERRIES-FROZEN-UNSW	1 cup	151.0	97.00	1.780	23.70	0.650	0.000	—	2.000	211.0	33.00
BLACKBERRIES-RAW	1 cup	144.0	74.00	1.040	18.40	0.560	0.000	0.000	0.000	282.0	29.00
BLUEBERRIES-FROZEN-UNSWEET	1 cup	155.0	78.00	0.650	18.90	0.990	0.000	—	1.000	83.00	8.000
BLUEBERRIES-RAW	1 cup	145.0	82.00	0.970	20.50	0.550	0.000	0.000	9.000	129.0	7.000
CHERRIES-SOUR-CAN/SIRUP	1 cup	256.0	232.0	1.860	59.60	0.240	0.000	0.054	18.00	238.0	14.00
CHERRIES-SWEET-RAW	1 item	6.8	4.900	0.082	1.130	0.065	0.000	0.015	0.000	15.20	0.800
CRANAPPLE JUICE-CAN	1 cup	253.0	180.0	0.177	45.90	0.127	0.000	—	17.70	70.80	5.060
CRANBERRY SAUCE-CAN-SWEET	1 cup	277.0	419.0	0.550	108.0	0.420	0.000	—	80.00	71.00	8.000
DATES-NATURAL-DRIED-CHOP	1 cup	178.0	489.0	3.500	131.0	0.800	0.000	—	5.000	1161	63.00
FIGS-DRIED-UNCOOKED	1 cup	199.0	508.0	6.060	130.0	2.320	0.000	0.466	22.00	1418	118.0
FRUIT COCKTAIL-CAN/SYRUP	1 cup	255.0	186.0	1.000	48.20	0.180	0.000	0.026	15.00	224.0	14.00
FRUIT COCKTAIL-CAN/JUICE	1 cup	248.0	113.0	1.130	29.40	0.030	0.000	0.005	9.000	235.0	17.00
FRUIT ROLL UP-CHERRY	1 item	14.4	50.00	0.000	12.00	1.000	—	—	5.000	45.00	—
GRAPEFRUIT-CAN/LIGHT SYRUP	1 cup	254.0	152.0	1.430	39.20	0.250	0.000	0.036	4.000	328.0	25.00
GRAPEFRUIT-RAW-PINK & RED	1 item	246.0	74.00	1.360	18.50	0.240	0.000	0.034	0.000	312.0	20.00
GRAPEFRUIT-RAW-WHITE	1 item	236.0	78.00	1.620	19.80	0.240	0.000	0.034	0.000	350.0	22.00
GRAPEFRUIT JUICE-CAN-SWEET	1 cup	250.0	116.0	1.450	27.80	0.230	0.000	0.030	4.000	405.0	24.00
GRAPEFRUIT JUICE-CAN-UNSW	1 cup	247.0	93.00	1.290	22.10	0.240	0.000	0.032	3.000	378.0	24.00
GRAPEFRUIT JUICE-FROZ-DILU	1 cup	247.0	102.0	1.370	24.00	0.330	0.000	0.047	2.000	337.0	26.00
GRAPEFRUIT JUICE-RAW	1 cup	247.0	96.00	1.240	22.70	0.250	0.000	0.035	2.000	400.0	30.00
GRAPES-RAW-AMERICAN TYPE	1 cup	92.0	58.00	0.580	15.80	0.320	0.000	0.027	2.000	176.0	5.000
GRAPE DRINK-CANNED	1 cup	250.0	135.0	0.000	35.00	0.000	0.000	—	2.000	88.00	—
GRAPE JUICE-CAN & BOTTLE	1 cup	253.0	155.0	1.410	37.90	0.190	0.000	0.063	7.000	334.0	24.00
GRAPE JUICE-FROZ-DILUTED	1 cup	250.0	128.0	0.470	31.90	0.230	0.000	0.073	5.000	53.00	11.00
KIWIFRUIT-RAW	1 item	76.0	46.00	0.750	11.30	0.340	0.000	0.000	4.000	252.0	23.00
LEMONADE-FROZ-DILUTED	1 cup	248.0	105.0	0.000	28.00	0.000	0.000	0.000	0.000	40.00	—
LEMONS-RAW-PEELED	1 item	58.0	17.00	0.640	5.410	0.170	0.000	0.023	1.000	80.00	—

Continued.

IRON Mg	ZINC Mg	V-A IU	V-ET Mg	V-C Mg	THIA Mg	RIBO Mg	NIAC Mg	V-B6 Mg	FOL Ug	VB12 Ug	CALC Mg	PHOS Mg	SEL Mg	FIBD Gm
—	—	—	—	—	—	—	—	—	—	—	—	—	—	—
—	—	—	—	—	—	—	—	—	—	—	—	—	—	—
—	—	—	—	—	—	—	—	—	—	—	—	—	—	—
—	—	—	—	—	—	—	—	—	—	—	—	—	—	—
—	—	—	—	—	—	—	—	—	—	—	—	—	—	—
2.330	—	682.0	—	0.000	0.078	0.155	3.880	—	—	—	0.000	—	—	—
3.150	—	1239	—	0.000	0.210	0.420	4.200	—	—	—	410.0	—	—	—
—	—	—	—	—	—	—	—	—	—	—	—	—	—	—
—	—	—	—	—	—	—	—	—	—	—	—	—	—	—
0.250	0.190	—	—	0.180	0.760	0.020	0.290	0.030	2.900	0.100	5.900	15.70	—	—
2.300	—	617.0	—	6.400	0.300	0.380	6.800	—	—	—	97.00	—	—	—

IRON Mg	ZINC Mg	V-A IU	V-ET Mg	V-C Mg	THIA Mg	RIBO Mg	NIAC Mg	V-B6 Mg	FOL Ug	VB12 Ug	CALC Mg	PHOS Mg	SEL Mg	FIBD Gm
0.320	0.070	75.00	—	0.300	0.027	0.021	0.162	0.075	1.000	0.000	8.000	13.00	0.001	4.100
0.250	0.050	74.00	0.911	7.800	0.023	0.019	0.106	0.066	3.900	0.000	10.00	10.00	0.001	3.200
0.920	0.070	2.000	—	2.300	0.052	0.042	0.248	0.074	0.200	0.000	16.00	18.00	0.002	0.520
0.610	0.090	—	—	1.400	0.001	0.036	0.091	0.079	0.700	0.000	14.00	16.00	0.002	0.000
0.890	0.100	28.00	—	4.400	0.033	0.071	0.479	0.066	1.500	0.000	9.000	17.00	0.001	4.340
0.290	0.060	70.00	—	2.900	0.032	0.061	0.459	0.063	1.400	0.000	7.000	18.00	0.001	4.150
0.740	0.270	4195	—	12.20	0.045	0.047	0.853	—	—	0.000	30.00	50.00	0.001	2.810
4.170	0.660	5909	—	3.900	0.015	0.075	2.360	0.285	0.000	0.000	40.00	104.0	—	6.700
6.110	0.970	9412	—	3.100	0.010	0.196	3.900	0.203	13.40	0.000	59.00	152.0	—	10.50
0.191	0.092	922.0	—	3.530	0.011	0.014	0.212	0.019	3.040	0.000	4.940	6.710	—	0.670
2.040	0.730	1059	—	13.70	0.187	0.211	3.320	0.484	113.0	0.000	19.00	73.00	—	6.130
0.350	0.190	92.00	0.365	10.30	0.051	0.114	0.616	0.659	21.80	0.000	7.000	22.00	0.001	2.650
1.210	0.370	172.0	—	4.700	0.044	0.069	1.820	0.092	51.30	0.000	44.00	46.00	0.001	7.550
0.830	0.390	237.0	—	30.20	0.043	0.058	0.576	0.084	18.00	0.000	46.00	30.00	0.001	8.930
0.280	0.110	126.0	—	3.800	0.050	0.057	0.806	0.091	10.40	0.000	12.00	18.00	0.001	4.940
0.240	0.160	145.0	—	18.90	0.070	0.073	0.521	0.052	9.300	0.000	9.000	15.00	0.001	3.920
3.320	0.160	1827	—	5.100	0.041	0.100	0.430	0.113	19.40	0.000	26.00	24.00	0.001	0.614
0.026	0.004	14.60	—	0.480	0.003	0.004	0.027	0.002	0.286	0.000	1.000	1.300	0.000	0.100
0.304	0.455	—	—	81.00	0.025	0.051	0.152	—	—	—	12.70	5.060	0.001	0.000
0.610	0.140	55.00	—	5.500	0.042	0.058	0.277	0.039	—	0.000	10.00	16.00	0.001	3.200
2.050	0.520	89.00	—	0.000	0.160	0.178	3.920	0.342	22.40	0.000	58.00	70.00	—	15.50
4.450	1.000	264.0	—	1.700	0.141	0.175	1.380	0.446	15.00	0.000	286.0	136.0	—	14.00
0.730	0.210	522.0	—	4.900	0.046	0.048	0.954	0.128	—	0.000	16.00	28.00	—	1.560
0.530	0.210	757.0	—	6.800	0.030	0.040	0.999	—	—	0.000	20.00	34.00	0.001	1.510
—	—	—	—	—	—	—	—	—	—	—	—	—	—	—
1.020	0.210	0.000	0.457	54.10	0.097	0.051	0.617	0.051	21.60	0.000	36.00	25.00	0.001	1.650
0.300	0.180	636.0	0.627	91.00	0.098	0.050	0.492	0.104	23.20	0.000	36.00	22.00	0.001	3.200
0.070	0.160	24.00	0.614	78.60	0.088	0.048	0.634	0.102	23.60	0.000	28.00	18.00	0.001	2.500
0.890	0.150	0.000	0.450	67.30	0.100	0.058	0.798	0.050	25.90	0.000	20.00	27.00	0.001	0.000
0.500	0.210	18.00	0.445	72.00	0.104	0.049	0.571	0.049	25.60	0.000	18.00	27.00	0.001	0.000
0.340	0.130	22.00	0.440	83.40	0.101	0.054	0.536	0.109	8.900	0.000	19.00	34.00	0.001	0.000
0.490	0.130	24.70	0.440	93.90	0.099	0.049	0.494	—	51.20	0.000	22.00	37.00	0.001	0.500
0.270	0.040	92.00	—	3.700	0.085	0.052	0.276	0.101	3.600	0.000	13.00	9.000	0.001	1.500
0.300	—	—	—	0.000	0.030	0.030	0.300	—	—	—	8.000	10.00	0.001	0.000
0.600	0.130	20.00	—	0.200	0.066	0.094	0.663	0.164	6.580	0.000	22.00	27.00	0.001	0.000
0.260	0.100	19.00	—	59.70	0.038	0.065	0.310	0.105	3.100	0.000	9.000	11.00	0.001	0.000
0.310	—	133.0	—	74.50	0.015	0.038	0.380	—	—	0.000	20.00	31.00	—	2.900
0.100	—	10.00	—	17.00	0.010	0.020	0.200	—	12.00	—	2.000	3.000	0.001	—
0.350	0.040	17.00	—	30.70	0.023	0.012	0.058	0.046	6.200	0.000	15.00	9.000	0.001	0.580

Continued.

Nutritive Components for Fruits—cont'd

Food Name	Serving	Gm wt	KCAL Kc	PROT Gm	CARB Gm	FAT Gm	CHOL Mg	SAFA Gm	SOD Mg	POT Mg	MAG Mg
LEMON JUICE-CAN & BOTTLE	1 cup	244.0	52.00	0.980	15.80	0.700	0.000	0.093	50.00	248.0	20.00
LEMON JUICE-RAW	1 cup	244.0	60.00	0.920	21.10	0.000	0.000	0.000	2.000	303.0	16.00
LIMES-RAW	1 item	67.0	20.00	0.470	7.060	0.130	0.000	0.015	1.000	68.00	—
LIME JUICE-CAN & BOTTLE	1 cup	246.0	51.00	0.610	16.50	0.570	0.000	0.064	39.00	185.0	16.00
LIME JUICE-RAW	1 cup	246.0	66.00	1.080	22.20	0.250	0.000	0.027	2.000	268.0	14.00
MELONS-CANTALOUPE-RAW	1 cup	160.0	57.00	1.400	13.40	0.440	0.000	0.000	14.00	494.0	17.00
MELONS-CASABA-RAW	1 cup	170.0	45.00	1.530	10.50	0.170	0.000	0.000	20.00	357.0	14.00
MELONS-HONEYDEW-RAW	1 cup	170.0	60.00	0.770	15.60	0.170	0.000	0.000	17.00	461.0	12.00
NECTARINES-RAW	1 item	136.0	67.00	1.280	16.00	0.620	0.000	—	0.000	288.0	11.00
ORANGES-RAW-ALL VARIETIES	1 item	131.0	62.00	1.230	15.40	0.160	0.000	0.020	0.000	237.0	13.00
ORANGE JUICE-CAN	1 cup	249.0	104.0	1.460	24.50	0.360	0.000	0.045	6.000	436.0	27.00
ORANGE JUICE-FROZ-DILUTED	1 cup	249.0	112.0	1.680	26.80	0.140	0.000	0.017	2.000	474.0	24.00
ORANGE JUICE-RAW	1 cup	248.0	111.0	1.740	25.80	0.500	0.000	0.060	2.000	496.0	27.00
PAPAYAS-RAW	1 cup	140.0	54.00	0.860	13.70	0.200	0.000	0.060	4.000	359.0	14.00
PEACHES-CAN/HEAVY SYRUP	1 cup	256.0	190.0	1.160	51.00	0.250	0.000	0.026	16.00	235.0	13.00
PEACHES-CAN/WATER PACK	1 cup	244.0	58.00	1.070	14.90	0.140	0.000	0.015	8.000	241.0	12.00
PEACHES-DRIED-COOKED-UNSW	1 cup	258.0	198.0	2.990	50.80	0.630	0.000	0.067	6.000	825.0	35.00
PEACHES-DRIED-UNCOOKED	1 cup	160.0	383.0	5.770	98.10	1.220	0.000	0.131	12.00	1594	67.00
PEACHES-FROZ-SLICED-SWEET	1 cup	250.0	235.0	1.560	59.90	0.330	0.000	0.035	16.00	325.0	12.00
PEACHES-RAW-SLICED	1 cup	170.0	73.00	1.190	18.90	0.160	0.000	0.017	1.000	334.0	11.00
PEACHES-RAW-WHOLE	1 item	87.0	37.00	0.610	9.650	0.080	0.000	0.009	0.000	171.0	6.000
PEARS-CAN/HEAVY SYRUP	1 cup	255.0	188.0	0.510	48.90	0.330	0.000	0.018	13.00	165.0	11.00
PEARS-CAN/JUICE	1 cup	248.0	123.0	0.850	32.10	0.160	0.000	0.010	10.00	238.0	17.00
PEARS-RAW-BARTLET-UNPEELED	1 item	166.0	98.00	0.650	25.10	0.660	0.000	0.037	1.000	208.0	9.000
PINEAPPLE-CAN/JUICE	1 cup	250.0	150.0	1.040	39.20	0.210	0.000	0.015	4.000	304.0	35.00
PINEAPPLE-CAN/SYRUP-BITS	1 cup	252.0	131.0	0.900	33.90	0.290	0.000	0.023	3.000	266.0	40.00
PINEAPPLE-RAW-DICED	1 cup	155.0	77.00	0.600	19.20	0.660	0.000	0.050	1.000	175.0	21.00
PINEAPPLE JUICE-CAN	1 cup	250.0	139.0	0.800	34.40	0.200	0.000	0.013	2.000	334.0	34.00
PINEAPPLE JUICE-FROZ-DILU	1 cup	250.0	129.0	1.000	31.90	0.080	0.000	0.005	3.000	340.0	23.00
PRUNES-DRIED-UNCOOKED	1 cup	162.0	385.0	4.200	101.0	0.830	0.000	0.066	6.000	1200	73.00
RAISINS-SEEDLESS	1 cup	145.0	434.0	4.670	115.0	0.670	0.000	0.218	17.00	1089	48.00
RAISINS-SEEDLESS-PACKET	1 item	14.0	42.00	0.451	11.10	0.064	0.000	0.021	1.680	105.0	4.620
RASPBERRIES-RAW	1 cup	123.0	61.00	1.110	14.20	0.680	0.000	0.023	0.000	187.0	22.00
STRAWBERRIES-FROZ-UNSWEET	1 cup	149.0	52.00	0.630	13.60	0.160	0.000	0.009	3.000	220.0	16.00
STRAWBERRIES-RAW-WHOLE	1 cup	149.0	45.00	0.910	10.50	0.550	0.000	0.030	2.000	247.0	16.00
TANGERINES-RAW-PEELED	1 item	84.0	37.00	0.530	9.400	0.160	0.000	0.018	1.000	132.0	10.00
WATERMELON-RAW	1 cup	160.0	50.00	0.990	11.50	0.680	0.000	0.000	3.000	186.0	17.00
POMEGRANATES-RAW	1 item	154.0	104.0	1.470	26.40	0.460	0.000	—	5.000	399.0	—
PRUNE JUICE-CAN & BOTTLE	1 cup	256.0	181.0	1.550	44.70	0.080	0.000	0.008	11.00	706.0	36.00
PLUMS-RAW-PRUNE TYPE	1 item	28.0	20.00	0.000	6.000	0.000	0.000	0.000	0.000	48.00	1.960
PAPAYA NECTAR-CAN	1 cup	250.0	142.0	0.430	36.30	0.380	0.000	0.118	14.00	78.00	8.000
RHUBARB-RAW-COOKED-SUGAR	1 cup	270.0	380.0	1.000	97.00	0.000	0.000	0.000	5.000	548.0	32.40
BOYSENBERRIES-FROZEN-UNSW	1 cup	132.0	66.00	1.460	16.10	0.350	0.000	—	2.000	183.0	21.00

Nutritive Components for Grains

Food Name	Serving	Gm wt	KCAL Kc	PROT Gm	CARB Gm	FAT Gm	CHOL Mg	SAFA Gm	SOD Mg	POT Mg	MAG Mg
MUFFIN-SOY	1 item	40.0	119.0	3.900	16.70	4.400	—	—	—	—	52.00
BISQUICK MIX-DRY	1 cup	112.0	480.0	8.000	76.00	16.00	—	—	1400	—	—
CORN CHIPS	1 srvg	28.4	155.0	1.700	16.90	9.140	0.000	1.500	164.0	43.30	21.90
CORNMEAL-DEGERM-ENR-COOKED	1 cup	240.0	120.0	3.000	26.00	0.000	0.000	0.000	264.0	38.00	16.80
CORNSTARCH-STIRRED	1 cup	128.0	463.0	0.400	112.0	0.000	—	0.000	0.000	0.000	—
CRACKERS-ANIMAL	1 item	1.9	8.670	0.127	1.470	0.200	—	—	7.530	1.670	0.267
CRACKERS-CHEDDAR SNACKS	1 item	1.6	7.220	0.144	1.110	0.261	—	—	14.30	2.170	0.278

Continued.

IRON Mg	ZINC Mg	V-A IU	V-ET Mg	V-C Mg	THIA Mg	RIBO Mg	NIAC Mg	V-B6 Mg	FOL Ug	VB12 Ug	CALC Mg	PHOS Mg	SEL Mg	FIBD Gm
0.310	0.150	37.00	—	60.40	0.100	0.022	0.481	0.105	24.60	0.000	26.00	21.00	0.001	0.732
0.080	0.120	49.00	—	112.0	0.073	0.024	0.244	0.124	31.50	0.000	18.00	14.00	0.001	0.732
0.400	0.070	7.000	—	19.50	0.020	0.013	0.134	—	5.500	0.000	22.00	12.00	0.001	—
0.560	0.150	40.00	—	15.70	0.081	0.007	0.401	0.066	19.50	0.000	30.00	24.00	0.001	0.000
0.080	0.150	25.00	—	72.10	0.049	0.025	0.246	0.106	—	0.000	22.00	18.00	—	0.000
0.340	0.250	5158	0.496	67.50	0.058	0.034	0.918	0.184	27.30	0.000	17.00	27.00	0.001	1.400
0.680	—	51.00	0.527	27.20	0.102	0.034	0.680	—	—	0.000	9.000	12.00	0.001	2.000
0.120	—	68.00	0.527	42.10	0.131	0.031	1.020	0.100	—	0.000	10.00	17.00	0.001	1.530
0.210	0.120	1001	—	7.300	0.023	0.056	1.350	0.034	5.100	0.000	6.000	22.00	0.001	2.990
0.130	0.090	269.0	0.314	69.70	0.114	0.052	0.369	0.079	39.70	0.000	52.00	18.00	0.002	2.620
1.100	0.170	437.0	0.498	85.70	0.149	0.070	0.782	0.219	136.0	0.000	21.00	36.00	0.001	0.260
0.240	0.130	194.0	0.498	96.90	0.197	0.045	0.503	0.110	109.0	0.000	22.00	40.00	0.001	0.700
0.500	0.130	496.0	0.496	124.0	0.223	0.074	0.992	0.099	136.0	0.000	27.00	42.00	0.001	1.980
0.140	0.100	2819	—	86.50	0.038	0.045	0.473	0.027	—	0.000	33.00	7.000	0.001	1.270
0.690	0.220	849.0	—	7.100	0.028	0.061	1.570	0.049	8.200	0.000	8.000	29.00	0.001	1.140
0.770	0.220	1298	—	7.000	0.020	0.046	1.270	0.046	8.200	0.000	6.000	25.00	0.001	1.080
3.370	0.470	508.0	—	9.500	0.013	0.054	3.920	0.098	0.200	0.000	23.00	99.00	0.001	6.700
6.500	0.920	3461	—	7.700	0.003	0.339	7.000	0.107	10.60	0.000	45.00	191.0	0.001	14.00
0.930	0.130	709.0	—	235.0	0.033	0.088	1.630	0.045	—	0.000	6.000	28.00	0.001	—
0.190	0.230	910.0	—	11.20	0.029	0.070	1.680	0.031	5.800	0.000	9.000	21.00	0.001	3.910
0.100	0.120	465.0	—	5.700	0.015	0.036	0.861	0.016	3.000	0.000	5.000	11.00	0.001	2.000
0.560	0.210	0.000	—	2.900	0.026	0.056	0.617	0.036	3.000	0.000	12.00	17.00	0.001	2.350
0.710	0.220	14.00	—	4.000	0.027	0.027	0.496	—	—	0.000	21.00	29.00	0.001	4.710
0.410	0.200	33.00	—	6.600	0.033	0.066	0.166	0.030	12.10	0.000	19.00	18.00	0.001	4.650
0.700	0.240	95.00	0.250	23.80	0.238	0.048	0.710	—	—	0.000	34.00	16.00	0.002	1.880
0.980	0.290	37.00	0.255	19.00	0.229	0.063	0.736	0.189	11.90	0.000	36.00	17.00	0.003	1.940
0.570	0.120	35.00	0.155	23.90	0.143	0.056	0.651	0.135	16.40	0.000	11.00	11.00	0.001	2.390
0.650	0.290	12.00	—	26.70	0.138	0.055	0.643	0.240	57.80	0.000	42.00	20.00	0.002	0.250
0.750	0.290	25.00	—	30.00	0.175	0.050	0.500	0.185	—	0.000	28.00	20.00	0.002	0.300
3.990	0.850	3199	—	5.400	0.130	0.261	3.160	0.425	5.900	0.000	82.00	127.0	0.001	11.00
3.020	0.380	11.00	—	4.800	0.226	0.128	1.190	0.361	4.800	0.000	71.00	140.0	0.001	12.60
0.291	0.039	1.120	—	0.462	0.022	0.012	0.115	0.035	0.462	0.000	6.860	13.60	0.000	1.220
0.700	0.570	160.0	—	30.80	0.037	0.111	1.110	0.070	6.000	0.000	27.00	15.00	0.001	5.500
1.120	0.190	66.00	0.596	61.40	0.033	0.055	0.688	0.042	25.00	0.000	23.00	20.00	0.001	3.900
0.570	0.190	41.00	0.387	84.50	0.030	0.098	0.343	0.088	26.40	0.000	21.00	28.00	0.001	3.200
0.090	—	773.0	—	25.90	0.088	0.018	0.134	0.056	17.10	0.000	12.00	8.000	0.001	1.680
0.280	0.110	585.0	—	15.40	0.128	0.032	0.320	0.230	3.400	0.000	13.00	14.00	0.001	0.300
0.460	—	—	—	9.400	0.046	0.046	0.462	0.162	—	0.000	5.000	12.00	0.001	1.100
3.030	0.520	9.000	—	10.60	0.041	0.179	2.010	—	1.000	0.000	30.00	64.00	0.001	0.100
0.100	0.028	80.00	—	1.000	0.010	0.010	0.100	0.023	0.616	0.000	3.000	5.000	0.000	0.588
0.860	0.380	277.0	—	7.500	0.015	0.010	0.375	0.023	5.200	0.000	24.00	1.000	0.001	0.125
1.600	0.216	220.0	—	16.00	0.050	0.140	0.800	0.054	14.30	0.000	211.0	41.00	0.001	5.400
1.120	0.290	89.00	—	4.100	0.070	0.049	1.010	0.074	83.60	0.000	36.00	36.00	0.001	5.150

IRON Mg	ZINC Mg	V-A IU	V-ET Mg	V-C Mg	THIA Mg	RIBO Mg	NIAC Mg	V-B6 Mg	FOL Ug	VB12 Ug	CALC Mg	PHOS Mg	SEL Mg	FIBD Gm
0.900	—	196.0	—	0.000	0.080	0.100	0.500	—	—	—	35.00	56.00	—	—
—	—	—	2.780	—	—	—	—	—	—	—	—	—	—	—
0.376	0.435	—	—	—	0.048	0.026	0.554	0.054	—	0.000	37.10	54.60	—	1.660
1.000	—	140.0	1.010	0.000	0.140	0.100	1.200	0.600	57.60	0.000	2.000	34.00	0.006	0.700
0.000	—	0.000	0.000	0.000	0.000	0.000	0.000	—	—	—	0.000	0.000	—	—
0.059	0.009	0.000	0.035	0.000	0.005	0.009	0.073	0.000	0.200	0.001	0.200	1.200	0.000	0.027
0.068	0.012	0.900	0.029	0.000	0.009	0.007	0.067	0.001	0.222	0.009	1.220	1.890	0.001	—

Continued.

Nutritive Components for Grains—cont'd

Food Name	Serving	Gm wt	KCAL Kc	PROT Gm	CARB Gm	FAT Gm	CHOL Mg	SAFA Gm	SOD Mg	POT Mg	MAG Mg
CRACKERS-CHEESE	1 item	1.0	5.380	0.091	0.520	0.327	—	0.090	12.00	1.860	0.220
CRACKERS-GRAHAM-PLAIN	1 item	7.0	27.50	0.500	5.000	0.500	0.000	0.100	33.00	27.50	3.570
CRACKERS-GRAHAM-SUG/HONEY	1 item	7.0	30.10	0.519	5.400	0.732	—	0.300	32.90	11.70	2.310
CRACKERS-RITZ	1 item	3.3	18.00	0.233	2.130	0.967	—	—	32.30	2.670	—
CRACKERS-RY KRISP-NATURAL	1 item	2.1	7.500	0.250	1.670	0.033	0.000	—	18.50	10.20	2.500
CRACKERS-RYE WAFERS	1 item	6.5	22.50	1.000	5.000	0.000	0.000	—	57.00	39.00	—
CRACKERS-SALTINES	1 item	2.8	12.50	0.250	2.000	0.250	0.750	0.100	36.80	3.250	0.770
CRACKERS-TRISCUITS	1 item	4.5	21.00	0.400	3.100	0.750	—	—	—	—	—
CRACKERS-WHEAT THINS	1 item	1.8	9.000	0.125	1.250	0.350	—	—	—	—	—
CROUTONS-HERB SEASONED	1 cup	30.0	100.0	4.290	20.00	0.000	—	0.000	372.0	38.60	11.40
FLOUR-BUCKWHEAT-LIGHT-SIFT	1 cup	98.0	340.0	6.000	78.00	1.000	0.000	0.200	0.000	314.0	47.00
FLOUR-WHEAT-ENR-SIFTED	1 cup	115.0	420.0	12.00	88.00	1.000	0.000	0.200	2.000	109.0	28.80
FLOUR-WHOLE WHEAT-STIRRED	1 cup	120.0	400.0	16.00	85.00	2.000	0.000	0.400	3.000	444.0	136.0
FRENCH TOAST-HOME RECIPE	1 slice	65.0	153.0	5.670	17.20	6.730	—	—	257.0	85.80	11.70
MACARONI-COOKED-FIRM-HOT	1 cup	130.0	190.0	7.000	39.00	1.000	0.000	—	1.000	103.0	26.00
NOODLES-CHOW MEIN-CANNED	1 cup	45.0	220.0	6.000	26.00	11.00	5.000	—	0.000	—	—
NOODLES-EGG-ENR-COOKED	1 cup	160.0	200.0	7.000	37.00	2.000	50.00	—	3.000	70.00	43.20
PANCAKES-BUCKWHEAT-MIX	1 item	27.0	55.00	2.000	6.000	2.000	20.00	0.800	160.0	66.00	5.130
PANCAKES-PLAIN-HOME RECIPE	1 item	27.0	60.00	2.000	9.000	2.000	20.00	0.500	160.0	33.00	5.130
PANCAKES-PLAIN-MIX	1 item	27.0	58.90	1.850	19.00	2.170	20.00	0.700	160.0	43.20	5.130
POPCORN-POPPED-PLAIN	1 cup	6.0	25.00	1.000	5.000	0.000	0.000	0.000	0.000	—	—
POPCORN-POPPED-SUGAR COAT	1 cup	35.0	135.0	2.000	30.00	1.000	0.000	0.500	0.000	—	—
PRETZEL-THIN-STICK	1 item	0.3	1.190	0.028	0.242	0.011	0.000	—	4.830	0.303	0.072
RICE-BROWN-LONG-COOKED-HOT	1 cup	195.0	232.0	4.900	49.70	1.200	0.000	—	0.000	137.0	—
RICE CAKE-REGULAR	1 item	9.3	35.00	0.700	7.600	0.280	—	—	10.80	27.20	—
RICE-SPANISH-HOME RECIPE	1 cup	245.0	213.0	4.400	40.70	4.200	—	—	774.0	566.0	—
RICE-WHITE-INSTANT-HOT	1 cup	165.0	180.0	4.000	40.00	0.000	0.000	0.000	13.00	—	13.20
RICE-WHITE-LONG GRAIN-COOK	1 cup	205.0	225.0	4.000	50.00	0.000	0.000	0.000	6.000	57.00	16.40
RICE-WHITE-PARBOIL-COOKED	1 cup	175.0	185.0	4.000	41.00	0.000	0.000	0.000	4.000	75.00	—
SHAKE'N BAKE	1 srvg	28.4	116.0	2.440	17.70	4.260	—	—	984.0	56.80	—
SPAGHETTI-COOK-TENDER-HOT	1 cup	140.0	155.0	5.000	32.00	1.000	0.000	—	1.000	85.00	23.80
STUFFING-MIX-DRY FORM	1 cup	30.0	111.0	3.900	21.70	1.100	—	—	399.0	52.00	—
STUFFING-MIX-PREPARED	1 cup	140.0	501.0	9.100	49.80	30.50	—	—	1254	126.0	—
TACO SHELLS	1 item	11.0	49.80	0.967	7.240	2.150	—	—	—	—	11.40
TORTILLA CHIPS-DORITOS	1 srvg	28.4	139.0	2.000	18.60	6.600	0.000	1.430	180.0	51.00	21.00
TORTILLA-CORN	1 item	30.0	67.20	2.150	12.80	1.140	—	—	53.40	52.20	19.50
TORTILLA-FLOUR	1 item	30.0	95.00	2.500	17.30	1.800	—	—	—	—	7.000
WAFFLES-FROZEN	1 item	37.0	103.0	2.150	15.90	3.520	—	—	256.0	77.70	7.770
WAFFLES-ENR-HOME RECIPE	1 item	75.0	245.0	6.930	25.70	12.60	45.00	2.300	445.0	129.0	16.50
NOODLES-RAMEN-ORIENTAL	1 cup	227.0	207.0	5.900	30.70	8.600	—	—	829.0	—	—
RICE-BROWN-UNCLE BEN'S	1 cup	146.0	220.0	5.000	46.40	1.820	0.000	—	2.400	172.0	—

Nutritive Components for Meats

Food Name	Serving	Gm wt	KCAL Kc	PROT Gm	CARB Gm	FAT Gm	CHOL Mg	SAFA Gm	SOD Mg	POT Mg	MAG Mg
BACON-PORK-BROILED/FRIED	1 slice	6.3	36.30	1.930	0.036	3.120	5.330	1.100	101.0	30.70	1.670
BACON BITS	1 tbsp	6.0	26.60	1.920	1.720	1.550	0.000	—	165.0	—	—
BEEF-DRIED-CHIPPED-JAR	1 item	71.0	117.0	20.70	1.110	2.770	650.0	1.130	2464	315.0	22.70
BEEF-LIVER-FRIED/MARG	1 slice	85.0	184.0	22.70	6.680	6.800	410.0	2.400	90.00	309.0	20.00
BOLOGNA-PORK	1 slice	23.0	57.00	3.520	0.170	4.570	14.00	1.580	272.0	65.00	3.000
BRAUNSCHWEIGER-SAUS-PORK	1 slice	18.0	65.00	2.430	0.560	5.780	28.00	1.960	206.0	36.00	2.000
CANADIAN BACON-PORK-GRILL	1 slice	23.3	43.00	5.640	0.315	1.960	13.50	0.660	360.0	90.50	5.000
CORNED BEEF HASH-CANNED	1 cup	220.0	400.0	19.00	24.00	25.00	50.00	11.90	1188	440.0	—
DEVILED HAM-CANNED	1 tbsp	13.0	45.00	2.000	0.000	4.000	10.00	1.500	160.0	—	1.690

Continued.

IRON Mg	ZINC Mg	V-A IU	V-ET Mg	V-C Mg	THIA Mg	RIBO Mg	NIAC Mg	V-B6 Mg	FOL Ug	VB12 Ug	CALC Mg	PHOS Mg	SEL Mg	FIBD Gm
0.035	0.010	—	0.018	0.000	0.004	0.004	0.082	—	—	—	1.050	2.100	0.000	0.025
0.250	0.053	0.000	0.128	0.000	0.010	0.040	0.250	0.006	0.910	0.000	3.000	10.50	0.001	0.200
0.183	0.053	0.000	0.127	0.000	0.024	0.019	0.218	0.006	0.910	0.000	2.660	8.260	0.001	0.200
0.100	—	—	—	—	0.013	0.013	0.100	—	—	—	5.000	8.000	—	—
0.092	0.057	—	0.038	—	0.006	0.005	0.033	0.007	0.833	—	0.833	6.830	0.001	0.280
0.250	—	0.000	0.118	0.000	0.020	0.015	0.100	—	—	—	3.500	25.00	0.001	0.866
0.125	0.017	0.000	0.050	0.000	0.125	0.013	0.100	0.001	0.495	0.000	0.500	2.500	0.004	0.039
—	—	—	0.082	—	—	—	—	—	—	—	—	—	0.001	—
—	—	—	0.033	—	—	—	—	—	—	—	—	—	0.000	—
1.540	0.300	0.000	—	—	0.129	0.200	1.720	0.000	0.000	—	—	—	—	—
1.000	—	0.000	7.750	0.000	0.080	0.040	0.400	0.566	43.10	0.000	11.00	86.00	0.004	—
3.300	0.800	0.000	0.265	0.000	0.740	0.460	6.100	0.069	24.20	0.000	18.00	100.0	0.005	3.230
4.000	2.900	0.000	4.740	0.000	0.660	0.140	5.200	0.408	64.80	0.000	49.00	446.0	0.006	15.20
1.340	0.553	111.0	—	0.000	0.124	0.163	1.010	0.038	17.60	0.291	72.20	84.50	—	—
1.400	0.700	0.000	0.351	0.000	0.230	0.130	1.800	0.083	15.60	0.000	14.00	85.00	0.032	1.040
—	—	—	—	—	—	—	—	—	—	—	—	—	—	0.810
1.400	—	110.0	—	0.000	0.220	0.130	1.900	0.141	19.20	0.000	16.00	94.00	0.094	1.440
0.400	0.192	60.00	—	0.000	0.040	0.050	0.200	0.057	2.970	0.355	59.00	91.00	0.002	—
0.400	0.192	30.00	—	0.000	0.060	0.070	0.500	0.057	2.970	0.355	27.00	38.00	0.002	—
0.265	0.192	38.30	—	0.000	0.038	0.059	0.254	0.057	2.970	0.355	35.60	70.70	0.003	—
0.200	0.500	—	—	0.000	—	0.010	0.100	0.012	—	0.000	1.000	17.00	0.001	0.400
0.500	—	—	—	0.000	—	0.020	0.400	—	—	—	2.000	47.00	0.007	—
0.006	0.003	0.000	0.002	0.000	0.001	0.001	0.013	0.000	0.048	0.000	0.078	0.273	—	—
1.000	—	0.000	3.980	0.000	0.180	0.040	2.700	—	—	—	23.00	—	0.076	6.440
—	—	—	—	—	—	—	—	—	—	—	—	—	—	—
1.500	—	1620	—	37.00	0.100	0.070	1.700	—	—	—	34.00	96.00	—	—
1.300	0.700	0.000	0.644	0.000	0.210	0.000	1.700	0.056	16.50	0.000	5.000	31.00	0.033	1.710
1.800	0.700	0.000	0.800	0.000	0.230	0.020	2.100	0.871	22.60	0.000	21.00	57.00	0.041	2.130
1.400	0.700	0.000	0.683	0.000	0.190	0.020	2.100	0.744	19.30	0.000	33.00	100.0	0.035	1.820
0.710	—	620.0	—	0.284	0.162	0.184	2.190	—	—	—	13.90	43.50	—	—
1.300	0.700	0.000	1.680	0.000	0.200	0.110	1.500	0.090	16.80	0.000	11.00	70.00	0.085	0.980
1.000	—	0.000	—	0.000	0.070	0.080	1.000	—	—	—	37.00	57.00	—	—
2.200	—	910.0	—	0.000	0.130	0.170	2.100	—	—	—	92.00	136.0	—	—
0.286	0.142	—	—	—	0.032	0.017	0.189	—	—	0.000	15.60	25.40	—	—
0.500	0.240	52.00	—	0.000	0.030	0.030	0.040	0.100	4.000	—	30.00	59.00	—	1.850
0.570	0.426	—	—	0.000	0.048	0.030	0.384	0.091	5.700	0.000	42.00	54.90	—	1.090
1.100	—	2.000	—	0.000	0.010	0.080	1.000	—	—	—	46.00	25.00	—	—
1.800	0.303	474.0	—	0.000	0.167	0.200	1.930	0.098	0.740	—	30.00	141.0	—	—
1.480	0.653	140.0	—	0.000	0.180	0.240	1.460	0.054	14.30	0.365	154.0	135.0	—	—
—	—	—	—	—	—	—	—	—	—	—	—	—	—	2.040
0.900	—	0.000	2.980	0.000	0.180	0.040	4.200	—	—	—	16.00	222.0	0.057	4.820

IRON Mg	ZINC Mg	V-A IU	V-ET Mg	V-C Mg	THIA Mg	RIBO Mg	NIAC Mg	V-B6 Mg	FOL Ug	VB12 Ug	CALC Mg	PHOS Mg	SEL Mg	FIBD Gm
0.103	0.206	0.000	0.037	2.130	0.044	0.018	0.464	0.017	0.333	0.110	0.667	21.30	0.002	0.000
0.300	—	0.000	—	0.180	0.025	0.018	0.138	—	—	—	8.400	18.10	—	—
3.200	3.720	—	—	0.000	0.050	0.230	2.700	—	—	1.310	4.260	124.0	0.038	0.000
5.340	4.630	30690	1.380	19.40	0.179	3.520	12.30	1.220	187.0	95.00	9.000	392.0	0.042	0.000
0.180	0.470	—	0.112	8.100	0.120	0.036	0.897	0.060	1.000	0.210	3.000	32.00	0.003	0.000
1.680	0.510	2529	0.124	2.000	0.045	0.275	1.510	0.060	—	3.620	2.000	30.00	0.002	0.000
0.190	0.395	0.000	—	5.000	0.192	0.046	1.610	0.105	1.000	0.180	2.500	69.00	0.003	0.000
4.400	—	—	0.088	—	0.020	0.200	4.600	—	—	—	29.00	147.0	—	0.000
0.300	0.238	0.000	0.068	—	0.020	0.010	0.200	0.042	—	0.091	1.000	12.00	0.002	0.000

Continued.

Nutritive Components for Meats—cont'd

Food Name	Serving	Gm wt	KCAL Kc	PROT Gm	CARB Gm	FAT Gm	CHOL Mg	SAFA Gm	SOD Mg	POT Mg	MAG Mg
FRANKFURTER-HOT DOG-NO BUN	1 item	57.0	183.0	6.430	1.460	16.60	29.00	6.130	639.0	95.00	6.000
HAM-REG-LUNCH MEAT-11% FAT	1 slice	28.4	52.00	4.980	0.880	3.000	16.00	0.960	373.0	94.00	5.000
HAM-REG-ROASTED-PORK	1 cup	140.0	249.0	31.70	0.000	12.60	83.00	4.360	2100	573.0	30.00
HAMBURGER-GROUND-REG-BAKED	1 srvg	85.0	244.0	19.60	0.000	17.80	74.00	6.990	51.00	188.0	13.00
HAMBURGER-GROUND-REG-FRIED	1 srvg	85.0	260.0	20.30	0.000	19.20	75.00	7.530	71.00	255.0	17.00
HAMB PATTY-BEEF-10% FAT	1 item	85.0	217.0	21.60	0.000	13.90	71.00	5.450	59.00	266.0	18.00
HAMB PATTY-BEEF-21% FAT	1 item	85.0	231.0	21.00	0.000	15.70	74.00	6.160	65.00	256.0	18.00
ITALIAN SAUSAGE-PORK-LINK	1 item	67.0	217.0	13.40	1.010	17.20	52.00	6.050	618.0	204.0	12.00
KIELBASA-PORK/BEEF	1 slice	26.0	81.00	3.450	0.560	7.060	17.00	2.580	280.0	70.00	4.000
KNOCKWURST-PORK/BEEF-LINK	1 item	68.0	209.0	8.080	1.200	18.90	39.00	6.940	687.0	136.0	8.000
LIVERWURST/LIVER SAUS-PORK	1 slice	18.0	59.00	2.540	0.400	5.140	28.00	1.910	215.0	—	—
LAMB-CHOP-LEAN/FAT-BROILED	1 item	89.0	360.0	18.00	0.000	32.00	86.00	14.80	62.00	200.0	15.10
LAMB-CHOP/RIB-LEAN-BROILED	1 item	57.0	120.0	16.00	0.000	6.000	56.00	2.500	39.00	174.0	12.50
LAMB-LEG-LEAN/FAT-ROASTED	1 slice	85.0	235.0	22.00	0.000	16.00	82.00	7.300	59.00	241.0	17.00
MORTADELLA-PORK/BEEF	1 slice	15.0	47.00	2.460	0.460	3.810	8.000	1.430	187.0	24.00	2.000
POLISH SAUSAGE-PORK	1 item	227.0	740.0	32.00	3.700	65.20	159.0	23.40	1989	538.0	31.80
PORK-CHOP-LEAN/FAT-BROILED	1 item	82.0	284.0	19.30	0.000	22.30	77.00	8.060	54.00	287.0	20.00
PORK-CHOP-LEAN-BROILED	1 item	66.0	169.0	18.40	0.000	10.10	63.00	3.480	49.00	276.0	19.00
PORK-LOIN-LEAN/FAT-ROAST	1 item	88.0	268.0	22.40	0.000	19.10	80.00	6.920	56.00	284.0	17.00
PORK-LOIN-LEAN-ROASTED	1 slice	72.0	180.0	21.40	0.000	9.810	68.00	3.380	52.00	271.0	16.00
PORK-TENDERLOIN-LEAN-ROAST	1 srvg	28.4	47.00	8.160	0.000	1.360	26.30	0.470	19.00	152.0	7.000
POT ROAST-ARM-BEEF-COOKED	1 slice	100.0	231.0	33.00	0.000	9.980	101.0	3.790	66.00	289.0	24.00
ROAST BEEF-RIB-LEAN/FAT	1 slice	85.0	308.0	18.30	0.000	25.50	73.00	10.80	52.00	257.0	17.00
ROAST BEEF-RIB-LEAN	1 slice	51.0	122.0	13.90	0.000	7.030	41.30	2.960	37.70	192.0	12.80
ROAST BEEF-HEEL-LEAN/FAT	1 slice	85.0	222.0	25.30	0.000	12.60	81.00	4.810	43.00	248.0	20.00
ROAST BEEF-HEEL-LEAN	1 slice	78.0	173.0	24.60	0.000	7.530	74.90	2.680	39.80	240.0	19.50
SALAMI-COOKED-BEEF	1 slice	23.0	58.00	3.380	0.570	4.620	14.00	1.940	266.0	52.00	3.000
SALAMI-DRY OR HARD-PORK	1 slice	10.0	41.00	2.260	0.160	3.370	8.000	1.190	226.0	—	2.000
SAUSAGE-LINK-PORK-COOKED	1 item	13.0	48.00	2.550	0.130	4.050	11.00	1.400	168.0	47.00	2.000
SAUSAGE-PATTY-PORK-COOKED	1 item	27.0	100.0	5.310	0.280	8.410	22.00	2.920	349.0	97.00	5.000
SPARERIBS-PORK-BRAISED	1 srvg	28.4	113.0	8.230	0.000	8.580	34.30	3.330	26.30	90.70	7.000
STEAK-CHICKEN FRIED	1 item	100.0	389.0	17.90	12.30	30.00	—	—	815.0	126.0	—
STEAK-RIB-COOKED	1 item	100.0	225.0	28.00	0.000	11.60	80.00	4.930	69.00	394.0	27.00
STEAK-ROUND-LEAN/FAT	1 srvg	85.0	179.0	26.20	0.000	7.490	72.00	2.800	51.00	365.0	26.00
STEAK-ROUND-LEAN-BRAISED	1 srvg	68.0	130.0	21.50	0.000	4.210	55.00	1.470	45.10	295.0	21.10
STEAK-SIRLOIN-LEAN/FAT	1 item	85.0	271.0	22.70	0.000	19.40	77.00	8.070	52.00	297.0	23.00
STEAK-SIRLOIN-LEAN-BROILED	1 item	56.0	133.0	17.00	0.000	6.630	50.00	2.710	37.00	226.0	17.90
STEAK-TENDERLOIN-COOKED	1 item	100.0	204.0	28.40	0.000	9.280	84.00	3.630	63.00	419.0	30.00
VEAL-CUTLET-MED FAT-BROIL	1 item	85.0	185.0	23.00	0.000	9.000	87.00	4.000	68.00	258.0	15.30
VEAL-RIB-ROASTED-NO BONE	1 srvg	85.0	230.0	23.00	0.000	14.00	87.00	6.100	68.00	259.0	17.00

Nutritive Components for Miscellaneous

Food Name	Serving	Gm wt	KCAL Kc	PROT Gm	CARB Gm	FAT Gm	CHOL Mg	SAFA Gm	SOD Mg	POT Mg	MAG Mg
BAKING POWDER-HOME USE	1 tsp	3.0	5.000	0.000	1.000	0.000	0.000	0.000	339.0	5.000	—
BAKING POWD/CALC SULFATE	1 tsp	2.9	5.000	0.000	1.000	0.000	0.000	0.000	328.0	—	—
BAKING POWDER/PHOSPHATE	1 tsp	3.8	5.000	0.000	1.000	0.000	0.000	0.000	429.0	6.000	—
BAKING POWDER-LOW SODIUM	1 tsp	4.3	5.000	0.000	2.000	0.000	0.000	0.000	0.000	471.0	—
BAKING SODA	1 tsp	3.0	0.000	0.000	0.000	0.000	0.000	0.000	821.0	—	—
CHEWING GUM-CANDY COATED	1 item	1.7	5.000	—	1.600	—	—	—	—	—	—
CHEWING GUM-WRIGLEYS	1 item	3.0	10.00	0.000	2.300	—	0.000	—	0.000	0.000	0.000
GELATIN-DRY-ENVELOPE	1 item	7.0	25.00	6.000	0.000	0.000	0.000	0.000	8.000	180.0	—
GELATIN DESSERT-PREP	1 cup	240.0	140.0	4.000	34.00	0.000	0.000	0.000	0.000	—	—
GEL-D ZERTA-LOW CAL-PREP	1 cup	240.0	16.00	4.000	0.000	0.000	0.000	0.000	—	—	—

Continued.

IRON Mg	ZINC Mg	V-A IU	V-ET Mg	V-C Mg	THIA Mg	RIBO Mg	NIAC Mg	V-B6 Mg	FOL Ug	VB12 Ug	CALC Mg	PHOS Mg	SEL Mg	FIBD Gm
0.660	1.050	—	0.080	15.00	0.113	0.068	1.500	0.080	2.000	0.740	6.000	49.00	0.013	0.000
0.280	0.610	0.000	0.146	8.000	0.244	0.071	1.490	0.100	1.000	0.240	2.000	70.00	0.013	0.000
1.880	3.460	0.000	0.728	31.70	1.020	0.462	8.610	0.430	—	0.980	12.00	393.0	0.066	0.000
2.050	4.160	—	—	0.000	0.026	0.136	4.040	0.200	7.000	1.990	8.000	117.0	—	0.000
2.080	4.310	—	—	0.000	0.026	0.170	4.960	0.200	8.000	2.300	10.00	145.0	—	0.000
2.000	4.630	20.00	0.536	0.000	0.051	0.230	4.220	0.230	8.000	1.840	6.000	137.0	0.020	0.000
1.790	4.560	30.00	0.517	0.000	0.043	0.179	4.390	0.220	8.000	2.000	9.000	134.0	0.020	0.000
1.010	1.590	—	—	1.300	0.417	0.156	2.790	0.220	—	0.870	16.00	114.0	0.022	0.000
0.380	0.520	—	0.083	6.000	0.059	0.056	0.749	0.050	—	0.420	11.00	38.00	0.004	0.000
0.620	1.130	—	0.388	18.00	0.233	0.095	1.860	0.110	—	0.800	7.000	67.00	0.010	0.000
1.150	—	—	0.124	—	0.049	0.185	—	0.030	5.000	2.420	5.000	41.00	0.003	0.000
1.000	3.500	—	0.285	—	0.110	0.190	4.100	0.245	2.670	1.800	8.000	139.0	0.016	0.000
1.100	2.480	—	0.182	—	0.090	0.150	3.400	0.157	1.710	1.230	6.000	121.0	0.010	0.000
1.400	3.500	—	—	—	0.130	0.230	4.700	0.234	2.550	1.830	9.000	177.0	0.015	0.000
0.210	0.320	—	0.048	4.000	0.018	0.023	0.401	0.019	—	0.220	3.000	15.00	0.002	—
3.270	4.380	—	0.726	2.270	1.140	0.336	7.820	0.431	—	2.220	27.20	309.0	0.066	0.000
0.660	2.010	7.000	0.492	0.200	0.690	0.294	4.320	0.310	4.000	0.810	5.000	193.0	0.014	0.000
0.610	1.930	5.000	0.396	0.200	0.641	0.278	3.930	0.300	4.000	0.710	5.000	184.0	0.011	0.000
0.870	1.800	7.000	0.527	0.300	0.727	0.210	4.440	0.350	1.000	0.530	5.000	173.0	0.028	0.000
0.820	1.710	6.000	0.431	0.300	0.681	0.196	4.090	0.340	0.000	0.450	4.000	164.0	0.023	0.000
0.437	0.850	2.000	0.210	0.100	0.266	0.111	1.330	0.120	1.670	0.157	2.330	81.70	0.009	0.000
3.790	8.660	—	—	0.000	0.081	0.289	3.720	0.330	11.00	3.400	9.000	268.0	0.006	0.000
1.770	4.270	69.90	—	0.000	0.065	0.146	2.650	0.250	5.000	2.370	10.00	140.0	0.020	0.000
1.330	3.540	10.00	—	0.000	0.042	0.107	2.100	0.153	4.080	1.490	5.100	109.0	0.012	0.000
2.760	4.360	10.00	—	0.000	0.060	0.208	3.290	0.290	9.000	2.040	5.000	217.0	0.020	0.000
2.700	4.270	0.000	—	0.000	0.059	0.203	3.180	0.281	8.580	1.930	3.900	212.0	0.019	0.000
0.460	0.490	—	0.156	3.000	0.029	0.059	0.785	0.050	0.000	1.110	2.000	23.00	0.004	0.000
0.130	0.420	—	0.068	—	0.093	0.033	0.560	0.060	—	0.280	1.000	23.00	0.002	0.000
0.160	0.330	—	0.042	0.000	0.096	0.033	0.587	0.040	—	0.220	4.000	24.00	0.004	0.000
0.340	0.680	—	0.086	0.000	0.200	0.069	1.220	0.090	—	0.470	9.000	50.00	0.003	0.000
0.527	1.300	3.000	0.170	—	0.116	0.108	1.550	0.100	1.330	0.307	13.30	74.00	0.005	0.000
2.300	—	26.00	0.550	—	0.110	0.140	2.700	—	—	—	11.00	110.0	—	—
2.570	6.990	—	—	0.000	0.105	0.216	4.800	0.400	8.000	3.320	13.00	208.0	0.006	0.000
2.390	4.590	20.00	0.468	0.000	0.097	0.221	4.980	0.460	10.00	2.080	5.000	203.0	0.029	0.000
1.960	3.790	10.00	0.374	0.000	0.076	0.184	3.720	0.134	5.950	1.990	4.000	182.0	0.023	0.000
2.490	4.730	50.00	0.468	0.000	0.092	0.218	3.210	0.330	7.000	2.220	9.000	180.0	0.029	0.000
1.880	3.650	10.00	0.308	0.000	0.071	0.165	2.400	0.252	5.600	1.600	6.160	137.0	0.019	0.000
3.580	5.590	—	—	0.000	0.130	0.298	3.920	0.440	7.000	2.570	7.000	238.0	0.006	0.000
2.700	3.500	—	0.204	—	0.060	0.210	4.600	—	—	1.360	9.000	196.0	—	0.000
2.900	3.500	—	0.204	—	0.110	0.260	6.600	—	—	1.400	10.00	211.0	—	0.000

IRON Mg	ZINC Mg	V-A IU	V-ET Mg	V-C Mg	THIA Mg	RIBO Mg	NIAC Mg	V-B6 Mg	FOL Ug	VB12 Ug	CALC Mg	PHOS Mg	SEL Mg	FIBD Gm
—	—	0.000	—	0.000	0.000	0.000	0.000	—	—	—	58.00	87.00	0.000	0.000
—	—	0.000	—	0.000	0.000	0.000	0.000	—	—	—	183.0	45.00	0.000	0.000
—	—	0.000	—	0.000	0.000	0.000	0.000	—	—	—	239.0	359.0	0.000	0.000
—	—	0.000	—	0.000	0.000	0.000	0.000	—	—	—	207.0	314.0	0.000	0.000
—	—	—	0.000	0.000	0.000	0.000	0.000	0.000	0.000	0.000	—	—	—	0.000
—	—	—	—	0.000	0.000	0.000	0.000	—	—	—	—	—	—	—
0.000	0.000	0.000	—	0.000	0.000	0.000	0.000	0.000	0.000	0.000	3.000	0.000	—	—
0.400	—	—	—	4.000	0.000	0.000	0.000	0.000	—	—	0.000	0.000	—	0.000
—	—	—	—	—	—	—	—	—	—	—	—	—	—	0.000
—	—	—	—	—	—	—	—	—	—	—	—	—	—	0.000

Continued.

Nutritive Components for Miscellaneous—cont'd

Food Name	Serving	Gm wt	KCAL Kc	PROT Gm	CARB Gm	FAT Gm	CHOL Mg	SAFA Gm	SOD Mg	POT Mg	MAG Mg
JELLO-GEL-SUGAR FREE-PREP	1 cup	240.0	16.00	2.000	0.000	0.000	0.000	0.000	120.0	—	—
OLIVES-GREEN-PICKLED-CAN	1 item	4.0	3.750	0.100	0.100	0.500	0.000	0.050	80.80	1.750	—
OLIVES-MISSION-RIPE-CAN	1 item	3.0	5.000	0.100	0.100	0.667	0.000	0.067	19.20	0.667	—
PICKLE-DILL-CUCUMBER-MED	1 item	65.0	5.000	0.000	1.000	0.000	0.000	0.000	928.0	130.0	7.800
PICKLE-FRESH PACK-CUCUMBER	1 item	7.5	5.000	0.000	1.500	0.000	0.000	0.000	50.00	—	—
PICKLE-SWEET/GHERKIN-SMALL	1 item	15.0	20.00	0.000	5.000	0.000	0.000	0.000	128.0	—	0.150
PICKLE/HAMBURGER RELISH	1 srvg	28.4	30.00	0.000	7.000	0.000	0.000	0.000	325.0	—	—
PICKLE/HOT DOG RELISH	1 srvg	28.4	35.00	0.000	8.000	0.000	0.000	0.000	200.0	—	—
PICKLE RELISH-SWEET	1 tbsp	15.0	20.00	0.000	5.000	0.000	0.000	0.000	124.0	—	—
POPSICLE	1 item	95.0	70.00	0.000	18.00	0.000	0.000	0.000	0.000	—	—
VINEGAR-CIDER	1 tbsp	15.0	0.000	0.000	1.000	0.000	0.000	0.000	0.125	15.00	—
VINEGAR-DISTILLED	1 cup	240.0	29.00	0.000	12.00	0.000	—	0.000	2.000	36.00	0.000
YEAST-BAKER-DRY-ACT-PACKET	1 srvg	7.0	20.00	3.000	3.000	0.000	0.000	0.000	1.000	140.0	3.780
YEAST-BREWERS-DRY	1 tbsp	8.0	25.00	3.000	3.000	0.000	0.000	—	9.000	152.0	18.40

Nutritive Components for Nuts & Seeds

Food Name	Serving	Gm wt	KCAL Kc	PROT Gm	CARB Gm	FAT Gm	CHOL Mg	SAFA Gm	SOD Mg	POT Mg	MAG Mg
NUTS-ALMOND-SHELLED-SLIVER	1 cup	115.0	677.0	22.90	23.50	60.00	0.000	5.690	12.70	842.0	340.0
NUTS-BRAZIL-DRIED-SHELLED	1 cup	140.0	919.0	20.10	17.90	92.70	0.000	22.60	2.000	840.0	315.0
NUTS-CASHEWS-DRY ROASTED	1 cup	137.0	787.0	21.00	44.80	63.50	0.000	12.50	21.00	774.0	356.0
NUTS-COCONUT CREAM-RAW	1 cup	240.0	792.0	8.700	16.00	83.20	0.000	73.80	10.00	781.0	—
NUTS-COCONUT-DRI-FLAKE-CAN	1 cup	77.0	341.0	2.580	31.50	24.40	0.000	21.60	15.00	249.0	38.00
NUTS-COCONUT-DRIED-SHRED	1 cup	93.0	466.0	2.680	44.30	33.00	0.000	29.30	244.0	313.0	47.00
NUT-FILBERT/HAZEL-DRI-CHOP	1 cup	115.0	727.0	15.00	17.60	72.00	0.000	5.300	3.000	512.0	328.0
NUTS-MACADAMIA-DRIED	1 cup	134.0	940.0	11.10	18.40	98.80	0.000	14.80	6.000	493.0	155.0
NUTS-MIXED-DRY ROASTED	1 cup	137.0	814.0	23.70	34.70	70.50	0.000	9.450	16.00	817.0	308.0
NUTS-MIXED-OIL ROASTED	1 cup	142.0	876.0	23.80	30.40	80.00	0.000	12.40	16.00	825.0	333.0
NUTS-PEANUTS-SPANISH-DRIED	1 cup	146.0	827.0	37.50	23.60	71.80	0.000	9.960	23.00	1047	262.0
NUTS-PEANUTS-OIL ROASTED	1 cup	145.0	840.0	38.80	26.70	71.30	0.000	9.900	22.00	1020	273.0
NUTS-PEANUTS-OIL-SALTED	1 cup	145.0	841.0	38.80	26.80	71.30	0.000	9.930	626.0	1020	273.0
NUTS-PECANS-DRIED-HALVES	1 cup	108.0	721.0	8.370	19.70	73.10	0.000	5.850	1.000	423.0	138.0
NUTS-PECANS-OIL ROASTED	1 cup	110.0	754.0	7.650	17.70	78.30	0.000	6.270	1.000	395.0	142.0
NUTS-PISTACHIO-DRIED	1 cup	128.0	739.0	26.30	31.80	61.90	0.000	7.840	7.000	1399	203.0
NUTS-PISTACHIO-DRY ROASTED	1 cup	128.0	776.0	19.10	35.20	67.60	0.000	8.560	8.000	1242	166.0
NUTS-WALNUT-BLACK-DRI-CHOP	1 cup	125.0	759.0	30.40	15.10	70.70	0.000	4.540	2.000	655.0	252.0
NUT-WALNUT-PERSIAN/ENGLISH	1 cup	120.0	770.0	17.20	22.00	74.20	0.000	6.700	12.00	602.0	203.0
PEANUT BUTTER-CHUNK STYLE	1 cup	258.0	1520	62.00	55.70	129.0	0.000	24.70	1255	1928	409.0
PEANUT BUTTER-LOW SODIUM	1 tbsp	16.0	95.00	5.000	2.500	8.500	0.000	—	5.000	—	—
PEANUT BUTTER-OLD FASHION	1 cup	16.0	95.00	4.200	2.700	8.100	0.000	1.500	75.00	110.0	30.00
PEANUT BUTTER-SMOOTH TYPE	1 tbsp	16.0	95.00	4.560	2.530	8.180	0.000	1.360	75.00	110.0	28.00
SEEDS-PUMPKIN/SQUASH-ROAST	1 cup	64.0	285.0	11.90	34.40	12.40	0.000	2.350	12.00	588.0	168.0
SEEDS-SESAME-ROASTED-WHOLE	1 srvg	28.4	161.0	4.820	7.310	13.60	0.000	1.910	3.000	135.0	101.0
SEEDS-SUNFLOWER-OIL ROAST	1 cup	135.0	830.0	28.80	19.90	77.60	0.000	8.130	4.000	652.0	171.0

IRON Mg	ZINC Mg	V-A IU	V-ET Mg	V-C Mg	THIA Mg	RIBO Mg	NIAC Mg	V-B6 Mg	FOL Ug	VB12 Ug	CALC Mg	PHOS Mg	SEL Mg	FIBD Gm
—	—	—	—	—	—	—	—	—	—	—	—	—	—	0.000
0.050	—	10.00	—	—	—	—	—	—	0.040	0.000	2.000	0.500	0.000	0.080
0.033	0.010	3.330	—	—	0.000	0.000	—	0.000	0.033	0.000	3.000	0.333	0.000	0.060
0.700	0.176	70.00	—	4.000	0.000	0.010	0.000	0.005	0.650	0.000	17.00	14.00	0.000	—
0.150	0.020	10.00	—	0.500	0.000	0.000	0.000	0.001	0.075	0.000	2.500	2.000	0.000	—
0.200	0.020	10.00	—	1.000	0.000	0.000	0.000	0.001	0.150	0.000	2.000	2.000	0.000	—
0.189	—	—	—	—	—	—	—	—	—	—	5.670	3.780	0.000	—
0.189	—	—	—	—	—	—	—	—	—	—	5.600	3.700	0.000	—
0.100	0.010	—	—	—	—	—	—	—	—	—	3.000	2.000	0.000	—
0.000	—	0.000	—	0.000	0.000	0.000	0.000	—	—	—	0.000	—	—	—
0.100	0.020	—	—	—	—	—	—	0.000	—	—	1.000	1.000	—	0.000
—	—	—	—	—	—	—	—	—	—	—	—	—	0.074	—
1.100	—	0.000	—	0.000	0.160	0.380	2.600	0.140	286.0	0.000	3.000	90.00	0.000	—
1.400	—	0.000	—	0.000	1.250	0.340	3.000	0.200	313.0	0.000	17.00	140.0	0.000	—

IRON Mg	ZINC Mg	V-A IU	V-ET Mg	V-C Mg	THIA Mg	RIBO Mg	NIAC Mg	V-B6 Mg	FOL Ug	VB12 Ug	CALC Mg	PHOS Mg	SEL Mg	FIBD Gm
4.210	3.360	0.000	28.20	0.690	0.243	0.896	3.870	0.130	67.50	0.000	306.0	598.0	0.005	10.70
4.760	6.420	—	—	1.000	1.400	0.171	2.270	0.351	5.600	0.000	246.0	840.0	0.144	10.80
8.220	7.670	0.000	15.00	0.000	0.274	0.274	1.920	0.351	94.80	0.000	62.00	671.0	0.007	10.00
5.470	2.300	0.000	—	6.700	0.072	0.000	2.140	—	—	0.000	26.00	293.0	—	—
1.420	1.230	0.000	—	0.000	0.023	0.015	0.235	—	—	0.000	11.00	79.00	—	4.400
1.780	1.690	0.000	—	0.600	0.029	0.019	0.441	—	—	0.000	14.00	99.00	0.016	3.900
3.760	2.760	77.00	—	1.200	0.575	0.127	1.300	0.704	82.60	0.000	216.0	359.0	0.002	9.770
3.230	2.290	0.000	—	—	0.469	0.147	2.870	—	—	0.000	94.00	183.0	0.007	12.40
5.070	5.210	21.00	16.40	0.600	0.274	0.274	6.440	0.406	69.00	0.000	96.00	596.0	0.007	11.60
4.560	7.220	28.00	17.00	0.700	0.707	0.315	7.190	0.341	118.0	0.000	153.0	659.0	0.007	10.90
4.710	4.780	0.000	17.30	0.000	0.969	0.191	20.70	0.432	147.0	0.000	85.00	560.0	0.007	13.60
2.780	9.600	0.000	16.70	0.000	0.425	0.146	21.50	0.576	153.0	0.000	125.0	733.0	0.055	11.10
2.780	9.600	0.000	16.80	0.000	0.425	0.146	21.50	0.577	153.0	0.000	125.0	733.0	0.055	11.20
2.300	5.910	138.0	21.40	2.100	0.916	0.138	0.958	0.203	42.30	0.000	39.00	314.0	0.003	8.300
2.330	6.050	—	21.90	—	—	—	—	—	—	0.000	37.00	324.0	0.006	8.470
8.670	1.710	299.0	—	—	1.050	0.223	1.380	—	74.20	0.000	173.0	644.0	0.007	9.900
4.060	1.740	—	—	—	0.541	0.315	1.800	—	—	0.000	90.00	609.0	0.007	9.900
3.840	4.280	370.0	24.50	—	0.271	0.136	0.863	—	—	—	72.00	580.0	0.024	11.80
2.930	3.280	148.0	23.50	3.900	0.458	0.178	1.250	0.670	79.20	0.000	113.0	380.0	0.023	—
4.900	7.170	0.000	—	0.000	0.323	0.289	35.30	1.160	237.0	0.000	105.0	817.0	—	9.800
—	—	—	3.200	—	—	—	—	—	—	—	—	—	0.002	1.700
0.300	0.500	—	—	—	0.010	0.010	2.300	—	—	—	5.000	60.00	—	—
0.290	0.470	—	3.200	0.000	0.024	0.017	2.150	0.062	13.10	0.000	5.000	60.00	0.002	1.400
2.120	6.590	—	—	—	—	—	—	—	—	0.000	35.00	59.00	—	—
4.190	2.030	—	6.450	—	—	—	—	—	—	0.000	281.0	181.0	—	5.320
9.050	7.040	—	70.40	1.900	0.432	0.378	5.580	—	316.0	0.000	76.00	1538	—	—

Nutritive Components for Poultry

Food Name	Serving	Gm wt	KCAL Kc	PROT Gm	CARB Gm	FAT Gm	CHOL Mg	SAFA Gm	SOD Mg	POT Mg	MAG Mg
CHICKEN-BREAST-FRI/BATTER	1 item	280.0	728.0	69.60	25.20	36.90	238.0	9.860	770.0	564.0	68.00
CHICKEN-BREAST-FRIED/FLOUR	1 item	196.0	436.0	62.40	3.220	17.40	176.0	4.800	150.0	506.0	58.00
CHICKEN-BREAST-ROASTED	1 item	196.0	386.0	58.40	0.000	15.30	166.0	4.300	138.0	480.0	54.00
CHICKEN-BREAST-STEWED	1 item	220.0	404.0	60.30	0.000	16.30	166.0	4.580	136.0	390.0	48.00
CHICKEN-BREAST-NO SKIN-FRI	1 item	172.0	322.0	57.50	0.880	8.100	156.0	2.220	136.0	474.0	54.00
CHICK-BREAST-NO SKIN-ROAST	1 item	172.0	284.0	53.40	0.000	6.140	146.0	1.740	126.0	440.0	50.00
CHICKEN-DRUMSTICK-FRIED	1 item	49.0	120.0	13.20	0.800	6.720	44.00	1.790	44.00	112.0	11.00
CHICKEN-FRANKFURTER	1 item	45.0	116.0	5.820	3.060	8.760	45.00	2.490	617.0	—	—
CHICKEN-GIBLETS-FRI/FLOUR	1 cup	145.0	402.0	47.20	6.310	19.50	647.0	5.500	164.0	478.0	37.00
CHICKEN-GIBLETS-SIMMERED	1 cup	145.0	228.0	37.50	1.370	6.920	570.0	2.160	85.00	229.0	30.00
CHICKEN-LIVER PATE-CAN	1 tbsp	13.0	26.00	1.750	0.850	1.700	—	—	—	—	—
CHICKEN-LIVER-SIMMERED	1 cup	140.0	219.0	34.10	1.230	7.630	883.0	2.580	71.00	196.0	29.00
CHICKEN-LEG-ROASTED	1 item	114.0	265.0	29.60	0.000	15.40	105.0	4.240	99.00	256.0	26.00
CHICKEN-LEG-NO SKIN-ROAST	1 item	95.0	182.0	25.70	0.000	8.010	89.00	2.180	87.00	230.0	23.00
CHICKEN-LEG-NO SKIN-STEWED	1 item	101.0	187.0	26.50	0.000	8.140	90.00	2.220	78.00	192.0	21.00
CHICKEN ROLL-LIGHT	1 slice	28.4	45.00	5.540	0.695	2.090	14.00	0.575	166.0	64.50	5.000
CHICKEN SPREAD-CANNED	1 tbsp	13.0	25.00	2.000	0.700	1.520	—	—	—	—	—
CHICKEN-THIGH-FRIED/FLOUR	1 item	62.0	162.0	16.60	1.970	9.290	60.00	2.540	55.00	147.0	15.00
CHICK-THIGH-NO SKIN-ROAST	1 item	52.0	109.0	13.50	0.000	5.660	49.00	1.570	46.00	124.0	12.00
CHICKEN-WING-FRIED/FLOUR	1 item	32.0	103.0	8.360	0.760	7.090	26.00	1.940	25.00	57.00	6.000
CHICKEN-WING-ROASTED	1 item	34.0	99.00	9.130	0.000	6.620	29.00	1.850	28.00	62.00	7.000
CHICKEN-WING-STEWED	1 item	40.0	100.0	9.110	0.000	6.730	28.00	1.880	27.00	56.00	6.000
DUCK-FLESH & SKIN-ROASTED	1 item	764.0	2574	145.0	0.000	217.0	640.0	73.90	454.0	1560	124.0
DUCK-NO SKIN-ROASTED	1 item	442.0	890.0	104.0	0.000	49.50	396.0	18.40	286.0	1114	88.00
TURK-BREAST-NO SKIN-ROAST	1 item	612.0	826.0	184.0	0.000	4.500	510.0	1.440	318.0	1784	178.0
TURKEY-DARK MEAT-NO SKIN	1 cup	140.0	262.0	40.00	0.000	10.10	119.0	3.400	110.0	406.0	34.00
TURKEY-LIGHT/DARK-NO SKIN	1 cup	140.0	238.0	41.00	0.000	6.950	107.0	2.290	99.00	418.0	37.00
TURKEY-LIGHT-NO SKIN-ROAST	1 cup	140.0	219.0	41.90	0.000	4.500	97.00	1.440	89.00	426.0	39.00
TURK HAM-CURED THIGH MEAT	1 slice	28.4	36.50	5.370	0.105	1.440	—	0.485	283.0	92.00	—
TURKEY LOAF-BREAST	1 srvg	28.4	31.20	6.380	0.000	0.447	11.50	0.137	406.0	78.80	5.670
TURKEY PASTRAMI	1 slice	28.4	40.00	5.210	0.470	2.060	—	1.030	297.0	73.50	4.000
TURKEY ROLL-LIGHT	1 srvg	28.4	42.00	5.300	0.150	2.050	12.00	0.570	139.0	71.00	5.000

Nutritive Components for Sauces & Dips

Food Name	Serving	Gm wt	KCAL Kc	PROT Gm	CARB Gm	FAT Gm	CHOL Mg	SAFA Gm	SOD Mg	POT Mg	MAG Mg
DIP-FRENCH ONION-KRAFT	1 tbsp	15.0	30.00	0.500	1.500	2.000	0.000	—	120.0	—	—
DIP-GUACAMOLE-KRAFT	1 tbsp	15.0	25.00	0.500	1.500	2.000	0.000	—	108.0	—	—
GRAVY-BEEF-CANNED	1 cup	233.0	124.0	8.730	11.20	5.490	7.000	2.750	117.0	189.0	—
GRAVY-CHICKEN-CANNED	1 cup	238.0	189.0	4.590	12.90	13.60	5.000	3.360	1375	260.0	—
GRAVY-TURKEY-CANNED	1 cup	238.0	122.0	6.200	12.20	5.010	5.000	1.480	—	—	—
HORSERADISH-PREPARED	1 tbsp	15.0	6.000	0.200	1.400	0.000	0.000	0.000	165.0	44.00	—
MUSTARD-BROWN-PREPARED	1 cup	250.0	228.0	14.80	13.30	15.80	—	—	3268	325.0	—
MUSTARD-YELLOW-PREPARED	1 tsp	5.0	5.000	0.100	0.100	0.100	0.000	0.000	65.00	7.000	2.000
SAUCE-BARBECUE	1 cup	250.0	188.0	4.500	32.00	4.500	0.000	0.670	2032	435.0	—
SAUCE-BEARNAISE-MIX/MILK	1 cup	255.0	701.0	8.320	17.50	68.20	189.0	41.80	1265	—	—
SAUCE-CHILI-BOTTLED	1 tbsp	15.0	16.00	0.400	3.700	0.000	0.000	0.000	201.0	56.00	—
SAUCE-CURRY-MIX/MILK	1 cup	272.0	270.0	10.70	25.70	14.70	35.00	6.050	1276	—	—
SAUCE-HEINZ 57	1 tbsp	15.0	15.00	0.400	2.700	0.200	0.000	0.000	265.0	—	—
SAUCE-MARINARA-CANNED	1 cup	250.0	171.0	4.000	25.50	8.380	0.000	1.200	1572	1061	59.00
SAUCE-MUSHROOM-MIX/MILK	1 cup	267.0	228.0	11.30	23.80	10.30	34.00	5.400	1533	—	—
SAUCE-PICANTE-CANNED	1 fl oz	16.0	9.000	0.300	1.900	0.500	0.000	0.000	218.0	77.00	—
SAUCE-SALSA/CHILIES-CANNED	1 fl oz	16.0	10.00	0.400	2.000	0.700	0.000	0.000	111.0	87.00	—
SAUCE-SPAGHETTI-CANNED	1 cup	249.0	272.0	4.530	39.70	11.90	0.000	1.700	1236	957.0	60.00

Continued.

IRON Mg	ZINC Mg	V-A IU	V-ET Mg	V-C Mg	THIA Mg	RIBO Mg	NIAC Mg	V-B6 Mg	FOL Ug	VB12 Ug	CALC Mg	PHOS Mg	SEL Mg	FIBD Gm
3.500	2.660	188.0	1.540	0.000	0.322	0.408	29.50	1.200	16.00	0.820	56.00	516.0	0.030	—
2.340	2.140	98.00	1.080	0.000	0.160	0.256	26.90	1.140	8.000	0.680	32.00	456.0	0.021	—
2.080	2.000	182.0	1.080	0.000	0.130	0.234	24.90	1.080	6.000	0.640	28.00	420.0	0.053	0.000
2.020	2.120	180.0	1.210	0.000	0.090	0.254	17.20	0.640	6.000	0.460	28.00	344.0	0.053	0.000
1.960	1.860	40.00	0.946	0.000	0.136	0.216	25.40	1.100	8.000	0.620	28.00	424.0	0.031	0.000
1.780	1.720	36.00	0.946	0.000	0.120	0.196	23.60	1.020	6.000	0.580	26.00	392.0	0.046	0.000
0.660	1.420	41.00	0.270	0.000	0.040	0.110	2.960	0.170	4.000	0.160	6.000	86.00	0.005	—
0.900	—	—	—	—	0.030	0.052	1.390	—	—	—	43.00	—	0.010	—
15.00	9.090	17300	2.090	12.70	0.141	2.210	15.90	0.880	550.0	19.30	26.00	414.0	0.025	—
9.340	6.630	10770	2.090	11.60	0.126	1.380	5.950	0.490	545.0	14.70	18.00	331.0	0.025	0.000
1.190	—	94.00	0.046	1.300	0.007	0.182	0.977	—	—	—	1.000	—	—	—
11.90	6.070	22930	2.020	22.20	0.214	2.450	6.230	0.820	1077	27.10	20.00	437.0	0.099	0.000
1.520	2.960	154.0	0.627	0.000	0.078	0.243	7.060	0.370	8.000	0.350	14.00	199.0	0.016	0.000
1.240	2.710	60.00	0.523	0.000	0.071	0.220	6.000	0.350	8.000	0.310	12.00	174.0	0.013	0.000
1.410	2.810	60.00	0.556	0.000	0.060	0.218	4.850	0.220	8.000	0.230	11.00	151.0	0.013	0.000
0.275	0.205	—	0.148	—	0.019	0.037	1.500	—	—	—	12.00	44.50	—	—
0.300	—	—	0.068	—	0.001	0.015	0.357	—	—	—	16.00	—	—	—
0.930	1.560	61.00	0.341	0.000	0.058	0.151	4.310	0.210	5.000	0.190	8.000	116.0	0.011	0.040
0.680	1.340	34.00	0.286	0.000	0.038	0.120	3.390	0.180	4.000	0.160	6.000	95.00	0.021	0.000
0.400	0.560	40.00	0.176	0.000	0.019	0.044	2.140	0.130	1.000	0.090	5.000	48.00	0.006	0.000
0.430	0.620	54.00	0.187	0.000	0.014	0.044	2.260	0.140	1.000	0.100	5.000	51.00	0.006	0.000
0.450	0.650	53.00	0.220	0.000	0.016	0.041	1.850	0.090	1.000	0.070	5.000	48.00	0.006	0.000
20.60	14.20	1608	5.350	0.000	1.330	2.060	36.90	1.400	50.00	2.260	86.00	1190	—	0.000
11.90	11.50	342.0	3.090	0.000	1.150	2.080	22.50	1.100	44.00	1.760	52.00	898.0	—	0.000
9.360	10.60	0.000	—	0.000	0.264	0.802	45.90	3.420	38.00	2.360	76.00	1370	—	0.000
3.270	6.250	0.000	—	0.000	0.088	0.347	5.110	0.500	13.00	0.520	45.00	286.0	—	0.000
2.490	4.340	0.000	—	0.000	0.087	0.255	7.620	0.640	10.00	0.520	35.00	298.0	—	0.000
1.880	2.850	0.000	—	0.000	0.085	0.181	9.570	0.750	8.000	0.520	27.00	307.0	—	0.000
0.785	—	—	—	—	0.015	0.070	1.000	—	—	—	2.500	54.00	—	—
0.113	0.318	0.000	—	0.000	0.011	0.030	2.360	0.100	—	0.572	2.000	64.80	—	0.000
0.470	0.610	—	—	—	0.016	0.071	1.000	—	—	—	2.500	56.50	—	—
0.360	0.440	—	—	—	0.025	0.064	1.990	—	—	—	11.00	52.00	—	—

IRON Mg	ZINC Mg	V-A IU	V-ET Mg	V-C Mg	THIA Mg	RIBO Mg	NIAC Mg	V-B6 Mg	FOL Ug	VB12 Ug	CALC Mg	PHOS Mg	SEL Mg	FIBD Gm
—	—	—	—	—	—	—	—	—	—	—	—	—	—	—
—	—	—	—	—	—	—	—	—	—	—	—	—	—	—
1.630	2.330	0.000	—	0.000	0.074	0.084	1.540	0.023	—	0.230	14.00	70.00	—	—
1.120	1.910	880.0	—	0.000	0.041	0.103	1.060	0.024	—	—	48.00	69.00	—	—
1.670	—	0.000	—	0.000	0.048	0.191	3.100	—	—	0.000	10.00	—	—	—
0.100	—	—	—	—	—	—	—	—	—	—	9.000	5.000	—	—
4.500	—	—	10.40	—	—	—	—	—	—	—	310.0	335.0	—	—
0.100	—	—	0.208	—	—	—	—	—	—	—	4.000	4.000	0.000	0.060
2.250	—	2170	—	17.50	0.075	0.050	2.250	0.188	—	0.000	48.00	50.00	—	2.300
—	—	—	—	—	—	—	—	—	—	—	—	—	—	0.090
0.100	—	210.0	—	2.000	0.010	0.010	0.200	—	—	—	3.000	8.000	0.000	—
—	—	—	—	—	—	—	—	—	—	—	485.0	280.0	—	0.900
—	—	—	—	—	—	—	—	—	—	—	—	—	0.000	—
2.000	0.670	2403	—	31.90	0.113	0.148	3.980	—	—	0.000	44.00	88.00	—	—
—	—	—	—	—	—	—	—	—	—	—	—	—	—	0.500
0.250	—	230.0	—	8.800	0.020	0.010	0.220	—	—	—	3.800	8.000	—	—
0.280	—	395.0	—	9.100	0.020	0.010	0.290	—	—	—	4.200	9.300	—	—
1.620	0.530	3055	—	27.90	0.137	0.147	3.750	—	—	0.000	70.00	90.00	—	—

Continued.

Nutritive Components for Sauces & Dips—cont'd

Food Name	Serving	Gm wt	KCAL Kc	PROT Gm	CARB Gm	FAT Gm	CHOL Mg	SAFA Gm	SOD Mg	POT Mg	MAG Mg
SAUCE-SOUR CREAM-MIX/MILK	1 cup	314.0	509.0	19.10	45.40	30.30	91.00	16.10	1007	733.0	—
SAUCE-SOY	1 tbsp	18.0	11.00	1.560	1.500	0.000	0.000	0.000	1029	64.00	8.000
SAUCE-SWEET/SOUR-MIX/PREP	1 cup	313.0	294.0	0.760	72.70	0.080	0.000	0.010	779.0	66.00	—
SAUCE-TABASCO	1 tsp	5.0	0.000	0.100	0.100	0.000	—	0.000	22.00	3.000	—
SAUCE-TACO-CANNED	1 fl oz	16.0	11.00	0.400	2.200	0.700	0.000	—	128.0	88.00	—
SAUCE-TERIYAKI-BOTTLED	1 tbsp	18.0	15.00	1.070	2.870	0.000	0.000	0.000	690.0	41.00	11.00
SAUCE-TOMATO-CAN-LOW SOD	1 cup	226.0	90.00	4.000	18.00	0.000	—	0.000	65.00	—	—
SAUCE-TOMATO-CAN-SALT ADD	1 cup	245.0	74.00	3.250	17.60	0.410	0.000	0.059	1481	908.0	46.00
SAUCE-TOMATO-SPANISH-CAN	1 cup	244.0	80.00	3.520	17.70	0.640	0.000	0.092	1152	—	—
SAUCE-WORCESTERSHIRE	1 tbsp	15.0	12.00	0.300	2.700	0.000	—	0.000	147.0	120.0	—
TOMATO CATSUP	1 tbsp	15.0	15.00	0.000	4.000	0.000	0.000	0.000	156.0	54.00	3.600
SAUCE-CHEESE-MIX/MILK	1 cup	279.0	307.0	16.00	23.20	17.10	53.00	9.320	1566	554.0	47.00

Nutritive Components for Soups

Food Name	Serving	Gm wt	KCAL Kc	PROT Gm	CARB Gm	FAT Gm	CHOL Mg	SAFA Gm	SOD Mg	POT Mg	MAG Mg
SOUP-VEGETABLE BEEF-CAN	1 cup	245.0	79.00	5.580	10.20	1.900	5.000	0.850	957.0	173.0	6.000
SOUP-BEAN/BACON-CAN-WATER	1 cup	253.0	173.0	7.890	22.80	5.940	3.000	1.530	952.0	403.0	44.00
SOUP-BEEF BROTH-CAN-READY	1 cup	240.0	16.00	2.740	0.100	0.530	0.605	0.260	782.0	130.0	—
SOUP-BEEF-CHUNKY-CAN	1 cup	240.0	171.0	11.70	19.60	5.140	14.00	2.550	867.0	336.0	—
SOUP-BLACK BEAN-CAN-WATER	1 cup	247.0	116.0	5.640	19.80	1.510	0.000	0.400	1198	273.0	42.00
SOUP-CREAM/CELERY-CAN-MILK	1 cup	248.0	165.0	5.690	14.50	9.680	32.00	3.950	1010	309.0	22.00
SOUP-CHEESE-CAN-MILK	1 cup	251.0	230.0	9.450	16.20	14.60	48.00	9.120	1020	340.0	20.00
SOUP-CHICK BROTH-CAN/WATER	1 cup	244.0	39.00	4.930	0.930	1.390	1.000	0.410	776.0	210.0	2.000
SOUP-CHICKEN-CHUNKY-CAN	1 cup	251.0	178.0	12.70	17.30	6.630	30.00	1.980	887.0	176.0	—
SOUP-CREAM/CHICK-CAN-MILK	1 cup	248.0	191.0	7.460	15.00	11.50	27.00	4.630	1046	273.0	18.00
SOUP-CHICKEN NOODLE-CAN	1 cup	241.0	75.00	4.040	9.350	2.450	7.000	0.650	1107	55.00	5.000
SOUP-CHICKEN/RICE-CAN	1 cup	240.0	127.0	12.30	13.00	3.190	12.00	0.950	888.0	—	—
SOUP-CLAM-MANHATTAN-WATER	1 cup	244.0	78.00	4.180	12.20	2.310	2.000	0.440	1808	262.0	10.00
SOUP-CLAM-NEW ENGLAND-MILK	1 cup	248.0	163.0	9.460	16.60	6.600	22.00	2.950	992.0	300.0	23.00
SOUP-BEEF BROTH-DEHY-CUBED	1 item	4.0	6.000	0.620	0.580	0.140	0.144	0.070	864.0	15.00	2.000
SOUP-ONION-DEHY-PACKET	1 srvg	39.0	115.0	4.520	20.90	2.330	2.000	0.540	3493	260.0	25.00
SOUP-MINESTRONE-CAN-WATER	1 cup	241.0	83.00	4.260	11.20	2.510	2.000	0.540	911.0	312.0	7.000
SOUP-CREAM/MUSHROOM-MILK	1 cup	248.0	203.0	6.050	15.00	13.60	20.00	5.120	1076	270.0	20.00
SOUP-ONION-CAN-WATER	1 cup	241.0	57.00	3.750	8.180	1.740	0.000	0.260	1053	69.00	2.000
SOUP-PEA-GREEN-CAN-WATER	1 cup	250.0	164.0	8.590	26.50	2.940	0.000	1.410	987.0	190.0	39.00
SOUP-PEA-SPLIT-CAN-WATER	1 cup	253.0	189.0	10.30	28.00	4.400	8.000	1.760	1008	399.0	48.00
SOUP-CREAM/POTATO-CAN-MILK	1 cup	248.0	148.0	5.780	17.20	6.450	22.00	3.760	1060	323.0	17.00
SOUP-TOMATO-CAN-MILK	1 cup	248.0	160.0	6.090	22.30	6.010	17.00	2.910	932.0	450.0	23.00
SOUP-TOMATO-CAN-WATER	1 cup	244.0	86.00	2.060	16.60	1.920	0.000	0.360	872.0	263.0	8.000
SOUP-TOMATO RICE-CAN-WATER	1 cup	247.0	120.0	2.110	21.90	2.720	2.000	0.520	815.0	330.0	5.000
SOUP-TURKEY-CHUNKY-CAN	1 cup	236.0	136.0	10.20	14.10	4.410	9.000	1.220	923.0	361.0	—
SOUP-TURKEY NOODLE-CAN	1 cup	244.0	69.00	3.900	8.630	1.990	5.000	0.560	815.0	75.00	5.000
SOUP-TURKEY VEGETABLE-CAN	1 cup	241.0	74.00	3.090	8.640	3.020	2.000	0.900	905.0	175.0	4.000
SOUP-VEGETARIAN-CAN-WATER	1 cup	241.0	72.00	2.100	12.00	1.930	0.000	0.290	823.0	209.0	7.000

IRON Mg	ZINC Mg	V-A IU	V-ET Mg	V-C Mg	THIA Mg	RIBO Mg	NIAC Mg	V-B6 Mg	FOL Ug	VB12 Ug	CALC Mg	PHOS Mg	SEL Mg	FIBD Gm
0.610	1.370	—	—	—	—	0.704	0.556	—	—	—	546.0	—	—	—
0.490	0.036	0.000	—	0.000	0.009	0.023	0.605	0.031	1.900	0.000	3.000	38.00	—	—
1.620	0.091	—	—	—	—	0.097	—	—	—	0.000	41.00	—	—	—
—	—	—	—	—	0.000	0.010	0.000	—	—	—	—	—	—	—
0.300	—	437.0	—	6.200	0.020	0.010	0.270	—	—	—	5.900	9.800	—	—
0.310	0.018	0.000	—	0.000	0.005	0.013	0.229	0.018	3.600	0.000	4.000	28.00	—	—
—	—	—	—	—	—	—	—	—	—	—	—	—	0.002	—
1.880	0.600	2399	—	32.10	0.162	0.142	2.820	—	—	0.000	34.00	78.00	—	—
8.500	—	2404	—	21.00	0.180	0.152	3.150	—	—	0.000	40.00	—	—	—
0.900	—	51.00	—	27.00	0.000	0.030	0.000	—	—	—	15.00	9.000	—	—
0.100	0.034	210.0	—	2.000	0.010	0.010	0.200	0.016	0.750	0.000	3.000	8.000	0.000	—
0.270	0.972	—	—	2.300	0.148	0.564	0.318	—	—	—	570.0	437.0	—	0.100

IRON Mg	ZINC Mg	V-A IU	V-ET Mg	V-C Mg	THIA Mg	RIBO Mg	NIAC Mg	V-B6 Mg	FOL Ug	VB12 Ug	CALC Mg	PHOS Mg	SEL Mg	FIBD Gm
1.110	1.550	1891	—	2.400	0.037	0.049	1.030	0.076	10.60	0.310	17.00	40.00	0.008	0.980
2.050	1.030	889.0	—	1.600	0.089	0.033	0.567	0.040	31.90	—	81.00	132.0	0.008	3.200
0.410	—	0.000	—	0.000	0.005	0.050	1.870	—	—	—	15.00	31.00	0.008	0.000
2.320	2.640	2611	—	7.000	0.058	0.151	2.710	0.132	13.40	0.610	31.00	120.0	0.008	—
2.160	1.410	506.0	—	0.800	0.077	0.054	0.534	0.094	24.70	0.020	45.00	107.0	0.008	—
0.690	0.196	461.0	—	1.400	0.074	0.248	0.436	0.064	8.500	—	186.0	151.0	0.008	0.770
0.810	0.688	1243	—	1.200	0.063	0.334	0.502	0.078	—	0.440	288.0	250.0	0.008	—
0.510	0.249	0.000	—	0.000	0.010	0.071	3.350	0.024	—	0.240	9.000	73.00	0.008	0.000
1.730	1.000	1299	—	1.300	0.085	0.173	4.420	0.050	4.600	0.250	24.00	113.0	0.008	—
0.670	0.675	715.0	—	1.300	0.074	0.258	0.923	0.067	7.700	—	180.0	152.0	0.008	0.500
0.780	0.395	711.0	—	0.200	0.053	0.060	1.390	0.027	2.200	—	17.00	36.00	0.008	—
1.870	—	5858	—	3.800	0.024	0.098	4.100	—	3.800	—	35.00	—	0.008	—
1.890	0.927	920.0	—	3.200	0.063	0.049	1.340	0.083	9.500	2.190	34.00	57.00	0.008	—
1.480	0.799	164.0	—	3.500	0.067	0.236	1.030	0.126	9.700	10.30	187.0	157.0	0.008	—
0.080	0.008	—	—	—	0.007	0.009	0.119	—	—	—	—	8.000	0.000	—
0.580	0.231	8.000	—	0.900	0.111	0.238	1.990	—	6.300	—	55.00	126.0	0.000	2.200
0.920	0.735	2337	—	1.100	0.053	0.043	0.942	0.099	16.10	0.000	34.00	56.00	0.008	1.900
0.590	0.640	154.0	—	2.300	0.077	0.280	0.913	0.064	—	—	178.0	156.0	0.008	—
0.670	0.612	0.000	—	1.200	0.034	0.024	0.600	0.048	15.20	0.000	26.00	11.00	0.008	—
1.950	1.710	202.0	—	1.700	0.108	0.068	1.240	0.053	1.800	0.000	27.00	124.0	0.008	—
2.280	1.320	444.0	—	1.400	0.147	0.076	1.480	0.068	2.500	0.000	22.00	213.0	0.008	—
0.540	0.675	443.0	—	1.100	0.082	0.236	0.642	0.089	9.200	—	166.0	160.0	0.008	—
1.820	0.290	849.0	—	67.70	0.134	0.248	1.520	0.164	20.90	0.440	159.0	148.0	0.008	0.800
1.760	0.244	688.0	—	66.50	0.088	0.051	1.420	0.112	14.70	0.000	13.00	34.00	0.008	0.900
0.790	0.514	755.0	—	14.80	0.062	0.049	1.060	0.077	—	0.000	23.00	33.00	0.008	1.700
1.910	2.120	7156	—	6.400	0.035	0.106	3.590	0.307	11.10	2.120	50.00	104.0	0.008	2.500
0.940	0.583	292.0	—	0.200	0.073	0.063	1.400	0.037	—	—	12.00	48.00	0.008	0.700
0.760	0.612	2445	—	0.000	0.029	0.039	1.010	0.048	—	0.170	17.00	40.00	0.008	0.964
1.080	0.460	3005	—	1.400	0.053	0.046	0.916	0.055	10.60	0.000	21.00	35.00	0.008	1.210

Nutritive Components for Sugars & Sweets

Food Name	Serving	Gm wt	KCAL Kc	PROT Gm	CARB Gm	FAT Gm	CHOL Mg	SAFA Gm	SOD Mg	POT Mg	MAG Mg
CANDY-ALMOND JOY	1 srvg	28.0	151.0	1.700	18.50	7.800	—	—	—	—	—
CANDY-BIT O HONEY	1 srvg	28.0	121.0	0.900	21.20	3.600	—	—	—	—	—
CANDY-CARAMELS-PLAIN/CHOC	1 srvg	28.0	115.0	1.000	22.00	3.000	0.000	1.600	74.00	54.00	1.000
CANDY-MILK CHOC/ALMONDS	1 srvg	28.0	151.0	2.600	14.50	10.10	—	—	23.00	125.0	—
CANDY-MILK CHOC/PEANUTS	1 srvg	28.0	154.0	4.000	12.60	10.80	—	—	19.00	138.0	—
CANDY-CHOC COATED PEANUTS	1 srvg	28.0	160.0	5.000	11.00	12.00	0.000	4.000	16.00	143.0	—
CANDY-MILK CHOCOLATE-PLAIN	1 srvg	28.0	145.0	2.000	16.00	9.000	0.000	5.500	28.00	109.0	16.00
CANDY-CHOCOLATE-SEMISWEET	1 cup	170.0	860.0	7.000	97.00	61.00	0.000	36.20	3.000	553.0	—
CANDY-FONDANT-UNCOATED	1 srvg	28.0	105.0	0.000	25.00	1.000	0.000	0.100	60.00	1.000	—
CANDY-FUDGE-CHOC-PLAIN	1 srvg	28.0	115.0	1.000	21.00	3.000	0.000	1.300	54.00	42.00	12.60
CANDY-GUM DROPS	1 srvg	28.0	100.0	0.000	25.00	0.000	25.00	0.000	10.00	1.000	—
CANDY-HARD	1 srvg	28.0	110.0	0.000	28.00	0.000	0.000	0.000	9.000	1.000	—
CANDY-JELLY BEANS	1 item	2.8	6.600	0.000	1.670	0.000	—	0.000	0.300	0.000	—
CANDY-KIT KAT BAR	1 item	43.0	210.0	3.000	25.00	11.00	—	—	38.00	129.0	19.00
CANDY-LIFE SAVERS	1 item	2.0	7.800	0.000	1.940	0.020	—	0.000	0.600	0.000	—
CANDY-LOLLIPOP	1 item	28.0	108.0	0.000	28.00	0.000	0.000	0.000	—	—	—
CANDY-M & M'S-PACKAGE	1 item	45.0	220.0	3.000	31.00	10.00	—	—	—	—	—
CANDY-MILKY WAY BAR	1 item	60.0	260.0	3.000	43.00	9.000	—	—	—	—	—
CANDY-PEANUT BRITTLE	1 srvg	28.0	123.0	2.400	20.40	4.400	—	—	9.000	43.00	—
CANDY-PEANUT BUTTER CUP	1 piece	17.0	92.00	2.200	8.700	5.350	2.500	3.000	54.50	68.00	14.50
CANDY-SNICKERS BAR	1 item	57.0	270.0	6.000	33.00	13.00	—	—	—	—	—
HONEY-STRAINED/EXTRACTED	1 tbsp	21.0	65.00	0.000	17.00	0.000	0.000	0.000	1.000	11.00	0.630
ICING-CAKE-WHITE-BOILED	1 cup	94.0	295.0	1.000	75.00	0.000	0.000	0.000	134.0	17.00	—
ICING-CAKE-WHITE/COCO-BOIL	1 cup	166.0	605.0	3.000	124.0	13.00	0.000	11.00	195.0	277.0	—
ICING-CAKE-CHOC-MIX/PREP	1 cup	275.0	1035	9.000	185.0	38.00	0.000	23.40	882.0	536.0	—
ICING-CAKE-FUDGE-MIX/WATER	1 cup	245.0	830.0	7.000	183.0	16.00	0.000	5.100	568.0	238.0	—
ICING-CAKE-WHITE-UNCOOKED	1 cup	319.0	1200	2.000	260.0	21.00	0.000	12.70	156.0	57.00	—
JAMS/PRESERVES-REGULAR	1 tbsp	20.0	55.00	0.000	14.00	0.000	0.000	0.000	2.000	18.00	—
MARSHMALLOWS	1 srvg	28.0	90.00	1.000	23.00	0.000	0.000	0.000	11.00	2.000	—
MOLASSES-CANE-BLACKSTRAP	1 tbsp	20.0	45.00	0.000	11.00	—	0.000	—	18.00	585.0	—
MOLASSES-CANE-LIGHT	1 tbsp	20.0	50.00	0.000	13.00	—	0.000	—	3.000	183.0	—
SYRUP-CHOC FLAVORED-FUDGE	1 fl oz	38.0	125.0	2.000	20.00	5.000	0.000	3.100	26.60	107.0	—
SYRUP-CORN-TABLE-LIGH/DARK	1 tbsp	21.0	60.00	0.000	15.00	0.000	0.000	0.000	14.70	1.000	0.420
SYRUP-PANCAKE-KARO	1 tbsp	20.5	60.00	0.000	14.90	0.000	—	0.000	35.00	1.000	—
SUGAR-EQUAL-PACKET	1 item	1.0	4.000	0.000	1.000	0.000	—	0.000	0.000	0.000	0.000
SUGAR-SWEET & LOW-PACKET	1 item	1.0	4.000	—	0.900	—	—	—	4.000	3.000	—
SUGAR-BROWN-PRESSED DOWN	1 cup	220.0	820.0	0.000	212.0	0.000	0.000	0.000	66.00	757.0	—
SUGAR-WHITE-GRANULATED	1 tbsp	12.0	45.00	0.000	12.00	0.000	0.000	0.000	0.120	0.000	—
SUGAR-WHITE-POWDER-SIFTED	1 cup	100.0	385.0	0.000	100.0	0.000	0.000	0.000	0.830	3.000	—

Nutritive Components for Vegetables

Food Name	Serving	Gm wt	KCAL Kc	PROT Gm	CARB Gm	FAT Gm	CHOL Mg	SAFA Gm	SOD Mg	POT Mg	MAG Mg
NUTS-CHESTNUTS-ROASTED	1 srvg	28.4	68.00	1.270	14.90	0.340	0.000	0.050	1.000	135.0	26.00
ALFALFA SEEDS-SPROUTED-RAW	1 cup	33.0	10.00	1.320	1.250	0.230	0.000	0.023	2.000	26.00	9.000
ARTICHOKES-BOIL-DRAIN	1 item	120.0	53.00	2.760	12.40	0.200	0.000	0.048	79.00	316.0	47.00
ASPARAGUS-FROZ-BOIL-SPEARS	1 cup	180.0	50.40	5.310	8.770	0.756	0.000	0.171	7.200	392.0	23.40
BEANS-BAKED BEANS-CANNED	1 cup	254.0	235.0	12.20	52.10	1.140	0.000	0.295	1008	752.0	82.00
BEANS-GARBANZO-CAN	1 srvg	28.4	27.80	1.310	4.660	0.511	0.000	—	113.0	54.80	9.370
BEANS-LIMA-CAN	1 cup	248.0	186.0	11.30	34.40	0.740	0.000	0.168	618.0	668.0	84.00
BEANS-LIMA-FROZ-BOIL-DRAIN	1 cup	170.0	170.0	10.30	32.00	0.580	0.000	0.130	90.00	694.0	58.00
BEANS-MUNG-SPROUTED-BOIL	1 cup	125.0	26.00	2.520	5.200	0.110	0.000	0.031	12.00	125.0	18.00
BEANS-NAVY PEA-DRY-COOKED	1 cup	190.0	225.0	15.00	40.00	1.000	0.000	—	13.00	790.0	—
BEANS-PINTO-FROZ-BOIL	1 srvg	28.4	46.00	2.640	8.770	0.135	0.000	0.017	—	—	—

Continued.

IRON Mg	ZINC Mg	V-A IU	V-ET Mg	V-C Mg	THIA Mg	RIBO Mg	NIAC Mg	V-B6 Mg	FOL Ug	VB12 Ug	CALC Mg	PHOS Mg	SEL Mg	FIBD Gm
—	—	—	1.180	—	—	—	—	—	—	—	—	—	0.001	—
0.250	—	—	—	—	0.000	0.130	1.400	—	—	—	13.00	—	0.001	—
0.400	—	0.000	—	0.000	0.010	0.050	0.100	—	—	—	42.00	35.00	0.001	—
0.500	—	70.00	1.180	0.000	0.020	0.120	0.200	—	—	—	65.00	77.00	0.001	—
0.400	—	50.00	1.180	0.000	0.070	0.070	1.400	—	—	—	49.00	83.00	0.001	—
0.400	—	0.000	—	0.000	0.100	0.050	2.100	—	—	—	33.00	84.00	0.001	—
0.300	—	80.00	1.570	0.000	0.020	0.100	0.100	—	1.960	—	65.00	65.00	0.001	—
4.400	—	30.00	—	0.000	0.020	0.140	0.900	—	—	—	51.00	255.0	0.006	—
0.300	—	0.000	—	0.000	0.000	0.000	0.000	—	—	—	4.000	2.000	0.001	0.000
0.300	—	0.000	—	0.000	0.010	0.030	0.100	—	—	—	22.00	24.00	0.001	—
0.100	—	0.000	—	0.000	0.000	0.000	0.000	—	—	—	2.000	0.000	0.001	0.000
0.500	—	0.000	—	0.000	0.000	0.000	0.000	—	—	—	6.000	2.000	0.001	0.000
0.030	—	0.000	—	0.000	0.000	—	—	—	—	—	0.300	0.100	0.000	0.000
0.560	0.430	30.00	—	—	0.030	0.110	0.100	—	—	—	65.00	78.00	0.002	—
0.040	—	0.000	—	0.000	0.000	0.000	0.000	—	—	—	0.400	0.200	0.000	0.000
0.000	—	0.000	—	0.000	0.000	0.000	0.000	—	—	—	0.000	0.000	0.001	0.000
—	—	—	1.890	—	—	—	—	—	—	—	—	—	0.002	—
—	—	—	2.520	—	—	—	—	—	—	—	—	—	0.002	—
0.560	—	8.000	—	0.000	0.020	0.010	1.300	—	—	—	11.00	35.00	0.001	—
0.240	0.240	3.500	0.714	—	0.050	0.030	0.800	—	—	—	14.50	41.00	0.001	—
—	—	—	2.390	—	—	—	—	—	—	—	—	—	0.002	—
0.100	0.020	0.000	—	0.000	0.000	0.010	0.100	0.004	—	0.000	1.000	1.000	0.001	0.060
0.000	—	0.000	—	0.000	0.000	0.030	0.000	—	—	—	2.000	2.000	0.001	0.000
0.800	—	0.000	—	0.000	0.020	0.070	0.300	—	—	—	10.00	50.00	0.002	—
3.300	—	580.0	—	1.000	0.060	0.280	0.600	—	—	—	165.0	305.0	0.003	—
2.700	—	0.000	—	0.000	0.050	0.200	0.700	—	—	—	96.00	218.0	0.003	—
0.000	—	860.0	—	0.000	0.000	0.060	0.000	—	—	—	48.00	38.00	0.003	0.000
0.200	—	0.000	—	0.000	0.000	0.010	0.000	0.004	1.600	0.000	4.000	2.000	0.000	—
0.500	0.010	0.000	—	0.000	0.000	0.000	0.000	—	—	—	5.000	2.000	0.000	0.000
3.200	—	—	—	—	0.020	0.040	0.400	0.040	—	0.000	137.0	17.00	0.026	0.000
0.900	—	—	—	—	0.010	0.010	0.000	0.040	—	0.000	33.00	9.000	0.026	0.000
0.500	0.300	60.00	—	0.000	0.020	0.080	0.200	—	—	—	48.00	60.00	—	—
0.800	0.010	0.000	—	0.000	0.000	0.000	0.000	—	—	—	9.000	3.000	0.003	0.000
0.800	—	0.000	—	0.000	0.000	0.000	0.000	—	—	—	9.000	3.000	0.000	0.000
0.000	0.000	0.000	—	0.000	0.000	0.000	0.000	0.000	0.000	0.000	0.000	0.000	0.000	—
—	—	—	—	—	—	—	—	—	—	—	—	—	0.000	—
7.500	—	0.000	—	0.000	0.020	0.070	0.400	—	—	—	187.0	42.00	0.003	0.000
0.000	0.006	0.000	—	0.000	0.000	0.000	0.000	—	—	—	0.000	0.000	0.000	0.000
0.100	—	0.000	—	0.000	0.000	0.000	0.000	—	—	—	0.000	0.000	0.001	0.000

IRON Mg	ZINC Mg	V-A IU	V-ET Mg	V-C Mg	THIA Mg	RIBO Mg	NIAC Mg	V-B6 Mg	FOL Ug	VB12 Ug	CALC Mg	PHOS Mg	SEL Mg	FIBD Gm
0.430	0.260	1.000	—	—	0.043	0.026	0.426	—	—	0.000	5.000	29.00	0.002	2.190
0.320	0.300	51.00	—	2.700	0.025	0.042	0.159	0.011	12.20	0.000	10.00	23.00	—	0.726
1.620	0.430	172.0	—	8.900	0.068	0.059	0.709	0.104	53.40	0.000	47.00	72.00	—	4.000
1.150	1.000	1472	2.860	43.90	0.117	0.185	1.870	0.036	242.0	0.000	41.40	99.00	0.007	2.160
0.740	3.550	434.0	—	—	0.389	0.152	1.090	0.340	60.70	0.000	128.0	264.0	—	6.600
0.710	0.264	5.680	0.871	1.420	0.003	0.011	0.085	—	—	—	11.10	30.10	—	1.400
3.940	1.580	428.0	—	21.60	0.072	0.106	1.320	0.154	—	0.000	70.00	176.0	—	10.40
2.320	0.740	324.0	13.00	21.80	0.120	0.104	1.800	0.208	111.0	0.000	38.00	153.0	0.001	8.330
0.810	0.580	17.00	2.460	14.10	0.062	0.126	1.010	—	166.0	0.000	15.00	34.00	—	2.700
5.100	1.800	0.000	4.290	0.000	0.270	0.130	1.300	1.060	66.50	0.000	95.00	281.0	—	9.310
0.770	—	0.000	—	0.190	0.078	0.031	0.180	—	—	0.000	14.90	—	—	1.390

Continued.

Nutritive Components for Vegetables—cont'd

Food Name	Serving	Gm wt	KCAL Kc	PROT Gm	CARB Gm	FAT Gm	CHOL Mg	SAFA Gm	SOD Mg	POT Mg	MAG Mg
BEANS-RED KIDNEY-CAN	1 cup	255.0	230.0	15.00	42.00	1.000	0.000	—	833.0	673.0	9.940
BEANS-REFRIED BEANS	1 cup	253.0	270.0	15.80	46.80	2.700	—	1.040	1071	994.0	99.00
BEANS-SHELLIE-CAN	1 cup	245.0	75.00	4.300	15.20	0.470	0.000	0.056	819.0	268.0	—
BEANS-SNAP-GREEN-RAW-BOIL	1 cup	125.0	44.00	2.360	9.860	0.360	0.000	0.080	4.000	373.0	32.00
BEANS-SNAP-GREEN-CAN-CUTS	1 cup	135.0	27.00	1.550	6.000	0.135	0.000	0.030	339.0	147.0	17.50
BEANS-GREEN-FROZ-FRENCH	1 cup	135.0	36.00	1.840	8.260	0.180	0.000	0.041	17.00	151.0	29.00
BEANS-SNAP-YELLOW/WAX-CAN	1 cup	136.0	26.00	1.560	6.120	0.140	0.000	0.030	340.0	148.0	18.00
BEANS-SNAP-WAX-RAW-BOIL	1 cup	125.0	44.00	2.360	9.860	0.360	0.000	0.080	4.000	373.0	32.00
BEETS-CAN-SLICED-DRAIN	1 cup	170.0	54.00	1.560	12.20	0.240	0.000	0.040	479.0	284.0	22.10
BROCCOLI-FROZ-BOIL-DRAIN	1 cup	185.0	51.00	5.710	9.850	0.210	0.000	0.030	44.00	332.0	37.00
BROCCOLI-RAW	1 cup	88.0	24.00	2.620	4.620	0.300	0.000	0.048	24.00	286.0	22.00
BROCCOLI-RAW-BOIL-DRAIN	1 cup	155.0	46.00	4.640	8.680	0.440	0.000	0.068	16.00	254.0	94.00
BRUSSEL SPROUTS-FROZ-BOIL	1 cup	155.0	65.00	5.640	12.90	0.610	0.000	0.126	36.00	504.0	37.00
BRUSSEL SPROUTS-RAW-BOIL	1 cup	156.0	60.00	3.980	13.50	0.800	0.000	0.164	34.00	494.0	32.00
CABBAGE-CELERY-RAW	1 cup	76.0	12.00	0.910	2.460	0.150	0.000	0.033	7.000	181.0	10.00
CABBAGE-WHITE MUSTARD-BOIL	1 cup	170.0	20.00	2.650	3.030	0.270	0.000	0.036	57.00	630.0	18.00
CABBAGE-WHITE MUSTARD-RAW	1 cup	70.0	9.000	1.050	1.530	0.140	0.000	0.018	45.00	176.0	13.00
CABBAGE-COMMON-BOIL-DRAIN	1 cup	145.0	30.50	1.390	6.920	0.363	0.000	0.046	27.60	297.0	21.80
CABBAGE-COMMON-RAW-SHRED	1 cup	90.0	21.60	1.090	4.830	0.162	0.000	0.021	16.20	221.0	13.50
CABBAGE-RED-RAW-SHREDDED	1 cup	70.0	19.00	0.970	4.290	0.180	0.000	0.024	7.000	144.0	11.00
CARROT-RAW-SHRED-SCRAPED	1 cup	110.0	48.00	1.120	11.20	0.200	0.000	0.034	38.00	356.0	16.00
CARROTS-BOIL-DRAIN-SLICED	1 cup	156.0	70.00	1.700	16.30	0.280	0.000	0.054	104.0	354.0	20.00
CARROTS-CAN-SLICED-DRAIN	1 cup	146.0	34.00	0.940	8.080	0.280	0.000	0.052	352.0	262.0	12.00
CARROTS-FROZEN-BOIL-DRAIN	1 cup	146.0	52.00	1.730	12.00	0.160	0.000	0.031	86.00	230.0	14.00
CARROT-RAW-WHOLE-SCRAPED	1 item	72.0	31.00	0.740	7.300	0.140	0.000	0.022	25.00	233.0	11.00
CAULIFLOWER-FROZ-BOIL	1 cup	180.0	34.00	2.900	6.760	0.390	0.000	0.060	32.00	250.0	16.00
CAULIFLOWER-RAW-CHOPPED	1 cup	100.0	24.00	1.990	4.920	0.180	0.000	0.000	15.00	355.0	14.00
CAULIFLOWER-RAW-BOIL-DRAIN	1 cup	124.0	30.00	2.320	5.740	0.220	0.000	0.046	8.000	400.0	14.00
CELERY-PASCAL-RAW-DICED	1 cup	120.0	18.00	0.800	4.360	0.140	0.000	0.038	106.0	340.0	14.00
CELERY-PASCAL-RAW-STALK	1 item	40.0	6.000	0.260	1.450	0.050	0.000	0.013	35.00	114.0	5.000
CHIVES-RAW-CHOPPED	1 tbsp	3.0	1.000	0.080	0.110	0.020	0.000	0.003	0.000	8.000	2.000
COLLARDS-FROZEN-BOIL-DRAIN	1 cup	170.0	61.00	5.040	12.10	0.690	0.000	—	85.00	427.0	52.00
COLLARDS-RAW-BOIL-DRAIN	1 cup	190.0	27.00	2.100	5.020	0.290	0.000	—	36.00	177.0	21.00
CORN-KERNELS FROM 1 EAR	1 item	77.0	83.00	2.560	19.30	0.980	0.000	0.152	13.00	192.0	24.00
CORN-SWEET-CREAM STYLE-CAN	1 cup	256.0	186.0	4.460	46.40	1.080	0.000	0.166	730.0	344.0	44.00
CORN-SWEET-CAN-DRAINED	1 cup	165.0	132.0	4.300	30.50	1.640	0.000	0.254	470.0	160.0	28.00
CORN-KERNELS&COB-FROZ-BOIL	1 item	228.0	118.0	3.920	28.10	0.920	0.000	0.144	6.000	316.0	36.00
CORN-FROZ-BOIL-KERNELS	1 cup	165.0	134.0	4.940	33.70	0.120	0.000	0.018	8.000	228.0	30.00
COWPEAS-BLACKEYE-FROZ-BOIL	1 cup	170.0	224.0	14.40	40.40	1.130	0.000	0.298	9.000	638.0	85.00
COWPEAS-BLACKEYE-RAW-BOIL	1 cup	165.0	179.0	13.40	29.90	1.320	0.000	0.345	7.000	693.0	83.00
CUCUMBER-RAW-SLICED	1 cup	104.0	14.00	0.560	3.020	0.140	0.000	0.034	2.000	156.0	12.00
EGGPLANT-BOILED-DRAINED	1 cup	96.0	27.00	0.800	6.370	0.220	0.000	0.042	3.000	238.0	13.00
ENDIVE-RAW-CHOPPED	1 cup	50.0	8.000	0.620	1.680	0.100	0.000	0.024	12.00	158.0	8.000
GARLIC-RAW-CLOVE	1 item	3.0	4.000	0.190	0.990	0.020	0.000	0.003	1.000	12.00	1.000
LEEKS-BOIL-DRAIN	1 item	124.0	38.00	1.010	9.450	0.250	0.000	0.033	13.00	108.0	18.00
LETTUCE-BUTTERHEAD-LEAVES	1 slice	15.0	2.000	0.190	0.350	0.030	0.000	0.004	1.000	39.00	1.650
LETTUCE-ICEBERG-RAW-CHOP	1 cup	55.0	7.150	0.556	1.150	0.105	0.000	0.014	4.950	86.90	4.950
LETTUCE-ICEBERG-RAW-LEAVES	1 srvg	135.0	17.60	1.360	2.820	0.257	0.000	0.034	12.20	213.0	12.20
LETTUCE-LOOSELEAF-RAW	1 cup	55.0	10.00	0.720	1.960	0.160	0.000	0.022	6.000	148.0	6.000
LETTUCE-ROMAINE-RAW-SHRED	1 cup	56.0	8.000	0.900	1.320	0.120	0.000	0.014	4.000	162.0	4.000
MISO-FERMENTED SOYBEANS	1 cup	275.0	565.0	32.50	76.90	16.70	0.000	2.420	10030	451.0	116.0
MUSHROOMS-BOIL-DRAIN	1 item	12.0	3.000	0.260	0.620	0.060	0.000	0.007	0.000	43.00	1.000
MUSHROOMS-CAN-DRAIN	1 item	12.0	3.000	0.220	0.600	0.040	0.000	0.005	—	—	—
MUSHROOMS-RAW-CHOPPED	1 cup	70.0	18.00	1.460	3.260	0.300	0.000	0.040	2.000	260.0	8.000
ONIONS-MATURE-BOIL-DRAIN	1 cup	210.0	58.00	1.900	13.20	0.340	0.000	0.056	16.00	318.0	22.00
ONIONS-MATURE-RAW-CHOPPED	1 cup	160.0	54.00	1.880	11.70	0.420	0.000	0.070	4.000	248.0	16.00
ONIONS-YOUNG GREEN	1 item	5.0	1.250	0.087	0.278	0.007	0.000	0.001	0.200	12.80	1.000
ONION RINGS-FROZ-PREP-HEAT	1 item	10.0	40.70	0.534	3.820	2.670	0.000	0.858	37.50	12.90	1.900
PARSLEY-RAW-CHOPPED	1 tbsp	4.0	1.200	0.088	0.276	0.012	0.000	0.000	1.600	21.60	1.600

Continued.

IRON Mg	ZINC Mg	V-A IU	V-ET Mg	V-C Mg	THIA Mg	RIBO Mg	NIAC Mg	V-B6 Mg	FOL Ug	VB12 Ug	CALC Mg	PHOS Mg	SEL Mg	FIBD Gm
4.600	1.910	10.00	0.128	7.650	0.130	0.100	1.500	1.120	35.70	0.000	74.00	278.0	—	12.50
4.470	3.450	—	—	15.20	0.124	0.139	1.230	—	—	—	118.0	214.0	—	—
2.430	—	559.0	—	7.500	0.078	0.132	0.502	—	—	0.000	72.00	—	—	12.00
1.600	0.450	833.0	0.138	12.10	0.093	0.121	0.768	0.070	41.60	0.000	58.00	46.00	0.001	2.250
1.200	0.390	471.0	0.068	6.500	0.020	0.075	0.270	0.054	43.00	0.000	35.00	34.00	0.001	1.760
1.110	0.840	713.0	0.325	11.10	0.065	0.100	0.563	0.076	44.20	0.000	61.00	33.00	0.001	2.160
1.220	0.400	474.0	—	6.400	0.020	0.076	0.274	0.057	43.00	0.000	36.00	26.00	0.001	1.770
1.600	0.450	833.0	—	12.10	0.093	0.121	0.768	0.070	41.60	0.000	58.00	48.00	0.001	2.250
3.100	0.360	30.00	—	5.000	0.020	0.050	0.200	0.085	40.80	0.000	32.00	31.00	0.001	3.200
1.130	0.560	3482	1.180	73.70	0.101	0.150	0.843	0.239	104.0	0.000	94.00	101.0	—	7.300
0.780	0.360	1356	0.563	82.00	0.058	0.104	0.562	0.140	62.40	0.000	42.00	58.00	—	3.170
1.780	0.240	2198	0.992	98.00	0.128	0.322	1.180	0.308	107.0	0.000	178.0	74.00	—	6.400
1.150	0.550	912.0	1.320	70.80	0.160	0.175	0.832	0.448	157.0	0.000	38.00	84.00	0.001	4.500
1.880	0.500	1122	1.320	96.80	0.166	0.124	0.946	0.278	93.60	0.000	56.00	88.00	0.001	4.520
0.230	0.170	912.0	0.098	20.50	0.030	0.038	0.304	0.176	59.80	0.000	58.00	22.00	0.002	1.630
1.770	—	4365	1.190	44.20	0.054	0.107	0.728	—	—	0.000	158.0	49.00	0.004	2.100
0.560	—	2100	0.091	31.50	0.028	0.049	0.350	—	—	0.000	74.00	26.00	0.002	1.300
0.566	0.232	125.0	2.420	35.20	0.083	0.080	0.330	0.093	29.40	0.000	47.90	36.30	0.003	4.000
0.504	0.162	113.0	1.500	42.60	0.045	0.027	0.270	0.086	51.00	0.000	42.30	20.70	0.002	1.800
0.350	0.150	28.00	0.140	39.90	0.035	0.021	0.210	0.147	14.50	0.000	36.00	29.00	0.002	1.700
0.540	0.220	30940	0.561	10.20	0.106	0.064	1.020	0.162	15.40	0.000	30.00	48.00	0.002	3.100
0.960	0.460	38300	0.713	3.600	0.054	0.088	0.790	0.384	21.60	0.000	48.00	48.00	0.002	5.770
0.940	0.380	20110	0.672	4.000	0.026	0.044	0.806	0.164	13.40	0.000	38.00	34.00	0.002	2.480
0.690	0.350	25850	0.672	4.100	0.039	0.054	0.639	0.188	15.80	0.000	41.00	39.00	0.003	5.400
0.360	0.140	20250	0.367	6.700	0.070	0.042	0.668	0.106	10.10	0.000	19.00	32.00	0.002	2.030
0.740	0.240	40.00	0.162	56.40	0.066	0.096	0.558	0.158	73.80	0.000	30.00	44.00	0.001	3.240
0.580	0.180	16.00	0.090	71.50	0.076	0.057	0.633	0.231	66.10	0.000	29.00	46.00	0.001	2.670
0.520	0.300	18.00	0.113	68.60	0.078	0.064	0.684	0.250	63.40	0.000	34.00	44.00	0.001	2.230
0.580	0.200	152.0	0.876	7.600	0.036	0.036	0.360	0.036	10.60	0.000	44.00	32.00	0.000	1.200
0.190	0.070	51.00	0.292	2.500	0.012	0.012	0.120	0.012	3.600	0.000	14.00	10.00	0.000	0.400
0.050	—	192.0	—	2.400	0.003	0.005	0.021	0.005	—	0.000	2.000	2.000	—	—
1.900	0.460	10170	—	44.90	0.080	0.196	1.080	0.194	129.0	0.000	357.0	46.00	0.001	5.200
0.780	1.220	4218	—	18.60	0.032	0.082	0.448	0.080	12.40	0.000	148.0	19.00	0.001	2.100
0.470	0.370	167.0	0.868	4.800	0.166	0.055	1.240	0.046	35.70	0.000	2.000	79.00	0.001	6.600
0.980	1.360	248.0	1.590	11.80	0.064	0.136	2.460	0.162	115.0	0.000	8.000	130.0	0.001	—
1.400	0.640	256.0	1.020	7.000	0.050	0.080	1.500	0.330	59.40	0.000	8.000	81.00	0.001	2.150
0.780	0.800	266.0	1.470	6.000	0.220	0.086	1.910	0.282	38.40	0.000	4.000	94.00	0.001	2.650
0.500	0.560	408.0	1.060	4.200	0.114	0.120	2.100	0.164	33.40	0.000	4.000	78.00	0.001	3.470
3.600	2.420	128.0	1.110	4.500	0.442	0.109	1.240	0.162	240.0	0.000	40.00	208.0	—	9.800
2.360	1.300	1051	4.470	2.600	0.112	0.177	1.770	0.083	173.0	0.000	46.00	197.0	—	11.00
0.280	0.240	46.00	0.322	4.800	0.032	0.020	0.312	0.054	14.40	0.000	14.00	18.00	0.001	1.460
0.340	0.140	61.00	—	1.300	0.073	0.019	0.576	0.083	13.80	0.000	5.000	22.00	—	2.690
0.420	0.400	1026	—	3.200	0.040	0.038	0.200	0.010	71.00	0.000	26.00	14.00	—	—
0.050	—	0.000	—	0.900	0.006	0.003	0.021	—	0.100	0.000	5.000	5.000	0.000	—
1.360	—	57.00	—	5.200	0.032	0.025	0.248	—	30.10	0.000	37.00	21.00	—	3.970
0.040	0.030	146.0	0.113	1.200	0.010	0.010	0.045	0.008	11.00	0.000	5.000	4.000	0.000	0.207
0.275	0.121	182.0	0.413	2.150	0.025	0.017	0.103	0.022	30.80	0.000	10.50	11.00	0.000	0.600
0.675	0.297	446.0	1.010	5.270	0.062	0.041	0.252	0.054	75.60	0.000	25.70	27.00	0.001	1.600
0.780	0.121	1064	0.413	10.00	0.028	0.044	0.224	0.030	76.00	0.000	38.00	14.00	0.000	0.760
0.620	—	1456	0.420	13.40	0.056	0.056	0.280	—	76.00	0.000	20.00	26.00	0.000	0.773
7.520	9.130	240.0	—	0.000	0.267	0.688	2.370	0.591	90.80	0.570	183.0	420.0	—	9.900
0.210	0.100	0.000	0.035	0.500	0.009	0.036	0.535	0.011	2.200	0.000	1.000	10.00	0.001	0.216
0.100	0.090	0.000	0.035	—	—	—	—	—	1.500	0.000	—	—	0.005	0.216
0.860	0.344	0.000	0.203	2.400	0.072	0.314	2.880	0.068	14.80	0.000	4.000	72.00	0.009	1.260
0.420	0.380	0.000	0.651	12.00	0.088	0.016	0.168	0.378	26.60	0.000	58.00	48.00	0.007	1.680
0.580	0.280	0.000	0.496	13.40	0.096	0.016	0.160	0.252	31.80	0.000	40.00	46.00	0.003	2.640
0.095	0.022	250.0	0.016	2.250	0.004	0.007	0.001	—	0.685	0.000	3.000	1.650	0.000	0.083
0.169	0.042	22.50	—	0.140	0.028	0.014	0.361	0.008	1.300	0.000	3.100	8.100	—	—
0.248	0.028	208.0	0.101	3.600	0.003	0.004	0.028	0.006	7.320	0.000	5.200	1.600	0.000	0.152

Continued.

Nutritive Components for Vegetables—cont'd

Food Name	Serving	Gm wt	KCAL Kc	PROT Gm	CARB Gm	FAT Gm	CHOL Mg	SAFA Gm	SOD Mg	POT Mg	MAG Mg
PEAS-GREEN-CAN-DRAINED	1 cup	170.0	118.0	7.520	21.40	0.580	0.000	0.106	372.0	294.0	30.00
PEAS-GREEN-FROZ-BOIL-DRAIN	1 cup	160.0	126.0	8.240	22.80	0.440	0.000	0.078	140.0	268.0	46.00
PEAS-SPLIT-DRY-COOKED	1 cup	200.0	230.0	16.00	42.00	1.000	0.000	—	8.000	592.0	—
PEPPERS-HOT-RED-DRIED	1 tsp	2.0	5.000	0.000	1.000	0.000	0.000	0.000	20.00	20.00	3.400
PEPPERS-JALAPENO-CAN-CHOP	1 cup	136.0	33.00	1.090	6.660	0.820	0.000	0.084	1990	185.0	16.00
POTATO-AU GRATIN-HOME REC	1 cup	245.0	322.0	12.40	27.60	18.60	58.00	11.60	1060	970.0	48.00
POTATO-BAKE-PEEL AFTER	1 item	156.0	145.0	3.060	33.60	0.160	0.000	0.041	8.000	610.0	39.00
POTATO-FLESH & SKIN-BAKE	1 item	202.0	220.0	4.650	51.00	0.200	0.000	0.052	16.00	844.0	55.00
POTATO-FRENCH FRIED-FROZ	1 item	5.0	11.10	0.173	1.700	0.438	0.000	0.208	1.500	22.90	1.100
POTATO-FRENCH FRIED-RAW	1 item	5.0	13.50	0.200	1.800	0.700	0.000	0.170	11.10	42.70	—
POTATO-HASHED BROWN-FROZ	1 cup	156.0	340.0	4.920	43.80	17.90	—	7.010	54.00	680.0	26.00
POTATO-HASH BROWN-PREP-RAW	1 cup	156.0	326.0	3.770	33.30	21.70	—	8.480	38.00	501.0	32.00
POTATO-MASHED-DEHY-PREP	1 cup	210.0	166.0	4.200	27.50	4.620	4.000	1.430	491.0	704.0	—
POTATO-MASHED-MILK/BUTTER	1 cup	210.0	222.0	3.950	35.10	8.870	4.000	2.170	619.0	607.0	37.00
POTATO PANCAKES-HOME REC	1 item	76.0	495.0	4.630	26.40	12.60	93.00	3.420	388.0	538.0	24.00
POTATO-SCALLOP-MIX-PREP	1 srvg	28.4	26.40	0.602	3.630	1.220	—	0.748	96.80	57.70	3.980
POTATO-SCALLOP-HOME REC	1 cup	245.0	210.0	7.030	26.40	9.020	29.00	5.530	821.0	925.0	46.00
POTATO CHIPS-SALT ADDED	1 item	2.0	10.50	0.128	1.040	0.708	0.000	0.181	9.400	26.00	1.200
POTATO SKIN-BAKED	1 item	58.0	115.0	2.490	26.70	0.060	0.000	0.015	12.00	332.0	25.00
PUMPKIN-CAN	1 cup	245.0	83.00	2.700	19.80	0.690	0.000	0.358	12.00	504.0	56.00
PUMPKIN PIE MIX-CAN	1 cup	270.0	282.0	2.930	71.30	0.340	0.000	0.176	561.0	372.0	43.00
RADISHES-RAW	1 item	4.5	0.700	0.027	0.161	0.024	0.000	0.001	1.100	10.40	0.400
RUTABAGAS-BOIL-DRAIN	1 cup	170.0	58.00	1.880	13.20	0.320	0.000	0.042	30.00	488.0	36.00
SAUERKRAUT-CANNED	1 cup	236.0	44.00	2.150	10.10	0.330	0.000	0.083	1561	401.0	31.00
SEAWEED-WAKAME-RAW	1 srvg	28.4	12.80	0.860	2.600	0.182	0.000	0.037	248.0	14.20	30.40
SPINACH-RAW-BOIL-DRAIN	1 cup	180.0	41.00	5.350	6.750	0.470	0.000	0.076	126.0	838.0	157.0
SPINACH-CAN-SOLIDS/LIQUIDS	1 cup	234.0	44.00	4.930	6.840	0.870	0.000	0.140	747.0	539.0	132.0
SPINACH-FROZ-BOIL-CHOPPED	1 cup	205.0	57.40	6.440	10.90	0.431	0.000	0.068	176.0	611.0	141.0
SPINACH-RAW-CHOPPED	1 cup	56.0	12.00	1.600	1.960	0.200	0.000	0.032	44.00	312.0	44.00
SQUASH-ACORN-BAKED	1 cup	205.0	115.0	2.290	29.90	0.290	0.000	0.059	9.000	896.0	87.00
SQUASH-BUTTERNUT-BAKED	1 cup	205.0	83.00	1.840	21.50	0.180	0.000	0.039	7.000	583.0	59.00
SQUASH-HUBBARD-BOIL-MASH	1 cup	236.0	70.00	3.500	15.20	0.880	0.000	0.179	12.00	504.0	32.00
SQUASH-SUMMER-BOIL-SLICED	1 cup	180.0	36.00	1.630	7.760	0.560	0.000	0.115	2.000	346.0	44.00
SQUASH-WINTER-BAKE-MASH	1 cup	205.0	79.00	1.810	17.90	1.290	0.000	0.267	3.000	895.0	16.00
SQUASH-ZUCCHINI-FROZ-BOIL	1 cup	223.0	37.00	2.560	7.940	0.290	0.000	0.060	5.000	434.0	28.00
SQUASH-ZUCCHINI-ITALIA-CAN	1 cup	227.0	65.00	2.330	15.60	0.250	0.000	0.052	850.0	622.0	31.00
SQUASH-ZUCCHINI-RAW-BOIL	1 cup	180.0	28.00	1.140	7.080	0.100	0.000	0.018	4.000	456.0	38.00
SQUASH-ZUCCHINI-RAW-SLICED	1 cup	130.0	19.00	1.500	3.780	0.180	0.000	0.038	3.000	322.0	28.00
SUCCOTASH-BOIL-DRAIN	1 cup	192.0	222.0	9.730	46.80	1.530	0.000	0.284	32.00	787.0	102.0
SWEET POTATO-BAKE-PEEL	1 item	114.0	118.0	1.960	27.70	0.130	0.000	0.027	12.00	397.0	23.00
SWEET POTATO-BOIL-MASHED	1 cup	328.0	344.0	5.400	79.60	0.970	0.000	0.210	42.00	602.0	32.00
SWEET POTATO-CAN-MASHED	1 cup	255.0	258.0	5.050	59.20	0.510	0.000	0.110	191.0	536.0	61.00
SWEET POTATO-CANDIED	1 piece	105.0	144.0	0.910	29.30	3.410	0.000	1.420	73.00	198.0	12.00
TOFU-SOYBEAN CURD	1 piece	120.0	86.00	9.400	2.900	5.000	0.000	—	8.000	50.00	—
TOMATO-RED-RAW-BOIL	1 cup	240.0	60.00	2.680	13.50	0.650	0.000	0.091	25.00	624.0	33.00
TOMATO-CAN-LOW SODIUM-DIET	1 cup	240.0	47.00	2.240	10.30	0.590	0.000	0.084	31.20	529.0	29.00
TOMATO-RED-CAN-STEWED	1 cup	255.0	68.00	2.370	16.50	0.360	0.000	0.051	647.0	611.0	29.00
TOMATO-RED-CAN-WHOLE	1 cup	240.0	47.00	2.240	10.30	0.590	0.000	0.084	390.0	529.0	29.00
TOMATO-RAW-RED-RIPE	1 item	135.0	24.00	1.090	5.340	0.260	0.000	0.037	10.00	254.0	14.00
TOMATO-STEW-COOK-HOME REC	1 cup	101.0	59.00	1.770	10.40	2.210	0.000	0.400	374.0	170.0	13.00
TOMATO JUICE-CAN	1 cup	244.0	42.00	1.860	10.30	0.140	0.000	0.020	882.0	536.0	28.00
TOMATO JUICE-LOW SODIUM	1 cup	244.0	42.00	1.860	10.30	0.140	0.000	0.010	24.40	536.0	28.00
TOMATO PASTE-CAN-SALT ADD	1 cup	262.0	220.0	9.900	49.30	2.330	0.000	0.332	2070	2442	134.0
TOMATO PASTE-CAN-LOW SOD	1 cup	262.0	220.0	9.900	49.30	2.330	0.000	0.332	172.0	2442	134.0
TOMATO POWDER	1 srvg	28.4	85.80	3.670	21.20	0.125	0.000	0.018	38.10	547.0	50.60
TOMATO PUREE-CAN-SALT ADD	1 cup	250.0	102.0	4.180	25.10	0.290	0.000	0.040	998.0	1051	60.00
TOMATO PUREE-CAN-LOW SOD	1 cup	250.0	102.0	4.180	25.10	0.290	0.000	0.040	49.00	1051	60.00
V-8 VEG JUICE-LOW SODIUM	1 cup	243.0	51.00	0.000	9.720	0.000	0.000	0.000	58.30	571.0	—
VEGETABLE JUICE-CAN	1 cup	242.0	44.00	1.520	11.00	0.220	0.000	0.032	884.0	468.0	26.00
YAMS-BOIL OR BAKE-DRAIN	1 cup	136.0	158.0	2.020	37.50	0.180	0.000	0.039	11.00	911.0	25.00
SOYBEAN-DRY-COOKED	1 cup	180.0	234.0	19.80	19.40	10.30	—	—	4.000	972.0	—

IRON Mg	ZINC Mg	V-A IU	V-ET Mg	V-C Mg	THIA Mg	RIBO Mg	NIAC Mg	V-B6 Mg	FOL Ug	VB12 Ug	CALC Mg	PHOS Mg	SEL Mg	FIBD Gm
1.620	1.200	1306	4.470	16.20	0.206	0.132	1.240	0.108	75.40	0.000	34.00	114.0	0.001	6.970
2.520	1.500	1068	1.040	15.80	0.452	0.160	2.370	0.180	93.80	0.000	38.00	144.0	0.001	6.080
3.400	2.100	80.00	4.540	—	0.300	0.180	1.800	—	—	—	22.00	178.0	0.003	—
0.300	0.054	1300	—	0.000	0.000	0.020	0.200	—	—	0.000	5.000	4.000	0.000	—
3.810	0.260	2312	—	17.70	0.041	0.068	0.680	—	—	0.000	35.00	23.00	—	—
1.560	1.690	646.0	—	24.30	0.157	0.284	2.430	0.426	19.90	0.492	292.0	278.0	—	4.410
0.550	0.450	—	0.094	20.00	0.164	0.033	2.180	0.470	14.20	0.000	8.000	78.00	0.001	3.740
2.750	0.650	—	0.121	26.10	0.216	0.067	3.320	0.701	22.20	0.000	20.00	115.0	0.001	4.850
0.067	0.021	0.000	—	0.550	0.006	0.002	0.115	0.012	0.830	0.000	0.400	4.300	0.000	0.160
0.070	—	0.000	—	1.100	0.007	0.004	0.160	0.009	1.100	0.000	0.800	5.600	0.000	0.160
2.340	0.500	—	—	9.800	0.174	0.032	3.780	0.196	38.80	0.000	24.00	112.0	0.001	1.500
1.270	0.460	—	—	8.900	0.115	0.031	3.120	0.434	12.00	0.000	13.00	65.00	—	—
1.260	—	189.0	—	6.300	0.063	0.105	1.680	—	—	—	65.00	92.00	0.001	1.200
0.550	0.580	355.0	0.126	12.90	0.176	0.084	2.270	0.470	16.70	0.000	54.00	97.00	0.001	—
1.210	0.680	89.00	—	0.400	0.104	0.095	1.610	0.290	21.50	0.217	21.00	78.00	—	—
0.108	0.071	—	—	0.937	0.005	0.016	0.292	0.012	0.312	—	10.20	15.90	—	0.540
1.410	0.980	332.0	—	26.10	0.169	0.225	2.580	0.436	21.30	0.348	140.0	154.0	—	4.410
0.024	0.021	0.000	0.146	0.830	0.003	0.000	0.084	0.010	0.900	0.000	0.500	3.100	0.000	0.029
4.080	0.280	—	—	7.800	0.071	0.061	1.780	0.356	12.50	0.000	20.00	59.00	—	3.020
3.410	0.410	54040	—	10.20	0.059	0.132	0.899	0.137	30.10	0.000	64.00	85.00	—	—
2.870	0.720	22410	—	9.500	0.043	0.319	1.010	—	—	0.000	99.00	120.0	—	—
0.013	0.013	0.300	—	1.030	0.000	0.002	0.014	0.003	1.220	0.000	0.900	0.800	0.000	0.100
0.800	0.520	0.000	—	37.20	0.122	0.062	1.070	0.154	26.40	0.000	72.00	84.00	—	2.500
3.470	0.440	42.00	—	34.80	0.050	0.052	0.337	0.307	7.050	0.000	72.00	46.00	—	—
0.619	0.108	102.0	—	0.852	0.017	0.065	0.454	—	—	0.000	42.60	22.70	—	1.200
6.420	1.370	14740	5.400	17.70	0.171	0.425	0.882	0.436	262.0	0.000	244.0	100.0	0.002	3.420
3.700	0.990	15050	0.140	31.60	0.042	0.248	0.634	0.187	136.0	0.000	195.0	74.00	0.003	5.080
3.120	1.440	15960	6.150	25.20	0.123	0.344	0.859	0.299	220.0	0.000	299.0	98.40	0.002	4.510
1.520	0.300	3760	1.650	15.80	0.044	0.106	0.406	0.110	108.0	0.000	56.00	28.00	0.001	1.760
1.910	0.350	878.0	—	22.10	0.342	0.027	1.810	0.398	38.40	0.000	90.00	93.00	0.002	4.300
1.220	0.270	14350	—	30.90	0.148	0.035	1.990	0.254	39.30	0.000	84.00	55.00	0.002	3.500
0.670	0.220	9452	—	15.40	0.099	0.066	0.788	0.243	23.00	0.000	23.00	33.00	0.002	4.200
0.640	0.710	517.0	—	10.00	0.079	0.074	0.923	0.117	36.20	0.000	48.00	69.00	0.006	3.160
0.670	0.540	7292	—	19.70	0.174	0.049	1.440	0.148	57.40	0.000	28.00	41.00	0.006	3.460
1.080	0.440	962.0	—	8.200	0.091	0.089	0.861	0.100	17.50	0.000	38.00	55.00	0.007	3.230
1.550	0.580	1225	—	5.200	0.095	0.091	1.200	—	—	0.000	38.00	66.00	—	—
0.640	0.320	432.0	—	8.400	0.074	0.074	0.770	0.140	30.20	0.000	24.00	72.00	0.006	2.300
0.550	0.260	442.0	—	11.70	0.091	0.039	0.520	0.116	28.80	0.000	20.00	42.00	0.004	2.000
2.930	1.220	564.0	—	15.70	0.323	0.184	2.550	0.223	—	0.000	32.00	224.0	—	—
0.520	0.330	24880	5.240	28.00	0.083	0.145	0.689	0.275	25.70	0.000	32.00	62.00	0.001	2.050
1.830	0.870	55940	15.10	55.90	0.174	0.459	2.100	0.800	36.30	0.000	70.00	88.00	0.002	5.580
3.390	0.540	38570	—	13.30	0.069	0.230	2.440	0.168	—	0.000	76.00	133.0	0.002	6.120
1.190	0.160	4399	—	7.000	0.019	0.044	0.414	0.043	12.00	0.032	27.00	27.00	0.001	1.100
2.300	—	0.000	—	0.000	0.070	0.040	0.100	—	—	—	154.0	151.0	—	—
1.440	0.320	3245	1.180	50.30	0.170	0.144	1.720	0.086	22.60	0.000	20.00	70.00	0.001	1.920
1.450	0.380	1450	—	36.30	0.108	0.074	1.760	0.216	—	0.000	63.00	46.00	0.002	1.690
1.860	0.420	1415	1.810	33.80	0.117	0.089	1.820	—	7.400	0.000	84.00	51.00	0.002	2.040
1.450	0.380	1450	—	36.30	0.108	0.074	1.760	0.216	7.000	0.000	63.00	46.00	0.002	1.930
0.590	0.130	1394	0.603	21.60	0.074	0.062	0.738	0.059	11.50	0.000	8.000	29.00	0.001	2.100
0.780	0.170	1017	0.495	14.80	0.067	0.064	0.750	0.031	9.900	0.000	19.00	32.00	0.001	—
1.420	0.360	1356	1.730	44.60	0.114	0.076	1.640	0.270	48.40	0.000	20.00	46.00	0.001	2.900
1.420	0.360	1356	1.730	44.60	0.114	0.076	1.640	0.270	48.40	0.000	20.00	46.00	0.001	2.800
7.830	2.100	6468	—	111.0	0.406	0.498	8.440	0.996	—	0.000	91.70	207.0	0.003	—
7.830	2.100	6468	—	111.0	0.406	0.498	8.440	0.996	—	0.000	91.70	207.0	0.003	—
1.300	0.486	4898	—	33.10	0.259	0.216	2.590	0.130	34.10	0.000	47.10	83.80	—	—
2.320	0.540	3402	1.780	88.20	0.178	0.135	4.290	0.380	—	0.000	37.00	99.00	0.003	—
2.320	0.540	3402	1.780	88.20	0.178	0.135	4.290	0.380	—	0.000	37.00	99.00	0.003	—
1.460	—	4374	—	53.00	0.049	0.073	1.940	—	—	—	38.90	—	0.001	2.700
1.020	0.480	2832	—	67.00	0.104	0.068	1.760	0.339	—	0.000	26.00	40.00	0.001	2.700
0.700	0.270	0.000	—	16.50	0.129	0.038	0.751	0.310	21.80	0.000	19.00	66.00	0.001	—
4.900	—	50.00	—	0.000	0.380	0.160	1.100	—	—	—	131.0	322.0	—	—

Appendix B
Physiological Values of Fuel Nutrients

	Carbohydrate	Protein	Fat
Gross kcalories per gram from bomb calorimetry studies	4.10	5.65	9.45
Adjustments needed to account for urea, creatinine, and uric acid in protein		−1.25	
SUBTOTAL	4.10	4.4	9.45
Digestibility	98%	92%	95%
Net kcalories per gram available to the body	4	4	9

Appendix C
Clinical and Biochemical Measures of Nutritional Status

Clinical Signs and Symptoms of Various Nutrient Deficiencies

Area of examination	Sign/symptom	Potential nutrient deficiency	Area of examination	Sign/symptom	Potential nutrient deficiency
Hair	Alopecia	Zinc, essential fatty acids	**Skin**	Follicular hyperkeratosis	Vitamin A, essential fatty acids
	Easy pluckability	Protein, essential fatty acids		Nasolabial seborrhea	Niacin, pyridoxine, riboflavin
	Lackluster	Protein, zinc		Bilateral dermatitis	Niacin, zinc
	"Corkscrew" hair	Vitamin C, Vitamin A	**Extremities**	Subcutaneous fat loss	kcalories
	Decreased pigmentation	Protein, copper		Muscle wastage	kcalories, protein
Eyes	Xerosis of conjunctiva	Vitamin A		Edema	Protein
	Corneal vascularization	Riboflavin		Osteomalacia, bone pain, rickets	Vitamin D
	Keratomalacia	Vitamin A		Arthralgia	Vitamin C
	Bitot's spots	Vitamin A	**Hematologic**	Anemia	Vitamin B-12, iron, folate, copper, vitamin E, vitamin K
GI tract	Nausea, vomiting	Pyridoxine		Leukopenia, neutropenia	Copper
	Diarrhea	Zinc, niacin		Low prothrombin, prolonged clotting time	Vitamin K
	Stomatitis	Pyridoxine, riboflavin, iron	**Neurologic**	Disorientation	Niacin, thiamin
	Cheilosis	Pyridoxine, iron		Confabulation	Thiamin
	Glossitis	Pyridoxine, zinc, niacin, folate, vitamin B-12		Neuropathy	Thimain, pyridoxine, chromium
	Magenta tongue	Riboflavin		Parasthesia	Thiamin, pyridoxine, Vitamin B-12
	Swollen, bleeding gums	Vitamin C	**Cardiovascular**	Congestive heart failure, cardiomegaly, tachycardia	Thiamin
	Fissured tongue	Niacin		Cardiomyopathy	Selenium
	Hepatomegaly	Protein			
Skin	Dry and scaling	Vitamin A, essential fatty acids, zinc			
	Petechiae/ecchymoses	Vitamin C, vitamin K			

From: Ross Laboratories

Biochemical indicators of good nutrition status

Nutrient or measurement	Test		Normal or acceptable levels: Men	Women
Iron	Hemoglobin (g/100 ml)		≥14.0	≥12.0
		Infants (under 2 years)	≥10.0	≥10.0
		Children (6-12 years)	≥11.5	≥11.5
		Pregnancy (2nd trimester)		≥11.0
		(3rd trimester)		≥10.5
Protein	Serum albumin (g/100 ml)		≥3.5	≥3.5
Normal lipid metabolism	Serum cholesterol (mg/100 ml)		<200	<200
	Serum triglyceride (mg/100 ml)		<250	<250
Normal carbohydrate metabolism	Serum glucose (mg/100 ml)		75-110	75-110
Sodium	Serum sodium (mEq/l)		130-150	130-155
Potassium	Serum potassium (mEq/l)		3.5-5.3	3.5-5.3
Vitamin A	Plasma vitamin A (μg/100 ml)		>20	>20
Vitamin C	Serum vitamin C (mg/100 ml)		≥0.3	≥0.3
Riboflavin	Erythrocyte glutathione peroxidase (% stimulation of activity by added riboflavin cofactor)		<20	<20
Vitamin B-6	Trytophan load test—increase in excretion of xanthurenic acid (mg/day)		<25	<25
Folate	Serum folate (nanogram/ml)		>6.0	>6.0
Thiamin	Urinary thiamin (μg/g creatinine)		>65	>65
Zinc	Plasma zinc (μg/100 ml)		80-115	80-115

Some information obtained from: Roe, D.A.: Drug-induced nutritional deficiencies, AVI Press, Westport, Conn., 1976, and Sauberlich, H.E., Skala, H.H., and Dowdy, R.P.: Laboratory tests for the assessment of nutritional status, CRC Press, Inc., Cleveland, 1974.

Appendix D
Periodic Table of the Elements

Key to Abbreviations

Name	Symbol	Name	Symbol	Name	Symbol	Name	Symbol
Actinium	Ac	Erbium	Er	Molybdenum	Mo	Samarium	Sm
Aluminum	Al	Europium	Eu	Neodymium	Nd	Scandium	Sc
Americium	Am	Fermium	Fm	Neon	Ne	Selenium	Se
Antimony	Sb	Fluorine	F	Neptunium	Np	Silicon	Si
Argon	Ar	Francium	Fr	Nickel	Ni	Silver	Ag
Arsenic	As	Gadolinium	Gd	Niobium	Nb	Sodium	Na
Astatine	At	Gallium	Ga	Nitrogen	N	Strontium	Sr
Barium	Ba	Germanium	Ge	Nobelium	No	Sulfur	S
Berkelium	Bk	Gold	Au	Osmium	Os	Tantalum	Ta
Beryllium	Be	Hafnium	Hf	Oxygen	O	Technetium	Tc
Bismuth	Bi	Helium	He	Palladium	Pd	Tellurium	Te
Boron	B	Homium	Ho	Phosphorus	P	Terbium	Tb
Bromine	Br	Hydrogen	H	Platinum	Pt	Thallium	Tl
Cadmium	Cd	Indium	In	Plutonium	Pu	Thorium	Th
Calcium	Ca	Iodine	I	Polonium	Po	Thulium	Tm
Californium	Cf	Iridium	Ir	Potassium	K	Tin	Sn
Carbon	C	Iron	Fe	Praseodymium	Pr	Titanium	Ti
Cerium	Ce	Krypton	Kr	Promethium	Pm	Tungsten	W
Cesium	Cs	Lanthanum	La	Protactinium	Pa	Uranium	U
Chlorine	Cl	Lead	Pb	Radium	Ra	Vanadium	V
Chromium	Cr	Lithium	Li	Radon	Rn	Xenon	Xe
Cobalt	Co	Lutetium	Lu	Rhenium	Re	Ytterbium	Yb
Copper	Cu	Magnesium	Mg	Rhodium	Rh	Yttrium	Y
Curium	Cm	Manganese	Mn	Rubidium	Rb	Zinc	Zn
Dysprosium	Dy	Mendelevium	Md	Ruthenium	Ru	Zirconium	Zr
Einsteinium	Es	Mercury	Hg				

H																	He
Li	Be											B	C	N	O	F	Ne
Na	Mg											Al	Si	P	S	Cl	Ar
K	Ca	Sc	Ti	V	Cr	Mn	Fe	Co	Ni	Cu	Zn	Ga	Ge	As	Se	Br	Kr
Rb	Sr	Y	Zr	Nb	Mo	Tc	Ru	Rh	Pd	Ag	Cd	In	Sn	Sb	Te	I	Xe
Cs	Ba	* 57-71	Hf	Ta	W	Re	Os	Ir	Pt	Au	Hg	T1	Pb	Bi	Po	At	Rn
Fr	Ra	† 89-102															

*	La	Ce	Pr	Nd	Pm	Sm	Eu	Gd	Tb	Dy	Ho	Er	Tm	Yb	Lu
†	Ac	Th	Pa	U	Np	Pu	Am	Cm	Bk	Cf	Es	Fm	Md	No	

The periodic table of elements.
The frequency of elements that occur in the earth's crust
in more than trace amounts is indicated in the vertical dimension.

Appendix E
Chemical Structures

Carbohydrates and sugar alcohols

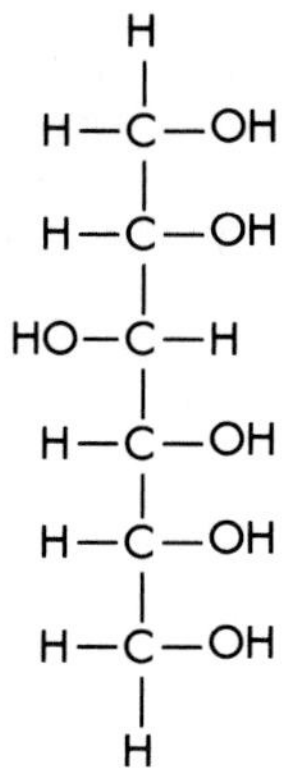

H
H—C—OH
H—C—OH
HO—C—H
H—C—OH
H—C—OH
H—C—OH
H

Sorbitol

H
H—C—OH
HO—C—H
HO—C—H
H—C—OH
H—C—OH
H—C—OH
H

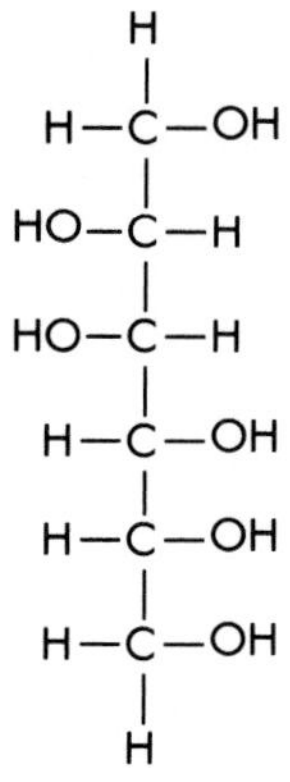

Mannitol

Sugar Substitutes

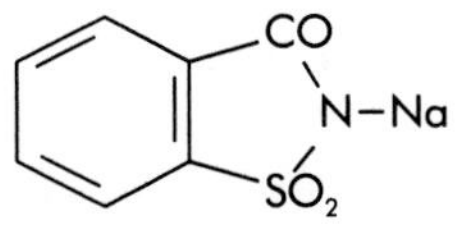

CO
N-Na
SO_2

Sodium saccharin

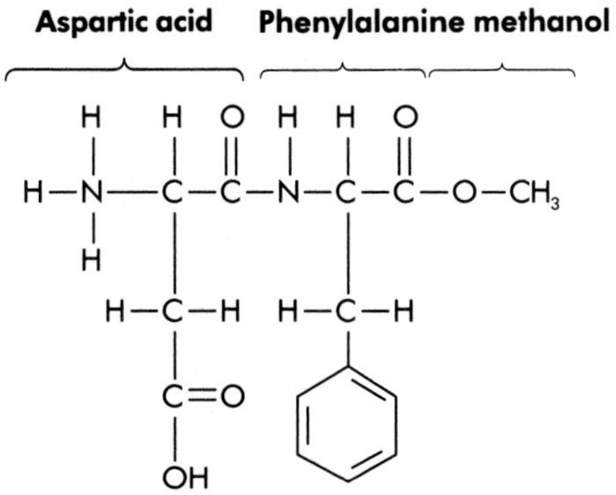

Aspartic acid **Phenylalanine methanol**

H H O H H O
H—N—C—C—N—C—C—O—CH_3
H
H—C—H H—C—H
C=O
OH

Aspartame

CH_3
O
O
N—SO_2
K^+

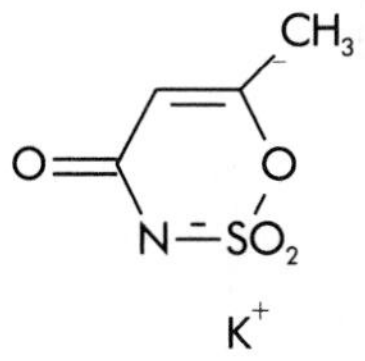

Acesulfame (potassium salt)

Proteins

With one amino group and one carboxyl group

$CH_2 < ^{NH_2}_{COOH}$

Glycine

$CH_3\ CH < ^{NH_2}_{COOH}$

Alanine

$HOCH_2\ CH < ^{NH_2}_{COOH}$

Serine

$^{CH_3}_{CH_3} > CH\ CH_2\ CH < ^{NH_2}_{COOH}$

Leucine

(essential)

$^{CH_3}_{CH_3} > CH\ CH < ^{NH_2}_{COOH}$

Valine

(essential)

$^{C_2H_5}_{CH_3} > CH\ CH < ^{NH_2}_{COOH}$

Isoleucine

(essential)

$^{CH_3}_{HO} > CH\ CH < ^{NH_2}_{COOH}$

Threonine

(essential)

$SH{-}CH_2\ CH < ^{NH_2}_{COOH}$

Cysteine

$CH_3\ SCH_2\ CH_2\ CH < ^{NH_2}_{COOH}$

Methionine

(essential)

With two amino groups and two carboxyl groups

$^{H_2N}_{HOOC} > CH\ CH_2{-}S{-}S{-}CH_2\ CH < ^{NH_2}_{COOH}$

Cystine

With one heterocyclic group

(indole ring, N–H)$-CH_2\ CH < ^{NH_2}_{COOH}$

Tryptophan

(essential)

N—CH ‖ ‖ HC C—CH_2 CH $< ^{NH_2}_{COOH}$ (ring closed through N–H)

Histidine

(essential)

H_2C——CH_2 | | H_2C C $< ^{H}_{COOH}$ (ring closed through N–H)

Proline

H HOC——CH_2 | | H_2C C $< ^{H}_{COOH}$ (ring closed through N–H)

Hydroxyproline

With two amino acid groups (one carboxyl)

$NH_2CH_2\ (CH_2)_3\ CH(NH_2)COOH$

Lysine

(essential)

$H_2N{-}C(=NH)\ NH\ (CH_2)_3\ CH(NH_2)COOH$

Arginine

(essential in some species)

With two carboxyl groups (one amino acid)

$HOOC{-}CH_2\ CH(NH_2)COOH$

Aspartic acid

$HOOC{-}CH_2\ CH_2\ CH(NH_2)COOH$

Glutamic acid

With benzene ring

$C_6H_5{-}CH_2\ CH(NH_2)COOH$

Phenylalanine

(essential)

$OH{-}C_6H_4{-}CH_2\ CH(NH_2)COOH$

Tyrosine

Ketones

$CH_3{-}C(=O){-}CH_2{-}C(=O){-}OH$

Acetoacetic Acid

Spontaneous

CO_2

$CH_3{-}C(=O){-}CH_3$

Acetone

H^+

$CH_3{-}CH(OH){-}CH_2{-}C(=O){-}OH$

ß-Hydroxybutyric Acid

Tryptophan and Serotonin

$CH_2{-}C(H)(NH_2){-}C(=O){-}OH$ (indole, N–H)

Tryptophan

HO–, $CH_2{-}C(H)(NH_2){-}C(=O){-}OH$ (indole, N–H)

5-Hydroxytryptophan (5-HT)

HO–, $CH_2{-}C(H)(H){-}NH_2$ (indole, N–H)

5-Hydroxytryptamine or Serotonin

Important metabolites

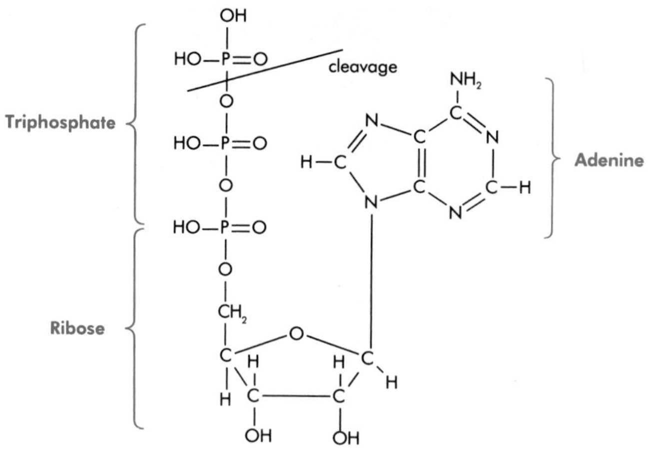

Triphosphate
cleavage
Adenine
Ribose

ATP

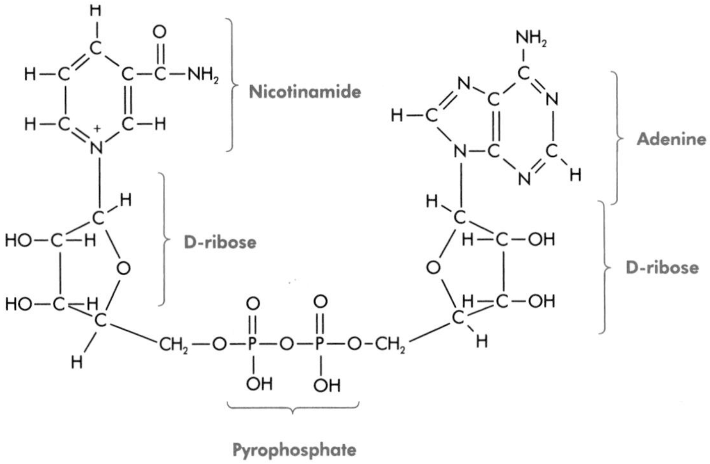

Nicotinamide
Adenine
D-ribose
D-ribose
Pyrophosphate

NAD

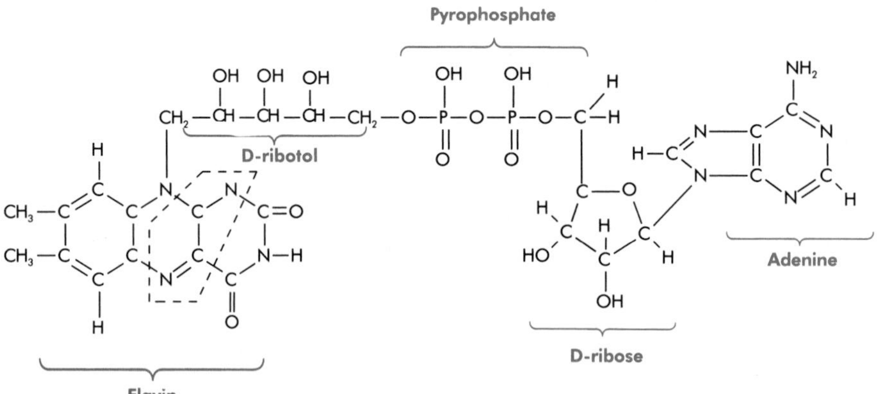

Pyrophosphate
D-ribotol
Adenine
D-ribose
Flavin

FAD

Appendix F
Recommended Dietary Intakes*

Category	Age	Vitamin A† (RE)	Vitamin K‡ (μg)	Vitamin C§ (mg)	Vitamin B-12‖ (μg)	Folate¶ (μg/kg)	Iron# (mg)
Infants	0-2.9 months	375	10**	25	0.3	16††	‡‡
	3-5.9 months	375	10	25	0.4	24††	6.6
	6-11.9 months	375	10	25	0.5	32††	8.8
Children	1-1.9 years	375	15(1-3 years)	25	0.7	3.3	10
	2-5.9 years	400	20(4-6 years)	25	1.0	3.3	10
	6-9.9 years	500	25(7-10 years)	25	1.5	3.3	10
Males	10-11.9 years	600	30	30	2	3	12
	12-14.9 years	700	30	40	2	3	12
	15-17.9 years	700	35	40	2	3	12
	18-70+ years	700	45	40	2	3	10
Females	10-14.9 years	600	30	30	2	3	15
	15-49.9 years	600	35	30	2	3	15
	50-70 years	600	35	30	2	3	10
	70+ years	600	35	30	2	3	10
Pregnant	0-2.9 months	0	+10	0	0	500††	15 + 30 add'l
	3-5.9 months	0	+10	+5	+0.5	500††	15 + 30 add'l
	6-9.0 months	+200	+10	+10	+0.5	500††	15 + 30 add'l
Lactating	0-6+ months	+400	+20	+25	+0.5	adult dose +100 μg/day	15
	6+ months	+320	+20	+20	+0.5	adult dose +100 μg/day	15

*Nutrient recommendations from the original RDA committee formed in 1980 to develop the tenth edition. Some of these recommendations appear in the final tenth edition of the RDA published in 1989, while other recommendations were not adopted by the final RDA committee.

†From Olson, JA: Am J Clin Nutr 45:704-716, 1987, RE = retinol equivalents. One RE equals 1 μg retinol, 6 μg β-carotene, or 12/μg of other provitamin A carotenoids. Because IU are not employed in defining the RDI, the assumed distribution of carotenoids and vitamin A in the diet is no longer of key importance. Nonetheless, the present average intake, as REs, is approximately 25% provitamin A carotenoids and 75% preformed vitamin A.

‡From Olson JA: Am J Clin Nutr 45:687-692, 1987. To convert μg of vitamin K (phylloquinone) to nmol, multiply by 2.219.

§From Olson JA and Hodges RE: Am J Clin Nutr 45:693-703, 1987. To convert mg of vitamin C to μmol, multiply by 5.679.

‖From Herbert V: Am J Clin Nutr 45:671-678, 1987. To convert μg of vitamin B_{12} to nmol, multiply by 1.4.

¶From Herbert V: Am J Clin Nutr 45:661-760, 1987. To convert μg of folate to nmol, multiply by 2.266.

#From Herbert V: Am J Clin Nutr 45:679-868, 1987. To convert mg of iron to nmol, multiply by 18.

**Provided as a daily supplement or as an intramuscular injection (1 mg) at birth.

††Total per day.

‡‡Because of storage iron present at birth, the normal-term infant, for the first 3 months of life, does not require exogenous iron beyond that provided by breast milk or by formulas containing iron of bioavailability equivalent to that of breast milk.

Appendix G

Recommended Nutrient Intakes for Canadians

Average energy requirements and summary examples of recommended nutrient intakes

Age	Sex	Average height (cm)[c]	Average weight (kg)[c]	Requirements[a,b] kcal/kg[c,d]	MJ/kg[d]	kcal/day[e]	MJ/day[f]	kcal/m[g]	MJ/cm[f]
Months									
0-4	Both	55	6.0	120-100	0.50-0.42	500	2.0	9	0.04
5-12	Both	63	9.0	100-95	0.42-0.40	700	2.8	11	0.05
Years									
1	Both	82	11	101	0.42	1100	4.8	13.5	0.06
2-3	Both	95	14	94	0.39	1300	5.6	13.5	0.06
4-6	Both	107	18	100	0.42	1800	7.6	17	0.07
7-9	M	126	25	88	0.37	2200	9.2	17.5	0.07
	F	125	25	76	0.32	1900	8.0	15	0.06
10-12	M	141	34	73	0.30	2500	10.4	17.5	0.07
	F	143	36	61	0.25	2200	9.2	15.5	0.06
13-15	M	159	50	57	0.24	2800	12.0	17.5	0.07
	F	157	48	46	0.19	2200	9.2	14	0.06
16-18	M	172	62	51	0.21	3200	13.2	18.5	0.08
	F	160	53	40	0.17	2100	8.8	13	0.05
19-24	M	175	71	42	0.18	3000	12.4		
	F	160	58	36	0.15	2100	8.8		
25-49	M	172	74	36	0.15	2700	11.2		
	F	160	59	32	0.13	1900	8.0		
50-74	M	170	73	31	0.13	2300	9.6		
	F	158	63	29	0.12	1800	7.6		
75+	M	168	69	29	0.12	2000	8.4		
	F	155	64	23	0.10	1500	6.0		
Pregnancy (additional)[h]									
First trimester									
Second trimester									
Third trimester									
Lactation (additional)[h]									

[a]Recommended nutrient intakes for Canadians, 1990—Committee for the revision of the Dietary Standard for Canada, Bureau of Nutritional Sciences, Department of National Health and Welfare. Recommended intakes of energy and of certain nutrients are not listed in this table because of the nature of the variables upon which they are based. The figures for energy are estimates of average requirements for expected patterns of activity. For nutrients not shown, the following amounts are recommended: thiamin, 0.4 mg/100 kcal (0.48 mg/5000 kJ); riboflavin, 0.5 mg/1000 kcal (0.6 mg/5000 kJ); niacin, 6.6 NE/1000 kcal (7.9 NE/5000 kJ); vitamin B-6, 15 μg, as pyridoxine, per gram of protein intake; phosphorus, same as calcium. Recommended intakes during periods of growth are taken as appropriate for individual representative of the mid-point in each age group. All recommended intakes are designed to cover individual variations in essentially all of a healthy population subsisting upon a variety of common foods available in Canada. It is emphasized that these are *examples* of the application of the recommended nutrient intakes to particular classes of individuals and/or particular situations.

[b]Requirements can be expected to vary within a range of ±30%.

[c]Figures rounded to the closest whole number when ≥10 and to the closest 0.5 when <10.

[d]First and last figures are averages at the beginning and at the end of the 3-month period.

[e]Figures rounded to the nearest 50 when <1000 and to the nearest 100 when ≥1000.

[f]Figures include two decimal fractions if value is <1 and one decimal fraction if ≥1.

[e]Figures rounded to the nearest 50 when <1000 and to the nearest 100 when ≥1000.

[f]Figures include two decimal fractions if value is <1 and one decimal fraction if ≥1.

Average energy requirements and summary examples of recommended nutrient intakes—cont'd

	Fat-soluble vitamins			Water-soluble vitamins			Minerals				
Protein (g/day)[i]	Vitamin A (RE/day)[j]	Vitamin D (μg/day)[k]	Vitamin E (mg/day)[l]	Vitamin C (mg/day)	Folacin (μg/day)[m]	Vitamin B-12 (μg/day)	Ca (mg/day)	Mg (mg/day)	Fe (mg/day)	I (μg/day)	Zn (mg/day)
12[n]	400	10	3	20	50	0.3	250	20	0.3[o]	30	2[p]
12[n]	400	10	3	20	50	0.3	400	32	7	40	3
19	400	10	3	20	65	0.3	500	40	6	55	4
22	400	5	4	20	80	0.4	550	50	6	65	4
26	500	5	5	25	90	0.5	600	65	8	85	5
30	700	2.5	7	25	125	0.8	700	100	8	110	7
30	700	2.5	6	25	125	0.8	700	100	8	95	7
38	800	2.5	8	25	170	1.0	900	130	8	125	9
40	800	5	7	25	180	1.0	1100	135	8	110	9
50	900	5	9	30	150	1.5	1100	185	10	160	12
42	800	5	7	30	145	1.5	1000	180	13	160	9
55	1000	5	10	40[r]	185	1.9	900	230	10	160	12
43	800	2.5	7	30[r]	160	1.9	700	200	12	160	9
58	1000	2.5	10	40[r]	210	2.0	800	240	9	160	12
43	800	2.5	7	30[r]	175	2.0	700	200	13	160	9
61	1000	2.5	9	40[r]	220	2.0	800	250	9	160	12
44	800	2.5	6	30[r]	175	2.0	700	200	13[q]	160	9
60	1000	5	7	40[r]	220	2.0	800	250	9	160	12
47	800	5	6	30[r]	190	2.0	800	210	8	160	9
57	1000	5	6	40[r]	205	2.0	800	230	9	160	12
47	800	2.5	5	30[r]	190	2.0	800	210	8	160	9
5	100	2.5	2	0	300	1.0	500	15	0	25	6
20	100	2.5	2	10	300	1.0	500	45	5	25	6
24	100	2.5	2	10	300	1.0	500	45	10	25	6
20	400	2.5	3	25	100	0.5	500	65	0	50	6

[g]Figures rounded to the nearest 0.5.

[h]Pregnancy: Add 100 kcal during the first trimester and 300 for the second and third trimesters. Lactation: Add 450 kcal/day.

[i]The primary units are of g/kg body weight. The figures shown here are only examples.

[j]One retinol equivalent (RE) corresponds to the biological activity of 1 μg of retinol, 6 μg of β-carotene or 12 μg of other carotenes.

[k]Expressed as cholecalciferol or ergocalciferol.

[l]Expressed as *d*-α-tocopherol equivalent, relative to which β- and γ-tocopherol and α-tocotrienol have activities of 0.5, 0.1 and 0.3 respectively.

[m]Expressed as total folate.

[n]Assumption that the protein is from breast milk or is of the same biological value as that of breast milk and that between 3 and 9 months adjustment for the quality of the protein is made.

[o]For the infant, it is assumed that breast milk is the source of iron up to 2 months of age.

[p]Based on the assumption that breast milk is the source of zinc up to 2 months of age.

[q]After the menopause the recommended intake is 7 mg/day.

[r]Smokers should increase vitamin C by 50%.

[p]Based on the assumption that breast milk is the source of zinc up to 2 months of age.

[q]After the menopause the recommended intake is 7 mg/day.

Appendix H
Exchange-System Lists—United States

Milk exchange list ***Skim milk*** (12 grams carbohydrate, 8 grams protein, 0 grams fat, 90 kcalories)	
1 cup	skim or nonfat milk (½% and 1%)
⅓ cup	powdered (nonfat dry, before adding liquid)
½ cup	canned, evaporated skim milk
1 cup	buttermilk made from skim milk
1 cup	yogurt made from skim milk (plain, unflavored)
Low-fat milk (12 grams carbohydrate, 8 grams proteins, 5 grams fat, 120 kcalories)	
1 cup	2% fat fortified milk
1 cup	plain nonfat yogurt (added milk solids)
Whole milk (12 grams carbohydrate, 8 grams protein, 8 grams fat, 150 kcalories)	
1 cup	whole milk
½ cup	buttermilk made from whole milk
1 cup	custard-style yogurt made from whole milk (plain, unflavored)

Vegetable exchange list

(5 grams carbohydrate, 2 grams protein, 0 grams fat, 25 kcalories)

1 exchange is
½ cup cooked vegetables or vegetable juice
1 cup raw vegetables

artichoke (½ medium)	celery	sauerkraut
asparagus	eggplant	spinach, cooked
beans (green, wax)	green pepper	squash, summer, zucchini
beets	greens	string beans (green, yellow)
broccoli	mushrooms, cooked	tomatoe
brussels sprouts	onions	tomato juice
cabbage, cooked	pea pods	turnips
carrots	rhubarb	vegetable juice
cauliflower		

Fruit exchange list

(15 grams carbohydrate, 0 grams protein, 0 grams fat, 60 kcalories)
1 fruit exchange

1	apple (2 inches in diameter)
4 rings	dried apple
½ cup	apple juice
½ cup	applesauce (unsweetened)
4	apricots, fresh
½ cup	apricots, canned
7 halves	apricots, dried
½	banana, 9 inches
¾ cup	blackberries
¾ cup	blueberries
1 cup	raspberries
1¼ cup	strawberries
⅓ melon	cantaloupe (5-inches in diameter)
12 large	cherries (large, raw)

Fruit exchange list—cont'd

½ cup	cherries, canned
½ cup	cider
⅓ cup	cranberry juice
2½ medium	dates
2	figs, fresh (2-inches in diameter)
1½	figs, dried
½	grapefruit
½ cup	grapefruit juice
15	grapes
⅓ cup	grape juice
⅛	honeydew melon (7-inches in diameter; cubes=1 cup)
1	kiwi (large)
¾ cup	mandarin oranges
½ small	mango
1 small	nectarine (1½-inches in diameter)
1 small	orange (2½-inches in diameter)
½ cup	orange juice
1 medium or ¾ cup	peach, fresh (2¾-inches in diameter)
½ cut or 2 halves	peach, canned
1 small or ½ large	pear, fresh
½ cup or 2 halves	pear, canned
¾ cup	pineapple, raw
⅓ cup	pineapple, canned
½ cup	pineapple juice
2	plums (2 inches in diameter)
3	prunes, dried
⅓ cup	prune juice
2 T	raisins
2	tangerine (2½-inches in diameter)
1¼ cups	watermelon (cubes)

Starch/bread exchange list

(15 grams carbohydrate, 3 grams protein, 0 grams fat, 80 kcalories)
1 starch/bread exchange

Bread	
1 slice	white (including French and Italian)
1 slice	whole wheat
1 slice	rye or pumpernickel
1 slice	raisin (unfrosted)
2 (⅔ ounces)	bread sticks (crisp, 4 inches long, ½-inch wide)
½ (1 ounce)	bagel, small
½	English muffin
1	plain roll
½ (1 ounce)	frankfurter bun
½ (1 ounce)	hamburger bun
3 tablespoons	dried bread crumbs
1	tortilla (6 inches in diameter)
½	pita (6 inches in diameter)
Cereal/grains/pasta	
½ cup	bran flakes
¾ cup	other ready-to-eat unsweetened cereal
1½ cup	puffed cereal (unfrosted)
½ cup	cereal (cooked)
⅓ cup	rice or barley (cooked)
3 tablespoons	grapenuts
½ cup	shredded wheat
3 tablespoons	wheat germ
½ cup	pasta (cooked spaghetti, noodles, macaroni)
2½ tablespoons	cornmeal (dry)

Starch/bread exchange list—cont'd

Cereal/grains/pasta

2½ tablespoons	flour (dry)

Crackers/snacks

3	graham (2½ inch square)
¾ ounce	matzo (4 inches × 6 inches)
24	oyster
4	rye crisp (2 inches × 3½ inches)
6	saltines
8	animal
5 slices	melba toast
3 cups	popcorn (popped with no added fat)
¾ ounce	pretzels

Dried beans/peas/lentils

⅓ cup	dried beans, such as kidney, white, split, blackeye (cooked)
⅓ cup	lentils (cooked)
¼ cup	baked beans

Starchy vegetables

½ cup	corn
1 cup	corn on the cob (6 inches)
½ cup	lima beans
½ cup	peas, green
1 small	potato, white (3 ounces baked)
½ cup	potato, mashed
¾ cup	winter squash, acorn or butternut
⅓ cup	yarn or sweet potato

Starch group (with fat)

1 starch/bread exchange
1 fat exchange

1	biscuit
½ cup	chow mein noodles
1 (2 ounce)	corn bread (2-inch cube)
6	cracker, round butter type
10 (1½ ounce)	french fries (2 inches to 3½ inches)
1	muffin, plain, small
2	pancake (4 inches in diameter)
¼ cup	stuffing, bread (prepared)
2	taco shell (6 inches across)
1	waffle (4½ inches square)
4-6 (1 ounce)	whole-wheat crackers (such as Triscuits)

Meat exchange list

Lean (0 grams carbohydrate, 7 grams protein, 3 grams fat, 55 kcalories)

Beef	1 ounce	baby beef (lean, chipped beef, chuck, flank steak, tenderloin, plate ribs, round (bottom, top), all cuts rump, spare ribs, tripe
Pork	1 ounce	leg (whole rump, center shank), ham (center slices), USDA good or choice grades such as round, sirloin, flank, and tenderloin
Veal	1 ounce	leg, loin, rib, shank, shoulder, chops, roasts, all cuts except cutlets (ground or cubed)
Poultry	1 ounce	chicken, turkey, cornish hen
Fish	2 ounce	fresh or frozen, any type canned salmon, tuna, mackerel, crab, or lobster

Meat exchange list—cont'd

Fish	1 ounce	clams, oysters, scallops, shrimp
	3 ounce	sardines, drained
Cheeses	1 ounce	cottage, farmer's, or pot (low-fat)
Dried beans and peas	½ ounce	cooked

Medium fat (0 grams carbohydrate, 7 grams protein, 5 grams fat, 75 kcalories)

Beef	1 ounce	all ground beef, roast (rib, chuck, rump), steak (cubed, porterhouse, T-bone), meat loaf
Lamb	1 ounce	leg, rib, sirloin, loin (roast and chops), shank, shoulder
Pork	1 ounce	loin (all cuts tenderloin), chops, roast, Boston butt, cutlets
Poultry	1 ounce	capon, duck (domestic), goose, ground turkey
Veal	1 ounce	cutlets
Organ meats	1 ounce	all types
Fish	¼ cup	tuna (canned in oil); salmon (canned)
Cheeses	¼ cup or 1 ounce	cottage (creamed), mozzarella (made with skim milk), ricotta, farmer's, Neufchatel
Egg	1	egg

High-fat (0 grams carbohydrate, 7 grams protein, 8 grams fat, 100 kcalories)

Beef	1 ounce	brisket, corned beef, ground beef (commercial), chuck (ground commercial), roasts (rib), steaks (club and rib); most USDA prime cuts of beef
Lamb	1 ounce	patties (ground lamb)
Pork	1 ounce	spare ribs, loin (back ribs), pork (ground), country style ham, deviled ham, pork sausage
Cheeses	1 ounce	all regular cheeses (American, blue, brick, Camembert, cheddar, Gouda, Limburger, Muenster, Swiss, Monterey), all processed cheeses
Cold cuts	1 ounce	bologna, salami, pimento loaf
Frankfurter	1 ounce	(turkey or chicken)
Peanut butter	1 tablespoon	
Sausage	1 ounce	(Polish, Italian)

Fat exchange list

(0 grams carbohydrate, 0 grams protein, 5 grams fat, 45 kcalories)

⅛ medium	avocado	***Nuts,*** 6	almonds, whole, dry roasted
1 strip	bacon, crisp	2 large	pecans, whole
1 teaspoon	butter, margarine	20 small or 10 large	peanuts, Spanish, whole
2 tablespoons	cream, light	10	peanuts, Virginia, whole
2 tablespoons	cream, sour	2 whole	walnuts
1 tablespoon	cream, heavy	1 tablespoon	cashews, dry roasted
1 tablespoon	cream cheese	1 tablespoon	seeds (pine, sunflower)
Dressing		2 teaspoons	pumpkin seeds
1 tablespoon	all varieties	1 tablespoon	other
2 teaspoons	mayonnaise type	***Oil***	
1 tablespoon	reduced calorie (mayonnaise type)	1 teaspoon	corn, cottonseed, safflower, soy, sunflower, olive, peanut,
1 tablespoon	gravy, meat		

Fat exchange list—cont'd

Dressing

2 tablespoons reduced kcalorie

Oil

canola

Olives 10 small or 5 large

Free Foods

A free food is any food or drink that contains less than 20 kcalories per serving. You can eat as much as you want of those items that have no serving size specified. You may eat two or three servings per day of those items that have a specific serving size. Be sure to spread them out through the day.

Drinks:
- Bouillon or broth without fat
- Bouillon, low-sodium
- Carbonated drinks, sugar-free
- Carbonated water
- Club soda
- Cocoa powder, unsweetened (1 tablespoon)
- Coffee/Tea
- Drink mixes, sugar-free
- Tonic water, sugar-free

Nonstick pan spray

Fruit:
- Cranberries, unsweetened (½ cup)
- Rhubarb, unsweetened (½ cup)

Vegetables:
(raw, 1 cup)
- Cabbage
- Celery
- Chinese cabbage
- Cucumber
- Green onion
- Hot peppers
- Mushrooms
- Radishes
- Zucchini

Salad greens:
- Endive
- Escarole
- Lettuce
- Romaine
- Spinach

Sweet Substitutes:
- Candy, hard, sugar-free
- Gelatin, sugar-free
- Gum, sugar-free
- Jam/Jelly, sugar-free (2 teaspoons)
- Pancake syrup, sugar-free (1-2 tablespoons)
- Sugar substitutes (saccharin, aspartame)
- Whipped topping (2 tablespoons)

Condiments:
- Catsup (1 tablespoon)
- Horseradish
- Mustard
- Pickles, dill, unsweetened
- Salad dressing, low-calorie (2 tablespoon)
- Taco sauce (1 tablespoon)
- Vinegar

Seasonings:
- Basil (fresh)
- Celery seeds
- Cinnamon
- Chili powder
- Chives
- Curry
- Dill
- Flavoring extracts (vanilla, almond, walnut, peppermint, butter, lemon, etc.)
- Garlic
- Garlic powder
- Herbs
- Hot pepper sauce
- Lemon
- Lemon juice
- Lemon pepper
- Lime
- Lime juice
- Mint
- Onion powder
- Oregano
- Paprika
- Pepper
- Pimento
- Spices
- Soy sauce
- Soy sauce, low sodium ("lite")
- Wine, used in cooking (¼ cup)
- Worcestershire sauce

Appendix I

Fatty Acids, Including Omega-3 Fatty Acids in Foods

Chain length and number of double bonds for common fatty acids

Common name of fatty acids	Number of carbon atoms and site of double bond starting from methyl end ($-CH_3$)
Saturated fatty acids	
Formic	1
Acetic	2:0
Propionic	3:0
Butyric	4:0
Valeric	5:0
Caproic	6:0
Caprylic	8:0
Capric	10:0
Lauric	12:0
Myristic	14:0
Palmitic	16:0
Stearic	18:0
Arachidic	20:0
Unsaturated fatty acids	
Oleic	18:1(9) w-9
Linoleic	18:2(6,9) w-6
Linolenic	18:3 (3,6,9) w-3
Arachidonic	20:4(6,9,12,15) w-6
Eicosapentaenoic	20:5 (3,6,9,12,15) w-3
Docosahexaenoic	22:6 (3,6,9,12,15,18) w-3

Fatty acid composition of selected foods*

Food item	Fatty acid†									
	<C12:0	C12:0	C14:0	C16:0	C18:0	C18:1 w-9	C18:2 w-6	C18:3 w-3	C20:5 w-3	C22:6 w-3
Fats and oils		**Lauric acid**	**Mysistic acid**	**Palmitic acid**	**Stearic acid**	**Oleic acid**	**Linoleic acid**	**Alpha linolenic acid**	**EPA‡**	**DHA‡**
Beef tallow	—	0.9	3.7	24.9	18.9	36.0	3.1	0.6	—	—
Butter	7.0	2.3	8.2	21.3	9.8	20.4	1.8	1.2	—	—
Cocoa butter	—	—	0.1	25.4	33.2	32.6	2.8	0.1	—	—
Corn oil	—	—	—	12.0	2.0	25.0	60.0	0.5	—	—
Cottonseed oil	—	—	0.8	22.7	2.3	17.0	51.5	0.2	—	—
Lard	0.1	0.2	1.3	23.8	13.5	41.2	10.2	1.0	—	—
Olive oil	—	—	—	13.0	2.5	74.0	9.0	0.5	—	—
Palm kernel oil	7.2	47.0	16.4	8.1	2.8	11.4	1.6	—	—	—
Palm oil	—	0.1	1.0	43.5	4.0	36.6	9.1	0.2	—	—
Safflower oil	—	—	—	6.5	2.5	11.5	79.0	0.5	—	—
Shortening§	0.2	0.4	0.4	19.3	9.9	50.6	13.5	0.6	—	—
Margarine, stick	2	1	10	23	9	31	7	1	—	—
Margarine, tub	1	1	1	12	8	22	52	1	—	—
Canola oil	—	—	—	5	1	62	22	9	—	—
Soybean oil	—	—	—	10	4	24	53	7	—	—
Coconut oil	14	45	17	8	3	6	2	—	—	—
Meat, fish, and poultry										
Beef, lean only, uncooked	—	—	0.17	1.4	0.74	2.4	0.2	0.01	—	—
Chicken, white meat, uncooked	—	—	0.01	0.3	0.1	0.4	0.2	0.01	—	—
Salmon, coho, raw	—	—	0.3	0.6	0.2	1.2	0.3	0.2	0.3	0.5
Tuna, light, canned in oil	—	—	0.03	1.4	0.1	2.8	2.7	0.07	0.03	0.1

*Only major fatty acids are presented
†Values resent %/100 edible portion
‡EPA eicosapentaenoic acid, DHA docosahexaenoic acid (fish oil)
§Soybean and palm oils, hydrogenated

From: USDA Agriculture Handbook No. 8-4 (28)

Omega-3 fatty acids in foods

Food item	Edible portion, raw (grams/100 grams)
Fish oils	
Cod liver oil	19.2
Herring oil	12.0
Menhaden oil	21.7
Salmon oil	20.9
Finned Fish	
Anchovy, European	1.4
Bluefish	1.2
Dogfish, spiny	1.9
Herring, Atlantic	1.7
Herring, Pacific	1.8
Mackerel, Atlantic	2.6
Mackerel, king	2.2
Mullet, unspecified	1.1
Sablefish	1.5
Salmon, Atlantic	1.4
Salmon, Chinook	1.5
Scad, Muroaji	2.1
Sprat	1.3
Sturgeon, Atlantic	1.5
Trout, lake	2.0
Tuna, albaccore	1.5
Tuna, bluefin	1.6
Whitefish, lake	1.3
Fats and oils	
Butter	1.2
Butter oil	1.5
Chicken fat	1.0
Duck fat	1.0
Lard	1.0
Linseed oil	53.3
Margarine, hard, soybean	1.5
Margarine, hard, soybean oil and hydrogenated soybean oil	1.9
Margarine, hard, hydrogenated soybean oil and palm oil	2.3
Margarine, hard, hydrogenated soybean oil and cottonseed oil	2.8
Margarine, hard, hydrogenated soybean oil and hydrogenated palm oil	3.0
Margarine, liquid, hydrogenated soybean oil, soybean oil and cottonseed oil	2.4
Margarine, soft, hydrogenated soybean oil and cottonseed oil	1.6
Margarine, soft, hydrogenated soybean boil and palm oil	1.9
Fats and oils—cont'd	
Margarine, soft, soybean oil, hydrogenated soybean oil and hydrogenated cottonseed oil	2.8
Rapeseed oil (canola)	11.1
Rice bran oil	1.6
Salad dressing, commmercial, blue cheese, regular	3.7
Salad dressing, commercial, Italian, regular	3.3
Salad dressing, commercial, mayonnaise (imitation), soybean, without cholesterol	4.6
Salad dressing, commercial, mayonnaise, safflower and soybean	3.0
Salad dressing, commercial, mayonnaise, soybean	4.2
Salad dressing, commercial, mayonnaise-type	2.0
Salad dressing, commercial, Thousand Island, regular	2.5
Salad dressing, home recipe, French	1.9
Salad dressing, home recipe, vinegar and soybean oil	1.4
Shortening, special purpose, for bread, soybean (hydrogenated) and cottonseed	4.0
Shortening, special purpose, heavy-duty, frying, soybean (hydrogenated)	2.4
Soybean lecithin	5.1
Soybean oil	6.8
Walnut oil	10.4
Legumes	
Soybeans, dry	1.6
Nuts and Seeds	
Beechnuts, dried	1.7
Butternuts, dried	1.7
Butternuts, dried	8.7
Chia seeds, dried	3.9
Walnuts, black	3.3
Walnuts, English/Persian	6.8
Vegetables	
Soybeans, green, raw	3.2
Soybeans, mature seeds, sprouted, cooked	2.1

From Hepburn, F.N., Exler, J., and Weihrauch, J.L.: Provisional tables on the content of omega-3 fatty acids and other fat components of selected foods, Journal of the American Dietetic Association 86:788, 1986.

Appendix J

Energy Expenditure in Household, Recreational, and Sports Activities (in kcal × min^{-1})

		Total kcal/min						
Activity	**kcal × min^{-1} × kg^{-1}**	**kg** / **lb**	**50** / **110**	**53** / **117**	**56** / **123**	**59** / **130**	**62** / **137**	**65** / **143**	**68** / **150**
Archery	0.065		3.3	3.4	3.6	3.8	4.0	4.2	4.4
Badminton	0.097		4.9	5.1	5.4	5.7	6.0	6.3	6.6
Bakery, general (F)	0.035		1.8	1.9	2.0	2.1	2.2	2.3	2.4
Basketball	0.138		6.9	7.3	7.7	8.1	8.6	9.0	9.4
Billiards	0.042		2.1	2.2	2.4	2.5	2.6	2.7	2.9
Bookbinding	0.038		1.9	2.0	2.1	2.2	2.4	2.5	2.6
Boxing									
in ring	0.222		6.9	7.3	7.7	8.1	8.6	9.0	9.4
sparring	0.138		11.1	11.8	12.4	13.1	13.8	14.4	15.1
Canoeing									
leisure	0.044		2.2	2.3	2.5	2.6	2.7	2.9	3.0
racing	0.103		5.2	5.5	5.8	6.1	6.4	6.7	7.0
Card playing	0.025		1.3	1.3	1.4	1.5	1.6	1.6	1.7
Carpentry, general	0.052		2.6	2.8	2.9	3.1	3.2	3.4	3.5
Carpet sweeping (F)	0.045		2.3	2.4	2.5	2.7	2.8	2.9	3.1
Carpet sweeping (M)	0.048		2.4	2.5	2.7	2.8	3.0	3.1	3.3
Circuit-training	0.185		9.3	9.8	10.4	10.9	11.5	12.0	12.6
Cleaning (F)	0.062		3.1	3.3	3.5	3.7	3.8	4.0	4.2
Cleaning (M)	0.058		2.9	3.1	3.2	3.4	3.6	3.8	3.9
Climbing hills									
with no load	0.121		6.1	6.4	6.8	7.1	7.5	7.9	8.2
with 5 kg load	0.129		6.5	6.8	7.2	7.6	8.0	8.4	8.8
with 10 kg load	0.140		7.0	7.4	7.8	8.3	8.7	9.1	9.5
with 20 kg load	0.147		7.4	7.8	8.2	8.7	9.1	9.6	10.0
Coal mining									
drilling coal, rock	0.094		4.7	5.0	5.3	5.5	5.8	6.1	6.4
erecting supports	0.088		4.4	4.7	4.9	5.2	5.5	5.7	6.0
shoveling coal	0.108		5.4	5.7	6.0	6.4	6.7	7.0	7.3
Cooking (F)	0.045		2.3	2.4	2.5	2.7	2.8	2.9	3.1
Cooking (M)	0.048		2.4	2.5	2.7	2.8	3.0	3.1	3.3
Cricket									
batting	0.083		4.2	4.4	4.6	4.9	5.1	5.4	5.6
bowling	0.090		4.5	4.8	5.0	5.3	5.6	5.9	6.1
Croquet	0.059		3.0	3.1	3.3	3.5	3.7	3.8	4.0
Cycling									
leisure, 5.5 mph	0.064		3.2	3.4	3.6	3.8	4.0	4.2	4.4
leisure, 9.4 mph	0.100		5.0	5.3	5.6	5.9	6.2	6.5	6.8
racing	0.169		8.5	9.0	9.5	10.0	10.5	11.0	11.5
Dancing									
ballroom	0.051		2.6	2.7	2.9	3.0	3.2	3.3	3.5
choreographed			8.4	8.9	9.4	9.9	10.4	10.9	11.4
"twist," "wiggle"	0.168		5.2	5.5	5.8	6.1	6.4	6.7	7.0
Digging trenches	0.145		7.3	7.7	8.1	8.6	9.0	9.4	9.9
Drawing (standing)	0.036		1.8	1.9	2.0	2.1	2.2	2.3	2.4
Eating (sitting)	0.023		1.2	1.2	1.3	1.4	1.4	1.5	1.6

71 **157**	**74** **163**	**77** **170**	**80** **176**	**83** **183**	**86** **190**	**89** **196**	**92** **203**	**95** **209**	**98** **216**
4.6	4.8	5.0	5.2	5.4	5.6	5.8	6.0	6.2	6.4
6.9	7.2	7.5	7.8	8.1	8.3	8.6	8.9	9.2	9.5
2.5	2.6	2.7	2.8	2.9	3.0	3.1	3.3	3.4	
9.8	10.2	10.6	11.0	11.5	11.9	12.3	12.7	13.1	13.5
3.0	3.1	3.2	3.4	3.5	3.6	3.7	3.9	4.0	4.1
2.7	2.8	2.9	3.0	3.2	3.3	3.4	3.5	3.6	3.7
9.8	10.2	10.6	11.0	11.5	11.9	12.3	12.7	13.1	13.5
15.8	16.4	17.1	17.8	18.4	19.1	19.8	20.4	21.1	21.8
3.1	3.3	3.4	3.5	3.7	3.8	3.9	4.0	4.2	4.3
7.3	7.6	7.9	8.2	8.5	8.9	9.2	9.5	9.8	10.1
1.8	1.9	1.9	2.0	2.1	2.2	2.2	2.3	2.4	2.5
3.7	3.8	4.0	4.2	4.3	4.5	4.6	4.8	4.9	5.1
3.2	3.3	3.5	3.6	3.7	3.9	4.0	4.1	4.3	4.4
3.4	3.6	3.7	3.8	4.0	4.1	4.3	4.4	4.6	4.7
13.1	13.7	14.2	14.8	15.4	15.9	16.5	17.0	17.6	18.1
4.4	4.6	4.8	5.0	5.1	5.3	5.5	5.7	5.9	6.1
4.1	4.3	4.5	4.6	4.8	5.0	5.2	5.3	5.5	5.7
8.6	9.0	9.3	9.7	10.0	10.4	10.8	11.1	11.5	11.9
9.2	9.5	9.9	10.3	10.7	11.1	11.5	11.9	12.3	12.6
9.9	10.4	10.8	11.2	11.6	12.0	12.5	12.9	13.3	13.7
10.4	10.9	11.3	11.8	12.2	12.6	13.1	13.5	14.0	14.4
6.7	7.0	7.2	7.5	7.8	8.1	8.4	8.6	8.9	9.2
6.2	6.5	6.8	7.0	7.3	7.6	7.8	8.1	8.4	8.6
7.7	8.0	8.3	8.6	9.0	9.3	9.6	9.9	10.3	10.6
3.2	3.3	3.5	3.6	3.7	3.9	4.0	4.1	4.3	4.4
3.4	3.6	3.7	3.8	4.0	4.1	4.3	4.4	4.6	4.7
5.9	6.1	6.4	6.6	6.9	7.1	7.4	7.6	7.9	8.1
6.4	6.7	6.9	7.2	7.5	7.7	8.0	8.3	8.6	8.8
4.2	4.4	4.5	4.7	4.9	5.1	5.3	5.4	5.6	5.8
4.5	4.7	4.9	5.1	5.3	5.5	5.7	5.9	6.1	6.3
7.1	7.4	7.7	8.0	8.3	8.6	8.9	9.2	9.5	9.8
12.0	12.5	13.0	13.5	14.0	14.5	15.0	15.5	16.1	16.6
3.6	3.8	3.9	4.1	4.2	4.4	4.5	4.7	4.8	5.0
11.9	12.4	12.9	13.4	13.9	14.4	15.0	15.5	16.0	16.5
7.3	7.6	7.9	8.2	8.5	8.9	9.2	9.5	9.8	10.1
10.3	10.7	11.2	11.6	12.0	12.5	12.9	13.3	13.8	14.2
2.6	2.7	2.8	2.9	3.0	3.1	3.2	3.3	3.4	3.5
1.6	1.7	1.8	1.8	1.9	2.0	2.0	2.1	2.2	2.3

Activity	kcal × min^{-1} × kg^{-1}	kg lb	50 110	53 117	56 123	59 130	62 137	65 143	68 150
Electrical work	0.058		2.9	3.1	3.2	3.4	3.6	3.8	3.9
Farming									
barn cleaning	0.135		6.8	7.2	7.6	8.0	8.4	8.8	9.2
driving harvester	0.040		2.0	2.1	2.2	2.4	2.5	2.6	2.7
driving tractor	0.037		1.9	2.0	2.1	2.2	2.3	2.4	2.5
feeding cattle	0.085		4.3	4.5	4.8	5.0	5.3	5.5	5.8
feeding animals	0.065		3.3	3.4	3.6	3.8	4.0	4.2	4.4
forking straw bales	0.138		6.9	7.3	7.7	8.1	8.6	9.0	9.4
milking by hand	0.054		2.7	2.9	3.0	3.2	3.3	3.5	2.7
milking by machine	0.023		1.2	1.2	1.3	1.4	1.4	1.5	1.6
shoveling grain	0.085		4.3	4.5	4.8	5.0	5.3	5.5	5.8
Field hockey	0.134		6.7	7.1	7.5	7.9	8.3	8.7	9.1
Fishing	0.062		3.1	3.3	3.5	3.7	3.8	4.0	4.2
Food shopping (F)	0.062		3.1	3.3	3.5	3.7	3.8	4.0	4.2
Food shopping (M)	0.058		2.9	3.1	3.2	3.4	3.6	3.8	3.9
Football	0.132		6.6	7.0	7.4	7.8	8.2	8.6	9.0
Forestry									
ax chopping, fast	0.297		14.9	15.7	16.6	17.5	18.4	19.3	20.2
ax chopping, slow	0.085		4.3	4.5	4.8	5.0	5.3	5.5	5.8
barking trees	0.123		6.2	6.5	6.9	7.3	7.6	8.0	8.4
carrying logs	0.186		9.3	9.9	10.4	11.0	11.5	12.1	12.6
felling trees	0.132		6.6	7.0	7.4	7.8	8.1	8.6	9.0
hoeing	0.091		4.6	4.8	5.1	5.4	5.6	5.9	6.2
planting by hand	0.109		5.5	5.8	6.1	6.4	6.8	7.1	7.4
sawing by hand	0.122		6.1	6.5	6.8	7.2	7.6	7.9	8.3
sawing, power	0.075		3.8	4.0	4.2	4.4	4.7	4.9	5.1
stacking firewood	0.088		4.4	4.7	4.9	5.2	5.5	5.7	6.0
trimming trees	0.129		6.5	6.8	7.2	7.6	8.0	8.4	8.8
weeding	0.072		3.6	3.8	4.0	4.2	4.5	4.7	4.9
Furriery	0.083		4.2	4.4	4.6	4.9	5.1	5.4	5.6
Gardening									
digging	0.126		6.3	6.7	7.1	7.4	7.8	8.2	8.6
hedging	0.077		3.9	4.1	4.3	4.5	4.8	5.0	5.2
mowing	0.122		5.6	5.9	6.3	6.6	6.9	7.3	7.6
raking	0.054		2.7	2.9	3.0	3.2	3.3	3.5	3.7
Golf	0.085		4.3	4.5	4.8	5.0	5.3	5.5	5.8
Gymnastics	0.066		3.3	3.5	3.7	3.9	4.1	4.3	4.5
Horse-grooming	0.128		6.4	6.8	7.1	7.6	7.9	8.2	8.7
Horse-racing									
galloping	0.137		6.9	7.3	7.7	8.1	8.5	8.9	9.3
trotting	0.110		5.5	5.8	6.2	6.5	6.8	7.2	7.5
walking	0.041		2.1	2.2	2.3	2.4	2.5	2.7	2.8
Ironing (F)	0.033		1.7	1.7	1.8	1.9	2.0	2.1	2.2
Ironing (M)	0.064		3.2	3.4	3.6	3.8	4.0	4.2	4.4
Judo	0.195		9.8	10.3	10.9	11.5	12.1	12.7	13.3
Knitting, sewing (F)	0.022		1.1	1.2	1.2	1.3	1.4	1.4	1.5
Knitting, sewing (M)	0.023		1.2	1.2	1.3	1.4	1.4	1.5	1.6
Locksmith	0.057		2.9	3.0	3.2	3.4	3.5	3.7	3.9
Lying at ease	0.022		1.1	1.2	1.2	1.3	1.4	1.4	1.5
Machine-tooling									
machining	0.048		2.4	2.5	2.7	2.8	3.0	3.1	3.3
operating lathe	0.052		2.6	2.8	2.9	3.1	3.2	3.4	3.5

71	74	77	80	83	86	89	92	95	98
157	163	170	176	183	190	196	203	209	216
4.1	4.3	4.5	4.6	4.8	5.0	5.2	5.3	5.5	5.7
9.6	10.0	10.4	10.8	11.2	11.6	12.0	12.4	12.8	13.2
2.8	3.0	3.1	3.2	3.3	3.4	3.6	3.7	3.8	3.9
2.6	2.7	2.8	3.0	3.1	3.2	3.3	3.4	3.5	3.6
6.0	6.3	6.5	6.8	7.1	7.3	7.6	7.8	8.1	8.3
4.6	4.8	5.0	5.2	5.4	5.6	5.8	6.0	6.2	6.4
9.8	10.2	10.6	11.0	11.5	11.9	12.3	12.7	13.1	13.5
3.8	4.0	4.2	4.3	4.5	4.6	4.8	5.0	5.1	5.3
1.6	1.7	1.8	1.8	1.9	2.0	2.0	2.1	2.2	2.3
6.0	6.3	6.5	6.8	7.1	7.3	7.6	7.8	8.1	8.3
9.5	9.9	10.3	10.7	11.1	11.5	11.9	12.3	12.7	13.1
4.4	4.6	4.8	5.0	5.1	5.3	5.5	5.7	5.9	6.1
4.4	4.6	4.8	5.0	5.1	5.3	5.5	5.7	5.9	6.1
4.1	4.3	4.5	4.6	4.8	5.0	5.2	5.3	5.5	5.7
9.4	9.8	10.2	10.6	11.0	11.4	11.7	12.1	12.5	12.9
21.1	22.0	22.9	23.8	24.7	25.5	26.4	27.3	28.2	29.1
6.0	6.3	6.5	6.8	7.1	7.3	7.6	7.8	8.1	8.3
8.7	9.1	9.5	9.8	10.2	10.6	10.9	11.3	11.7	12.1
13.2	13.8	14.3	14.9	15.4	16.0	16.6	17.1	17.7	18.2
9.4	9.8	10.2	10.6	11.0	11.4	11.7	12.1	12.5	12.9
6.5	6.7	7.0	7.3	7.6	7.8	8.1	8.4	8.6	8.9
7.7	8.1	8.4	8.7	9.0	9.4	9.7	10.0	10.4	10.7
8.7	9.0	9.4	9.8	10.1	10.5	10.9	11.2	11.6	12.0
5.3	5.6	5.8	6.0	6.2	6.5	6.7	6.9	7.1	7.4
6.2	6.5	6.8	7.0	7.3	7.6	7.8	8.1	8.4	8.6
9.2	9.5	9.9	10.3	10.7	11.1	11.5	11.9	12.3	12.6
5.1	5.3	5.5	5.8	6.0	6.2	6.4	6.6	6.8	7.1
5.9	6.1	6.4	6.6	6.9	7.1	7.4	7.6	7.9	8.1
8.9	9.3	9.7	10.1	10.5	10.8	11.2	11.6	12.0	12.3
5.5	5.7	5.9	6.2	6.4	6.6	6.9	7.1	7.3	7.5
8.0	8.3	8.6	9.0	9.3	9.6	10.0	10.3	10.6	11.0
3.8	4.0	4.2	4.3	4.5	4.6	4.8	5.0	5.1	5.2
6.0	6.3	6.5	6.8	7.1	7.3	7.6	7.8	8.1	8.3
4.7	4.9	5.1	5.3	5.5	5.7	5.9	6.1	6.3	6.6
9.1	9.5	9.9	10.2	10.6	11.0	11.4	11.8	12.2	12.5
9.7	10.1	10.6	11.0	11.4	11.8	12.2	12.6	13.0	13.4
7.8	8.1	8.5	8.8	9.1	9.5	9.8	10.1	10.5	10.8
2.9	3.0	3.2	3.3	3.4	3.5	3.6	3.8	3.9	4.0
2.3	2.4	2.5	2.6	2.7	2.8	2.9	3.0	3.1	3.2
4.5	4.7	4.9	5.1	5.3	5.5	5.7	5.9	6.1	6.3
13.8	14.4	15.0	15.6	16.2	16.8	17.4	17.9	18.5	19.1
1.6	1.6	1.7	1.8	1.8	1.9	2.0	2.0	2.1	2.2
1.6	1.7	1.8	1.8	1.9	2.0	2.0	2.1	2.2	2.3
4.0	4.2	4.4	4.6	4.7	4.9	5.1	5.2	5.4	5.6
1.6	1.6	1.7	1.8	1.8	1.9	2.0	2.0	2.1	2.2
3.4	3.6	3.7	3.8	4.0	4.1	4.3	4.4	4.6	4.7
3.7	3.8	4.0	4.2	4.3	4.5	4.6	4.8	4.9	5.1

Activity	kcal × min^{-1} × kg^{-1}	kg lb	50 110	53 117	56 123	59 130	62 137	65 143	68 150
Machine-tooling—cont'd									
operating punch press	0.088		4.4	4.7	4.9	5.2	5.5	5.7	6.0
tapping and drilling	0.065		3.3	3.4	3.6	3.8	4.0	4.2	4.4
welding	0.052		2.6	2.8	2.9	3.1	3.2	3.4	3.5
working sheet metal	0.048		2.4	2.5	2.7	2.8	3.0	3.1	3.3
Marching, rapid	0.142		7.1	7.5	8.0	8.4	8.8	9.2	9.7
Mopping floor (F)	0.062		3.1	3.3	3.5	3.7	3.8	4.0	4.2
Mopping floor (M)	0.058		2.9	3.1	3.2	3.4	3.6	3.8	3.9
Music playing									
accordion (sitting)	0.032		1.6	1.7	1.8	1.9	2.0	2.1	2.2
cello (sitting)	0.041		2.1	2.2	2.3	2.4	2.5	2.7	2.8
conducting	0.039		2.0	2.1	2.2	2.3	2.4	2.5	2.7
drums (saitting)	0.066		3.3	3.5	3.7	3.9	4.1	4.3	4.5
flute (sitting)	0.035		1.8	1.9	2.0	2.1	2.2	2.3	2.4
horn (sitting)	0.029		1.5	1.5	1.6	1.7	1.8	1.9	2.0
organ (sitting)	0.053		2.7	2.8	3.0	3.1	3.3	3.4	3.6
piano (sitting)	0.040		2.0	2.1	2.2	2.4	2.5	2.6	2.7
trumpet (standing)	0.031		1.6	1.6	1.7	1.8	1.9	2.0	2.1
violin (sitting)	0.045		2.3	2.4	2.5	2.7	2.8	2.9	3.1
woodwind (sitting)	0.032		1.6	1.7	1.8	1.9	2.0	2.1	2.2
Painting, inside	0.034		1.7	1.8	1.9	2.0	2.1	2.2	2.3
Painting, outside	0.077		3.9	4.1	4.3	4.5	4.8	5.0	5.2
Planting seedings	0.070		3.5	3.7	3.9	4.1	4.3	4.6	4.8
Plastering	0.078		3.9	4.1	4.4	4.6	4.8	5.1	5.3
Printing	0.035		1.8	1.9	2.0	2.1	2.2	2.3	2.4
Running, cross-country	0.163		8.2	8.6	9.1	9.6	10.1	10.6	11.1
Running, horizontal									
11 min, 30 s per mile	0.135		6.8	7.2	7.6	8.0	8.4	8.8	9.2
9 min per mile	0.093		9.7	10.2	10.8	11.4	12.0	12.5	13.1
8 min per mile	0.208		10.8	11.3	11.9	12.5	13.1	13.6	14.2
7 min per mile	0.228		12.2	12.7	13.3	13.9	14.5	15.0	15.6
6 min per mile	0.252		13.9	14.4	15.0	15.6	16.2	16.7	17.3
5 min, 30 s per mile	0.289		14.5	15.3	16.2	17.1	17.9	18.8	19.7
Scraping paint	0.063		3.2	3.3	3.5	3.7	3.9	4.1	4.3
Scrubbing floors (F)	0.109		5.5	5.8	6.1	6.4	6.8	7.1	7.4
Scrubbing floors (M)	0.108		5.4	5.7	6.0	6.4	6.7	7.0	7.3
Shoe repair, general	0.045		2.3	2.4	2.5	2.7	2.8	2.9	3.1
Sitting quietly	0.021		1.1	1.1	1.2	1.2	1.3	1.4	1.4
Skiing, hard snow									
level, moderate speed	0.119		6.0	6.3	6.7	7.0	7.4	7.7	8.1
level, walking	0.143		7.2	7.6	8.0	8.4	8.9	9.3	9.7
uphill, maximum speed	0.274		13.7	14.5	15.3	16.2	17.0	17.8	18.6
Skiing, soft snow									
leisure (F)	0.111		4.9	5.2	5.5	5.8	6.1	6.4	6.7
leisure (M)	0.098		5.6	5.9	6.2	6.5	6.9	7.2	7.5
Skindiving, as frogman									
considerable motion	0.276		13.8	14.6	15.5	16.3	17.1	17.9	18.8

71 **157**	**74** **163**	**77** **170**	**80** **176**	**83** **183**	**86** **190**	**89** **196**	**92** **203**	**95** **209**	**98** **216**
6.2	6.5	6.8	7.0	7.3	7.6	7.8	8.1	8.4	8.6
4.6	4.8	5.0	5.2	5.4	5.6	5.8	6.0	6.2	6.4
3.7	3.8	4.0	4.2	4.3	4.5	4.6	4.8	4.9	5.1
3.4	3.6	3.7	3.8	4.0	4.1	4.3	4.4	4.6	4.7
10.1	10.5	10.9	11.4	11.8	12.2	12.6	13.1	13.5	13.9
4.4	4.6	4.8	5.0	5.1	5.3	5.5	5.7	5.9	6.1
4.1	4.3	4.5	4.6	4.8	5.0	5.2	5.	5.5	5.7
2.3	2.4	2.5	2.6	2.7	2.8	2.8	2.9	3.0	3.1
2.9	3.0	3.2	3.3	3.4	3.5	3.6	3.8	3.9	4.0
2.8	2.9	3.0	3.1	3.2	3.4	3.5	3.6	3.7	3.8
4.7	4.9	5.1	5.3	5.5	5.7	5.9	6.1	6.3	6.6
2.5	2.6	2.7	2.8	2.9	3.0	3.1	3.2	3.3	3.4
2.1	2.1	2.2	2.3	2.4	2.5	2.6	2.7	2.8	2.8
3.8	3.9	4.1	4.2	4.4	4.6	4.7	4.9	5.0	5.2
2.8	3.0	3.1	3.2	3.3	3.4	3.6	3.7	3.8	3.9
2.2	2.3	2.4	2.5	2.6	2.7	2.8	2.9	1.9	2.0
3.2	3.3	3.5	3.6	3.7	3.9	4.0	4.1	4.3	4.4
2.3	2.4	2.5	2.6	2.7	2.8	2.8	2.9	3.0	3.1
2.4	2.5	2.6	2.7	2.8	2.9	3.0	3.1	3.2	3.3
5.5	5.7	5.9	6.2	6.4	6.6	6.9	7.1	7.3	7.5
5.0	5.2	5.4	5.6	5.8	6.0	6.2	6.4	6.7	6.9
5.5	5.8	6.0	6.2	6.5	6.7	6.9	7.2	7.4	7.6
2.5	2.6	2.7	2.8	2.9	3.0	3.1	3.2	3.3	3.4
11.6	12.1	12.6	13.0	13.5	14.0	14.5	15.0	15.5	16.0
9.6	10.0	10.5	10.9	11.3	11.7	12.1	12.5	12.9	13.3
13.7	14.3	14.9	15.4	16.0	16.6	17.2	17.8	18.3	18.9
14.8	15.4	16.0	16.5	17.1	17.7	18.3	18.9	19.4	20.0
16.2	16.8	17.4	17.9	18.5	19.1	19.7	20.3	20.8	21.4
17.9	18.5	19.1	19.6	20.2	20.8	21.4	22.0	22.5	23.1
20.5	21.4	22.3	23.1	24.0	24.9	25.7	26.6	27.5	28.3
4.5	4.7	4.9	5.0	5.2	5.4	5.6	5.8	6.0	6.2
7.7	8.1	8.4	8.7	9.0	9.4	9.7	10.0	10.4	10.7
7.7	8.0	8.3	8.6	9.0	9.3	9.6	9.9	10.3	10.6
3.2	3.3	3.5	3.6	3.7	3.9	4.0	4.1	4.3	4.4
1.5	1.6	1.6	1.7	1.7	1.8	1.9	1.9	2.0	2.1
8.4	8.8	9.2	9.5	9.9	10.2	10.6	10.9	11.3	11.7
10.2	10.6	11.0	11.4	11.9	12.3	12.7	13.2	13.6	14.0
19.5	20.3	21.1	21.9	22.7	23.6	24.4	25.2	26.0	26.9
					—				
7.0	7.3	7.5	7.8	8.1	8.4	8.7	9.0	9.3	9.6
7.9	8.2	8.5	8.9	9.2	9.5	9.9	10.2	10.5	10.9
19.6	20.4	21.3	22.1	22.9	23.7	24.6	25.4	26.2	27.0

Activity	kcal × min^{-1} × kg^{-1}	kg / lb	50 / 110	53 / 117	56 / 123	59 / 130	62 / 137	65 / 143	68 / 150
Skindiving, as frogman—cont'd									
moderate motion	0.206		10.3	10.9	11.5	12.2	12.8	13.4	14.0
Snowshoeing, soft snow	0.166		8.3	8.8	9.3	9.8	10.3	10.8	11.3
Squash	0.212		10.6	11.2	11.9	12.5	13.1	13.8	14.4
Standing quietly (F)	0.025		1.3	1.3	1.4	1.5	1.6	1.6	1.7
Standing quietly (M)	0.027		1.4	1.4	1.5	1.6	1.7	1.8	1.8
Steel mill, working in									
fettling	0.089		4.5	4.7	5.0	5.3	5.5	5.8	6.1
forging	0.100		5.0	5.3	5.6	5.9	6.2	6.5	6.8
hand rolling	0.137		6.9	7.3	7.7	8.1	8.5	8.9	9.3
merchant mill rolling	0.145		7.3	7.7	8.1	8.6	9.0	9.4	9.9
removing slag	0.178		8.9	9.4	10.0	10.5	11.0	11.6	12.1
tending furnace	0.126		6.3	6.7	7.1	7.4	7.8	8.2	8.6
tipping molds	0.092		4.6	4.9	5.2	5.4	5.7	6.0	6.3
Stock clerking	0.054		2.7	2.9	3.0	3.2	3.3	3.5	3.7
Swimming									
backstroke	0.169		8.5	9.0	9.5	10.0	10.5	11.0	11.5
breast stroke	0.162		8.1	8.6	9.1	9.6	10.0	10.5	11.0
crawl, fast	0.156		7.8	8.3	8.7	9.2	9.7	10.1	10.6
crawl, slow	0.128		6.4	6.8	7.2	7.6	7.9	8.3	8.7
side stroke	0.122		6.1	6.5	6.8	7.2	7.6	7.9	8.3
treading, fast	0.170		8.5	9.0	9.5	10.0	10.5	11.1	11.6
treading, normal	0.062		3.1	3.3	3.5	3.7	3.8	4.0	4.2
Table tennis	0.068		3.4	3.6	3.8	4.0	4.2	4.4	4.6
Tailoring									
cutting	0.041		2.1	2.2	2.3	2.4	2.5	2.7	2.8
hand-sewing	0.032		1.6	1.7	1.8	1.9	2.0	2.1	2.2
maching sewing	0.045		2.3	2.4	2.5	2.7	2.8	2.9	3.1
pressing	0.062		3.1	3.3	3.5	3.7	3.8	4.0	4.2
Tennis	0.109		5.5	5.8	6.1	6.4	6.8	7.1	7.4
Typing									
electric	0.027		1.4	1.4	1.5	1.6	1.7	1.8	1.8
manual	0.031		1.6	1.6	1.7	1.8	1.9	2.0	2.1
Volleyball	0.050		2.5	2.7	2.8	3.0	3.1	3.3	3.4
Walking, normal pace									
asphalt road	0.080		4.0	4.2	4.5	4.7	5.0	5.1	5.4
fields and hillsides	0.082		4.1	4.3	4.6	4.8	5.1	5.3	5.6
grass track	0.081		4.1	4.3	4.5	4.8	5.0	5.3	5.5
plowed field	0.077		3.9	4.1	4.3	4.5	4.8	5.0	5.2
Wallpapering	0.048		2.4	2.5	2.7	2.8	3.0	3.1	3.3
Watch repairing	0.025		1.3	1.3	1.4	1.5	1.6	1.6	1.7
Window cleaning (F)	0.059		3.0	3.1	3.3	3.5	3.7	3.8	4.0
Window cleaning (M)	0.058		2.9	3.1	3.2	3.4	3.6	3.8	3.9
Writing (sitting)	0.029		1.5	1.5	1.6	1.7	1.8	1.9	2.0

*Data from E.W. Bannister and S.R. Brown: The relative energy requirements of physical activity in H.B. Falls, ed., *Exercise Physiology,* Academic Press, New York; 1968; E.T. Howley and M.E. Glover, The Caloric costs of running and walking one mile for men and women, *Medicine and Science in Sports* 6:235, 1974; R. Passmore and J.V.G.A. Durnin, Human energy expenditure, *Physiologic Reviews* 35:801, 1955.

Note: Symbols (M) and (F) denote experiments for males and females, respectively.

From Katch and McArdle: Nutrition, weight control and exercise, 1983, Lea & Febiger.

71	**74**	**77**	**80**	**83**	**86**	**89**	**92**	**95**	**98**
157	**163**	**170**	**176**	**183**	**190**	**196**	**203**	**209**	**216**
14.6	15.2	15.9	16.5	17.1	17.7	18.3	19.0	19.6	20.2
11.8	12.3	12.8	13.3	13.8	14.3	14.8	15.3	15.8	16.2
15.1	15.7	16.3	17.0	17.6	18.2	18.9	19.5	20.1	20.8
1.8	1.9	1.9	2.0	2.1	2.2	2.2	2.3	2.4	2.5
1.9	2.0	2.1	2.2	2.2	2.3	2.4	2.5	2.6	2.6
6.3	6.6	6.9	7.1	7.4	7.7	7.9	8.2	8.5	8.7
7.1	7.4	7.7	8.0	8.3	8.6	8.9	9.2	9.5	9.8
9.7	10.1	10.6	11.0	11.4	11.8	12.2	12.6	13.0	13.4
10.3	10.7	11.2	11.6	12.0	12.5	12.9	13.3	13.8	14.2
12.6	13.2	13.7	14.2	14.8	15.3	15.8	16.4	16.9	17.4
8.9	9.3	9.7	10.1	10.5	10.8	11.2	11.6	12.0	12.3
6.5	6.8	7.1	7.4	7.6	7.9	8.3	8.5	8.7	9.0
3.8	4.0	4.2	4.3	4.5	4.6	4.8	5.0	5.1	5.3
12.0	12.5	13.0	13.5	14.0	14.5	15.0	15.5	16.1	16.6
11.5	12.0	12.5	13.0	13.4	13.9	14.4	14.9	15.4	15.9
11.1	11.5	12.0	12.5	12.9	13.4	13.9	14.4	14.8	15.3
9.1	9.5	9.9	10.2	10.6	11.0	11.4	11.8	12.2	12.5
8.7	9.0	9.4	9.8	10.1	10.5	10.9	11.2	11.6	12.0
12.1	12.6	13.1	13.6	14.1	14.6	15.1	15.6	16.2	16.7
4.4	4.6	4.8	5.0	5.1	5.3	5.5	5.7	5.9	6.1
4.8	5.0	5.2	5.4	5.6	5.8	6.1	6.3	6.5	6.7
2.9	3.0	3.2	3.3	3.4	3.5	3.6	3.8	3.9	4.0
2.3	2.4	2.5	2.6	2.7	2.8	2.8	2.9	3.0	3.1
3.2	3.3	3.5	3.6	3.7	3.9	4.0	4.1	4.3	4.4
4.4	4.6	4.8	5.0	5.1	5.3	5.5	5.7	5.9	6.1
7.7	8.1	8.4	8.7	9.0	9.4	9.7	10.0	10.4	10.7
1.9	2.0	2.1	2.2	2.2	2.3	2.4	2.5	2.6	2.6
2.2	2.3	2.4	2.5	2.6	2.7	2.8	2.9	2.9	3.0
3.6	3.7	3.9	4.0	4.2	4.3	4.5	4.6	4.8	4.9
5.7	5.9	6.2	6.4	6.6	6.9	7.1	7.4	7.6	7.8
5.8	6.1	6.3	6.6	6.8	7.1	7.3	7.5	7.8	8.0
5.8	6.0	6.2	6.5	6.7	7.0	7.2	7.5	7.7	7.9
5.5	5.7	5.9	6.2	6.4	6.6	6.9	7.1	7.3	7.5
3.4	3.6	3.7	3.8	4.0	4.1	4.3	4.4	4.6	4.7
1.8	1.9	1.9	2.0	2.1	2.2	2.2	2.3	2.4	2.5
4.2	4.4	4.5	4.7	4.9	5.1	5.3	5.4	5.6	5.8
4.1	4.3	4.5	4.6	4.8	5.0	5.2	5.3	5.5	5.7
2.1	2.1	2.2	2.3	2.4	2.5	2.6	2.7	2.8	2.8

Appendix K
Metabolic Pathways

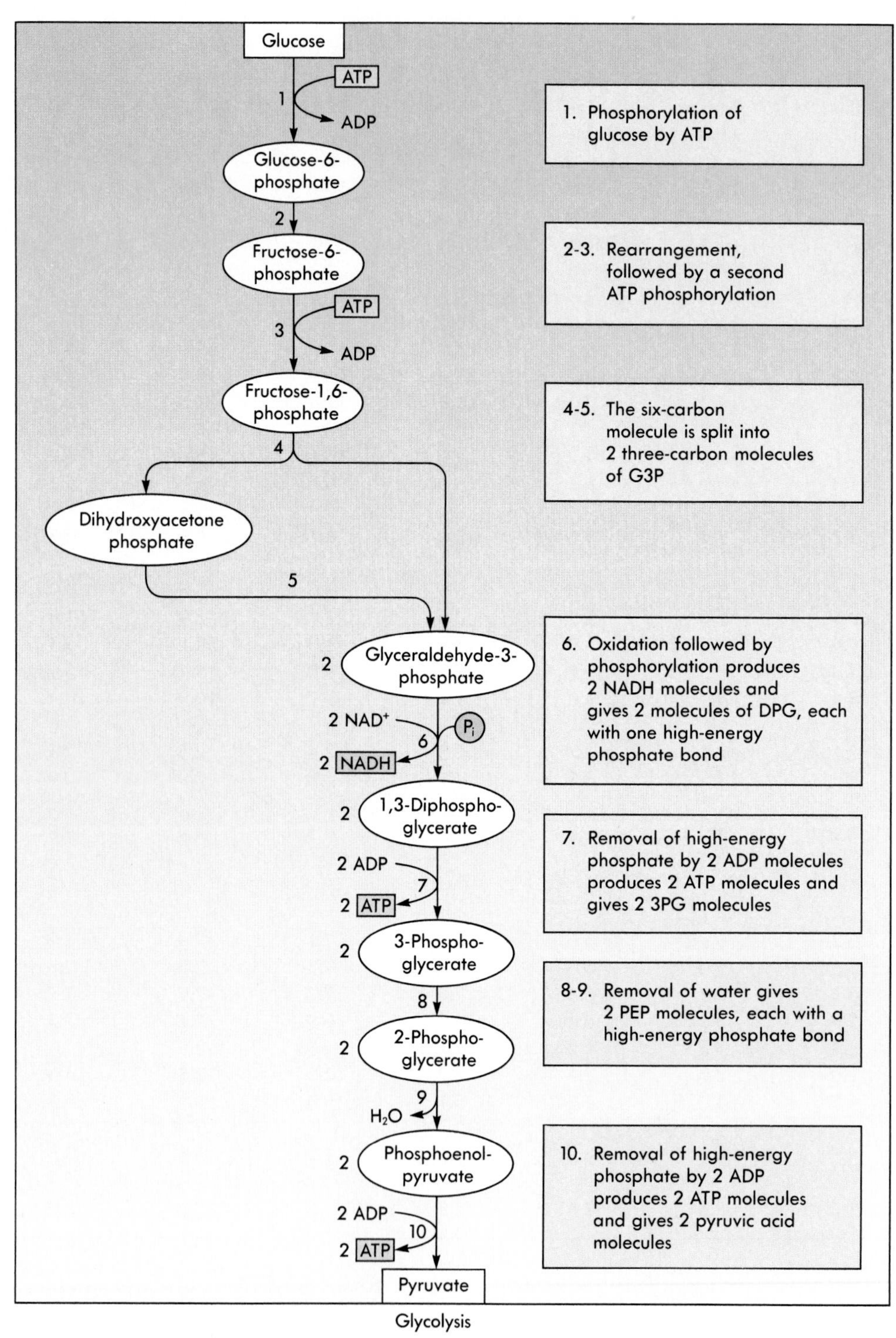

Glycolysis

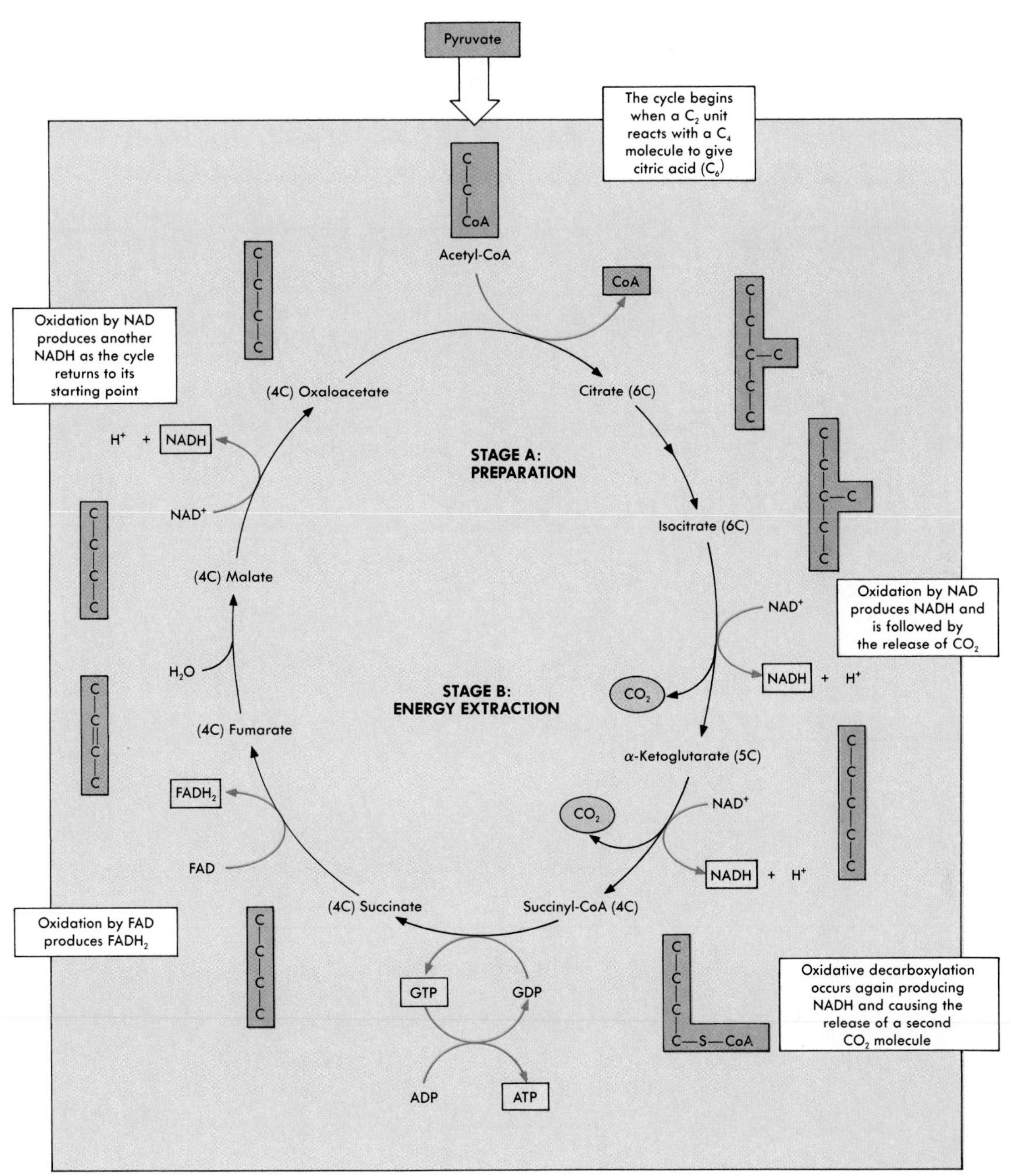

The citric acid cycle

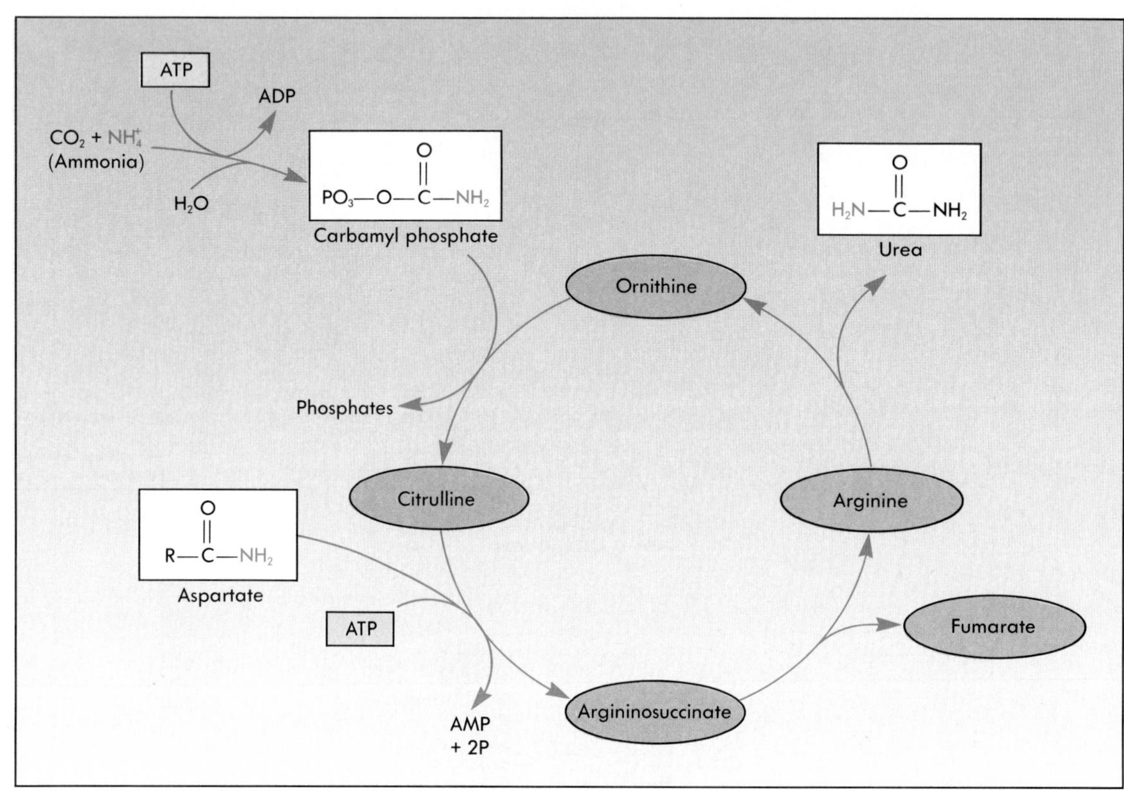

The urea cycle

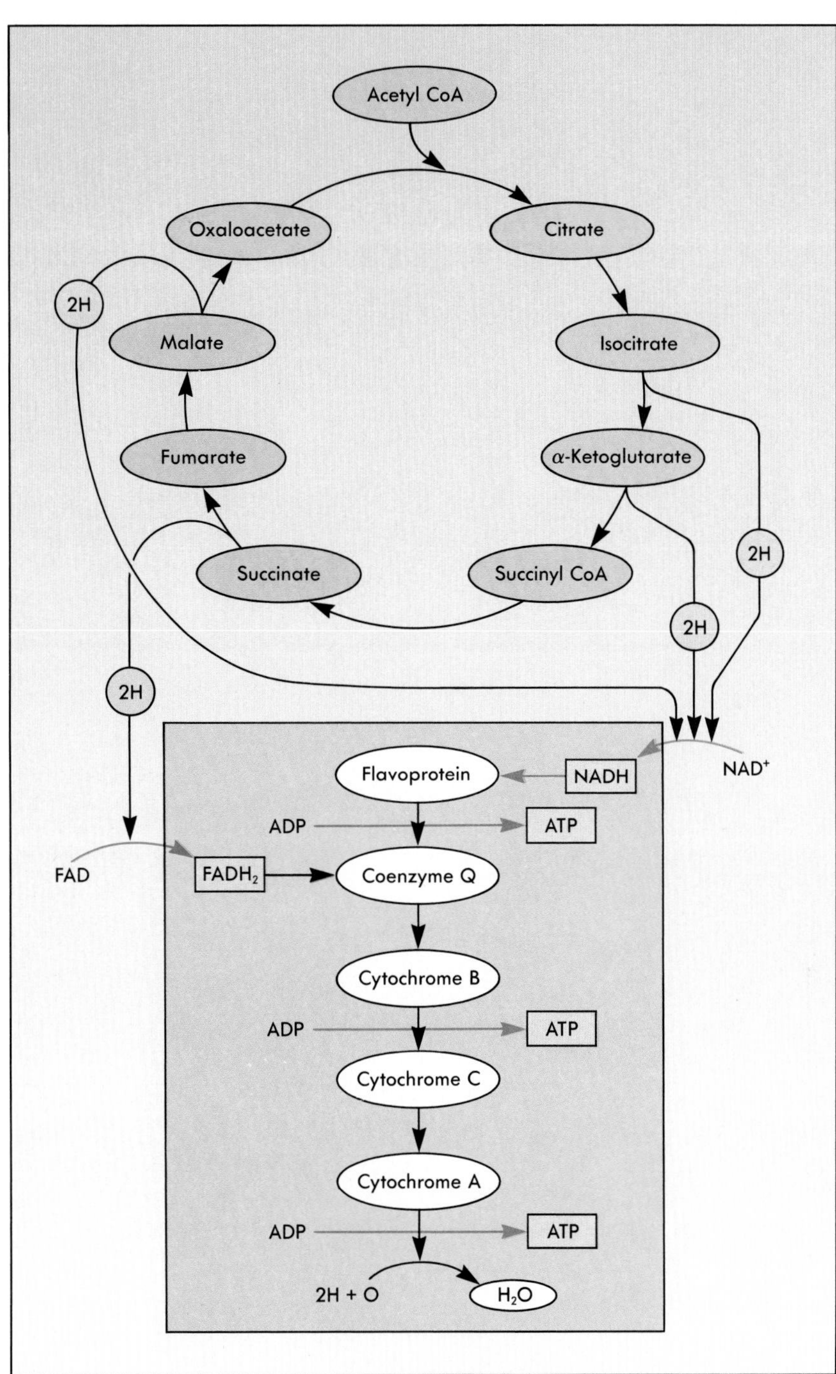

The electron transport chain

Appendix L
Height-Weight Tables

1983 Metropolitan Life Insurance Company height-weight table in metric units

	Males				Females		
Height (cm)	Small frame (kg)	Medium frame (kg)	Large frame (kg)	Height (cm)	Small frame (kg)	Medium frame (kg)	Large frame (kg)
157.5	58.2—60.9	59.4—64.1	62.7—68.2	147.5	46.4—50.5	49.5—55.0	53.6—59.5
160	59.1—61.8	60.5—65.0	63.6—69.5	150	46.8—51.4	50.5—55.9	54.5—60.9
162.5	60.0—62.7	61.4—65.9	64.5—70.9	152.5	47.3—52.3	51.4—57.3	55.5—62.3
165	60.9—63.7	62.3—67.3	65.5—72.7	155	48.2—53.6	52.3—58.6	56.8—63.6
167.5	61.8—64.5	63.2—68.6	66.4—74.5	157.5	49.1—55.0	53.6—60.0	58.2—65.0
170	62.7—65.9	64.5—70.0	67.7—76.4	160	50.5—56.4	55.0—61.4	59.5—66.8
173	63.6—67.3	65.9—71.4	69.1—78.2	162.5	51.8—57.7	56.4—62.7	60.9—68.6
175	64.5—68.6	67.3—72.7	70.5—80.0	165	53.2—59.1	57.7—64.1	62.3—70.5
178	65.4—70.0	68.6—74.1	71.8—81.8	167.5	54.5—60.5	59.1—65.5	63.6—72.3
180	66.4—71.4	70.0—75.5	73.2—83.6	170	55.9—61.8	60.5—66.8	65.0—74.1
183	67.7—72.7	71.4—77.3	74.5—85.6	173	57.3—63.2	61.8—68.2	66.4—75.9
185.5	69.1—74.5	72.7—79.1	76.4—87.3	175	58.6—64.5	63.2—69.5	67.7—77.3
188	70.5—76.4	74.5—80.9	78.2—89.5	178	60.0—65.9	64.5—70.9	69.1—78.6
190.5	71.8—78.2	75.9—82.7	80.0—91.8	180	61.4—67.3	65.9—72.3	70.5—80.0
193	73.6—80.0	77.7—85.0	82.3—94.1	183	62.3—68.6	67.3—73.6	71.8—81.4

Andres table for adults and the elderly—age-specific weight-for-height tables* (Gerontology Research Center)

Height	Weight range for men and women by age (years) in pounds†				
	25	35	45	55	65
ft—in					
4—10	84—111	92—119	99—127	107—135	115—142
4—11	87—115	95—123	103—131	111—139	119—147
5—0	90—119	98—127	106—135	114—143	123—152
5—1	93—123	101—131	110—140	118—148	127—157
5—2	96—127	105—136	113—144	122—153	131—163
5—3	99—131	108—140	117—149	126—158	135—168
5—4	102—135	112—145	121—154	130—163	140—173
5—5	106—140	115—149	125—159	134—168	144—179
5—6	109—144	119—154	129—164	138—174	148—184
5—7	112—148	122—159	133—169	143—179	153—190
5—8	116—153	126—163	137—174	147—184	158—196
5—9	119—157	130—168	141—179	151—190	162—201
5—10	122—162	134—173	145—184	156—195	167—207
5—11	126—167	137—178	149—190	160—201	172—213
6—0	129—171	141—183	153—195	165—207	177—219
6—1	133—176	145—188	157—200	169—213	182—225
6—2	137—181	149—194	162—206	174—219	187—232
6—3	141—186	153—199	166—212	179—225	192—238
6—4	144—191	157—205	171—218	184—231	197—244

*Values in this table are in pounds for height without shoes and weight without clothes. To convert inches to centimeters, multiply by 2.54; to convert pounds to kilograms, multiply by 0.455. †Data from Andres R: Gerontology Research Center, National Institute of Aging, Baltimore, Md.

Desireable weights* for men and women aged 20 to 74 years by height: United States, 1971-74, HANES, 1979

Height (inches)†	Weight (pounds)	
	Men	Women
57	—	113
58	—	117
59	—	120
60	—	123
61	—	127
62	136	130
63	140	134
64	145	137
65	150	140
66	155	144
67	159	147
68	163	151
69	168	154
70	173	158
71	178	—
72	182	—
73	187	—
74	192	—

*Based on average weights estimated from regression equation of weight on height for men and women aged 20 to 29 years. †Height measured without shoes. Clothing ranged from 0.20 to 0.62 pounds, which was not deducted from weight shown.

A quick way to determine body mass index (BMI)

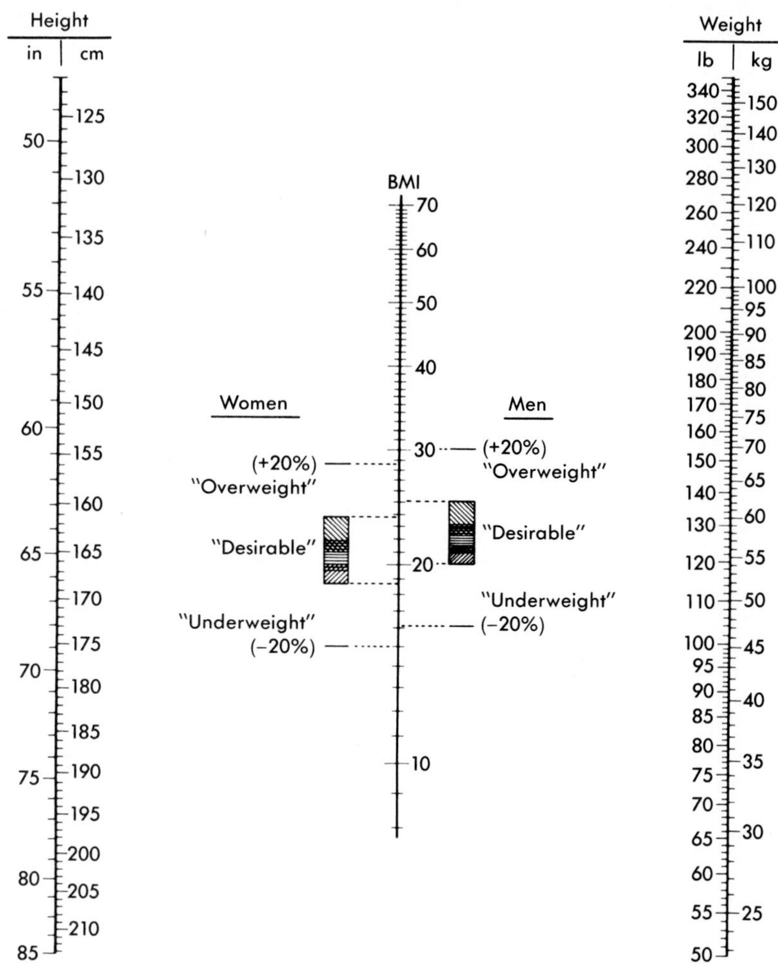

Nomograph for body mass index (kg/m^2). The ratio weight/height^2 is read from the central scale. The ranges suggested as "desirable" are from life insurance data.

*From Thomas AE, McKay DA, and Cutlip MB: Am J Clin Nutr 29:302, 304, 1976.

Appendix M
Estimating Energy Needs

Harris-Benedict Equations

Women:

$655 + 9.56 \times$ weight (in kilograms) $+ 1.85 \times$ height (in centimeters) $- 4.68 \times$ age (in years)

Men:

$66.5 + 13.8 \times$ weight (in kilograms) $+ 5 \times$ height (in centimeters) $- 6.76 \times$ age (in years)

Owen equations

Women:

$795 + 7.18 \times$ weight (in kilograms)

Men:

$879 + 10.2 \times$ weight (in kilograms)

Boothby and Berkson nomogram for estimation of caloric requirements

Food nomogram

Directions for Estimating Caloric Requirement: To determine the desired allowance of calories, proceed as follows: 1. Locate the ideal weight on Column 1 by means of a common pin. 2. Bring edge of one end of a 12- or 15-inch ruler against the pin. 3. Swing the other end of the ruler to the patient's height on Column II. 4. Transfer the pin to the point where the ruler crosses Column III. 5. Hold the ruler against the pin in Column III. 6. Swing the left hand end of the ruler to the patient's sex and age (measured from last birthday) given in Column IV (these positions correspond to the Mayo Clinic's metabolism standards for age and sex). 7. Transfer the pin to the point where the ruler crosses Column V. This gives the basal caloric requirement (basal calories) of the patient for 24 hours and represents the calories required by the fasting patient when resting in bed. 8. To provide the extra calories for activity and work, the basal calories are increased by a percentage. To the basal calories for adults add: 50 to 80 percent for manual laborers, 30 to 40 percent for light work or 10 to 20 percent for restricted activity such as resting in a room or in bed. To the basal calories for children add 50 to 100 percent for children ages 5 to 15 years. This computation may be done by simple arithmetic or by the use of Columns VI and VII. If the latter method is chosen, locate the "percent above or below basal" desired in Column VI. By means of the ruler connect this point with the pin on Column V. Transfer the pin to the point where the ruler crosses Column VII. This represents the calories estimated to be required by the patient.

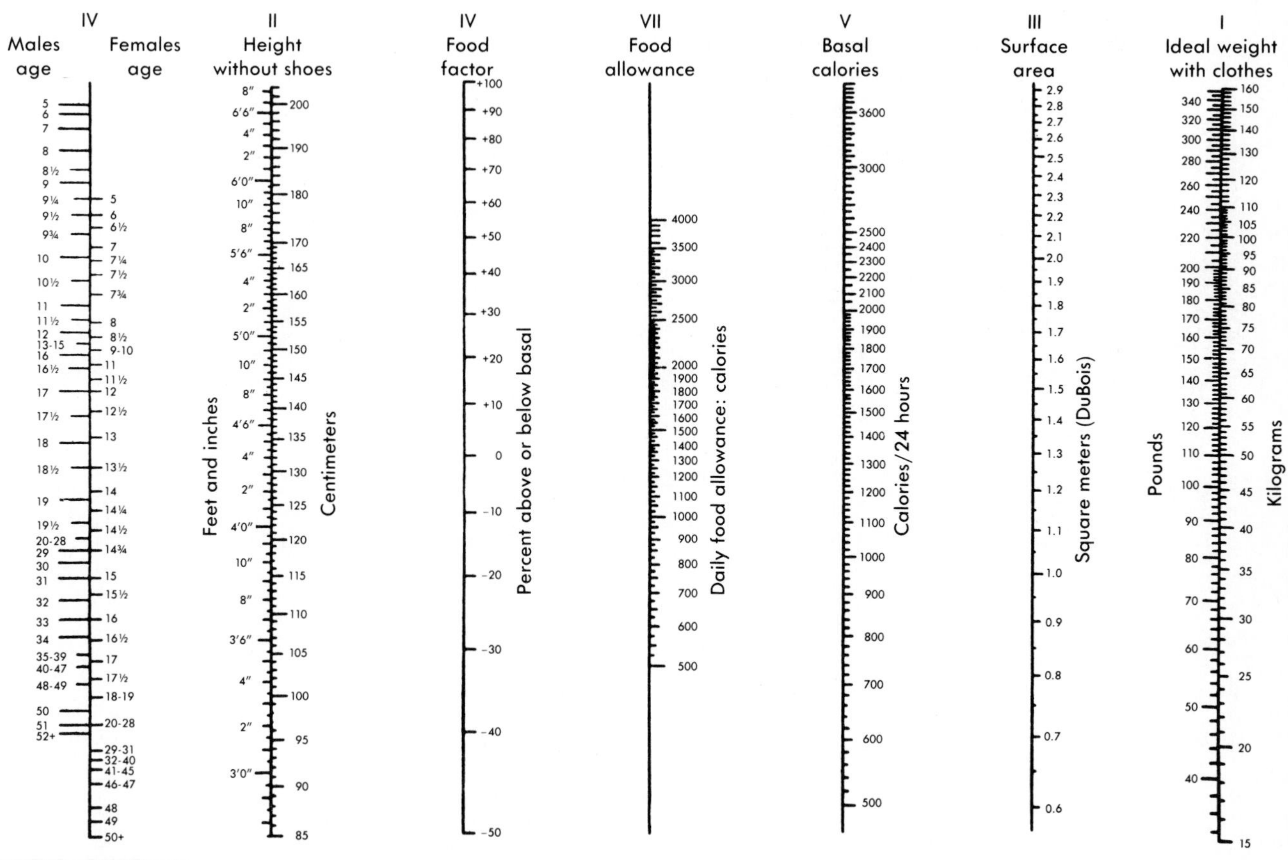

The error in some published versions of the nomogram devised by Boothby and Sandiford for determining body surface area (see Turcotte G. Erroneous nomograms for body surface area [letter to the editor]. N Engl J Med 1979;300:1339), does not occur in this nomogram.

Appendix N
Nutrient Conversion Formulas for Vitamins A and E

Formulas for converting forms of vitamin A into retinol equivalents (REs)

1. If retinol and beta-carotene are given in micrograms,

$$\mu\text{g retinol} + \frac{\mu\text{g beta-carotene}}{6} = \text{RE}$$

2. If retinol and beta-carotene are given in IUs,

$$\frac{\text{IU retinol}}{3.3} + \frac{\text{IU beta-carotene}}{10} = \text{RE}$$

3. If beta-carotene and other carotenoids are given in μg,

$$\frac{\mu\text{g beta-carotene}}{6} + \frac{\mu\text{g other carotenoids}}{12} = \text{RE}$$

4. If retinol, beta-carotene, and other carotenoids are given in μg,

$$\mu\text{g retinol} + \frac{\mu\text{g beta-carotene}}{6} + \frac{\mu\text{g carotenoids}}{12} = \text{RE}$$

Formula for converting forms of vitamin E into alpha-tocopherol equivalents

Alpha-tocopherol equivalents = mg alpha-tocopherol
+ mg beta-tocopherol/2
+ mg gamma-tocopherol/10
+ mg alpha-tocotrienol/3.3

Appendix O

An Example of Prenatal Vitamin/Mineral Supplements and Prenatal Weight Gain Chart

Natalins® Rx

INGREDIENTS	NATALINES RX	
Vitamins	**Units**	**%RDA**
Vitamin A, IU	8000	100
Vitamin D, IU	400	100
Vitamin E, IU	30	100
Vitamin C, mg	90	150
Folic Acid, mg	1	125
Thiamin (B_1), mg	2.55	150
Riboflavin (B_2), mg	3	150
Niacin, mg	20	100
Vitamin B_6, mg	10	400
Vitamin B_{12}, mcg	8	100
Biotin, mg	0.05	16
Pantothenic Acid, mg	15	150
Minerals		
Calcium, mg	200	15
Iodine, mcg	150	100
Iron, mg	60	333
Magnesium, mg	100	22
Copper, mg	2	100
Zinc, mg	15	100
Artificial color	none	
Artificial flavor	none	

Natalins Rx is a multivitamin, multimineral supplement for pregnant or lactating women. Daily dose: 1 tablet or as prescribed.

Contraindications: Natalins Rx should not be prescribed in patients with hemochromatosis or patients with Wilson's disease.

Caution: Pernicious anemia should be excluded before using this product. In patients with kidney stones, the calcium content of Natalins Rx tablets should be considered before prescribing.

From: Mead Johnson & Company

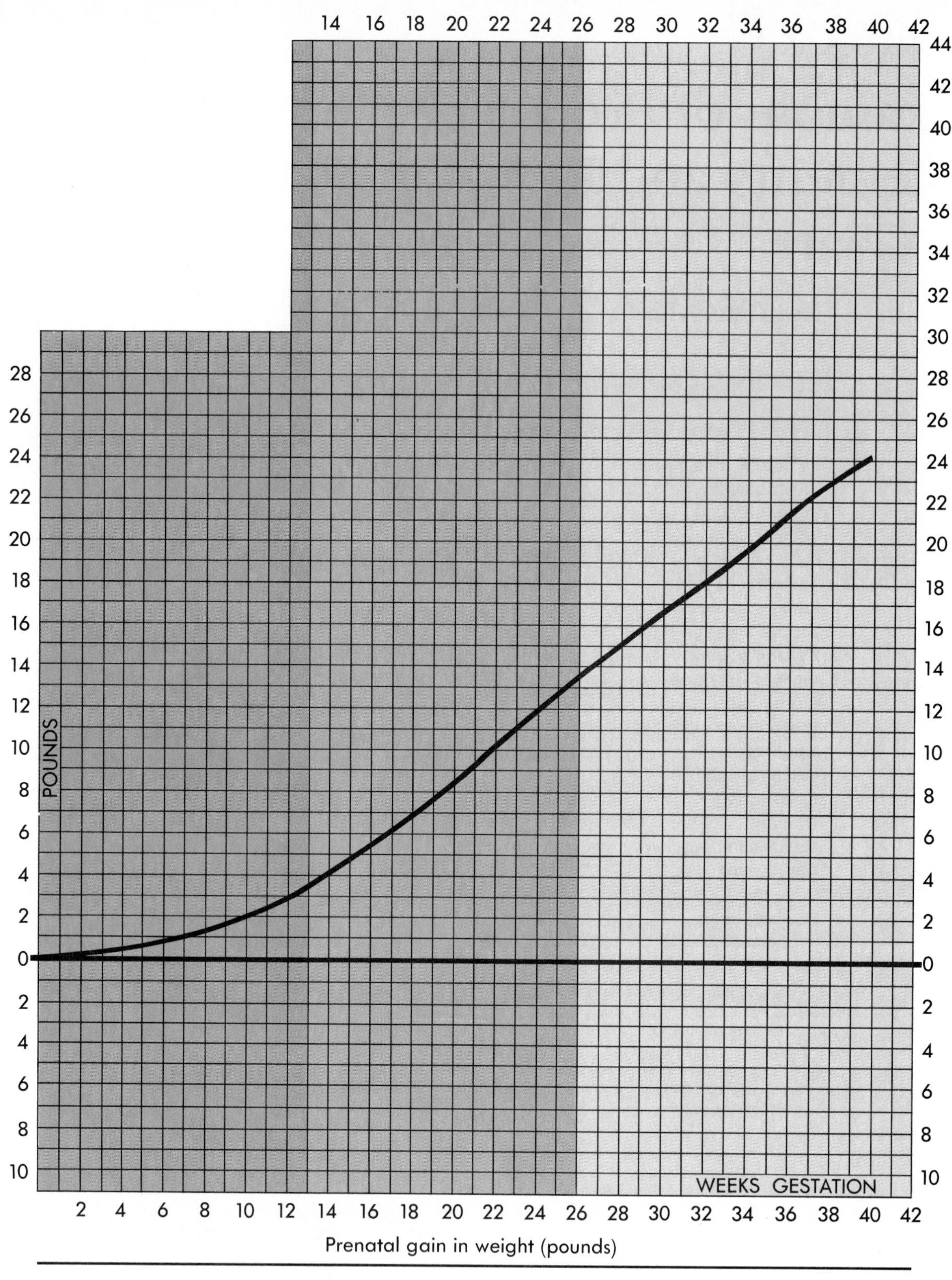

Immediate pregravid weight: ______________

Height in inches without shoes (plus one inch): ______________

Standard weight: ______________

(Record weight *with* shoes) ______________

Appendix P

Infant and Child Growth Charts

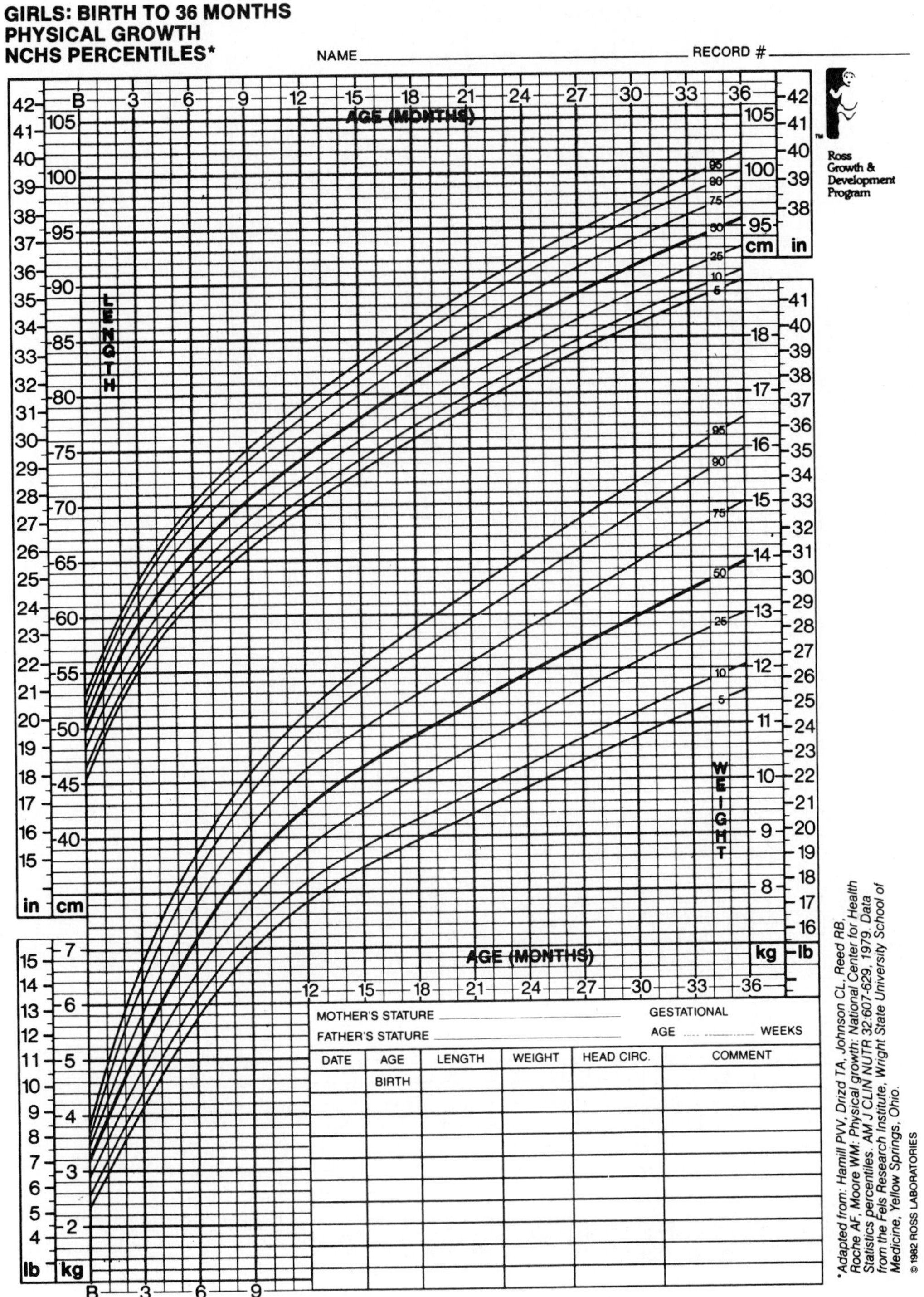

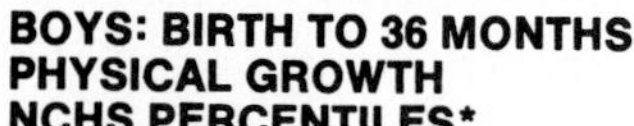

BOYS: BIRTH TO 36 MONTHS
PHYSICAL GROWTH
NCHS PERCENTILES*

NAME ______________________ RECORD # ______________

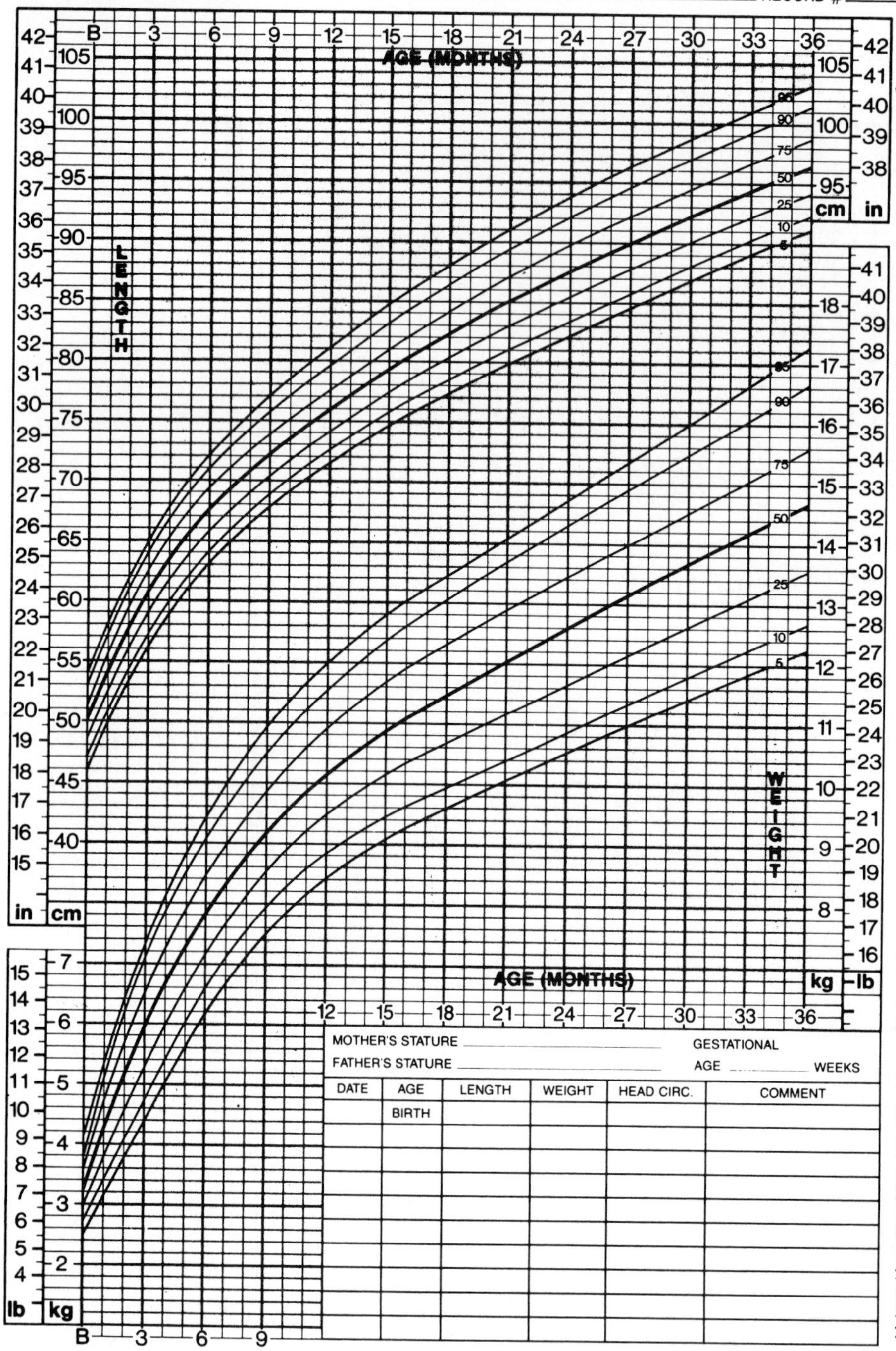

MOTHER'S STATURE ______________ GESTATIONAL
FATHER'S STATURE ______________ AGE ______ WEEKS

DATE	AGE	LENGTH	WEIGHT	HEAD CIRC.	COMMENT
	BIRTH				

*Adapted from: Hamill PVV, Drizd TA, Johnson CL, Reed RB, Roche AF, Moore WM: Physical growth: National Center for Health Statistics percentiles. AM J CLIN NUTR 32:607-629, 1979. Data from the Fels Research Institute, Wright State University School of Medicine, Yellow Springs, Ohio.

GIRLS: BIRTH TO 36 MONTHS
PHYSICAL GROWTH
NCHS PERCENTILES*

NAME __________ RECORD # __________

AGE (MONTHS): B 3 6 9 12 15 18 21 24 27 30 33 36

HEAD CIRCUMFERENCE

LENGTH: cm 50 55 60 65 70 75 80 85 90 95 100; in 19 20 21 22 23 24 25 26 27 28 29 30 31 32 33 34 35 36 37 38 39 40

WEIGHT

DATE	AGE	LENGTH	WEIGHT	HEAD CIRC.	COMMENT

*Adapted from: Hamill PVV, Drizd TA, Johnson CL, Reed RB, Roche AF, Moore WM: Physical growth: National Center for Health Statistics percentiles. AM J CLIN NUTR 32:607-629, 1979. Data from the Fels Research Institute, Wright State University School of Medicine, Yellow Springs, Ohio.

BOYS: BIRTH TO 36 MONTHS
PHYSICAL GROWTH
NCHS PERCENTILES*

NAME________________ RECORD #________

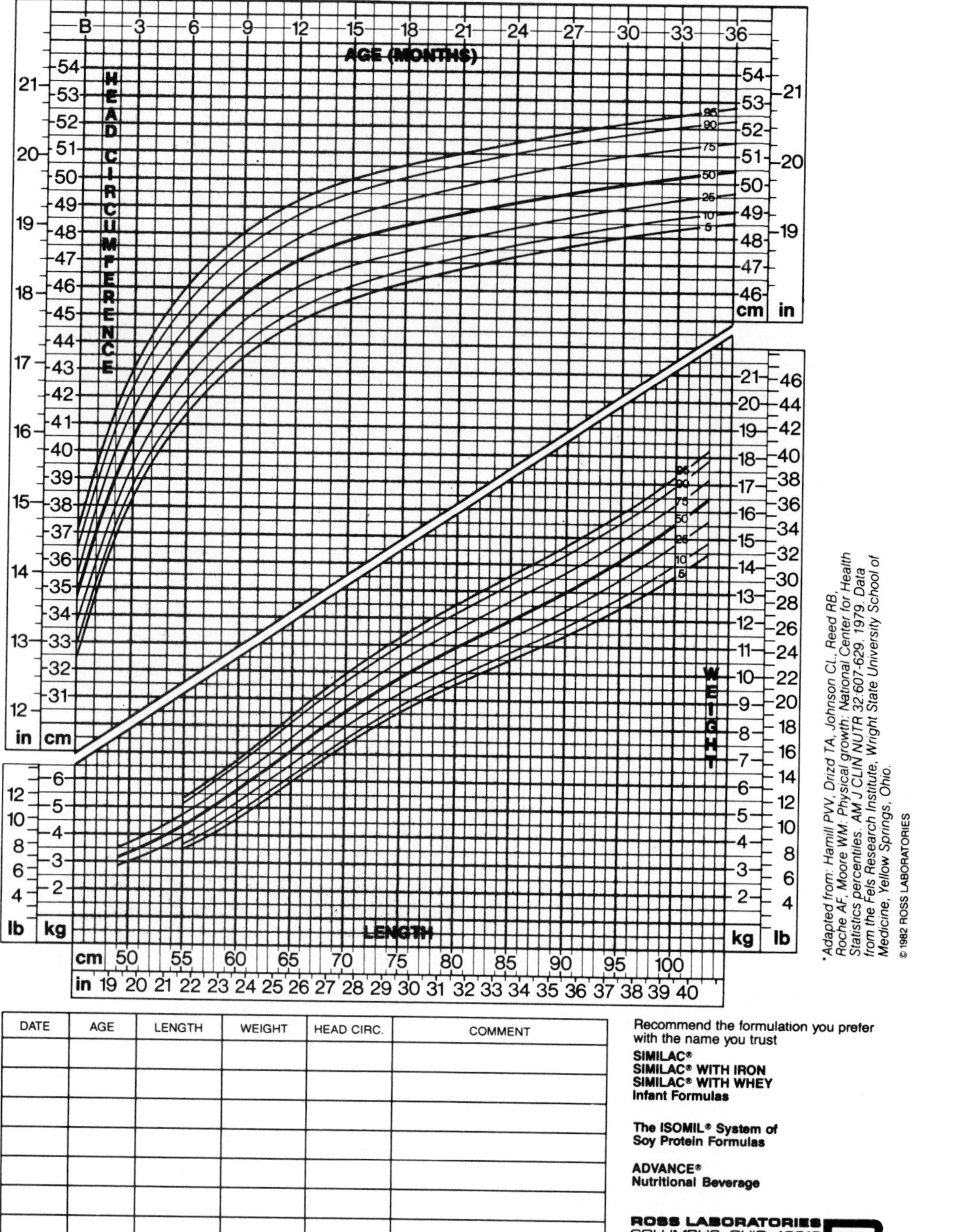

DATE	AGE	LENGTH	WEIGHT	HEAD CIRC.	COMMENT

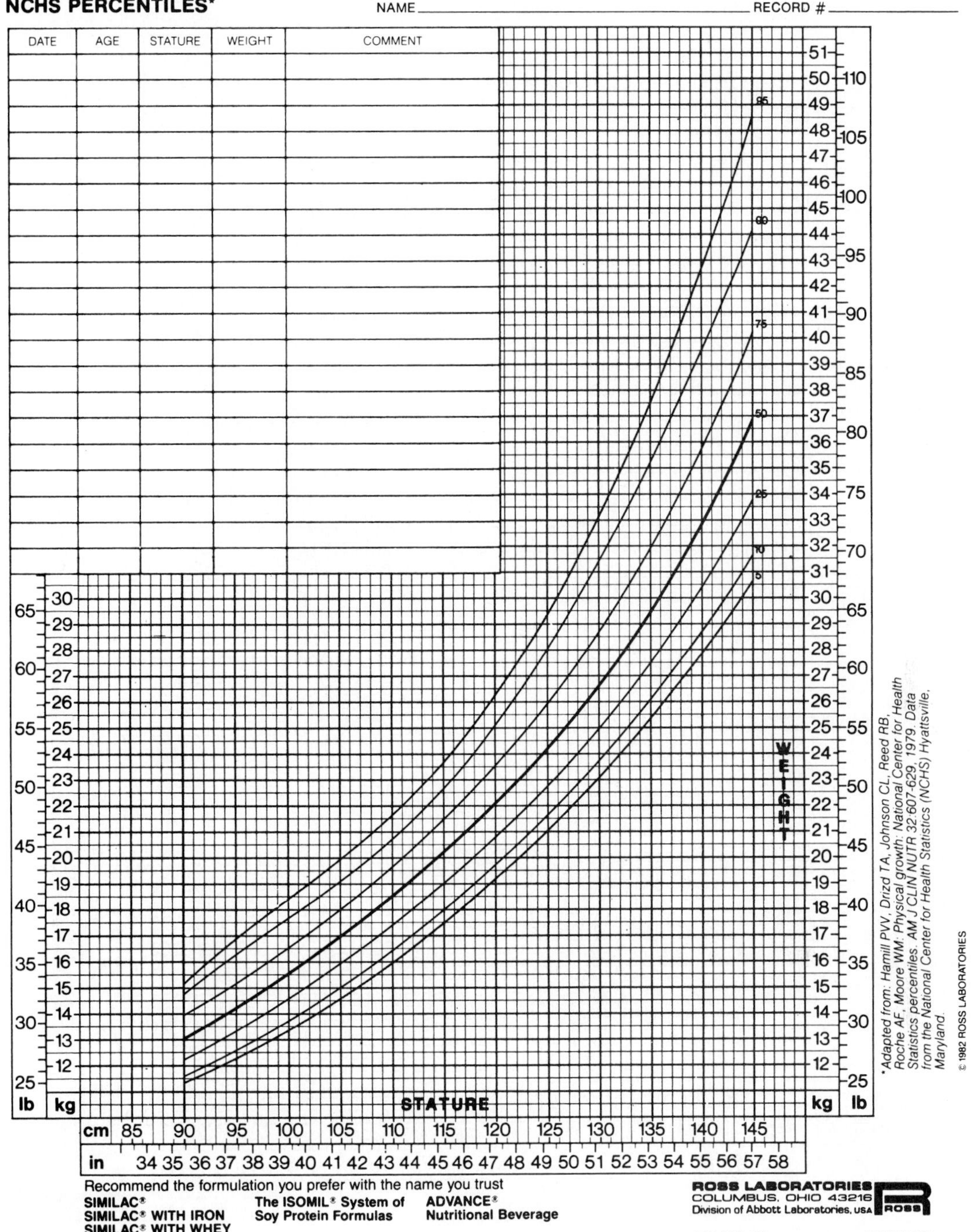
BOYS: PREPUBESCENT
PHYSICAL GROWTH
NCHS PERCENTILES*
NAME
RECORD #
DATE
AGE
STATURE
WEIGHT
COMMENT
95
90
75
50
25
10
5
WEIGHT
STATURE
lb
kg
cm
in
*Adapted from: Hamill PVV, Drizd TA, Johnson CL, Reed RB, Roche AF, Moore WM: Physical growth: National Center for Health Statistics percentiles. AM J CLIN NUTR 32:607-629, 1979. Data from the National Center for Health Statistics (NCHS) Hyattsville, Maryland.
© 1982 ROSS LABORATORIES
Recommend the formulation you prefer with the name you trust
SIMILAC®
SIMILAC® WITH IRON
SIMILAC® WITH WHEY
Infant Formulas
The ISOMIL® System of
Soy Protein Formulas
ADVANCE®
Nutritional Beverage
ROSS LABORATORIES
COLUMBUS, OHIO 43216
Division of Abbott Laboratories, USA
ROSS
G107/JUNE 1983
LITHO IN USA

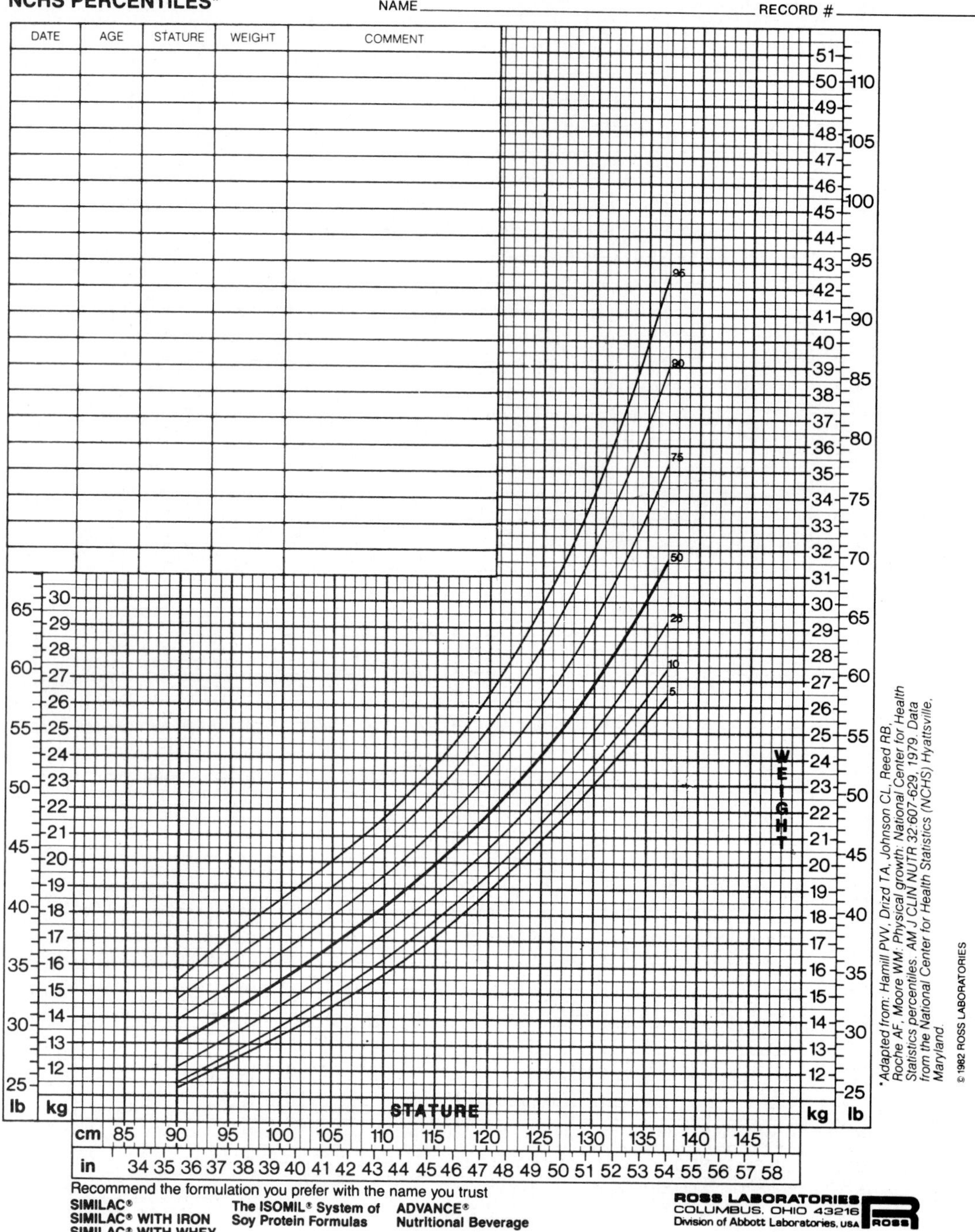

Recommend the formulation you prefer with the name you trust

SIMILAC®
SIMILAC® WITH IRON
SIMILAC® WITH WHEY
Infant Formulas

The ISOMIL® System of Soy Protein Formulas

ADVANCE® Nutritional Beverage

ROSS LABORATORIES
COLUMBUS, OHIO 43216
Division of Abbott Laboratories, USA

G108/JUNE 1983

LITHO IN USA

GIRLS: 2 TO 18 YEARS
PHYSICAL GROWTH
NCHS PERCENTILES*

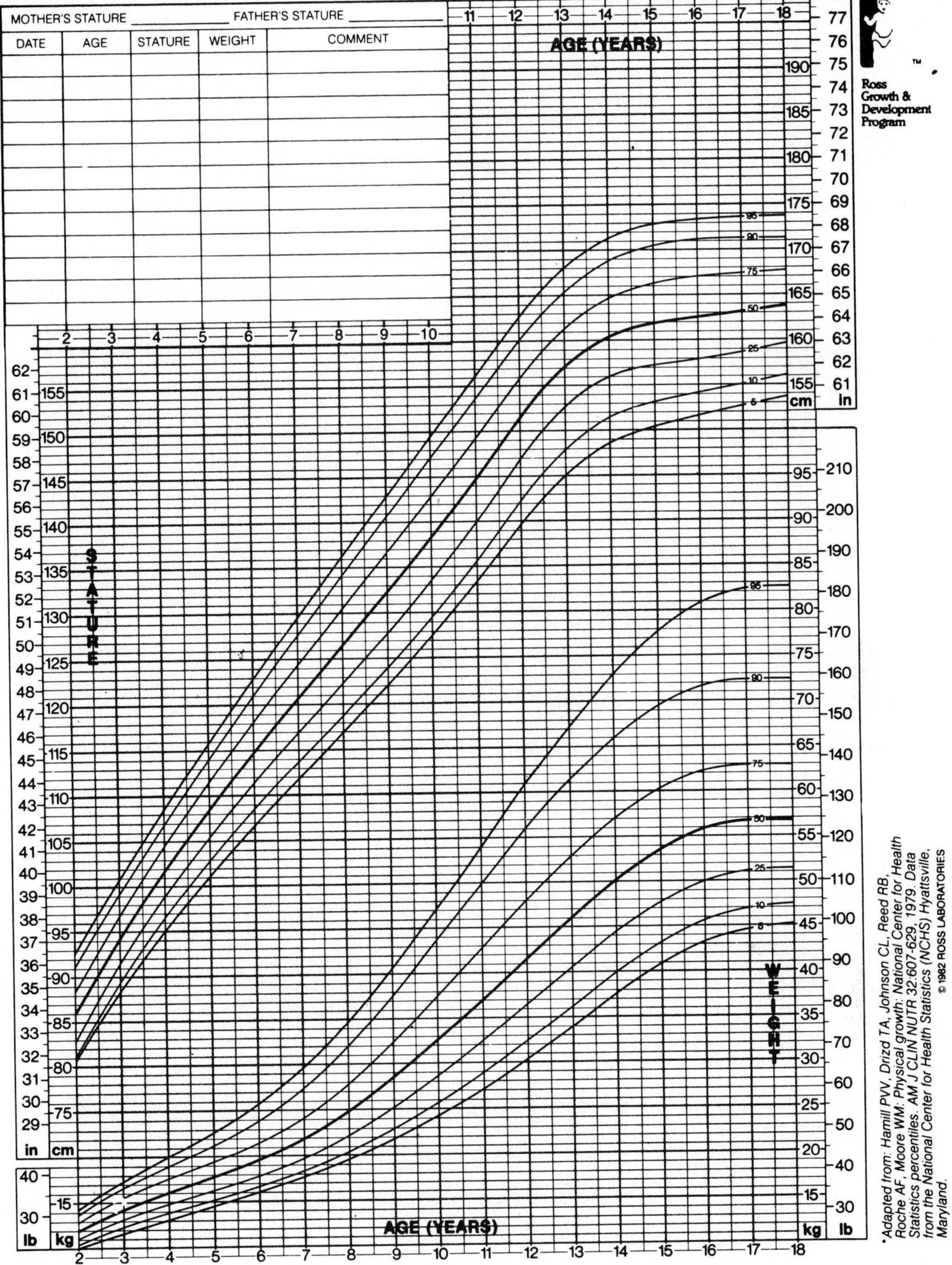

BOYS: 2 TO 18 YEARS
PHYSICAL GROWTH
NCHS PERCENTILES*

NAME ____________________ RECORD # ________

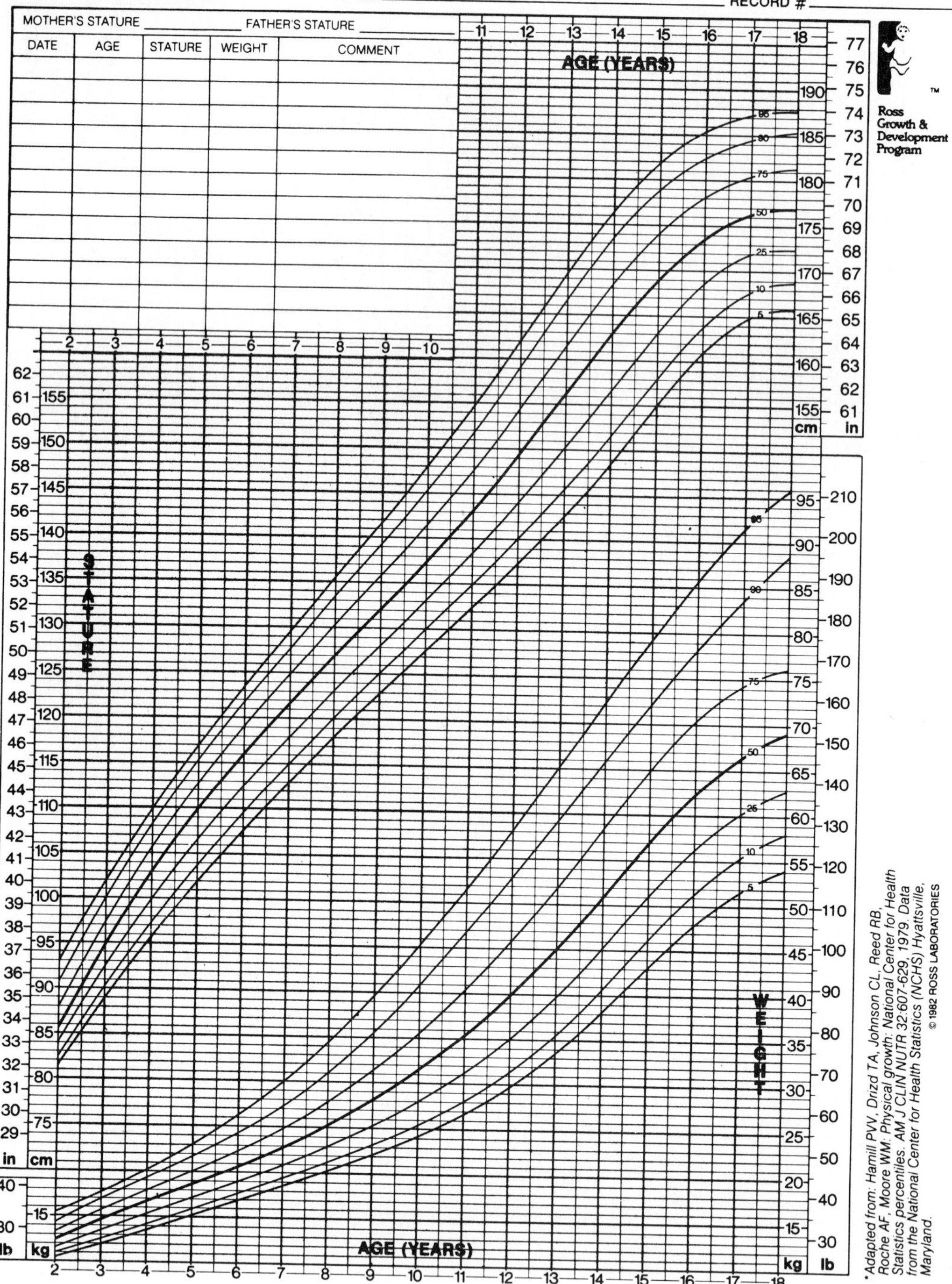

Appendix Q
Dietary Intake Assessment

Though it may seem overwhelming at first, it is actually very easy to track the foods you eat. One tip is to record foods and beverages consumed as close as possible to the actual time of consumption.

Fill in the food record form that follows. We supply a blank copy (see the completed example in Table 9-4). Then, to estimate the nutrient values of the foods you are eating, consult food labels and the food composition table in Appendix A or use your Mosby Diet Simple nutrition software package. If these resources do not have the serving size you need, adjust the value. If you drink ½ cup of orange juice, for example, but a table has values for only 1 cup, halve all values before you record them. Then, consider pooling all the same food to save time; if you drink a cup of 1% milk three times throughout the day, enter your milk consumption only once as 3 cups. As you record your intake of the nutrient analysis form that follows, use the nutrient values you found to complete this nutrient analysis form.

I. Consider the following tips as you record the types of foods and beverages you eat in one day:

- Measure and record the amounts of food eaten in portion sizes of cups, teaspoons, tablespoons, ounces, slices, or inches. (Or convert metric units to these units)
- Record brand names of all food products, such as "Quick Quaker Oats"
- Measure and record all those little extras, such as gravies, salad dressings, taco sauces, pickles, jelly, sugar, ketchup, and margarines
- Beverages—
  —List the type of milk, such as whole, skim, 2%, evaporated, chocolate, or reconstituted dry
  —Indicate whether fruit juice is fresh, frozen, or canned
  —Indicate type for other beverages, such as fruit drink, fruit-flavored drink, Kool-Aid, and hot chocolate made with water or milk
- Fruits—
  —Indicate whether fresh, frozen, dried, or canned
  —If whole, record as number eaten and size with approximate measurements (such as 1 apple—3 inches in diameter)
  —Indicate whether processed in water, light syrup, heavy syrup, or other medium
- Vegetables—
  —Indicate fresh, frozen, canned, dried
  —Record as portion of cup, teaspoon, or tablespoon or as pieces (such as 2 carrot sticks—4 inches long, ½ inch thick)
  —Record preparation method
- Cereals—
  —Record cooked cereals in portions of tablespoon or cup, (a level measurement after cooking)
  —Record dry cereal in level portions of cup or tablespoons
  —If margarine, milk, sugar, fruit, or something else is added, then measure and record amount and type
- Breads—
  —Indicate whether whole wheat, rye, white, and so on
  —Measure and record number and size of portion (biscuit—2 inches

across, 1 inch thick; slice of homemade rye bread—3 inches by 4 inches, ¼ inch thick).

—Sandwiches: list **ALL** ingredients (lettuce, mayonnaise, tomato, and so on) with amounts

- Meats, Fish, Poultry, Cheese—

—Give size (length, width, thickness) in inches or weight in ounces after cooking for meats, fish, and poultry (such as cooked hamburger patty—3 inches across, ½ inch thick)

—Give size (length, width, thickness) in inches or weight in ounces for cheese

—Record measurements only on the cooked edible part—without bone or fat that is left on the plate

—Describe how meat was prepared

- Eggs—

—Record as soft or hard cooked, fried, scrambled, poached, or omelet

—If milk, butter, or drippings are used, specify kinds and amount

- Desserts—

—List commercial brand or "homemade" or "bakery" under brand

—Purchased candies, cookies, and cakes: Specify kind and size

—Measure and record portion size of cakes, pies, and cookies by specifying thickness, diameter, and width or length, depending on the item

I. Complete the food record form (see Table 9-4 for a completed example).

Time	Minutes spent eating	Meals or Snack	Hunger (1-3; 3=max.)	Activity while eating	Place of eating	Food and quantity	Others present	Feeling before eating

II. Now complete the nutrient analysis form as shown using your food record. A blank copy of this form also follows for your use.

Nutrient analysis form (sample)

Food or beverage	Approximate measure	Food energy (kcalories)	Protein (grams)	Total fat (grams)	Unsaturated fat (grams)	Carbohydrate (grams)
Egg bagel	1	180	7	1	1	35
Jelly	1 T.	49	tr	tr	tr	13
Orange pop	12 oz.	170	0	0	0	42
McDonald's cheeseburgers	2	636	30	32	14	58
French fries	regular	220	3	12	8	26
McDonald's cookies	small box	308	4	10	6	49
Cola drink	12 oz.	151	0	0	0	39
Pork chop-lean only	2½ oz.	172	21	9	6	0
Baked potato	1 avg.	145	3	tr	tr	34
Frozen peas	½ c.	63	4	tr	tr	11
Butter	2 t.	68	0	8	0	0
Iceberg lettuce	2 c.	14	2	0	0	2
French dressing	2 oz.	165	tr	18	15	2
2% milk	½ c.	61	4	3	1	6
Graham crackers	2 squares	60	1	2	1	11
Totals		2462	79	95	51	328
Your RDA			46			
% of Your RDA			170			

*Values are from the inside cover. Some are Estimated Safe & Adequate Daily Dietary Intakes or Minimum Requirements—not true RDAs.
†For vitamin A, use the number from the RDA table in this text that represents International Units (IUs), since that is the type of unit the food composition tables use to describe vitamin A quantities. Do not use the value for retinol equivalents (REs).

Calcium (milligrams)	Phosphorus (milligrams)	Sodium (milligrams)	Potassium (milligrams)	Iron (milligrams)	Zinc (milligrams)	Vitamin A (IU)	Thiamin (milligrams)	Riboflavin (milligrams)	Niacin (milligrams)	Vitamin B-6 (milligrams)	Vitamin B-12 (micrograms)	Folate (micrograms)	Vitamin C (micrograms)
20	61	300	65	2.1	.6	0	.26	.20	2.4	.03	0	16	0
2	1	4	16	.1	0	2	tr	tr	tr	tr	0	2	1
15	2	48	20	.3	.3	0	0	0	tr	0	0	0	0
338	410	1460	314	5.6	5.2	706	.60	.48	8.6	.24	1.82	42	4
9	101	109	564	.6	.3	17	.12	.02	2.3	.22	.03	19	13
12	74	358	52	1.5	.3	27	.23	.23	2.9	.03	.03	6	1
9	46	15	4	.1	.1	0	0	0	0	0	0	0	0
3	177	56	303	.7	1.6	5	.83	.22	2.5	.34	.52	4	tr
8	78	8	610	.6	.5	0	.16	.03	2.2	.47	0	14	20
19	72	70	134	1.3	.8	534	.23	.14	1.2	.09	0	47	8
2	2	78	2	0	0	289	0	0	0	0	tr	0	0
22	22	10	178	.6	.2	370	.06	.04	.2	.04	0	62	4
4	.2	367	2	.1	tr	tr	tr	tr	tr	tr	0	0	tr
149	116	61	189	.1	.5	250	.05	.20	.1	.06	.45	6	1
6	20	86	36	.4	.1	0	.02	.03	.6	.01	0	2	0
618	1184	3030	2489	14.1	10.5	2200†	2.56	1.59	23.0	1.53	2.85	220	52
800	800	500	2000	15	12	4000	1.1	1.3	15	1.6	2	180	60
77	148	600		94	88	55	233	122	153	96	143	122	87

†Intakes greater than 2000 milligrams per day are fine.

Nutrient analysis form

Food or beverage	Approximate measure	Food energy (kcalories)	Protein (grams)	Total fat (grams)	Unsaturated fat (grams)	Carbohydrate (grams)
TOTALS						
Your RDA						
% of your RDA						

*Values are from the inside cover. Some are Estimated Safe & Adequate Daily Dietary Intakes or Minimum Requirements—not true RDAs.

†For vitamin A, use the number from the RDA table in this text that represents International Units (IUs), since that is the type of unit the food composition tables use to describe vitamin A quantities. Do not use the value for retinol equivalents (REs).

Calcium (milligrams)	Phosphorus (milligrams)	Sodium (milligrams)	Potassium (milligrams)	Iron (milligrams)	Zinc (milligrams)	Vitamin A (IU)	Thiamin (milligrams)	Riboflavin (milligrams)	Niacin (milligrams)	Vitamin B-6 (milligrams)	Vitamin B-12 (micrograms)	Folate (micrograms)	Vitamin C (micrograms)

‡ Intakes greater than Minimum Requirements are fine.

III. For this same day you keep your food record, also keep a 24-hour record of your activities. Include sleeping, sitting, and walking, as well as the obvious forms of exercise. Calculate your kcalorie expenditure for these activities using Appendix J. Try to substitute a similar activity if your particular activity is not listed in Appendix J. (Note: To determine your weight in kilograms, 1 kg = 2.2 lbs; 24-hours = 1440 minutes). Calculate the total kcalories you used for the day (Total for column 3). Here is an example of an activity record. A blank form follows for your use.

WEIGHT (KG): **HEIGHT (IN):**

		ENERGY COST		
Activity	Time (minutes); Convert hours to minutes	Column 1 kcal/kg/min (from table)	Column 2 (Column 1 × Time)	Column 3 (Column 2 × Weight in Kg.)
Example for 70 Kg. man:				
Brisk Walking	60 minutes	.0857	(×60) = 5.142	(×70) = 360
Calculate total kcalories used for the day:				

WEIGHT (KG): **HEIGHT (IN):**

		ENERGY COST		
Activity	Time (minutes); Convert hours to minutes	Column 1 kcal/kg/min (from table)	Column 2 (Column 1 × Time)	Column 3 (Column 2 × Weight in Kg.)
Total kcalories used (from adding all of column 3)				

This Appendix is now completed. Return to Take Action for Chapter 17 to perform some final calculations.

Appendix R
Common Food Additives

This list identifies the functions of some of the more than 2800 additives allowed in the U.S. food supply.

Additive	Function
A	
Acetic acid	pH control‡
Acetone peroxide	mat-bleach-condit§
Adipic acid	pH control‡
Ammonium alginate	stabil-thick-tex*
Annatto extract	color
Arabinogalactan	stabil-thick-tex*
Ascorbic acid	nutrient preservative antioxidant
Azodicarbonamide	mat-bleach-condit§
B	
Benzoic acid	preservative
Benzoyl peroxide	mat-bleach-condit§
Beta-apo-8′ carotenal	color
Beta carotene	nutrient color
BHA (butylated hydroxyanisole)	antioxidant
BHT (butylated hydroxytoluene)	antioxidant
Butylparaben	preservative
C	
Calcium alginate	stabil-thick-tex*
Calcium bromate	mat-bleach-condit§
Calcium lactate	preservative
Calcium phosphate	leavening†
Calcium propionate	preservative
Calcium silicate	anticaking‖
Calcium sorbate	preservative
Canthaxanthin	color
Caramel	color
Carob bean gum	stabil-thick-tex*
Carrageenan	emulsifier stabil-thick-tex*
Carrot oil	color
Cellulose	stabil-thick-tex*
Citric acid	preservative antioxidant pH control‡
Citrus Red No. 2	color
Cochineal extract	color
Corn endosperm	color
Corn syrup	sweetener
D	
Dehydrated beets	color
Dextrose	sweetener
Diglycerides	emulsifier
Diocytl sodium sulfosuccinate	emulsifier
Disodium guanylate	flavor enhancer
Disodium inosinate	flavor enhancer
Dried algae meal	color
E	
EDTA (ethylenediaminetetraacetic acid)	antioxidant
F	
FD&C Colors:	
Blue No. 1	color
Red No. 3	color
Red No. 40	color
Yellow No. 5	color
Fructose	sweetener
G	
Gelatin	stabil-thick-tex*
Glucose	sweetener
Glycerine	humectant
Glycerol monostearate	humectant
Grape skin extract	color
Guar gum	stabil-thick-tex*
Gum arabic	stabil-thick-tex*
Gum ghatti	stabil-thick-tex*
H	
Heptylparaben	preservative
Hydrogen peroxide	mat-bleach-condit§
Hydrolyzed vegetable protein	flavor enhancer
I	
Invert sugar	sweetener
Iodine	nutrient
Iron	nutrient
Iron-ammonium citrate	anticaking‖
Iron oxide	color

Additive	Function
K	
Karaya gum	stabil-thick-tex*
L	
Lactic acid	pH control‡ preservative
Larch gum	stabil-thick-tex*
Lecithin	emulsifier
Locust bean gum	stabil-thick-tex*
M	
Mannitol	sweetener anticaking‖ stabil-thick-tex*
Methylparaben	preservative
Modified food starch	stabil-thick-tex*
Monoglycerides	emulsifier
MSG (monosidium glutamate)	flavor enhancer
N	
Niacinamide	nutrient
P	
Paprika (and oleoresin)	flavor color
Pectin	stabil-thick-tex*
Phosphates	pH control‡
Phosphoric acid	pH control‡
Polysorbates	emulsifiers
Potassium alginate	stabil-thick-tex*
Potassium bromate	mat-bleach-condit§
Potassium iodide	nutrient
Potassium propionate	preservative
Potassium sorbate	preservative
Propionic acid	preservative
Propyl gallate	antioxidant
Propylene glycol	stabil-thick-tex* humectant
Propylparaben	preservative
R	
Riboflavin	nutrient color
S	
Saccharin	sweetener
Saffron	color
Silicon dioxide	anticaking‖
Sodium acetate	pH control‡
Sodium alginate	stabil-thick-tex*
Sodium aluminum sulfate	leavening†
Sodium benzoate	preservative
Sodium bicarbonate	leavening†
Sodium calcium alginate	stabil-thick-tex*
Sodium citrate	pH control‡
Sodium diacetate	preservative
Sodium erythorbate	preservative
Sodium nitrate	preservative
Sodium nitrite	preservative
Sodium propionate	preservative
Sodium sorbate	preservative
Sodium stearyl fumarate	mat-bleach-condit§
Sorbic acid	preservative
Sorbitan monostearate	emulsifier
Sorbitol	humectant sweetener
Spices	flavor
Sucrose (table sugar)	sweetener
T	
Tagetes (Aztec Marigold)	color
Tartaric acid	pH control‡
TBHQ (tertiary butyl hydroquinone)	antioxidant
Thiamine	nutrient
Titanium dioxide	color
Toasted, partially defatted cooked cottonseed flour	color
Tocopherols (vitamin E)	nutrient antioxidant
Tragacanth gum	stabil-thick-tex*
Turmeric (oleoresin)	flavor color
U	
Ultramarine blue	color
V	
Vanilla, vanillin	flavor
Vitamin A	nutrient
Vitamin C (ascorbic acid)	nutrient preservative antioxidant
Vitamin D (D-2, D-3)	nutrient
Vitamin E (tocopherols)	nutrient
Y	
Yeast-malt sprout extract	flavor enhancer
Yellow prussiate of soda	anticaking‖

Key to abbreviations: *stabil-thick-tex = stabilizers-thickeners-texturizers; †leavening = leavening agents; ‡pH control = pH control agents; §mat-bleach-condit = maturing and bleaching agents, dough conditioners; ‖anticaking = anticaking agents.

From Lehmann P: More than you ever thought you would know about food additives, FDA Consumer reprint, Health and Human Services Publication No. (FDA) 79-2115, 1979.

Appendix S
Safe Food Storage

Safe Food Storage & Handling Chart
—Refrigerator Storage—

The suggested storage time aims at maintaining good eating quality and minimizing loss of nutritive value. Suggested maximum times for storing food in refrigerator at 34° to 40° F

Food	Time	Special handling
Canned food after opening		
Baby food	2–3 days	*Store covered. Don't feed baby from jar; saliva may liquefy food.*
Fish, seafood, and poultry	1 day	
Fruit	1 week	*Store all canned foods tightly covered. It is not necessary to remove food from can.*
Meats, gravy, broths	2 days	
Pickles, olives	1 month	
Sauce, tomato based	5 days	
Vegetables	3 days	
Cured and smoked meats		
Bacon, corned beef	5–7 days	*Keep wrapped. Store in coldest part of refrigerator or in a meat keeper. Times are of opened packages of sliced meats. Unopened vacuum packs keep about 2 weeks.*
Bologna loaves	4–6 days	
Dried beef	10–12 days	
Dry and semi-dry sausage (salami, etc)	2–3 weeks	
Frankfurters, liver sausage	4–5 days	
Hams (whole, halves)	1 week	
Hams, canned (unopened)	6 months	
Luncheon meat	3 days	
Sausage, fresh or smoked	2-3 days	
Dairy products		
Butter, margarine	1–2 weeks	*Keep tightly wrapped or covered.*
Buttermilk, sour cream, or yogurt	5–14 days	
Cheese		
cottage, ricotta	5 days	*Keep all cheese tightly packaged in moisture-resistant wrap. If outside of hard cheese gets moldy, just cut away mold—it won's affect flavor.*
cream, Neufchatel	2 weeks	
hard and wax-coated cheeses		
large pieces (unopened)	3–6 months	
(opened)	3–4 weeks	
(sliced)	2 weeks	
process (opened)	3–4 weeks	*Unopened process cheese need not be refrigerated.*
Cream—light, heavy, half-and-half	3 days	*Keep tightly covered. Don't return unused cream to original container. This would spready any bacteria present in leftover cream*
Dips—sour cream, etc		
commercial	2 weeks	
homemade	2 days	
Eggs: in shell	3 weeks	

whites	3 days	*Store in covered container.*
yolks	3 days	*Cover yolks with water; cover container.*
Milk		
evaporated (opened)	4–5 days	
pasteurized, reliquefied nonfat dry, skimmed	3–4 days	*Keep containers tightly closed. Do not return unused milk to original container.*
sweetened condensed	4–5 days	*Remove entire lid of can to make pouring easier. Keep covered.*
Fruits and vegetables—fresh		
Fruits		
apples, melons, citrus fruits	1 week	*Do not wash fruit before storing—moisture encourages spoilage. Store in crisper or moisture-resistant bags or wrap. Wrap uncut cantaloupe, honeydew, etc., to prevent odor spreading to other foods.*
berries, cherries	1–2 days	
other fruit	3–5 days	
citrus juices, bottled, frozen, canned	6 days	
Vegetables		
beets, carrots, radishes	2 weeks.	*Remove leafy tops; keep in crisper.*
mushrooms	1–2 days	*Do not wash before storing.*
shredded salad greens	1–2 days	*Keep in moisture-resistant wrap or bags.*
peas (in the pod), corn in husks	3–5 days	*Keep in crisper or moisture-resistant wrap or bags.*
other vegetables	3–5 days	*Keep in crisper or moisture-resistant wrap or bags.*
Meat, fish, and poultry—fresh uncooked		
Meats—beef, lamb, pork, and veal—chops	3–4 days	
ground meat, stew meat	1–2 days	
roasts	5–6 days	
steaks	3–5 days	
variety meats (liver, heart, etc.)	1–2 days	
Fish and shellfish		
fresh cleaned fish including steaks and fillets	1 day	*Store loosely wrapped. Keep in coldest part of refrigerator or in meat keeper.*
clams, crab, lobster in shell	2 days	*Cook only live shellfish.*
seafood including shucked clams, oysters, scallops, shrimp	1 day	
Poultry		
ready-to-cook chicken, duck or turkey	2 days	*Store loosely wrapped. Keep fresh poultry in coldest part of refrigerator or in meat keeper.*
Other foods		
Coffee, regular	2 weeks	
Honey, jams, jellies		*Refrigeration not needed but storage life is lengthened if refrigerated.*
Nuts	2 weeks.	*Refrigerate nuts after opening.*
Refrigerated biscuits, rolls, pastries, cookie dough	date on label	*Products keep better if stored in back of refrigerator where it is colder.*
Salad dressings (opened)	3 months	*Keep covered.*
Wines, table	2–3 days	*Keep tightly closed.*
cooking	2–3 months.	*Keep tightly closed.*

Safe Food Storage & Handling Chart
—Freezer Storage—

Suggested maximum times for storing foods in freezer at 0° F.
Longer than recommended storage is not dangerous, but flavors and textures begin to deteriorate.

Food	Time	Special handling
Dairy products		
Butter, margarine	9 months	*Store in airtight freezer containers or wrapped in freezer wrap.*
Cheese		
cream cheese	1 month	*Thaw in refrigerator.*
hard cheeses	3 months	*Thaw in refrigerator.*
Roquefort, blue, process	3 months	*Thaw in refrigerator.*
Cream—light, heavy, half-and-half	2 months	*Heavy cream may not whip after thawing. Use for cooking. Thaw in refrigerator.*
Cream, whipped	1 month	
Eggs: whites	1 year	*Store in covered container. Freeze in amounts for favorite recipes.*
yolks	1 year	
Ice cream, ice milk, sherbet	1 month	*Cover surface with plastic wrap or foil after each use to keep from drying*
Milk	3 months	*Freezing affects flavor and appearance. Use in cooking and baking. Thaw in refrigerator.*
Fruits and vegetables		
Fruits		
berries, cherries, peaches, pears, pineapple, etc.	1 year	
citrus fruit and juice, frozen at home	6 months	
fruit juice concentrates	1 year	
Vegetables		
home frozen	10 months	*Cabbage, celery, salad greens, tomatos do not freeze successfully.*
purchased frozen	8 months	
Meat, fish, and poultry		
Meats—home frozen		
bacon, frankfurters, ham slices, luncheon meats	1 month	*If meat is purchased fresh on trays and in plastic wrap, check for holes. If none, freeze in this wrap for up to 1 month. For longer storage, over-wrap with foil, plastic wrap or freezer wrap.*
corned beef	2 weeks	
ground beef, lamb and veal	4 months	
ground pork	3 months	
ham, whole	2 months	
roasts		
beef	1 year	
lamb, veal	9 months	
pork	6 months	
sausage, dry, smoked	1 month	*Keep meat purchased frozen in original package. Thaw and cook according to label instructions.*
sausage, fresh	2 months	
steaks		
beef	1 year	
lamb, veal	9 months	
pork	6 months	
Fish		
fillets and steaks from "lean" fish—cod, flounder, haddock, sole	6 months	*To home-freeze fish, wrap in foil, plastic wrap or freezer wrap. Make packages as airtight as possible. Freeze in coldest part of freezer.*
"fatty" fish—bluefish, mackerel, perch, salmon	3 months	

Food	Storage time	Notes
breaded fish	3 months	*Keep fish purchased frozen in original wrapping. Thaw and cook according to label directions.*
clams, lobster, scallops	3 months	
cooked fish or seafood	3 months	
king crab	10 months	
oysters	4 months	
shrimp, unbreaded	1 year	
shrimp, breaded	4 months	
Poultry		
chicken, whole or cut-up	1 year	*Cook all thawed poultry within 1 day.*
chicken livers	3 months	
cooked poultry	3 months	
duck, turkey	6 months	
Miscellaneous		
Baked goods		
breads, baked	3 months	*Package foods tightly in foil, plastic wrap, freezer wrap or watertight freezer containers.*
breads, unbaked	2 months	
cakes		
cheesecake	3 months	
chocolate	4 months	
fruitcake	1 year	
spongecake	2 months	
yellow or pound	6 months	
pies		
cream, custard	8 months	
fruit	8 months	
Main dishes		
meat, fish and poultry pies and casseroles	3 months	*For casseroles, allow head room for expansion. Freeze in coldest part of freezer.*
TV dinners	6 months	
Nuts	3 months	

Safe Food Storage & Handling Chart
—Pantry Shelf Storage—

Suggested maximum times for storing foods in coldest cabinets

Food	Time	Special handling
Canned and dried food		
Canned pineapple, tomato or sauerkraut	8 months	
Fruits, canned	1 year	
dried	6 months	*Put in airtight container.*
Gravies	1 year	
Meat, fish, poultry	1 year	
Pickles, olives	1 year	*Refrigerate after opening.*
Soups, canned, dried	1 year	
Vegetables, canned, dried	1 year	
Herbs, spices and condiments		
Catsup (opened)	1 month	
Herbs and spices		
whole spices, herbs	1 year	
ground spices, herbs	6 months	
Tabasco, Worcestershire	2 years+	
Mixes and packaged foods		
Cakes, prepared	1–2 days	*If butter-cream, whipped-cream or custard frostings, fillings, refrigerate.*
Cake mixes	1 year	
Casserole mixes	1 year	
Cookies, homemade	1 week	*Put in airtight container.*
packaged	4 months	*Keep box tightly closed.*
Crackers	3 months	*Keep box tightly closed.*
Frosting, in cans or mixes	8 months	
Hot roll mix	18 months	*If opened, put in airtight container.*
Pancake mix	6 months	*Put in airtight container.*
Piecrust mix	8 months	
Pie and pastries	2–3 days	*Refrigerate whipped cream, custard, chiffon fillings.*
Potatoes, instant	18 months	
Toaster pop-ups	3 months	
Staples		
Baking powder	18 months	
Boullion cubes	1 year	
Bread crumbs, dried	6 months	
Cereals, ready-to-eat	4 months	
ready to cook	6 months	
Chocolate, premelted	1 year	
semi-sweet	2 years	
unsweetened	18 months	
Coffee, cans (unopened)	1 month	*Refrigerate after opening.*
Coffee, instant (opened)	2 weeks	*Keep lid tightly closed.*
(unopened)	6 months	
Coffee lighteners (dry) (opened)	6 months	
Condensed and evaporated milk	1 year	*Refrigerate after opening.*
Flour (all types)	1 year	*Put in airtight container.*
Gelatin (all types)	18 months	
Honey, jams, syrups	1 year	
Nonfat dry milk	6 months	*Put in airtight container.*

Pasta	2 years+	*Keep tightly closed.*
Pudding mixes	1 year	
Rice, white	2 years+	*Keep tightly closed.*
Rice mixes	6 months	
Salad dressing (all types)	3 months	*Refrigerate after opening.*
Salad oil	1–3 months	
Shortening, solid.	8 months	
Sugar, brown	4 months	*Put in airtight container.*
confectioners'	4 months	*Put in airtight container.*
granulated, molasses	2 years+	*Keep tightly covered.*
Tea, bags	18 months	*Put in airtight container.*
instant	3 years	*Keep tightly covered.*
loose	2 years	*Put in airtight container.*
Miscellaneous		
Coconut	1 year	*Refrigerate after opening.*
Metered-calorie products, instant breakfasts	6 months	
Nuts	9 months	*Refrigerate after opening.*
Onions, potatoes, sweet potatoes	2 weeks.	*For longer storage, keep below 50° F, but not refrigerated. Keep dry, out of sun.*
Parmesan cheese	2 months	
Peanut butter (opened)	2 months	
(unopened)	9 months	
Soft drinks	3 months	
Whipped topping mix	1 year	

Appendix T
Sources of nutrition information

Consider the following reliable sources of food and nutrition information:

Journals that regularly cover nutrition topics:

*American Family Physician**
American Journal of Clinical Nutrition
American Journal of Epidemiology
American Journal of Medicine
American Journal of Nursing
American Journal of Obstetrics and Gynecology
American Journal of Physiology
American Journal of Public Health
American Scientist
Annals of Internal Medicine
Annual Reviews of Medicine
Annual Reviews of Nutrition
Archives of Disease in Childhood
Archives of Internal Medicine
British Journal of Nutrition
British Medical Journal
Cancer
Cancer Research
Circulation
Diabetes
Diabetes Care
Disease-a-Month
Ecology of Food and Nutrition
FASEB Journal
*FDA Consumer**
Food Chemical Toxicology
Food Engineering
Geriatrics
Gastroenterology
Gut
Human Nutrition: Applied Nutrition
Human Nutrition: Clinical Nutrition
*Journal of The American Dietetic Association**
Journal of The American Geriatric Society
Journal of The American Medical Association
Journal of Applied Physiology
*Journal of Canadian Dietetic Association**
Journal of Clinical Investigation
Journal of Food Science
Journal of Food Technology
Journal of The National Cancer Institute
Journal of Nutrition
*Journal of Nutrition Education**
Journal of Nutrition for the Ederly
Journal of Nutrition Research
Journal of Pediatrics
Lancet
Mayo Clinic Proceedings
Medicine and Science in Sports and Exercise
Nature
New England Journal of Medicine
Nutrition
Nutrition Reviews
*Nutrition Today**
Pediatrics
The Physician and Sports Medicine
*Postgraduate Medicine**
Proceedings of the Nutrition Society
Science
*Science News**
*Scientific American**

The majority of these journals will be available in a university's main library, or in a specialty library on campus, much as one designated for health sciences or home economics. Have a reference librarian help you locate these sources. The asterisked (*) journals are ones we feel you will find especially interesting and useful because the number of nutrition articles presented each month or the less technical nature of the presentation.

Magazines for the nonmedical person that cover nutrition topics:

American Health
Better Homes and Gardens
Consumer Reports
Good housekeeping
Parents
Self

Textbooks for advanced study of nutrition topics:

Food and Nutrition Board: Recommended dietary allowances, ed 10, Washington, DC, 1989, National Academy of Sciences.
Linder MC: Nutritional biochemistry and metabolism with clinical applications, New York, 1985, Elsevier Science Publishing Co, Inc.
Murray RK and others: Harper's biochemistry, ed 21, Norwalk, 1988, Appleton & Lange.
Pike RL and Brown ML: Nutrition: an integrated approach, ed 3, New York, 1984, John Wiley & Sons, Inc.
Present knowledge in nutrition, ed 5, 1984, The Nutrition Foundation.
Schils ME and Young ER: Modern nutrition in health and disease, ed 7, Philadelphia, 1988, Lea & Febiger.

Newsletters that cover nutrition issues on a regular basis:

Contemporary Nutrition
General Mills, Inc.
Production Manager
P.O. Box 1112, Department 65
Minneapolis, MN 55440
(inexpensive)

CNI Nutrition Week
Community Nutrition Institute
2001 S. St. NW
Washington, D.C. 20009

Dairy Council Digest
National Dairy Council
6300 River Rd.
Rosemont, IL 60018
(inexpensive)

Dietetic Currents
Ross Laboratories
Director of Professional Services
625 Cleveland Ave.
Columbus, OH 43216
(free)

Environmental Nutrition
52 Riverside Dr.
New York, NY 10024

Food and Nutrition News
National Livestock and Meat Board
444 Michigan Ave.
Chicago, IL 60610
(free)

Harvard Medical School Health Letter
Department of Continuing Education
25 Shattuck St.
Boston, MA 02115

Healthline
1149 Chestnut St. #10
Menlo Park, CA 94025

National Council Against Health Fraud Newsletter
NCAHF
P.O. Box 1276
Loma Linda, CA 92354

Nutrition & the M.D.
P.O. Box 2160
Van Nuys, CA 91404

Nutrition Forum
George Stickley Co.
210 Washington Square
Philadelphia, PA 19106

Nutrition Research Newsletter
P.O. Box 700
Pallisades, NY 10964

Tufts University Diet & Nutrition Letter
P.O. Box 10948
Des Moines, IA 50940

Professional organizations with a commitment to nutrition issues:

American Academy of Pediatrics
P.O. Box 1034
Evanston, IL 60204

American Cancer Society
777 Third Ave.
New York, NY 10017

American Dental Association
211 E. Chicago Ave.
Chicago, IL 60611

American Diabetes Association
2 Park Ave.
New York, NY 10016

American Dietetic Association
216 W. Jackson Blvd.
Suite 800
Chicago, IL 60606

American Geriatrics Society
770 Lexington Ave.
Suite 400
New York, NY 10021

American Heart Association
7320 Greenville Ave.
Dallas, TX 75231

American Home Economics Association
2010 Massachusetts Ave. N.W.
Washington, DC 20036

American Institute of Nutrition
9650 Rockville Pike
Bethesda, MD 20014

American Medical Association
Nutrition Information Section
535 N. Dearborn St.
Chicago, IL 60610

American Public Health Association
1015 Fifteenth St. N.W.
Washington, DC 20005

American Society for Clinical Nutrition
9650 Rockville Pike
Bethesda, MD 20014

The Canadian Diabetes Association
123 Edward St.
Suite 601
Toronto, Ontario M5G 1E2 Canada

The Canadian Dietetic Association
480 University Ave.
Suite 601
Toronto, Ontario M5G 1V2 Canada

The Canadian Society
for Nutritional Sciences
Department of Foods and Nutrition
University of Manitoba
Winnipeg, Manitoba, Canada R3T 2N2

Food and Nutrition Board
National Research Council
National Academy of Sciences
2101 Constitution Ave. N.W.
Washington, DC 20418

Institute of Food Technologies
221 N. LaSalle St.
Chicago, IL 60601

National Council on the Aging
1828 L St. N.W.
Washington, DC 20036

National Institute of Nutrition
1335 Carling Ave.
Suite 210
Ottawa, Ontario, Canada K1Z 0L2

Nutrition Foundation, Inc.
1126 Sixteenth St. N.W.
Suite 111
Washington, D.C. 20036

Nutrition Today Society
428 E. Preston St.
Baltimore, MD 21202

Society for Nutrition Education
1736 Franklin St.
Oakland, CA 94612

Professional or lay organizations concerned with nutrition issues:

Bread for the World
802 Rhode Island Ave. N.E.
Washington, DC 20018

Center for Science in the Public Interest (CSPI)
1755 S. Street N.W.
Washington, DC 20009

Children's Foundation
1420 New York Ave. N.W.
Suite 800
Washington, D.C. 20005

California Council Against Health Fraud, Inc.
P.O. Box 1276
Loma Linda, CA 92354

Food Research and Action Center (FRAC)
2011 I Street N.W.
Washington, D.C. 20006

Institute for Food and Development Policy
1885 Mission St.
San Francisco, CA 94103

La Leche League International, Inc.
9616 Minneapolis Ave.
Franklin Park, IL 60131

March of Dimes Birth Defects Foundation
(national headquarters)
1275 Mamaroneck Ave.
White Plains, NY 10605

Overeaters Anonymous (OA)
2190 190th St.
Torrance, CA 90504

Oxfam America
115 Broadway
Boston, MA 02116

Local resources for advice on nutrition issues:

Cooperative extension agents in county extension offices
Dietitians (Contact the state or local Dietetics Association.)
Nutrition faculty affiliated with departments of food and nutrition, home economics, and dietetics
Nutritionists (RDs) in city, county, or state agencies

Government agencies that are concerned with nutrition issues or that distribute nutrition information:

United States

Department of Agriculture (USDA)
Extension Services
3 South Building
Room 6007
Washington, DC 20250

The Consumer Information Center
Department 609K
Pueblo, CO 81009

Food and Drug Administration (FDA)
5600 Fishers Lane
Rockville, MD 20852

National Agricultural Library
10301 Baltimore Blvd.
Room 304
Beltsville, MD 20705

Food and Nutrition Information and Education Resources Center
National Library of Congress
Beltsville, MO 20705

Human Nutrition Research Division
Agricultural Research Center
Beltsville, MD 20705

Office of Cancer Communications
National Cancer Institute
Building 31
Room 10A18
900 Rockville Pike
Bethesda, MD 20205

National Center for Health Statistics
3700 East-West
Hyattsville, MD 20782

U.S. Government Printing Office
The Superintendent of Documents
Washington, DC 20402

Canada

Nutrition Programs
446 Jeanne Mance Building
Tunney's Pasture
Ottawa, Ontario K1A 1B4

Nutrition Services
P.O. Box 488
Halifax, Nova Scotia B3J 3R8

Nutrition Services
P.O. Box 6000
Fredericton, New Brunswick E3B 5H1

Department of Community Health
1075 Ste-Foy Rd.
Seventh Floor
Quebec, Quebec G1S 2M1

Public Health Resource Service
15 Overlea Blvd.
Fifth Floor
Toronto, Ontario M4H 1A9

Home Economics Directorate
880 Portage Ave.
Second Floor
Winnipeg, Manitoba R3G 0P1

United Nations

Food and Agriculture Organization (FAO)
North American Regional Office
1325 C St. S.W.
Washington, D.C. 20025
Via della Terma di Caracella
0100 Rome, Italy

World Health Organization (WHO)
1211 Geneva 27
Switzerland

Trade organizations and companies that distribute nutrition information:

American Egg Board
1460 Renaissance St.
Park Ridge, IL 60068

American Institute of Banking
P.O. Box 1148
Manhattan, KS 66502

American Meat Institute
P.O. Box 3556
Washington, D.C. 20007

Best Foods
Consumer Service Department
Division of CPC International
Internation Plaza
Englewood Cliffs, NY 07623

Borden Farm Products
Bordon Co.
Consumer Affairs
180 E. Broad St.
Columbus, OH 43215

Campbell Soup Co.
Food Service Products Division
375 Memorial Ave.
Camden, NJ 08101

Del Monte Teaching Aids
P.O. Box 9075
Clinton, IA 52736

Fleischman's Margarines
Standard Brands, Inc.
625 Madison Ave.
New York, NY 10022

General Foods Consumer Center
250 North St.
White Plains, NY 10625

General Mills
P.O. Box 113
Minneapolis, MN 55440

Gerber Products Co.
445 State St.
Fremont, MI 49412

H.J. Heinz
Consumer Relations
P.O. Box 57
Pittsburgh, PA 15230

Hunt-Wesson Foods
Educational Services
1645 W Valencia Dr.
Fullerton, CA 92634

Kellogg Co.
Department of Home Economics Services
Battle Creek, MI 49016

Mead Johnson Nutritionals
2404 Pennsylvania Ave.
Evansville, IN 47721

National Dairy Council
6300 N. River Rd.
Rosemont, IL 60018-4233

Oscar Mayer Co.
Consumer Service
P.O. Box 1409
Madison, WI 53701

Pillsbury Co
1177 Pillsbury Building
608 Second Ave. S.
Minneapolis, MN 55402

The Potato Board
1385 S. Colorado Blvd.
Suite 512
Denver, CO 80222

Rice Council
P.O. Box 22802
Houston, TX 77027

Ross Laboratories
Director of Professional Services
625 Cleveland Ave.
Columbus, OH 43216

Sunkist Growers Consumer Service
Division BB, P.O. Box 7888
Valley Annex
Van Nuys, CA 91409

Vitamin Nutrition Information Service (VNIS)
Hoffmann-LaRoche
340 Kingsland Ave.
Nutley, NJ 07110

United Fresh Fruit and Vegetable Association
727 N Washington St.
Alexandria, VA 22314

Glossary

Medical Terminology to Aid in the Study of Nutrition

Term	Meaning
a-	without, from
acyl	a carbon chain
aden-, adeno-	gland
-algia	pain
aliment	food
-amine	containing nitrogen
andr-, andro-	man or male
apo- or ap-	detached
arteri-, arterio-	artery
arthr-, arthro-	joint
-ase	enzyme
-blast	immature form, embryonic
brady-	slow
buli-	ox
canc-, carcino-	malignant tumor
cardi-, cardio-	heart
centi-	divided into one hundred parts
chol-, chole-, cholo-	bile, gall
cholecyst-	gallbladder
chondr-, chondri-, chondro-	cartilage
chrom-, chromo-	color, colored
-clast	something that breaks
col-, coli, colo-	colon
cyano-, cyan-	blue
cyt-, cyto-	cell
derm-, dermato-	skin
dextr-, dextro-	right, on or toward the right
duoden-, duodeno-	duodenum
dys-	difficult, painful
ect-, ecto-	without, outside, external
-ectomy	excision of
-ein	a protein
em-	blood
-emia	in blood
encephal- encephalo-	brain
endo-, ento- end-, ento-	within
enter- entero-	intestine
erythr-, erythro-	red

esophag- esophago-	esophagus
eu-	well, easy, good
gastr-, gastro- gastri-	stomach
gen-	to become or produce
gloss-, glosso-	tongue
glyco- glyc-	sugar
gynec-, gyn-, gyne-	woman or female (especially female reproductive organs)
hem-, hemat-	blood
hepat-, hepato-	liver
hexa-, hex-	six
histo- hist-	tissue
homeo-, homoeo, homoio	sameness, similarity
hydr-, hydro-	water
hyper-	excessive, above, beyond
hypo-, hyp-	under, beneath, deficient
hyster-, hystero-	uterus
idio-	one's own, peculiar to, separate, distinct
ile- ileo-	ileum
inter-	between, among
intra-	within, during, between layers of
-itis	inflammation of
jejun- jejuno-	jejunum
kilo-	One thousand times
lact-, lacti- lacto-	milk
leuc-, leuk-	white, colorless
lev-, levo-	left, levorot
lip- lipo-	fat, lipid
litho- lith-	stone
lymph-, lympho-	waterlike
-lysis	destruction
mal-	bad, badly
malac-, malaco-	soft a condition of abnormal softness
mega- meg-	large, great
meta-	after, later; change, exchange
metallo-	containing metal
micro-	divided into one million parts
milli-	divided into one thousand parts
mono-	one
morph-, morpho-	form, shape
my-, myo-	muscle
myel-, myelo-	marrow, spinal cord
nas- naso-	nose, nasal
necr- necro-	dead
nephr-, nephro-	kidney
neur- neuro-	nerve
-oid	formed like
olig- oligo-	few, scant
-ol	alcohol
-oma	tumor
ophthalmo- ophthalm-	eye, eyeball
-orex	mouth
-orexis	desire, appetite
ost-, osteo-, oste-	bone
-ose	sugar, carbohydrate

-osis	action, process, result, usually discussed
ot-	ear
ovari-, ovario-	ovary
ovo-, ovi	eggs
pan-	all,
pancreat- pancreato-	pancreas
para-	beside
parieto-	wall of a cavity, parietal bone
patho- path-	disease
ped-	child, foot
-penia	without, lack of
-phobia	fear of
-plasm, -plasma	formative, formed, cell or tissue substance
pneum-, pneumo-, pneumono-	lung
-poiesis	production, format
poly-	many, much
post-	after
pre-	before
prot- proto-	first
pseud-, pseudo-	false
pulmo-, pulmon-, pulmono-	lung
pyel-, pyelo-	pelvis
pyr-	fever, fire
rect-, recto-	rectum
reni-, reno-	kidney
rhin-, rhino-	nose
-rrhagia	rupture, excessive fluid discharge
-rrhea	flow, discharge
sate	to fill
scler- sclero-	hard, hardness
-scopy	viewing
seb-, sebi, sebo-	hard fat sebum, sebaceous glands
semi-	half
-soma somat-, somato-	body
-stasia, -stasis	slowing or stopping of
stenosis	narrowing of
stomat-, stomato-	mouth, stoma
-stomy	surgical opening
sub-	under, below
super-	over, above
tachy-	swift, fast
thi-, thio-	containing sulfur
thromb- thrombo-	blood clot
tox-, toxi-, toxo-	poison
trache-, tracheo-	trachea
-trophy	growth or mutation
ure-, urea-, ureo-	urine
uter-, utero-	uterus
vas- vaso-	blood vessel
ven-, veni-, veno-	vein
vita-	life
xer- xero-	dry

Glossary Terms

absorptive cells (ab-SORP-tiv) A class of cells that line the villi finger projections in the small intestine and participate in nutrient absorption.

acesulfame (ay-see-SUL-fame) An artificial sweetener that yields no energy to the body; it is 200 times sweeter than sucrose.

achlorhydria (ay-clor-HIGH-dre-ah) A state of reduced acid production by the stomach, primarily resulting from loss of the acid-producing cells in the stomach associated with aging.

acid ash Acid compounds that form from the residue of metabolized sulfur- and phosphorus-containing foods, such as protein foods.

acid pH A pH less than 7. Lemon juice has an acid pH.

active absorption Absorption in which a carrier is used and ATP energy is expended. In this way, the absorptive cell can absorb nutrients, such as glucose, against a concentration gradient.

adenosine triphosphate (ATP) (ah-DEN-o-sin try-FOS-fate) The main energy currency for cells. ATP energy is used to promote ion pumping, enzyme activity, and muscular contraction.

adipose (fat) cells (ADD-ih-pos) Fat-storing cells.

adipsin (ah-DIP-sin) A protein that appears to be made by adipose cells and acts as a communication link between adipose cells and the brain.

adult-onset obesity Obesity that develops in adulthood; characterized by a normal number of adipose cells, but each cell is enlarged because of fat storage.

aerobic (air-ROW-bic) Requiring oxygen.

alcohol Ethyl alcohol or ethanol, CH_3-CH_2OH.

alcohol dehydrogenase (dee-high-DRO-jen-ase) The enzyme used in alcohol (ethanol) breakdown; the major enzyme used in the liver when alcohol is in low concentrations.

aldosterone (al-DOS-ter-own) A powerful hormone produced by the adrenal glands that acts on the kidney to cause sodium reabsorption and, in turn, water conservation.

alimentary canal (al-ih-MEN-tah-ree) Gastrointestinal tract.

alkaline ash (AL-kah-line) Alkaline compounds that form in the body from residue of metabolized potassium-and sodium-containing foods, such as fruits and vegetables.

alkaline (basic) pH (AL-kah-line) A pH greater than 7. Baking soda in water yields an alkaline pH.

allergy (AL-ler-jee) An immune response when antibodies react with a foreign substance (antigen).

alpha bond (AL-fa) A type of carbohydrate bond that can be digested by human intestinal enzymes.

alpha-linolenic bond (AL-fah-lin-oh-LE-nik) A fatty acid with 18 carbon atoms and 3 double bonds (omega-3).

alveoli (al-VE-o-lye) Small air sacs of the lung.

amino acid (ah-MEE-noh AH-sid) The building block for proteins containing a central carbon atom with a nitrogen atom and other atoms attached.

amniotic fluid (am-nee-OTT-ik) The fluid that surrounds and protects the fetus in the uterus.

amylase (AM-uh-lace) Starch-digesting enzymes from the salivary glands or pancreas.

amylopectin (am-ih-low-PEK-tin) A branched-chain polysaccharide made of glucose units.

amylose (AM-uh-los) A straight-chain digestible polysaccharide made of glucose units.

anabolism (an-AH-bol-iz-um) The process of building compounds.

anaerobic (AN-ah-ROW-bic) Not requiring oxygen.

anaphylactic shock (an-ah-fih-LAK-tic) A severe allergic response that results in greatly lowered blood pressure, as well as respiratory and gastrointestinal distress.

androgen (AN-dro-jen) A general term for hormones that stimulate development in male sex organs; for example, testosterone.

android obesity (AN-droyd) Obesity in which fat storage is located primarily in the abdominal area; defined as a waist-to-hip circumference ratio greater than 0.9 in men and 0.8 in women. Android obesity is closely associated with a high risk of heart disease, hypertension, and diabetes.

anergy (AN-er-jee) Lack of an immune response to foreign compounds entering the body.

angiotensin I (an-jee-oh-TEN-sin) An intermediary compound produced during the body's attempt to conserve water and sodium; it is converted to angiotensin II.

angiotensin II A compound, produced in response to low blood pressure, that increases blood vessel constriction and triggers production of the hormone aldosterone.

animal model Study of disease in animals that duplicates human disease. This can be used to understand more about the human disease.

anorexia nervosa (an-oh-REX-ee-uh ner-VOH-sah) An eating disorder involving a psychological loss of appetite and self-starvation, resulting in part from a distorted body image and various social pressures associated with puberty.

anthropometry (an-throw-po-MEH-tree) The measurement of weight, lengths, circumferences, and thicknesses of the body.

antibody (AN-tih-bod-ee) Blood proteins that inactivate foreign proteins found in the body. This helps prevent infections.

antidiuretic hormone (ADH) (an-tie-dye-URET-ik) A hormone, secreted by the pituitary gland, that acts on the kidney to cause a decrease in water excretion.

antioxidant (an-tie-OX-ih-dant) A compound that can donate electrons to electron-seeking compounds.

apoferritin (ape-oh-FERR-ih-tin) A protein in the intestinal cell that binds with the ferric form of iron (Fe^{+3}) to form ferritin.

apolipoproteins (APE-oh-lip-oh-PRO-teens) Proteins inbedded in the outer shell of lipoproteins.

appetite (AP-peh-tight) The psychological drive to find and eat food, often in the absence of hunger.

arachidonic acid (ar-a-kih-DON-ik) A fatty acid with 20 carbon atoms and four double bonds (omega-6).

areola (ah-REE-oh-lah) The circular dark area of skin at the center of the breast.

ariboflavinosis (aH-rih-bo-flay-vih-NOH-sis) A condition resulting from a lack of riboflavin. The "a" stands for "without", and the "osis" stands for "a condition of".

aseptic processing (ah-SEP-tik) A method by which food and container are simultaneously sterilized. It allows manufacturers to produce boxes of milk that can be stored at room temperature. Variations of this process are also known as ultra high temperature (UHT) packaging.

aspartame (AH-spar-tame) A sweetener made of two amino acids and methanol; it is 200 times sweeter than sucrose.

atherosclerosis (ath-e-roh-scle-ROH-sis) A build-up of fatty material in the arteries, including those surrounding the heart.

atom Smallest combining unit of an element.

autodigestion Literally, self-digestion. The stomach limits autodigestion by covering itself with a thick layer of mucous and producing enzymes and acid only when needed for digestion of foodstuffs.

autoimmune Immune reactions against normal body cells; self against self.

avidin (AV-ih-din) A protein found in raw egg whites that can bind biotin and inhibit its absorption. Avidin is destroyed by cooking.

baryophobia (bear-ee-oh-FO-bee-ah) A disorder associated with a poor rate of growth in children because the parents underfeed them in an attempt to prevent development of obesity and/or heart disease.

basal metabolism (BAY-sal) The minimum energy the body requires to support itself when resting and awake. To have basal metabolic rate (BMR) measured, a person must not have eaten in the previous 12 hours and be maintained in a warm, quiet environment during the measurement.

beriberi (BEAR-ee-BEAR-ee) The thiamin deficiency disorder characterized by muscle weakness, loss of appetite, nerve degeneration, and sometimes edema.

beta bond (BAY-tuh) A type of carbohydrate bond that is not digested by human intestinal enzymes when it is part of a long chain of monosaccharides.

beta-oxidation The breakdown of a fatty acid into numerous acetyl-CoA molecules.

BHA and BHT (Butylated hydroxyanisole and butylated hydroxytoluene) Two common synthetic antioxidants added to foods

bile A substance made in the liver and stored in the gallbladder; it is released into the small intestine to aid fat absorption.

bile acids Emulsifiers synthesized by the liver and released by the gallbladder during digestion to aid in fat digestion.

bioavailability The degree to which the amount of an ingested nutrient actually gets absorbed and so is available to the body.

biochemical lesion (LEE-zhun) Nutritional deficiency symptoms observed in the blood or urine, such as low levels of nutrient byproducts or low enzyme activities, indicating reduced body function.

bioelectrical impedance (im-PEE-dance) A method to estimate total body fat that uses a low-energy electrical current. The more fat storage a person has, the more impedance (resistance) to electrical flow will be exhibited.

biological value of a protein The body's ability to retain protein absorbed from a food.

B-lymphocytes (LIM-fo-site) White blood cells synthesized by lymph tissues and responsible for antibody production.

body mass index Weight (in kilograms) divided by height squared (in meters). A value of 25 or greater shows obesity-related health risks.

bomb calorimeter (kal-oh-RIM-eh-ter) An instrument used to determine the kcalorie content of a food.

bond A sharing of electrons, charges, or attractions. This links two atoms.

brown adipose tissue (ADD-ih-pos) A specialized form of adipose tissue that produces large amounts of heat by metabolizing energy-yielding nutrients without synthesizing much ATP. The energy released simply forms heat.

buffer Compounds that can take up or release hydrogen ions to maintain a certain pH value in a solution.

bulimia (boo-LEEM-ee-uh) An eating disorder in which large quantities of food are eaten at one time (bingeing) and then purged from the body by vomiting, use of laxatives, or other means.

cafeteria-fed animal A laboratory animal that is fed a high fat and sugary diet to encourage it to overeat and become obese.

calcitriol (kal-sih-TRIH-ol) The active hormone form of vitamin D. It contains a derivative of cholesterol as part of its structure.

calmodulin (kal-MOD-you-lin) A cell protein that, once it binds calcium, can influence the activity of certain enzymes in the cell.

cancer A condition characterized by uncontrolled growth of body cells.

carbohydrate (kar-bow-HIGH-drate) A compound containing carbon, hydrogen, and oxygen atoms; most are known as sugars and starches.

carbohydrate-loading A process in which a 600-gram carbohydrate intake (or 70% of total energy, whichever is larger) is consumed for 7 days before an athletic event in an attempt to increase muscle glycogen stores.

cardiac output (CARD-ee-ack) Amount of blood pumped by the heart.

cariogenic (CARE-ee-oh-jen-ik) A substance, often carbohydrate-rich, that promotes dental caries, such as caramels and raisins.

carnitine (CAR-nih-teen) A compound used to shuttle fatty acids from the cytosol of the cell into mitochrondria.

carotenes (CARE-oh-teens) Pigments substances in plants that can often form vitamin A. Beta-carotene is the most active form.

carpal tunnel syndrome (CAR-pull) (SIN-drom) A disease where nerves that travel to the wrist are pinched as they pass through a narrow opening in a bone in the wrist.

casein (KAY-seen) Proteins in milk that form hard curds. These are difficult for infants to digest.

catalyst (CAT-ul-ist) A compound that speeds reaction rates but is not altered by the reaction.

catabolic (cat-ah-BOL-ik) Breaking down compounds.

celiac disease Also known as gluten-induced enteropathy. It is caused by an allergy to protein found in wheat, rye, oats, and barley. If untreated, it causes a severe flattening of the villi in the intestine, leading to severe malabsorption of nutrients.

cell (SELL) A minute structure, the living basis of plant and animal organization. In animals it is composed of a cell membrane. Cells contain both genetic material and systems for synthesizing energy-yielding compounds. Cells have the ability to both take up compounds from and excrete compounds into their surroundings.

cellulose (SELL-you-los) A straight-chain polysaccharide of glucose molecules that is undigestible because of the presence of beta carbohydrate bonds.

Celsius A centigrade measure of temperature:

(degrees in Fahrenheit − 32) × 5⁄9 = °C

(degrees in centigrade × 9/5) + 32 = °F.

cerebrovascular accident (CVA) (se-REE-bro-VAS-cue-lar) Death of part of the brain tissue due to a blood clot.

ceruloplasmin (se-RUE-low-PLAS-min) A copper-containing protein component of plasma that changes iron to Fe^{+3} (ferric form) so it can bind with apoferritin.

chain-breaking Breaking the link between two or more behaviors that encourage problem behaviors, such as snacking while watching television.

chemical reaction An interaction between two chemicals that changes both participants.

chemical score A ratio comparing the essential amino acid content of the protein in a food with the essential amino acid content in a reference protein, such as one established by the Food and Agriculture Organization. The lowest ratio for an essential amino acid is the chemical score.

cholecystokinin (CCK) (ko-la-sis-toe-KY-nin) A hormone that stimulates enzyme release from the pancreas and bile release from the gallbladder

cholesterol (ko-LES-te-rol) A waxy lipid; it has a structure containing multiple chemical rings.

chronic (KRON-ik) Long-standing, developing over time; slow to develop or resolve. When referring to disease, this indicates that the disease progress, once developed is slow and tends to remain; a good example is heart disease.

chylomicrons (kye-lo-MY-krons) Dietary fat surrounded by a shell of cholesterol, phospholipids, and protein. These are made in the intestine after fat absorption and travel through the lymphatic system to the bloodstream.

chyme (KIME) A mixture of stomach secretions and partially digested food.

cirrhosis (see-ROH-sis) A loss of functioning liver cells, which are replaced by nonfunctioning connective tissue. Any substance that poisons liver cells can lead to cirrhosis. The most common cause is a long-standing, excessive alcohol intake.

cis isomer (sis I-so-mer) An isomer form seen in compounds with double bonds, such as fat, where the hydrogens on both sides of the double bond lie on the same side of that bond.

citric acid cycle (SIT-rik) A pathway that breaks down acetyl-CoA, yielding carbon dioxide, $FADH_2$, NADH, and GTP. The pathway can also be used to synthesize compounds.

clinical lesion (LEE-zhun) Nutritional deficiency sign seen on physical examination.

clostridium botulinum (klo-STRID-ee-um BOT-you-LY-num) A bacterium that can cause a fatal type of food poisoning.

cognitive restructuring Changing one's attitude regarding eating; for example, no longer using a difficult day as an excuse to overeat, but instead, substituting other pleasures or activities, such as a relaxing walk with a friend.

colic (KOL-ik) Periodic crying in a healthy infant, apparently resulting from gastrointestinal gas build-up.

colostrum (ko-LAHS-trum) The first milk secreted during late pregnancy and the first few days after birth. This thick fluid is rich in immune factors and protein.

complement A group of serum proteins involved in immune responses, such as phagocytosis and the destruction of bacteria.

complete proteins Proteins that contain ample amounts of all nine essential amino acids.

compound A group of different types of atoms bonded together in definite proportion (see **molecule**)

compression of morbidity Using good health practices to delay the onset of disabilities caused by chronic disease.

condensation reaction A reaction that forms a bond between two compounds by removing a water molecule.

contingency management Forming a plan of action to respond to an environment where overeating is likely, such as when snacks are within arms' reach at a party.

conditioning The process through which an originally neutral stimulus repeatedly paired with a reinforcing agent elicits a predictable response.

conjugase (KON-ju-gase) Enzyme systems in the intestine that enhance folate absorption.

connective tissue Tissue that holds different structures in the body together.

control group Participants in an experiment whose habits are not altered.

coordinated program in dietetics A baccalaureate program that integrates the 900 hours of supervised professional practice that are needed to qualify for the RD credential examination within the junior and senior years of college course work.

cortical bone (KORT-ih-kal) Dense, compact bone that comprises the outer surface and shafts of bone.

cortisol (KORT-ih-sol) A hormone made by the adrenal gland that, among other functions, stimulates the production of glucose from amino acids.

covalent bond (ko-VAY-lent) A union of two atoms formed by the sharing of electrons.

cretensim (KREET-in-ism) Stunting of body growth and poor mental development in an infant that results from inadequate maternal intake of iodine during pregnancy.

Crohn's disease (Krown) A disease of unknown cause in which the small intestine becomes severly inflamed and its absorptive capacity limited.

crude fiber What remains of dietary fiber after acid and alkaline treatment. This consists of primarily cellulose and lignin.

cystic fibrosis (SIS-tik figh-BRO-sis) A disease that often leads to overproduction of mucus. Mucus can invades the pancreas, decreasing enzyme output. The lack of lipase enzyme output then contributes to severe fat malabsorption.

cytochromes (SITE-o-krome) Electron-accepting compounds that participate in the electron transport chain.

cytotoxic test (SITE-o-TOX-ik) An unreliable test to define food allergies that involves mixing whole blood with food proteins.

deamination (dee-am-ih-NA-shun) The removal of an amine group from an amino acid.

Delaney clause This clause to the 1958 Food Additives Amendment of the Pure Food and Drug Act prevents the intentional (direct) addition to foods of a compound introduced after that date that has been shown to cause cancer in animals or man.

denature (dee-NAY-ture) Alteration of the tertiary structure of a protein, usually as a result of treatment by heat, acid, base, or agitation.

dental caries (KARE-ees) Erosions in the surface of a tooth caused by acids made by bacteria as they metabolize sugars.

depolarize To create a neutral or uncharged condition.

diabetes mellitus (DYE-uh-BEET-eez MELL-uh-tus) A disease characterized by high blood sugar levels (hyperglycemia), resulting from either an insufficient insulin release by the pancreas or a general inability for insulin to act on certain body cells, such as adipose cells (see **insulin-dependent diabetes mellitus** and **noninsulin-dependent diabetes mellitus**).

diastolic blood pressure (dye-ah-STOL-ik) The pressure in the bloodstream found when the heart is between beats.

dietary fiber Substances in food (essentially all from plants) that are not digested by the processes present in the stomach and small intestine.

dietary goals Specific goals for nutrient intakes set in 1977 by a Committee of the U.S. Senate.

dietary guidelines General goals for nutrient intake and diet composition, set by government agencies—USDA and DHHS.

dietitian See **registered dietitian.**

digestibility (dye-JES-tih-bil-it-ee) The proportion of food substances eaten that can be broken down in the intestinal tract and absorbed into the bloodstream.

direct calorimetry (kal-oh-RIM-eh-tree) A method to determine energy use by the body by measuring heat that emanates from the body, usually using an insulated chamber.

disaccharides (dye-SACK-uh-rides) Class of sugars formed by the chemical bonding of two monosaccharides.

diuretic (dye-URET-ik) A substance that, when ingested, increases the flow of urine.

diverticula (DYE-ver-TIK-you-luh) Pouches that protrude through the wall of the large intestine to the outside of the intestine.

diverticulitis (DYE-ver-tik-you-LITE-us) An inflammation of the diverticula caused by acids produced by bacterial metabolism inside the diverticula.

diverticulosis (DYE-ver-tik-you-LOH-sis) The condition of having many diverticula in the colon.

double-blind study An experiment in which the subjects and researchers are unaware of the outcome of the study until it is completed.

duodenum (doo-oh-DEE-num, or doo-ODD-num) The first 12 inches (30 centimeters) of the small intestine.

ectomorph (EK-tuh-morf) A body type associated with very long, thin bones and very long, thin fingers.

edema (uh-DEE-muh) The build-up of fluid in extracellular spaces.

eicosanoids (eye-KOH-san-oyds) Hormone-like compounds synthesized from polyunsaturated fatty acids. Within this class of compounds are prostaglandins, thromboxanes, and leukotrienes.

eicosapenteanoic acid (EPA) (eye-KOH-sah-pen-tah-NO-ik) An omega-3 fatty acid with 20 carbon atoms and 5 double bonds; present in fish oils.

electrolytes (ih-LEK-tro-lites) Compounds that break down into ions in water and, in turn, are able to conduct an electrical current.

electron A part of an atom that is negatively charged. Electrons orbit the nucleus.

electron transport chain A series of reactions using oxygen that converts NADH and $FADH_2$ into free NAD and FAD, yielding water and ATP.

elements Substances that cannot be broken down further by using ordinary chemical procedures.

elimination diet A restrictive diet that systematically tests foods that may cause an allergic response by first eliminating suspected foods, and then adding them back, one at a time.

embryo (EM-bree-oh) The developing infant during the second to eighth week after conception.

emulsify (ee-MULL-sih-fye) To suspend fat in water by isolating individual fat drops using sheets of water molecules or other substances to prevent the fat from coalescing.

endocrine-onset obesity (EN-doh-krin) Obesity caused by rare hormonal abnormalities or rare genetic disorders. This is the cause of less than 10% of obesity in North America.

endometrium (en-doh-ME-tree-um) A layer of cells that line the wall of the uterus.

endomorph (EN-doh-morf) A body type characterized by short, stubby bones, a short trunk, and short fingers.

endorphins (en-DOR-fins) Natural body tranquilizers that may be involved in the feeding response and function in pain reduction.

enterohepatic circulation (EN-ter-oh-heh-PAT-ik) Recycling of compounds between the small intestine circulation and the liver over and over again, as happens with bile acids.

enzyme (EN-zime) A compound that speeds the rate of a chemical reaction but is not altered by the chemical reaction. Almost all enzymes are proteins.

epidemiology (ep-uh-dee-me-OLL-uh-gee) The study of how disease rates vary between different population groups, such as the rate of stomach cancer in Japan compared with that in Canada.

epigenetic carcinogens (promoters) (ep-ih-je-NET-ik car-SIN-oh-jens) Compounds that increase cell division, and thereby increase the chance that a cell with altered DNA will develop into cancer.

epinephrine (ep-ih-NEF-rin) Also known as adrenaline. This hormone is released by the adrenal gland and various nerve endings in the body. It acts to increase glycogen breakdown in the liver, among other functions.

epithelial cells (ep-ih-THEE-lee-ul) The surface cells that line the outside of the body and all external passages within it.

equilibrium (ee-kwih-LIB-ree-um) A state in which nutrient intake equals nutrient losses. Thus the body maintains a stable condition.

erythropoietin (eh-REE-throw-POY-eh-tin) A protein secreted by the kidneys that enhances red blood cell synthesis and stimulates red blood cell release from bone marrow.

essential Having no obvious, external cause.

essential amino acids Amino acids not efficiently synthesized by humans and that must therefore be included in the diet. There are nine essential amino acids.

essential fatty acids Fatty acids that must be present in the diet to maintain health. These are linoleic acid and alpha-linolenic acid.

esterification (e-ster-ih-fih-KAY-shun) The process of attaching fatty acids to a glycerol molecule, creating an ester bond. Removing a fatty acid is called deesterification; reattaching a fatty acid is called reesterification.

estimated safe and adequate daily dietary intake (ESADDI) Nutrient intake recommendations first made in 1980 by the Food and Nutrition Board. A range for intake of some nutrients was given as not enough information was available to set a Recommended Dietary Allowance (RDA).

eustachian tubes (you-STAY-shun) Thin tubes connected to the middle ear that open into the throat.

exchange The serving size of a food within a specific exchange system group.

exchange system A grouping of foods in six lists. When the proper serving size for any food in a list is consumed, all foods within the list yield a similar amount of carbohydrate, fat, protein, and energy.

experiment A test made to examine the validity of a hypothesis.

extracellular fluid Fluid present outside the cells; this includes intravascular and interstitial fluids.

extracellular space The space between cells.

facilitated absorption Absorption where a carrier is used to shuttle substances into the absorptive cells, but no energy is expended. A concentration gradient higher in the intestinal lumen than in the absorptive cell drives the absorption.

failure to thrive Inadequate gains in height and weight in infancy, often due to an inadequate food intake.

fasting hypoglycemia (HIGH-po-gligh-SEE-me-uh) Low blood sugar that follows a day or so of fasting.

fatty acids Acids found in lipids, composed of carbon atoms bonded by hydrogen atoms, with an acid group ($-\overset{\overset{\displaystyle O}{||}}{C}-OH$) at one end.

feeding center A group of cells in the hypothalamus that, when stimulated, causes hunger. These cells are also known as the lateral feeding centers.

ferritin (FERR-ih-tin) A protein compound that serves as the storage form of iron in the blood and tissues.

fetal alcohol syndrome (FAS) (FEET-al) A group of physical and mental abnormalities in the infant that result from the mother consuming alcohol during pregnancy.

fetus (FEET-us) The developing life form from 8 weeks until birth.

flavin adenine dinucleotide (FAD) (FLAY-vin ADD-eh-neen dye-NUK-lee-oh-tide) A hydrogen carrier in the cell; synthesized from the vitamin riboflavin.

fluoroapatite (fleur-oh-APP-uh-tite) Tooth crystals containing fluoride ions that are relatively acid-resistant.

food intolerance An adverse reaction to food that does not involve an immune response.

food sensitivity A mild reaction to a substance in a food that might be expressed as slight itching or redness of the skin.

fore milk (FOR) The first breast milk delivered in the nursing session.

fraternal twins Fetuses that develop from two separate ova and sperm and, therefore have separate genetic identities, although they develop simultaneously in the mother.

free erythrocyte protoporphyrins (FEP) (eh-RITH-row-sight pro-tow-POR-fy-rins) Immature forms of red blood cells released from the bone marrow. An increased serum level of FEP reflects a decreased ability to make red blood cells and suggests iron-deficiency anemia. Lead poisoning also raises blood FEP levels.

free radical Short-lived form of compounds that exist with an unpaired electron in their outer electron shell. This causes it to have an electron-seeking nature, which can be very destructive to electron-dense areas of a cell, such as DNA and cell membranes.

fructose (FROOK-tose) A monosaccharide with six carbons that form a five-membered ring with oxygen in the ring; found in fruits and honey.

fruitarian (froot-AIR-een-un) A person who eats primarily fruits, nuts, honey, and vegetable oils.

galactose (gah-LAK-tose) A six-carbon monosaccharide; an isomer of glucose.

galactosemia (gah-LAK-toh-SEE-mee-ah) A disease characterized by the build-up of the monosaccharide, galactose, in the bloodstream resulting from the inability of the liver to metabolize it. If present at birth and left untreated, this causes severe growth and mental retardation in the infant.

gastric balloon (GAS-trik) A balloon about the size of a soft drink can that is inserted surgically into the upper part of the stomach to stimulate feelings of satiety.

gastric inhibitory peptide (GAS-trik in-HIB-ih-tor-ee PEP-tide) A hormone that slows gastric motility and stimulates insulin release from the pancreas.

gastrin (GAS-trin) A hormone that stimulates enzyme and acid secretion in the stomach.

gastrointestinal (GI) tract (GAS-troh-in-TES-tin-al) The main sites in the body used for digestion and absorption of nutrients. It consists of the mouth, esophagus, stomach, small intestine, large intestine, rectum, and anus.

gastroplasty (GAS-troh-plas-tee) Surgery performed on the stomach to limit its volume to approximately 50 milliliters, the size of a shot glass.

gene (JEAN) The genetic material on chromosomes that provides the blueprint for the production of cell proteins.

generally recognized as safe (GRAS) A group of food additives that in 1958 were considered safe, therefore allowing manufacturers to use them from then on when needed in food products. The FDA bears responsibility for proving they are not safe.

genotoxic carcinogen (initiator) (JEH-no-TOK-sik car-SIN-oh-jen) A compound that alters DNA in a cell, in turn providing the potential for cancer to develop.

gestation (jes-TAY-shun) The time between conception and birth of the fetus.

gestational diabetes (jes-TAY-shun-al) A high blood glucose level that develops during pregnancy but returns to normal after birth. One cause is production of hormones by the placenta that antagonize the action of the hormone insulin.

glucagon (GLOO-kuh-gon) A hormone made by the pancreas that stimulates the breakdown of glycogen in the liver into glucose; this raises the blood glucose level. Glucagon also performs other functions.

gluconeogenesis (gloo-ko-nee-oh-JEN-uh-sis) The production of new glucose molecules by metabolic pathways in the cell. The source of the carbon atoms for these new glucose molecules is usually amino acids.

glucose (GLOO-kos) A six-carbon atom carbohydrate found as such in blood, and in table sugar bound to fructose; also known as dextrose, it is one of the simple sugars.

glutathione peroxidase (gloo-tah-THIGH-own per-OX-ih-dase) A selenium-containing enzyme that can break down peroxides.

glycemic index (gligh-SEE-mik) A ratio used to measure the relative ability of a carbohydrate to raise blood glucose levels as opposed to the ability of white bread (or glucose) to raise blood glucose levels.

glycerol (GLISS-er-ol) A carbohydrate containing three hydroxyl groups (—OH); used to help form triglycerides.

glycogen (GLIGH-ko-jen) A carbohydrate made of multiple units of glucose containing a highly branched structure; the storage form of carbohydrate for muscle and liver; sometimes known as animal starch.

glycolysis (gligh-COLL-ih-sis) The pathway that results in the breakdown of glucose into pyruvate (lactate) molecules.

glycosidic bond (gligh-coh-SID-ik) The covalent bond formed between two monosaccharides when a water molecule is lost.

goiter (GOY-ter) An enlargement of the thyroid gland often caused by a lack of iodide in the diet.

goitregens (GOY-troh-jens) Substances in food that interfere with thyroid hormone metabolism and so may cause goiter if consumed in large amounts.

gram Measure of weight in the metric system. One gram equals 1/28 of an ounce

gum A dietary fiber containing chains of galactose, glucuronic acid, and other monosaccharides; characteristically found in exudates from plant stems.

gynecoid obesity (GIGH-nih-coyd) Obesity in which fat storage is located primarily in the buttocks and thigh area.

H_2 blockers Medications, such as cimetidine, that block the stimulation of stomach acid production caused by histamine.

Harris-Benedict equation An equation that predicts resting metabolic rate based on a person's weight, height, and age.

heartburn A pain emanating from the esophagus, caused by stomach acid backing up into the esophagus and irritating the esophageal tissue.

heart disease Disease usually caused by the deposition of fatty material in the blood vessels in the heart. This in turn reduces blood flow to the heart, thereby reducing heart function.

heat-labile (LAY-bile) A structure or activity that is changed by heating.

hematocrit (hee-MAT-oh-krit) The percentage of total blood volume occupied by red blood cells.

heme iron (HEEM) Iron provided from animal tissues as products of hemoglobin and myoglobin. Approximately 40% of the iron in meat is heme iron. This is readily absorbed.

hemicellulose (hem-ih-SELL-you-los) A dietary fiber containing xylose, galactose, glucose, and other monosaccharides bonded together.

hemosiderin (heem-oh-SID-er-in) An insoluble iron-protein compound found in the liver. Hemosiderin stores increase as the amount of iron in the liver exceeds the storage capacity of ferritin.

hemochromatosis (heem-oh-krom-ah-TOS-sis) A disorder of iron metabolism characterized by increased iron absorption, increased saturation of iron-binding proteins, and deposition of hemosiderin in the liver tissue.

hemoglobin (HEEM-oh-glow-bin) The iron-containing protein in the red blood cell that carries oxygen to the cells and carbon dioxide away from the cells. It is also responsible for the red color of blood.

hemolysis (hee-MOL-ih-sis) A breakdown of red blood cells caused by the destruction of the red blood cell membranes.

hemorrhoids (HEM-or-oyds) A pronounced swelling in a large vein, particularly veins found in the anal region.

hexose (HEK-sos) A general term describing a carbohydrate containing six carbon atoms.

high density lipoprotein (HDL) The lipoprotein synthesized by the liver and intestine that picks up cholesterol from dying cells and other sources and transfers it to the other lipoproteins in the bloodstream. A low HDL level increases the risk for heart disease.

high-fructose corn syrup A corn syrup that has been manufactured to contain between 40% and 90% fructose.

hind milk (HYND) The milk secreted at the end of a nursing session; it is higher in fat than fore milk.

histamine (HISS-tuh-meen) A breakdown product of the amino acid histidine that stimulates acid secretion by the stomach and other effects on the body, such as contraction of smooth muscles, increased nasal secretions, relaxation of blood vessels, and changes in relaxation of airways.

hormone A compound secreted into the bloodstream that acts to control the function of distant cells. Hormones can be either protein-like or fat-like, such as insulin or estrogen.

hunger The physiological drive to find and eat food.

hydrogenation (high-dro-jen-AY-shun) The addition of hydrogen atoms to the double bonds of polyunsaturated and monounsaturated fatty acids to reduce the extent of unsaturation. This process turns liquid vegetable oils into solid fats.

hydroloysis reaction (high-DROL-ih-sis) A reaction in which a compound is split into parts, releasing water in the process.

hydrophilic (high-dro-FILL-ik) Attracts water (literally, "water-loving").

hydrophobic (high-dro-FO-bik) Repels water (literally, "water-fearing").

hydroxyapatite (high-drox-ee-APP-uh-tite) A compound composed of calcium and phosphate that is deposited into the bone protein matrix to give bone strength and rigidity.

hyperactivity A poorly defined term generally used to label inattention, irritability, and excessively active behavior in children.

hypercalcemia (high-per-kal-SEE-mee-ah) A high level of calcium in the bloodstream. This can lead to loss of appetite, calcium deposits in organs, and other health problems.

hypercarotenemia (high-per-car-oh-teh-NEEM-ee-ah) High level of carotene in the bloodstream, usually caused by a diet high in carrots or yellow squash.

hyperglycemia (HIGH-per-gligh-SEE-me-uh) High blood glucose levels, above 140 milligrams per 100 milliliters of blood.

hyperplasia (high-per-PLAY-zee-uh) An increase in cell number.

hypertension (high-per-TEN-shun) A condition in which blood pressure remains persistently elevated, especially when the heart is between beats.

hypertrophy (high-PURR-tro-fee) An increase in cell size.

hypochromic (high-po-KROME-ik) Pale red blood cells lacking sufficient hemoglobin (often caused by an iron deficiency).

hypoglycemia (HIGH-po-gligh-SEE-mee-uh) Low blood glucose levels, below 40 to 50 milligrams per 100 milliliters of blood.

hypothalamus (high-po-THALL-uh-mus) A part of the brain that contains cells that play a role in the regulation of hunger, respiration, body temperature, and other body functions.

hypothesis (high-POTH-eh-sis) An "educated guess" by a scientist to explain a phenomenon.

identical twins Two fetuses that develop from a single ovum and sperm and, consequently, have the same genetic makeup.

ileum (ILL-ee-um) The last half of the small intestine.

incidental food additives Additives that gain access to food products indirectly from environmental contamination of food ingredients or during the manufacturing process.

incomplete proteins Lack of an ample amount of one or more essential amino acids to support human protein needs.

index of nutritional quality (INQ) The numerical value for nutrient density.

indirect calorimetry (kal-oh-RIM-eh-tree) A method to measure the energy output by the body by measuring oxygen uptake and/or carbon dioxide output. Formulas are then used to convert these gas exchange values into kcalorie use.

infectious disease (in-FEK-shus) Any disease caused by an invasion of the body by microorganisms, such as bacteria or fungi. Viruses also cause infections.

inorganic Free of carbon atoms bonded to hydrogen atoms.

insensible losses Fluid losses which are not perceptible to the senses, such as losses through lungs, feces, and skin (an exception is heavy perspiration).

insoluble fibers (in-sol-you-bul) Fibers that, for the most part, do not dissolve in water nor are digested by bacteria in the large intestine. These include cellulose, some hemicelluloses, and lignin.

insulin (IN-suh-lin) A hormone produced by the beta cells of the pancreas. Insulin increases the synthesis of glycogen in the liver and the movement of glucose from the bloodstream into muscle and adipose cells, among other processes.

insulin-dependent diabetes mellitus A form of diabetes prone to ketosis and that requires insulin therapy.

intentional food additives Additives knowingly (directly) incorporated into food products by manufacturers.

intermediate density lipoprotein (IDL) (lip-oh-PRO-teen) The product formed after a very low density lipoprotein (VLDL) has most of its triglyceride removed.

international unit (IU) A crude measure of vitamin activity, often based on the growth rate of animals. Today these units have been replaced by more precise milligram and microgram quantities.

internship A program offered by a hospital or other health- or foodservice-related organization that provides 900 hours of supervised professional practice for dietetic students.

interstitial fluid (in-ter-STISH-ul) Fluid between cells.

intestinal bypass A surgical procedure that causes intentional malabsorption of food by shortening the length of the intestine by about 12 of its normal 15 feet. This procedure is no longer used to treat obesity because of the many medical problems that result.

intracellular fluid Fluid contained within a cell.

intravascular fluid Fluid within the bloodstream (that is, in the arteries, veins, and capillaries).

intraveneous (in-tra-VEEN-us) Introduced directly into the bloodstream.

intrinsic factor A protein-like compound produced by the stomach that enhances vitamin B-12 absorption.

in utero (in YOU-ter-oh) "In the uterus" or, in other words, during pregnancy.

ion An atom with an unequal number of electrons and protons. If the number of electrons exceeds the number of protons, the ion is negative. If the number of protons exceeds the number of electrons, the ion is positive.

ionic bond (eye-ON-ik) A union between two atoms formed by an attraction of a positive ion to a negative ion, as seen in table salt (Na^+Cl^-).

irradiation (ir-RAY-dee-AY-shun) A process in which radiation energy is applied to foods. This then creates compounds (free radicals) in the food that destroy cell membranes, break down DNA, link proteins together, limit enzyme activity, and alter a variety of other proteins and cell function that can lead to food spoilage. The net result is less food spoilage.

isomer (EYE-so-mer) Different chemical structures for compounds that share the same chemical formula.

isotope (EYE-so-towp) An alternate form of a chemical element. It differs from other atoms of the same element in the number of neutrons in its nucleus.

jaundice (JAWN-diss) A yellow staining of the skin and sclerae (white of the eye) resulting from a build-up of bile pigments in the bloodstream. Liver or gallbladder disease is often the cause.

jejunem (je-JOON-um) The first half of the small intestine (minus the first 12 inches, which is the duodenum).

juvenile-onset obesity Obesity that develops in childhood; often characterized by an excess number of adipose cells that are also very large because of abundant fat storage.

kcalories (kay-KAL-oh-rees) The heat needed to raise 1,000 grams (1 liter) of water 1 degree Celsius.

ketone bodies (KEE-tone) Products of acetyl-CoA (fat) metabolism containing three to four carbon atoms: acetoacetic acid, beta-hydroxybutyric acid, and acetone. These contain a ketone group, hence, the name.

ketosis (kee-TOE-sis) The condition of having high levels of ketones in the bloodstream.

kidney nephrons (NEF-rons) Cells of the kidney that filter waste out of the bloodstream.

kjoule (KAY-jool) A measure of work in which one kjoule equals the work needed to move one kilogram a distance of one meter with the force of one newton. 1 kcalorie equals 4.8 kjoules.

kwashiorkor (kwash-ee-OR-core) A disease, seen primarily in young children, in which sufficient kcalories are consumed, but not a sufficient amount of protein. The child will suffer from edema, poor growth, weakness, and an increased susceptibility to infections.

lactic acid (LAK-tik AS-id) A three-carbon acid formed during anaerobic cell metabolism; a partial breakdown of glucose.

lactovegetarian (lak-toe vej-eh-TEAR-ree-an) A person who consumes only plant products and dairy products.

lactobacillus bifidus factor (lak-toe-bah-SIL-us BIFF-id-us) A protective factor secreted in human milk that encourages growth of beneficial bacteria in the intestine of the infant.

lacto-ovo-vegetarian A person who consumes only plant products, dairy products, and eggs.

lacto-ovo-pesco vegetarian A person who consumes only plant products, dairy products, eggs, and fish.

lactose intolerance (primary and secondary) Primary lactose intolerance takes place when lactase production declines for no apparent reason. Secondary lactose intolerance takes place when a specific cause, like long-standing diarrhea, results in a decline in lactase production.

lanugo (lah-NEW-go) Down-like hair that appears after one has lost much body fat during semistarvation. The hair stands erect and traps air, which acts as insulation to the body, replacing that usually supplied by body fat. Fetuses also show lanugo.

larvae (LAR-vee) An early developmental stage in the life history of some microorganisms, such as parasites.

laxative A medication or other substance that stimulates evacuation of the intestinal tract.

lecithin (LESS-uh-thin) A phospholipid containing two fatty acids, a phosphate group, and a choline molecule.

lean body mass The part of the human body which is free of all but essential body fat. About 2% of body fat is essential to retain. The rest of the fat in the body represents storage and so is not part of lean body mass. Lean body mass includes muscle, bone, organs, connective tissue, skin, and other body parts.

"let-down reflex" A reflex stimulated by infant suckling that causes the release (ejection) of milk from milk ducts in the mother's breasts.

license Established by a state legislature, a professional license confers on its owner the right to use specific titles or practice specific activities. In some instances, people who are not licensed are prevented from using certain titles and/or practicing some activities.

life expectancy Average length of life for a given group of people.

life span Potential oldest age to which a person can survive.

lignin (LIG-nin) An insoluble fiber made up of a multiringed alcohol (noncarbohydrate) structure.

limiting amino acid The essential amino acid in the lowest concentration in a food in comparison with the body's need.

linoleic acid (lin-oh-LEE-ik) A fatty acid with 18 carbon atoms and two double bonds; omega-6.

lipase (LYE-pase) Fat digesting enzymes; linguinal lipase is produced by the tongue, gastric lipase by the stomach, and pancreatic lipase by the pancreas.

lipid (LIP-id) A compound containing carbon, hydrogen, oxygen, and, sometimes, other atoms. Lipids dissolve in ether or benzene and are known as fat and oils.

lipofuscin (ceroid pigments) (lip-oh-FEW-shun SER-oyd) Signs of accumulation of lipid breakdown products, often seen as brown spots on the skin.

lipogenesis (lye-poh-JEN-eh-sis) The building of fatty acids using derivatives of acetyl-CoA molecules.

lipogenic (lye-poh-JEN-ik) Means creating lipid. The liver is the major lipogenic organ in the human body.

lipolysis (lye-POL-ih-sis) The breakdown of lipid.

lipoprotein (lye-poh-PRO-teen) A compound found in the bloodstream containing a core of lipids with a shell of protein, phospholipid, and cholesterol.

lipoprotein lipase (lye-poh-PRO-teen LYE-pase) An enzyme attached to the outsides of the cells that line the bloodstream; it breaks down triglycerides into free fatty acids and glycerol.

liter (LEE-ter) A measure of volume in the metric system. One liter equals 0.96 quarts.

lobules (LOB-you-els) Sack-like structures in the breast that store milk.

long-chain fatty acids Fatty acids that contain more than 12 carbon atoms.

low birth weight (LBW) Infant weight at birth of less than 2,500 grams, (5.5 pounds); caused by either prematurity or growth retardation during pregnancy. These infants are at higher risk for health problems.

low density lipoprotein (LDL) The product of the intermediate density lipoprotein (IDL) containing primarily cholesterol. An elevated level is strongly linked to heart disease.

lumen (LOO-men) The inside cavity of a tube, such as the GI tract

lymphatic system (lim-FAT-ick) A system of vessels in the body that can accept large particles, such as chylomicrons, and eventually pass them into the bloodstream.

lysosome (LYE-so-som) A cellular body that contains digestive enzymes for use inside the cell.

lysozyme (LYE-so-zime) A substance produced by a variety of cells in the body that can destroy bacteria.

macrocyte (MAC-row-site) A greatly enlarged mature red blood cell having a short lifespan.

major mineral A mineral vital to health that is required in the diet in amounts greater than 100 milligrams per day.

malnutrition Failing health that results from a long-standing dietary intake that fails to meet nutritional needs.

maltose (MAWL-tose) Glucose bonded to glucose; a simple sugar.

mannitol (MAN-it-tol) An alcohol derivative of fructose.

marasmus (mah-RAZ-mus) Results in a person consuming insufficient protein and kcalories; usually seen in infancy. It is the equivalent of protein-energy malnutrition in adults. The person will have little or no fat stores and show muscle wasting and weakness. Death from infections is common.

mass movement A peristaltic wave that simultaneously coordinates contraction over a large area of the colon. Mass movements move material from one portion of the colon to another and from the colon into the rectum.

mast cells Cells in the body that contain histamine and are responsible for some aspects of allergic and inflammatory reactions.

maximum volume of oxygen consumption (Vo_2 max) The maximum amount of oxygen consumption a person can achieve during exercise, such as when riding a bicycle or running on a treadmill.

meconium (mee-KOH-nee-um) The first thick, mucousy stool passed after birth.

medium-chain fatty acids Fatty acids that contain 8-12 carbon atoms.

megaloblast (MEG-ah-low-blast) A large, immature red blood cell that results from an inability for cell division during red blood cell development.

menaquinones (men-AH-kwih-nones) Forms of vitamin K that come from animal food sources or bacterial synthesis.

menarche (men-AR-kee) Onset of menses in women, usually between ages 10 to 13 years.

menopause (MEN-oh-paws) The cessation of menses in women, usually beginning at about 50 years of age.

mesomorph (mez-oh-morf) A body type associated with average bone size, trunk size, and finger length.

metabolism (meh-TAB-oh-lizm) Chemical reactions that occur in the body, enabling cells to release energy from foods, convert one substance into another, and prepare end products for excretion.

metallothionein (meh-TAL-oh-THIGH-oh-neen) Protein that binds and regulates the release of zinc and copper (and other positive ions) in intestinal and liver cells.

meter (MEET-er) A measure of length in the metric system. One meter equals 39.4 inches.

micelles (MY-sells) An emulsification product in which individual emulsifiers organize with their hydrophobic parts to the center of the micelle and their hydrophilic parts to the outside. Lipids are attracted to the center area and water is attracted to the outside periphery.

microcytic my-kro-SIT-ik) Literally, "small cell". Red blood cells that are smaller than normal.

microfractures Small fractures, undetectable by x-rays or other bone scans, that may occur frequently in bones.

microsomol ethanol oxidizing system (my-kro-SO-mol ETH-an-ol) An alternative pathway for alcohol metabolism when it is in high concentrations in the liver; uses rather than yields energy.

minerals Elements used in the body to promote chemical reactions and help form body structures.

miscarriage Loss of pregnancy that occurs before 28 weeks of gestation; also called spontaneous abortion.

modified food starch Starch molecules that have been chemically linked together to increase stability.

molecule A group of like or unlike atoms chemically combined (see **compound**).

monoglyceride (mon-oh-GLIS-er-ide) A breakdown product of a triglyceride consisting of one fatty acid bonded to the carbohydrate glycerol.

monosaccharide (mon-oh-SACK-uh-ride) A single sugar, such as glucose, that is not broken down further during digestion.

monounsaturated fatty acid A fatty acid containing one C=C double bond.

mortality Death rate. The term morbidity refers to the rate/amount of sickness present.

mottling (MOT-ling) Discoloration or marking of the surface of teeth caused by a high fluoride content.

mucilage (MYOO-sih-laj) A dietary fiber consisting of chains of galactose, mannose, and other monosaccharides; characteristically found in seaweed.

mucopolysaccharides (MYOO-ko-POL-ee-SAK-ah-rides) Substances containing protein and carbohydrate parts; found in bone and other organs.

mucus (MYOO-cuss) A thick fluid secreted by glands throughout the body. It contains a compound that has both carbohydrate and protein parts (glycoprotein). It acts as a lubricant and means of protection for cells.

mycotoxins (MY-ko-tok-sins) A group of toxic compounds produced by molds, such as aflatoxin B-1 found on moldy grains.

myocardial infarction (MY-oh-CARD-ee-ahl in-FARK-shun) Death of part of the heart muscle.

myoglobin (my-oh-GLOW-bin) Iron-containing compound that transports oxygen and CO_2 in muscle.

net protein utilization Biological value of a protein multiplied by digestibility of that protein.

neutron (NEW-tron) The part of an atom that has no charge.

neutrophil (NEW-tro-fil) The major form for white blood cells, comprising 55 to 65% of the total.

nicotinamide adenine dinucleotide (NAD) (nik-oh-TIN-ah-mide AD-en-een dye-NUK-lee-oh-tide) A hydrogen carrier that represents a potential form of energy; made from the vitamin niacin.

nonessential amino acids Amino acids that can be readily made by the body. There are 11 nonessential amino acids found in foods.

non-heme iron Iron provided from plant sources and animal tissues other than part of hemoglobin and myoglobin. Non-heme iron needs to be changed to Fe^{+2} before absorption; less efficiently absorbed than heme iron.

noninsulin-dependent diabetes mellitus A form of diabetes in which ketosis is not commonly seen. Insulin therapy can be used, but often is not required.

nonpolar A compound with no charges present; no positive or negative poles present.

no observable effect level (NOEL) The highest dose of an additive that, when fed, produces no deleterious health effect in animals.

nucleus (NEW-klee-us) The core of an atom; it consists of protons and neutrons.

nutrient density The ratio formed by dividing a food's contribution to the needs for a nutrient by its contribution to kcalorie needs. When the contribution to nutrient needs exceeds that of kcalorie needs, the food is considered to have a favorable nutrient density.

nutrients Chemical substances in food that nourish the body by providing energy, building materials, and factors to regulate needed chemical reactions in the body. The body either can't make these nutrients or can't make them fast enough for its needs.

nutrition label A label format that must be included on foods under certain circumstances, such as when nutrients are added to foods, or when a nutritional claim is made for the food. The nutrition label follows specific guidelines set by the FDA.

nutritional status The nutritional health of a person as determined by anthropometric measures (height, weight, circumferences, and so on), biochemical measures of nutrients or their by-products in blood and urine, a clinical (physical) examination, and a dietary analysis (ABCD).

nutritionist A person who advises about nutrition and/or works in the field of food and nutrition. In many states in the United States a person does not need formal training to use this title. Some states reserve this title for Registered Dieticians.

obesity (oh-BEES-ih-tee) A condition characterized by excess body fat, usually defined as 20% above desirable weight.

oligosaccharides (ol-ih-go-SAK-ah-rides) Carbohydrates containing three to ten monosaccharide units

omega-3 fatty acid A fatty acid with its first double bond starting at the third carbon atom from the methyl end ($—CH_3$).

omega-6 fatty acid A fatty acid with its first double bonds starting at the sixth carbon atom from the methyl end ($—CH_3$).

oncogenes (ahn-ko-jeens) Genes that code for proteins that in turn cause growth.

oncotic force (ahn-KAH-tik) The osmotic potential exerted by blood proteins in the bloodstream.

organ A group of tissues designed to perform a specific function, for example, the heart. It contains muscle tissue, nerve tissue, and so on.

organic A compound that contains carbon atoms bonded to hydrogen atoms.

organism A living thing. The human body is an organism consisting of many organs that act in a coordinated manner to support life.

osmotic potential (oz-MOT-ik) The tendency to attract water across a semi-permeable membrane, usually to dilute some constituent in a fluid.

osmotic pressure The pressure needed to be exerted to keep particles in a solution from drawing liquid across a semipermeable membrane.

osteomalacia (OS-tee-oh-mal-AY-shuh) Adult rickets. A vitamin D deficiency disease that causes weak bones and increases fracture risk.

osteopenia (os-tee-oh-PEE-nee-ah) Decreased bone mass, resulting from cancer, hyperthyroidism, or other causes.

osteoporosis (os-tee-oh-po-ROH-sis) A bone disease that develops primarily after menopause in women and is characterized by a decrease in bone density.

ostomy (OSS-toh-mee) A surgically-created short circuit in intestinal flow where the exit point is usually through the abdomen, rather than at the anus.

outpatient A person treated by medical personnel outside the hospital setting; for example, in a clinic or a physician's office.

overnutrition A state in which nutritional intake exceeds the body's needs.

oxidize (OX-ih-dize) To lose an electron or gain an oxygen atom.

oxidizing agent A compound capable of capturing an electron from another compound or supplying an oxygen atom to a compound.

palatable (PAL-it-ah-bull) Pleasing to taste.

passive absorption Absorption that uses no energy. It requires permeability for the substance through the wall of the small intestine and a concentration gradient higher in the lumen of the small intestine than in the absorptive cell.

pasteurization (pas-tur-eye-ZAY-shun) The process of heating food products to kill pathogenic microorganisms. One method heats milk at 161° F for at least 20 seconds.

pathway A metabolic progression of individual steps from starting materials to ending products.

pectin (PEK-tin) A dietary fiber containing chains of galacturonic acid and other monosaccharides; characteristically found between plant cell walls.

peer-reviewed journal A journal that publishes research only after two or three scientists, who were not part of the study, agree it was well conducted and the results are fairly represented. Thus, the research has been approved by peers of the research team.

pellagra (peh-LAHG-rah) A disease characterized by inflammation of the skin, diarrhea, and eventual mental incapacity resulting from the lack of the vitamin niacin in the diet.

pepsin (PEP-sin) A protein-digesting enzyme produced by the stomach.

peptide bond A bond formed by the reaction of an amine group with an acid group while splitting off a water molecule. This is the main bond that links amino acids in a protein.

peptides A few amino acids bonded together; often two to four.

peptones A partial breakdown product of proteins.

percentile Classification of a measurement of a group into divisions of 100.

peristalsis (per-ih-STALL-sis) A coordinated muscular contraction that is used to propel food down the gastrointestinal tract.

pernicious anemia (per-NISH-us ah-NEE-mee-ah) The anemia that results from a lack of vitamin B-12 absorption. It is pernicious (deadly) because of the associated nerve degeneration that can result in eventual paralysis and death.

pH A measure of the hydrogen ion concentration in a solution.

phagocytosis/pinocytosis (FAG-oh-sigh-TOW-sis/PIN-oh-sigh-TOW-sis) A form of active absorption in which the absorptive cell forms an indentation, and particles or fluids entering the indentation are then engulfed by the cell.

phenylketonuria (PKU) (fen-ihl-kee-toh-NEW-ree-ah) A disease caused by a defect in the ability of the person's liver to metabolize the amino acid phenylalanine into the amino acid tyrosine.

phenylpropanolamine (fen-ihl-pro-pan-OL-ah-meen) An over-the-counter decongestant that has a mild appetite-reducing effect.

psyllium (SIL-ee-um) A mostly soluble type of dietary fiber found in the seeds of the plantain plant.

phylloquinone (fil-oh-KWIN-own) A form of vitamin K that comes from plants.

physiological anemia The normal increase in blood volume in pregnancy that ends up diluting the quantity of red blood cells, resulting in anemia; also called hemodilution.

phytic acid (phytate) (FY-tick, FY-tate) A constituent of plant fibers that binds positive ions to its multiple phosphate groups.

phytobezoars (fy-tow-BEE-zors) A pellet of fiber characteristically found in the stomach.

pica (PIE-kah) The practice of eating non-food items such as dirt, laundry starch, or clay.

placebo (plah-SEE-bo) A fake medicine used to disguise the roles of participants in an experiment; if fake surgery is performed, that is called a sham operation.

placenta (plah-SEN-tah) An organ formed only during pregnancy that secretes hormones and makes possible the transfer of oxygen and nutrients from the mother's blood to the fetus and the removal of fetal wastes.

plaque (PLACK) A cholesterol-rich substance deposited in the blood vessels. It also contains various white blood cells, other lipids, and eventually calcium.

polar A compound with distinct positive and negative charges (poles) on it. These charges act like poles on a magnet.

polyglutamate form (POL-ee-GLOO-tah-mate) Folate with more than one glutamate molecule attached.

polypeptide (POL-ee-PEP-tide) Fifty to 100 amino acids bonded together.

polysaccharides (POL-ee-SACK-uh-rides) Carbohydrates containing many glucose units, up to 3000 or more.

polyunsaturated fatty acid A fatty acid containing two or more C=C double bonds.

pool The amount of a mineral stored within the body that can be readily mobilized when needed.

portal vein A large vein that distributes blood from the intestine to the liver through capillaries.

positive balance A state in which a nutrient intake exceeds losses. This causes a net gain of the nutrient in the body, such as when tissue protein is gained during growth. The opposite of this would be negative balance, where losses exceed intake, as in cases of starvation.

pregnancy-induced hypertension A serious disorder that can involve high blood pressure, kidney failure, convulsion, and even death of the mother and the fetus. Although the exact cause is not known, good nutrition and prenatal care can prevent or limit its severity. Protein in the urine is an early sign, also know as preeclampsia.

premature An infant born before 38 weeks of gestation.

premenstrual syndrome A disorder (also referred to as PMS) found in some women a few days before the onset of menses and characterized by depression, headache, bloating, and mood swings.

preservatives Compounds that extend the shelf-life of foods by inhibiting microbial growth or minimizing the destructive effect of oxygen and metals.

primary structure of a protein The order of amino acids in the protein molecule.

progestins (pro-JES-tins) Hormones, including progesterone, that are necessary for pregnancy and lactation.

prognosis (prog-NO-sis) A forecast of the probable course of a disease.

prolactin (pro-LACK-tin) A hormone secreted by the mother that stimulates the synthesis of milk.

prostaglandin prostaglandin I_2 (pros-tah-GLAN-din) An inhibitor of blood clotting made by blood vessel cells.

prostate A gland located near the urinary tract in males that produces a fluid used for the discharge of semen.

protein Compounds made of amino acids, containing carbon, hydrogen, oxygen, nitrogen, and sometimes sulfur atoms, in a specific configuration.

protein efficiency ratio A measure of protein quality determined by the ability of a protein to support the growth of a young rat.

protein-energy malnutrition (PEM) This results when a person regularly consumes insufficient amounts of kcalories and protein. The deficiency eventually results in body wasting and an increased susceptibility to infections.

prothrombin (pro-THROM-bin) A blood protein needed for blood clotting that requires vitamin K for its synthesis.

proton (PRO-ton) The part of an atom that is positively charged.

proto-oncogenes (PRO-tow-ahn-ko-jeens) Growth-promoting genes found naturally in human cells.

raffinose (RAF-ih-nos) An indigestible oligosaccharide containing three monosaccharide units.

rancid (RAN-sid) Containing products of decomposed fatty acids; these yield off-flavors and odors.

reactive hypoglycemia (HIGH-po-gligh-SEE-mee-uh) Low blood sugar that follows a meal high in simple sugars, with corresponding symptoms of irritability, headache, nervousness, and sweating.

receptive framework The process by which a person opens oneself to learning more about a problem; it usually involves seeking more information about the issue from books and people. In the case of seeking behavior changes, it involves examining one's own background experiences to evaluate whether a behavior change is feasible.

receptor A site in a cell at which compounds (such as hormones) bind. Cells that contain receptors for a specific compound are partially controlled by that compound.

receptor pathway for cholesterol uptake A process by which LDL molecules (cholesterol-containing) are bound by cell receptors, with the incorporation of the LDL molecule into the cell.

Recommended Dietary Allowances (RDA) Recommended intakes for nutrients that meet the needs of almost all people of similar age and gender. These are established by the Food and Nutrition Board of the National Academy of Sciences.

Recommended Dietary Intake (RDI) Recommendations from the original tenth edition RDA Committee that were published in 1987 in the American Journal of Clinical Nutrition after the National Academy of Sciences refused to publish the original tenth edition of the RDA.

Recommended Nutritional Intakes (RNI) The Canadian version of the RDA.

reduction To gain an electron or hydrogen atom.

Registered Dietitian (RD) (dye-eh-TISH-shun) A person who has completed both a baccalaureate degree program approved by The American Dietetic Association and at least 900 hours of supervised professional practice and passed a registration examination.

requirement The amount of a nutrient required by one person to maintain health. This varies between individuals. We do not know our individual requirements for each nutrient.

renin (REN-in) An enzyme formed in the kidney in response to low blood pressure; it acts on a blood protein to produce angiotensin I.

reserve capacity The extent to which an organ can preserve essentially normal function despite the loss of cells or reduction in cell activity.

resting metabolic rate Essentially the same as the basal metabolic rate, but the subject does not need to meet the strict conditions used for a basal metabolic rate determination. Today, both terms are often used interchangeably.

retinoids (RET-ih-noyds) Forms of preformed vitamin A; one source is animal foods, like liver.

reverse transport of cholesterol The process by which cholesterol is picked up by HDL molecules and transferred to other lipoproteins that can dispose of it in the liver.

rhodopsin (row-DOP-sin) A protein involved in vision; it is made in the eye and incorporates a protein called opsin and a form of vitamin A; especially important in night vision.

ribose (RIGH-bos) A five carbon sugar found in genetic material, specifically RNA.

rickets A disease characterized by softening of the bones because of poor calcium deposition. This deficiency disease arises from lack of vitamin D activity in the body.

risk factor A characteristic or a behavior that contributes to the chances of developing an illness.

R-protein A protein produced by the salivary glands that enhances vitamin B-12 absorption.

runner's anemia (ah-NEE-mee-ah) A decrease in the blood's ability to carry oxygen that may be caused by iron loss through perspiration, red blood cell destruction resulting from the impact of exercise, or increased blood volume; found in athletes.

saccharin (SACK-ah-rin) An artificial sweetener that yields no energy to the body; it is 500 times sweeter than sucrose.

saliva (sah-LIGH-vah) A watery fluid produced by the salivary glands in the mouth that contains lubricants, enzymes, and other substances.

salt Generally refers to a mixture of sodium and chloride in a 40:60 ratio.

satiety (suh-TIE-uh-tee) A state in which there is no longer a desire to eat.

satiety center A group of cells in the hypothalamus that, when stimulated, causes satiety. These cells are also known as the ventromedial satiety center.

saturated fatty acid A fatty acid containing no C=C double bonds.

scavenger pathway for cholesterol uptake A process by which LDL molecules (cholesterol-containing) are taken up by scavenger cells imbedded in the blood vessels.

scurvy (SKER-vee) The deficiency disease that results after a few weeks of consuming a diet free of vitamin C; pinpoint hemorrhages are an early clinical sign.

sebaceous glands (seh-BAY-shus) Glands surrounding hair follicles on the face, back, and elsewhere that secrete fatty substances.

sebum (SEE-bum) Secretion of the sebaceous glands, consisting of lipids, waxes, and other triglycerides.

secondary deficiency A deficiency caused not by lack of the vitamin in question, but by lack of a substance that is needed for that vitamin to function.

secondary structure of a protein The interactions (bonds) formed between amino acids placed close together in the primary structure.

secretin (SEE-kreh-tin) A hormone that causes bicarbonate ion release from the pancreas.

self-monitoring A process of tracking foods eaten and conditions affecting eating; actions are usually recorded in a diary, along with location, time, and state of mind. This is a tool to help a person understand more about his or her eating habits.

semi-essential amino acids Amino acids that, when consumed, spare the need to use an essential amino acid for their synthesis. Tyrosine in the diet, for example, spares the need to use phenylalanine for its synthesis.

sequesterants (see-KWES-ter-ants) Compounds that bind free metal ions. By so doing, they reduce the ability of ions to cause rancidity in compounds containing fat.

serotonin (ser-oh-TONE-in) A neurotransmitter synthesized from the amino acid tryptophan that appears to both decrease the desire to eat carbohydrates and induce sleep.

set point Often refers to the close regulation of body weight. It is not known what cells control this set point nor how it actually functions in weight regulation. There is no doubt, however, that there are mechanisms that help regulate weight.

short-chain fatty acids Fatty acids that contain fewer than eight carbon atoms.

sickle cell anemia An anemia that results from a malformation of the red blood cell protein hemoglobin because of an incorrect primary structure in part of its protein chains. The disease can lead to episodes of severe bone and joint pain, abdominal pain, headache, convulsions, paralysis, and even death.

sign A change in health status that is apparent on physical examination.

small-for-gestational age (SMA) (jes-TAY-shun-al) Infants born after normal gestation length (38 weeks), but weighing less than 2500 grams (about 5.5 pounds).

soluble fibers (SOL-you-bull) Fibers that either dissolve or swell when put into water or are metabolized (fermented) by bacteria in the large intestine. These include pectins, gums, mucilages, and some hemicelluloses.

solvent A substance that other substances dissolve in.

sorbitol (SOR-bih-tol) An alcohol derivative of glucose.

sphincter (SFINK-ter) A muscular valve that controls flow of foodstuffs in the GI tract.

stable isotope (I-so-tope) An isotope form of an element that does not emit radiation.

stachyose (STAK-ee-os) An indigestible oligosaccharide with four monosaccharide units.

Standard of Identity If a food is produced according to a specific recipe on file with the FDA, the label does not have to list its ingredients. In that case, the manufacturer is using its Standard of Identity to avoid disclosing its ingredients.

starch A carbohydrate made of multiple units of glucose attached together in a form the body can digest; also known as complex carbohydrate.

stroke The loss of body function that results from a blood clot in the brain, which in turn causes the death of brain tissue.

subclinical disease Disease or disorder that is present, but not severe enough to produce symptoms that can be detected or diagnosed.

subjects Participants in an experiment.

sucrose (SOO-kros) Fructose bonded to glucose; table sugar.

superoxide dismutase (soo-per-OX-ide DISS-myoo-tase) An enzyme that can neutralize a superoxide free radical.

symptom A change in health status noted by the person with the problem, such as a stomach pain.

systolic blood pressure (sis-TOL-ik) The pressure in the arteries associated with the pumping of blood from the heart.

tertiary structure of a protein (TER-she-air-ee) The three-dimensional structure of a protein, formed by interactions of amino acids placed far apart in the primary structure.

tetany (TET-ah-nee) A syndrome marked by sharp contraction of muscles with failure to relax afterward; usually caused by abnormal calcium metabolism.

theory An explanation for a phenomenon that has numerous lines of evidence to support it.

thermic effect of food The increase in kcalorie use that occurs during the digestion, absorption, and metabolism of energy-yielding nutrients.

"thrifty" metabolism A metabolism that characteristically uses less kcalories than normal, such that the risk of weight gain and obesity is enhanced.

thromboxane A_2 (throm-BOX-ane) A stimulus for blood clotting made by particles (platelets) in the bloodstream.

thyroid-stimulating hormone A hormone that regulates the uptake of iodide by the thyroid gland and is secreted in response to low levels of circulating thyroid hormone.

tissue A group of cells designed to perform a specific function; nerve tissue is an example.

t-lymphocyte (tee-LYMF-oh-site) White blood cells synthesized by the thymus gland and responsible for recognition of foreign substances (for example, bacterial cells) in the body.

tocopherols (tuh-KOFF-er-alls) The chemical name for some forms of vitamin E.

trabecular bone (trah-BEK-you-lar) The spongy, inner matrix of bone, found primarily in the spine, pelvis, and ends of bones.

trace mineral A mineral vital to health that is required in the diet in amounts less than 100 milligrams per day.

transamination (trans-am-ih-NAT-shun) The transfer of an amine group from an amino acid to a carbon skeleton to form a new amino acid.

trans isomer (EYE-so-mer) An isomer form found in compounds with double bonds, such as fatty acids, where the hydrogens of both carbon atoms forming the double bond lie on opposite sides of that bond.

triglyceride (try-GLISS-uh-ride) The major form of lipid in food. It is composed of three fatty acids bonded to the carbohydrate glycerol.

trimester The normal pregnancy of 38 to 42 weeks is divided into three 13 to 14 week periods called trimesters.

trypsin (TRIP-sin) A protein-digesting enzyme secreted by the pancreas (in a zymogen form) that acts in the small intestine.

ulcer (UL-sir) Erosion of the tissue lining usually in the stomach or the upper small intestine. These are generally referred to as a peptic ulcer.

uncoupling The dissociation between the liberation of energy from energy-yielding substances and the formation of ATP.

U.S. Recommended Daily Allowances (U.S. RDA) Standards established by the FDA for use on nutrition labels. For the most part, the four existing versions use the highest nutrient recommendation in the appropriate age and gender category from the 1968 publication of the RDA. The version that includes children over 4 years of age and adults is most commonly seen on nutrition labels.

variability The variation one would expect to see within a group of individuals, as with nutrient requirements.

vegan (VEE-gun) A person who eats only plant foods.

very low calorie diet (VLCD) Known also as a protein-sparing, modified fast (PSMF), this diet allows a person 400 to 700 kcalories per day, often in liquid form. Of this, 30 grams or so are carbohydrate; the rest is high biological value protein.

very low density lipoprotein (VLDL) The lipoprotein that initially leaves the liver. It carries both the cholesterol and lipid newly synthesized by the liver.

villi (VIL-eye) Finger-like protrusions into the small intestine that participate in digestion and absorption of foodstuffs.

vitamins Compounds needed in very small amounts in the diet to help regulate and support chemical reactions in the body.

water activity A measure of the amount of free water in a food. Most bacteria need a water activity greater than 0.9 to grow, while molds can grow in water activity as low as 0.6.

whey (WAY) Proteins, such as lactalbumin, that are found in great amounts in human milk and are easy to digest.

whole grains Grains containing the entire seed of the plant, including the bran, germ, and endosperm (starchy interior).

xanthinine dehydrogenase (ZAN-thin-een dh-HY-droj-eh-nase) An enzyme, containing molydenum and iron, that functions in the formation of uric acid and the mobilization of iron from liver ferritin stores.

xerophthalmia (zer-op-THAL-mee-uh) A cause of blindness that results from infection of the eye resulting from a vitamin A deficiency. The specific cause is a lack of mucus production by the eye, which then leaves it more vulnerable to surface dirt and bacterial infections.

xylitol (ZIGH-lih-tol) An alcohol derivative of the five-carbon monosaccharide, xylose.

yo-yo dieting The practice of losing weight and then regaining it, only to lose it and regain it again. This practice in animals (and probably humans) can make it more difficult to succeed in further attempts to lose weight because thyroid hormone levels may drop very low in subsequent dieting, thereby slowing basal metabolism significantly.

zymogen (zigh-MO-gin) An inactive form of an enzyme.

Index

CREDITS

Chapter 1

P. 3, Four By Five; p. 5, (left) from Estimates from the National Center for Health Statistics, Monthly Vital Statistics Report, 37:1, April 25, 1988, (right) Jeff Dunn/The Picture Cube; p. 7, modified from Guthrie, Helen A: *Introductory Nutrition,* ed. 7, Times Mirror/Mosby College Publishing, 1989; p. 8, William C. Ober; p. 12, (top) L. Fritz/H. Armstrong Roberts, (bottom) Jeffry W. Myers/Stock Boston; p. 13, from Healthline, Menlo Park, CA; p. 15, Pelto, used with permission, *Journal of Nutrition Education* (13) 1, 1981 (c) Society for Nutrition Education; p. 16 (left) Ray Block/H. Armstrong Roberts, (right) from USDA, Determinants of Food Consumption in American Households, December 1982, Marketing Science Institute, Cambridge, Massachusetts, in conjunction with Community Nutrition Institute, Washington, D.C., 1982; p. 17, John H. Anderson/Photographic Resources; p. 18, Courtesy of Dorman-Roth Foods, Inc; p. 19, Tom Ebenhoh/Photographic Resources; p. 22, adapted from Raven, Peter H. and Johnson, George B: *Understanding Biology,* ed. 1, Times Mirror/Mosby College Publishing, 1988.

Chapter 2

P. 27, Wolff Communications; p. 29, (top right) H. Armstrong Roberts, (bottom left), Ed Reschke, illustrations, William C. Ober, from Raven, Peter H. and Johnson, George B: *Understanding Biology,* ed. 1, Times Mirror/Mosby College Publishing, 1988; p. 30, William C. Ober; p. 31, (top right) William C. Ober, (bottom right) J.D. Sloan/The Picture Cube; p. 33, William C. Ober; p. 36, Dave Schaefer/The Picture Cube; p. 37, William C. Ober; p. 38, Richard Pasley/Stock, Boston; p. 39, from Guthrie, Helen A: *Introductory Nutrition,* ed. 7, Times Mirror/Mosby College Publishing, 1989; p. 40, Wolff Communications; p. 41, *Recommended Dietary Allowances,* 10th Edition, National Academy Press, 1989; pp. 43-44, "Hassle-free Daily Food Guide," USDA; p. 45 from "Canada's Food Guide," Health and Welfare, Canada, 1983 and Reproduced with permission of the Minister of Supply and Services, Canada; p. 46, from USDA Home and Garden Bulletin, Number 232-1, 1986; p. 47, Don Katchusky/The Picture Cube; p. 49, U.S. Senate Select Committee on Nutritional and Human Needs; Dietary Goals for the United States, ed. 2, 1977; pp. 50-53, International Diabetes Center, Minneapolis, MN; p. 51, the American Diabetes Association and the American Dietetics Association, Exchange Lists for Meal Planning, 1986; p. 59, from *Healthline,* Menlo Park, CA; p. 61, Wolff Communications.

Chapter 3

P. 63, Cecil Fox/Photo Researchers; p. 65 (top) William C. Ober; p. 65, (bottom) Ron Ervin, from Raven, Peter H. and Johnson, George B: *Understanding Biology,* ed. 1, Times Mirror/Mosby College Publishing, 1988; p. 66, William C. Ober; p. 67, (top) Science Photo Library/Photo Researchers; p. 69, William C. Ober; p. 70, (top) International Diabetes Center, Minneapolis, MN, (bottom) William C. Ober, from Raven, Peter H. and Johnson, George B: *Understanding Biology,* ed. 1, Times Mirror/Mosby College Publishing, 1988; p. 72, William C. Ober; p. 73, (top) William C. Ober, (bottom) Trent D. Stephens, from Seeley, Rod R., Stephens, Trent D., and Tate, Philip: *Anatomy and Physiology,* ed. 1, Times Mirror/Mosby College Publishing, 1989; p. 74, William C. Ober; p. 75, Courtesy of the American Dairy Association; p. 78 (top) William C. Ober, (bottom right) William C. Ober, from Raven, Peter H. and Johnson, George B: *Understanding Biology,* ed. 1, Times Mirror/Mosby College Publishing, 1988; p. 78, (bottom left) From Guthrie, Helen A: *Introductory Nutrition,* ed. 7, Times Mirror/Mosby College Publishing, 1989; p. 79, (top) William C. Ober, from Raven, Peter H. and Johnson, George B: *Understanding Biology,* ed. 1, Times Mirror/Mosby College Publishing, 1988; p. 80, William C. Ober; p. 81 Joan M. Beck/Donna Odle, from Seeley, Rod R., Stephens, Trent D., and Tate, Philip: *Anatomy and Physiology,* ed. 1, Times Mirror/Mosby College Publishing, 1989; p. 82, William C. Ober; p. 85, from *Healthline,* Menlo Park, CA; p. 88, Photographic Resources; p. 89, The Picture Cube.

Chapter 4

P. 93, Wolff Communications; p. 95, William C. Ober; p. 96 (top) William C. Ober, (bottom) Eve Lowry/Nutrivisuals; p. 98, William C. Ober; p. 101, (top) Jeffry W. Myers/Stock, Boston; p. 103, William C. Ober; p. 105, from *Healthline,* Menlo Park, CA; p. 107, (top) Steve Hansen/Stock, Boston, (bottom) Wolff Communications; p. 110, modified from Jenkins, D.A. and others: The Glycemaemic Response to Carbohydrate Foods, Lancet 2:388, 1984; p. 111, modified from USDA Home and Garden Bulletin No. 232-5, 1986; p. 113, courtesy of the Rice Council; p. 115, Wolff Communications; p. 119, Richard Hutchings/Photo Researchers.

Chapter 5

P. 123, William Curtsinger/Photo Researchers; p. 125, William C. Ober; p. 126, courtesy of Proctor & Gamble; p. 127, from Deitel, Mervyn: *Nutrition in Clinical Surgery,* ed. 2, 1985, the Williams & Wilkins Co., Baltimore; p. 128, (bottom) courtesy of the Pacific Kitchens Division, Evans Food Group p. 129, from *Healthline,* Menlo Park, CA; p. 130, Nutrivisuals; p. 132, (bottom) William C. Ober; p. 134 (bottom) William C. Ober, from Raven, Peter H. and Johnson, George B: *Understanding Biology,* ed. 1, Times Mirror/Mosby College Publishing, 1988; p. 135, (top) William C. Ober; p. 137, William C. Ober; p. 139, Courtesy of National Institutes of Health, National Heart, Lung, and Blood Institute; p. 141, (top) from Circulation 77: 721A, 1988; p. 142, (left) courtesy of the National Livestock and Meat Board; p. 146, William C. Ober, from Raven, Peter H. and Johnson, George B: *Understanding Biology,* ed. 1, Times Mirror/Mosby College Publishing, 1988; p. 148, Wolff Communications; p. 151, William C. Ober.

Chapter 6

P. 155, National Cancer Institute, Bethesda, MD; p. 159, William C. Ober; p. 161, William C. Ober; p. 162, (top) William C. Ober; (bottom) Bill Longcore, Science Source; p. 164, William C. Ober; p. 165, Lennart Nilsson (c) Boehringer Ingelheim International GmbH; p. 167, From Williams, Sue Rodwell: *Nutrition and Diet Therapy,* ed. 6, Times Mirror/Mosby College Publishing, 1988; p. 167, Bob Daemmrich/Stock Boston; pp. 172-173, from *Healthline,* Menlo Park, CA; p. 174, Courtesy of the National Cancer Institute, Bethesda, MD; p. 178, Wad Kowli, Sudan Thomas S. England/Science Source; p. 179, David Burnett/Contact Press Images.

Chapter 7

P. 189, Michael P. Gadomski/Photo Researchers; p. 191, K.G. Murti/Visuals Unlimited, from Raven, Peter H. and Johnson, George B: *Understanding Biology,* ed. 1, Times Mirror/Mosby College Publishing; p. 191, from Flickinger, Charles: *Medical Cell Biology,* W.B. Saunders, 1979; p. 192, Jerry Howard/Stock Boston; p. 193, William C. Ober; p. 195, from Raven, Peter H., and Johnson, George B.: *Understanding Biology,* ed. 1, Times Mirror/Mosby College Publishing; p. 196, William C. Ober; p. 197, (c) 1989 M.C. Escher Heirs/Cordon Art—Baarn—Holland; p. 198, William C. Ober; p. 199, From Raven, Peter H., and Johnson, George B: *Understanding Biology,* ed. 1, Times Mirror/Mosby College Publishing; p. 202, William C. Ober; p. 205, (top) Richard Stockton/Photographic Resources, (bottom) William C. Ober; pp. 206-207, from *Healthline,* Menlo Park, CA; p. 208, William C. Ober, from Raven, Peter H. and Johnson, George B: *Understanding Biology,* ed. 1, Times Mirror/Mosby College Publishing; p. 209, William C. Ober; p. 212, Bruce Kliewe/The Picture Cube; p. 213, adapted from "Caffeine," A Scientific Status Summary by the Institute of Food Technologists, April, 1983; p. 214, from Guthrie, Helen A: *Introductory Nutrition,* ed. 7, Times Mirror/Mosby College Publishing, 1989; p. 215 (bottom) Nik Kleinberg/Stock Boston; p. 216, William C. Ober; pp. 217-219, Clark, Nancy, Developing a Sports Nutrition Practice, Nutrition Today, 24:No. 3, pp. 35-37.

Chapter 8

P. 221, Robert Jones, Jr; p. 226, Richard Stockton/Photographic Resources; p. 227, William C. Ober; p. 230, Mike Mazzaschi/Stock Boston; p. 231, from Guthrie, Helen A: *Introductory Nutrition,* ed. 7, Times Mirror/Mosby College Publishing, 1989; p. 232, From the NCHS report "Anthropometric Reference Data and Prevalence of Overweight United States, 1976-1980," data from the second National Health and Nutrition Examination Survey (NHANES II), conducted 1976-1980; p. 235, courtesy of Metropolitan Life Insurance Company; p. 236, (top) Grant, J.P: Handbook of Total Parenteral Nutrition, Philadelphia, 1980, W.B. Saunders Co., (bottom) From Metropolitan Life Insurance Company, 1983; p. 237, adapted from Gray, David: Diagnosis and Prevalence of Obesity, Medical Clinics of North America, Vol. 73, pp. 1-13, 1989; p. 238, Diana Linsley, from Payne, Wayne A. and Payne, Dale B: *Understanding Your Health,* ed. 2, Times Mirror/Mosby College Publishing, 1989; p. 240, (top) Chris Bryant/Photographic Resources; pp. 242-243, from *Healthline,* Menlo Park, CA; p. 245, H. Armstrong Roberts; p. 247, Wasye Szkodzinsky/Photo Researchers.

Chapter 9

P. 253, Wolff Communications; p. 256, Ron Blakely/Photographic Resources; p. 257, adapted from USDA Home and Garden Bulletin No. 232-2, 1986; p. 258, adapted from USDA Home and Garden Bulletin No. 232-2, 1986; p. 258, adapted from Christian, Janet L. and Greger, Janet L.: *Nutrition for Living,* ed. 2, Benjamin-Cummings Publishing Company, Inc., 1988; p. 260, W. Metzen/H. Armstrong Roberts p. 263, From Laquatra I. and Danish, S.J., A Primer for Nutrition Counselling, in Frankle, R.T., and Yang M. eds: *Obesity and Weight Control,* Rockville, M.D. Aspen Publishers, Inc. 1988; p. 263, R.C. Paulson/H. Armstrong Roberts; p. 264, William C. Ober; p. 264, Bob Peterson/West Stock; p. 265, From McArdle, W.D. et al: *Exercise Physiology, Energy, Nutrition and Human Performance,* (c) Lea and Febiger, 1986; p. 268, from *Healthline,* Menlo Park, CA; p. 269, From Hechtlinger, Adelaide: *The Great Patent Medicine Era,* Grosset & Dunlap, Inc., 1970; p. 273, (top) Wolff Communications; p. 273, (bottom) Reprinted with special permission of King Features Syndicate, Inc., 1989; pp. 274-275, from *Healthline,* Menlo Park, CA; pp. 280-281, from *Healthline,* Menlo Park, CA

Chapter 10

P. 283, Paul Buddle/H. Armstrong Roberts; p. 285, Diagnostic and Statistical Manual of Mental Disorders DSM 111R (14) American Psychiatric Association, ed. 3; p. 286, adapted from Christian, Janet L., and Greger, Janet L: *Nutrition for Living,* ed. 2, Benjamin-Cummings Publishing Company, Inc., 1988; p. 287, Paul Buddle/H. Armstrong Roberts; p. 288, Bruce Fields/Bruce Fields Studio, Inc; p. 289, Cathy Lander-Goldberg/Lander Photographics; p. 290, Jeffrey Myers/Stock Boston; p. 291, Bob Daemmrick/Stock Boston; p. 292, Cathy Lander-Goldberg/Lander Photographics; p. 293, Paul S. Casamassimo, D.D.S., M.S; pp. 294-295, from *Healthline,* Menlo Park, CA; p. 286, from Story M: Nutrition Management and Dietary Treatment of Bulemia, Journal of the American Dietetic Association 86:517, 1986; p. 300, A) Culver Pictures, Inc., B) Kobal Collection, Superstock International Inc; C) Caron/Gamma Liason D) 1989, Sports Illustrated; p. 301, John Held/The Granger Collection.

Chapter 11

P. 305, Wolff Communications; pp. 310, 311, William C. Ober; p. 312, from McLaren, Donald S.: *A Colour Atlas of Nutritional Disorders,* ed. 1, Wolfe Medical Publications, Ltd., 1981; p. 314, Don Katchusky/The Picture Cube; p. 314, D Cody p. 315, adapted from Hegarty, Vincent: *Decisions in Nutrition,* ed. 1, Times Mirror/Mosby College Publishing, 1988; pp. 316-317, from *Healthline,* Menlo Park, CA; p. 319, William C. Ober; p. 320, (top) from McLaren, Donald S.; *A Colour Atlas of Nutritional Disorders,* ed. 1, Wolfe Medical Publications, Ltd., 1981; p. 320, (bottom) Wally McNamee/Woodfin Camp and Associates, Inc.; p. 321, Mike Mazzaschi, Stock Boston; p. 322, (top) C. Mehrtens/Photographic Resources, (bottom) William C. Ober; p. 324, (left) R.J. Bennett/H. Armstrong Roberts; p. 325, (bottom) Wolff Communications; p. 326, (top right) William C. Ober; p. 326, (bottom) M. Glanzman/FPG International.

Chapter 12

P. 335, Frank Oberle/Photographic Resources; p. 337, (top) From Guthrie, Helen A: *Introductory Nutrition,* ed. 7, Times Mirror/Mosby College Publishing, 1989; p. 337, International Diabetes Center, Minneapolis, MN; p. 339, (bottom) from McLaren, Donald S: *A Colour Atlas of Nutritional Disorders,* ed. 1, Wolfe Medical Publications, Ltd., 1981; p. 340 (bottom) J. Minnihan/Photographic Resources; p. 342, from McLaren, Donald S.: *A Colour Atlas of Nutritional Disorders,* ed. 1, Wolfe Medical Publications, Ltd., 1981; p. 345, (bottom) Gary D. McMichael/Photographic Resources; p. 350, from Powers, Lawrence W.: *Diagnostic Hematology: Clinical and Technical Principles,* ed. 1, The C.V. Mosby Company, 1989; p. 351, (top) David C. Bitters/The Picture Cube; p. 352, from *Healthline,* Menlo Park, CA; p. 355, William C. Ober; p. 357, (bottom) J. Nettis/H. Armstrong Roberts; p. 359, from McLaren, Donald S: *A Colour Atlas of Nutritional Disorders,* ed. 1, Wolfe Medical Publications, Ltd., 1981; p. 360, (top) Peter Vandermark/Stock Boston.

Chapter 13

P. 373, M. Thonig/H. Armstrong Roberts; p. 375, from Linder, M., ed., *Nutritional Biochemistry and Metabolism,* Elsevier, New York, NY, 1985; p. 376, D. Rawcliff/FPG International; p. 377, from Guthrie, Helen A: *Introductory Nutrition,* ed. 7, Times Mirror/Mosby College Publishing, 1989; p. 380, (center) Wolff Communications, (bottom) William C. Ober; p. 382, from Ross, E.M., Compendium of Human Responses to Aerospace Environment, Vol. 3, Section 15, 1962; p. 384, (bottom) Stanley Rowin/The Picture Cube; p. 385, 386-87, from USDA Home and Garden Bulletin No. 232-6, April 1986; p. 387, (bottom) Bob Peterson/West Stock; p. 389, FPG International; p. 391, William C. Ober; p. 392, Courtesy of Lunar, Madison, WI; p. 393, (left and right) from Williams, Sue Rodwell: *Nutrition and Diet Therapy,* ed. 6, Times Mirror/Mosby College Publishing, 1989; (center) David Mascaro and Associates; pp. 396-397, from *Healthline,* Menlo Park, CA; p. 398, H. Armstrong Roberts; p. 400, Courtesy of the National Cancer Institute; p. 407, Chet Hanchett/Photographic Resources.

Chapter 14

P. 413, CNRI/Science Photo Library/Photo Researchers; p. 415, Norm Thomas/Photo Researchers; p. 417, (top) R. Pleasant/FPG International; p. 417, (bottom) William C. Ober; p. 419, (bottom left), from Powers, Lawrence W: Diagnostic Hematology: The C.V. Mosby Company, 1989; p. 420, (top) Frank Oberle/Photographic Resources; p. 420, (bottom left) Wolff Communications; p. 422, Four By Five; p. 424, (left) Anada S. Prasad, M.D., Ph.D., American Journal of Medicine, 31:532–546, 1961; pp. 426-427, from *Healthline,* Menlo Park, CA; p. 430, Martin Rogers/FPG International; p. 432, from McLaren, Donald S.: *A Colour Atlas of Nutritional Disorders,* ed. 1, Wolfe Medical Publications, Ltd., 1981; p. 433, Paul Buddle/H. Armstrong Roberts; p. 435, Photographic Resources; p. 443, William C. Ober; p. 444, (c) 1988, TIME, Inc. Reprinted by permission, photographs by Mario Ruiz/TIME Magazine.

Chapter 15

P. 449, Lennart Nilsson/*Behold Man,* Little, Brown and Company, Boston; p. 451, (top) William C. Ober; p. 452, Lennart Nilsson/*Behold Man,* Little, Brown and Company, Boston; p. 453, William C. Ober; p. 454 (top) Wolff Communications, p. 454, (bottom) Tom Tracy/FPG International; p. 455, (bottom) Zefa - U.K./H. Armstrong Roberts; pp. 456-457, from *Healthline,* Menlo Park, CA; p. 458, from Kennedy, E.T: A Prenatal Screening System for Use in a Community-Based Setting, Journal of the American Dietetic Association, 86:1372, 1986; p. 459, Guy Marcie/FPG International; p. 460, (top) Jim Pickerell/FPG International; p. 461, Steven Jones/Steven Jones Photography; pp. 462, 463, from Maternal Nutrition and the Course of Pregnancy, Washington, DC, 1970, National Academy of Sciences—National Research Council; p. 465, (bottom) Zefa-U.K./H. Armstrong Roberts; p. 469, (right) FPG International; p. 470, adapted from Guthrie, Helen A: *Introductory Nutrition,* ed. 7, Times Mirror/Mosby College Publishing, 1989; p. 474, courtesy of Gerber Products Company, Fremont, MI; p. 478, from Streissguth, A., and others: Science 109:353, 1980 Copyright 1980 American Association for the Advancement of Science; p. 480, Patrick Donahue/Photo Researchers.

Chapter 16

P. 481, H. Armstrong Roberts; p. 482, Don Mason/West Stock; p. 484, courtesy of Ross Laboratories, Columbus, OH; p. 486, (top) Peter Pearson/H. Armstrong Roberts; p. 487, FPG International; p. 488, E. Masterson/H. Armstrong Roberts; p. 490, adapted from Pipes, P.L: *Nutrition in Infancy and Childhood,* ed. 4, Times Mirror/Mosby College Publishing, 1989; p. 492, (top) Paul S. Casamassimo, D.D.S., M.S., (bottom) Four By Five; p. 495, (top) Junebug Clark/Photo Researchers, (bottom) John Fogle/The Picture Cube; p. 496, Edward Lettau/FPG International; p. 497, Calvin and Hobbes, copyright 1988 Universal Press Syndicate, reprinted with permission, all rights reserved; p. 498, adapted from Endres, J. and Rockwell, R: *Food, Nutrition and the Young Child,* The C.V. Mosby Company, 1980, and the National Livestock and Meat Board, 444 North Michigan Avenue, Chicago, IL 60611; p. 499, from "A Food Guide for the First Five Years," National Live Stock and Meat Board, 444 North Michigan Avenue, Chicago, IL 60611; p. 501, (top) Photographic Resources, (bottom) Edward Lettau, FPG International; p. 502, from *Healthline,* Menlo Park, CA; p. 504, Jeffrey Myers/West Stock; p. 505, From the "Hassle-Free Daily Food Guide." USDA; p. 506, (top) Four By Five; p. 515, D. Logan/H. Armstrong Roberts.

Chapter 17

P. 517, K. Reno/H. Armstrong Roberts; p. 519, (top) Michael Philip Manheim/West Stock; p. 519, (bottom) Cathy Lander-Goldberg/Lander Photographics; p. 521, from National Academy of Sciences Report on Diet and Health, Nutrition Reviews, 47:142, 1989; pp. 524-525, 526-527, from *Healthline,* Menlo Park, CA; p. 529, (top) from Fries, J.F., and Crapo, L.M: Elimination of Premature Disease, from Dychtwald, K., *Wellness and Health Promotion for the Elderly,* Aspen Publishers, Rockville, MD, 1986; p. 529 (bottom) From Insel, P.M. and Roth, W.T.: *Core Concepts in Health,* Mayfield Publishing Co., Mountain View, CA 1988; p. 530, From Hegarty, Vincent: *Decisions in Nutrition,* ed. 1, Times Mirror/Mosby College Publishing, 1988; p. 533, (left) From Davies, L: Practical Nutrition for the Elderly, Nutrition Reviews 46:83, 1988; p. 533 (right) Zefa/H. Armstrong Roberts; p. 535, Richard Hutchings, Photo Researchers, Inc; p. 537, (right) H. Armstrong Roberts; p. 538 (top) J. Nettes/H. Armstrong Roberts; p. 539, Miro Vintoniv/The Picture Cube; p. 545, from Fitness Fundamentals, USDHHS, 1985, U.S. Government Printing Office; p. 546, From Rippe, J.M: 29 Tips for Staying With It, American Health, p. 43, June, 1988; p. 549, Susan Van Etten/The Picture Cube.

Chapter 18

P. 553, Ellis Herwig/The Picture Cub; p. 555, from *Healthline,* Menlo Park, CA; p. 557, (top) Wolff Communications; p. 557, (bottom) From Snook, J.T: *Nutrition: A Guide to Decision Making,* Prentice-Hall, Inc. Englewood Cliffs, N.J., 1984; p. 560, adapted from Nash, J.D: *Maximize Your Body Potential,* Bull Publishing, Co., Palo Alto, CA, 1986; p. 561, Cathy, copyright 1989 Universal Press Syndicate, reprinted with permission, all rights reserved; p. 562, from Davis, T.M: Instructor's Resource Guide to accompany *Core Concepts in Health,* Mayfield Publishing Co. Mountain View, CA, 1988; p. 564, from Ferguson, J.: *Habits, Not Diets:* The Secret to Lifetime Weight Control, Bull Publishing Co., Palo Alto, CA, 1988; p. 565, (top) Jeffrey Myers/Stock Boston, (bottom) Jeffrey Myers/H. Armstrong Roberts; p. 566, Wolff Communications; p. 570 Gabor Demjen/Stock Boston; p. 571, from Thrifty Meals for Two, USDA Home and Garden Bulletin 244, December 1985; p. 573, David Bill/The Picture Cube.

Chapter 19

P. 575, Stacey Pick/Stock Boston; p. 577, (top) Wolff Communications; p. 577, (bottom), Herman, copyright 1986 Universal Press Syndicate, reprinted with permission, all rights reserved; p. 581, Wolff Communications; p. 582, adapted from Temperature Guide to Food Safety: Food and Home Notes, No. 25, Washington, USDA, June 20, 1977; p. 583, from Boyd, Robert F.: *General Microbiology,* ed. 2, Times Mirror/Mosby College Publishing, 1988; p. 584, (top) Wolff Communications; p. 584, (bottom), P.D. Walker, Welcome Research Laboratories, Kent, England; p. 585, H. Armstrong Roberts; p. 587, Don Mason/West Stock; p. 589, from Hegarty, Vincent: *Decisions in Nutrition,* ed. 1, Times Mirror/Mosby College Publishing, 1988; pp. 592, 593, Nutrivisuals; p. 594, from *Healthline,* Menlo Park, CA; p. 596, Steven R. Krous/Stock Boston.

Chapter 20

P. 605, courtesy of the American Dietetic Association; p. 606, Robert Jones, Jr; p. 607, courtesy of the American Dietetic Association; p. 609, (top and bottom) Robert Jones, Jr; p. 610, (top and bottom) courtesy of the American Dietetic Association; p. 611, (top) courtesy of the American Dietetic Association, (bottom), Robert Jones, Jr; p. 612, courtesy of the American Dietetic Association; p. 614, from *Healthline,* Menlo Park, CA; p. 617, Robert Jones, Jr.

Median Heights and Weights and Recommended Energy Intake
10th edition RDA

Category	Age (years) or Condition	Weight (kg)	Weight (lb)	Height (cm)	Height (in)	Ree[a] (kcal/day)	Average Energy Allowance (kcal)[b] Multiples of REE	Per kg	Per day[c]
Infants	0.0–0.5	6	13	60	24	320		108	650
	0.5–1.0	9	20	71	28	500		98	850
Children	1–3	13	29	90	35	740		102	1,300
	4–6	20	44	112	44	950		90	1,800
	7–10	28	62	132	52	1,130		70	2,000
Males	11–14	45	99	157	62	1,440	1.70	55	2,500
	15–18	66	145	176	69	1,760	1.67	45	3,000
	19–24	72	160	177	70	1,780	1.67	40	2,900
	25–50	79	174	176	70	1,800	1.60	37	2,900
	51 +	77	170	173	68	1,530	1.50	30	2,300
Females	11–14	46	101	157	62	1,310	1.67	47	2,200
	15–18	55	120	163	64	1,370	1.60	40	2,200
	19–24	58	128	164	65	1,350	1.60	38	2,200
	25–50	63	138	163	64	1,380	1.55	36	2,200
	51 +	65	143	160	63	1,280	1.50	30	1,900
Pregnant	1st Trimester								+0
	2nd Trimester								+300
	3rd Trimester								+300
Lactating	1st 6 months								+500
	2nd 6 months								+500

[a] Resting energy expenditure (REE); calculation based on FAO equations, then rounded. This is the same as RMR.

[b] In the range of light to moderate activity, the coefficient of variation is ±20%.

[c] Figure is rounded.

Metropolitan Life Insurance Company Height-Weight Data, Revised 1983

Height-Weight Tables for Adults (1983)

WOMEN Height Ft	In	Frame* Small	Medium	Large	MEN Height Ft	In	Frame* Small	Medium	Large
4	10	102-111	109-121	118-131	5	2	128-134	131-141	138-150
4	11	103-113	111-123	120-134	5	3	130-136	133-143	140-153
5	0	104-115	113-126	122-137	5	4	132-138	135-145	142-156
5	1	106-118	115-129	125-140	5	5	134-140	137-148	144-160
5	2	108-121	118-132	128-143	5	6	136-142	139-151	146-164
5	3	111-124	121-135	131-147	5	7	138-145	142-154	149-168
5	4	114-127	124-138	134-151	5	8	140-148	145-157	152-172
5	5	117-130	127-141	137-155	5	9	142-151	148-160	155-176
5	6	120-133	130-144	140-159	5	10	144-154	151-163	158-180
5	7	213-136	133-147	143-163	5	11	146-157	154-166	161-184
5	8	126-139	136-150	146-167	6	0	149-160	157-170	164-188
5	9	129-142	139-153	149-170	6	1	152-164	160-174	168-192
5	10	132-145	142-156	152-173	6	2	155-168	164-178	172-197
5	11	135-148	145-159	155-176	6	3	158-172	167-182	176-202
6	0	138-151	148-162	158-179	6	4	162-176	171-187	181-207

Based on a weight-height mortality study conducted by the Society of Actuaries and the Association of Life Insurance Medical Directors of America, Metropolitan Life Insurance Company, revised 1983.

*Weights at ages 25 to 59 based on lowest mortality. Height includes 1-in heel. Weight for women includes 3 lb. for indoor clothing. Weight for men includes 5 lb. for indoor clothing. (See p. 479 for controversy surrounding the use and abuse of these tables over the years.)